EDITION 2

Community and Public Health Nursing

EVIDENCE FOR PRACTICE

• **Gail A. Harkness,** DrPH, RN, FAAN
Professor Emeritus
University of Connecticut School of Nursing
Storrs, Connecticut
and
Contract Public Health Nurse
Department of Health and the Environment
Barnstable County, Massachusetts

• **Rosanna F. DeMarco,** PhD, RN, PHCNS-BC, APHN-BC, FAAN
Chair and Professor, Department of Nursing
College of Nursing and Health Science
University of Massachusetts, Boston
Boston, Massachusetts

Wolters Kluwer
Philadelphia • Baltimore • New York • London
Buenos Aires • Hong Kong • Sydney • Tokyo

Acquisitions Editor: Christina C. Burns
Product Development Editor: Annette Ferran
Editorial Assistant: Zack Shapiro
Marketing Manager: Dean Karampelas
Production Project Manager: Cynthia Rudy
Design Coordinator: Steve Druding
Artist/Illustrator: Karen Harkness
Manufacturing Coordinator: Karin Duffield
Prepress Vendor: S4Carlisle Publishing Services

Second edition

9 8 7 6 5 4 3 2 1

Printed in China

Library of Congress Cataloging-in-Publication Data
Harkness, Gail A., author.
Community and public health nursing : evidence for practice / Gail A. Harkness, Rosanna F. DeMarco. — Second edition.
p. ; cm.
Includes bibliographical references and index.
ISBN 978-1-4511-9131-8 (alk. paper)
I. DeMarco, Rosanna F., author. II. Title.
[DNLM: 1. Community Health Nursing—United States. 2. Evidence-Based Nursing—United States. 3. Nursing Theory—United States. 4. Public Health Nursing—United States. WY 108]
RT98
610.73'43—dc23

2014045143

CCS0115

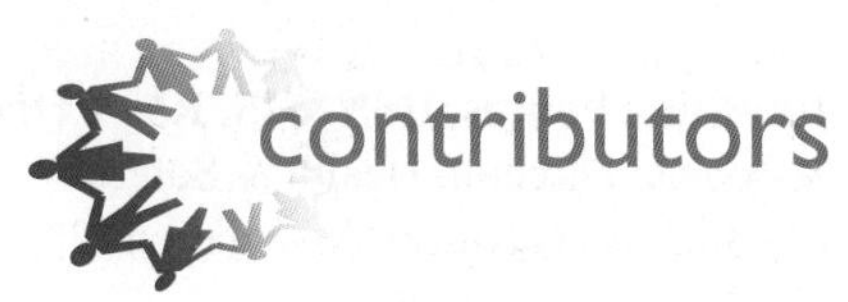

Stephanie M. Chalupka, EdD, RN, PHCNS-BC, FAAOHN
Associate Dean for Nursing
Worcester State University
Worcester, Massachusetts
Chapter 9: Planning for Community Change

Susan K. Chase, EdD, ARNP, FNP-BC, FNAP
Professor and Associate Dean for Graduate Affairs
University of Central Florida
Orlando, Florida
Chapter 23: Faith-Oriented Communities and Health Ministries in Faith Communities

Karen Conley, DNP, RN, AOCN, NEA-BC
Chief Associate Nursing
Brigham and Women's Hospital
Boston, Massachusetts
Chapter 16: Violence and Abuse

Sabreen A. Darwish, BScN, MScN, RN
PhD student /Research assistant
College of Nursing and Health Sciences
University of Massachusetts, Boston
Boston, Massachusetts
Chapter 3: Health Policy, Politics, and Reform

Rosanna F. DeMarco, PhD, RN, PHCNS-BC, APHN-BC, FAAN
Chair and Professor, Department of Nursing
College of Nursing and Health Science
University of Massachusetts, Boston
Boston, Massachusetts
Chapter 2: Public Health Systems
Chapter 5: Frameworks for Health Promotion, Disease Prevention, and Risk Reduction
Chapter 11: Community Assessment
Chapter 12: Care Management, Case Management, and Home Healthcare
Chapter 18: Underserved Populations

Pamela DiNapoli, PhD, RN, CNL
Associate Professor of Nursing
University of New Hampshire
Durham, New Hampshire
Chapter 22: School Health

Barbara A. Goldrick, MPH, PhD, RN
Epidemiology Consultant
Chatham, Massachusetts
Chapter 8: Gathering Evidence for Public Health Practice
Chapter 14: Risk of Infectious and Communicable Diseases
Chapter 15: Emerging Infectious Diseases

Susan L. Hamilton, PhD, RN
Assistant Professor
MGH Institute of Health Professions
Boston, Massachusetts
Chapter 9: Planning for Community Change

Gail A. Harkness, DrPH, RN, FAAN
Professor Emeritus
University of Connecticut School of Nursing
Storrs, Connecticut
and
Contract Public Health Nurse
Department of Health and the Environment
Barnstable County, Massachusetts
Chapter 1: Public Health Nursing: Present, Past, and Future
Chapter 6: Epidemiology: The Science of Prevention
Chapter 7: Describing Health Conditions: Understanding and Using Rates
Chapter 15: Emerging Infectious Diseases
Chapter 20: Community Preparedness: Disaster and Terrorism
Chapter 25: Occupational Health Nursing

Anahid Kulwicki, DNS, RN, FAAN
Dean of College of Nursing and Health Sciences
University of Massachusetts
Boston, Massachusetts
Chapter 3: Health Policy, Politics, and Reform

Annie Lewis-O'Connor, PhD, NP-BC, MPH, FAAN
Founder and Director
Women's After CARE Clinic
Boston, Massachusetts
Chapter 16: Violence and Abuse

Christine Pontus, BSN, MS, RN, COHN-S/CCM
Associate Director, Health & Safety
Massachusetts Nurses Association
Canton, Massachusetts
Chapter 25: Occupational Health Nursing

Joyce Pulcini, PhD, PNP-BC, FAAN, FAANP
Professor
Director of Community and Global Initiatives
George Washington University
Washington, DC
Chapter 4: Health and the Global Environment

Teresa E. Roberts, PhD, RN, ANP-BC
Clinical Assistant Professor
University of Massachusetts
Boston, Massachusetts
Chapter 10: Cultural Diversity and Values

Mary Margaret Segraves, PhD, RN
School Health Nurse
School Health Program, Cambridge Department of Health
Cambridge, Massachusetts
Chapter 13: Family Assessment

Judith Shindul-Rothschild, PhD, RNPC
Associate Professor
Boston College
Chestnut Hill, Massachusetts
Chapter 17: Substance Abuse
Chapter 21: Community Mental Health

Tarah S. Somers, BSN, MSN/MPH, RN
Regional Director, Agency for Toxic Substances and Disease Registry, New England Office
U.S. Public Health Service Commissioned Corps
Boston, Massachusetts
Chapter 19: Environmental Health

Joy Spellman, MSN, RN
Director, Center for Public Health Preparedness
Burlington County College
Mount Laurel, New Jersey
Chapter 20: Community Preparedness: Disasters and Terrorism

Patricia Tabloski, PhD, GNP-BC, FGSA, FAAN
Associate Professor
William F. Connell School of Nursing
Chestnut Hill, Massachusetts
Chapter 24: Palliative and End-of-Life Care

Lynda Tyer-Viola, PhD, RNC, FAAN
Associate Professor
MGH Institute of Health Professions
Charlestown, Massachusetts
Chapter 4: Health and the Global Environment

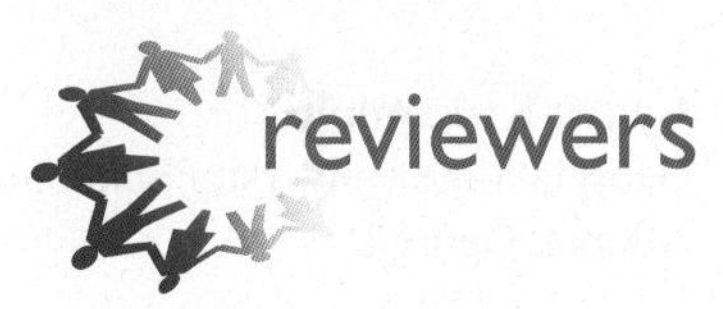

Nancy Ballard
University of Texas, Tyler
Tyler, Texas

Christina Barrick
Towson University
Towson, Maryland

Joan Bickes
Wayne State University
Detroit, Michigan

Lynn Blanchette
Rhode Island College
Providence, Rhode Island

Victoria Britson
National American University
Sioux Falls, South Dakota

Esther Brown
Widener University School of Nursing
Chester, Pennsylvania

Chesanny Butler
Saginaw Valley State University
Utica, Michigan

Kathy Cervasio
Long Island University
Brooklyn, New York

Colleen Clark
Minnesota State University, Mankato
Mankato, Minnesota

Sarah Cloud
State College of Florida
Sarasota, Florida

Jennifer Chilton
University of Texas, Tyler
Tyler, Texas

Cathleen Colleran-Santos
Curry College
Milton, Massachusetts

Sally Dampier
Confederation College
Thunder Bay, Ontario

Yolanda R. Davila
University of Texas Medical Branch, Galveston
Galveston, Texas

Teresa Decker
Widener University
Chester, Pennsylvania

Carolynn DeSandre
University of North Georgia
Dahlonega, Georgia

Lori Edwards
Johns Hopkins University School of Nursing
Baltimore, Maryland

Aida L. Egues
New York City College of Technology
Brooklyn, New York

Maria Fletcher
St. Joseph's College
Brooklyn, New York

Debra A. Grosskurth
Salve Regina University
Newport, Rhode Island

Kay Gurtz
Kent State University
Burton, Ohio

Elizabeth Heavey
State University of New York, Brockport
Brockport, New York

Lynn van Hofwegen
California State University, East Bay
Hayward, California

Vicky P. Kent
Towson University
Towson, Maryland

Kenya Kirkendoll
Georgia State University School of Nursing
Atlanta, Georgia

Michelle Kluka
Oakland University School of Nursing
Rochester, Michigan

Jamie Koonmen
University of Michigan, Flint
Flint, Michigan

Kathleen M. Lamaute
Molloy College
Rockville Centre, New York

Mary Lashley
Towson University
Towson, Maryland

Susan Lindner
Virginia Commonwealth University School of Nursing
Richmond, Virginia

Janet LoVerde
Aurora University
Aurora, Illinois

Bette Mariani
Villanova University
Villanova, Pennsylvania

Nancy Michela
The Sage Colleges
Troy, New York

Dorothy Miller
College of Coastal Georgia
Brunswick, Georgia

Geraldine Moore
Molloy College
Rockville Centre, New York

Vicki Moran
Saint Louis University
St. Louis, Missouri

Shirley Newberry
Winona State University
Winona, Minnesota

Liz Nims
Lourdes University
Sylvania, Ohio

Chastity Osborn
Lakeview College of Nursing
Danville, Illinois

Nanci R. Peek
Lewis University College of Nursing
Romeoville, Illinois

Jennan A. Phillips
University of Alabama, Birmingham
Birmingham, Alabama

Ursula A. Pritham
Georgia Southern University
Statesboro, Georgia

Barbara B. Puryear
Holmes Community College
Ridgeland, Mississippi

Judith Quaranta
Decker School of Nursing
Binghamton, New York

Cindy Rieger
University of Oklahoma College of Nursing
Oklahoma City, Oklahoma

Sherrie Rubio-Wallace
University of Wyoming
Laramie, Wyoming

Cathleen Santos
Curry College
Milton, Massachusetts

Kathleen Saunders
University of California Irvine Program in Nursing
Irvine, California

Marjorie Schaffer
Bethel University
St. Paul, Minnesota

John Schmidt
Cuyahoga Community College
Cleveland, Ohio

Leigh Shaver
Texas A&M University, Corpus Christi
Corpus Christi, Texas

Sheila Shipley
William Jewell College
Liberty, Missouri

Kellie Smith
Thomas Jefferson University, Jefferson School of Nursing
Philadelphia, Pennsylvania

Barbara E. Stanley
University of Massachusetts, Amherst
Amherst, Massachusetts

Teresa Taylor
Missouri Valley College
Marshall, Missouri

Jane A. Tiedt
Gonzaga University
Spokane, Washington

Cindy Versteeg
Algonquin College
Ottawa, Ontario

Nancy Wagner
Youngstown State University
Youngstown, Ohio

Jane Weilert
Newman University
Wichita, Kansas

Kim W. White
Southern Illinois University, Edwardsville
Edwardsville, Illinois

Robin White
Ohio Northern University
Ada, Ohio

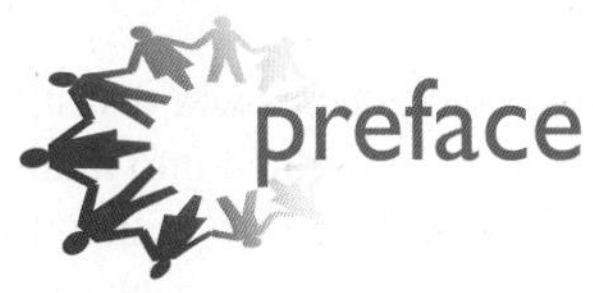

preface

There is no more vulnerable human combination than an undergraduate.

John Sloan Dickey, President of Dartmouth College

You're only given a little spark of madness. You mustn't lose it.

Robin Williams

Only the wisest and stupidest of men never change.

Confucius

We are experiencing extraordinary changes in healthcare in this century—changes that call upon the most creative, analytical, and innovative skills available. While the world has the resources to reduce healthcare disparities and eliminate the gaps in healthcare that exist between various population groups across the globe, accomplishing this is a long-term and complicated task. Improvement in the social structure within which people live, and a redistribution of resources so that all people have access to the basic necessities of life, require an unprecedented global consciousness and political commitment.

Ultimately, reducing health disparities occurs within the local community where people reside. Nurses are by far the largest group of healthcare providers worldwide and, as such, have the ability and responsibility to be change agents and leaders in implementing change in their communities. They can be the primary participants in the development of health policy that specifically addresses the unique needs of their communities. Through implementation and evaluation of culturally appropriate, community-based programs, nurses can use their expertise to remedy the conditions that contribute to health disparities. People need to be assured that their healthcare needs will be assessed and that healthcare is available and accessible.

In the United States, public health is a national priority. Through *Healthy People 2020*, national goals have been set to promote a healthy population and address the issue of health disparities. The process of implementing the *Healthy People 2020* objectives rests with regional and local practitioners, with nurses having a direct responsibility in the implementation process. The nurse practicing in the community has a central role in providing direct care for the ill as well as promoting and maintaining the health of groups of people, regardless of the circumstances that exist. Today, there are unparalleled challenges to the nurse's problem-solving skills in carrying out this mission.

Whether caring for the individual or the members of a community, it is essential that nurses incorporate evidence from multiple sources in the analysis and solution of public health issues. *Community and Public Health Nursing: Evidence for Practice* focuses on evidence-based practice, presenting multiple formats designed to develop the abstract critical thinking skills and complex reasoning abilities necessary for nurses becoming generalists in community and public health nursing. The unique blend of both the nursing process and the epidemiologic process provides a framework for gathering evidence about health problems, analyzing the information, generating diagnoses or hypotheses, planning for resolution, implementing plans of action, and evaluating the results.

To every complex question there is a simple answer …
and it is wrong.

H. L. Mencken (writer and wit, 1880–1956)

CONTENT ORGANIZATION

It is the intention of *Community and Public Health Nursing: Evidence for Practice* to present the core content of community and public health nursing in a succinct, logically organized, but comprehensive manner. The evidence for practice focus not only includes chapters on epidemiology, biostatistics, and research but also integrates these topics throughout the text in multiple formats. Concrete examples assist students in interpreting and applying statistical data. *Healthy People* goals and measurable objectives serve as an illustration of the use of rates throughout the text. Groups with special needs, such as refugees and the homeless, have been addressed in several chapters; however, tangential topics that can be found in adult health and maternal–child health textbooks have been omitted. A chapter on environmental health concerns has been included, along with a chapter on community preparedness for emergencies and disasters. Also, a global perspective has been incorporated into many chapters.

Challenges to critical thinking are presented in multiple places throughout each chapter. Case studies are integrated into the content of each chapter and contain critical thinking questions imbedded in the case study content. Also, a series of critical thinking questions can be found at the end of each chapter. (Please see the description of features below.) Considering the onus presented by Mark Twain: "Be careful about reading health books. You may die of a misprint," every attempt has been made to present correct, meaningful, and current evidence for practice.

Part One presents the context within which the community or public health nurse practices. An overview of the major drivers of healthcare change leads to a discussion of evolving trends, such as the emphasis on patient/client-centered care, the effects of new technology upon the delivery of care, and the need for people to assume more responsibility for maintaining their health. Community and public health nursing as it presently exists is analyzed and reviewed from a historical base, and issues foreseen for both the present and immediate future are discussed. The nursing competencies necessary for community and public health practice are also presented.

A more in-depth discussion of the complex structure, function, and outcomes of public health and healthcare systems follows. National and international perspectives regarding philosophical and political attitudes, social structures, economics, resources, financing mechanisms, and historical contexts are presented, highlighting healthcare organizations and issues in several developed countries. Stressing the importance of the nurse engaging in the political process to advance healthcare, a new Chapter 3 addressing health policy, politics, and reform has been added to this edition.

The World Health Organization's commitment to improving the public's health in developing countries follows, with an emphasis on refugees and disaster relief. With the burden of disease growing disproportionately in the world, largely due to climate, public policy, socioeconomic conditions, age, and an imbalance in distribution of risk factors, the countries burdened by disease often have the least capacity to institute change. Part One concludes with examination of the indicators of health, health and human rights, factors that affect health globally, and a framework for improving world health.

Part Two provides the frameworks and tools necessary to engage in evidence-based practice focused on the population's health. Concepts of health promotion, disease prevention, and risk reduction are explored, and a variety of conceptual frameworks are presented with a focus on both the epidemiologic and ecologic models. Epidemiology is presented as the science of prevention, and nurses are shown how epidemiologic principles are applied in practice, including the use of rates and other statistics as community health indicators. Specific research designs are also explored, including the application of epidemiologic research to practice settings.

Part Three is designed to develop the skills necessary to implement nursing practice effectively in community settings. Since healthcare is in a unique state of transformation, planning for community change is paramount. The health planning process is described, with specific attention given to the social and environmental determinants of change. Lewin's change theory, force field analysis, and the effective use of leverage points identified in the force field analysis demonstrate the change process in action.

Changes directed at decreasing health disparities must be culturally sensitive, client-centered, and community-oriented. A chapter on cultural diversity and values fosters the development of culturally competent practitioners, and the process of cultural health assessment is highlighted. Frameworks of community assessment are presented, and various approaches are explored. Management of care and the case management process follows. The role and scope of home care nursing practice and the provision of services are presented along with the challenges inherent with interdisciplinary roles, advances in telehealth, and other home care services.

Although content on family assessment can be found in other texts, it is an integral component of community and public health practice. Therefore, nursing theory in relation to the nursing care of families has been presented along with the influence of diversity on family health patterns. Indicators of family health, family dynamics, and coping styles are addressed, and the impact of stress is discussed, particularly in relation to vulnerable families.

Part Four presents the common challenges in community and public health nursing. The chapter addressing the risk of infectious and communicable diseases explores outbreak investigation with analysis of data experience provided by the case studies. Public health surveillance, the risk of common food-borne and waterborne illnesses, and sexually transmitted diseases are followed by a discussion of factors that influence the emergence/reemergence of infectious diseases, examples of recent outbreaks, and means of prevention and control. The ongoing epidemic of Ebola is explored.

The challenge presented by violence in the community is presented with an emphasis on intimate partner violence and the role of the healthcare provider. Owing to the cultural variations in substance abuse, multifaceted approaches to the problem are discussed, with the recommendation that evidence-based prevention and treatment protocols for substance abuse are incorporated by community health nurses in all practice settings. Meeting the healthcare needs of vulnerable and underserved populations is another challenge. Health priorities for people who live in rural areas; who are gay, lesbian, bisexual, or transgender; who are homeless; or who live in correctional institutions are reviewed. The issues of access to quality care, chronic disease management, interaction with health personnel, and health promotion in hard-to-reach populations are also presented.

The environmental chapter demonstrates how to assess contaminants in the community by creation of an exposure pathway. The health effects of the exposure pathway can then be ascertained. Individual assessment of contaminant exposures, interventions, and evaluations are also explored, ending with a focus on maintaining healthy communities. The final chapter in Part Four presents the issue of community preparedness. The types of disasters, along with classification of agents, are described, disaster management is outlined, and the public health response is explained. The role and responsibility of nurses in disasters and characteristics of the field response complete the content.

Part Five describes five common specialty practices within community and public health nursing. All have frameworks that define practice and reflect the competencies necessary for competent evidence-based practice in a variety of community settings. These include application of the principles of practice to community mental health, school health, faith-oriented communities, palliative care, and occupational health nursing.

Features Found in Each Chapter

• chapter highlights

Brief outline of the content and direction of the chapter

• key terms

Essential concepts and terminology required for comprehension of chapter content

• objectives

Observable changes expected following completion of the chapter

Case Study

Vignettes presented at the beginning and throughout each chapter, designed to stimulate critical thinking and analytic skills

• EVIDENCE FOR PRACTICE

Examples of objective evidence obtained from research studies that provide direction for practice

• PRACTICE POINT

Highlighting of essential facts relevant to practice

○ STUDENT REFLECTION

Student stories of their own experience and reflections

key concepts

Summary of important concepts presented in the chapter

critical thinking questions

Problems requiring critical analysis that combines research, context, and judgment

community resources

List of resources that support the content of selected chapters

I didn't fail the test, I just found 100 ways to do it wrong.

Benjamin Franklin

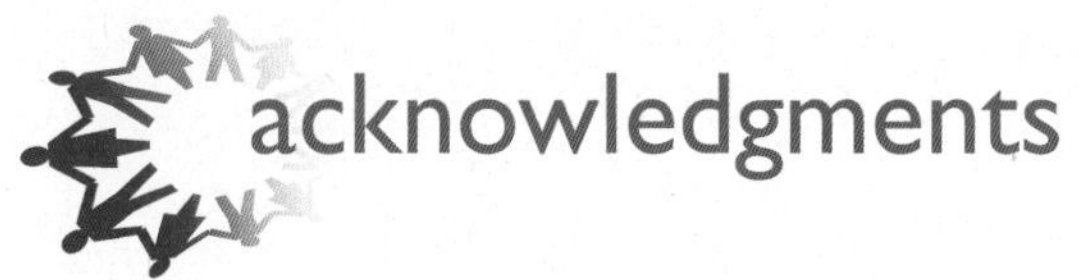

acknowledgments

The support of colleagues, family, and friends was instrumental in the development of the second edition of *Community and Public Health Nursing: Evidence for Practice.* A special thanks belongs to our contributors who were willing to share their expertise by writing chapters filled with passion and commitment to public health. All contributors to the first edition remained with us in developing its sequel. Karen Harkness worked closely with us in creating the colorful, detailed illustrations found throughout the text. She assisted in solving graphic design issues and in editing chapters at various stages throughout the development of the second edition. Her talents were especially helpful in copyediting of page proofs. Ann Napier was an indispensable editor of newly submitted chapters. She provided the consistency found both within and among chapters. Jean Steel and Ann Dylis deserve a special thank-you for providing consultation, encouragement, support, and a means of escape in pressing times.

Students from Boston College and the University of Massachusetts, Boston, shared their insights of nursing practice in community settings, contributing to the student reflections contained in each chapter. In addition, we are thankful for the invaluable experiences we obtained from our public health work that interfaced and informed the production of this book. Those experiences ranged from developing interventions with and for women living with HIV/AIDS in Boston, to leadership roles on local boards of health that are responsible for the health of our local communities, to the hands-on practice of primary, secondary, and tertiary preventions. Our Product Development Editor, Annette Ferran, was so very helpful in setting schedules, editing, answering questions, calming frustrations, providing moral support, and solving problems. Thank you all for helping us create this unique approach to public health nursing!

Gail A. Harkness
Rosanna F. DeMarco

contents

PART one
The Context of Public Health Nursing 1

CHAPTER 1
Public Health Nursing: Present, Past, and Future 3

HEALTHCARE CHANGES IN THE TWENTY-FIRST CENTURY 4
PUBLIC HEALTH NURSING TODAY 9
ROOTS OF PUBLIC HEALTH NURSING 12
CHALLENGES FOR PUBLIC HEALTH NURSING IN THE TWENTY-FIRST CENTURY 19

CHAPTER 2
Public Health Systems 26

IMPORTANCE OF UNDERSTANDING HOW PUBLIC HEALTH SYSTEMS ARE ORGANIZED 27
STRUCTURE OF PUBLIC HEALTHCARE IN THE UNITED STATES 27
FUNCTIONS OF PUBLIC HEALTH IN THE UNITED STATES 30
TRENDS IN PUBLIC HEALTH IN THE UNITED STATES 32
HEALTHCARE SYSTEMS IN SELECTED DEVELOPED NATIONS 34
PUBLIC HEALTH COMMITMENTS TO THE WORLD: INTERNATIONAL PUBLIC HEALTH AND DEVELOPING COUNTRIES 40

CHAPTER 3
Health Policy, Politics, and Reform 46

HEALTHCARE POLICY AND THE POLITICAL PROCESS 47
HEALTHCARE FINANCES AND COST–BENEFIT 50
ACCESS TO CARE AND HEALTH INSURANCE 51
HEALTHCARE WORKFORCE DIVERSITY 52
NURSING'S ROLE IN SHAPING HEALTHCARE POLICY 53
QUALITY OF CARE 54
INFORMATION MANAGEMENT 55
EQUITY IN HEALTHCARE ACCESS AND QUALITY 55
ETHICAL CONSIDERATION 56
HEALTH ADVOCACY AND HEALTHCARE REFORM 57
HEALTH SERVICES RESEARCH 58
CONCLUSION 58

CHAPTER 4
Health and the Global Environment 62

DEFINITIONS OF HEALTH 63
CRITICAL GLOBAL HEALTH CONCEPTS 64
THE MILLENNIUM DEVELOPMENT GOALS 71
OTHER FACTORS THAT AFFECT GLOBAL HEALTH 74
ROLE OF NURSES 77

PART two
Evidence-Based Practice and Population Health 81

CHAPTER 5
Frameworks for Health Promotion, Disease Prevention, and Risk Reduction 83

HEALTH PROMOTION, DISEASE PREVENTION, AND RISK REDUCTION AS CORE ACTIVITIES OF PUBLIC HEALTH 85
HEALTHY PEOPLE INITIATIVES 86
ROAD MAPS TO HEALTH PROMOTION 87
BEHAVIOR MODELS 92
USE OF THE ECOLOGIC MODEL: EVIDENCE FOR HEALTH PROMOTION INTERVENTION 98
HEALTH PROMOTION AND SECONDARY/TERTIARY PREVENTION FOR WOMEN LIVING WITH HIV/AIDS 100
ROLE OF NURSES 100

CHAPTER 6
Epidemiology: The Science of Prevention 105

DEFINING EPIDEMIOLOGY 107
DEVELOPMENT OF EPIDEMIOLOGY AS A SCIENCE 108
EPIDEMIOLOGIC MODELS 110
APPLYING EPIDEMIOLOGIC PRINCIPLES IN PRACTICE 113

CHAPTER 7
Describing Health Conditions: Understanding and Using Rates 121

UNDERSTANDING AND USING RATES 123
SPECIFIC RATES: DESCRIBING BY PERSON, PLACE, AND TIME 127
TYPES OF INCIDENCE RATES 133
SENSITIVITY AND SPECIFICITY 134
USE OF RATES IN DESCRIPTIVE RESEARCH STUDIES 135

CHAPTER 8
Gathering Evidence for Public Health Practice 137

OBSERVATIONAL STUDIES 139
INTERVENTION (EXPERIMENTAL) STUDIES 144

PART three
Implementing Nursing Practice in Community Settings 149

CHAPTER 9
Planning for Community Change 151

HEALTH PLANNING 152
COMMUNITY ASSESSMENT 154
SYSTEMS THEORY 155
WORKING WITH THE COMMUNITY 155
SOCIAL ECOLOGIC MODEL 157
HEALTH IMPACT PYRAMID 157
MULTILEVEL INTERVENTIONS 158
SOCIAL DETERMINANTS OF HEALTH 159
CHANGE THEORY 161
PLANNING COMMUNITY-LEVEL INTERVENTIONS 164
COLLABORATION AND TEAMWORK 166
EVALUATING COMMUNITY-LEVEL INTERVENTIONS 167
FUNDING COMMUNITY-LEVEL INTERVENTION PROGRAMS 168
SOCIAL MARKETING 170
NURSE-MANAGED HEALTH CENTERS 170

CHAPTER 10
Cultural Diversity and Values 174

CULTURE AND NURSING 175
WESTERN BIOMEDICINE AS "CULTURED" 180
ASPECTS OF CULTURE DIRECTLY AFFECTING HEALTH AND HEALTHCARE 180
CULTURAL HEALTH ASSESSMENT 184

CHAPTER 11
Community Assessment 187

DEFINING THE COMMUNITY AND ITS BOUNDARIES 189
FRAMEWORKS FOR COMMUNITY ASSESSMENT 192

CHAPTER 12
Care Management, Case Management, and Home Healthcare 204

CARE MANAGEMENT 205
CASE MANAGEMENT 206
HOME HEALTHCARE 207
CASE MANAGEMENT, HOME HEALTHCARE, AND CURRENT HEALTHCARE REFORM 221

CHAPTER 13
Family Assessment 225

FAMILIES IN COMMUNITIES 226
NURSING PERSPECTIVES ON THE FAMILY AND APPLICATIONS FOR ASSESSMENT 228
DIVERSITY AND FAMILY 234
FAMILIES AND HEALTH RISK 237
COMMUNITY HEALTH NURSES' RESPONSIBILITY TO FAMILIES 244

PART four
Challenges in Community and Public Health Nursing 249

CHAPTER 14
Risk of Infectious and Communicable Diseases 251

EPIDEMIOLOGY OF THE INFECTIOUS PROCESS: THE CHAIN OF INFECTION 255
OUTBREAK INVESTIGATION 258
HEALTHCARE-ASSOCIATED INFECTIONS 260
PUBLIC HEALTH SURVEILLANCE 261
SPECIFIC COMMUNICABLE DISEASES 262
PREVENTION AND CONTROL OF SPECIFIC INFECTIOUS DISEASES 276

CHAPTER 15
Emerging Infectious Diseases 281

FACTORS THAT INFLUENCE EMERGING INFECTIOUS DISEASES 282
RECENT EMERGING AND REEMERGING INFECTIOUS DISEASES 287
CONCLUSIONS 303

CHAPTER 16
Violence and Abuse 307

OVERVIEW OF VIOLENCE 308
INTIMATE PARTNER VIOLENCE 311
MANDATORY REPORTING OF ABUSE 317
INTERVENTION 319
MODEL OF CARE FOR VICTIMS OF INTENTIONAL CRIMES 320
FORENSIC NURSING 320

CHAPTER 17
Substance Use 325

INTERNATIONAL ASPECTS OF SUBSTANCE ABUSE 326
HEALTH PROFILES AND INTERVENTIONS FOR -HIGH-RISK POPULATIONS 331
IMPACT ON THE COMMUNITY 343
PUBLIC HEALTH MODELS FOR POPULATIONS AT RISK 343

TREATMENT INTERVENTIONS FOR SUBSTANCE ABUSE 348
GOALS OF *HEALTHY PEOPLE 2010* 351

CHAPTER 18
Underserved Populations 357

THE CONTEXT OF HEALTH RISKS 358
RURAL POPULATIONS 360
CORRECTIONAL HEALTH: UNDERSERVED POPULATIONS IN JAILS AND PRISONS 367
GAY, LESBIAN, BISEXUAL, AND TRANSGENDER PEOPLE 371
HOMELESS POPULATIONS 373

CHAPTER 19
Environmental Health 378

HUMAN HEALTH AND THE ENVIRONMENT 379
ASSESSMENT 382
INTERVENTIONS 395
EVALUATION 397
ENVIRONMENTAL EPIDEMIOLOGY 397
WORKING TOWARD HEALTHY ENVIRONMENTS 399
CHILDREN'S HEALTH AND THE ENVIRONMENT 399
ENVIRONMENTAL JUSTICE 401
GLOBAL ENVIRONMENTAL HEALTH CHALLENGES 401

CHAPTER 20
Community Preparedness: Disaster and Terrorism 405

EMERGENCIES, DISASTERS, AND TERRORISM 407
DISASTER PREPAREDNESS IN A CULTURALLY DIVERSE SOCIETY 409
DISASTER MANAGEMENT 410
ROLES OF NURSES IN DISASTER MANAGEMENT 414
BIOTERRORISM 419
CHEMICAL DISASTERS 425
RADIOLOGIC DISASTERS 429
BLAST INJURIES 430
PUBLIC HEALTH DISASTER RESPONSE 431

PART five
Specialty Practice 437

CHAPTER 21
Community Mental Health 439

CULTURAL CONTEXT OF MENTAL ILLNESS 440
DEFINITIONS OF MENTAL ILLNESS 441
SCOPE OF MENTAL ILLNESS 441
SOME MAJOR MENTAL ILLNESSES 442
EVOLUTION OF COMMUNITY MENTAL HEALTH 458
LEGISLATION FOR PARITY IN MENTAL HEALTH INSURANCE BENEFITS 459
ROLES AND RESPONSIBILITIES OF THE COMMUNITY MENTAL HEALTH PRACTITIONER 460
PSYCHOLOGICAL FIRST AID 461

CHAPTER 22
School Health 469

HISTORICAL PERSPECTIVES 470
ROLE OF THE SCHOOL NURSE 471
COMMON HEALTH CONCERNS 475
THE SCHOOL NURSE AS A CHILD ADVOCATE 482
THE FUTURE OF SCHOOL HEALTH: THE COMMUNITY SCHOOL MODEL 483

CHAPTER 23
Faith-Oriented Communities and Health Ministries in Faith Communities 486

NURSING IN FAITH COMMUNITIES 487
HISTORY OF FAITH COMMUNITY NURSING 488
MODELS OF FAITH COMMUNITY PRACTICE 488
THE UNIQUENESS OF FAITH COMMUNITIES 489
ROLES OF THE FAITH COMMUNITY NURSE 492
HEALTHY PEOPLE 2020 PRIORITIES 492
SCOPE AND STANDARDS OF PRACTICE 493
THE NURSING PROCESS IN FAITH COMMUNITY NURSING 494
ETHICAL CONSIDERATIONS 497
EDUCATION FOR FAITH COMMUNITY NURSING 498

CHAPTER 24
Palliative and End-of-Life Care 501

NURSING AND PATIENTS WITH CHRONIC DISEASE 502
DEATH IN THE UNITED STATES 505
NURSING CARE WHEN DEATH IS IMMINENT 507
PALLIATIVE CARE 511
HOSPICE CARE 511
CARING FOR PATIENTS AT THE END OF LIFE 512
NURSING CARE OF PATIENTS WHO ARE CLOSE TO DEATH 520
COMPLEMENTARY AND ALTERNATIVE THERAPIES 522

CHAPTER 25
Occupational Health Nursing 525

THE WORKER AND THE WORKPLACE 526
OCCUPATIONAL HEALTH NURSING 530
CONCEPTUAL FRAMEWORKS 532
OCCUPATIONAL HEALTH NURSING: PRACTICE 535
IMPLEMENTING HEALTH PROMOTION IN THE WORKPLACE 540
IMPLEMENTING A PROGRAM: EXAMPLE, SMOKING CESSATION 541
EPIDEMIOLOGY AND OCCUPATIONAL HEALTH 542
EMERGENCY PREPAREDNESS PLANNING AND DISASTER MANAGEMENT 544

Index 549

The Context of Public Health Nursing

PART
one

CHAPTER 1

Public Health Nursing: Present, Past, and Future

Gail A. Harkness

Nursing is based on society's needs and therefore exists only because of society's need for such a service. It is difficult for nursing to rise above society's expectations, limitations, resources, and culture of the current age.

Patricia Donahue, Nursing, the Finest Art: An Illustrated History

I believe the history of public health might be written as a record of successive redefinings of the unacceptable.

George Vicker

Some people think that doctors and nurses can put scrambled eggs back into the shell.

Dorothy Canfield Fisher, social activist and author

The only way to keep your health is to eat what you don't want, drink what you don't like, and do what you'd rather not.

Mark Twain

chapter highlights

- Healthcare changes in the 21st century
- Characteristics of public health nursing
- Public health nursing roots
- Challenges for practice in the 21st century

objectives

- Outline three major changes in healthcare in the 21st century.
- Identify the eight principles of public health nursing practice.
- Explain the significance of the standards and their related competencies of professional public health nursing practice.
- Discuss historical events and relate them to the principles that underlie public health nursing today.
- Consider the challenges for public health nurses in the 21st century.

key terms

Aggregate: Population group with common characteristics.

Competencies: Unique capabilities required for the practice of public health nursing.

District nurses: Public health nurses in England who provide visiting nurse services; historically, they cared for the people in the poorest parish districts.

Electronic Health Records: Digital computerized versions of patients' paper medical records.

Epidemiology: Study of the distribution and determinants of states of health and illness in human populations; used both as a research methodology to study states of health and illness, and as a body of knowledge that results from the study of a specific state of health or illness.

Evidence-based nursing: Integration of the best evidence available with clinical expertise and the values of the client to increase the quality of care.

Evidence-based public health: A public health endeavor wherein there is judicious use of evidence derived from a variety of science and social science research.

Healthcare disparities: Gaps in healthcare experienced by one population compared with another.

Health information technology: Comprehensive management of health information and its secure exchange between consumers, providers, government and quality entities, and insurers.

Public health: What society does collectively to ensure that conditions exist in which people can be healthy.

Public health interventions: Actions taken on behalf of individuals, families, communities, and systems to protect or improve health status.

Public health nursing: Focuses on population health through continuous surveillance and assessment of the multiple determinants of health with the intent to

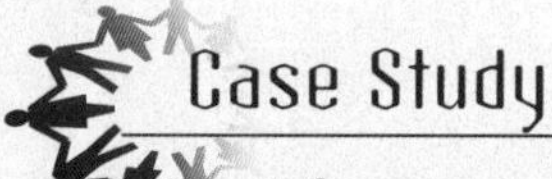

Case Study

References to the case study are found throughout this chapter (look for the case study icon). Readers should keep the case study in mind as they read the chapter.

The Department of Health and Human Services (HHS) in a southeastern state has begun implementing the recommendations from both the U.S. Institute of Medicine's publication *The Future of the Public's Health in the 21st Century* and the 10-year national objectives for promoting health and preventing disease in the United States established by *Healthy People 2020*. A task force is developing a new vision for **public health** in the state. Sandy is a program developer in the state's Department of Public Health, with the primary responsibility of assisting local public health departments in developing, implementing, and evaluating public health nursing initiatives. Sandy represents public health nursing on the task force. (Adapted from Jakeway, Cantrell, Cason, & Talley, 2006).

key terms (continued)

promote health and wellness; prevent disease, disability, and premature death; and improve neighborhood quality of life (American Nurses Association [ANA], 2013).

Telehealth: Use of electronic information and telecommunications technologies to support long-distance clinical healthcare, patient and professional health-related education, public health, and health administration.

Social determinants of health: Social conditions in which people live and work.

HEALTHCARE CHANGES IN THE TWENTY-FIRST CENTURY

A worldwide phenomenon of unprecedented change is occurring in healthcare. There are new innovations to test, ethical dilemmas to confront, puzzles to solve, and rewards to be gained as healthcare systems develop, refocus, and become more complex within a multiplicity of settings. Nurses, the largest segment of healthcare providers in the world, are on the frontline of that change.

Demographic characteristics indicate that people in developed countries are living longer and healthier lives, yet tremendous health and social disparities exist. The social conditions in which people live, their income, their social status, their education, their literacy level, their home and work environments, their support networks, their gender, their culture, and the availability of health services are the **social determinants of health**. These conditions have an impact on the extent to which a person or community possesses the physical, social, and personal resources necessary to attain and maintain health. Some population groups, having fewer resources to offset these effects, are affected disproportionately. The results are **healthcare disparities**, or gaps in care experienced by one population compared with another.

For example, the World Health Organization (WHO) estimates that almost half of all countries surveyed have access to less than half the essential medicines they need for basic healthcare in the public sector. These essential medicines include vaccines, antibiotics, and painkillers. Children in low-income countries are 16 times more likely to die before reaching the age of 5 years, often because of malnourishment, than children in high-income countries. The double burden of both undernutrition and overweight conditions causes serious health problems and affects survival (WHO, 2013). Globally, resources exist to remedy these circumstances, but does the political commitment exist?

> *The development of society, rich or poor, can be judged by the quality of its population health, how fairly health is distributed across the social spectrum, and the degree of protection provided from disadvantage as a result of ill health.*
>
> **World Health Organization**

Role of the Government in Healthcare

A government has three core functions in addressing the health of its citizens: (1) it assesses healthcare problems; (2) it intervenes by developing relevant healthcare policy that provides access to services; and (3) it ensures that services are delivered and outcomes achieved. The United States, the United Kingdom, the European community, and some newly industrialized countries have embraced these principles. However, governments in other countries struggle to build any semblance of a health system. Unstable governments do not have the concern, motivation, or resources to address healthcare issues.

There were unprecedented public health achievements in the United States during the 20th century. The Centers for Disease Control and Prevention (CDC) has listed the Ten Great **Public Health** Achievements based on supportive epidemiologic analyses and comparisons of health factors over 30 years (Box 1.1). However, healthcare expenditures are now more than $2.6 trillion per year (CDC, 2013). Infant mortality, longevity, and other health indicators still fall behind those of many other industrialized nations. The current U.S. healthcare system faces serious challenges on multiple

box 1.1 Ten Great Public Health Achievements in the United States, 1900–1999

Vaccination
Motor vehicle safety
Safer workplaces
Control of infectious diseases
Decline in coronary heart disease and stroke deaths
Safer and healthier foods
Healthier mothers and babies
Family planning
Fluoridation of drinking water
Recognition of tobacco as a health hazard

Source: Centers for Disease Control and Prevention. (1999). Ten Great Public Health Achievements — United States, 1900–1999. *Morbidity Mortality Weekly Report, 48*(12), 241–243.

fronts. Although the United States is considered the best place for people to obtain accurate diagnoses and high-quality treatment, until 2014 nearly 45 million Americans lacked health insurance and therefore access to care. These uninsured Americans were primarily young people, low-income single adults, small-business owners, self-employed adults, and others who did not have access to employer-sponsored health insurance.

The Patient Protection and Affordable Care Act (PPACA) was signed into law by President Barack Obama in 2010. The goal of the PPACA is to help provide affordable health insurance coverage to most Americans, lower costs, improve access to primary care, add to preventive care and prescription benefits, offer coverage to those with pre-existing conditions, and extend young adults' coverage under their parents' insurance policies. It is estimated that 95% of legal U.S. residents will ultimately be covered by health insurance, although implementation will evolve over time (Doherty, 2010). The passage of the PPACA was the first step in providing Americans with the security of affordable and lifelong access to high-quality healthcare. More information about the Affordable Care Act, unofficially known as "Obamacare," is found in Chapter 3.

It is cheaper to promote health than to maintain people in sickness.

Florence Nightingale

PRACTICE POINT

Making healthcare a right rather than a privilege has global implications.

The United States assesses and monitors people's health through an intricate system of surveillance surveys conducted by the HHS, the CDC, and the state and local governments. Health policy development focuses on cost, access to care, and quality of care. *Access* is defined as the ability to get into the healthcare system, and *quality care* is defined as receiving appropriate healthcare in time for the services to be effective. Outcomes are ensured by a continual evaluation system linked in part with the CDC surveys. Despite this elaborate healthcare system, health disparities related to race, ethnicity, and socioeconomic status still pervade the healthcare system. Health disparities vary in magnitude by condition and population, but they are observed in almost all aspects of healthcare, in quality, access, healthcare utilization, preventive care, management of chronic diseases, clinical conditions, and settings, and within many subpopulations.

The *National Healthcare Quality Report* (NHQR) and the *National Healthcare Disparities Report* (NHDR) measure trends in the effectiveness of care, patient safety, timeliness of care, patient centeredness, and efficiency of care. The reports present, in chart form, the latest available findings on quality of and access to healthcare (Agency for Healthcare Research and Quality, 2014). For example, Figure 1.1 indicates that although quality is improving slowly for all groups, significant health disparities continue to exist in many populations.

The challenge for the United States in the 21st century is to create a dynamic, streamlined healthcare system that produces not only the finest technology and research but also the most accessible, efficient, low-cost, and high-quality healthcare in the world. The current healthcare system also must be transformed to become one of the most competitive and successful systems in the world. Innovative and creative changes will be needed to create a patient/client–centered, provider-friendly healthcare system that is consumer-driven. The political will does exist to create a better future: patient/client–centered care is evolving, new technology is shaping delivery of care, and people are assuming more responsibility for maintaining their health.

Patient/Client–Centered Care

Healthcare has been evolving toward a multifaceted system that empowers patients and clients rather than providers, as was common in the past. This transformation is considered the best way to ensure that patients have access to high-quality care, regardless of their income, where they live, the color of their skin, or how old or ill they are.

Patient/client–centered care considers cultural traditions, personal preferences, values, families, and lifestyles. People requiring healthcare, along with their families or significant others, become an integral part of the healthcare team, and clinical decisions are made collaboratively with professionals. Clients become active participants in their own care, and monitoring health becomes the client's responsibility. Support, advice, and counsel from health professionals are available, along with the tools that are needed to carry out that responsibility. The shift toward patient/client–centered care means that a broader range of outcomes needs to be measured from the patient's

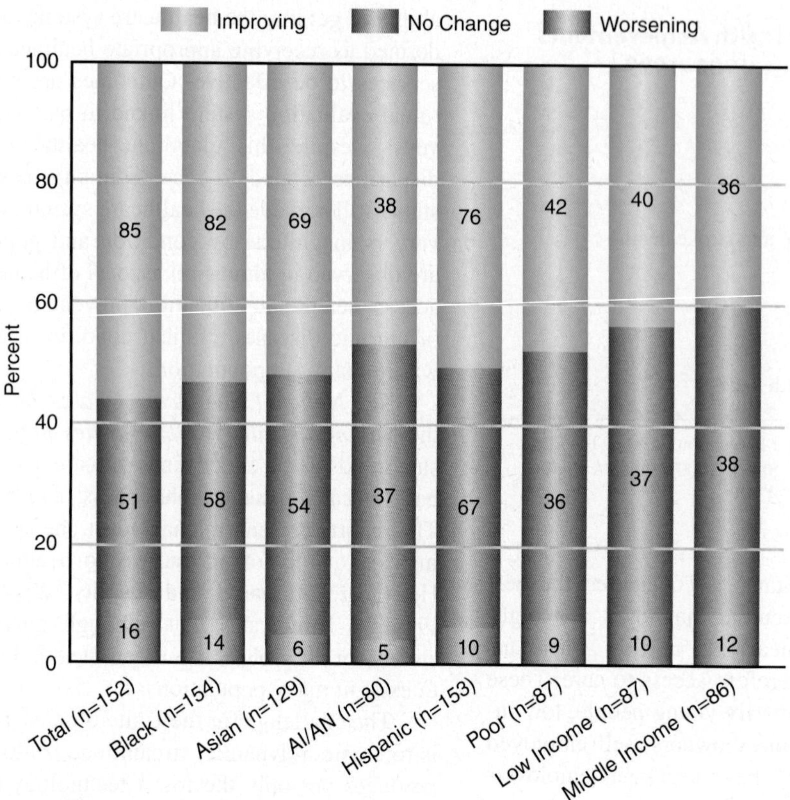

Key:

AI/AN = American Indian or Alaska Native

n = number of measures

Improving = Quality is moving in a positive direction at an average annual rate greater than 1% per year

No Change = Quality is not changing or is changing at an average annual rate less than 1% per year

Worsening = Quality is moving in a negative direction at an average annual rate greater than 1% per year

Note: For each measure, the earliest and most recent data available to our team were analyzed; for the vast majority of measures, this represents trend data from 2000–2002 to 2008–2010.

figure 1.1 Number and proportion of all quality measures that are improving, not changing, or worsening, overall and for select populations.

perspective to understand the true benefits and risks of healthcare interventions.

PRACTICE POINT

The Agency for Healthcare Research and Quality (AHRQ) has developed a series of tools to assist clients in making healthcare decisions.

To help clients and their healthcare providers make better decisions, the AHRQ has developed a series of tools that empower clients and assist providers in achieving desired outcomes. Tools include questionnaires to help determine important treatment preferences and decisions, symptom severity indexes, client fact sheets, client-reported functional status indicators, and other helpful decision-making guidelines. These are available to both consumers and healthcare providers at the AHRQ website.

For the system to work effectively, transitions between providers, departments, various healthcare settings, and the home must be coordinated and efficient so that unneeded or unwanted services can be reduced. Americans are sophisticated, empowered consumers in almost every aspect of their lives and will make the best decisions both for themselves and, collectively, for the healthcare economy and society itself.

Technology

Rapidly advancing forms of technology are dramatically improving lives. Thousands of new ideas are investigated each year, with hundreds of new medical devices submitted to the U.S. Food and Drug Administration annually. Medical devices vary considerably, such as computer-assisted robotic surgical techniques, artificial cervical disks, new diagnostic techniques, implantable microchip-containing devices that control dosing from drug reservoirs, continuous glucose-monitoring systems for detecting trends and tracking patterns in people with diabetes, and many more.

> *The benefits of biomedical progress are obvious, clear, and powerful. The hazards are much less well appreciated.*
>
> **Leon Kass, physician**

Although massive investments in medical research have been made, there has been an underinvestment in both research and the infrastructure necessary to translate basic research into results. For example, studies indicate that it takes physicians an average of 17 years to adopt widely the findings from basic research. The healthcare sector invests nearly 50% less in information technology than any other major sector of the U.S. economy. More comprehensive knowledge bases of healthcare information, computerized decision support, and a health information technology (HIT) infrastructure with national standards of interoperability to promote data exchange are necessary.

Health Information Technology

Health information technology is defined as the comprehensive management of health information and its exchange between consumers, providers, government, and insurers in a secure manner. HIT makes it possible for healthcare providers to better manage patient care through secure use and sharing of health information. It is viewed as the most promising tool for improving the overall quality, safety, and efficiency of the health delivery system.

> *Health information technology and electronic health information exchange have emerged as a primary means of shaping a healthcare system that is effective, safe, transparent, and affordable. When linked with other health system reforms, technology can support better quality healthcare, reduce errors . . . and improve population health.*
>
> **State Alliance for e-Health**

Health information technology includes the use of **electronic health records** (EHRs), digital computerized versions of patients' paper medical records, to maintain people's health information. EHRs and other HIT systems are powerful tools that are having a significant impact on healthcare. Consumers are empowered with more information, choices, and control, and providers have reliable access to complete personal health information that can help them make the right decisions. All necessary health information, from medical histories to billing information, will be accessible from the Internet and readily available to all appropriate healthcare facilities and providers of care (with permission of the client). With faster diffusion of medical knowledge through the Internet, decision-making will be expedited, medical errors reduced, and duplication of tests and misdiagnosis decreased. However, to protect these records from unauthorized, inappropriate, or unethical use, national privacy laws must be in place.

In the United States, The Office of the National Coordinator for Health Information Technology (ONC) is the principal federal entity responsible for the coordination and safety of information technology issues. It is a resource to the entire health system to support the adoption of HIT and to promote nationwide health information exchange to improve healthcare. ONC is organizationally located within the Office of the Secretary for the U.S. HHS. The ONC has developed SAFER guides for EHRs, consisting of nine guides organized into three broad groups that enable healthcare organizations to address EHR safety in a variety of areas. The guides identify recommended practices to optimize the safety and safe use of EHRs and can be found on the ONC website (see Web Resources on thePoint®).

The ONC funds the Nationwide Health Information Network (NwHIN), a collaborative organization of federal, local, regional, and state agencies. Its mission is to develop the envisioned secure, nationwide, interoperable health information infrastructure to connect providers, consumers, and organizations involved in supporting health and healthcare. The major goals of NwHIN are to enable health information to follow the consumer, to be available for clinical decision-making, and to support appropriate use of healthcare information beyond direct client care to improve the health of communities. The conceptual model that guides NwHIN is illustrated in Figure 1.2. The NwHIN has developed a set of standards, services, and policies that enable the secure exchange of health information nationwide over the

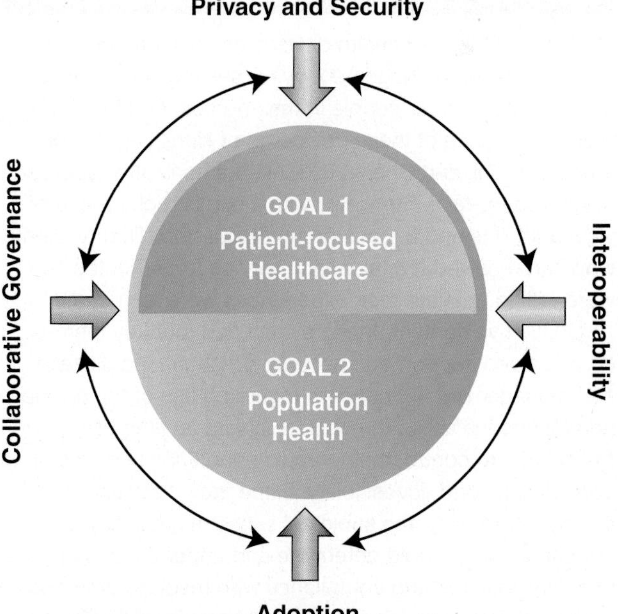

figure 1.2 The nationwide health information network conceptual model. (From Nationwide Health Information Network [NwHIN]. Retrieved from http://www.ahrq.gov/research/findings/nhqrdr/nhdr12/highlights.html).

Internet. Health information will follow the patient and be available for clinical decision-making as well as for uses beyond direct patient care, such as measuring quality of care. It is proposed that the NwHIN will be the vehicle through which health information will be exchanged.

Telehealth

Telehealth is the use of electronic information and telecommunications technologies to support long-distance clinical healthcare, patient and professional health-related education, public health, and health administration (Health Resources and Services Administration, 2014). Telehealth is becoming a necessity, due in part to the aging population, the rising number of people with chronic conditions, and the need to increase healthcare delivery to medically underserved populations.

Advances in technology, specifically those involving videoconferencing, medical devices, sensors, high-speed telecommunication networks, store-and-forward imaging, streaming media, and terrestrial and wireless communications have made it possible to assess clients' conditions remotely in their homes. Information can be stored for later access or assessments can be performed in real time using Internet video systems. It is also possible to obtain the advice of expert specialty consultants without meeting in person. The increasing complexity of telehealth requires ongoing communication, training, cultural sensitivity, and customization for individual clients. However, access, availability, and cost issues can be barriers to use of this technology (Ackerman, Filart, Burgess, Lee, & Poropatich, 2010).

EVIDENCE FOR PRACTICE

The use of home telehealth devices as an alternative for chronic disease management by nurses has the potential to assist many older people in their homes, and therefore, their acceptance of these devices is of significant importance. Lu, Chi, and Chen (2013) used a qualitative approach using face-to-face interviews with a semistructured interview guideline and a focus group discussion. Twenty clients who had received the telehealth service for 3 months and were willing to share their experiences were recruited.

Qualitative content analysis identified four key themes: (1) perceived support and security, (2) enhanced disease self-management, (3) concern regarding use of the devices, and (4) worries about the cost. Subjects favored using the service to control their chronic conditions because of convenience and accessibility. Since their condition could be measured daily, the subjects' sense of security was enhanced. They could determine and understand changes in their condition, and compliance with medical regimens improved. Subjects felt empowered to revise their lifestyles for better disease self-management. Since telehealth was in the stage of pilot testing, concerns were related to being unfamiliar with operation of the equipment and doubts about quality of the home health-monitoring equipment. Users also expressed concerns about future costs and policy changes in the future.

The authors concluded that most users perceived telehealth care as a convenient and useful model for healthcare delivery. It increased the availability of healthcare and improved the self-care ability of clients. Concern about the home monitoring devices suggests a need for further consumer education regarding use of home-monitoring devices and systems, a function normally performed by public health nurses (PHNs). Proper training and support for any problems when adopting the system will foster clients' willingness to use telehealth services. Further research is recommended to assess client perceptions of their current health status and their functional limitations in relation to their use of monitoring devices in the home.

Personal Responsibility for Health

Increased personal responsibility for preventing disease and disability is a vital component of healthcare change. The underlying premise holds that if people have a vested interest in their health, they will do more to maintain it. However, if a person is healthy, he or she may not focus on maintaining individual health, yet no one is more seriously affected when illness or disability occurs. Preventing or modifying unhealthy behaviors can save both lives and money, but can personal responsibility regarding one's health be truly mandated and regulated?

Personal responsibility for health involves active participation in one's own health through education and lifestyle changes. It includes responsibility for reviewing one's own medical records, including laboratory test results, and monitoring both the positive and negative effects of prescription and over-the-counter medications. It means showing up for scheduled tests and procedures, following dietary recommendations, losing weight if needed, avoiding tobacco and recreational drug use, engaging in exercise programs, and educating oneself about one's own conditions. Ultimately, people must take the responsibility for making their own choices and healthcare decisions

> *The...patient should be made to understand that he or she must take charge of his own life. Don't take your body to the doctor as if he were a repair shop.*
>
> **Quentin Regestein, psychiatrist, Harvard University**

U.S. government initiatives have been implemented to encourage personal responsibility for health. *Healthy People 2020* is a national, science-based plan designed to reduce certain illnesses and disabilities by reducing disparities in healthcare services in people of different economic groups. Since 1979, *Healthy People* programs have measured and tracked national health objectives to encourage collaboration, guided people toward making informed health decisions, and assessed the impact of prevention activity. Specific objectives with baseline values for measurement are devel-

box 1.2 Healthy People 2020 Overarching Goals

1. Attain high-quality, longer lives free of preventable disease, disability, injury, and premature death.
2. Achieve health equity, eliminate disparities, and improve the health of all groups.
3. Create social and physical environments that promote good health for all.
4. Promote quality of life, healthy development, and healthy behaviors across all life stages.

oped, setting specific targets to be achieved by 2020. The four major overarching goals that incorporate these objectives are listed in Box 1.2 (*Healthy People 2020,* n.d.)

PUBLIC HEALTH NURSING TODAY

The shorter length of stay in acute care facilities, as well as the increase in ambulatory surgery and outpatient clinics, has resulted in more acute and chronically ill people residing in the community who need professional nursing care. Fortunately, these people can have their care needs met cost-effectively outside of expensive acute care settings. As a result, demand has increased for nurses in ambulatory clinics, home care, and care management.

Hospitals remain the most common workplace for RNs in the United States (62.2%). However, the number of RNs working in home health service units or agencies is increasing (6.4%) (Department of Health and Human Services, Health Resources and Service Administration, 2014). Public health, ambulatory care, and other noninstitutional settings have historically had the largest increases in RN employment. These statistics indicate a shift in the roles of nurses, particularly for those working in public health settings.

Nursing is the protection, promotion, and optimization of health and abilities, prevention of illness and injury, alleviation of suffering through the diagnosis and treatment of human response, and advocacy in the care of individuals, families, communities, and populations.

American Nurses Association

Public Health Nursing

A decades-long debate about terminology has fostered confusion regarding the roles of nurses who serve the community. However, public health professionals nationwide have come together to define the principles of public health (Box 1.3). Embracing these fundamental principles for all public health professionals, the Quad Council of Public Health Nursing Organizations established eight principles of public health nursing practice (Box 1.4). The Quad Council of Public Health Nursing Organizations is an alliance of four national nursing organizations that address public health nursing issues in the United States, comprising the following:

- Association of Community Health Nurse Educators (ACHNE)
- ANA's Congress on Nursing Practice and Economics (CNPE)
- American Public Health Association (APHA)—Public Health Nursing Section
- Association of State and Territorial Directors of Nursing (ASTDN)

box 1.3 Principles of Public Health

Focus on the **aggregate.**
Promote prevention.
Encourage community organization.
Practice the ethical theory of the greater good.
Model leadership in health.
Use epidemiologic knowledge and methods.

box 1.4 Principles of Public Health Nursing: The public health nurse is guided by adherence to all of the following principles

The client or unit of care is the population.
The primary obligation is to achieve the greatest good for the greatest number of people or number of people as a whole.
Public health nurses collaborate with the client as an equal partner.
Primary prevention is the priority in selecting appropriate activities.
Public health nursing focuses on strategies that create health environmental, social, and economic conditions in which populations may thrive.
A public health nurse is obligated to actively identify and reach out to all who might benefit from a specific activity or service.
Optimal use of available resources and creation of new evidence-based strategies is necessary to assure the best overall improvement in the health of populations.
Collaboration with other professions, populations, organizations, and stakeholder groups is the most effect way to promote and protect the health of the people.

Source: American Nurses Association. (2013). *Public health nursing: Scope and standards of practice*. Silver Spring, MD: Nursesbooks.

Public health is what we, as a society, do collectively to assure the conditions in which people can be healthy.

Institute of Medicine, 1988

Scope and Standards of Practice

The American Nurses Association sets the scope and standards for all professional nursing practice. The publication *Public Health Nursing: Scope and Standards of Practice* establishes the characteristics of competent public health nursing practice and is the legal standard of practice. It defines the essentials of public health nursing, the activities, and the accountabilities that are characteristic of practice at all levels and settings. An important component of this document is the designation of **competencies** required to meet each standard of practice. This scope and standards document can be used by PHNs from entry-level to senior management in a variety of practice settings and is an indispensable publication reference for every practicing PHN (ANA, 2013).

Competencies for Public Health Nursing Practice

The Core Competencies for Public Health Nurses (CCPHN) defined in the ANA (2013) publication are aligned with core competencies developed by other public health organizations. The CCPHN reflect the unique capabilities required for the practice of public health nursing. Three tiers of practice are defined, along with competencies associated with that level of practice. Tier 1 core competencies apply to entry-level public health professionals at the basic or generalist level. For example, individuals who have limited experience working in the public health field and are not in management positions would be considered practicing at Tier 1. Tier 2 core competencies apply to individuals with management and/or supervisory responsibilities and are considered specialists or mid-level practitioners. Tier 3 core competencies apply to senior managers and leaders at the executive level who deal with multisystems. Essentially, these competencies underlie the wide variety of roles and responsibilities that PHNs accept in the workplace.

The CCPHN are integrated into the Standards of Practice for Public Health Nursing (ANA, 2013). Each standard of practice is followed by the essential competencies required to meet that standard. Following each standard of practice, additional competencies are presented for practice as an advanced PHN.

Public Health Nursing Interventions

The **public health nursing intervention** (wheel) model, illustrated in Figure 1.3, is (1) a population-based model that (2) is applied to individuals, families, communities, or within systems and (3) defines 17 public health interventions focusing upon prevention. It is a way of defining public health nursing by the type of actions taken on behalf of clients to protect or improve health status. The interventions in the wheel model complement the competencies that each PHN must demonstrate for safe practice. The competencies define what should be done while the interventions provide a means to accomplish those actions. Table 1.1 describes the 17 interventions illustrated in the wheel. Other interventions have been suggested, such as that of change agent, culture

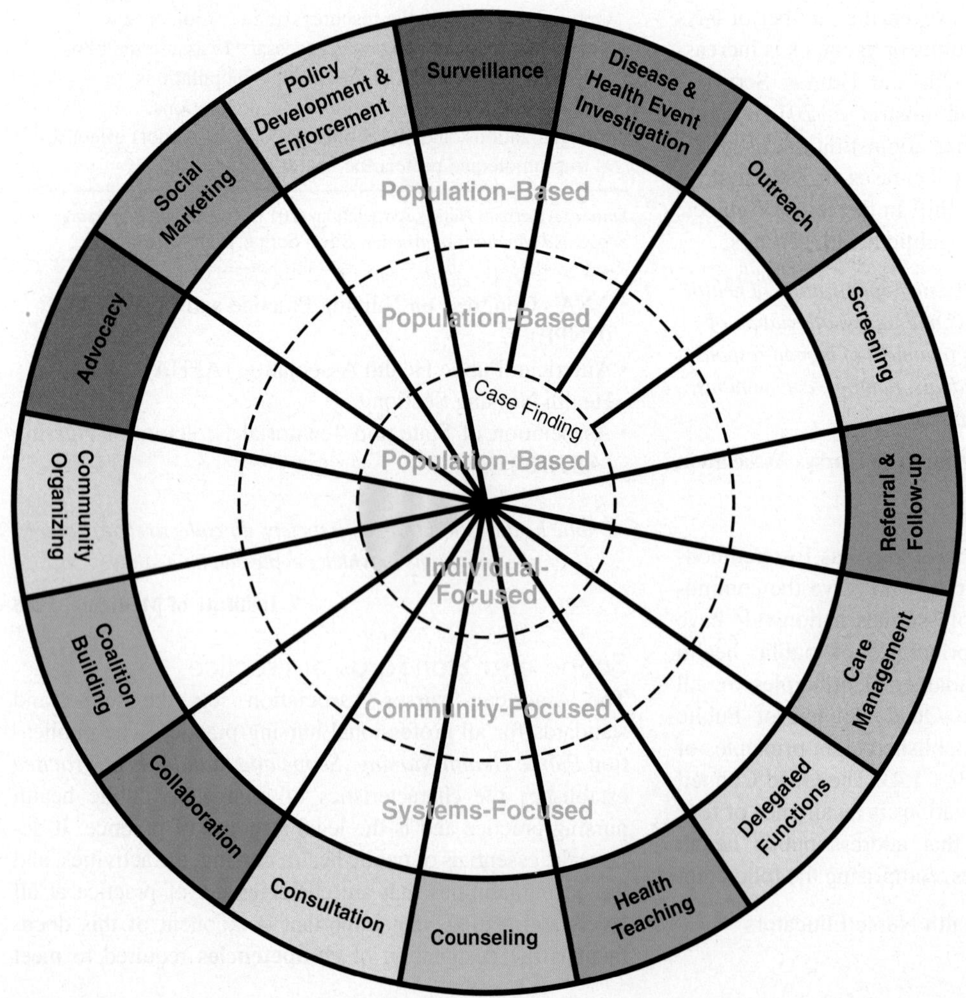

figure 1.3 Public health intervention wheel.

table 1.1 **Public Health Nursing Interventions**

Intervention	Definition
Surveillance	Monitors health events through ongoing, systematic collection, analysis and interpretation of health data for planning, implementing, and evaluating public health interventions
Investigation of disease and other health events	Systematically gathers and analyzes data about threats to population health, determines the source, identifies cases and those at risk, and determines control measures
Outreach	Locates populations at risk, provides information, identifies possible actions, and identifies access to services
Screening	Identifies individuals with unrecognized risk factors or asymptomatic conditions
Case-finding	Locates individuals and families with identified risk factors and connects them with resources
Referral and follow-up	Assists in identifying and accessing necessary resources to prevent or resolve concerns
Case management	Coordination of a plan or process to bring health services, and the self-care capabilities of the client, together as a common whole in a cost-effective way
Delegation	Direct care tasks an RN entrusts to other appropriate personnel
Teaching	Develop a health education plan and teach clients and other caregivers leading to behavior change
Counseling	Develops an interpersonal relationship with the client to increase their capabilities to address or solve issues
Consultation	Seeks information and generates solutions to health problems or issues through interactive problem-solving
Collaboration	Work with people or representatives of organizations to achieve a common goal
Coalition building	Foster, mobilize, and participate in community-wide alliances to achieve a specific goal
Community organizing	Help community groups to identify common problems or goals, mobilize resources, and develop and implement strategies for reaching those goals
Advocacy	Act on behalf of clients who have lost control of factors that affect their health and a need is unmet; strengthen clients' capacity to act
Social marketing	Use marketing principles and technology to design programs to address needs of the client
Policy development	Promote beneficial social changes that influence the health of groups and populations
Policy enforcement	Compels others to comply with the laws, rules, regulations, and ordinances created in conjunction with policy development

Source: Adapted from *Public Health Interventions: Application for Nursing Practice*. Retrieved from www.health.state.mn.us/divs/opi/cd/phn/wheel.html

broker, and researcher. The wheel creates a structure for identifying and documenting interventions, thereby capturing the nature of public health nursing practice.

Two years ago, Sandy participated in a statewide survey of both the public health nurses in the state as well as their employers. The purpose of the survey was to determine the characteristics of public health nursing practice, especially the use of principles of population health. Results indicated that the majority of the public health nurse's time is spent in the provision of primary care and clinical services to individual clients. The major factors that contribute to this finding include the number of uninsured people (16%) and a large population of medically underserved people.

Define the type of practice (Tier) that the public health nurses were performing.

The new vision for public health being designed by the task force promotes a shift from a predominantly individual and clinic-based care model to a population health practice model. The public health nurses in the state were unprepared for this transition and lacked a strong understanding of population health concepts and competencies. Using the standards of practice and associated competencies outlined in *Public Health Nursing: Scope and Standards of Practice*, and with assistance from faculty members at the state university, the task force is helping to develop an online population-based health course to meet the needs of the public health nurses in the state. The priorities of the online course are as follows:

- Community assessment and diagnosis
- Interpreting and presenting health information
- Using computer technology in health planning and policy development
- Building community coalitions

Using *Public Health Nursing: Scope and Standards of Practice*, choose the appropriate standards and competencies that the public health nurses should demonstrate to meet the priorities listed above.

Education for Public Health Nursing Practice

The educational credential for entry into public health nursing practice is the baccalaureate degree in nursing. This can be a baccalaureate in nursing (BS or BSN) or a generalist master's degree as a clinical nurse leader (CNL). Public health nursing specialists in population health may have a master of science in nursing (MSN), master of public health (MPH), a joint MSN/MPH, or a doctoral degree. Doctoral degrees may be doctor of philosophy (PhD), doctor of nursing practice (DNP), or doctor of public health (DrPH). Diploma- and associate degree–prepared RNs and licensed practical nurses may practice in some public health settings. In these positions, nurses provide care for individuals or families, but not for populations (ANA, 2013).

Certification for Public Health Nursing Specialty Practice

Advanced nursing practice at the master's level is considered a specialty practice in public health nursing, and the standard credential awarded for passing the American Nurses Credentialing Center (ANCC) certification examination is Advanced Public Health Nurse–Board Certified (APHN–BC). The advanced practice student must study pathophysiology, physical assessment, and pharmacology, with an emphasis on caring for people in communities to affect public health interests positively, to qualify for the examination. The ANCC website explains eligibility criteria, the application process, steps to maintain certification, and the process for renewal.

ROOTS OF PUBLIC HEALTH NURSING

Exploring the roots of the healing professions provides the background for understanding the characteristics of nursing practice today (Table 1.2). Since the beginning of civilization, people in all cultures have focused on birth, health, illness, and death. Historical records indicate that early societies engaged in public health measures by burying wastes away from water supplies, developing sewage systems, and draining marshes to control communicable disease. In these times, people spent their lives with their family and community, especially when they were ill and needed care. Early caregivers, usually women, cultivated healing herbs, applied poultices, applied heat and cold, immobilized fractures, delivered babies, and attended the dead.

In the Middle Ages, care of ill people was based in the household. Care was haphazard. The few hospitals that existed were run by monks and nuns, primarily for residents of monasteries, and only the wealthy could afford assistance with their care. Changes in social structures encouraged the development of cities, but overcrowding, lack of sanitation, and an ever-increasing susceptible population contributed to recurring epidemics. During the 14th century, the Black Plague alone killed approximately one-fourth of the population of Europe. From the 1500s through the 1700s, the Renaissance in Europe stimulated the rise of scientific thought and inspired social consciousness.

The English Poor Law of 1601 marked the beginning of state-provided relief for the poor, placing a legal responsibility on each district to care for people within its boundaries who, either because of age or infirmity, were unable to work. The Sisters (or Daughters) of Charity, known as the "Grey Sisters," was founded in 1617 in France, with members taking vows to provide care to the sick poor. The organization was so successful that it spread from the rural districts to Paris, and a training program was established in 1633 for young women who were devoted to serving people in need. From that time through the 19th century, this nursing community spread throughout the world. Today, the mother house is located in Paris.

In the 1800s, a variety of reforms were initiated to care for the sick poor throughout Europe that interacted and built on one another. Hospitals were established. By 1825, there were 154 in England alone. However, the fatality rates in these institutions were high, particularly for newborns and people with open wounds; the hospitals were called "death houses." So-called "ward maids," equivalent to housekeepers, provided care.

In Holland, Mennonites recruited women of the church to form deaconess groups to care for the poor. In 1836, Theodore Fliedner, a German Lutheran pastor, established a 3-year training school for deaconesses, which was associated with a new hospital. Fliedner also founded parish districts by dividing towns geographically into smaller areas to provide care to residents.

In Victorian times, poorhouses or workhouses existed for chronically ill poor people who were often elderly, without families. The primary reason for poverty was illness, and tuberculosis was rampant. Each parish had its own poorhouse. "Pauper nurses" were poor residents themselves, given the responsibility to care for the destitute. Conditions in many of these poor houses were deliberately harsh and often abysmal. Unfortunately, some pauper nurses were illiterate, irresponsible drunks who were vicious to residents, prolonging their illness (The Public Health [Scotland] Act, 1897). One of the most famous comical, fictional characters in Charles Dickens' works is nurse Sairey Gamp in *The Life and Adventures of Martin Chuzzlewit.* She was a nurse of sorts who dealt with the "lying in and the laying out" extremities of life, representing some of the more questionable characteristics of the so-called nurses at the time (Fig. 1.4).

During the latter part of the 19th century, when **district nursing** was established, meeting the needs of the ill became more organized in England. At that time, William Rathbone, a Quaker merchant and philanthropist in Liverpool, England, organized help for the poor. In 1859, he hired Mary Robinson, a nurse who previously had cared for his terminally ill wife, to provide care for the people in one of the poorest parish districts in Liverpool. Mary became the first **district nurse** in England. Box 1.5 lists the duties of district nurses in Liverpool. District nursing soon sprang up in other towns, cities, and rural areas in England, funded by local philanthropists.

Rathbone devoted the rest of his life to expanding services for the sick poor, with assistance from his friend Florence Nightingale and others. Nightingale, the daughter

table 1.2 **Milestones in Public Health and Public Health Nursing**

1601	Poor Law instituted in England; beginning of state-supported assistance for the poor
1617	Sisters (or Daughters) of Charity founded in France
1789	First local permanent health department in the United States founded in Baltimore, Maryland
1798	Marine Hospital Service established in the United States; later became the Public Health Service
1809	Sisters of Charity founded by Elizabeth Ann Seton in Maryland
1813	Ladies' Benevolent Society of Charleston, South Carolina, established to provide home care to the sick
1825	154 hospitals had been established in England
1836	Training school for deaconesses established by Theodore Fliedner, a German Lutheran pastor
1840/1841	Dorothea Dix began her lifelong campaign to improve the life of the mentally ill
1850	Shattuck Report published by the Massachusetts Sanitary Commission; recommended the establishment of a state health department and local health boards in every town, collection of vital statistics, sanitation, disease control, health education, town planning, and teaching of prevention in medical schools
1851	Florence Nightingale attended Fliedner's school for deaconesses
1859	William Rathbone established district nursing in England
1860	Florence Nightingale established the first school for nurses at St. Thomas Hospital in London
1861	Soldiers in the American Civil War attended by visiting nurses
1870s	First nursing schools opened in the United States based on the Nightingale model
1872	American Public Health Association established
1882	Clara Barton convinced the U.S. Congress to establish the American Red Cross with an extended mission to provide aid for natural disasters
1885/1886	Visiting nurse associations established in Boston, Philadelphia, and Buffalo
1893	Lillian Wald established the Henry Street Settlement in New York City for the sick poor
1895	Ada Steward employed by Vermont Marble Works as the first occupational health nurse
1898	Significant use of trained nurses in military hospitals
1901	U.S. Army Nurse Corps established
1908	U.S. Navy Nurse Corps established
1912	National Organization for Public Health Nursing established, with Lillian Wald the first President; U.S. Children's Bureau established; Marine Hospital Service changed to U.S. Public Health Service
1914	First postgraduate program in public health nursing at Teachers College in New York City, affiliated with the Henry Street Settlement, established by Mary Adelaide Nutting
1920	90% of the ill were cared for at home with assistance from the community
1925	Frontier Nursing Service in the United States established by Mary Breckinridge to provide access to healthcare in remote Appalachian regions of southeastern Kentucky
1933	Pearl McIver became the first nurse employed by the U.S. Public Health Service
1935	U.S. Social Security Act passed
1943	Frances Payne Bolton was instrumental in founding the Cadet Nurse Corps as a part of the Public Health Service to train nurses during World War II
1953	U.S. Department of Health, Education, and Welfare established
1957	Nationalized Canadian healthcare system established
1965	Public health pediatric nurse practitioner program established at University of Colorado
1966	Medicare for the elderly established in the United States
1967	Medicaid for the medically indigent established in the United States
1970	Occupational Safety and Health Administration established
1974	National Health Planning and Resources Development Act passed
1975	Certification for community health nurses established by the American Nurses Association (ANA)
1979	Smallpox eradication worldwide certified by the WHO[a]
1980	First national health objectives for the United States established: *Promoting Health/Preventing Disease: Objectives for the Nation*
1980	Direct reimbursement through Medicaid for nurse practitioner in rural health clinics, United States
1984	Behavioral Risk Factor Surveillance System (BRFSS) established
1989	*Guide to Clinical Preventive Services* (standardizing screening and prevention strategies) published by the U.S. Public Health Services Task Force
1990	*Healthy People 2000: National Health Objectives for Health Promotion and Illness Prevention* published
1991	*Nursing's Agenda for Health Care Reform* published by a coalition of more than 60 nursing organizations
1998	*The Public Health Workforce: An Agenda for the 21st Century* published by U.S. Public Health Service
2000	*Healthy People 2010* published
2002	European region of WHO declared free of polio
2002	U.S. Office of Homeland Security established
2003	U.S. Institute of Medicine recommends that undergraduate nursing students understand the ecological model of health and core competencies of population-based practice
2010	Patient Protection and Affordable Care Act (PPACA) passed

[a]WHO = World Health Organization.

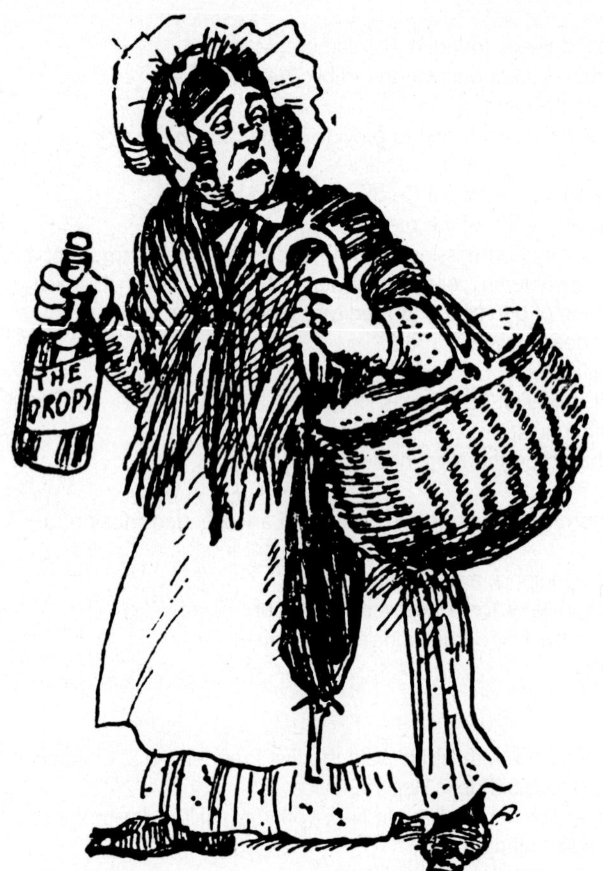

figure 1.4 Dickens' character, Sairey Gamp. (From Kalisch, P. A., & Kalisch, B. J. [2004]. *American nursing: A history.* Philadelphia, PA: Lippincott Williams & Wilkins.)

box 1.5 Duties of District Nurses in Liverpool, England: 1865

Investigate new referrals as soon as possible.
Report to the superintendent situations in which additional food or relief would improve recovery.
Report neglect of patients by family or friends to the superintendent.
Assist physicians with surgery in the home.
Maintain a clean, uncluttered home environment and tend fires for heat.
Teach the patient and family about cleanliness, ventilation, giving of food and medications, and obedience to the physician's orders.
Set an example for "neatness, order, sobriety, and obedience."
Hold family matters in confidence.
Avoid interference with the religious opinions and beliefs of patients and others.
Report facts to and ask questions of physicians.
Refer acutely ill to hospitals and the chronically ill, poor without family to infirmaries.

Source: Brainard, M. (1985). *The evolution of public health nursing* (pp. 120–121). New York, NY: Garland. (Original work published in 1922. Philadelphia, PA: W.B. Saunders.)

of a wealthy English landowner, devoted her life to the prevention of needless illness and death. In 1851, she attended Theodore Fliedner's program for deaconesses—for nurse training—in Kaiserwerth, Germany. She formed a team of nurses that assisted soldiers during the Crimean War (1854–1856) and statistically documented her successes saving lives through prevention of infections and improving environmental conditions (Fig. 1.5). In 1860, following the war, Nightingale opened the first school of nursing, and Rathbone hired several graduates as district nurses. Two years later, with Nightingale's assistance, he established a nursing school in Liverpool (see Chapter 6).

Public Health Initiatives in Early America

American social values were strongly influenced by British traditions, including care for the sick poor. Care of destitute and infirm residents was the responsibility of the town or county, similar to the English Poor Law of 1601. In the 1700s, early public health efforts in the colonies were focused on sanitation, collection of vital statistics, and control of infectious diseases. People with contagious diseases were isolated in "pesthouses," and home quarantines were instituted. Women of the house were responsible for care of the ill, and treatments consisted of home remedies that were often passed down through generations.

Occasionally, a board of health would be established to address a specific problem, but it was then disbanded. In 1789, the first local health department with a permanent board of health was formed in Baltimore, Maryland. In 1798, the Marine Hospital Service was established by Congress to provide for the temporary relief and maintenance of sick and disabled seamen, as a means to protect the public from contagious diseases brought into port by the sailors. This was the first prepaid medical care program in the United States, financed through compulsory employer tax and federally administered.

At the beginning of the 1800s, people recognized that they needed a more organized public health system. In 1809, Elizabeth Ann Seton founded the Sisters of Charity in Maryland. The Sisters of Charity (also called Daughters of Charity) established and operated many hospitals, orphanages, and educational institutions over the years. In 1813, the Ladies' Benevolent Society of Charleston, South Carolina, was established to provide organized home care to the sick. Knowing the threats that sick merchant seamen posed to the general population, Congress passed the Act for the Relief of Sick and Disabled Seamen in 1798 (amended in 1802) to establish hospitals for merchant seamen. However, conditions in many cities remained nearly intolerable.

The Industrial Revolution resulted in the transformation of primarily agricultural economies to large industrial centers. Large numbers of people migrated into cities, living in crowded tenement houses. Working conditions were poor,

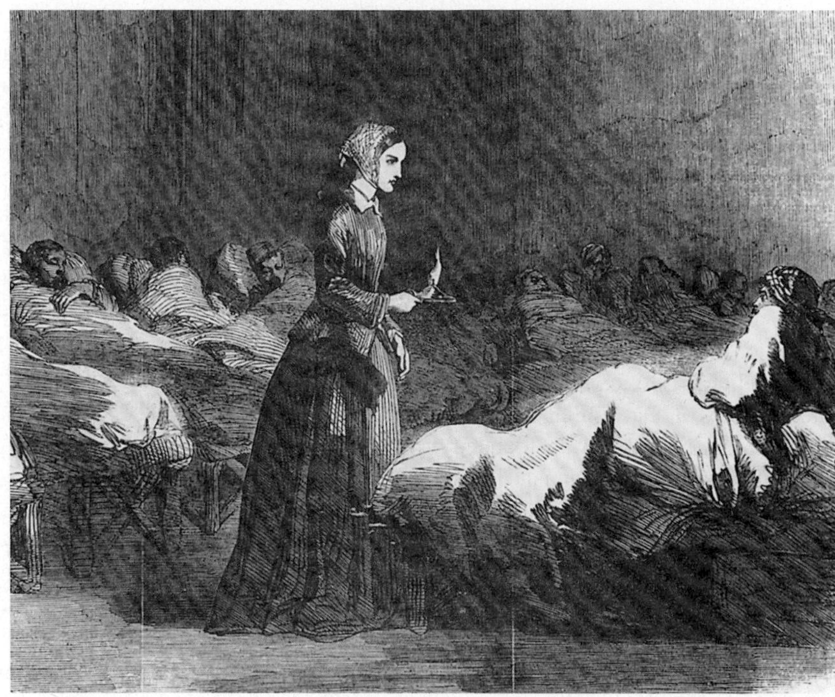

figure 1.5 Florence Nightingale, the "Lady with the Lamp." (From Kalisch, P. A., & Kalisch, B. J. [2004]. *American nursing: A history*. Philadelphia, PA: Lippincott Williams & Wilkins.)

people were overworked and underpaid, and child labor was prevalent. Poor nutrition and overcrowded living conditions led to the rapid spread of communicable diseases. For example, New York City's streets were piled with garbage and sewage, and tenements were filthy and crowded, providing breeding grounds for tuberculosis, smallpox, and typhus. Although initial attempts were made to protect residents from infectious diseases by providing healthcare to merchant seamen, diseases became epidemic and quarantine became inadequate. Few advances in public health were made other than scattered smallpox regulations until the Shattuck Report was published.

Lemuel Shattuck

Lemuel Shattuck prepared a report for the Massachusetts Sanitary Commission that pointed out that much of the ill health and disability in American cities in 1850 could be traced to unsanitary conditions. The report is now considered one of the fundamental documents in public health in the United States. It provided for the first systematic use of birth and death records and demographic data to describe the health of a population. The recommendations became the foundation of the sanitation movement in the United States, which laid the framework for the dramatic increase in life expectancy that occurred in the next 150 years. In 1850, the average life span was 25 years, and by 2000, it was more than 75 years. The Shattuck Report recommended the establishment of a state health department and local health boards in every town, and resulted in the first attempt to write a comprehensive public health code. Following the Civil War, many states and localities adopted these recommendations, ultimately resulting in the public health system that exists today.

Perhaps the most significant single document in the history of public health—I know of no single document in the history of that science quite so remarkable in its clarity and completeness and in its vision of the future.

C.-E. A. Winslow, bacteriologist and public health expert, on the Shattuck Report

Dorothea Dix

Dorothea Dix was also an American political activist in the 19th century who became aware of the dreadful conditions in prisons and mental hospitals, and she vigorously lobbied state and federal officials to remedy the situation. She had traveled to England in 1836, and during her time there, she met William Rathbone, who was spending a year as a guest at the family estate in Liverpool. In addition, she met political activists who believed that government should take an active role in social welfare. The lunacy reform movement was underway in England at the time, and the detailed investigations of the madhouses were published, resulting in legislative changes. After returning from England in 1840, Dix traveled the state of Massachusetts, visiting jails and insane asylums. She was appalled by conditions there and compiled a report that she presented to the Massachusetts Legislature. Considered the most progressive state in the union, Massachusetts quickly allocated funds to establish the first hospitals for the mentally ill. After making changes in Massachusetts, Dorothea moved on to other states and other countries, establishing hospitals and improving life for the mentally ill.

I proceed, Gentlemen, briefly to call your attention to the present state of Insane Persons confined within this Commonwealth, in cages, stalls, pens! Chained, naked, beaten with rods, and lashed into obedience.

Dorothea Lynde Dix

Clara Barton

Clara Barton achieved widespread recognition during the Civil War, distributing supplies to wounded soldiers and caring for the casualties with the help of her team of nurses. As a result of these experiences, she recognized the need for a neutral relief society in the United States that could be activated in times of war, similar to the International Committee of the Red Cross that was founded in 1863 in Geneva, Switzerland, by Henry Dunant. Barton lobbied tirelessly, and in 1882, she convinced Congress to ratify the Treaty of Geneva, and the American Red Cross was established with an extended mission—to provide aid for natural disasters.

Lillian Wald

In the 1880s, 20 years following the establishment of district nursing in England, a similar movement began in the United States. Urban tenement houses in the large American cities across the country were crowded and unsanitary, and infectious diseases such as tuberculosis, typhoid fever, smallpox, and scarlet fever were prevalent. A number of initiatives were undertaken in the major cities to improve the life of residents. An increased understanding of communicable disease indicated that education about prevention of infections would reduce these illnesses. Teaching methods to prevent infectious disease, implementing sanitary reforms, and fostering better nutrition became the foundations of community nursing practice in the United States.

Lillian Wald, the founder of public health nursing, was born into a life of privilege (as was Florence Nightingale) (Fig. 1.6). At the age of 22, Wald attended the New York Hospital School of Nursing. While taking classes at the Women's Medical College, she became involved in organizing a class in home nursing for poor immigrants on New York's Lower East Side. Distressed by the living conditions in the dingy multistory flats, Wald moved to the neighborhood, and she and her classmate Mary Brewster volunteered their services. With the aid of several patrons, they founded the Henry Street Settlement in 1893; fees were based on the patient's ability to pay. In addition to providing acute and long-term care for the sick, Wald and Brewster taught health and hygiene to the immigrant women, stressing the importance of preventive care. Wald called her services "public health nursing." Similar settlement houses in other American cities developed rapidly.

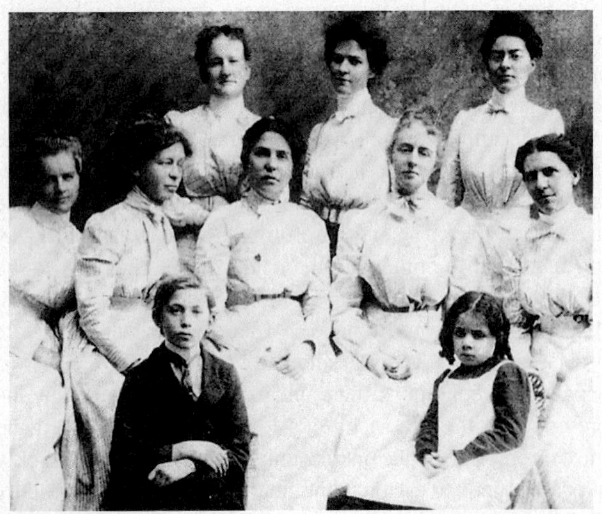

figure 1.6 Lillian Wald (center, second row) and nurses of the Henry Street Settlement. (From Kalisch, P. A., & Kalisch, B. J. [2004]. *American nursing: A history*. Philadelphia, PA: Lippincott Williams & Wilkins.)

The vermin in these old houses are terribly active at night… there is nothing harder to endure than to watch by a night sickbed in these old worn houses and see the crawling creatures, and the babes so accustomed to them that their sleep is scarcely disturbed.

Lillian Wald, *The House on Henry Street*

Wald devoted herself full time to the Lower East Side community, ultimately becoming one of the most influential and respected social reformers and humanitarians of the 20th century. Within a decade, the Henry Street Settlement included a team of 20 nurses, and it offered an astonishing array of innovative and effective social, recreational, and educational services. Eventually, the organization incorporated housing, employment, educational assistance, and recreational programs. It also placed nurses in public schools and businesses. Later, the Henry Street Settlement became the Visiting Nurse Association of New York City (Henry Street Settlement, 2004).

Nursing is love in action, and there is no finer manifestation of it than the care of the poor and disabled in their own homes.

Lillian Wald

In 1912, Wald helped found the National Organization for Public Health Nursing, which set the first professional standards for the practice of public health nursing. These standards were a precursor to ANA's *Public Health Nursing: Scope and Standards of Practice*, which guides the practice of public health nursing today. As a founder of Columbia University's School of Nursing, she persuaded the administration to appoint the first professor of nursing in the country, laying the foundation for nursing education in institutions of higher learning. Wald also was an advocate for children and women's rights, helping with the establishment of the United States Children's Bureau, National Child Labor Committee, and the National Women's Trade Union League.

Public Health Initiatives in the Twentieth Century

Public Health in the First Half of the Century

Public health and nursing initiatives grew exponentially in the 1900s, a century dominated by two world wars and an astounding increase in scientific knowledge. Recognition of public health nursing as a necessary function of government came about gradually in the early part of the 20th century. Local health departments, charged with control of communicable diseases, sanitation, maintaining a safe water supply, food inspection, health education, and other functions, began hiring more nurses. Although there was a rapid growth in the number of hospitals, few resources were available to people who had to be cared for in their homes. The first PHNs focused on care at the bedside, but they soon realized that their efforts had little effect if conditions were unsanitary and if there was no food in the house. PHNs effectively served as sanitary inspectors, tenement house inspectors, probation officers, and social welfare service workers. Before long, it was clear that nursing practice demanded psychosocial and political skills, along with a broad understanding of the community.

As demand for services grew, the role of PHNs became more focused on teaching and counseling, showing others how to care for the sick, instructing them on how to prevent illness, and promoting maternal and child health (Kalisch & Kalisch, 1978). Health promotion and disease prevention began with the need for health education during home visits to the poor living in large cities and expanded over time to schools, employees, and the rural population.

Mary Breckinridge

An innovation in the provision of health services occurred when Mary Breckinridge founded the Frontier Nursing Service in 1925 (Fig. 1.7). Following the death of her two children, she decided to devote her life to improving the health of children and developing a system of rural healthcare in the remote regions of Kentucky and throughout the world. Traveling on horseback, Breckinridge studied the health needs of the mountain people. She found that women lacked prenatal care, gave birth to an average of nine children, and primarily had self-taught midwives in attendance at their delivery. Maternal and infant mortality were high. Breckinridge realized that children's healthcare must begin before birth with care of the mother and continue throughout childhood, while including care for the entire family. She founded the Frontier Nursing Service, which continues to provide family-oriented healthcare to rural and underserved populations today. In 1939, she helped establish the Frontier Graduate School of Midwifery, one of the first midwifery programs in the country (Frontier Nursing Service Inc., n.d.)

Our aim is to see ourselves surpassed.

Mary Breckinridge

Early Twentieth-Century Federal Healthcare Initiatives

The Spanish–American War of 1898 led to a significant use of trained nurses in military hospitals. For the first time, the graduates of nearly 200 nurse training schools throughout the country were incorporated into a single nursing corps. These nurses were the forerunners of women in the armed services. A permanent Army Nurse Corps was established in February, 1901, followed by creation of a Navy Nurse Corps in 1908 (Kalisch & Kalisch, 1978).

Prior to the 20th century, government involvement in healthcare was left to the states. By 1900, health departments had been established in the majority of states, but their function was limited. By 1912, there was a growing acceptance that the U.S. government should take an active role in the health and welfare of the people. The need for a permanent federal agency that was responsible for the health of citizens was recognized, and the Marine Hospital Service, originally established in 1798 for seamen, was reorganized to form the U.S. Public Health Service (USPHS). The office of the U.S. Surgeon General was also founded that year. Federal programs focused on the health of mothers and children, the poor, the mentally ill, and those with sexually

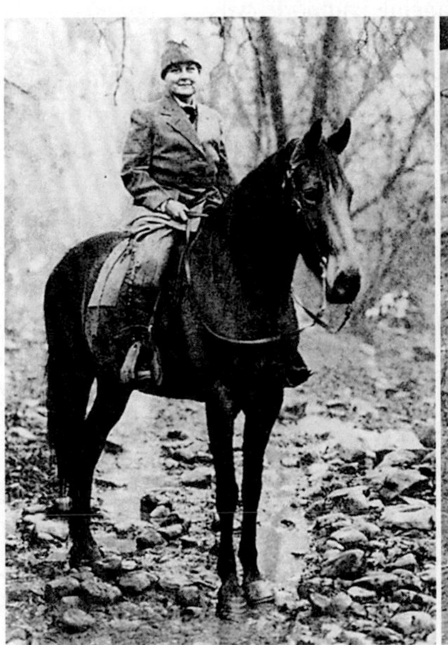
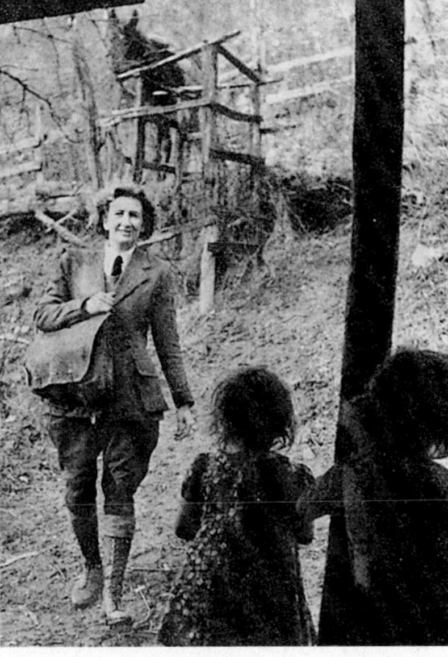

figure 1.7 Mary Breckinridge and a frontier nursing visit. (From Kalisch, P. A., & Kalisch, B. J. [2004]. *American nursing: A history*. Philadelphia, PA: Lippincott Williams & Wilkins.)

transmitted diseases were implemented. For example, the Maternal and Infancy Act (Sheppard–Towner Act), passed in 1921, provided matching funds to states that developed maternal and child divisions in their health departments. Home visits by PHNs encouraged prenatal care and health promotion for mother and child, and maternity centers and child health clinics were established (Kalisch & Kalisch, 2004).

World War I (1914–1918) was a military conflict centered in Europe that involved most of the world's great powers. Although the Army Nurse Corps and the Navy Nurse Corps had expanded, care of the wounded was still insufficient, and civilian nurses were in short supply. The types of wounds from modern weapons and the use of poisonous gases required new nursing skills, and wound infections were rampant. Then, in late 1918, when the armistice occurred, an influenza pandemic spread throughout the world, with soldiers becoming vectors of the viral infection.

By 1920, there was a significant shortage of nurses, and patient care suffered. It was estimated that 90% of ill people were cared for at home with assistance from the community (Kalisch & Kalisch, 1978). The Great Depression began in 1929, resulting in widespread unemployment, including nurses. At the same time, the need for health services expanded, especially for charity cases. The federal government became even more active in health and social welfare programs, employing nurses through the Federal Emergency Relief Act, the Civil Works Administration, and other agencies. In 1933, Pearl McIver became the first nurse to be employed by the USPHS. Her primary role was to provide consultation services to state public health departments, resulting in an increase in local PHN employment.

The Social Security Act of 1935 was passed to help prevent a recurrence of the problems associated with the Depression, especially for poor elderly people. It provided a system of federal old-age benefits and enabled states to make more adequate provision for elderly people, the blind, dependent and crippled children, maternal and child welfare, public health, and the administration of state unemployment compensation laws. Financial support was provided to increase public health programs, particularly for mothers and children in rural areas. Local health departments designed their programs on the basis of the funding that was available, rather than directing their efforts toward a comprehensive community health program. A component of the federal approach to health policy today still directs funding to special population groups or to the prevention and control of specific diseases.

With the onset of the United States' involvement in World War II, it became clear that the United States would soon face a critical shortage of nurses nationwide. Through the work of Congresswoman Frances Payne Bolton, the Cadet Nurse Corps was founded as a part of the USPHS to train nurses during World War II. Applicants were granted subsidization of nursing school tuition and associated expenses, and schools were funded to provide expedited training. In exchange, applicants agreed to provide nursing services to the military or other essential civilian industries for the duration of the war. The number of PHNs employed by industry almost doubled during this time. Public health nursing also expanded in rural areas during World War II, and some official agencies began to offer bedside care.

Public Health in the Second Half of the Century

After the war, the increased demand for healthcare services led to increased opportunities for PHNs, changes in healthcare delivery and financing, and the growth of health insurance. Local health departments faced increases in demand for services related to community problems such as alcoholism and mental illness. Their services increased to include screening for tuberculosis and sexually transmitted diseases as well as treatment of infectious diseases, and services were extended to rural areas.

By mid-century, a number of social improvements resulted in an increased life span. Public health measures such as improved sanitation, provision of potable water, better nutrition, and better housing contributed to this phenomenon, along with medical developments such as immunizations and antibiotics. Childhood mortality decreased, and more Americans lived into middle and old age. Infectious diseases were the leading causes of mortality in 1900; by 1950, the leading causes of death were heart disease, cancer, and cerebrovascular disease, as they remain today. With the increased life span, new challenges related to chronic diseases emerged.

In 1966, the Social Security Act was amended and Medicare was created to provide healthcare funding to the elderly. The next year, Medicaid was established to provide funding for the indigent (see Chapter 2). These programs contributed to the continued increase in demand for services, and costs of healthcare escalated. Some people perceived these programs to be the first step toward universal healthcare coverage in the United States. To address increased demands, the federal government passed health planning legislation to meet differing needs throughout the country. Although this legislation had merit, it failed to produce expected results. Federal efforts to reform healthcare continued to focus on organization of services and financing, rather than implementing changes in the social conditions that led to health disparities.

The roles and responsibilities of PHNs continued to expand during the 1970s, and they contributed significantly to the improvement of the health of communities. A wide variety of programs were implemented according to need. Hospice services, day care centers for the disabled, alcohol and drug abuse programs, halfway houses, and rehabilitation centers are just a few of the public health initiatives that nurses helped create. Home nursing visits increased following Medicare's implementation of diagnosis-related groups (DRGs) that were designed to lower costs through reduced hospital stays. Medicaid also reimbursed some home care services, as did the Veterans Administration and private medical insurance. More and more acutely ill people were cared for in the home, creating an ongoing demand for PHNs.

Despite the increased need for nursing services, public health as a whole declined in the 1980s. The economic recession resulted in decreased funding for social programs. The Institute of Medicine (IOM) published *The Future of by Public Health* in 1988, finding that public health services varied considerably across the United States. The system was in disarray, controlled more by the political system than by public health professionals. This study set the stage for the development of the *Healthy People* initiative that designed a national strategy to improve the health of Americans. *Healthy People 2020*, discussed earlier in this chapter, is the most recent vision for the next decade. Many of these measurable objectives (see Box 1.2) are discussed throughout this text.

The task force decides that a written and pictorial presentation on the historical roots of public health nursing practice will be a component of the online course.

Describe three characteristics of population-based nursing practice that have been present since the first district nurse was appointed in England.

The First Decade of the Twenty-First Century

The Department of Homeland Security (DHS) was created by the Department of Homeland Security Act of 2002 and is an outgrowth of the Office of Homeland Security established by President George W. Bush shortly after the terrorist attacks of September 11, 2001. The primary mission of DHS is to lead the unified national effort to secure the United States, reducing the vulnerability of the United States to terrorism and protecting against and responding to threats and hazards to the United States.

The DHS fosters an all-hazards, all-disciplines approach to emergency management that allows effective response to all emergencies, whether natural or human-made, or caused by terrorists. To meet this mission, the DHS builds collaboration and partnerships with all levels of government, the private sector, academia, and the general public. Because all disaster response begins at the local level, all cities and towns in the United States are now required to have all-hazards local emergency preparedness plans (see Chapter 20). The National Response Framework, established by DHS, guides the overall conduct and coordination of all-hazards incident responses when the scope of a disaster extends beyond the capability of local and state governments to respond.

Through education and outreach, homeland security expertise is fostered across multiple disciplines to serve as an indispensable resource for the United States. The Federal Emergency Management Agency, as the lead agency for emergency management, offers courses for first responders. The CDC also offers many online training sessions, and many states and localities have developed their own training programs.

The aftermath of the destruction of the World Trade Center in 2001 also identified a lack of trained leaders and workers in all areas of public health service. In an era in which public health threats range from pandemics of emerging infectious diseases to obesity epidemics to bioterrorism, the need for an effective public health workforce is paramount. PHNs constitute the single largest group of professionals practicing public health; however, all nurses, to some degree, are involved in public health. Therefore, the IOM (2003) has recommended that undergraduate nursing students have an understanding of the ecological model of health (see Chapter 5) and the core competencies of population-based practice discussed earlier in this chapter.

Some of the issues that were characteristic of public health nursing in the past are still prevalent today, and a multitude of new challenges exists. To provide the most comprehensive care to clients, whether individual people, families, or groups, PHNs must be flexible, be politically active, embrace change, and refresh their knowledge of public health issues on a continual basis.

CHALLENGES FOR PUBLIC HEALTH NURSING IN THE TWENTY-FIRST CENTURY

Many yet-unknown challenges will develop during the 21st century. Communities will evolve and change, cultures will merge, environments worldwide will undergo transformation, and advances in technology and therapeutic techniques will result in dramatic changes to healthcare. The following are some of the challenges for PHNs foreseen at present.

Engaging in Evidence-Based Practice

Nurses have always used the knowledge gained through education and experience in making decisions about the care of clients—accentuated by a dose of intuition. The challenge today and for the future is to document and use the best evidence available in making decisions with clients about their care. **Evidence-based nursing** is the integration of the best evidence available with clinical expertise and the values of the client to increase the quality of care. Similarly, **evidence-based public health** is a public health endeavor in which there is judicious use of evidence derived from a broad variety of science and social science research. In addition to published research, PHNs can gather information from interviews and through observation of specific population groups and gather pertinent information about the geographic locale.

Epidemiology is the science of prevention. Epidemiologic research has provided knowledge of the natural history of diseases and identified the (risk) factors that increase a person's susceptibility to illness. Nurses use the evidence that epidemiologic research has established when assessing clients and using data for planning and implementing interventions. Using the epidemiologic body of knowledge that has been developed for specific conditions, nurses can determine the stage of the illness in question and decide with the client what type of interventions are most appropriate for preventive or therapeutic purposes (see Chapters 5 and 6 for discussions of primary, secondary, and tertiary prevention strategies). Nurses engaging in community assessment also use epidemiologic methods to determine the assets and health needs of populations, and the evidence is used to create a variety of intervention programs. The public health approach to problem-solving is illustrated in Figure 1.8.

Sandy and other members of the task force think that evidence-based practice should be part of the online population-based health course. What activities could be assigned that would foster evidence-based practice?

PRACTICE POINT

Systematic reviews of research evidence, such as those included in the Cochrane Database of Systematic Reviews, are instrumental in implementing evidence-based practice.

Helping Eliminate Health Disparities in Underserved Populations

Eliminating health disparities is a combined effort of health professionals in all settings, but PHNs deal directly with these issues, often on a personal basis. Ultimately, the most important changes occur at the local level. By participating in the development, implementation, and evaluation of culturally appropriate, community-based programs, nurses use their expertise to remedy the conditions that contribute to health disparities.

Demonstrating Cultural Competence

Countless cultures in the world are constantly changing. The shared cultural symbols and meanings that are a part of people's daily social interactions have an impact on their acceptance or rejection of actions taken to promote their health. Therefore, nursing strategies that are focused on people with little attention as to how they think, feel, and interact with their world are not sufficient.

Cultural competency is an expected component of nursing practice, but it will become even more essential as interaction and integration among cultures increases. The characteristics of the major cultural groups that make up a community must be understood, along with those aspects of the community that give it its own unique subculture. It is necessary for nurses to be aware of cultural interpretations of healthcare activities so that they know what questions to ask and interventions to suggest. To achieve cultural competence, nurses should respect differences, understand their own beliefs, and not let personal beliefs have an undue influence on others. Nurses need to communicate curiosity and openness to others' ideas and ways of life, respect their decisions, and demonstrate patience and humility (see Chapter 10).

Misunderstanding a culture's symbols is a common root of prejudice.

Dan Brown, *The Lost Symbol*

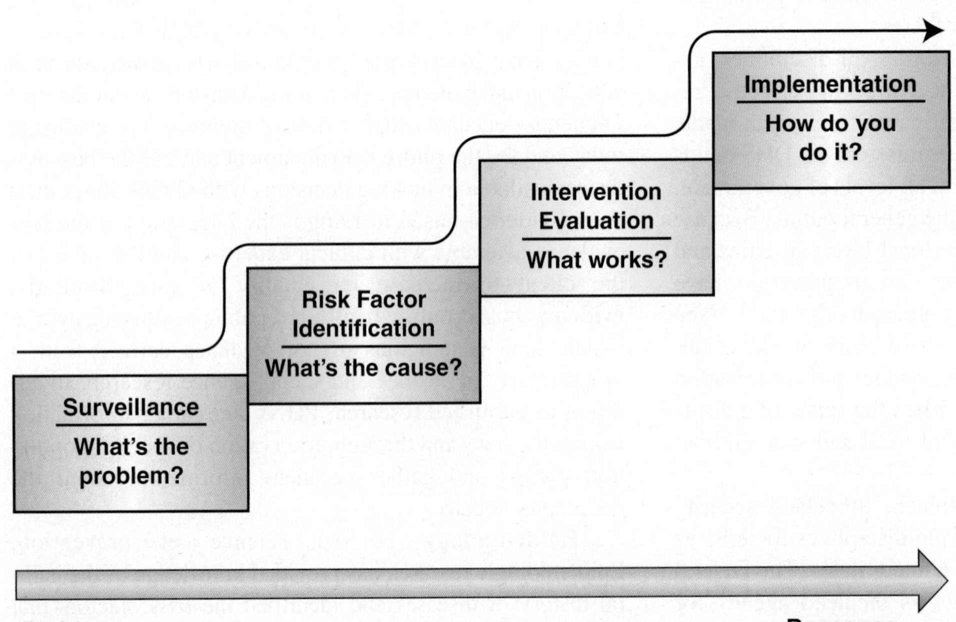

figure 1.8 The public health approach to problem-solving.

EVIDENCE FOR PRACTICE

The delivery of culturally competent public health nursing that can address health disparities depends on competent nursing practice. Understanding the nurse characteristics, care situations, and training associated with culturally competent awareness and behavior provides a basis for planning and developing interventions to ensure competent nursing care. To meet this objective, a cross-sectional, descriptive, and exploratory study was conducted among 31 PHNs in a southeastern U.S. public health department using a cultural competence assessment tool with an internal consistency reliability of 0.90.

The self-reported study findings showed moderate competence in awareness and sensitivity. Although nursing care was consistent with guidelines and mandates found in the National Standards for Culturally and Linguistically Appropriate Services in Health Care (U.S. Office of Minority Health), the nurses did not assess their behaviors at comparable levels. While providing care, the nurses encountered multiple racial/ethnic and special population groups, including many that are at risk for or experiencing health disparities and poor outcomes. Therefore, being culturally competent in both thought and actions is necessary and important for these nurses. These nurses felt frustrated in their attempts to provide care that was consistent with their perceptions of culturally competent care. Lack of human or financial resources, interpreters, gender-specific providers, and time were the most common barriers. In addition, the nurses expressed a desire for additional diversity training.

To meet the goals of a culturally competent workforce, formal courses, continuing education programs, and practical experiences should focus on awareness, sensitivity, and behaviors consistent with culturally competent care. To develop additional evidence-based knowledge for practice, additional studies of clients' perceptions and evidence of culturally competent care is needed. This information is necessary for the development of practice interventions with measurable outcomes that can be evaluated for effectiveness in addressing health disparities (Starr & Wallace, 2009).

Planning for Community Change

Change in healthcare at all levels can occur through behavior change, or through modifications in the environment, public policy, social or cultural norms, or healthcare delivery. Often, interventions at institutional or societal levels may lead to significant changes in public health without the need for behavior change on the part of individual people; fluoridation of water is an example. Even small changes in health behavior at the community or population level have the potential to significantly affect health status. The use of gel alcohol in hospitals and the availability of disinfectant wipes in grocery stores and other public places are examples.

Change should be planned and should meet specific needs to be the most effective. The impetus for change varies considerably. For example, installation of home monitoring devices may require new responsibilities, an influx of immigrants may increase the healthcare needs of a community, data may indicate that drug abuse and violence are increasing in specific groups, or new state regulations may require the establishment of new programs. On a community basis, health planning occurs on both an ongoing and an episodic basis depending on the need, and usually is a collaborative effort between multiple groups and organizations. A good example is the development of emergency preparedness plans in cities and towns (see Chapter 20).

Monitoring and evaluating the health status of individual people, families, and community groups are primary components of nursing practice in the community, as is the investigation of emerging health and environmental problems. Therefore, accepting responsibility for contributing to community health change as a policy advocate and political activist is essential. Few practitioners are as well prepared to address community health issues as PHNs. See Chapter 9 for more information on planning for community change.

The state department of public health recognizes that increasing the knowledge base of PHNs in population-based practice is just one step in implementing the new vision of public healthcare delivery. Knowledge alone cannot change practice from a clinical focus to a population-based focus if the work environment does not support the transition. Sandy is preparing another survey to determine current practices that need to be discontinued, strengthened, or developed within the next 5 years. Although the new vision for PHNs will include primary care, the majority of skills in the new model of practice will focus on population-based competencies.

Design a simple public health nursing model that incorporates the basic principles of population-based nursing.

EVIDENCE FOR PRACTICE

Domestic abuse and neglect have escalated in the United States to the point of overwhelming health and social service agencies that are attempting to address the safety of their clients. To address the need for a screening method that would identify people at risk, with funding from the U.S. Department of Commerce, investigators used a Home Health Visiting Nurse Association (HHVNA) in the Merrimack River valley to conduct a project that demonstrated innovative use of screening technology in clients' homes, followed by appropriate interventions through the use of community resources (Hawkins, Pearce, Skeith, Dimitruk, & Roche, 2009).

(continued on page 22)

Researchers adapted an initial risk screening tool and a follow-up risk assessment tool from several existing tools and research findings. All healthcare providers received training in the use of these screening tools via their personal digital assistants (PDA). The sample consisted of clients served by HHVNA during the study period. When a person screened positive on the initial risk screening tool, resources were mobilized for a same-day follow-up risk assessment and referrals were made to appropriate community agencies. Through the combination of technology and the skills and knowledge of healthcare professionals, the screening for domestic abuse and neglect has been mainstreamed into routine care at the agency, providing a new level of efficacy in prevention and early intervention.

Contributing to a Safe and Healthy Environment

Where people live, work, and spend their time can have direct consequences on their health. In every community in the world, clients are part of the environment, which has a direct impact on their health and well-being. The WHO (2014) reports that 23% of the global burden of disease is attributable to the environment. There are two ways to examine the effects of the environment on human health. The first focuses on how contaminants in the environment, such as asbestos, lead, or radon, influence human health. The second focuses on how the entire environment surrounding the community, such as the climate, neighborhood safety, access to grocery stores, and the physical layout of the community, affects health. Often, the two types of environmental effects interact.

The challenge for environmental health nurses is to use the best science available to assess how the local environment affects human health, to formulate evidence-based or best-practice interventions, and to evaluate the effectiveness of those interventions. Nurses are in a strong position to advocate for healthier environments in both the workplace and community (see Chapter 19).

Responding to Emergencies, Disasters, and Terrorism

All disaster response begins at the local level, and PHNs have always responded to community emergencies and disasters. They play an important role in all phases of the disaster management continuum, whether anticipating potential emergencies, developing appropriate community preparedness plans, building system-wide partnerships, practicing implementation of disaster management plans and skills on a regular basis, or evaluating outcomes (see Chapter 20).

Disaster preparedness plans are proactive planning efforts that are developed in anticipation of disaster scenarios, providing structure to a response before the disaster occurs. In an all-hazards event plan, the response must be a coordinated community effort, in which members of the community are engaged in ongoing preparedness activities focused on a variety of disaster situations. The capacity to respond to threats depends in part on the ability of healthcare professionals and public health officials to rapidly and effectively detect, manage, and communicate during an event. The terrorist attacks in 2001 identified a lack of workers in all areas of public health, as well as a growing appreciation of the first responders, primarily firemen, police, and healthcare personnel. Increased competency in disaster response added a new dimension to nursing practice. The public health workforce continues to be mobilized to ensure the training and education of communities across the nation regarding biological, chemical, and radiological attacks. It is necessary to learn how to prepare for events that are difficult to imagine, and it is even more challenging to mount a response.

Responding to the Global Environment

The burden of disease is growing disproportionately in the world and is largely affected by climate, public policy, age of the population, socioeconomic conditions, and factors that place people at risk for illness. Most of the countries burdened by disease have the least amount of human and economic capacity to effect change. Extreme poverty is the driving force behind increased mortality, and women are disproportionately affected.

Although maternal deaths have dropped worldwide by almost 50% in the last decade, maternal mortality is still unacceptably high. On any given day, approximately 800 women die from preventable causes related to pregnancy and childbirth, nearly all (99%) occurring in developing countries. Many of the complications resulting from childbirth can be prevented by skilled care before, during, and after childbirth by midwives and nurses. When a mother dies or is disabled, her children may be forced to live in poverty. Presently, about 6.6 million children younger than 5 die each year; poor nutrition is the underlying cause of death (WHO, 2014).

The leading causes of mortality and global burden of disease worldwide have shifted from communicable to noncommunicable, chronic diseases as a result of population aging and better control of infectious diseases. Cardiovascular disease is already the leading cause of death in the world, followed by stroke. Figure 1.9 shows the 10 leading causes of death worldwide. Only lower respiratory infections, diarrheal diseases, and HIV/AIDS are infectious diseases remaining in the top 10. Chronic diseases such as trachea, bronchus, and lung cancers and diabetes mellitus are causing increased numbers of deaths worldwide. Traffic injuries worldwide are expected to grow from the ninth leading cause of death in 2004 to the fifth in 2030. The global burden of disease and methods to improve global quality of care are discussed in Chapter 4.

With the world becoming a global village, problems that affect people in other countries also affect people in their own countries. Nurses and community healthcare providers need to be knowledgeable about the needs of all people, as well as their patients, in the global society. Opportunities

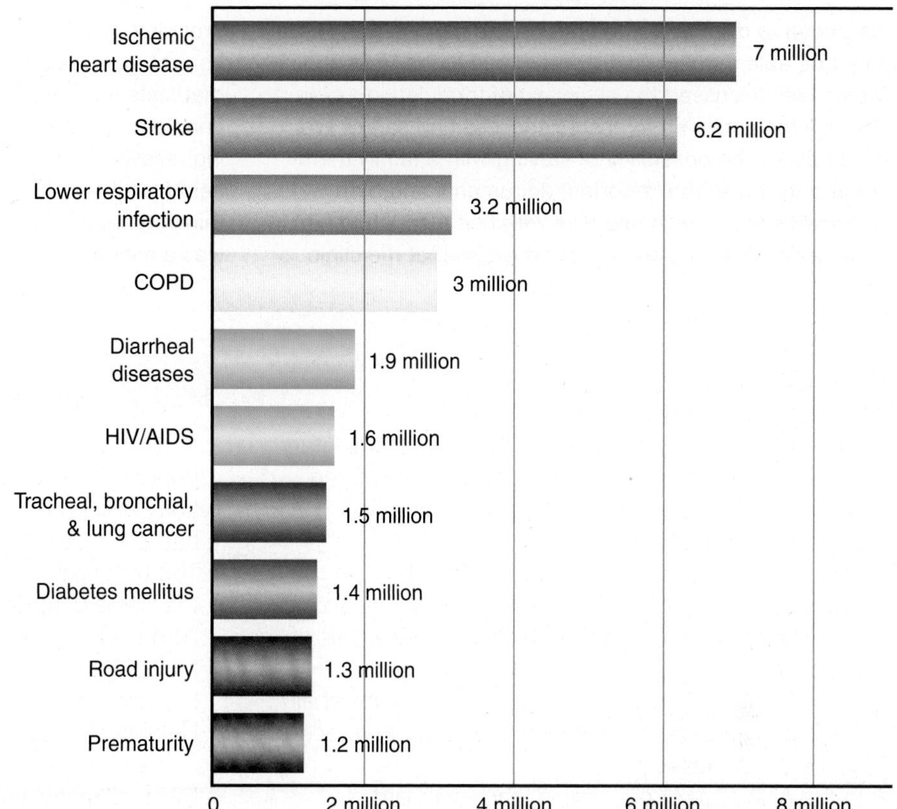

Figure 1.9 The 10 leading causes of death in the world.

have expanded for nurses to work internationally in a wide variety of roles: working side by side with local people in healthcare, initiating health education programs, establishing local primary healthcare programs, and participating in countless other activities. Advanced technology and knowledge transfer techniques will allow rapid transfer of information from electronic monitoring equipment, presenting exciting opportunities to improve health in remote locations. New cooperative healthcare ventures will occur throughout the world in the 21st century.

PRACTICE POINT

In this dynamic time, care will be transformed as needs rapidly evolve. Newly prepared nurses will experience events never before thought possible.

STUDENT REFLECTION

Over the spring vacation, a group of eight undergraduate nursing students, three graduate students, and three faculty members flew to Nicaragua to work in a clinic for the week. There was one person who stands out in my mind. She was a 25-year-old woman who came to the clinic complaining of diarrhea, accompanied by her 6-year-old son and 3-year-old daughter. One of our nurse practitioners (NPs) cared for her while I observed. After the NP determined that the woman had a gastrointestinal parasite that was common in Nicaragua and prescribed treatment, the nurse asked the client about her wishes to have more children. The woman responded quietly that she did not want more children, but that her husband was adamant that she not use birth control. When the NP asked if birth control was a sensitive subject between them, the woman began to cry. She told us that after the birth of her daughter, she began birth control without consulting her husband, and when he found out, he became verbally and physically abusive. Since that point, their relationship had become increasingly violent and the woman said she feared for her life, along with the lives of her children. Her husband felt that if she used birth control she was cheating. He told her that he was not going to use a condom, and if she did not want to have his children, she didn't love him.

This situation made me realize just how dismal it can be for women in violent relationships. Because of lack of resources, it is very difficult for abused women to find help, and many lose hope, believing that nothing can be done. Their situation is complicated since the majority of women are financially dependent on their partners. Our client was in a similar situation. She was afraid of her husband, vulnerable financially, and had two children to protect. Her situation would be further complicated if she continued without birth control.

During the visit, the NP and I listened and provided the emotional support that she so desperately needed.

(continued on page 24)

We began to discuss some options and actions that she might be able to take. Just as we would in the United States, we discussed the necessity of formulating a plan before acting, helping to ensure success and safety. We talked about the possibility of staying with a family member and reviewed the important documents and birth certificates that she should take with her. Also, I told her about a domestic violence support group that the clinic provided. Finally, we discussed multiple forms of birth control that she could use, such as the hormone injection that lasts for 3 months to prevent pregnancy, if she were unable to leave for any reason. I think the woman left feeling relieved and somewhat hopeful for what the future held for her family. Even if I was only able to get my client thinking about her options, I feel that our time together was a success.

key concepts

- Three major changes in healthcare in the 21st century include the development of patient/client–centered care, increased use of technology, and increased personal responsibility for health.
- The practice of public health nursing is defined in the ANA (2013) publication *Public Health Nursing: Scope and Standards of Practice*. It defines the essentials of public health nursing, the activities, and the accountabilities that are characteristic of practice at all levels and settings. It is the legal standard of practice set by the profession.
- In the ANA (2013) publication, each standard of practice is followed by the essential competencies required to meet that standard.
- The Public Health Intervention Wheel defines 17 interventions—actions taken on behalf of individuals, families, communities, and systems to protect or improve health status.
- Entry into public health nursing practice requires a baccalaureate degree.
- The historical roots of public health nursing have set the framework for current nursing practice in the community.
- Multiple challenges face PHNs in the 21st century:
  Engaging in evidence-based practice
  Helping eliminate health disparities in underserved populations
  Demonstrating cultural competence
  Planning for community change
  Contributing to a safe and healthy environment
  Responding to emergencies, disasters, and terrorism
  Responding to the global environment

critical thinking questions

1. Review the public health milestones presented in Box 1.1. What potential health successes might be cited in the next decade?
2. Identify a new role for nursing that will most likely evolve in the first half of the 21st century.
3. Analyze the roots of public health nursing and its influence on practice today.

references

Ackerman, M. J., Filart, R., Burgess, L. P., Lee, I., & Poropatich, R. K. (2010). Developing next-generation telehealth tools and technologies: Patients, systems, and data perspectives. *Telemedicine Journal and E-Health, 16*(1), 93–95.

Agency for Healthcare Research and Quality. (2014). *National healthcare quality report, 2012, National health disparities report, 2012*. U.S. Department of Health and Human Services. Retrieved from http://nhqrnet.ahrq.gov/inhqrdr/reports/index

American Nurses Association. (2013). *Public health nursing: Scope and standards of practice*. Silver Spring, MD: Nursesbooks.

Centers for Disease Control and Prevention. (1999). 10 great public health achievements—United States, 1900–1999. *Morbidity Mortality Weekly Report, 48*(12), 241–243.

Centers for Disease Control and Prevention. (2013). *FastStats: Health expenditures*. Retrieved from http://www.cdc.gov/nchs/fastats/hexpense.htm

Department of Health and Human Services, Health Resources and Service Administration. (2014). *The registered nurse population findings from the March 2008 National Sample Survey of Registered Nurses*. Retrieved from http://bhpr.hrsa.gov/healthworkforce/rnsurvey2008.html

Doherty, R. B. (2010). The certitudes and uncertainties of health care reform. *Annals of Internal Medicine, 152*(10), 679–682.

Frontier Nursing Service Inc. (n.d.). *A brief history of the Frontier Nursing Service*. Retrieved from http://www.frontiernursing.org

Hawkins, J. W., Pearce, C. W., Skeith, J., Dimitruk, B., & Roche, R. (2009). Using technology to expedite screening and intervention for domestic abuse and neglect. *Public Health Nursing, 26*(1), 58–69.

Health Resources and Services Administration. (2014). Retrieved from http://www.hrsa.gov/ruralhealth/about/telehealth/

Healthy People 2020. (n.d.). Retrieved from http://www.healthypeople.gov/2020/about/default.aspx

Henry Street Settlement. (2004). *About our founder, Lillian Wald*. Retrieved from http://www.henrystreet.org/about/history/.org/

Institute of Medicine. (2003). *Who will keep the public healthy? Educating public health professionals for the 21st century.* Retrieved October 2, 2014, from http://books.nap.edu/openbook.php?record_id=10542&page=R2

Jakeway, C. C., Cantrell, E. E., Cason, J. B., & Talley, B. S. (2006). Developing population health competencies among public health nurses in Georgia. *Public Health Nursing, 23*(2), 161–167.

Kalisch, P. A., & Kalisch, B. J. (1978). *The advance of American nursing*. Boston, MA: Little Brown.

Kalisch, P. A., & Kalisch, B. J. (2004) *American nursing: A history*. Philadelphia, PA: Lippincott, Williams & Wilkins.

Lu, J. F., Chi, M. J., & Chen, C. M. (2013). Advocacy of home telehealth care among consumers with chronic conditions. *Journal of Clinical Nursing*. Advance online publication. doi:10.1111/jocn.12156

Nationwide Health Information Network (NwHIN). Retrieved from http://www.healthit.gov/policy-researchers-implementers/nationwide-health-information-network-nwhin

Starr, S., & Wallace, D. C. (2009). Self-reported cultural competence of public health nurses in a southeastern U.S. public health department. *Public Health Nursing, 26*(1), 48–57.

The Public Health (Scotland) Act. (1897). Pauper nurses. *The British Medical Journal, 2*, 104. Retrieved from http://www.ncbi.nlm.nih.gov/pmc/articles/PMC2407239/pdf/brmedj08725–0040 a.pdf

World Health Organization. (2013). *World health statistics 2013*. Retrieved from http://www.who.int/gho/publications/world_health_statistics/2013/en/index.html

World Health Organization. (2014). *Data and statistics*. Retrieved from http://www.who.int/research/en/

web resources

Please visit thePoint® (http://thepoint.lww.com/Harkness) for up-to-date web resources on this topic.

CHAPTER 2

Public Health Systems

Rosanna DeMarco

It is no measure of health to be well adjusted to a profoundly sick society.

Jiddu Krishnamurti

Without health life is not life; it is only a state of languor and suffering—an image of death.

Buddha

America's health care system is neither healthy, caring, nor a system.

Walter Cronkite

Everyone should have health insurance? I say everyone should have health care. I'm not selling insurance.

Dennis Kucinich

chapter highlights

- Public health and healthcare systems as a complex organization of institutions and structures
- National and international perspectives on public health structure, function, and outcomes differ by fiscal support and philosophical attitudes concerning health.
- Public health administration as a reflection of health, politics, economics, and social structures
- Influences of history, resources, financing mechanisms, interest groups, and environmental conditions on public health
- Governmental and nongovernmental organizations and public health

objectives

- Understand and describe the challenges in reducing the gap between healthcare expenditures and healthcare disparities.
- Compare and contrast differences across international public health systems.
- Explain the different contributions of governmental and nongovernmental structures in public health systems in different countries.

key terms

Bilateral agency: Refers to two agencies that conduct business within one country.

Department of Health and Human Services: U.S. branch of government responsible for health and welfare of citizens.

Health disparities: Difference in the quality of healthcare delivered or obtainable, often tied to race or ethnicity or socioeconomic status.

Healthy People 2020: A U.S. national consensus plan with specific health goals.

International Council of Nurses (ICN): A federation of more than 130 national nurses associations (NNAs), representing the more than 16 million nurses worldwide.

Millennium Development Goals (United Nations): Eight goals that all 191 UN member states have agreed to try to achieve by the year 2015 to combat poverty, hunger, disease, illiteracy, environmental degradation, and discrimination against women.

Multilateral agencies: Agencies that use both governmental and nongovernmental resources.

National Health Expenditure Accounts (NHEA): Comprised of measures of costs of healthcare goods and services in the United States.

Nongovernmental organization (NGO): Agency that acquires resources to help others from private (vs. public) sources.

Organization for Economic Cooperation and Development: A group that collects data related to healthcare use across a variety of professional and service parameters.

Philanthropic organization: An organization that uses endowments or private funding to address the needs of individuals, families, and populations.

Refugee: Person who leaves his or her place of origin and cannot return because of a well-founded fear of being persecuted for reasons that include race, religion, nationality, membership of a particular social group, or political opinion.

World Bank: International organization that uses funds from developed countries to help initiatives of developing countries.

World Health Organization: International center that collects data, advances initiatives, and offers support related to public health.

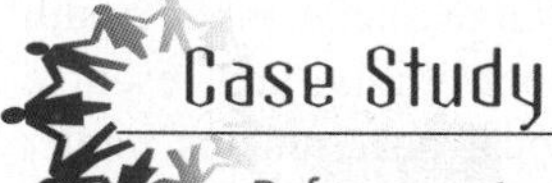

Case Study

References to the case study are found throughout this chapter (look for the case study icon). Readers should keep the case study in mind as they read the chapter.

When Clara arrived in the United States as a refugee* after surviving many years of violence and brutality in her native Sudan, she was barely 20 years of age (an estimate). Many girls like Clara do not know their age; they often do not know the year in which they were born. Clara represents a community or population of women who have experienced hard realities related to the genocide in Sudan. War between the North and the South, which still continues, results from different religious views and ethnicity, and it puts all people, particularly some young women, in a vulnerable position. In their commitment to ethnic cleansing, men in the army have raped young girls without hesitation, leaving them to face pregnancy with no women's healthcare and with very little support to change their future circumstances in a patriarchal society.

Clara has found asylum in the United States through the generosity of a nongovernmental health organization. She now enters a healthcare system that offers screening, care, follow-up, and support as she learns that she and her child are human immunodeficiency virus (HIV) seropositive. Although Clara and her young child face the prospect of a life-threatening illness, she is supported by a system that seems to care about her progress and future health, as well as the health of the entire population.

*The United States provides refuge to persons who have been persecuted or have well-founded fear of persecution through two programs: one for refugees (persons outside the United States and their immediate relatives) and one for asylees (persons in the United States and their immediate relatives) (http://www.dhs.gov/refugees-and-asylees-2011).

Comparing healthcare systems allows for an examination of how these systems, which help ensure the health or wellness of populations, are organized and financed; cost control is important. Comparing helps develop standards and initiatives directed by organizations discussed in this chapter, such as the **World Health Organization** (WHO), the **World Bank**, and the **Organization for Economic Cooperation and Development** (OECD). In addition, such comparisons aid researchers who study specific healthcare interventions and outcomes internationally. The fundamental challenge in making comparisons is the difficulty in finding universal measures of health which can be compared fairly. In the final analysis, what should be of most interest is learning which healthcare system yields the highest quality of care and universal access at a reasonable cost.

IMPORTANCE OF UNDERSTANDING HOW PUBLIC HEALTH SYSTEMS ARE ORGANIZED

Public health involves organized efforts to improve the health of communities rather than individual people. Thus, the central goal of public health is the reduction of disease through prevention and the improvement of health in the community, both nationally and internationally (Schneider, 2014). As shown in Chapter 1, it has been the characteristics of population health and illness over time that have directed how public health is defined, organized, delivered, and evaluated. But it would be naive to believe that these characteristics are the only things that contribute to the ways in which public health initiatives and the structure behind them have developed. So, to understand how public health systems are organized in a city, state, or country, it seems logical and necessary to explore a variety of components to fully realize why public health systems exist and how they function. To that end, the following section explores a variety of general health and public health systems ranging from those in industrialized countries to those in developing countries. The text discusses the role of public health personnel in the context of how local and global communities organize their efforts to keep the population disease- and injury-free. For people who are committed to the ideals of prevention and access to care for all, public health is not without challenges.

STRUCTURE OF PUBLIC HEALTHCARE IN THE UNITED STATES

In the midst of many successes and challenges related to health and illness, the public health delivery system in the United States supports efforts to address significant healthcare concerns, which affect both citizens and refugees/asylees, through government agencies, nongovernmental organizations (NGOs), and **philanthropic organizations** (Office for Refugees and Immigrants [ORI], 2010). The following section describes the complexity of relationships among the agencies devoted to public health delivery at the local and state levels. The activities of these agencies vary widely because local priorities and values influence availability and operations.

Government Agencies and Public Health

Through public efforts, the U.S. government becomes involved with providing services that benefit the social welfare of citizens in terms of health at national, state, and local levels. The federal government creates policy, financing, and regulatory enforcement when a service that would benefit citizens is identified and available (Schneider, 2014). Good examples of government efforts to improve public health include providing free drug information on government-published databases, establishing disaster preparedness plans, and creating quality indicators for child health (Jesano, 2010; Kavanagh, Adams, & Wang, 2009; Sakauye et al., 2009).

The federal government plays an important role in regulation. Public health regulatory entities are often related to (1) food, (2) drugs, (3) devices, (4) occupational health, and (5) the environment through the **Department of Health and Human Services** (Health & Human Services, 2013). However, out of concern related to the quality of healthcare, the government can "step in" to assist private citizens on different occasions. Two examples are federal regulations related to women delivering children who need at least 48 hours (for) of inpatient care, and making sure that mental healthcare is in parity with medical care (Marth, 2009).

The federal government allocates tax funds to state governments in support of specific public health programs. For example, block grants give money to specific programs and providers based on of state health needs (Urban Institute, 2013). Some examples of block grants include Maternal and Child Health Services, and Prevention and Treatment of Substance Abuse Block Grants. Entitlement programs to support the healthcare needs of low-income families come from the federal government. Three important examples of entitlement programs are Medicare, Medicaid, and the Special Supplemental Food Program for Women, Infants, and Children (WIC; Jost, 2003). The Medicaid program requires matching funds from the states to provide for the healthcare needs of citizens (Centers for Medicare and Medicaid Services [CMS], 2013) (Fig. 2.1).

State governments also play a large role in public health regulatory activities, program responsibility, and resource allocation—to varying extents. Local governments implement the public health activities within communities.

Generally, from either an economic or theoretical perspective, the private sector often does not provide services that would improve social welfare, although in many ways private organizations often directly assist the common good of populations through their endowment funds (endowed with monies often directly assists the common good of populations); they direct their efforts to key initiatives that are altruistic and very helpful to community dwellers. Examples include philanthropies such as the Kellogg Foundation and the Robert Wood Johnson Foundation (WK Kellogg Foundation, 2013; Robert Wood Johnson Foundation, 2013).

Clara is a good example of a person who came to the United States with no resources. She has no income and is trying to find a way to sustain herself and her child while dealing with the trauma of her past life, and her future life with a chronic, life-threatening illness. She is receiving Medicaid from the state in which she now lives in the United States, WIC for her child, and support from the Ryan White HIV/acquired immunodeficiency syndrome (AIDS) Program. Since 1991, this program has provided supplemental support for medical care, medications, housing, and public health services for those living with HIV.

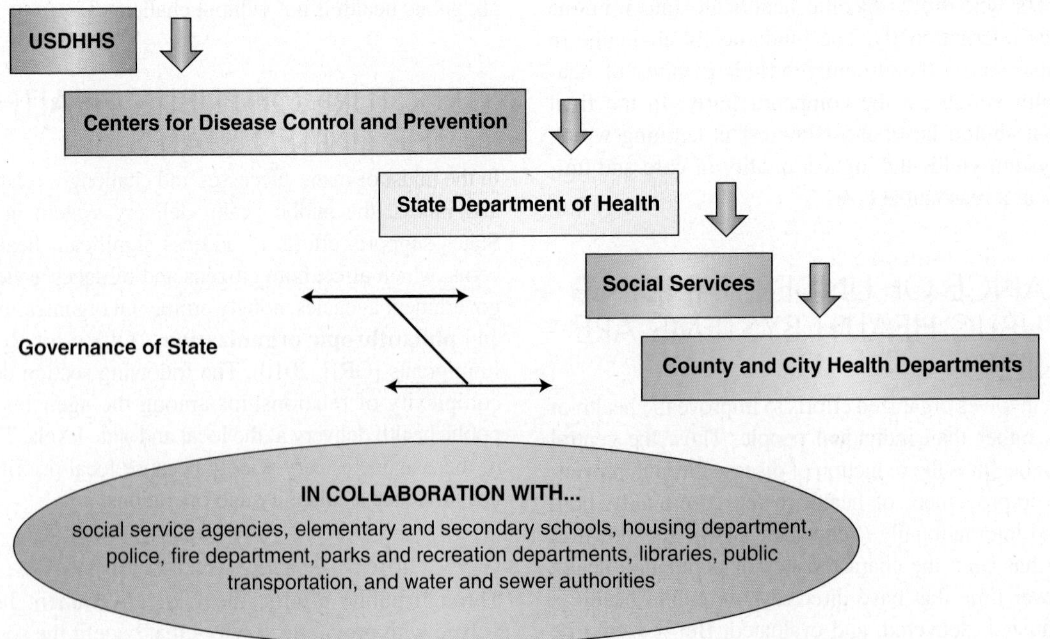

figure 2.1 Sample configuration of health department structures in the United States. USDHHS, U.S. Department of Health and Human Services. (From http://www.hhs.gov/about/orgchart.)

EVIDENCE FOR PRACTICE

The Ryan White Program funds networks of care, which include medical care providers and support services, for people living with HIV or AIDS (PLWHA) in 51 eligible metropolitan areas (EMAs). Researchers created a survey to measure characteristics of care networks and the quality, accessibility, and coordination of services from the perspective of case management and medical providers, administrators, and consumers (Hirschhorn et al., 2009), and they administered the surveys in 42 EMAs.

The investigators then rated the care networks highly on access, quality, and coordination between case management and primary care providers. However, there were frequent differences in ratings of quality and barriers by the type of respondents (consumer representatives, grantees, and providers). There were also substantial variations across EMAs in network characteristics, perceived effectiveness, performance measurement, and quality improvement activities. The results indicated that the Ryan White Program has been somewhat successful in developing networks of care. However, support is needed to strengthen the comprehensiveness and coordination of care.

Specific Agencies

United States Department of Health and Human Services

The U.S. Department of Health and Human Services or USDHHS (USDHHS, 2013a) is the federal agency that is directly involved with the health and healthcare of U.S. citizens or refugees/asylees. The office of the Secretary of Health and Human Services oversees the work of 11 agencies (Fig. 2.2). These agencies work in collaboration with state and local governments in the United States to provide (1) assessment information regarding the level of health or illness in the nation; (2) assurance that the infrastructure, including trained personnel, is available to all citizens and refugees/asylees; and (3) legislation and implementation of health policy. The federal government makes public health policy. By producing information gathered through research, it provides evidence that can effectively change public health practice (Parkhurst, Weller, & Kemp, 2010). Thus, the federal government supports research efforts that can help citizens improve their health significantly, and promotes ways to implement the evidence from a culturally relevant and sensitive perspective. For example, the National Institutes of Health (NIH, 2013), Agency for Healthcare Research and Quality (AHRQ, 2013), and the Centers for Disease Control and Prevention (CDC, 2013a) are three important organizations in which research is undertaken and used effectively to address healthcare concerns such as HIV screening and care, adverse events in hospital settings, and measures to decrease the rates of emerging infectious diseases (Health & Human Services, 2013).

State and Local Health Departments

State agencies, which administer specific federal public health activities throughout a particular state, are influenced from a structural and functional perspective by the federal government. However, state departments of health can be diverse for political and environmental reasons (CDC, 2013a), and they influence NGOs as well as local health departments.

According to Schneider (2014), there are several types of models of health department structure. Most commonly, a state health department is an independent organization that is in communication with the head of the executive branch of the state government (governor). (Within the health department are core public health areas, such as infectious disease control, preventive health, health institution licensing, and epidemiology, but they may relate to a political agenda or worldview of the state leadership.) The head of the state health department can be, but is not necessarily, a physician, although in some states, this is a statutory requirement. The state governor may choose the head of the department of health, or members of a state board of health may make the appointment. These boards of health are representative of the state demographics and may include residents who may be health professionals or may simply be healthcare consumers.

Another model is the state department of health and human services. This model focuses on public health, social service, and medical assistance programs. This relationship between public health and social services often helps bring together related expertise to address complex problems that frequently require coalition building with the public (Rosales, Coe, Stroupe, Hackman, & de Zapien, 2010).

Although local health departments (city or county) can be governed by state health departments, the local departments often create their own structure based on of the needs of the local community, and these local health departments implement programs that serve local citizens. In a county health department, it would not be unusual to see a functioning tuberculosis clinic and tuberculosis surveillance program that works in collaboration with the state health department to care for patients exposed to or infected with the tuberculosis bacillus.

Finally, many other contributors to public health initiatives have strong relationships and interagency affiliations with state and local health departments. They include social service agencies, elementary and secondary schools, housing departments, police and fire departments, parks and recreation departments, libraries, public transportation systems, and water and sewer authorities. Government authorities are often involved in these areas within the context of public health. Generally, localities create relationships and

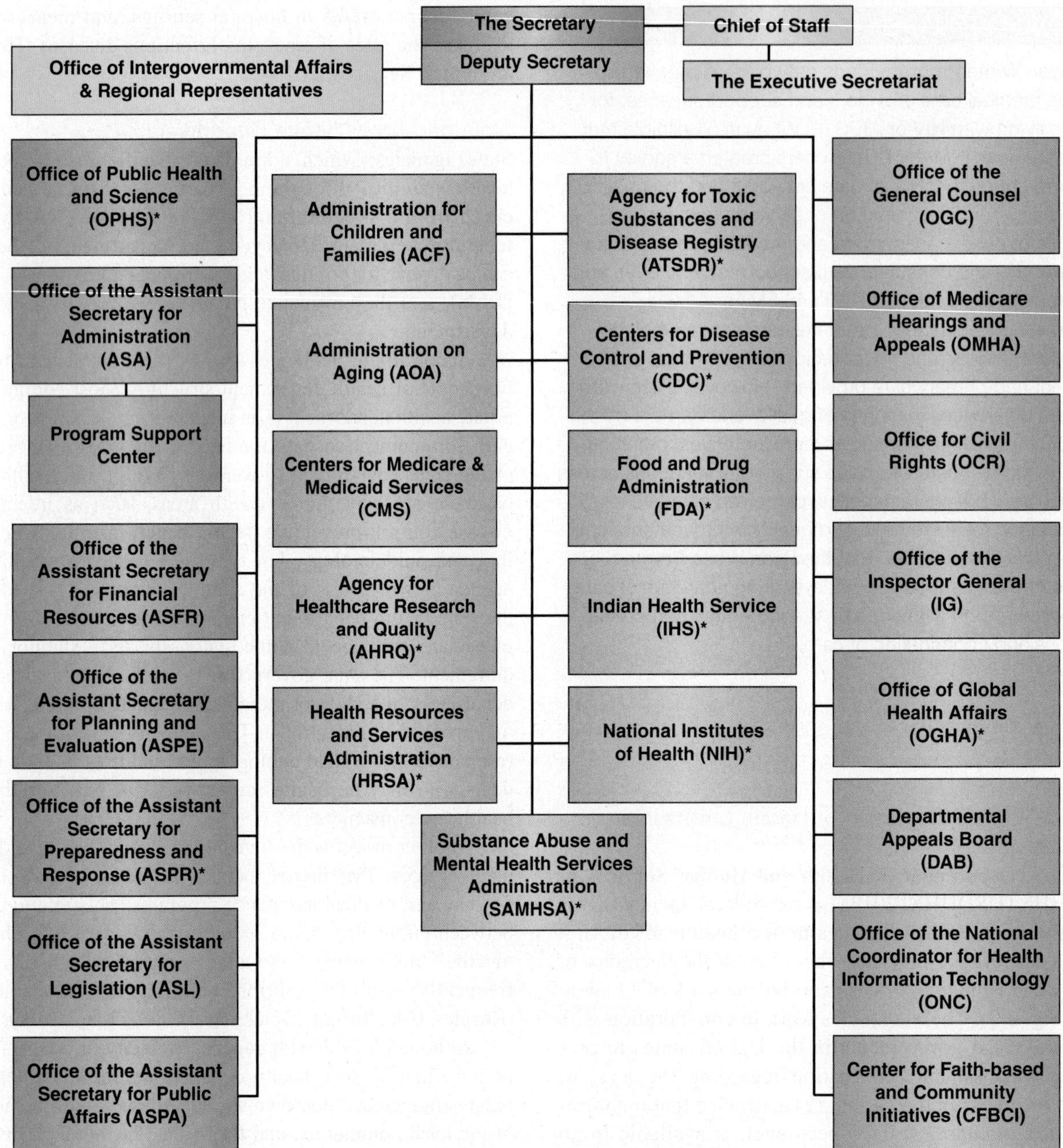

figure 2.2 Federal agencies with public health responsibilities. (Redrawn from: U.S. Department of Health and Human Services organizational chart.) *Designates components of the Public Health Service. (From http://www.hhs.gov/about/orgchart.)

lines of authority that make sense for the particular needs of their citizens (see Fig. 2.1).

FUNCTIONS OF PUBLIC HEALTH IN THE UNITED STATES

In the chapters that follow, there are specific explanations with examples of the functions that public health offers to people in the United States. However, it is important to review several key components of the function public health serves, including a national consensus on goals (USDHHS, 2013b); provision of systems of health insurance based on risk, not necessarily on health; and the role of nongovernmental entities in disease prevention and health promotion. In the United States, public healthcare includes disease prevention and health promotion based on science and cultural relevance. It is not focused on the health of the individual person, but on the population as a whole. The goal of public healthcare is to keep populations healthy through a broader "reach" than connection at the individual level.

One way to develop a system that advises people with backgrounds similar to Clara's involves strategically putting language-sensitive notices in places where these people live, congregate, or travel. They need to (1) go to their local healthcare centers to get tested for the HIV virus and (2) receive appropriate care. This "reach" may help more at-risk members of a community than discussing the HIV-testing program with people at healthcare facilities. This approach uses broad strategic planning, including the voices of community members, multidisciplinary teams, and nongovernmental not-for-profit sectors of health organizations, which focuses on key target objectives.

Public health goals and focused target objectives are identified and promulgated by a national publication called ***Healthy People 2020***. *Healthy People 2020* is a national consensus plan identifying focal areas which need active and specific plans and implementations, based on levels of illness (morbidity) and death (mortality) that account for the physical, psychosocial, and financial suffering of citizens (USDHHS, 2013a, 2013b). *Healthy People 2020* is mentioned throughout this book as a source of goals and indicators that should direct community healthcare at the local, state, and federal level. However, the United States and its system of healthcare have historically given, and continue to give, stronger support to (1) individual rather than community care and (2) cure rather than prevention. It involves highly specialized healthcare providers who have little contribution to community outreach.

Funding for the healthcare system in the United States comes primarily from privately-owned health insurance companies. Exceptions include programs that are publically funded, such as Medicare, Medicaid, TRICARE (civilian health benefits for military personnel, retirees, and dependents), Children's Health and Insurance Program (CHIP), and Veterans Health Administration (Center for Medicare and Medicaid Services, 2014; Children's Health Insurance Program, 2014; U. S. Department of Veterans Affairs Health Benefits, 2014). At least 15.7% of the U.S. population is completely uninsured (Kaiser Foundation, 2013), and a substantial portion of the population (35%) is underinsured. More is spent on healthcare in the United States than in any other nation in the world. Even though not all citizens have health insurance, according to the OECD, the United States has the third highest public healthcare expenditure per capita, and still lags behind in measures to decrease infant mortality and raise life expectancy, as compared with other nations in the world (OECD, 2013a) (Table 2.1). Active debate about healthcare in the United States includes serious ethical questions about whether health is a right or a privilege, and whether all people should have equal access to quality healthcare. In 2010, controversial federal legislation took positive steps to give access to healthcare to all citizens through private and public funding for health insurance. The difficult road ahead is to figure out how to follow through on this promise, taking into account the expense and the assurance of efficiency, effectiveness, and quality (The White House, 2010).

Beyond the system of public and private control and ownership of healthcare services in the United States, a vast array of NGOs helps keep people healthy through voluntary and philanthropic services. For example, private community hospitals are sometimes supported by community groups which ensure that vulnerable populations have access to healthcare. The care may be free. In addition, the community facility may sponsor community health education programs and prevention/screening clinics for underserved populations. Although many states provide communities with (community) municipal or neighborhood health centers and ambulatory/outpatient services through local or federal funding, health services can be offered through private groups who are interested in supporting specific areas of need, such as migrant or school-based health programs (Lutz, 2008). These programs are often run by

table 2.1 **Measures of Healthcare in Selected Developed Countries**

Country	Life Expectancy (years)	Infant Mortality	No. of Physicians/ 1,000 People	No. of Nurses/ 1,000 People	Per Capita Spending on Healthcare (U.S.$)	Healthcare Costs (GDP)[a]	Percentage of Government Revenue Spent on Health/ Percentage of Healthcare Costs Paid by the Government
Australia	81.4	4.2	2.8	9.7	3,137	8.7	17.7/67.0
Canada	80.7	5.0	2.2	9.0	3,895	10.1	16.7/69.8
France	81.0	4.0	3.4	7.7	3,601	11.0	14.2/79.0
Germany	79.8	3.8	3.5	9.9	3,588	10.4	17.6/76.9
Japan	82.6	2.6	2.1	9.4	2,581	8.1	16.8/81.3
Sweden	81.0	2.5	3.6	10.8	3,323	9.1	13.6/81.7
United Kingdom	79.1	4.8	2.5	10.0	2,992	8.4	15.8/81.7
United States	78.1	6.7	2.4	10.6	7,290	16.0	18.5/45.4

[a]GDP = gross domestic product.

Source: Organization of Economic Cooperation and Development. Retrieved from http://www.oecd.org/els/health-systems/49105858.pdf

altruistic, nonprofit organizations. Examples of some NGOs in the United States include the American Diabetes Association, Citizens for Global Solutions, Americorps, and the U.S. Fund for UNICEF (United Nations Children's Fund, 2013).

TRENDS IN PUBLIC HEALTH IN THE UNITED STATES

In the United States, the federal government expends time and effort every year to create a report of the trends in the following areas: (1) health status and what determines health (determinants), (2) how communities use healthcare services (health utilization) and healthcare resources to help communities stay healthy, (3) how much money is spent on healthcare (expenditures), and (4) which citizens are the most vulnerable. The following sections explain these four areas more specifically.

Health Status and Its Determinants

Measuring the health status of citizens in communities helps the U.S. public health system determine how to direct resources (money and services) to keep people healthy. Despite the fact that life expectancy is higher for both men and women in countries such as Japan, the overall health of people in the United States has improved over the years. However, in the United States, current data show a downward shift related to malignancies, obesity, and dental care (Organization of Economic Cooperation and Development [OECD], 2013b). It is believed that the health successes found in the United States result from money spent on health education programs, public health programs, health research, and healthcare itself. The trend has been toward using larger sums of money to help Americans keep healthy. Much of the funding currently spent on healthcare is spent on prescription drugs and care of chronic conditions, which often affect the elderly or disabled. A good example of how increases in funding have improved health is the significant improvement in mortality (numbers of deaths) and morbidity (numbers of recorded illnesses) statistics in a variety of health-related actions, such as the use of corticosteroids in acute lung injury or disease (Tang, Craig, Eslick, Seppelt, & McLean, 2009).

Mortality (death rates) and morbidity (illness rates) have improved for many reasons, but a primary reason is that an organized effort on the part of the American public health system has injected resources to study certain prominent problems in the United States. A good example is the provision of services to prevent progression of cardiac illness. Thus, the death rate from heart disease has decreased, primarily because health education has emphasized a healthier lifestyle and cholesterol screening (Myers, 2003). Another example is the decrease in mortality and morbidity rates of individuals living with HIV/AIDS. The use of highly active antiretroviral therapy, including protease inhibitors, has dramatically changed patterns of survival; these patterns now assume the trajectory of a chronic illness. Regardless of inequalities in gender, race, and socioeconomic status, people who once lived for 5 years after being diagnosed with HIV now live for 15 years, and children born with HIV from perinatal transmission are now teens who deal with HIV, safe sex behaviors, and disclosure issues with sexual partners (Regidor et al., 2009).

> **PRACTICE POINT**
>
> It is easy to receive morbidity and mortality information in the United States by going to the CDC website and electronically subscribing to the *Morbidity and Mortality Weekly Report (MMWR)* for free. The *MMWR* reports are very informative about trends in assessing the public health status of the United States. More specifically, the *MMWR* reports publicly, in a systematic way, the frequencies of diseases, disabilities, or health-related events, and it supplies information about trends provided by the CDC and other health officials.

Despite these successes, key social and behavioral determinants of health still need to be addressed. For example, obesity, diabetes, and cigarette smoking are significant risk factors for diseases that may interfere with healthy brain functioning (Desai, Grossberg, & Chibnall, 2010). Although much effort has been given to preventive education in these areas, a high percentage of adults and adolescents continue to make no effort to change their exercise, smoking, or eating patterns. In addition, rates of reportable childhood infectious diseases have decreased and cancer has declined in men, but there has been no significant change in the rates for women's cancers. In fact, many believe that there has been an epidemic of breast cancer in non-Hispanic White women in recent years (Sexton et al., 2011).

Utilization of Healthcare Resources

Changes in payment policies, which are intended to decrease direct and indirect costs, as well as losses from billing fraud/abuse, continue to change healthcare delivery in the United States. There is less use of institutions (i.e., hospitals). Highly complex diagnostic procedures and surgical interventions like cardiac surgery are more likely to take place in hospitals. However, emergency departments and office-based physician, and physician-group visits, as well as ambulatory surgical procedures, have increased. In particular, emergency department admissions have increased for those citizens who are asthmatic, especially children (Gorman & Chu, 2009). At the same time, there has been a significant decrease in Medicare-certified home health agencies. In 1997, there were 10,800 agencies, and in 2002, there were 6,800 agencies, primarily because the Balanced Budget Act of that year forced either consolidations or closing of existing services (Center of Budget and Policy Priorities, 2013).

Prevention-oriented approaches and services decrease morbidity and mortality rates (Friis & Sellers, 2009). For example, distribution of flu or pneumonia vaccines as a form of prevention and a common public health campaign demonstrates a commitment of public health to decreasing morbidity and mortality. However, the funding for such programs is often slashed when fiscal constraints cause fiscal interme-

PRACTICE POINT

Assurance is a word used in public health to identify an important concept: that individual people, families, and populations have the healthcare personnel and systems needed to address their respective healthcare needs. Assurance as a goal is highly related to the goal of maintaining healthcare professionals in the work force who are competent and stay in the work force. It is possible to think about schools of nursing as a way in which nursing programs are supporting assurance. To understand the level of commitment to healthcare education for nursing professionals in the state in which you live, determine the number of schools of nursing in the state, which ones specifically offer advanced practice specialties in community/public health, the number of schools of public health, and the number of medical schools. In addition, check labor statistics related to trends in the retirement of health professionals. Each of these efforts can help make it possible to understand trends in the preparation of healthcare providers, and also help assess needs for the future from the local perspective. Comparison among states gives a larger perspective and can be obtained by accessing the Health Resources and Services Administration (HRSA) website, which is the federal organization specifically responsible for health professional resources in the United States.

diaries to (address) pay for treatment of well-known illnesses and disabilities, rather than provide funding for prevention programs which have the potential to impact large populations. Despite decreases in financial support for vaccination programs, there have been increases in the number of children 19 to 35 months of age who have received combined vaccinations (Chidiac & Ader, 2009). In addition, the number of women older than 18 obtaining a Papanicolaou (Pap) smear screen has also increased. However, there is a link between this preventive intervention, some college training, and the vaccine that counters certain strains of human papillomavirus (CDC, 2013b).

Expenditures and Health: Trying to Improve Public Health Economically

Access to healthcare is critical for prevention and treatment of illness and injury. Health insurance and appropriate coverage often determine access. Lack of health insurance is related to poverty, and puts residents in a position of vulnerability. The Unites States spends more on healthcare than any industrialized country. Although hospital care accounts for the largest share of healthcare spending, prescription drugs are the fastest growing healthcare expenditure. Medicare pays for only a little of this expense, even though citizens aged 65 and older, who are the primary recipients of Medicare, have the greatest need for therapeutic drugs. Thus, people whose income is reduced through retirement, or death of a family member, may have a substantial out-of-pocket expense (Heisler et al., 2010).

National Health Expenditure Accounts (NHEAs) are a measure of expenditures on healthcare goods and services in the United States. These accounts are prepared by the National Health Statistics Group. Government public health activity constitutes an important service category in NHEAs. In the most recent set of estimates, expenditures totaled $56.1 billion in 2004, or 3.0% of total U.S. health spending (CMS, 2013). What becomes challenging is specifically identifying what is considered "public health" in an expenditure.

Vulnerable Populations and Healthcare

Key indicators in the United States reveal a healthcare gap between the overall American population and people of different genders and ethnicities. There is also a healthcare gap for those who have less education, lower socioeconomic status, and live in certain geographic areas in the United States. These disparities are characteristic of people who have been marginalized and oppressed. Marginalization often occurs in people who live below the poverty level in the United States, and these people frequently are poorly educated. In the chapters that follow, higher rates of morbidity, mortality, difficulty in accessing care, and negative outcomes when receiving care will be seen as key issues in such populations.

Clara is a good example of someone who has been courageous in coming to the United States, but is compromised in terms of literacy and socioeconomic needs. She also is unfamiliar, at a basic level, with how healthcare systems work, and how to access them effectively. She needs someone to advocate for her. Even if there are services available to help her, she may not know how to gain access to these services.

Historically, in 2002, the Institute of Medicine released a document called *Unequal Treatment: Confronting Racial and Ethnic Disparities in Healthcare* (Institute of Medicine, 2002). The report defines **health disparities** as "racial or ethnic difference in the quality of healthcare which is not due to access-related factors or clinical needs, preferences, and appropriateness of intervention" (Institute of Medicine, 2002, p. 3). Disparities are found in certain types of illness, such as cardiovascular disease, cancer, HIV, diabetes, end-stage renal disease, and certain surgical procedures. Surgical procedures such as amputations have been found to be more common within minority groups.

The Department of Health and Human Services has identified six areas for which it has oversight. These areas are (1) infant mortality, (2) cancer screening, (3) cardiovascular disease, (4) diabetes, (5) HIV/AIDS, and (6) immunizations. In addition, there are also several areas that need special emphasis, including mental health, hepatitis, syphilis, and tuberculosis.

HEALTHCARE SYSTEMS IN SELECTED DEVELOPED NATIONS

Overall, the commitment to prevention and the cost savings, whether a personal commitment or an economic commitment, is yet to become effective in the United States across a variety of parameters. However, other countries have been able to achieve success with their healthcare system structure, function, and outcomes. Figure 2.3 provides an overview of the relative rankings of six countries, including the United States, by outcomes. For purposes of comparison and contrast, the following section discusses how Canada, France, Germany, the Netherlands, and the United Kingdom keep their citizens healthy and well. These countries were chosen because they historically have had healthcare philosophies that are based on inclusivity of all citizens, lower cost, quality, and a perspective that healthcare is a right. No country is perfect, and many face the same escalating costs as the United States. However, a key international source, the OECD (OECD, 2013a), presents comparative data that demonstrate that these countries have better morbidity and mortality rates, as well as other health-related factors, than the United States. The approaches of these countries to the healthcare of their citizens can serve as important examples of goals which other countries may want to pursue. Key components to advancing public health and public health systems are (1) identifying indicators of health, (2) being committed to providing healthcare professionals and the public with a system that works, and (3) generating policy that allows for the production of positive outcomes. The following countries have been selected because of unique positive contributions they have made in healthcare outcomes, through creative funding and infrastructure adjustments, to meet the unique needs of their respective populations. In many cases, comparisons have been made to these countries because of the positive experiences that have been reported from health outcome data as it relates to costs.

Canada

According to Health Canada (2013) and the OECD Canada (2013c), Canada is the second largest country in the world, with 10 provinces and 2 territories. Its 31.5 million people have a life expectancy of 78 years (men) and 82 years (women). Seventeen percent of the population is older than 60 years of age. Cancer is the leading cause of mortality, followed by congestive heart failure.

Canada's healthcare system is a national health program; it is considered a single-payer system with universal coverage. This means that all Canadian citizens are covered for healthcare by one government-run system. Canadian Medicare, the healthcare insurance coverage for all, began in 1968 to eliminate financial barriers to care and to allow citizens to have choice in what physician they chose for their care (Health Canada, 2013). Culturally, Canada is made up

	AUSTRALIA	CANADA	GERMANY	NEW ZEALAND	UNITED KINGDOM	UNITED STATES
OVERALL RANKING (2007)	3.5	5	2	3.5	1	6
Quality Care	4	6	2.5	2.5	1	5
Right Care	5	6	3	4	2	1
Safe Care	4	5	1	3	2	6
Coordinated Care	3	6	4	2	1	5
Patient-centered Care	3	6	2	1	4	5
Access	3	5	1	2	4	6
Efficiency	4	5	3	2	1	6
Equity	2	5	4	3	1	6
Long, Healthy, and Productive Lives	1	3	2	4.5	4.5	6
Health Expenditures per Capita, 2004	$2,876*	$3,165	$3,005*	$2,083	$2,548	$8,102

Country Rankings: 1.0–2.66 | 2.67–4.33 | 4.34–6   * 2003 data

figure 2.3 Overall ranking of countries according to various healthcare indicators (2007). *2003 data. (From The Commonwealth Fund [2013]. International Health Policy Survey, the Commonwealth Fund 2005; International Health Policy Survey of Sicker Adults; the 2006 Commonwealth Fund International Health Policy Survey of Primary Care Physicians; and the Commonwealth Fund Commission on a High-performance Health System National Scorecard.)

of multicultural and multilingual populations because of high immigration rates over the years. Canadians view healthcare as a right, not a privilege, and more specifically, as a social responsibility.

Funding for the Canadian healthcare system comes from personal, sales, and corporate taxes, and federal transfer payments (<25%). The federal government provides healthcare only for special populations (military personnel, native Canadians, and federal prisoners [<2% of the population]). The government of Canada has the responsibility for what are considered the public health arms of the National Institutes of Health, occupational and environmental health, health promotion, Indian Health Service, and health protection.

Despite a single-payer reimbursement system, the 12 provinces determine the management, delivery, and financial arrangements for the Canadian Medicare services. Private insurance exists to cover services not covered under Medicare, such as vision needs, dental services, and pharmaceuticals for nonelderly people. This type of private insurance is acquired through employment contributions, and represents a small portion of total health expenditures (15%). Provinces raise money specifically for Medicare through taxes, corporate contributions, personal income, fuel taxes, and lottery profits.

The money allocated through these approaches supports the individual health costs of citizens in each unique province or territory, hospital payments, and physician salaries, which are capped and negotiated, drugs, long-term care and mental health institutions, and provincial healthcare planning. At the national level, there is oversight of the development and safety of pharmaceuticals, and reviews that survey physician production, practice, and quality.

The most powerful individuals in the healthcare system are health administrators, not physicians. These health administrators put an emphasis on cost, efficiency, and social responsibility. Unlike in the United States, most of the physicians are generalists who are reimbursed by provincial health plans (99%) through fee-for-service, capitation (maximal amount of money based on patient caseload), or salaries in health centers. Nevertheless, the majority of care occurs in the private physician's office. Nurses have little autonomy and often migrate to the United States to practice in order to gain higher salaries (Health Canada, 2013).

Capital expenditures are separate from operating expenditures, which gives provinces control over facility development and renovation. There is a trend toward delivering healthcare and performing medical and surgical procedures outside of hospital settings, with an increasing focus on health promotion and disease prevention. Most procedures are scheduled in advance and take place in outpatient or ambulatory areas. Although there may be long waits for care, it is important to remember that the wait time is not for emergency or life-threatening conditions. It is a way to distribute care more evenly and to control costs.

Individual provinces closely monitor quality of care, with strong emphasis on decreasing duplication of services across all levels of care. Hospitals, in particular, are used not just for acute care, but for long-term care of patients (23% of hospital beds). There have been reports of inequities between provinces (Health Canada, 2013) and fear that cost containment may limit the use of newer and developing technologies. The balanced benefit of this approach is that Canada has better health outcomes than the United States (30th vs. 37th) in OECD rankings (OECD Canada, 2013c) while spending less money per person on healthcare. Many people believe that it is far better to wait for nonemergent care than to be uninsured (see Table 2.1).

EVIDENCE FOR PRACTICE

Brehaut et al. (2009) used population-based data to evaluate whether caring for a child with health problems had implications for caregiver health after controlling for relevant covariants. They used data on 9,401 children and their caregivers from a population-based Canadian study to analyze and compare 3,633 healthy children with 2,485 children with health problems. Caregiver health outcomes included chronic conditions, activity limitations, self-reported general health, depressive symptoms, social support, family functioning, and marital satisfaction. Covariants included family (single-parent status, number of children, income adequacy), caregiver (gender, age, education, smoking status, biological relationship with child), and child (age, gender) characteristics. Their findings showed that caregivers of children with health problems had more than twice the odds of reporting chronic conditions, activity limitations, and elevated depressive symptoms, and had greater odds of reporting poorer general health than did caregivers of healthy children. This study points out that caregivers of children with health problems had substantially greater odds of also having health problems than did caregivers of healthy children. From a public health assurance perspective, this indicates that healthcare initiatives need be directed not only to individual children who are chronically ill but also to families. There is an important link between those with chronic illness and those who care for them.

STUDENT REFLECTION

We were asked in clinical seminar to think about and discuss the prejudices we may have heard about other healthcare systems in the world, and I immediately thought of Canada because it is our next-door neighbor. Everybody says that healthcare is rationed, there aren't enough doctors, the quality of care is poor, and that it is "socialized medicine." I have realized that although there may be a wait for specialist care, there is no wait for the most common need for care...primary care. There is rationing related to immediate need versus needs that can be delayed.

(continued on page 36)

The most important thing is that everybody has insurance, and nobody is denied care because they can't pay for it. Although there are some shortages of physicians, there is more of a sense of balance in having more physicians available to take care of the common illnesses of the population (primary care). From what I have read, the quality of care is acceptable, especially in light of the fact that in our own country some have no ability to obtain care. I guess the bottom line is, as I prepare to practice nursing, I am keenly aware of the need to ensure all populations of having access to get help for common problems and to have, most importantly, equal access to quality care.

France

Despite the French people's dissatisfaction with their healthcare system, many consider their system one of the best in the world (Bourdelais, 2010). According to the OECD (OECD, 2013f), France, a republic with a population of 61,000,000, is a healthy country in terms of infant mortality, life expectancy, and healthcare-related costs (see Table 2.1).

The Ministry of Health runs two large organizations that cover the funding and provision of health services in 22 regional services agencies: (1) General Health Management and (2) Hospital and Healthcare Management. The structure of the healthcare system in France includes the National Institute of Health, established in 1998; the French Agency of Health Safety of Health Products, which functions similarly to the Food and Drug Administration (FDA) of the United States, also established in 1998; the Agency of Environmental Health Safety (established in 2000); French Institute of Blood, established in 1992; French Institute of Transplants (established in 1994); and the Ministry for Health, Family and the Disabled.

The government presents a law to the parliament every year as a way to use public policy to finance a social security fund, which includes the national expenditure on health insurance. This public policy effort also specifies goals for the healthcare system, similar to the *Healthy People 2020* effort in the United States. The Ministry of Health delegates the planning and implementation of health initiatives to regions that make up the country, in order to decentralize and make care plans specific to each region. A National Health Insurance guarantees universal access to 80% of the French people by offering health coverage to wage earners through what is called the CNAMTS (Caisse Nationale d'Assurance Maladie des Travailleurs Salari or French National Health Insurance Agency for Wage Earners). The rest of the national funding is divided among other funds that are occupationally specific (physicians, agricultural workers, and students). Therefore, the French population is 100% covered by a public mandatory health insurance. Funds are financed by payroll taxes (60%) and, since 1990, by a proportional income tax (40%), called the CSG ("Contribution sociale généralisée"). The funds are governed by boards with representatives of the government, the main workers unions, and the association of French manufacturers.

France has an essential single payer system (Le Pen, 2014). More than 80% of French people carry a supplemental form of private insurance often linked to employment. Public payment covers 76% of French health expenditure. Patients pay physicians directly and apply for reimbursement, and 21% of expenditures are on pharmaceuticals. For 96% of the population, healthcare is entirely free; it is reimbursed up to 100%. Users of this system can select any physician—even a specialist and hospital (public or private)—with the belief that choice leads to successfully-managed competition and quality care.

In France, there are more than 1.2 million employees in the health service sector. Physicians consider public hospital jobs undesirable, and often foreign physicians fill these positions. The majority of physicians in private practice participate in a government-fixed fee-for-service scheme, and the remainder charge what they wish. Physicians accept what the government pays, and the patient pays the difference. French general practitioners earn the equivalent of about $55,000 per year. Other characteristics of physicians working in France are presented in Box 2.1.

The French healthcare system is made up of public, private, and not-for-profit sectors, which avoids the long-waiting lists characteristic of other socialized medicine systems. Health insurance supplies a large majority (91%) of the funds for the 1,032 (85% of total) public hospitals, which account for 65% of all hospital beds in France. Private, not-for-profit hospitals account for 15% of all hospital beds, and specialize in medium- to long-term care. Private, for-profit hospitals account for 20% of all hospital beds. The private hospitals conduct 50% of surgeries and 60% of cancer care.

A key ethic of this system is individual choice of physician and place of service, including a tradition of long-term care in the private home. France maintains strict boundaries between health and social services, and outcomes and performance are benchmarks for both home healthcare and nursing homes. Financial aid is given to people in the form of *allocation personnalisée d'autonomie*, or allocation for loss of autonomy, to purchase care—even

box 2.1 Characteristics of Physicians in France

- Physicians are unevenly distributed between rural and urban areas.
- About 50% of physicians are women.
- Physician visits can take 15 to 30 minutes.
- Physicians see about 10 patients per day.
- Medical education for physicians is publicly funded.
- Ratio of generalists to specialists is 1:1.
- Ranking system of hospital practitioners is nationwide.
- Physicians, biologists, and dentists are all salaried hospital practitioners.
- Advancement is based on seniority.

Source: Organization of Economic Cooperation and Development. (2006, January 16). *The supply of physician services in OECD countries* (OECD health working papers No. 21). Retrieved from http://www.oecd.org/els/health-systems/35987490.pdf

EVIDENCE FOR PRACTICE

The following two survey studies are examples of this commitment to the health of the French population.

1. Constant, Salmi, Lafont, Chiron, and Lagarde (2009) investigated behavioral changes in a cohort of car drivers to understand why there was a decrease in motor vehicle road casualties in France. Researchers offered self-report survey questions to more than 11,000 people between 2001 and 2004 to explore attitudes related to road safety and driving behaviors. Investigators found that adequate sleep was related to positive outcomes in road safety. Decreases in cell phone use and speeding over this time period demonstrated decreases in road mortality in France.
2. Nayaradou, Berchi, Dejardin, and Launoy (2010) elicited preferences of the population for willingness to participate in a mass colorectal cancer screening initiative in northwest France. (The implementation of a mass colorectal cancer screening program is a public health priority.) They interpreted the results of a survey conducted by mail from June 2006 to October 2006 on a representative random sample of 2,000 inhabitants, aged 50 to 74 years. On the questionnaire, each person made three or four discrete choices between hypothetical tests that differed in eight ways: how screening is offered, process, test sensitivity, rate of unnecessary colonoscopy, expected mortality reduction, method of screening, test result transmission, and cost. Results from the 32.8% of respondents indicated that expected mortality reduction, sensitivity, cost, and process were among the population preferences. Researchers found that the sensitivity of the test was most important in respondents with higher financial resources. Key implications included how adherence to screening could be accomplished in light of these data.

from family members or other unskilled labor—as a way to promote employment.

Clients in nursing homes pay for their room and board separately from nursing/healthcare, and these costs come from pension funds or welfare funds. The residents of nursing homes are legally entitled to be involved in the governance of their home, and in France, this system is highly respected and well run, with little inefficiency. Finally, there is a strong emphasis on prevention as a priority.

Germany

Germany, the largest country in Europe, is made up of 82.4 million people divided into 16 states. From a vital statistics perspective, life expectancy varies between men and women (76 and 82 years, respectively), and 19% of the population is older than 65 years of age. The leading causes of death include heart disease and lung cancer (OECD, 2013d).

Germany has a universal healthcare system (OECD, 2013d). Historically, health insurance was a requirement and directed at low-income workers and certain government employees. Eventually, all people were able to obtain insurance. Currently, physicians in private practice provide ambulatory care, and centralized nonprofit hospitals offer the majority of inpatient care. Most of the population has health insurance; individuals can obtain coverage from a variety of "sickness funds" financed by public and private sources. Funds for standard insurance come from a combination of employee/employer contributions and government subsidies, which are scaled on the basis of need. An option exists for individuals to choose to pay a tax and opt out of the standard plan, in favor of "private" insurance. Many people with higher salaries choose this option, but their premiums are linked to health status, not to income level.

Regional physician's associations negotiate provider reimbursement for specific services. A Commission, composed of representatives of business, labor, physicians, hospitals, and insurance and pharmaceutical industries, meets annually. The Commission takes into account government policies and makes recommendations on overall expenditure targets to regional associations. Although reimbursement of providers is on a fee-for-service basis, including copayments, the amount to be reimbursed for each service is determined retrospectively to ensure that spending targets are not exceeded. The average length of hospital stay in Germany has decreased in recent years from 14 to 9 days, still considerably longer than the 5- to 6-day average in the United States (Eco-Sante Databases, 2010). Drug costs have increased substantially each year, despite attempts to contain costs. Overall healthcare expenditures have risen, but costs are substantially less than those in the United States (OECD, 2013d).

The reunification of East and West Germany, which occurred in 1991, did increase variation in health statistics by lowering infant mortality and increasing life expectancy. However, differences continue to exist between the two parts of the country because of differences in philosophy and distribution of care in the past. Philosophically, the idea that all people should have health insurance, and that the nation is responsible to provide systems of healthcare to its citizens is common to both regions. Health insurance coverage is maintained by all citizens sharing in the effort to have an insurance pool, and payment is based on income, not risk. The healthcare benefits are extremely comprehensive and include medications, dental, vision, medical treatments, and even health spas. Decentralization of healthcare administration includes a federal institute for communicable and noncommunicable disease similar to the CDC in the United States. The organizations of a variety of institutes are grouped across a regional healthcare system which is managed by the sickness funds and physician associations.

Prevention has an important role in the German system, not only as an effort toward cost saving but also in increasing the quality of life of citizens. Public health efforts

EVIDENCE FOR PRACTICE

Stolle, Sack, and Thomasius (2009) have expressed concern about episodic excessive alcohol consumption (binge drinking) in children and adolescents as a serious public health problem in Germany because of its associated risks with further morbidities and mortality. An extensive literature search for evidence related to binge drinking from 1998 to 2008 revealed that episodic excessive alcohol consumption is associated not only with somatic complications, but also with traffic accidents and other types of accidents; violent behavior, and suicide. The more frequently a child or adolescent drinks to excess, and the younger he or she is, the greater is the risk of developing an alcohol-related disorder (alcohol misuse or dependence syndrome). Although in the United States, brief motivational interventions have been shown to have a small to medium-sized beneficial effect in reducing further binge drinking and its complications, the Germans use an intervention called HaLT ("stop," also an acronym for Hart am Limit—"near the limit"). Further types of brief motivating intervention could be integrated in this approach as another variable to decrease binge drinking behavior and prevent the development of alcohol-related disorders.

include not only primary prevention but also health screening, with a special emphasis on youth development.

Nurses in the German healthcare system, called sisters, are mostly diploma-educated individuals working with a physician. There has been a protracted history of shortages of nurses in the 831 public hospitals, 835 independent nonprofit hospitals, and 374 private hospitals. As a final comparison, Germany's healthcare system is 6th in financial fairness, 14th in overall goal attainment, and 14th in terms of overall performance. America's system is 54th in financial fairness, 15th in goal attainment, and 37th in overall performance.

STUDENT REFLECTION

It is stunning to me that when you explore different healthcare systems in the United States, the systems seem so wasteful or greedy or just not inclusive enough to allow everyone to have the same healthcare opportunities. One of the things I was thinking about is that, in the United States, we have accepted for a long time the necessity of education. Whether the quality of the education is there or not...the idea is that education is a significant predictor of success and gainful employment in life. Well, if that is the case why would we not have the same perspective for health? Isn't good health a predictor of future good health? Recently, some people in the United States were very worried about the effort to create opportunities for all people to have access to healthcare...not necessarily effective or efficient healthcare but healthcare, period. My sense was that people were divided about using tax money for healthcare. Some felt that the United States was becoming "socialized." I guess it made me sad to think about so many people I have met in poor, run-down neighborhoods who could use the benefits of a philosophy that does not forget them, that cares for them, and wants them to have an equal share of a quality life.

The Netherlands

According to the OECD (2013f), total health spending in the Netherlands accounted for 9.8% of the GDP, slightly more than the average of other OECD countries. The Netherlands also ranks above the OECD average in terms of health spending per capita, with current spending of US$3,52 (adjusted for purchasing power parity), compared with an OECD average of US$2,964. Health spending per capita in the Netherlands remains much lower than in the United States, Norway, Switzerland, and Luxembourg.

The Netherlands has a dual-level healthcare payment system. All primary and acute care is financed from private mandatory insurance. Long-term care for the elderly, the dying, long-term mentally ill, and so on is covered by money acquired from taxation and is considered a "social insurance." Insurance companies must offer a core universal insurance package for universal primary, curative care, which includes the cost of all prescription medicines at a fixed price without discrimination by age or levels of health or illness (AARP, 2010). Otherwise, they are considered to be operating illegally.

According to OECD health data (2013b), for people whose health expenses are higher because of illness, insurance companies receive more compensation if they have to pay out more than might be expected. This allows them to accept all patients in an ethically sound way and take care of their needs, rather than strategizing savings by not insuring those who have expensive, long trajectories of needed care. Insurance companies compete with each other on price for insurance premiums and negotiate deals with hospitals to keep costs low and quality high. There is formal regulation that includes checking for abuse and for acts that are against consumer interests. An insurance regulator ensures that all basic policies have identical coverage rules, so that no person is medically disadvantaged by his or her choice of insurer.

Payroll taxes paid by employers, and a fund controlled by the health regulator, or the "regulator's fund," finance the healthcare system. The government contributes 5% to the regulator's fund. The remaining money needed to cover the country's health expenses is collected as premiums paid by those insured. Insurance companies, many of which are private, can offer additional services, such as dental care, at extra cost over and above the universal system. The standard monthly premium for healthcare paid by individual adults is about €100 (currently about US$129) per month, and people with low incomes can get help from the government to pay for the premiums. The regulator's fund pays for all children's healthcare in the country.

Hospitals in the Netherlands, which have been advancing in quality over time, are regulated and inspected regularly. They are privately run and for-profit. People can choose where they want to be treated; on the Internet, they can obtain access to information about the performance and waiting times at each hospital. Those who are dissatisfied with their insurer and choice of hospital can cancel at any time, but they must make a new agreement with another insurer (Dückers, Makai, Vos, Groenewegen, & Wagner, 2009).

Physicians are primarily in private practice, and primary care physicians control use of the hospital systems. Nursing is considered a profession (12.8 per 1,000 of the population), but nurses are not paid well. They may be specialists in acute care in the hospital setting or in community care (with a direct emphasis on home-based care). Several universities offer undergraduate and graduate degrees (Nursing in the Netherlands, 2010).

The Netherlands primarily funds what is considered one of the best long-term care systems through non–means-tested social insurance programs financed by national premiums. The programs cover a broad range of institutional and noninstitutional services (Wiener, Tilly, & Cuellar, 2003). This system includes mental health and substance abuse care. Prescriptions are covered by insurers who use specific cost formularies. Generally, co-payments, with options to pay more for certain drugs, are available.

EVIDENCE FOR PRACTICE

Investigators in the Netherlands examined the association between dairy product intake and the risk of bladder cancer in 120,852 men and women 55 to 69 years of age (Keszei, Schouten, Goldbohm, & Van Den Brandt, 2009). By using a 150-item food frequency questionnaire, several researchers studied a cohort for 16 years and identified and examined 1,549 people. The findings suggested a positive correlation in women between butter intake and bladder risk.

United Kingdom

The National Health Service (NHS), which provides healthcare in the United Kingdom, began in 1948 (U.K. Department of Health, 2013). The system operates across the four countries that make up the United Kingdom (England, Scotland, Wales, and Northern Ireland). Although there are differences in how the health system is implemented, its basic organization and functions are detailed in a constitution which includes specific rights and governance.

The NHS constitution states that healthcare will be provided for all permanent residents of the United Kingdom, regardless of age, gender, disability, race, sexual orientation, religion, or belief, and access to healthcare is based only on need. People are able to choose their own physician; if necessary, this may involve traveling outside the United Kingdom to see other medical professionals for healthcare. About 36% of clients wait for hospital admission for treatment of nonacute conditions, and emergencies are addressed immediately. Two-thirds of patients are treated in less than 12 weeks (OECD, 2013e).

The NHS system is decentralized, with access to care and prevention provided by the Strategic Health Authorities. The primary treatment centers are structured like departments of health in the United States and are responsible for (1) assessing healthcare needs of communities, (2) commissioning health services needed by these communities based on this assessment, (3) identifying goals for improving the health of communities, (4) ensuring access to care, (5) assessing the interaction between healthcare organizations and social services organizations, and (6) assessing the quality of healthcare personnel.

Each of the foundation trusts, which are decentralized departments whose goal is the health of specific sectors of the population, acts as a department of health (U.K. Department of Health, 2014). There is also a central Department of Health which is not involved in day-to-day decision-making and implementation of care. This department makes policy decisions on a large scale, and local governments can define how they will uniquely carry out those policies for their citizens. The NHS provides primary, inpatient, long-term, psychiatric, and eye care free to many people, including children, the elderly, the unemployed, and low-income residents. Private healthcare does exist in the United Kingdom, but only a small percentage of the population use it, generally for specialty care. Private insurance does not cover the cost of pre-existing conditions, chronic conditions, or pregnancy.

Access to medications and healthcare personnel and facilities include prescriptions which are paid by either a flat rate or through annual capped charges. Physicians contract with the NHS to provide services and receive a salary. The majority of the hospitals are owned and run by the NHS trusts. Of the 2.1 physicians per 1,000 population, most are general practitioners. They can have both a public and private practice. They are paid by a mix of capitation, salary, and fees. Those physicians who are specialists are called "consultants," and they are based in hospitals. Nurses make up the largest group of NHS staff and are paid from 40% of the NHS budget. As in most parts of the world, there is a nursing shortage. Although most nurses work in hospital systems, they are educated as specialists, and focus on particular specialty areas such as maternal health.

Revenues for all NHS health services come from taxes (83%), employer–employee contributions (13%), and user fees or co-payments (4%). Expenditures come from the NHS (88%) and private insurance (12%). All people in the United Kingdom have health insurance; in comparison, 44 million in the United States are uninsured, with no access to healthcare. Although there are questions about the level of quality of care in the NHS when compared to the United States, there is much better cost control, and access to care for all people, which translates into better health for the U.K. population.

EVIDENCE FOR PRACTICE

The Royal College of Paediatrics and Child Health (RCPCH) in the United Kingdom introduced guidelines for reimmunization of children after completion of standard-dose chemotherapy and after hematopoietic stem cell transplant (HSCT) (Patel, Chisholm, & Health, 2008). To understand if the guidelines were properly applied and whether they created a positive standard, researchers offered an online anonymous survey to pediatric principal treatment center (PTC) consultants and shared care (SC) consultants. Results from 55 PTC consultants and 54 SC consultants demonstrated that most PTC and SC consultants recommend initiating reimmunization at 6 months after completion of standard-dose chemotherapy. Between 93% and 100% of respondents reported reimmunization at the recommended time after HSCT for each transplant type. (Physicians recommended pneumococcal conjugate vaccine after chemotherapy by 58.3% (35/60) of respondents and by 51.7% (30/58) after HSCT.) There were distinct differences between PTC and SC consultants in their choice of varicella postexposure prophylaxis.

PUBLIC HEALTH COMMITMENTS TO THE WORLD: INTERNATIONAL PUBLIC HEALTH AND DEVELOPING COUNTRIES

The following section addresses public health commitment from an organizational perspective. The WHO will be discussed, especially in relation to its current health goals, and the structures and processes which are intended to yield positive outcomes. Initiatives to address refugees internationally through the United Nations and other organizations across the globe (bilateral, multilateral, NGOs) will also be considered. In addition, the international face of nursing will be discussed, with its focus on offering nursing science and evidence-based practice internationally.

World Health Organization

When the United Nations was established in 1945, a key directive and commitment was to protect human rights, security, and the social development of all countries (United Nations, 2013). The WHO was established in 1946 as part of the United Nations to maximize health and wellness for all (World Health Organization [WHO], 2013a). The WHO is located in Geneva, Switzerland, and has six regional offices, including a U.S. branch located in Washington, DC (Pan American Health Organization, PAHO). The relationship of the United Nations to the WHO is similar to that of the USDHHS and the NIH to the CDC. For example, there is a keen focus on supplying current information about disease and disability, and establishing standards of care on the basis of evidence found in health research. In the WHO, efforts are directed primarily to safely conquer disease and to help advance professionals and healthcare systems which allow this to occur with efficiency and effectiveness. In addition, the WHO focuses on policy development through a process of supporting annual commissions and assemblies (e.g., World Health Assembly) as a means of advancing policies and guidelines to countries with common, or uniquely specific, healthcare problems. (WHO, 2013c) (Fig. 2.4). The development of the WHO's Child Growth Standards used data collected in the WHO Multicentre Growth Reference Study. The WHO provides international access to documentation on how physical growth curves and motor-skill milestones of achievement were developed, as well as application tools to support implementation of the standards (WHO, 2013b).

The 63rd session of the World Health Assembly in Geneva in May 2010 (WHO, 2013d) discussed a number of public health issues, including (1) implementation of the International Health Regulations (IHR), (2) monitoring of the achievement of the health-related Millennium Development Goals (MDGs), (3) strategies to reduce the harmful use of alcohol, and (4) counterfeit medical products.

The IHR document is a legal brief that addresses transnational control of infectious diseases, and which was developed as a response to the increase in international travel and trade. On June 15, 2007, the IHRs became international law; 194 countries have agreed to implement the regulations. The IHR requires nations to strengthen core surveillance and response capacities to infection control at the primary, intermediate, and national level, as well as at designated international ports, airports, and ground crossings. The regulations further introduce a series of health documents, including ship sanitation certificates, and an international certificate of vaccination or prophylaxis for travelers. The document is available at the WHO website.

The United Nations **Millennium Development Goals** are eight goals that all 189 UN member states at the time

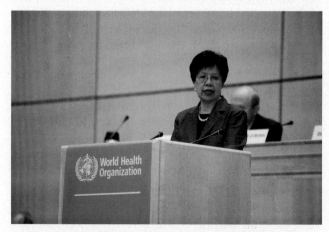

figure 2.4 Opening of the 63rd World Health Assembly. Dr. Margaret Chan, Director-General of the World Health Organization, opened the assembly by reminding all present that 30 years ago, the World Health Assembly declared that "the world and all its people have won freedom from smallpox."

agreed to try to achieve by the year 2015 (WHO, 2013d). The United Nations Millennium Declaration, signed in September 2000, commits world leaders to combat poverty, hunger, disease, illiteracy, environmental degradation, and discrimination against women. The MDGs are derived from this Declaration, and all have specific targets and indicators. The following are the specific goals:

1. To eradicate extreme poverty and hunger
2. To achieve universal primary education
3. To promote gender equality and empowering women
4. To reduce child mortality rates
5. To improve maternal health
6. To combat HIV/AIDS, malaria, and other diseases
7. To ensure environmental sustainability
8. To develop a global partnership for development

The World Bank, the International Monetary Fund, and the African Development Bank agreed to cancel debt of the poorest countries so that resources could be used to improve health. Key criticisms about this monetary support has been related to the fact that much of the money (at least 50%) was diverted to disaster relief and military aid, areas for which it was not intended (Waage et al., 2010).

Refugee and Disaster-Relief Assistance

A **refugee** is defined as "any person who is outside his or her country of origin and who is unwilling or unable to return there or to avail him- or herself of its protection because of a well-founded fear of being persecuted for reasons of race, religion, nationality, membership in a particular social group, or political opinion or a threat to life or security as a result of armed conflict and other forms of widespread violence which seriously disturb the public order" (UNHCR, 2013). The United Nations High Commissioner for Refugees (UNHCR) was established by the International Refugee Organization, an organization that was founded on April 20, 1946, to deal with the massive refugee problem created by World War II.

Internally-displaced persons are people who have been forced to flee their homes suddenly or unexpectedly in large numbers because of armed conflict, internal strife, systematic violations of human rights, or natural disasters, and who are *within* the territory of their own country (Office of the United Nations High Commissioner for Human Rights [OHCHR], 2013).

Most conflicts occur within rather than between countries. Compared with other continents, Africa and Asia have consistently registered high numbers of civil armed conflicts (Reliefweb, 2013). Some of the countries that have experienced violent conflicts and prominent humanitarian interventions in the past two decades include Liberia, Angola, Sierra Leone, Rwanda, Sudan, Chechnya, Bosnia and Herzegovina (formerly Yugoslavia), Somalia, Sri Lanka, Azerbaijan, Armenia, Democratic Republic of Congo (DRC), Kosovo, East Timor, Afghanistan, and Iraq (Reliefweb, 2013).

The health consequences experienced by populations affected by armed conflict are generally similar in nature. War-induced displacement is psychologically and physically traumatizing to everyone affected. People are rarely prepared for flight and have no time to gather clothes, food, or anything that can sustain their lives during displacement. Their search for safety can last for long periods, depending on the nature of war, prevailing geographical conditions, and the willingness of host communities to welcome them. Relatives and family members are often separated. Some are lost to capture, displacement, and/or death (Impact of armed conflict on children, 2013).

The health effects of armed conflict may be direct or indirect. The direct effects include injuries (e.g., due to land mines, weapons), sexual violence, human rights violations, psychological trauma, and death. Indirect effects include food scarcity, population displacement, high levels of morbidity and mortality, infectious disease, complications of chronic disease, reproductive health morbidities, malnutrition, and disruption of health services (Toole, Waldman, & Zwi, 2000). It is significant that the United Nations, in its human rights activities, works with bilateral and multilateral agencies, NGOs, and the World Bank to offer health assistance in addition to the many other competing direct and indirect needs related to refugees.

Multilateral, Bilateral, and Nongovernmental Organizations as International Organizations for Health

International health organizations are classified on the basis of their relationships with other distinguished organizations which match their commitment to specific aspects of population-based health, the specific implementation of health goals both directly and indirectly, and their particular resources, including financial contributions. **Multilateral agencies** and organizations receive funding from both governmental and nongovernmental sources. Examples of these multilateral agencies include the United Nations and the WHO, which were discussed previously. The World Bank is another multilateral organization. Its major goal is to lend money to countries in need of developing their infrastructure on a variety of fronts. Some of the projects undertaken by the World Bank and related to health include addressing access to safe drinking water, soil development so that healthy foods can be grown and eaten, building sanitation systems so that water drainage is not connected directly to sewage, and promotion of vaccination programs, as well as promoting primary healthcare, which includes screening programs. Specific programs include Roll Back Malaria, the Joint United Nations Programme on HIV/AIDS, the Global Alliance for Vaccines and Immunizations, Onchocerciasis Control Program (river blindness control), and the Global Water Project (World Bank, 2013). (See the earlier discussion of WHO, United Nations, and Millennium Development Goals for a critique of the use of promised monies to assist with health goals by World Bank and other funding organizations.)

Bilateral agencies and organizations conduct their services within one specific country. The U.S. Agency for

International Development (USAID) is a good example in the United States. It is a committed initiative which works with developing countries to enhance systems to fortify the health and welfare of international populations. USAID focuses specifically on support directed to sub-Saharan Africa, Asia, Latin America, the Caribbean, Eurasia, and the Middle East. Key health prevention initiatives focus on larger areas of child, maternal, and reproductive health, and have specific interests in HIV/AIDS, malaria, and tuberculosis care (USAID, 2013). Many of the healthcare systems in countries described earlier in this chapter have parallel organizations to USAID.

Nongovernmental organizations, discussed earlier in this chapter, are private agencies that voluntarily use their resources to address a variety of healthcare initiatives in the United States. Some of these organizations have specific goals or roles in global health. For example, the International Committee of the Red Cross (2013) is known most for its role in disaster relief. Some groups, such as Catholic Relief Services (2013), have a particular religious affiliation, and others, such as Oxfam International (2013), are directed specifically to issues related to hunger and nutritional health. Philanthropies are organizations that are similar to NGOs, but they receive funding through personal endowments. For example, the Bill and Melissa Gates Foundation (2013) focuses on health, poverty, and development in Africa, South America, Asia, and Australia. Specifically, The Living Proof Project supports vaccine and nutrition programs, as well as decreasing the incidence of diseases such as polio, HIV/AIDS, and tropical illnesses. In all cases, NGOs and philanthropies view human rights as a fundamental (motivation) basis for addressing the unseen and unfelt pain of many people in the world who suffer needlessly.

PRACTICE POINT

The United States offers a process of applying for tax-exempt status for not-for-profit NGOs, which are focused on national or international public health. This process requires filing specific forms with the Internal Revenue Service (IRS) and a fee, and there must be no involvement with or by any political campaigns. The organizational status acquired through this process is a tax-exempt, nonprofit corporation or association (a 501c3). It requires a board of directors be formed, with a stipulation in its by-laws which states the work intended to be done by the organization. In return, the IRS gives the organization tax exemption for purchases aligned with the mission of the organization, as well as other benefits and protections. Donations and contributions made to nonprofit organizations may be claimed as tax deductions on individual or corporate tax returns. Check out your local rules and regulations, or discuss this idea with any legal consultant you may know (perhaps a law student at your university or town).

International Council of Nurses

The International Council of Nurses (ICN) is a federation of more than 130 national nurses associations, representing more than 13 million nurses worldwide. Founded in 1899, ICN is the world's first and widest-reaching international organization for health professionals. Operated by internationally-prominent nurses, ICN works to ensure quality nursing care for all, sound health policies globally, the advancement of nursing knowledge, and the presence worldwide of a respected nursing profession and a competent and satisfied nursing work force (International Council of Nurses [ICN], 2013).

ICN advances nursing, nurses, and health through its policies, partnerships, advocacy, leadership development, networks, congresses, and special projects, and by its work in the arenas of professional practice, regulation, and socioeconomic welfare. ICN is particularly active in the following:

- International classification of nursing practice
- Advanced nursing practice
- Entrepreneurship
- HIV/AIDS, tuberculosis, and malaria
- Women's health
- Primary healthcare
- Family health
- Safe water

Despite the variation in healthcare structures between countries, and the varying degrees of both fiscal and health outcomes, nurses continue to advance the health of the public. Through (1) assessment of health across a variety of specialties and patient groups, (2) education of other nurses in health promotion and disease prevention, and (3) contributions to health policy development, nurses represent the voice of patients and clients worldwide.

key concepts

- Healthcare systems are organized based on philosophies of care, and are culturally influenced.
- The United States healthcare system includes structure and functions to support assessment, assurance, and health policy related to the health of populations.
- Despite the economic strength of the United States and other industrialized nations, many countries have found more efficient and effective ways to care for all by decreasing health disparities and giving equal access to care.
- Public, philanthropic, and nongovernmental agencies all contribute to the health of populations through diverse structures, financing, and personnel approaches to the health needs of citizens.

critical thinking questions

1. Give three reasons why you think that comparing healthcare systems between countries is an important approach to serving the healthcare needs of people.
2. In thinking about multilateral, bilateral, and nongovernmental organizations, where would you see the role of a community/public health nurse? Give some examples and explain why public health nurses provide a unique contribution.
3. How do cultural and philosophical factors play an important role in how healthcare systems are developed and supported? Give explicit examples.

community resources

- Local philanthropies and foundations with goals focused on healthcare
- State Department of Health
- Organizational chart of the (state house) legislative governance in your state (look for Health and Human Services)
- Insurance companies (private, HMOs)
- Departments of Social Services (Medicaid Division)

references

AARP. (2010). *AARP European Leadership Study: Cost containment*. Retrieved from http://assets.aarp.org/www.aarp.org_/cs/gap/ldrstudy_costcontain.pdf;

Agency for Healthcare Research and Quality (AHRQ) (2010). Retrieved from http://www.ahrq.gov/

Agency for Healthcare Research and Quality. (2013). Retrieved from http://www.ahrq.gov/

Bourdelais, P. (2010). *Improving public health in France. The local political mobilization in the nineteenth century*. Retrieved from http://www.ep.liu.se/ej/hygiea/ra/026/paper.pdf

Brehaut, J. C., Kohen, D. E., Garner, R. E., Miller, A. R., Lach, L. M., Klassen, A. F., & Rosenbaum, P. L. (2009). Health among caregivers of children with health problems: Findings from a Canadian population-based study. *American Journal of Public Health*, 99, 1254–1262. doi:10.2105/AJPH.2007.129817

Catholic Relief Services. (2013). Retrieved from http://crs.org/

Center on Budget and Policy Priorities. (2013). *Balance Budget Act 1997*. Retrieved from http://www.cbpp.org/cms/index.cfm?fa=view&id=2138

Centers for Disease Control and Prevention. (2013a). Retrieved from http://www.cdc.gov/

Centers for Disease Control and Prevention. (2013b). *HPV vaccine*. Retrieved from http://www.cdc.gov/hpv/vaccine.html

Centers for Medicare and Medicaid Services. (2013). *National health expenditures*. Retrieved from http://www.cms.gov/Research-Statistics-Data-and-Systems/Statistics-Trends-and-Reports/NationalHealthExpendData/index.html?redirect=/NationalHealthExpendData/

Centers for Medicare and Medicaid Services. (2014). Retrieved from http://cms.hhs.gov/

Chidiac, C., & Ader, F. (2009). Pneumococcal vaccine in the elderly: A useful but forgotten vaccine. *Aging Clinical & Experimental Research*, *21*(3), 222–228.

Children's Health Insurance Program. (2014). Retrieved from http://www.medicaid.gov/Medicaid-CHIP-Program-Information/By-Topics/Childrens-Health-Insurance-Program-CHIP/Childrens-Health-Insurance-Program-CHIP.html

Constant, A., Salmi, L. R., Lafont, S., Chiron, M., & Lagarde, E. (2009). Road casualties and changes in risky driving behavior in France between 2001 and 2004 among participants in the GAZEL cohort. *American Journal of Public Health*, 99, 1247–1253. doi:10.2105/AJPH.2007.126474

Desai, A. K., Grossberg, G. T., & Chibnall, J. T. (2010). Healthy brain aging: A road map. *Clinics in Geriatric Medicine*, *26*(1), 1–16.

Dückers, M., Makai, P., Vos, L., Groenewegen, P., & Wagner, C. (2009). Longitudinal analysis on the development of hospital quality management systems in the Netherlands. *International Journal for Quality in Health Care*, *21*(5), 330–340. doi:10.1093/intqhc/mzp031

Eco-Sante databases. (2010). Retrieved from http://www.ecosante.org

Friis, R. H., & Sellers, T. A. (2009). *Epidemiology for Public Health Practice* (4th ed.). Sudbury, MA: Jones & Bartlett.

Gates Foundation. (2013). Retrieved from http://www.gatesfoundation.org/Pages/home.aspx

Gorman, B. K., & Chu, M. (2009). Racial and ethnic differences in adult asthma prevalence, problems, and medical care. *Ethnicity & Health*, *14*(5), 527–552.

Health and Human Services. (2013). Retrieved from http://www.hhs.gov/about/whatwedo.html

Health Canada. (2013). Retrieved from http://www.hc-sc.gc.ca/index-eng.php

Heisler, M., Choi, H., Rosen, A. B., Vijan, S., Kabeto, M., Langa, K. M., & Piette, J. D. (2010). Hospitalizations and deaths among adults with cardiovascular disease who underuse medications because of cost: A longitudinal analysis. *Medical Care*, *48*(2), 87–94.

Hirschhorn, L. R., Landers, S., McInnes, D. K., Malitz, F., Ding, L., Joyce, R., & Cleary, P.D. (2009). Reported care quality in federal Ryan White HIV/AIDS Program supported networks of HIV/AIDS care. *AIDS Care*, *21*(6), 799–807.

Impact of armed conflict on children. (2013). Retrieved from http://www.un.org/rights/introduc.htm#contents

Institute of Medicine. (2002). *Unequal treatment: Confronting racial and ethnic disparities in healthcare*. Washington, DC: The National Academies Press.

International Committee of the Red Cross. (2013). Retrieved from http://www.icrc.org/

International Council of Nurses. (2013). Retrieved from http://www.icn.ch/

references (continued)

Jesano, R. (2010). Free drug information sources on the web: Government sites. *Journal of Hospital Librarianship*, *10*(2), 145–151.

Jost, T. S. (2003). The tenuous nature of the medicaid entitlement. *HealthAffairs*, *22*(1), 145–153. Retrieved from http://content.healthaffairs.org/content/22/1/145.full

Kaiser Foundation. (2013). *Uninsured*. Retrieved from http://kff.org/uninsured-3/

Kavanagh, P. L., Adams, W. G., & Wang, C. J. (2009). Quality indicators and quality assessment in child health. *Archives of Disease in Childhood*, *94*(6), 458–463.

Keszei, A. P., Schouten, L. J., Goldbohm, R. A., & Van Den Brandt, P. A. (2009). Dairy intake and the risk of bladder cancer in the Netherlands cohort study on diet and cancer. *American Journal of Epidemiology*, *171*(4), 436–446.

Le Pen, C. (2014). The French health care system. *ISPOR Connections Uniting Science and Practice*. Retrieved from http://www.ispor.org/news/articles/November09/tfhcs.asp

Lutz, S. (2008). Happy together: Consumer expectation for a public-private healthcare system. *Journal of Healthcare Management*, *53*(3), 149–152.

Marth, D. (2009). Mental Health Parity Act of 2007: An analysis of the proposed changes. *Mental Health*, *7*(6), 556–571.

Myers, J. (2003). Exercise and cardiovascular health. *Circulation*, *107*, e2–e5. Retrieved from http://circ.ahajournals.org/content/107/1/e2.full

National Institutes of Health. (2013). Retrieved from http://nih.gov

Nayaradou, M., Berchi, C., Dejardin, O., & Launoy, G. (2010). Eliciting population preferences for mass colorectal cancer screening organization. *Medical Decision Making*, *30*(2), 224–233.

Nursing in the Netherlands. (2010). Retrieved from http://ec.europa.eu/internal_market/qualifications/docs/nurses/2000-study/nurses_nederland_en.pdf

Office for Refugees and Immigrants. (2010). http://www.mass.gov/?pageID=eohhs2agencylanding&L=4&L0=Home&L1=Government&L2=Departments+and+Divisions&L3=Office+for+Refugees+and+Immigrants&sid=Eeohhs2

Office of the United Nations High Commissioner for Human Rights. (2013). *Questions and answers about IDP*. Retrieved from http://www2.ohchr.org/english/issues/idp/issues.htm

Organization of Economic Cooperation and Development. (2013a). Retrieved from http://www.oecd/

Organization of Economic Cooperation and Development. (2013b). *Better life index*. Retrieved from http://www.oecdbetterlifeindex.org/topics/health/

Organization of Economic Cooperation and Development. (2013c). *Canada*. Retrieved from http://www.oecd.org/health/health-systems/health-at-a-glance.htm

Organization of Economic Cooperation and Development. (2013d). *Health at a glance 2013: Key findings for Germany*. Retrieved from http://www.oecd.org/health/health-systems/health-at-aglance.htm

Organization of Economic Cooperation and Development. (2013e). *Health at a glance 2013: Key findings for the United Kingdom*. Retrieved from http://www.oecd.org/health/health-systems/healthat-a-glance.htm

Organization of Economic Cooperation and Development. (2013f). *Health data 2013*. Retrieved from http://www.oecd.org/health/health-systems/health-at-a-glance.htm

Oxfam International. (2013). Retrieved from http://www.oxfam.org/

Parkhurst, J., Weller, I., & Kemp, J. (2010). Getting research into policy, or out of practice, in HIV? *Lancet*, *375*(9724), 1414–1415.

Patel, S. R., Chisholm, J. C., & Health, P. T. (2008). Vaccinations in children treated with standard-dose cancer therapy or hematopoietic stem cell transplantation. *Pediatric Clinics of North American*, *55*(1), 169–186.

Regidor, E., Sánchez, E., de la Fuente, L., Luquero, F. J., de Mateo, S., & Domínguez, V. (2009). Major reduction in AIDS-mortality inequalities after HAART: The importance of absolute differences in evaluating interventions. *Social Science & Medicine*, *68*(3), 419–426.

Reliefweb. (2013). Retrieved from http://www.reliefweb.int/rw/dbc.nsf/doc100?OpenForm

Robert Wood Johnson Foundation. (2013). Retrieved from http://www.rwjf.org/

Rosales, C., Coe, M. K., Stroupe, N. R., Hackman, A., & de Zapien, J. G. (2010). The culture of health survey: A qualitative assessment of a diabetes prevention coalition. *Journal of Community Health*, *35*(1), 4–9.

Sakauye, K. M., Streim, J. E., Kennedy, G. J., Kirwin, P. D., Llorente, M. D., Schultz, S. K., & Srinivasan, S. (2009). AAGP position statement: Disaster preparedness for older Americans: Critical issues for the preservation of mental health. *American Journal of Geriatric Psychiatry*, *17*(11), 916–924.

Schneider, M. (2014). *Introduction to public health*. Burlington, MA: Jones & Barlett Learning.

Sexton, K. R, Franzini, L., Day, R. S., Brewster, A., Vernon, S. W., & Bondi, M. L. (2011). A review of body size and breast cancer risk in Hispanic and African American women. *Cancer*, *117*(23), 5271–5281.

Stolle, M., Sack, P., & Thomasius, R. (2009). Binge drinking in childhood and adolescence: Epidemiology, consequences, and interventions. *Deutsches Ärzteblatt International*, *106*(19), 323–328.

Tang, B. M., Craig, J. C., Eslick, G. D., Seppelt, I., & McLean, A. S. (2009). Use of corticosteroids in acute lung injury and acute respiratory distress syndrome: A systematic review and meta-analysis. *Critical Care Medicine*, *37*(5), 1594–1603.

Toole, M. J., Waldman, R. J., & Zwi, A. B. (2000). Complex humanitarian emergencies. In M. H. Merson, R. E. Black & A. J. Mills (Eds.), *International public health* (1st ed., pp. 439–513). Gaithersburg, MD: Aspen Publishers.

The White House. (2010). Retrieved from http://www.whitehouse.gov/healthreform

U.K. Department of Health. (2013). Retrieved from http://www.dh.gov.uk/en/index.htm

U.K. Department of Health. (2014) . Retrieved from https://www.gov.uk/government/organisations/department-of-health

United Nations. (2013). Retrieved from http://un.org/en

United Nations Children's Fund. (2013). Retrieved from http://www.unicef.org

United Nations High Commissioner for Refugees. (2013). Retrieved from http://www.unhcr.org/cgi-bin/texis/vtx/home

Urban Institute. (2013). *Block grants: Historical overview and lessons learned*. Retrieved from http://www.urban.org/publications/310991.html

U.S. Agency for International Development. (2013). Retrieved from http://www.usaid.gov/our_work/global_health/

U.S. Department of Health and Human Services. (2013a). Retrieved from http://www.hhs.gov/about/

U.S. Department of Health and Human Services. (2013b). *Healthy People 2020*. Retrieved from http://www.healthypeople.gov/hp2020/

U.S. Department of Veterans Affairs Health Benefits. (2014). Retrieved from http://www.va.gov/healthbenefits/online/

Waage, J., Banerji, R., Campbell, O., Chirwa, E., Collender, G., Dieltiens, V.,… Unterhalter, E. (2010). The millennium development goals: A cross-sectoral analysis and principles for goal setting after 2015. *The Lancet*, doi:10.1016/S0140-*6736*(10)61196-8

Wiener, J. M., Tilly, J., Cuellar, A.V. (2003) *Consumer directed home care, Netherlands, England, and Germany*. Retrieved from http://assets.aarp.org/rgcenter/health/2003_12_eu_cd.pdf
WK Kellogg Foundation. (2013). Retrieved from http://wkkf.org
World Bank. (2013). Retrieved from http://www.worldbank.org/
World Health Organization. (2013a). *History of WHO*. Retrieved from http://www.who.int/about/en/
World Health Organization. (2013b). *Child growth standards*. Retrieved from http://www.who.int/childgrowth/en/
World Health Organization. (2013c). *Governance*. Retrieved from http://www.who.int/governance/en/REF
World Health Organization. (2013d). *Millennium declaration*. Retrieved from http://www.wpro.who.int/countries/mdg/

web resources

Please visit thePoint® for up-to-date web resources on this topic.

CHAPTER 3

Health Policy, Politics, and Reform

Anahid Kulwicki and Sabreen A. Darwish

Healing is a matter of time, but it is sometimes also a matter of opportunity.

Hippocrates

chapter highlights

- Healthcare policy and the political process
- Healthcare finance and cost–benefit in relation to health policy
- Access to healthcare and insurance facts in the United States
- Healthcare workforce diversity and its effects on the quality of healthcare
- Nursing's role in shaping healthcare policy
- Quality of care and evaluation
- Information management facts
- Equity in healthcare access
- Ethical consideration in health policy
- Health advocacy and healthcare reform
- Health services research application to healthcare policy

objectives

- Define public health, policy, and politics while identifying the relationships between concepts.
- Explain the effect of politics in healthcare policy.
- Identify the steps of policy-making and understand them comprehensively.
- Apply the process of policy-making to explain daily decisions regarding health and health choices.
- Understand facts regarding the healthcare system, access to care, and insurance issues.
- Identify the basic economic and financial concepts in relation to healthcare services.
- Identify the definition and determinants of quality of care.
- Understand the role of nurses in informing healthcare policies.
- Explain the importance of workforce diversity, and the concept of cultural competency.
- Understand the information management involved in the healthcare system.
- Explain the ethical and legal considerations in the policy-making process.
- Explain the major reforms in the healthcare system in the United States.
- Understand the value of health services research in the healthcare system.

key terms

Cost–benefit: An economic approach or analysis tool used to evaluate the effectiveness of a treatment or intervention. Mathematically speaking, the net economic benefit can be calculated by subtracting the costs for a service from the benefits of this service. If this value is positive, it implies that the benefit from a specific intervention exceeds its cost. An intervention is judged to be unworthy if its cost exceeds the benefits gained from carrying it out.

Cultural competency: The knowledge, skills, attitudes, and behaviors that are learned in order to provide the optimal health service to individuals from a variety of ethnic, racial, and cultural backgrounds.

Economics: The study of how individuals, groups, organizations, and society allocate and utilize finances, personnel, time, and physical space as components of resources. Economic tools and other quantitative financial measures are used as a method of evaluating the existing governmental programs or public policy alternatives.

Equity: As applied to healthcare, the notion that healthcare does not vary in quality because of gender, race, ethnicity, geographic location, or socioeconomic status.

Gross domestic product (GDP): The main economic indicator used to evaluate the degree of economic growth in the United States. It is defined as the final and total output of goods and services produced in one year by labor input within the United States. The figure of GDP is reported quarterly.

Health policy: Policy that has an impact on the health of an individual, a family, a population, or a community and is created by the government, institution(s), or professional association(s).

Policy: Principles that govern an action to achieve a given outcome. Policies are guidelines that direct individuals' behavior toward a specific goal. They are deliberate courses of action chosen by an individual or group to confront problems.

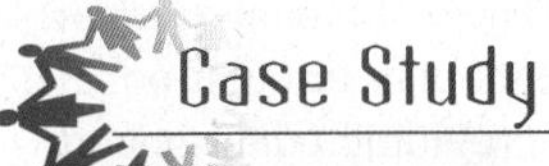

Case Study

References to the case study are found throughout this chapter (look for the case study icon). Readers should keep the case study in mind as they read the chapter.

You are caring for an 8-year-old African-American female patient on the general pediatrics floor. She was transferred from the PICU, where she was admitted for respiratory failure and status asthmaticus. She has a history of "wheezing" but has never been diagnosed with asthma. She receives the majority of her care in the emergency department (ED) and urgent care centers. She has never been on asthma medications. She lives at home with her mother and two siblings. Her mother is employed as a clerk at a hospital and earns $29,942 per year. Her mother's employer provides health insurance. However, she cannot afford to add all three of her children to her health insurance plan. As you read through the chapter, consider the following questions.

Lack of health insurance limits this patient's access to quality asthma care. Barriers to quality care exist even for those who are insured. What are some of those barriers? Are there differences in asthma prevalence by race and income? Are there differences in how children in minority groups access medical care? How do these differences affect asthma care? How are most children in the United States insured? Do you think it is common for a person to have a job yet not have health insurance coverage for their children? What are other health insurance options available to this family? How can you advocate for this child? How can you help ensure improved asthma care for all?

key terms (continued)

Politics: Process of influencing the allocation of scarce resources (financial, human, time, or physical space). Additionally, politics represents how conflicts are expressed and resolved in a society. Politics also may be a factor in deciding who participates or who influences governmental decision-making.

Public health policy: The set of policies (governing principles) that has a health-related mission and has an impact on the general population.

Quality of care: A concept used to evaluate the extent of how efficiently and effectively healthcare systems provide safe patient care at a reasonable cost to people in need. It is the degree to which health services for individuals and populations increase the likelihood of a desired health outcome.

National health expenditure: The total spending in dollars for the costs of healthcare goods and services in a one year period. National health spending is one of the many parts that constitute the GDP, and the growth in health expenditure is usually compared to the GDP growth.

Reform: Means form again; improvement of what is wrong or unsatisfactory. It is for the better, especially as a result of improvement of legal or political abuses or malpractices.

Workforce diversity: The presence of a variety of ethnic, racial, and cultural backgrounds of the workers in a specific area such as the health sector.

Being engaged in the healthcare system, as a healthcare professional providing care, as an administrator, or even as a client, it is important to have a general understanding of how the system works. What are the guiding principles that affect individuals' daily decisions regarding their health and health choices? Who is involved in the process of decision-making? What are the steps that are followed during this process? How can nurses be an active part in the process of developing or changing healthcare policies? Do patients have input into these policies? How does a policy affect an individual's access to healthcare? Is politics different from healthcare policies? Is politics isolated from any ethical or legal considerations? As healthcare providers, how can nurses be involved in reforming the healthcare system? How can they do so using research or evidence in reforming healthcare?

This chapter will answer these questions. Moreover, it will give the reader the opportunity to start thinking about the challenges and problems in the healthcare system in a broad and comprehensive manner, to analyze these problems critically, and to find solutions by considering the political process and policy actions. In other words, the reader will be able to better understand challenges addressed by health policies and understand researcher input that may improve the U.S. healthcare system.

HEALTHCARE POLICY AND THE POLITICAL PROCESS

Porche (2012) defines **policies** as a set of principles that govern an action to achieve a given outcome, or guidelines that direct individuals' behavior toward a specific goal. Kraft and Furlong (2013) define *policy* as decisions characterized by behavioral consistency, which reflect the values and beliefs of two parties, namely, policy-makers and policy followers. Moreover, they claim that *policy* refers to the goals, plans, and specific strategies or programs used in achieving a given outcome. Public policies address community problems and are developed by public or government officials (Anderson, 2006; Kraft & Furlong, 2013). **Public health policy** is defined as the decisions made in regard to the health of individuals and the community (Hewlett, Bleich, Cox, & Hoover, 2009).

Health policies are those policies that have an impact on the health of an individual, a family, and a population or community and are created within the government, institution, or professional association (Porche, 2012). Health policies are crafted to alleviate issues of health or healthcare (Mason, Leavitt, & Chaffee, 2012). "States use health policies to specify requirements for licensure in the health professions, to set criteria for eligibility for Medicaid, and to mandate immunization requirements for public university students" (Mason et al., 2012, p. 3). In addition to the state level, policies can be separated into local or national. An example of a state-level policy would be a school board crafting a policy in regard to contraceptive care, whereas an example of national policies would include laws and regulations in regard to access to care and reimbursement for advanced practice nurses (Anderson, 2006; Leavitt, 2009). Moreover, three main components of the public health policy were reported consistently in the literature, namely, (1) health-related decisions guided by the stated laws written by legislators, (2) rules and regulations designed to operate the health-related activities and programs, and (3) the judicial decisions related to health, which involve both federal and state governments (Porche, 2012).

PRACTICE POINT

As was previously discussed, politics cannot be separated from the process of policy-making. There are many different ways to describe the impact of politics. First, **politics** is concerned with the exercising of power and decision-making in a society (Kraft & Furlong, 2013). Second, politics is usually studied as the process of formulating and adopting policies along with focusing on the role of both governmental institutions and the public.

Involving Politics

Politics is the process of influencing the allocation of resources needed to enable policies, and involves the strategies needed to achieve the desired goals (Mason et al., 2012). Politics also reflects how conflicts and problems are expressed and resolved in the context of society, and involves choices and influences based on power dynamics (Leavitt, 2009). Additionally, politics helps in answering questions regarding who participates or who influences governmental decision-making, and who benefits or who does not. Therefore, it is impossible to understand health policy or any type of public policy without considering political factors, which affect every level of policy formulation.

Kraft and Furlong (2013) discussed many reasons to involve the government in the policy-making process. These reasons usually reflect political, moral, ethical, and economical responsibilities. The two latter reasons will be discussed later in this chapter. In reference to a political issue, the government should be interested in problems that affect a specific group or a whole population. This interest usually takes the form of legislations that provide substantial solutions for the health problems that threaten the safety of the citizens and/or their environment. There are many examples of the positive role that governments play through policies and legislations—to name a few: providing equal opportunity through universal provision of education, healthcare, and often, housing and nutrition programs (Grogan, 2012).

Solutions can be achieved by working at either the federal or the state level. However, Rice, Roseanau, Unruh, and Barnes (2013) explain that there is little agreement between the two major U.S. political parties (Democrats and Republicans) when it comes to how, when, to whom, and what kind of healthcare should be provided, and who should pay for it. Rice et al. (2013) concluded that in attempting to answer healthcare-related critical questions, disagreement between the two major political parties can create difficulty in finding solutions to the problems of the society, and hence to policies, including those of healthcare. Consequently, this can influence access to healthcare and the possibility of improving the **quality of care** provided (Rice et al., 2013).

Additionally, politics interferes with every aspect of healthcare in the United States (Morone, Litman, & Robins, 2008). Accordingly, U.S. politicians are interested in making decisions for the society that can be enforced by rules, laws, and regulations. Politics is sometimes perceived as a negative and unfavorable way to deal with social issues. However, politics provides the power needed to influence critical decisions regarding the allocation and distribution of resources in a society. Moreover, political actions are the tools used by politicians and the official representatives of the citizenry to shape decisions.

In summary, Mason et al. (2012) identified three common themes, which can be extracted from the different definitions of politics. First, the power of influence implies there is room for shaping desired outcomes by having an impact on the decisions made by governments, communities, or associations. Second, the most critical process for politics is to make decisions regarding the distribution and allocation of resources. Third, resources vary and include financial, human (personnel), time, and physical space. These resources are often found to be scarce. It is argued by Brownson, Fielding, and Maylahn (2009) that the availability of adequate resources can strongly affect the decision-making process. Accordingly, resources are believed to affect the desired outcome and outputs from a given policy.

While the previous themes of governmental power, decision-making, and resources are vital in understanding the political role in decision-making, it is crucial to acknowledge the fact that healthcare professionals have political skills and active roles in healthcare leadership. As highlighted by Mason et al. (2012), those skills are as follows:

1. Having social skills and the ability to understand, interpret, and represent one's own and others' behaviors
2. Having the ability, qualifications, and power to influence others and make changes
3. Networking ability to develop, connect, and use different social networks
4. Having a high level of integrity, sincerity, and genuineness

Politics is interconnected with policy-making because politicians can control and determine the allocation of resources. To put health policies in place, politicians must agree on the most prevalent health issues and on how to address these issues, as they greatly impact the nation's health (Porche, 2012). To best serve their patients and best understand their field, nurses and other healthcare professionals are encouraged to be involved in the political process and in the development of health policies. For these reasons, it is important for healthcare professionals to understand some of the important terms and concepts that are related to healthcare politics and policy.

Putting policies in place is a process. Policy-making takes a great deal of effort, time, and commitment. Porche (2012) laid out a dynamic series of events that take place in the policy-making process (Fig. 3.1).

Setting an agenda: the crucial basic phase where the problem of common interest is identified for a specific community or a group. Three factors were found to play a role in this stage and were identified by Porche (2012): (1) the significance of the problem, (2) the political support for addressing the problem, and (3) the ability to perceive the viability of proposed alternative solutions for the problem. For example, tobacco use is a major contributor to morbidity and mortality, which threaten populations globally. Consequently, governments play a critical role in encouraging or discouraging smoking behavior through different policies along with the role of nurses as political advocates for achieving health improvements.

Policy formulation: the stage in which the possible and available alternative policies are identified and a specific policy is selected. Continuing the discussion on tobacco use, all possible and effective policy measures, such as smoke-free indoor air laws, tobacco industry–regulating policies at all levels—state, local, and national—should be addressed and discussed to select the most effective policy in reducing the prevalence of smoking.

Policy adoption: the process of selecting the policy that should gain support, power, and directions for the legislators. In order to proceed in the process of fighting tobacco use, all proposed policies need to gain support from stakeholders at the different levels starting from state level and ending at the local level, along with nursing role in reflecting and directing the selection of policies.

Policy implementation: the stage in which the actual carrying out of the policy takes place by using the available human and financial resources. In terms of tobacco use, in this stage, real application of the anti-tobacco policies takes place where representatives at different political levels, including nurses, start to enhance and reinforce the application of smoke-free environments using all possible resources. Law enforcement is critical in this stage.

Policy assessment: evaluation of the implemented policy in terms of being compliant or congruent with the statutory requirements, and whether it really serves the goal of solving the problem. Because the goal of anti-tobacco policies and regulations is to prevent tobacco-related diseases through reducing smoking prevalence, the success of these policies can be evaluated mainly by assessing the extent of achieving these goals, along with consideration for cost containment and effectiveness of policy-based interventions.

Policy modification: depending on the prior step, the policy can be maintained, changed, or eliminated, according to its level of appropriateness. In this step, a decision takes place either to maintain working according to the anti-tobacco policies or to modify them and replace them, considering other alternative policies, where the process of policy-making repeats itself.

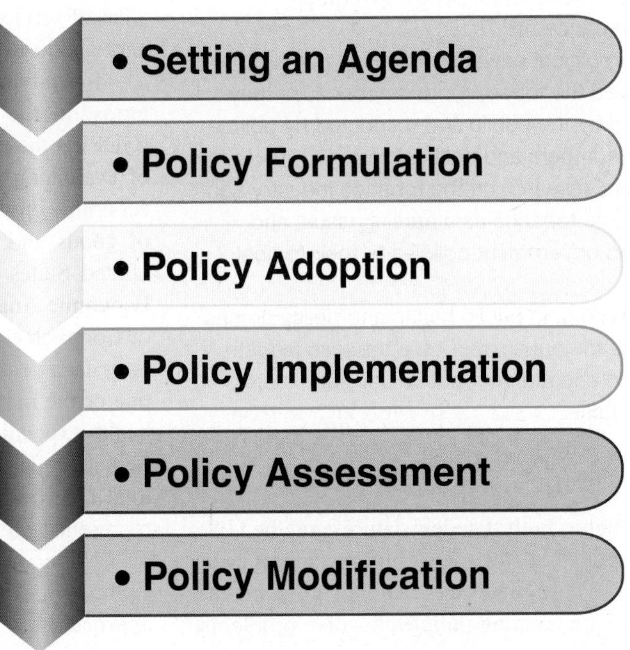

figure 3.1 Policy cycle.

EVIDENCE FOR PRACTICE

Tobacco use is a major global contributor to illness, which is projected to kill more than one billion people during this century if present trends continue (World Health Organization [WHO], 2008). Nurses are increasingly engaged in community- and policy-level activities to improve health and prevent disease and disability, by conducting research, which focuses on the tobacco industry and related policies. Malone (2009) conducted a literature review on research studies conducted by nurses on the tobacco industry. The epidemic of tobacco and its health consequences result primarily from the industry enhancing the addictiveness of cigarettes, marketing them aggressively to vulnerable groups, hiding or manipulating knowledge about the products' harmfulness, and undermining public health efforts. The efforts of the tobacco industry to perpetuate the idea that smoking is solely a problem of individual behavior still creates barriers to understanding the larger social and political context within which individuals use and attempt to quit tobacco.

Nurses have been among the researchers worldwide who are studying tobacco industry activities and their role in policy and public health. Much of the nursing research to date focuses on four broad areas: (1) the tobacco industry's influence on policy, (2) its strategic responses to public health efforts, (3) its targeting of marginalized groups, and (4) its influence on research processes and outcomes.

Recommendations:

1. Traditional tobacco prevention and cessation efforts must accompany understanding of the role of the tobacco industry in shaping and contextualizing counseling programs.
2. Nurses need to be prepared to intervene as clinicians, community health proponents, policy advocates, researchers, and educators.
3. Nurses have the political power to influence perceptions about tobacco and the tobacco industry because they are highly trusted by the public and respected by policymakers for their numbers and political savvy.
4. Innovative archival research on the tobacco industry can help nurses reframe tobacco as a nursing issue, and link practices and government policies to their clinical practice.
5. Finally, nurses working in public health and policy arenas can help educate the public about the tobacco industry's ongoing efforts to encourage tobacco use, with major health consequences.

In the United States, both state legislatures and the U.S. Congress are responsible for determining appropriate healthcare policies. These state and national government representatives work on creating policies to solve problems affecting a specific group, a geographic area, or the entire population (Kraft & Furlong, 2013). These policies usually take the form of legislation, which provides substantial solutions for the health problems that threaten the health and safety of the citizens. This legislation can be achieved by working at either the federal or the state level. Although state legislatures and members of Congress can work collaboratively to solve problems and distribute resources, there is often much delay and disagreement between major political parties such as the Democratic and Republican parties (Rice et al., 2013). Because of such disagreements, it is difficult to build an effective collaboration in healthcare policy-making, and this can influence the individual's access to care and the possibility of improving the quality of care (Rice et al., 2013).

HEALTHCARE FINANCES AND COST–BENEFIT

Economics is the study of how individuals, groups, organizations, and society allocate and utilize resources (Porche, 2012). Consequently, it is critical to apply economic tools and various quantitative measures as a method of evaluating the existing governmental programs or public policy alternatives (Kraft & Furlong, 2013). Politics and economics interact at either the microeconomics level, which concerns the allocation of resources at the individual decision-making level, or the macroeconomic level (Porche, 2012). Economically speaking, any process of allocating fiscal resources is usually directed to best meet the human need and to improve their well-being (Kraft & Furlong, 2013). In the health context, for example, if the government spends more on medical visits than is needed to benefit its populations, this will lead to a decrease in resources available for other services such as education. Hence, the role of economics is extremely vital to enforce appropriate, effective, and efficient allocation of resources on the different areas of services provided for populations, and to achieve balance and justice reinforced by policies, laws, and regulation.

In studying health finance, it is critical to understand key terms. In the United States, the **gross domestic product** (GDP) is the main economic indicator used in the processes of evaluating policies in terms of their contribution to the economic growth. GDP is defined as the final and total output of goods and services produced by labor input within the United States in one year as determined by the Bureau of Economic Analysis (USBEA, 2013) in the U.S. Department of Commerce. The GDP figure is reported and released quarterly each year by the BEA. **National health expenditure** is one of the many components of the GDP, and the growth in health expenditure is usually compared to the GDP. As highlighted by Hartman, Martin, Benson, and Catlin (2013), the total U.S. healthcare spending reached $2.7 trillion in 2011, representing a 3.9% increase from 2010.

There is a set of economic analysis processes used to evaluate economic policy outcomes. The cost–benefit approach has been considered pivotal in evaluating the effectiveness of a treatment or intervention (Sorbello, 2008).

It is the most frequently used approach because it serves to illustrate both the strengths and weaknesses of a given policy (Kraft & Furlong, 2013). Consequently, economists were found to be continuously interested in finding answers for the questions such as *who gets the benefit and who bears the burden of a policy? How should we measure the values, costs, and benefits of a specific policy?* In this type of analysis, economists are concerned with measuring the relative costs (in actual monetary value) against the benefits (both monetary and quality-of-life value) of a given program or any aspect of healthcare (Sorbello, 2008).

PRACTICE POINT

Mathematically speaking, the net economic benefit can be calculated by subtracting the costs from the benefits. If this value was positive, this implies that the benefit from a specific intervention exceeds its cost, so a decision is made to adopt such intervention. In contrast, an intervention is judged to be ineffective in terms of its costs if its cost exceeds the benefits gained from carrying it out. Although this process seems to be easily accomplished, it is a complicated process when it involves the healthcare system.

As described by Sorbello (2008), cost can be direct, in which the patient as a consumer is supposed to pay these costs at the time of service. For example, direct costs can be supplies or medications. Indirect costs are costs that are not assigned directly to the patient, but are related to the provision of services at the organizational level. Similarly, health benefits or outcomes can vary from simple, direct benefits to more complicated benefits. Outcomes should be objective, measurable, and representative of the treatment interventions, which is not an easy task to calculate, especially if the outcomes need to be expressed in dollars (Kraft & Furlong, 2013). However, less tangible outcomes, such as prevention of long-term suffering or disability, and quality of life, are more difficult to quantify. On the other hand, hospital days or dollars spent in a specific health service, for example, can be easily measured and evaluated.

There is one important process, which should not be ignored in **cost–benefit** analysis. Economists in their analysis of the costs and benefits must involve the perspectives of the different healthcare components that are participants in providing or receiving this service. Morone et al. (2008) explains there are many perspectives that should be considered and satisfied when providing a specific healthcare service. In other words, it is crucial for economists to consider the costs of the people who are counted, the type of costs involved, and the type of outcome that is desired. From the patients' perspective, patients usually are more interested in their own costs and benefits. In other words, they are interested in their own expenses and out-of-pocket (OOP) payment. Patients are also concerned about other types of costs, such as their psychological costs, suffering, and pain, which are difficult to quantify yet have long-lasting negative effects. Regarding the payer's perspective, the actual payment for the service is usually what matters. The providers are usually concerned with the actual and direct cost of providing a service. Finally, it is critical to consider the societal concern, which usually includes all direct and indirect costs and benefits at the broader community level regardless of who benefits from or pays for the services. However, using the cost–benefit analysis as the only criterion in evaluating the efficiency and effectiveness of a policy is restricted by the fact that cost and benefits are not distributed evenly among individuals, consumers, or providers (Kraft & Furlong, 2013). In other words, the economic analysis should involve the distribution of costs and accessibility of the benefits in their analysis. Equity will be discussed in the following sections.

In summary, health spending is a product of services and the cost associated with those services. When a policy is evaluated for its effectiveness, there is an interest in keeping the cost of a specific health program within reason. Moreover, there is consideration for the overall costs and benefits of the existing program, in the event a more efficient and effective service is identified.

ACCESS TO CARE AND HEALTH INSURANCE

Before discussing access to care and health insurance, it is important first to understand the nature of the U.S. healthcare system, which is a unique system of independent and collaborative powers of both federal and state governments (Morone et al., 2008).

EVIDENCE FOR PRACTICE

In a large exploratory study comparing the U.S. healthcare system with those of other countries, Rice et al. (2013), highlighted the following facts about the U.S. system:

1. Private sector stakeholders play a stronger role in the U.S. healthcare system than in other high-income countries.
2. The major federal government health insurance programs Medicare and Medicaid were established in the mid-1960s.
3. Medicare provides coverage for seniors and the disabled, while Medicaid covers healthcare services for qualified low-income individuals (also covering limited care needs for qualifying seniors).
4. Public sources constitute 48% of healthcare expenditures in the United States.
5. Private third-party payers pay 40%, with the remaining 12% being paid OOP by individuals.
6. Only a minority (30%) of the U.S. population is covered by the public financing system, mainly through

(continued on page 52)

Medicare and Medicaid. Currently, 54% of Americans receive their coverage from private health insurance, with most (36%) privately insured individuals obtaining coverage through an employer.

7. One in six Americans is uninsured and over 17% of the population are without health insurance.
8. Even among those with coverage, high OOP costs can be a barrier to receiving timely care and medications. Many others face high OOP expenses due to underinsurance.
9. The underinsured include elderly individuals who receive Medicare but cannot afford supplemental insurance or the OOP expenses associated with Medicare.
10. Those covered by Medicaid have insurance, but may experience problems accessing primary care due to their inability to find a private physician who accepts Medicaid patients. OOP expenses may also be a factor in inability to access care.
11. Patients in rural areas may find it impossible to get to primary care facilities. Medical costs are responsible for over 60% of personal bankruptcies in the country.

Concerns regarding racial/ethnic minorities, low-income groups, and uninsured groups overlap because of similar barriers these populations experience in accessing healthcare and obtaining quality services. Many low-income and uninsured populations are from diverse racial and ethnic minorities. National programs for improvement of access to quality healthcare for low-income and ethnic and racial minorities in United States are often addressed simultaneously. There are, of course, special issues within each population that need to be taken into consideration. Frequently, community health agencies play an important role in providing access to healthcare for underserved groups, especially those who are uninsured and with low income.

HEALTHCARE WORKFORCE DIVERSITY

The United States is a home for individuals from different ethnic backgrounds. Although the numbers are not growing as rapidly as the immigration of ethnically diverse populations, the United States has had an increase in the number of healthcare professionals immigrating to the United States from other countries (Morone, Litman, & Robins, 2008). Moreover, the shortage of healthcare providers in the United States and the higher pay of health professionals in high-income countries have led to the migration of healthcare professionals from developing countries. In addition to the higher wages in United States, the opportunities for advancement are an incentive for health professionals' migration to the United States. However, the migration of healthcare professionals from other countries has created some challenges to the U.S. healthcare workforce, mainly because of the inability to balance the needs of the low-income and/or developing countries who cannot compete with U.S. wages, the right of nurses to migrate for the sake of their personal needs, and the needs of healthcare professionals and workers in both the country of origin and the receiving countries.

EVIDENCE FOR PRACTICE

In the National Survey of Registered Nurses, the U.S. Department of Health and Human Services, Office of Health Resource Service Administration (HRSA) reported that the number of registered nurses (RNs) from minority or ethnic backgrounds has grown from 119,512 in 1980 to 513,860 in 2008 (USDHHS, HRSA, 2010). The survey also revealed that while only 65.6% of the U.S. population is White and non-Hispanic, 83.3% of RNs were White and non-Hispanic. RNs from Asian backgrounds were overrepresented, with 5.8%, compared to 4.5% of the U.S population. This imbalance of RNs from Asian ethnicity in the United States can be explained by the fact that United States recruits RNs primarily from the Philippines and/or India. In terms of languages spoken, most RNs spoke only English. Only 5.1% spoke Spanish, 3.6% spoke Filipino languages, 1.1% spoke French, and less than 1% spoke Chinese, German, or other languages. There are 165,539 RNs living in the United States who were educated in other countries. This number accounts for 5.6% of the entire licensed RNs workforce in the United States. Figure 3.2 shows the distribution of countries of origin of internationally educated RNs in the United States.

As the minority populations increase at rapid rates, there is an increasing need for a **diverse workforce** of healthcare providers who can provide culturally competent care.

Transcultural and **cultural competency** are very important terms to be addressed when addressing needs of diverse multicultural populations. Leininger (1999) defined transcultural nursing as a formal area of study, research, and practice focused on culturally based care beliefs, values, and practices to help achieving the goal of well-being, and prevention of disability in a culturally congruent and beneficial ways. Because culture is focused on the holistic way of human beings, religion, kinship, education, technology, language, environmental context, and worldviews are all considered, and need to be integrated into nursing care (Leininger, 1999).

As defined by Bearskin (2011), *cultural competence* refers to the skills, knowledge, and attitudes required to provide care with consideration for various cultural differences. HRSA (2010) acknowledged that the most dominant determinant in RN cultural competency is the language used to communicate with the population being served by the RN. Simialrily, a number of critical cultural competency interventions were proposed by Betancourt, Green, Carrillo, and Ananeh-Firempong (2003), which included minority recruitment into health professions,

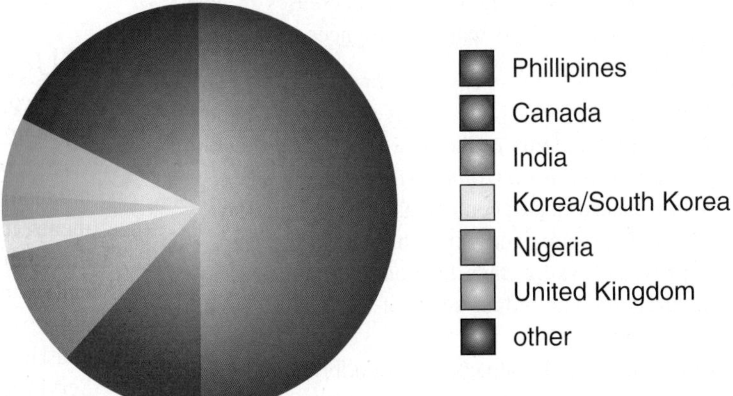

figure 3.2 2008 National Sample Survey of Registered Nurses. (From U.S. Department of Health and Human Services, Office of Health Resources and Services Administration. (2010). *Findings from the 2008 national survey of registered nurses (chap 8, p. 192).* Retrieved from http://www.hrsa.gov/about/news/pressreleases/2010/100922nursingworkforce.html)

development of interpreter services and language-appropriate health educational materials, and education of healthcare providers on cross-cultural issues in order to best address health and healthcare disparities.

It is also clear that cultural competency is required for achieving the aims of public health in the context of the client, individual, family, or community. Because healthcare professionals are involved in the process of policy formation, it is logical that the less diverse the work force is, the less appropriate and effective the healthcare policies will be for disadvantaged populations. Healthcare professionals continue to report that marginalized (minority) populations experience greater healthcare needs and receive lower quality of care (Bearskin, 2011). As a result, the U.S. Health and Human Services and the Office of HRSA have taken bold steps to increase workforce diversity by providing funds for programs that address this important issue.

Despite all national efforts to improve the diversity of the healthcare workforce, Hunt (2007) reported that managing a racially and culturally diverse workforce is complex and challenging for nurses. He stated, "There are no ready-made tools to show them how to do so…[A]chieving effective management of a culturally diverse workforce comes from an intrinsic motivation to develop the cultural competence to engage with them." (Hunt, 2007, p. 2252).

NURSING'S ROLE IN SHAPING HEALTHCARE POLICY

As highlighted by Porche (2012), nurses and other healthcare professionals have a rich preparation in knowledge, and personal, and professional experiences within the healthcare system that enable them to influence the development of health policy. Nurses are experts as clinicians, educators, researchers, and administrators and need to perceive that they have power in public policy. Nurses' expertise should be translated into the policy arena where they can utilize their knowledge, their perspective, their experiences, and their skills to be change agents for public policy at all levels of government (Leavitt, 2009). Nurses also represent communities and speak as trusted and respected professionals, evidenced by the annual surveys, which indicate that the public continues to rate RNs as the most trusted profession on the basis of their professional honesty and ethical standards (Spring, 2013).

In addition to their clinical expertise, nurses are being sought out to serve in a variety of leadership positions and develop policy recommendations related to a wide range of healthcare policy issues (Dean, 2011). Accordingly, policy-makers need to hear from nurses because they are in the best position to communicate citizens' problems, represent them, and be advocates for their rights and healthcare needs.

Nurses continuously demonstrate evidence-based care, and they share decision-making with patients and families, resulting in improved quality and reduced cost. Nurses have also been active in the development of public policies as members of the legislative and executive branches at national and state levels (Dean, 2011; Leavitt, 2009). Nurses as educators have a particular responsibility to teach students how to translate issues into health policy. They can serve as both role models and teachers where there is a need to include political competence and citizenship in the education system (Carnegie & Kiger, 2009). Because nursing roles are interrelated, educators can work with researchers, and administrators can work with clinicians to share their perspectives and diverse knowledge to make tremendous contributions to policy development (Hewlett et al., 2009).

In the research arena, all nurses engaged in research usually consider the policy implications of their work, and even if the researcher is not the advocate, those who are engaged in workplace and public policy can use research studies to propose policy alternatives and enhance policy modification accordingly (Leavitt, 2009). Nurses have many milestones in policy development, as addressed by Leavitt (2009), through their practice and research, which have contributed to (1) quality outcomes, (2) decreases in cost, (3) expanded access, and (4) major differences to the health of the nation. To name a few:

1. The magnet process, which was originated by the American Academy of Nursing (AAN), has been integrated into the Joint Commission's standards.
2. School-based health centers, as demonstrated by advanced practice and public health nurses, can improve access for underinsured and uninsured children and can reduce some of the disparities in healthcare access.
3. Linda Aiken and colleagues' groundbreaking research on nurse staffing and the effect on patient outcomes has resulted in laws and regulations that created guidelines for staffing criteria of hospital units in many states (Aiken, Xue, Clarke, & Sloane, 2006).

In terms of policy-making, nurses have the basic vital evidence either supporting or opposing a policy. They can be members of an organization or a group, which enables them to be involved in agenda setting and the introduction of a specific problem into the national agenda, identifying the goals and tools, and advocating and disseminating health issues through the media (Milstead, 2008). Myers (2010) pointed out that the American Nurses Association (ANA), which serves as the strongest nursing organization in the United States, has been engaged in helping its members play a significant role in advocating for their patients by closing the gaps in the healthcare access for patients and their families through testifying at congressional hearings, healthcare summits, and regional forums. Nurses can also serve on a personal and professional level in the process of political election to be instrumental in serving the nation's health (Porche, 2012). ANA works with coalitions and advocates for nurses to serve as members of governing boards in each state, to advance the role of and recognition of nurses, to prevent potential declines in quality, and to communicate with the Congress in the prevention of harmful changes in Medicare actions (Dean, 2011; Spring, 2013). However, Myers (2010) fears that too many nurses have been absent from policy deliberations despite ANA's calls for advocacy, minimizing the collective power of nurses in the legislative process. As indicated by Milstead (2008), nurses are experts who can address both the rational shaping of the policy, and the emotional aspects of the process, and should feel morally obligated to advocate for their patients.

In summary, the nursing profession is one of the largest sectors of the healthcare industry in the United States and has a rich history as a unique profession, with its own values, ethics, respect, integrity, and responsibility. Nurses' opportunities for contributions to healthcare policies are unlimited. As Fyffe (2009) pointed out, there is a need for greater coordination of action to ensure that nursing is represented and actively supported in influencing and shaping health and healthcare policy.

QUALITY OF CARE

The healthcare system in the United States is very complex, made up of diverse patients, healthcare providers, and healthcare payers. With patients, providers, and payers constantly interacting for varying reasons and in a variety of environments, it is extremely difficult to evaluate the complexities of the quality of care for the U.S. population. Despite the difficulties in evaluating the quality of healthcare, much is being done by the federal government, U.S. Department of Health and Human Services, the Center for Medicaid and Medicare Services, private institutions and organizations to examine the healthcare system in terms of quality, access, and cost. Mason et al. (2012) report several examples as to how efficiently and effectively healthcare systems provide safe patient care to people in need at a reasonable price and with equal distribution. Mason et al. (2012) references The Institute of Medicine report (2001), which lists the following dimensions of healthcare systems that should be considered when quality, cost, and access are examined:

1. Safety: avoiding injury and harm from care that is meant to aid patients
2. Effectiveness: assuring that "evidence-based" care is actually delivered, by avoiding overuse of medically unproven care, and underuse of medically sound care
3. Patient-centeredness: involving patients thoroughly in the decision-making process about their care, thereby respecting their culture, social circumstances, and needs
4. Timeliness: avoiding unwanted delays in treatment
5. Equality: closing racial, ethnic, gender, and socioeconomic gaps in care and outcomes

Quality of care is defined by the Institute of Medicine (2001) as the degree to which health services for individuals and populations increase the likelihood of desired outcomes, and are consistent with current knowledge. In demonstrating quality care, patients receive correct assessment and diagnosis, are given appropriate and effective treatment, and are monitored closely. The Commonwealth Fund Commission on a High Performance Health System (Mongan, 2006) states the following six drivers of high performance in healthcare systems: (1) patient information is available to patients and all providers through health record systems; (2) patient care is coordinated among multiple providers and managed accurately; (3) all providers have accountability to each other and to the patient and collaborate to reliably deliver high-quality care; (4) patients have access to appropriate and culturally competent care and information; (5) accountability is present for the care of patients; and (6) the system is working to improve the quality of healthcare.

EVIDENCE FOR PRACTICE

On the global level, quality of care is tracked based on attainment, equity of health outcomes across populations, and in terms of fairness of financial contributions. Additional measures include how investments in public health impact social objectives like reducing health disparities, improving health, and providing responsive services that best assist patients (Murray & Frenk, 2010). On the basis of these measures, the quality of care of the U.S. healthcare system was ranked 37th among the industrialized countries by the World Health Report 2000, *Health Systems: Improving Performance* (WHO, 2000). The World Health Organization (WHO) (2009) explained that Americans spend a significant amount for health insurance but receive little in terms of quality of care. For example, in 2006, Americans were ranked number 1 in terms of healthcare spending but were ranked very poorly in infant mortality (39th), adult female mortality (42nd), and life expectancy (36th). Comparative evidence has shown that the U.S. healthcare system is gradually slipping behind less-industrialized countries each year, and improvements in healthcare has been slower when compared to other industrialized or developed countries (Murray & Frenk, 2010). Furthermore, the U.S. healthcare system has been deemed broken by many people, with skyrocketing costs and plummeting coverage for middle-class and low-income families (Jacobs & Skocpol, 2012). To overcome this downward spiraling of quality and access to healthcare, it is essential that the United States better evaluate performance of healthcare and compare results with other countries (Murray & Frenk, 2010).

INFORMATION MANAGEMENT

As highlighted earlier in this chapter, information management of the U.S. healthcare system must be improved to advance the overall delivery of healthcare. Healthcare experts, the Congress, and the Obama administration overwhelmingly agree that implementing electronic information systems could greatly improve the efficiency of the healthcare system and the health of Americans (Blumenthal, 2009). In such efforts, U.S. policy-makers have adopted the health information technology (HIT), labeled HITECH in law, a high priority through the American Recovery and Reinvestment Act (ARRA) (Jha, DesRoches, Kralovec, and Joshi 2010). The ARRA offers significant incentives through Medicare and Medicaid funding to physicians and hospitals if they adopt effective HIT and electronic health records (EHRs). Through ARRA, $17 billion in financial aid was used as incentive for doctors and hospitals to utilize EHRs. Physicians who adopt and use EHRs meaningfully, can be reimbursed for their services up to $44,000 over 5 years. Similarly, hospitals that effectively utilize EHRs earn an incentive of $2 million through a one-time bonus. Furthermore, HITECH provides $2 billion in assistance to put systems in place and offers grants that assist providers' installation of EHRs. Physicians and hospitals refusing to implement EHRs face penalties, such as losing a percentage of their Medicare fees (Blumenthal, 2009; Fonkych & Taylor, 2005). HITECH "provisions created an essential foundation for restructuring healthcare delivery and for achieving the key goals of improving healthcare quality; reducing costs; and increasing access through better methods of storing, analyzing, and sharing health information" (Buntin, Jain, & Blumenthal, 2010, p.1).

Despite incentives offered through the ARRA, the majority of medical records in the United States are still stored on paper (IOM, 2012). An estimated 17% of doctors and 10% of hospitals utilize EHRs. Barriers to adopting systems include, but are not limited to, high costs, technical challenges in implementing and maintaining the system, and concerns of privacy (Blumenthal, 2009; Fonkych & Taylor, 2005). Providers who have not implemented an EHR system have difficulty in coordinating care, evaluating quality of care, and avoiding medical errors.

EQUITY IN HEALTHCARE ACCESS AND QUALITY

Equity is defined by the Institute of Medicine (2001) as healthcare that does not vary in quality because of gender, race, ethnicity, geographic location, or socioeconomic status. The U.S. Department of Research and Quality (U.S. Department of Health and Human Services, Agency for Healthcare Research and Quality, 2007) indicates that significant healthcare disparities exist and the progress in eliminating health disparities is limited. Eliminating health disparities has become a priority of the Obama administration as the U.S. population becomes increasingly diverse (Mason et al., 2012). Furthermore, insurance rates are rising more rapidly than wages, and middle- and low-income families and employers are having great difficulty affording insurance (Institute of Medicine, 2003).

Schoen, Davis, How, and Schoenbaum (2006) developed a scoring system of equity in the U.S. healthcare system, and have concluded that there are major inequities in health, quality, access, and efficiency. More researchers have reported that individuals living in low-income communities are associated with significant disparities. For example, researchers found that Whites, Blacks, and Hispanics with cancer, who lived in high-poverty geographic areas, experienced a systematically lower 5-year survival rate. In addition to disparities due to poverty, there were disparities found in terms of race and ethnicity as well. In terms of getting effective and appropriate care, White patients were more likely to receive timely, patient-centered care than African-Americans and Hispanics. Additionally, African-Americans and Hispanics had higher mortality rates than Whites. Researchers went further to explain, "Black, Hispanic, low-income and uninsured patients are less likely to have primary care providers to coordinate care, are more likely to experience test results/records delays and duplication, are more likely to go to the emergency departments when other care was not available, and more likely to be admitted to the hospital for potentially preventable conditions, than white, higher-income, and insured patients" (Schoen et al., 2006, p. 472). In summary, because there is an abundance of evidence indicating increased disparities in healthcare delivery when assessed by income, insurance, and race, it is imperative that appropriate efforts continue in reducing health disparities in the United States.

Because of such vast disparities in healthcare access and quality, President Obama has made healthcare his issue. Obama's presidential campaign promised affordable and adequate healthcare for all Americans, and in March of 2010, President Obama signed the Patient Protection and Affordable Care Act (ACA) into law (Jacobs & Skocpol, 2010). Efforts put forth through the ACA, such as the Community Transformation Grant (CTG) program, provide funds to organizations, health centers, and initiatives with goals of creating healthy communities and assisting vulnerable populations (Hennrikus, 2013). The CTG grants fund programs that promote tobacco-free living, physical activity, healthy eating, services to prevent and control high blood pressure and high cholesterol, social and emotional wellness, and health and safe environments. It is estimated the CTG program will affect 40% of the U.S. population with health promotion and disease prevention efforts, with vast opportunities for nurses to get involved.

Achieving health equity is, and must continue to be a priority for this country to move forward. It is critical that nurses stay involved and offer their expertise. Nurses' involvement with research, advocacy, community outreach, and policy efforts will help underserved populations receive the care that they need and deserve (Mason et al., 2012).

ETHICAL CONSIDERATION

Individuals have their own moral "lens" through which they view the world, and where they can judge what is right and wrong. No matter what nurses' personal moral views may be, employers establish policies regarding appropriate behavior in the workplace and these expectations are known as nurses' "organizational ethics," which are defined as expectations about the "right" behaviors for healthcare professionals in the work setting (Indiana State Nurse Association, 2013). An example of such ethics is the standards provided in the Code of Ethics for Nurses (American Nurses Association [ANA], 2010). The ANA Code of Ethics with Interpretive Statements (ANA, 2001) has addressed nine main nursing ethical principles:

1. Compassion and respect for the dignity, worth, and uniqueness of every individual
2. Primary commitment to patient (individual, family, group, or community)
3. Promotion and advocacy to protect patients' health, safety, and rights
4. Responsibility and accountability for individual nursing practice by appropriate delegation of tasks to provide optimum care
5. Responsibility to preserve integrity and safety, maintain competence, and continue personal/professional growth
6. Participation in establishing, maintaining, and improving healthcare environments and conditions
7. Participation in advancement of the profession through contributions to practice, education, administration, and research
8. Collaboration with other healthcare professionals and the public in promoting community, national, and international efforts to meet health needs
9. Responsibility for articulating values, maintaining integrity, and shaping social policy

Healthcare workers encounter complicated ethical issues in their practice, however, and nursing particularly is involved in infinite judgments regarding the morality and immorality of their actions or interventions toward their patient. This has resulted mainly from the radical progress in biomedical sciences and the technological piece of the healthcare, which affects the lives of billions of people throughout the world. Consequently, nurses are required to hold the responsibility of both safeguarding the values of their society and developing their own moral framework for dealing with the moral dilemmas. The role of the nurse, as a member of the interprofessional care team, is to identify potentially ethics-related situations, work with others to address these issues, and provide holistic support for patients, families, and colleagues. Thus, in order to guide the process of moral decision-making, for example, the Ohio Nurses Association (2013) developed a process to guide RNs in the process of working through ethical ambiguity or dilemmas, which includes the following:

1. Identifying the existence of the ethical dilemma (conflict in values)
2. Gathering and analyzing relevant information—including identification of stakeholders, interdisciplinary team members, and other sources of relevant information
3. Clarifying personal values and moral position, including the moral perspectives of other "players" in the scenario
4. Determining options, based on careful consideration of alternatives' benefits and risks
5. Making responsible decisions about actions or recommendations, in collaboration with other interested parties
6. Evaluating the impact of the action and outcomes.

EVIDENCE FOR PRACTICE

Technological and societal changes have created both ethical issues and new requirements for nursing education in the context of ethics (Ramos et al., 2013). However, there is reporting of a lack of ethical confidence among newly graduated nurses (Park, 2009). In a qualitative case study conducted by Ramos et al. (2013), the participants, who were nursing teachers, expressed that reflection on nurses' ethics education should take place and that this reflection should not be limited to discussing content or instructional methods but should be extended to engage the student in critical analysis of moral scenarios. Students should actively pursue the building of their professional values (Ramos et al., 2013).

As concluded by Park (2009), nursing students have not been prepared to encounter ethical dilemmas in their nursing practice. The author also proposes the need for pragmatic teaching methods as a solution. In other words, planned ethics content in the nursing curriculum is necessary to improve moral sensitivity and moral reasoning of students (Park et al., 2012). Students must also be prepared to adopt different ways of thinking, to be open to the ethical issues by utilizing their absolute professional values and their professional code of ethics, and to apply them by using the lenses of their clients in order to achieve moral sensitivity.

HEALTH ADVOCACY AND HEALTHCARE REFORM

The concept of advocacy is both a morally, and professionally important duty in nursing practice. This implies that nurses are required to help the patient make decisions according to their personal beliefs and values, and to protect the patient's right through communicating with other healthcare providers (Leavitt, 2009; Park, 2009). Advocacy is a requirement for nurses. Advocacy is collaborating with colleagues, or other healthcare professionals, and engaging in conversations with decision-makers (Carnegie & Kiger, 2009). Because nurses have the position of communicating, interacting with, and caring for individuals and communities, it is extremely important that they listen to the experiences of individuals, and offer them the opportunity to address, and contribute to policies that affect their health (Carnegie & Kiger, 2009).

Healthcare systems are dynamic. Overall, they have been changing worldwide for decades, particularly in the United States. O'Grady (2009) made it clear that as communities are engaging in complex and dynamic health **reforms**, nurses are required to develop the language for a healthcare delivery system that is patient centered, longitudinal and sustainable, relationship based, and evidence based. RNs are increasingly being recognized as leaders in transforming the healthcare system to meet the demand for illness prevention, wellness, and primary care services, with special attention to improving quality and managing costs (Dean, 2011).

President Barack Obama signed into law the Patient Protection and ACA on Tuesday, March 23, 2010, expressing, "The bill I am signing will set in motion reforms that generations of Americans have fought for and marched for and hungered to see; the core principle that everybody should have some basic security when it comes to healthcare," (Jacobs & Skocpol, 2010, p. 1). Prior to 2010, efforts were made for universal health insurance coverage dating back to the 1910s, during the presidential campaign of Theodore Roosevelt. Even though such coverage has been established in all other industrial or industrializing nations, healthcare reformers have faced daunting political opposition in attempts at universal coverage in the United States (Jacobs & Skocpol, 2010). Although halted on universal coverage, in the 1960s, reformers were able to establish Medicare to help cover costs for the elderly and Medicaid to help cover costs for low-income individuals. After incredible efforts that lasted over a decade, the ACA of 2010 rightfully became a monumental milestone.

Through the Patient Protection and ACA, the Obama administration's goals in improving the overall healthcare system and the quality of care include, but are not limited to, expanding health insurance coverage, shifting the focus of the healthcare delivery system from treatment to prevention, and reducing the costs and improving the efficiency of healthcare (Hellerstedt, 2013). The ACA was put in place to improve the quality, access, and affordability of healthcare. "The American College of Physicians hopes that the legislation will advance key priorities on coverage, workforce, and payment and delivery system reform" (Doherty, 2010, p. 679).

Additionally, the ACA expanded healthcare access to children (Oberg, 2013). Through the ACA, youth are allowed to remain on their parents' healthcare plan to the age of 26, insurers are no longer allowed to exclude children from coverage because of pre-existing conditions, and access has been expanded through state-based health insurance exchanges for uninsured families (Oberg, 2013). Medicaid and Children's Health Insurance Program (CHIP) provisions have been administered through the ACA with goals of enrolling uninsured children. Such reforms will work to insure vulnerable childhood populations like children aging out of the foster care system (Oberg, 2013). Furthermore, reforms in healthcare for children will help reduce the cost of healthcare for families so that more children will be covered.

The U.S. Department of Health and Human Services, Agency for Healthcare Research and Quality (2012) reported that although indicators have shown that quality of healthcare for the general population is improving, quality of care is still not up to par for minorities and low-income communities. Furthermore, although the ACA has made strides for healthcare for all, an estimated 49 million Americans are still without health insurance (Hellerstedt, 2013).

EVIDENCE FOR PRACTICE

In measuring the equity of healthcare and in working on reform, it is also important to review the effects of social determinants of health, which include early childhood education, employment opportunities, treatment of women, the effects of poverty, and individual empowerment on humans' health status and life expectancy (Wilensky & Satcher, 2009). The WHO's Commission on the Social Determinants of Health was created in 2005 to focus on the social determinants as a means of reducing health disparities (Wilensky & Satcher, 2009). The WHO's Commission on the Social Determinants of Health explains that healthcare reform must focus on nutrition, education, reducing substance abuse, and access to care. In the United States, the following four components have been, or need to be, addressed in the following ways:

1. Nutrition: Over the years, the federal government has put in place systems which work to improve nutrition for low-income communities such as the federal food stamp program and the Special Supplemental Nutrition Program for Women, Infants, and Children (WIC and SNAP)
2. Education: Programs like the No Child Left behind Act and the Action for Healthy Kids Program work to help low-income students by providing additional academic support, and proper nutrition and physical activity.
3. Reducing substance use: Because many children are born with medical challenges due to their mother's substance abuse, more aggressive intervention must be put in place to help pregnant women deal with substance abuse. Programs for mothers should be free to those who cannot afford them.
4. Access to care: Medicaid and the State Children's Health Insurance Program (SCHIP) were put in place to ensure low-income children were provided with appropriate care. Although such systems were put in place, many children who are eligible are not enrolled. More aggressive outreach campaigns must be established to educate families on the care they are eligible to receive.

HEALTH SERVICES RESEARCH

Although the ACA has been passed and efforts to improve healthcare are increasing, the quality of healthcare and services has not improved significantly. Researchers, healthcare professionals, and other advocacy groups continue to push for an improved healthcare system in the United States, with appropriate health services for all, and to do this, the healthcare system needs an accelerated transformation, which brings about quality care, proper information management, insurance for all, and equity to access (Dougherty & Conway, 2008). Dougherty and Conway (2008) proposed a model to transform the U.S. healthcare system, explaining how to deliver high-quality healthcare. Their plan outlines the activities, participants, investments, and fundamental shifts required to create and sustain a high-quality, patient-focused, healthcare system. Porter (2009) lists the following steps that must take place to improve the U.S. healthcare system:

1. Measurement and dissemination of health outcomes must be shared.
2. The delivery of prevention, wellness, screening, and routine health maintenance services must be fundamentally restructured.
3. Care delivery must be reorganized around medical conditions.
4. A reimbursement program for healthcare professionals as incentives to achieve better outcomes for patients should be introduced.
5. Providers must compete for patients, based on the quality of the care provided.
6. All providers must establish electronic medical records.
7. Patients' involvement in their health must improve and incentives for patient involvement should be considered.

Porter explains that all items must happen simultaneously to build an effective healthcare system. Conway and Clancy (2009), in speaking of improving the healthcare system on the front line, emphasize the importance of improving measurements, adopting information technology, accelerating the production and use of requisite research, improving collaborations and networks, and increasing clinical training. Taking such action, Conway and Clancy claim, may significantly improve clinician engagement and patient care.

CONCLUSION

At this moment in history, healthcare is at the forefront of the public's attention. As the president's platform, as the most popular topic on the news and radio, and as an issue greatly impacting individuals and employers, healthcare is an important topic, which is receiving attention from everyone. During this significant moment in the history of healthcare, nurses play an important role in providing quality healthcare, tracking patient progress, and being active members in healthcare reform. It is important that nurses are knowledgeable about health policy, politics, and healthcare reform because it will improve their understanding about where they work, the patients they care for, and government efforts that will impact both.

key concepts

- Because policy development and formulation is concerned with providing population-based interventions which will greatly impact the nation's health, the political process has a close relationship with health policies.
- Making health policy takes great time, effort, and commitment. This process is presented as a dynamic and cyclic series of six events, namely, agenda setting, policy formulation, policy adoption, policy implementation, policy assessment, and finally policy modification.
- When a policy is evaluated for its effectiveness, there is an interest in keeping the cost of a specific health program within reason, and it is critical to consider the overall costs and benefits of an existing program when a more efficient and effective service is identified and adopted.
- The U.S. healthcare system is a unique system of both independent and collaborative power and action by both federal and state governments.
- Healthcare issues of racial and ethnic minorities, low-income individuals, and the uninsured overlap. Community health agencies play an important role in providing access to healthcare for those who are underserved, whether from uninsured or low-income communities.
- The U.S. has an increasing healthcare professional immigration from other countries.
- There is an increasing need for a diverse workforce of healthcare providers who can provide culturally competent care for the growing minority population. The less diverse the workforce, the less representative and influential will be the impact of the healthcare providers on healthcare policies.
- Nursing has a rich history as a unique profession, with its own values, ethics, respect, integrity and responsibility. Nurses' contributions to the policies are unlimited; there is a need for greater coordination of action to ensure that nursing is actively supported and involved in influencing and shaping health and healthcare policy.
- It is extremely difficult to evaluate the complexities of the quality of care for the U.S. population.
- U.S. policy-makers have made the adoption of health information technology a priority so that health records can be kept electronically, assisting patients, providers, and insurers.
- Because of the vast disparities in healthcare access and quality, President Obama has made healthcare his top priority, promising affordable and adequate healthcare insurance for all Americans.
- Healthcare is closely linked with ethical issues and decisions and has implications for patients, providers, and healthcare leaders.
- Although most politicians agree a reform must take place, many cannot agree on what the change should look like. Consequently, healthcare reform in the United States has been a long political battle for quite some time.
- Research continues to be an influencing power by documenting the need for an accelerated reform in order to achieve quality care, proper information management, and insurance for all, and equity to access.

critical thinking questions

1. Consider that you are a nurse working with a patient who is from a different cultural and ethnic background from your own. Explain how you could translate the concept of cultural competency into practice. Do not forget ethical considerations.
2. After reading this chapter, you have learned about the six stages of the process of policy. Give at least one example showing how nurses can be engaged in each stage of the process.
3. You have heard a lot about President Obama's Patient Protection and Affordable Care Act.
   a. What are the major milestones of this act that represent the healthcare reform?
   b. Explain how this act helps in delivering better healthcare services.
   c. Explain why this act has been considered as a long political battle for a period of time.
4. You have learned about the health information technology (HIT) in this chapter:
   a. Give a few examples for the application of HIT in the clinical practice.
   b. Explain the main barriers of using HIT in the healthcare system.
   c. How has the American Recovery and Reinvestment Act (ARRA) reinforced the use of HIT in different healthcare settings?
5. How can research help in improving the U.S. healthcare system?
6. After carefully reading about Rice's exploratory study regarding the U.S. healthcare system, summarize in a short paragraph the major problems in this system.

references

Aiken, L. H., Xue, Y., Clarke, S. P., & Sloane, D. M. (2006). Supplemental nurse staffing in hospitals and quality of care. *The Journal of Nursing Administration, 37*(7–8), 335–342.

American Nurses Association. (2001). *The code of ethics for nurses with interpretive statements*. Washington, DC: Nursesbooks.org.

American Nurses Association. (2010). *Guide to the code of ethics for nurses: Interpretation and application*. Silver Spring, MD: Nursesbooks.org.

Anderson, J. (Ed.). (2006). *Public policymaking: An introduction*. Boston, MA: Houghton Mifflin.

Bearskin, R. (2011). A critical lens on culture in nursing practice. *Nursing Ethics, 18*(4), 548–559.

Betancourt, J. R., Green, A. R., Carrillo, J. E., & Ananeh-Firempong, II, O. (2003). Defining cultural competence: A practical framework for addressing racial/ethnic disparities in health and healthcare. *Public Health Reports, 118*(4), 293.

Blumenthal, D. (2009). Stimulating the adoption of health information technology. *New England Journal of Medicine, 360*(15), 1477–1479.

Brownson, R., Fielding, F., & Maylahn, C. (2009). Evidence-based public health: A fundamental concept for public health. *Annual Review of Public Health, 30*(1), 313–315.

Buntin, M. B., Jain, S. H., & Blumenthal, D. (2010). Health information technology: Laying the infrastructure for national health reform. *Health Affairs, 29*(6), 1214–1219.

Carnegie, E., & Kiger, A. (2009). Being and doing politics: An outdated model or 21st century reality? *Journal of Advanced Nursing, 65*(9), 1976–1984. doi:10.1111/j.1365-2648.2009.05084.x

Conway, P., & Clancy, C. (2009). Transformation of healthcare at the front line. *JAMA, 301*(7), 763–765.

Dean, E. (2011). Reforms forum fails to insist on nurse role in commissioning. *Nursing Standard*, 25(41), 9–9. Retrieved from http://ezproxy.lib.umb.edu/login?url=http://search.ebscohost.com/login.aspx?direct=true&db=ccm&AN=2011184887&site=ehost-live

Doherty, R. B. (2010). The certitudes and uncertainties of healthcare reform. *Annals of Internal Medicine, 152*(10), 679–682.

Dougherty, D., & Conway, P. (2008). The "3T's" road map to transform US healthcare: The "How" of high-quality care. *JAMA, 299*(19), 2319–2321.

Fonkych, K., & Taylor, R. (2005). *The state and pattern of health information technology adoption*. Santa Monica, CA: Rand Corporation.

Fyffe, T. (2009). Nursing shaping and influencing health and social care policy. *Journal of Nursing Management, 17*(6), 698–706.

Grogan, C. M. (2012). The murky relationship between ideology and the role of government in health policy. *Journal of Health Politics, Policy & Law, 37*(3), 361–364. doi:10.1215/03616878-1573058

Hartman, M., Martin, A., Benson, J., & Catlin, A. (2013). National health spending in 2011: Overall growth remains low, but some payers and services show signs of acceleration. *Health Affairs, 32*(1), 87–99.

Hellerstedt, W. L. (2013). *The Affordable Care Act: What are its goals and do we need it?* Retrieved from http://www.epi.umn.edu/mch/wp-content/uploads/2013/09/ACA-Overview.pdf

Hennrikus, D. (2013). The Community Transformation Grant Program. *Healthy Generations*, 16. Retrieved from http://www.epi.umn.edu/mch/wpcontent/uploads/2012/05/HG_Fall20132.pdf#page=18

Hewlett, P. O., Bleich, M., Cox, M. F., & Hoover, K. W. (2009). Changing times: The role of academe in health reform. *Journal of Professional Nursing, 25*(6), 322–328. doi:10.1016/j.profnurs.2009.10.008

Hunt, B. (2007). Managing equality and cultural diversity in the health workforce. *Journal of Clincial Nursing, 16*(12), 2252–2259.

Indiana State Nurse Association. (2013). *Public policy platform 2013*. Retrieved from http://www.IndianaNurses.org

Institute of Medicine. (2001). *Crossing the quality chasm: A new health system for the 21st century*. Washington, DC: National Academies Press.

Institute of Medicine. (2003). *Hidden Costs, Value Lost: Uninsurance in America*. Washington, DC: National Academies Press.

Institute of Medicine. (2012). *Best care at lower cost: The path to continuously learning healthcare in America*. Retrieved from http://www.iom.edu/~/media/Files/Report%20Files/2012/Best-Care/Best%20Care%20at%20Lower%20Cost_Recs.pdf

Jacobs, L. R., & Skocpol, T. (2012). *Health care reform and American politics: What everyone needs to know*. New York, NY: Oxford University Press.

Jha, A., DesRoches, C., Kralovec, P., & Joshi, M. (2010). A progress report on electronic health records in US hospitals. *Health Affairs, 29*(10), 1951–1957.

Kraft, M., & Furlong, S. (Ed.). (2013). *Public policy, politics, analysis and alternatives*. California: Sage Publication.

Leavitt, J. K. (2009). Leaders in health policy: A critical role for nursing. *Nursing Outlook, 57*(2), 73–77. doi:10.1016/j.outlook.2009.01.007

Leininger, M. M. (1999). What is transcultural nursing and culturally competent care? *Journal of Transcultural Nursing, 10*(1), 9.

Malone, R. E. (2009). The social and political context of the tobacco epidemic: Nursing research and scholarship on the tobacco industry. *Annual Review of Nursing Research, 27*, 63–90. doi:10.1891/0739-6686.27.63

Mason, D., Leavitt, J., & Chaffee, M. (2012). *Policy and politics in nursing and healthcare* (6th ed.). Missouri, MO: Elsevier Sauders.

Milstead, J. (Ed.). (2008). *Health policy and politics: A nurse's guide*. Boston, MA: Jones and Bartlett Publishers.

Mongan, J. (2006). *Commonwealth fund commission framework for a high performance health system for the United States*. Retrieved from http://www.commonwealthfund.org/publications/fund-reports

Morone, J., Litman, T., & Robins, L. (Eds.). (2008). *Health politics and policy*. New York, NY: Delmar.

Murray, C., & Frenk, J. (2010). Ranking 37th—measuring the performance of the US healthcare system. *New England Journal of Medicine, 362*(2), 98–99.

Myers, C. (2010). Being there: Policy making and nurses. *Tennessee Nurse, 73*(3), 9–10.

Oberg, C. N. (2013). The Affordable Care Act and children. *Healthy Generations*, 26. Retrieved from http://www.epi.umn.edu/mch/wp-content/uploads/2013/09/ACA-Children.pdf

O'Grady, E. (2009). Health policy and politics. Acknowledge the paradoxes and advance the profession. *Nursing Economics, 27*(5), 337. Retrieved from http://web.a.ebscohost.com.ezproxy.lib.umb.edu/ehost/pdfviewer/pdfviewer?sid=32b50468-22d0-47c3-ab5e-26cb8e67064b%40sessionmgr4001&vid=1&hid=4214

Ohio Nurses Association. (2013). What do I do now? Ethical dilemmas in nursing and healthcare. *ISNA Bulletin, 39*(2), 5–12. Retrieved from http://ezproxy.lib.umb.edu/login?url=http://search.ebscohost.com/login.aspx?direct=true&db=ccm&AN=2012007375&site=ehost-live

Park, M. (2009). The legal basis of nursing ethics education. *Journal of Nursing Law, 13*(4), 106–113. doi:10.1891/1073-7472.13.4.106

Park, M., Kjervik, D., Crandell, J., & Oermann, M. (2012). The relationship of ethics education to moral sensitivity and moral reasoning skills of nursing student. *Nursing Ethics, 19* (4), 568–580.

Porche, D. (2012). *Health policy, application for nurses and other healthcare professionals*. Canada: Jones and Bartlett Learning.

Porter, M. (2009). A strategy for healthcare reform—toward a value-based system. *New England Journal of Medicine, 361*(2), 109–112.

Ramos, F., de Pires, D., Brehmer, L., Gelbcke, F., Schmoeller, S., & Lorenzetti, J. (2013). The discourse of ethics in nursing education: Experience and reflection of Brazilian teachers-case study. *Nurse Education Today, 33*, 1124–1129.

Rice, T., Roseanau, P., Unruh, L., & Barnes, A. (2013). United States of America: Health system review. *Health Systems in Transition, 15*(3), 1–467.

Schoen, C., Davis, K., How, S., & Schoenbaum, S. C. (2006). US health system performance: A national scorecard. *Health Affairs, 25*(6), w457–w475.

Sorbello, B. (2008). Finance: It's not a dirty word. *American Nurse Today, 3*(8), 32–35.

Spring, S. (2013). Nurses earn highest ranking ever, remain most ethical of professions in poll: ANA urges policymakers to listen to nurses on healthcare policy, funding. *New Mexico Nurse*, 58(1), 13–13. Retrieved from http://web.b.ebscohost.com/ehost/pdfviewer/pdfviewer?vid=4&sid=52b6a79f-1e1b-434c-93d3-65b4aa885ea8%40session

U.S. Bureau of Economic Analysis. (2013). *GDP and the economy: Survey of current business*. Retrieved from http://www.bea.gov

U.S. Department of Health and Human Services, Agency for Healthcare Research and Quality. (2007). *National healthcare disparities report*.

U.S. Department of Health and Human Services, Office of Health Resources and Services Administration. (2010). *Findings from the 2008 national survey of registered nurses (chap 8, p. 192)*. Retrieved from http://www.hrsa.gov/about/news/pressreleases/2010/100922nursingworkforce.html.

U.S. Department of Health and Human Services, Agency for Healthcare Research and Quality. (2012). *2012 National healthcare disparities report*. Retrieved from http://www.ahrq.gov/research/findings/nhqrdr/nhdr12/

Wilensky, G., & Satcher, D. (2009). Don't forget about the social determinants of health. *Health Affairs, 28*(2), w194–w198.

World Health Organization. (2008). *World health report 2008*. Geneva, Switzerland: Author.

World Health Organization. (2009). WHO statistical information system (WHOSIS). *World Health Statistics 2009*.

http://www.advocacyoncall.org/docs/CaseStudy_HealthDisparities.pdf

web resources

Please visit thePoint® for up-to-date web resources on this topic.

CHAPTER 4

Health and the Global Environment

Joyce Pulcini and Lynda Tyer-Viola

It's immoral that people in Africa die like flies of diseases that no one dies of in the United States. And the more disease there is, the more political unrest there will be....

Bill Clinton

Of all the forms of inequality, injustice in health care is the most shocking and inhumane.

Martin Luther King Jr.

chapter highlights

- Definitions of global health and global burden of disease
- Indicators of health
- Health and human rights
- Factors that affect health globally
- Framework for improving world health
- Millennium Development Goals

objectives

- Identify critical determinants of global health and the intersection between health and the environment.
- Describe the approaches to achieving maximum health outcomes in poor countries and in affluent countries.
- Define the concept of burden of disease, how it is measured, and the ultimate effect on a population's health.
- Identify and explain the effects of political, economic, and sociodemographic risk factors on health.
- Describe the purpose of the Millennium Development Goals and their future impact on improving global health.
- Describe key indicators of health that can be measured or used as benchmarks to examine the health outcomes of a population.

key terms

Demographic and epidemiologic transitions: Progressive improvement in health from a global perspective.

Determinants of health: Factors that affect outcomes of health status, such as physical environment, social environment, health behaviors, and individual health, as well as broader factors such as access to health services and overall health policies and interventions.

Global burden of disease: The importance of risks to health and their outcomes in different demographic populations and social settings.

Global health: Health issues and concerns that transcend national boundaries and may best be addressed by cooperative actions and solutions. People may also define health differently on the basis of their culture, role in life, or even what is possible in their environment.

Health: A state of complete physical, mental, and social well-being, not merely the absence of disease or infirmity.

Health indicators: Descriptors of the general health of a nation that are grouped into four categories: morbidity and mortality, risk factors, health service coverage, and health system resources.

Noncommunicable disease: Diseases that afflict a population which are chronic in nature and may be due to lifestyle changes, sometimes as a result of modernization of societies. Examples include cardiovascular diseases, cancers, diabetes, obesity, and chronic respiratory diseases.

Primary Healthcare: "Essential health care based on practical, scientifically sound and socially acceptable methods and technology, made universally accessible to individuals and families in the community. It is through their full participation and at a cost that the community and the country can afford to maintain at every stage of their development in the spirit of self-reliance and self-determination" (World Health Organization, 1978).

Right to health: The right of all people to enjoy the highest attainable standard of physical and mental health.

Risk factors: Personal habits and behaviors, environmental conditions, or inborn or inherited characteristics that are known to affect a health-related condition which could be alleviated or managed.

Public health: Ensuring that every person in the community has a standard of living adequate for the maintenance of health. This involves the science and art of preventing disease, prolonging life, and promoting physical health and efficiency through organized community efforts. This includes the sanitation of the environment, the control of community infections, the education of the individual in principles of personal hygiene, the organization of medical and nursing services for the early diagnosis and preventive treatment of disease, and the development of the necessary social machinery.

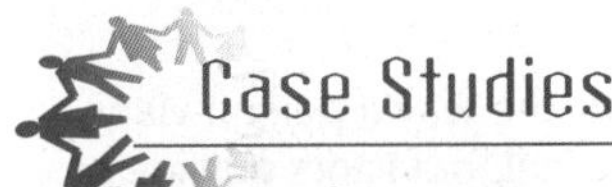

Case Studies

References to case studies are found throughout this chapter (look for the case study icon). Readers should keep the case studies in mind as they read the chapter.

CASE 1

Mumeka, a 19-year-old pregnant woman, has traveled to her mother's village in Zambia to give birth to her third child. She has had no prenatal care in the village where she lives. Mumeka realizes that this pregnancy is different from the others; so she seeks care from a community health worker (CHW). The health worker advises Mumeka to get a sonogram. However, Mumeka lacks access to these services. Now she is in labor. Her aunt and mother are attending to her in their home. The labor is progressing slowly, and there is bleeding present, yet the family is hesitant to seek the help of the CHW as they have seen this many times during childbirth and believe it is normal. Mumeka continues to labor and bleed and the health worker is called. Mumeka is examined, and it appears the infant is out of position and she may have a problem with the placement of her placenta. Arrangements are made to transfer Mumeka to the district hospital 60 km from her home. The CHW travels with her. Upon arrival, the infant's heart rate is slow and the bleeding increases. Finally, the baby is delivered stillborn with a placental abruption.

CASE 2

James, who is 95 years, has failing hearing, reduced vision, and a blood pressure of 140/88 mmHg, for which he takes no medications. He lives in a small village in Asia surrounded by his children and grandchildren. His family has little money but does own a small, sustainable farm. Members of the community view James as a wise elder. Is he healthy, given his age, and just subject to normal processes of aging? Or does he have disease, and can he be categorized as sick?

What does it mean to be healthy in a global context? A person's health status is highly dependent on his or her living environment, social norms, gender, and age, specifically in low-resourced settings. Access to and utilization of healthcare is highly dependent on where you live in the world and the community definition of health. In addition, the health of individuals depends on the social and economic conditions in which they live. Many factors affect the health and well-being of individuals. This chapter explores an array of factors that affect health and the global environment.

DEFINITIONS OF HEALTH

The World Health Organization (WHO) in 1947 defined **health** as "a state of complete physical, mental, and social well-being and not merely the absence of disease or infirmity" (WHO, 1947, p. 1). The WHO definition of health encompasses the highest level of health, involving self-actualization or reaching one's true potential. The more specific concepts of public health or global health may be important when the concept of an individual's health is considered. All are interrelated in a global context.

Primary healthcare is a broad term that is defined as "essential health care based on practical, scientifically sound and socially acceptable methods and technology, made universally accessible to individuals and families in the community. It is through their full participation and at a cost that the community and the country can afford to maintain at every stage of their development in the spirit of self-reliance and self-determination" (WHO, 1978). This term, coined at the Alma Alta conference of 1978, encompasses a goal of healthcare for all and a broad thinking about the healthcare that all individuals deserve.

Winslow (1920), often called the father of public health, defined **public health** as "the science and art of preventing disease, prolonging life, and promoting physical health and efficiency through organized community efforts for the sanitation of the environment, the control of community infections, the education of the individual in principles of personal hygiene, the organization of medical and nursing service for the early diagnosis and preventive treatment of disease, and the development of the social machinery which will ensure to every individual in the community a standard of living adequate for the maintenance of health" (p. 23). The identification of nursing in 1923 as a key participant in the social construct of health recognized the contribution that nurses could make to promote health and well-being of all humankind.

Halbert Dunn (1959) also placed health on a continuum, ranging from premature death to wellness to high-level wellness, which can be equated to self-actualization. In this model, the environment (i.e., factors outside of the person) plays a major role in health (Fig. 4.1)

In her classic work, Smith (1981) identified four models of health:

1. *Clinical model:* elimination of disease or symptoms. For example, some people feel that they are well when they have no symptoms or diagnosed diseases and would not classify themselves as sick otherwise.

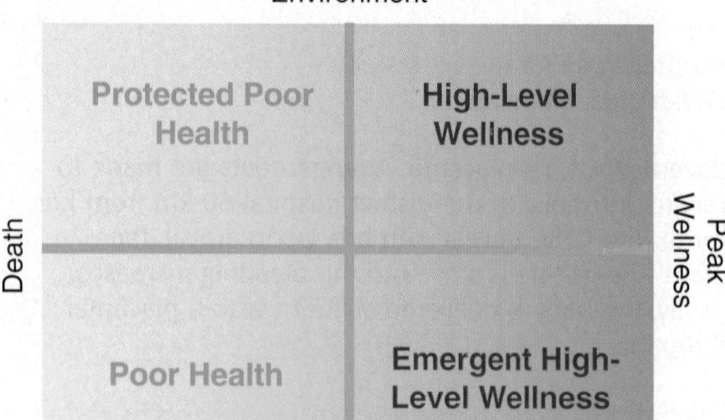

figure 4.1 The health grid: Its axes and quadrants. (From Dunn, H. [1959]. High-level wellness for man and society. *American Journal of Public Health*, *49*[6], 788.)

2. *Role-performance model:* health that involves a match between people and social roles. For example, some people, even if they have symptoms of disease, would classify themselves as unhealthy only if they could not fulfill their roles in life, such as mother or worker.
3. *Adaptive model:* health that involves adaptation to the environment. For example, some people consider health to be determined by their ability to adapt in the face of adversity or disease.
4. *Eudaimonistic model:* health that is the actualization or realization of human potential. In this model, for example, people would consider themselves to be healthy only if they are functioning not only physically but also emotionally and socially. The WHO definition of health (1947) actually strives for this level of health.

Global health was defined by the Institute of Medicine (IOM, 1997) as "health problems, issues, and concerns that transcend national boundaries and may best be addressed by cooperative actions and solutions" (p. 2). Each of Smith's four models can be viewed within the definition of the IOM and includes people's definition of health based on their culture, role in life, and environmental resources. A person's definition of health actually determines how and when he or she seeks assistance from the healthcare system and may ultimately affect the outcome of long-term health.

The evolution of the definition of health clearly shows an increased appreciation of the biophysical, sociodemographic, and environmental influences on individual, family, and community health. Health is a complex concept that can be conceptualized in many ways, from a broad to narrow disease-specific view. Further, complexity comes into play when the social, political, and economic conditions are factored into the equation.

In each of the case studies, the way a person views health and the environment, or factors outside of the individual, affects whether a person is viewed as healthy or unhealthy and at risk. The way women view health, and in particular pregnancy, can affect birth outcomes. The environment is the key in each case and ultimately changes the context in which the health or illness conditions are played out. When the dimensions of political and economic instability are added to the equation, it is possible to further understand the complexity of the concept of health and its determinants.

CRITICAL GLOBAL HEALTH CONCEPTS

Determinants of Health

Global health is a dynamic concept with many components. In examining this concept, several factors need to be considered. Skolnik (2008) identifies the key **determinants of health**, which encompass the following domains: (1) physical environment, (2) social environment, (3) health behaviors, and (4) individual health, in the context of the broader factors of access to health services, as well as health policies and interventions.

Demographic and Epidemiologic Transitions

When it comes to global health, there is no "them"... only "us."

Global Health Council

Demographic and epidemiologic transitions refer to the improvement in global health indicators (WHO, 2013a). Changes in these demographic indicators signify improvement in health over time. In addition, specific indicators provide a unique picture of community health: life expectancy and morbidity and mortality, selected infectious diseases, health service coverage, health systems expenditure and inequities, and demographic and socioeconomic statistics (WHO, 2014a). They include many factors, such as age, gender, socioeconomic status, and disease prevalence, and taken together, they can portray the health of a community and identify areas in need of intervention.

In addition, these indicators are tracked by the demographic and health survey (DHS) program, which is conducted at the household level to evaluate the health of a nation (United States Agency for International Development, 2014). Every 3 to 4 years, a DHS is conducted to describe the health of a country and define specific demographics that then can be compared to each other to determine specific transitions. These transitions are used as a measure of improvement of health of a nation.

Demographic transitions may progress from low to high levels:

1. High fertility and high mortality, resulting in slow population growth
2. Improvement in hygiene and nutrition, leading to a decreased burden of infectious disease
3. Mortality declines, and later fertility declines
4. Relative proportion of elderly population increases

Epidemiologic transitions include the following:

1. High and fluctuating mortality, due to poor health, epidemics, and famine
2. Progressive declines in mortality, as epidemics become less frequent
3. Further decline in mortality, increasing life expectancy, and predominance of noncommunicable diseases

As a country becomes more developed, levels of demographic or epidemiologic transitions shift upward. For example, as mortality rates decrease, more attention can be paid to increase the quality of life of all citizens, including the elderly. As the number of children involved in agrarian functions decreases and as the need for formal education increases, fertility rates tend to decrease. As more members of a population are educated, indicators of health, such as higher life expectancy and lower mortality rates, improve.

Global Burden of Disease

Every observer of human misery among the poor reports that disease plays the leading role.

Fisher (1909, p. 124)

Global burden of disease (GBD) is the risks to health and health outcomes in different demographic populations and social settings related to a set of diseases and injuries. There are 18 components of GBD that are interrelated and create the changing picture of burden related to specific communities (Institute for Health Metrics and Evaluation, 2014). The largest study of these indicators was published in 2012, revealing that women and men are living longer but spending more time living with illness and injury (Horton, 2013). The collection of specific data related to risk factors, health indicators, and health outcomes of 291 diseases and injuries in 20 regions of the world determines the GBD (Murray et al., 2012). Indicators include lower respiratory tract infection, diarrheal disease, malaria, and protein energy malnutrition as well as road injuries and pollution (Institute of Health Metrics and Evaluation, 2014). Changes in these factors can identify areas of improvement or the need for intervention. The goal of analyzing these data is to summarize measures of a population's health and to identify risk factors that affect health. The concept of disease burden first occurred in the early 1980s, when the World Bank signaled the need for a better understanding of disease control and mortality to set priorities for resource-limited countries. In an era of unmet needs, economic divisions, and health inequalities, the need for rigorous data for decision-making despite limited resources was, and still is, vital (Lopez, Mathers, Ezzati, Jamison, & Murray, 2006). Examining the effects of health indicators and risk factors on the overall health of a community can guide healthcare planners and providers in choosing those services and interventions that can improve health.

As health policy-makers and governments better understood the impact of disease, the need for an analysis of the circumstances grew. In 1990, the World Bank commissioned the first study on disease burden (World Bank, 1993). In 1994, Jamison and Jardel (1994) incorporated the concept of cost–benefit analysis related to disease burden to assist countries in decision-making about health interventions. In 1996, Murray and Lopez edited a publication called *The Global Burden of Disease*. All of these reports later influenced the ongoing analysis by the World Bank, as well as work by the Fogarty International Center at the U.S. National Institutes of Health and the Bill and Melinda Gates Foundation, to form the Disease Control Priorities Project (DCPP). The project's purpose has been "to review, generate, and disseminate information that contributes to the scientific evidence base for improving population health in developing countries" (DCPP, 2008, p. 1). Current data compare disease and injury from 1990 through 2010, providing a longitudinal assessment of effects of disease and injury on specific populations (Murray et al., 2012). The goal of integrating the process of collecting health data, evidence that supports the use of these data, and its application to the critical needs related to disease outcomes is paramount to improving global health.

Noncommunicable Diseases

In 2012, the World Health Assembly endorsed an important new health goal: to reduce avoidable mortality from **noncommunicable diseases** by 25% by 2025 (the 25 by 25 goal) (Alleyne et al., 2013). The Global Burden of Disease and Risk Factors study report built upon earlier versions, providing a comprehensive analysis of the health of the world's population, including health indicators for disease outcomes, as well as risk factors and monitoring strategies that can be used for program planning to improve health outcomes (Murray et al., 2012).

Four common behavioral risk factors that occur globally, to some degree (tobacco use, excessive alcohol consumption, poor diet, and lack of physical activity), are associated with four health deviations (cardiovascular diseases, cancers, chronic pulmonary diseases, and diabetes) that account for about 80% of deaths from noncommunicable diseases (Hunter & Reddy, 2013, p. 1336). Clearly, the leading causes of mortality and burden of disease worldwide are now shifting from communicable to noncommunicable diseases. This change represents an

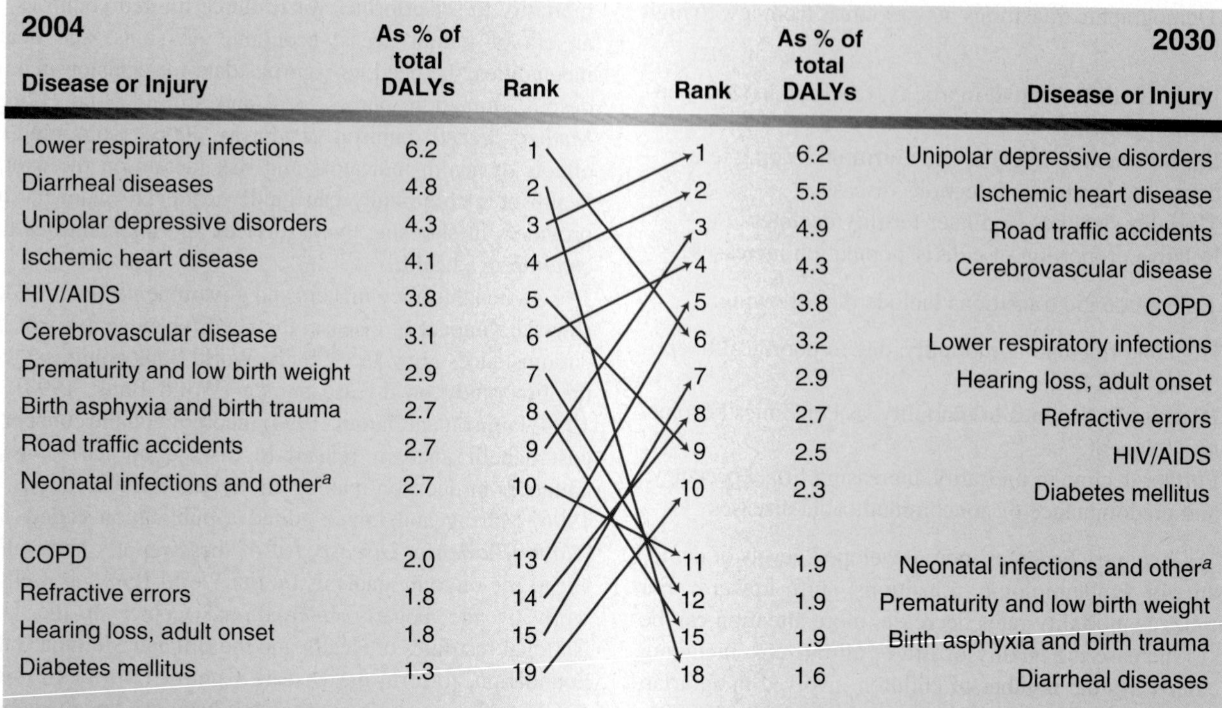

2004
Disease or Injury
As % of total DALYs
Rank
Lower respiratory infections 6.2 1
Diarrheal diseases 4.8 2
Unipolar depressive disorders 4.3 3
Ischemic heart disease 4.1 4
HIV/AIDS 3.8 5
Cerebrovascular disease 3.1 6
Prematurity and low birth weight 2.9 7
Birth asphyxia and birth trauma 2.7 8
Road traffic accidents 2.7 9
Neonatal infections and other[a] 2.7 10
COPD 2.0 13
Refractive errors 1.8 14
Hearing loss, adult onset 1.8 15
Diabetes mellitus 1.3 19
2030
Rank
As % of total DALYs
Disease or Injury
1 6.2 Unipolar depressive disorders
2 5.5 Ischemic heart disease
3 4.9 Road traffic accidents
4 4.3 Cerebrovascular disease
5 3.8 COPD
6 3.2 Lower respiratory infections
7 2.9 Hearing loss, adult onset
8 2.7 Refractive errors
9 2.5 HIV/AIDS
10 2.3 Diabetes mellitus
11 1.9 Neonatal infections and other[a]
12 1.9 Prematurity and low birth weight
15 1.9 Birth asphyxia and birth trauma
18 1.6 Diarrheal diseases
DALYs = Disability Adjusted Life Years
The sum of years of potential life lost due to premature mortality and the years of productive life lost due to disability.
[a] This category also includes other noninfectious causes arising in the perinatal period apart from prematurity, low birth weight, birth trauma, and asphyxia. These noninfectious causes are responsible for about 20% of DALYs shown in this category.

figure 4.2 The leading causes of death worldwide. COPD, chronic obstructive pulmonary disease. (From WHO. [2004]. Global burden of disease. Selected figures and tables. Retrieved from http://www.who.int/healthinfo/global_burden_disease/GBD2004ReportFigures.ppt#2)

opportunity for communities to address behaviors that can affect overall health (Fig. 4.2). When examining the GBD chart, many diseases can be ameliorated through health promotion, education, and the provision of skilled healthcare (Box 4.1).

According to the *WHO Global Status Report on Non-Communicable Diseases* (2011), of the 52.8 million global deaths in 2010, 34.5 million, or 65%, were due to noncommunicable diseases, the most prominent of which were cardiovascular diseases, diabetes, cancers, and chronic respiratory diseases. Nearly 80% of deaths from noncommunicable diseases occur in low- and middle-income countries (Lozano et al., 2012). Low-income countries are mostly situated in middle Africa, but middle-income countries include most of Central and South America, Eastern Europe, and Asia. While noncommunicable diseases are still not the most frequent causes of death in African nations, these diseases are rising rapidly and are projected to exceed communicable, maternal, perinatal, and nutritional diseases as the most common causes of death by 2030.

More than half of all cancer deaths occur in developing nations (Cancer Research UK, 2014). Noncommunicable diseases also cause death at younger ages in low- and middle-income countries. For example, 29% of deaths due

box 4.1 Top 10 Facts According to the Global Burden of Disease

1. Around 7 million children under the age of 5 die each year.
2. Cardiovascular diseases are the leading causes of death in the world.
3. HIV/AIDS is the leading cause of adult death in Africa.
4. Population aging is contributing to the rise in cancer and heart disease.
5. Lung cancer is the most common cause of death from cancer.
6. Complications of pregnancy account for almost 15% of deaths in women of reproductive age worldwide.
7. Mental disorders such as depression are among the 20 leading causes of disability worldwide.
8. Hearing loss, vision problems, and mental disorders are the most common causes of disability.
9. Nearly 3,500 people die from road traffic crashes every day.
10. Undernutrition is the underlying cause of death for at least one-third of all children under age 5.

Source: World Health Organization. (2012). *10 Facts on the state of global health.* Retrieved from http://www.who.int/features/factfiles/global_burden/facts/en/index.html

to noncommunicable diseases in low- and middle-income countries occur among people under the age of 60, compared to 13% in high-income countries. A WHO report (2011) states that the estimated percentage increase in cancer incidence by 2030, compared with 2008, will be greater in low-income (82%) and lower-middle-income countries (70%) compared with the upper-middle-income (58%) and high-income countries (40%).

Key factors in the rise of noncommunicable diseases are similar in all countries, and the diseases are often preventable (Box 4.2). In low- and middle-income countries that are now seeing increases in the rate of noncommunicable diseases, the process is accelerated by urbanization, culture change especially among the young, increasing sedentary lifestyles, and corporate marketing that targets these populations. One might see older populations still eating more healthy traditional foods, and younger populations lured in by fast food marketing, for example. Recommendations are being made, especially in low-resource settings, for increased surveillance and reporting of these diseases as well as increased efforts to educate the public on this important health area. Noncommunicable diseases play an important role not only on their effect on individuals but on social, economic, and environmental factors that affect human development (Alleyne et al., 2013; WHO, 2011).

An important factor in the increase in noncommunicable diseases is also the aging of the population, which is being seen in all countries around the world. As we look to the future, the combination of aging and increased noncommunicable diseases is likely to cause a higher disease burden.

Who Shoulders the Disease Burden?

The burden of disease is growing disproportionately in the world and is largely affected by climate, public policy, aging of the population, socioeconomic conditions, and risk factors (Fig. 4.3). Most of the countries burdened by disease have the least amount of human and economic capacity to effect change (Farmer, Furin, & Katz, 2004). Sub-Saharan Africa is unique in having an overwhelming share of the disease burden related to poverty and people living with HIV/AIDS (United Nations, 2012a).

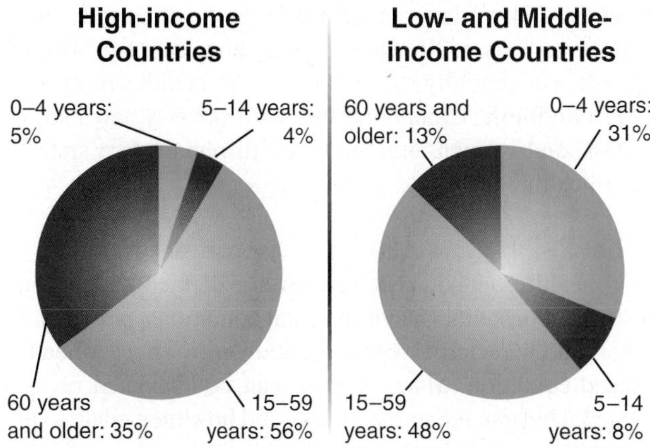

figure 4.3 Disease burden by age and income. (From WHO. [2004]. Global burden of disease. Selected figures and tables. Retrieved from http://www.who.int/healthinfo/global_burden_disease/GBD2004ReportFigures.ppt#2)

Women are disproportionately affected by the disease burden related to reproductive health and HIV infection (Hawkes & Buse, 2013). Globally, an estimated 800 women die daily from complications of childbirth (WHO, 2014b). Many of the complications resulting from childbirth can be prevented with the use of skilled midwives and nurses at birth. When a mother dies or is disabled, her children may be forced to live in poverty. Addressing the causes of these health discrepancies with education, specifically education for girls, and creating integrated health programs, such as HIV treatment and prenatal care, will improve the quality of care and thus decrease the disease burden (Potter et al., 2008). Girls and young women aged 15 to 24 years are twice as likely to become infected with HIV and account for 22% of new HIV infections (United Nations AIDS, 2013). Women now comprise 50% of individuals infected with HIV worldwide (United Nations, 2012b). Of adults living with HIV in sub-Saharan Africa, 58% are women, compared with 26% in North America.

Children younger than 5 years who may be malnourished shoulder a significant portion of the disease burden. Nutrition is related to access to a food source and the quality of the food. In many countries, the staple food such as rice, nshima, or millet, and other grain-based substances is abundant but lacks basic nutrients. Undernutrition and a diet of foods with poor nutritional content contribute to 45% of deaths in children younger than 5 years in developing countries (WHO, 2014c). Optimal breast-feeding could save more than 800,000 lives of children younger than 5 years each year. Lack of inclusion of the needs of underserved, poor people living in rural areas, especially women and children, has been recognized as an issue in the analysis of health data (Setel et al., 2007). This primarily results

box 4.2 Key Factors in Rise of Noncommunicable Diseases

Tobacco use
Insufficient physical activity
Harmful use of alcohol
Unhealthy diet
Raised blood pressure
Overweight and obesity
Raised cholesterol
Cancer-associated infections

Source: World Health Organization. (2011). *Global status report on noncommunicable diseases*. Retrieved from http://www.who.int/chp/ncd_global_status_report/en/

from the lack of national infrastructure to adequately measure the effects of ill health on the entire country. Women are often essentially "invisible" to the healthcare system after childbirth. Compound this with poverty and lack of access, and women and children will remain in a state of poor health.

What Risk Factors Affect the Disease Burden?

In a health context, **risk factors** are defined as personal habits and behaviors, environmental conditions, or inborn or inherited characteristics that are known to affect a health-related condition. Many of these can be alleviated or prevented. Understanding risk factors and how they relate to the population improves how the health status of a nation is understood. Risk factors occur in combination and change with age, creating different patterns of risk over a lifetime. Risk factor categories found to be associated with overall health include the following:

- *Childhood and maternal undernutrition:* Overall, underweight children and conditions related to iron, vitamin A, and zinc deficiencies contribute to poor health outcomes.
- *Other nutrition-related risk factors and inactivity:* Obesity and physical inactivity, coupled with high blood pressure and high cholesterol, affect adults as well as children worldwide.
- *Addictive substances:* Tobacco smoking and alcohol, as well as illicit drug use, affect the health of major portions of the world's population.
- *Sexual and reproductive health:* The generalized risk factors of unsafe sex, and no use or ineffective use of methods of contraception, contribute to decreased health of women and children.
- *Environmental risks:* Unsafe drinking water, unsanitary conditions, and poor hygiene, as well as urban air pollution and indoor smoke created by the burning of solid fuels, contribute to poor health.

The health of a nation is overwhelmingly affected by the presence of specific risk factors and the nation's capacity to support and implement health programs that will affect the major causes of morbidity and mortality. Risk factors such as tobacco use, nutritional status, alcohol consumption, and condom use can be modified with educational interventions and have an effect on the overall quality of life (WHO, 2004). Nurses can have a profound effect on risk factors by playing a major role in health promotion and education. The quality of health service coverage, even in settings with few resources or ones where an extreme nursing shortage exists, can be improved by nurses who target health-promotion issues within their community. One example is educating families on the daily use of insecticide-treated bed nets (ITNs) in regions where malaria is highly endemic, and use of artemisinin-based combination therapies (ACTs) in high-prevalence regions (WHO, 2013b). Artemisinin is a drug known for its ability to swiftly reduce the number of *Plasmodium* parasites in the blood of patients with malaria. In 2011 alone, 278 million courses of ACTs contributed to a 25% decrease in mortality from malaria. However, as cases of malaria have diminished, the use of bed nets has decreased. The public health sector needs to advocate that the nets are essential for all areas, and that they be retreated annually for efficacy. The Roll Back Malaria project of the WHO focuses on the community commitment to fight malaria (WHO, 2013b), and ITNs are one method of prevention. Promoting the proper use of ITNs would be an example of a program based on a specific demographic risk factor that nurses, as trustees of health, could promote.

Risk factors can be addressed both at the individual level and at the societal level. Often, the way in which various risk factors interact with one another, and the best approach to addressing each one, is not well understood or defined. If demographics and geographic patterns are applied to each of the risk categories, different patterns of need emerge. Using risk factors as a guide to which interventions will work (i.e., the package of interventions) greatly improves outcomes in specific communities. Removal of major risk factors, overall or in specific patterns, could improve healthy life expectancy worldwide. For example, for the GBD of lower respiratory tract infection, contributing risk factors are underweight children, zinc deficiency, and smoking, and Ezzati, Vander Hoorn, Rodgiers, Lopez, Mathers, and Murray (2003) predicted that if the individual risk of exposure was reduced by an alternative distribution of factors, theoretically the disease burden could be reduced by 55% to 62% (p. 274). Future studies on risk reduction and its effect on disease burden are critical to improving overall health.

PRACTICE POINT

Nurses can have a substantial effect on people's health by focusing their educational efforts on risk factors that can be modified, such as lifestyle behaviors.

Health Indicators

According to the WHO statistical information system, **health indicators** may be placed in four categories: morbidity and mortality, risk factors, health service coverage, and health system resources. Each category has a list of indicators and universal definitions. Morbidity and mortality are measured by life expectancy at birth and health-adjusted life expectancy (HALE) at birth. The effect of mortality on a population is reported as disability-adjusted life years (DALYs) (Box 4.3). These three indicators reflect the general health of a population. Secondary measures of mortality, such as maternal and neonatal rates, reflect at-risk groups that affect overall mortality. Risk factors focus on nutrition and health behaviors and environmental factors such as clean drinking water and burning of solid fuels. Health service coverage data identify uptake of specific services known to improve or promote health and well-being,

box 4.3 Health Indicator Descriptions

Life expectancy at birth (years): average number of years a newborn is expected to live if the current mortality rates continue to apply

HALE (health-adjusted life expectancy at birth [years]): average number of years that a person can expect to live in "full health" by taking into account years lived in less than full health due to disease and/or injury

DALYs (disability-adjusted life years): quantifying the burden of disease to a healthy life. The loss of years related to burden of disease. The gap in years reflects the current state of health versus an optimum state of health of a nation.

Source: World Health Organization (2014). *Health statistics and health information systems*. Retrieved from http://www.who.int/healthinfo/en

such as reproductive health services, infant and child health and immunization, HIV, and tuberculosis care. Health system resources focus on the capacity and supply of healthcare providers. These indicators in the aggregate provide valuable benchmarks that are used by health ministries and nongovernmental organizations (NGOs) as benchmarks for measuring target interventions.

Box 4.4 reflects the 10 highlights of the WHO Health Statistics Report for 2013 (WHO, 2013c). These highlights indicate that health discrepancies continue, and that interventions and benchmarks targeted at health indicators need to be based on the community-specific risk factors. Programs should focus on areas that have high impact on the overall health and well-being of the population they are intended to serve. These highlights suggest that global health continues to have an immense disease burden that is filled with opportunities for nurses to make a difference.

PRACTICE POINT

Culturally appropriate, community-driven, and community-based programs are critical for eliminating disparities; strategies directed at individuals are not sufficient.

From what you know about global risk factors that affect burden of disease, in reviewing the highlights of the WHO report, where do you see opportunity for improvement? What risk factors could be targeted that would address some of the issues highlighted within the report? For example, we know that unsafe sex practices is a major risk factor affecting reproductive health—maternal mortality is declining too slowly and cases of HIV infection are still on the rise in young women. Do you think addressing contraception and pregnancy in adolescents would be important? What other factors would we need to know within a global setting before we could conduct a community needs assessment about unsafe sex practices? For example, how should we optimally address ameliorating unsafe sex practices for men as well as women?

box 4.4 Ten Highlights of the WHO World Health Statistics Report for 2013

- Every day, about 800 women die due to complications of pregnancy and childbirth.
- In some countries, less than 10% of women who want to prevent pregnancy have access to any contraceptive methods.
- The government of Luxembourg spends more money on health per person than any other country in the world.
- 80% of deaths from malaria occur in just 14 countries.
- Children in low-income countries are 16 times more likely to die before reaching the age of 5 than children in high-income countries.
- China now has a higher life expectancy at birth than 7 out of 10 countries in Eastern Europe.
- Almost half of all countries surveyed have access to less than half of essential medicines they need for basic health-care in the public sector.
- Together with inadequate breast-feeding, vitamin A and zinc deficiencies contribute to more than a third of all child deaths.
- Almost 10% of the world's adult population has diabetes, measured by elevated fasting blood glucose (≥126mg/dL).
- The world had made significant progress in reducing child deaths by 40% from nearly 12 million deaths in 1990 to less than 7 million in 2011.

Source: World Health Organization (2013). *World health statistics report for 2013*. Retrieved from http://www.who.int/gho/publications/world_health_statistics/2013/en/

Statistics on population health indicators are used by governments and donor agencies. Health statistics will become vital to cost–benefit analysis for program development, with the shift in the developing world toward implementing a sector-wide approach program for health planning (WHO, 2008). A sector-wide approach promotes the collective agreement of the government entity (e.g., a ministry of health), donor countries, and other key stakeholders in the community such as physician and nurse organizations, NGOs, and researchers. The process ensures that the government assumes leadership in developing a common policy and program for health, including monitoring arrangements and instituting more coordinated procedures for funding and procurement (WHO, 2000). The challenge for ministries of health will be to administer, implement, and evaluate their annual healthcare goals and to work to identify ways and means to address the shortcomings that most affect the communities. Box 4.5 describes common shortcomings in many health delivery systems.

EVIDENCE FOR PRACTICE

Deaths from injuries and car accidents are about as prevalent as HIV/AIDS in the world. Bus accidents also cause many injuries in countries where safety laws are not well enforced. More than 90% of injury deaths occur in low- and middle-income countries, where preventive efforts are often nonexistent and healthcare systems are least prepared to meet the challenge, according to the WHO (2009). What kinds of interventions can nurses institute that would approach a solution to this problem?

Mumeka did not get her ultrasound because she could not afford it. Had she been able to secure the fees, she would have known that she had a deviation in her placenta that put her at risk for hemorrhage during delivery. This would have allowed for the health worker to contact her and her family to prepare to travel to the hospital prior to her going into labor. Fees for health services are a barrier to care. Although health policies regarding fees are slowly changing, the hidden costs of seeking maternal healthcare still create a barrier to receiving care. How can nurses act as strong community advocates to abolish all fees related to maternal and child health or assist communities in creating community spending accounts for all village people to access? The community funds could be used by any member of the community to access healthcare, such as paying for transportation or laboratory tests. If this proactive initiative had been in place, Mumeka might have received her ultrasound and her child might have lived.

box 4.5 United Nations Millennium Development Goals and Targets

Goal 1 Eradicate Extreme Poverty and Hunger
Halve the proportion of people whose income is less than $1.25 day and who suffer from hunger.

Goal 2 Achieve Universal Primary Education
All children will complete a full course of primary education.

Goal 3 Promote Gender Equality and Empower Women
Eliminate gender disparity in education.

Goal 4 Reduce Child Mortality
Reduce mortality rate of children younger than 5 years by two-thirds.

Goal 5 Improve Maternal Health
Reduce maternal mortality ratio by three-fourths.

Goal 6 Combat HIV/AIDS, Malaria and Other Diseases
Halt and begin to reverse the spread of HIV/AIDS, the incidence of malaria and other diseases.

Goal 7 Ensure Environmental Sustainability
Integrate the principles of sustainable development into policies and program development and reverse the loss of resources.

Goal 8 Develop a Global Partnership for Development
Develop a nondiscriminatory trade and finance system.

Source: http://www.un.org/millenniumgoals/

Poverty and Risk Factors

Low- and middle-income countries have an increased burden of the risk factor of poverty. Extreme poverty—the inability to meet the basic needs of adequate nutrition, safe drinking water, basic education, and primary health services, and a livelihood that can generate the means to secure these basic needs—is the driving force behind increased mortality (Sachs, 2005). Unlike those who are moderately and relatively poor, those who are extremely poor cannot access healthcare and are chronically hungry (Sachs, 2005). With a substantial segment of the world population existing on less than a dollar a day, the choices within the environment for sustenance create health risks. Approximately 1.9 billion people in sub-Saharan Africa rely on biomass energy sources, such as wood and dung, for cooking and heat, with estimated growth by 2030 in Sub-Saharan Africa from 593 to 996 million people (Venro, 2009). The continuous smoke from the burning of air-polluting solid fuels affects the population's health, which, in turn, affects economic prospects. Attention to achieving sustainable energy sources, particularly in Africa, will help to alleviate poverty, improve healthcare status, and address ever-expanding greenhouse gas emissions (Venro, 2009). This continued reliance on air-polluting fuels such as in China affects the population's health (which, in turn, affects their economic prospects).

Unclean water remains a major problem in reducing diarrheal illness and waterborne and water-related illnesses and their health consequences. Between 1990 and 2011, 1.9 million people gained access to improved sanitation facilities (United Nations, 2013a) and the proportion of people using an improved water source rose from 76% to 89%. Developing basic sanitation expectations for communities and decreasing reliance on traveling great distances to acquire water will improve health overall.

Only when (and if) the "haves" develop genuine empathy for the "have-nots," and come to acknowledge their own long-term interdependence with all other humans, will the global economy be improved to any significant advantage for the desperately poor.

Benatar in *PLOS Medicine* (2005)

The burden of disease associated with reproductive health affects the health indicators of a nation. Thompson (2007) described the deadly combination of poverty, the right to economic development, and the poor health of women as barriers to improving the health of the world's families. If maternal and child healthcare is left unattended, the rates of maternal and neonatal mortality will rise and national development in those nations with the fewest resources will be limited. The continued low status of women, despite years of policy development, increases the risk of disease and disability. The power imbalances within households around the world affect the health of women and young girls. Maternal, newborn, and child health affect population mortality and health in profound ways. An estimated three million unsafe abortions occur annually among girls and young women age 15 to 19 years (WHO, 2014b). Despite evidence of low-cost interventions that would improve reproductive health outcomes, scale-up for these interventions is lacking (Bhutta et al., 2008). The known interventions are focused on recognizing maternal and neonatal complications; procedures to prevent postpartum hemorrhage (PPH), such as active management of the third stage of labor; neonatal care at birth, such as drying the infant off and wrapping the infant immediately; and having a skilled provider examine the infant within 2 days of birth. Each of these interventions relies heavily on education of the mother and community and should be a primary focus of community-based programs to improve maternal and child health. As education increases in the community, evaluating the use of such interventions still remains low. Such low-cost, low-tech interventions can address the imbalances in maternal and child health, if used for every pregnancy and birth, and evaluated for quality of delivery and effectiveness. Refocusing efforts on the full cycle of quality improvement will greatly affect overall global health.

In case 1, Mumeka benefited from the presence of the trained CHW and her ability to influence the family regarding the need to seek a higher level of care. The locally trained worker was able to describe the needs for the complicated pregnancy and how moving to the hospital setting was important for the patient's well-being. What do you see as the role of the nurse when there is disagreement between family and care providers in seeking healthcare? How would you work with the family and a caregiver, to translate evidence into practice?

THE MILLENNIUM DEVELOPMENT GOALS

The Right to Health and the Millennium Development Goals

The political view of health as a right has been at the center of the debate on how to improve global health. The development of the Millennium Development Goals (MDGs) was a way for the world to join together in promoting health for all human beings. During the Millennium Development Summit of 2000, 147 nations agreed to an outline of a wide range of commitments in human rights, good governance, and democracy. The highlight of this summit was the universal framework for development, the eight MDGs (United Nations, 2000). To ensure success, the summit set health indicator targets to track success by 2015 (see Box 4.5). The goals addressed the barriers to health, including poverty and its dimensions—income, hunger, education, and disease—while promoting the abolition of gender inequalities, especially in education, and recognizing the need for sustainable environmental resources.

The MDG initiative was not the first time that the **right to health** had been mentioned as a human right. In 1978, the Alma Alta Declaration for Primary Healthcare reaffirmed that health is a fundamental human right (Lawn et al., 2008). This declaration, the first global consensus document, proposed a shift in philosophy that health is not just the result of interventions to ameliorate ill health, but is the result of social determinants such as economic development. Nations recognized that attainment of the highest possible status of health for all members requires the commitment of many social, political, and economic sectors (Lawn et al., 2008). The Safe Motherhood Initiative in 1988, the World Summit for Children in 1990, and follow-up initiatives in individual nations continued to foster the role of individuals and communities in improving health. The year 2008 marked the 60th anniversary of the Declaration for Human Rights. This international decree, which provided the first agreed-upon standards to guide and monitor governments in many sectors, has had a direct impact on the right to health and the need for a functioning health system (Marks, 2006). The right of all people to enjoy the highest attainable standard of physical and mental health, the right to health, is integral to each of these human rights documents. These integral steps to link human rights and health created the basis for the world to come together to form a foundation for health for humanity. Other international documents, including the International Covenant on Economic, Social, and Cultural Rights (ICESCR) (Sepúlveda, 2003) and the Convention on the Rights of the Child (CRC) (United Nations, 1989), are legally binding human rights treaties that have been adopted by almost all countries (Backman et al., 2008).

Impact of the Millennium Development Goals

The long-term results of the success of the MDGs may not be realized until well after 2015 (United Nations Economic and Social council, 2014). As of late 2013, many targets and countries have had great success in areas such as improved clean water sources, a decline in the number of slum dwellers related to the population of metropolises, and remarkable gains in preventing and treating malaria and tuberculosis. Conversely, despite best efforts, the environment continues to be under threat of deterioration, interventions to improve child survival need to be sustained, maternal mortality rates are still alarming, and too many children are still denied access to education (United Nations, 2013b). Many countries may never reach these global targets. The post-2015 agenda to sustain advances recognizes the need to empower countries to set their own goals (Cohen, Bishai, Alfonso, Kuruvilla, & Schweitzer, 2014). Table 4.1 highlights achievements and remaining challenges. Gains in areas of employment, poverty, and women's rights create the context for better health. Employment rates have increased, yet over 60% of workers in the developing world still live on less than $4 per day (United Nations, 2013a). Women are far

table 4.1 **Progress to Date: Millennium Development Goals Report, 2013**

Achievements	Barriers and Continued Focal Points
• Extreme poverty is falling in every region. People living on less than $.25 a day fell from 47% in 1990 to 22% in 2010. • In China, extreme poverty dropped from 60% in 1990 to 12% in 2010. • The number of people who are undernourished has decreased in the developing world from 23% in 1990 to 15% in 2010. • The number of children out of school worldwide decreased from 102 million to 57 million. • Literacy rates are on the rise, and gender gaps are narrowing. • Steady progress has been made toward equal access to education with gender disparities more evident at the tertiary level. • Forty out of 100 wage earners in the nonagricultural sector are women. • Child mortality has dropped 41% since 1990. • Measles vaccines have averted 10 million deaths in children since 2000. • Maternal mortality has declined by two-thirds in Eastern Asia, Northern Africa, and Southern Asia. • Skilled birth attended deliveries have risen from 55% in 1990 to 66% in 2011. • More women have access to and are using contraception and family planning. • Incidence of HIV is declining steadily with 230,000 fewer children under age 15 in 2011 infected than in 2001. • By the end of 2015, 15 million people will be receiving antiretroviral medicines. • With treatment improvements, more people are living with HIV than ever before. • In the last decade, 1.1 million deaths from Malaria were averted. • Tuberculosis treatment has saved 20 million lives between 1995 and 2011and has succeeded global targets. • More than 2.1 billion people have gained access to improved water sources and sanitation facilities since 1990. • The target of decreasing slum dwellers has been exceeded. • Development assistance was stagnant at $126 billion in 2012. • In 2010–2011, increasingly aid is being directed toward gender equality and women's empowerment. • Duty-free access is improving for least-developed countries.	• Measuring poverty is a barrier to policy-making. Abject poverty deprives people of health and education, limiting productive employment. • 870 million people still do not consume enough food to meet their nutritional energy requirements. • More than 100 million children are still undernourished and underweight. • The number of people uprooted by conflict and persecution is at its highest in 18 years. • Poverty, gender, and place of residence continue to be barriers to child school enrollment. • Of the 137 million children who start primary education, 34 million will most likely leave before completion. • Only 2 out of 130 countries have achieved gender parity at the primary level. • Women tend to hold less secure jobs than men. • Women have increased decision-making related to their health and social interactions yet still remain dependent on men related to monetary decision-making. • 6.9 million children under 5 died in 2011 from mostly preventable diseases. • One in nine children die before the age of 5 in sub-Saharan Africa, 16 times the average for the region. • Focusing on children in the first month of life will greatly improve child mortality rates globally. • 46 million women deliver their babies without the assistance of a skilled birth attendant. More than half of women in rural areas lack access to skilled care. • Adolescent childbearing continues to create risk for both mother and child. • 2.5 million people are newly infected with HIV each year. • Young people are vulnerable with more than 60% of new infections occurring in women. • The gap in education of HIV transmission knowledge and condom use is appallingly low considering efforts in this area. • Global emissions continue to grow at an alarming rate. • Overexploitation of fish stocks is resulting in continued diminished yield. • Open defecation continues to affect community health. • Urban residents living in slum conditions due to the fast pace of urbanization will continue. • The global economic crisis and subsequent rebound will need to be evaluated for sustainable effect on improving donor-spending plans. • Only 31% of the developing world population uses the Internet; improved access will affect all development goals.

Source: United Nations. (2013). *The Millennium Development Goals report 2013.* New York, NY: United Nations. Retrieved from http://www.un.org/millenniumgoals/pdf/report-2013/mdg-report-2013-english.pdf

more likely than men to be engaged in vulnerable employment that consists of shared or unpaid family work (United Nations, 2012a). This specific inequality disproportionately affects young women and children, along with the continued presence of poverty and hunger. Young people who live in poverty, combined with lack of food sources, create the context where acquiring and sustaining profit in the labor force is difficult. New methodologies for measuring food insecurity could help tackle hunger through the design of new interventions at the systems level.

MDGs 4 and 5, directed at child and maternal mortality, have received tremendous attention. Overall, the mortality rate for under-5 children has decreased by one-third (United Nations, 2013a). Children born into poverty, however, are almost two times more likely to die before the age of 5 years than their wealthier counterparts. The challenges continue in the area of infant mortality and during the vulnerable period of the first 28 days of life. The region still contributing to this high rate of infant mortality is sub-Saharan Africa, with 35 neonatal deaths per 1,000 births. A woman in Chad has a 1 in 15 chance of dying in childbirth, compared to 1 in 3,800 in the developing world (WHO, 2012b). These deaths, both neonate and mother, are often linked to the lack of care of the mother prior to and during childbirth. Although two-thirds of deliveries are now attended to by skilled health personnel, there is slow growth in this intervention, and assessment of the competency of personnel and the care delivered is lacking. Countries that have improved the quality of care have seen significant improvement in maternal and newborn health (Van Lerberghe et al., 2014). Significant advances have been made in child mortality, and with continued funding and support, many countries can achieve success. A refocus on the mother/baby couplet and newborn-specific needs could affect both of these goals and improve overall health (Houweling et al., 2014). A new focus on adolescent girls and the every newborn action plan by the United Nations creates a new platform for the future health of nations (United Nations, 2014).

The key limiting factor to achieving success is external aid. MDG 8 on sustainable global partnerships has been greatly influenced by the economic downturn between 2008 and 2012 (United Nations, 2013a). Jeffery Sachs, Millennium Village founder and global health economist, believes that "if high-income countries build on their (domestic programs) of the past decade, and deliver a mere 0.1% of the GDP for health sector official development aide as a part of a larger overall aide programme, they and their low-income partners will celebrate great MDG successes as of 2015" (Sachs, J. 2010, p. 951). Many challenges appear to be overwhelming, yet with a final push and commitment to success, many more goals can be achieved.

EVIDENCE FOR PRACTICE

The 2015 countdown report for maternal, newborn, and child survival outlines the progress that has been made in improving the lives of families. Yet more can be done with basic, low-cost interventions (United Nations, 2013a). Sustaining focused interventions on early detection and treatment of diarrhea and pneumonia will decrease mortality (Walker et al., 2013). Four interventions known to affect both diarrhea and pneumonia include the following (Bhutta et al., 2013):

- Breast-feeding. Not breast-feeding resulted in a 165% increased risk of acquiring diarrhea from 0 to 5 months of age (Lamberti, Walker, Noiman, Victora, & Black, 2011).
- Breast-feeding education on exclusive breast-feeding. Significant results, as high as 90%, were attributed to promotional interventions for children from 0 to 6 months of age (Bhutta et al., 2013).
- WASH interventions. Water, sanitation, and hygiene (WASH) interventions demonstrated a risk reduction of 17% with proper excreta disposal, and risk reductions of up to 48% with water and soap handwashing (Cairncross et al., 2010).
- Zinc supplementation. Supplementation resulted in a reduction in diarrhea and acute lower respiratory tract infection mortality (Yakoob et al., 2011).
- Postpartum hemorrhage. PPH is the leading cause of maternal death, claiming an estimated 140,000 lives in low-resource settings, with an additional 2 million women left to recover from anemia (Bradley, Prata, Young-Lin, & Bishai, 2007; Prata, Passano, Sreenivas, & Gerdts, 2010; Smith, Gubin, Holston, Fullerton, & Prata, 2013) The use of uterotonics such as oxytocin or misoprostol can have a profound effect on preventing and treating PPH. Several large randomized controlled trials (RCTs) have shown that the use of such medications will improve delivery of the placenta, decrease blood loss, and avert death and disability. Implementation of such treatments as a standard of care requires a reliable supply chain for medications, and the support of nurse leaders to implement the procedures for every delivery, since we know that long labors and multiple gestations increase the risk for PPH, but many women with no risk factors suffer hemorrhage.
- Creating political will is important to improving health. Countries that improved care by strengthening their health system with education and deployment of midwives reduced their maternal mortality ration by 2% to 5% and will have a median drop of maternal mortality ratio by 63% over 20 years (Van Lerberghe et al., 2014). Countries with sustainable changes focused on improving access as close to the family as possible, scaling up birth care in line with the population, decreasing fees and financial barriers to care, and making quality care a priority. In countries where these four elements have been most successful, nurse midwifery has become more visible and accepted.
- Preterm birth and stillbirth have been neglected in improving child mortality (WHO, 2012a). Investing in low-cost interventions, such as universal kangaroo care, and high-cost interventions, such as corticosteroid injections, could save up to 950,000 infants per year. Education of skilled health personnel, specifically nurses and midwives, on tools to support preterm care, and access to essential equipment and education, can have a profound effect on neonatal survival. The global action report by WHO *Born too Soon* (WHO, 2012a) outlines steps that can improve preterm birth and prevent causes of stillbirth, such as maternal malnutrition.

OTHER FACTORS THAT AFFECT GLOBAL HEALTH

Economics and Politics

The global environment is intricately intertwined with the economic and political status of a nation. As one area improves, so do others, and vice versa. It is known that health and education are clearly linked, in that the better educated the population is, the better the health of the population is (Ross & Wu, 1995). Political and economic instability, which leads to poverty, is a major barrier to achieving health for a population. When economies and political systems are stable, the health of a population also tends to get better.

Over the past 60 years, the world economy has increased, and yet has spawned greater disparities. For example, the global economy increased sevenfold since 1950, whereas the disparity in gross domestic product between the 20 richest and 20 poorest nations more than doubled between 1960 and 1997 (British Medical Journal, 1999). Extreme poverty is decreasing in every region of the world, according to the 2013 MDG Report of the United Nations. The proportion of people living on less than $1.25 a day fell from 43% in 1990 to 21% in 2010 (The World Bank, 2014). An estimated 2.4 billion people lived on less than $2 a day in 2010, with decreasing numbers of people living in conditions of extreme poverty. Yet living in poverty remains the driving economic condition that significantly affects health and well-being in sub-Saharan Africa and in southern Asia (United Nations, 2013a).

The current economic and political instability of many parts of the world only exacerbates the difficulties for the world's poor. The effects of a slowdown of the world economy on the incomes of other less wealthy nations have become evident. This ripple effect is felt by the poorest people of the world.

The first wealth is health.

Ralph Waldo Emerson

Even with these enormous disparities in health, poor countries can learn to become more economically self-sufficient by producing enough basic commodities and foods for their population to survive, and also by producing specific goods for export that are not readily available in wealthier countries. Poor countries must grow staple foods that lead to nutritionally balanced diets for the local people. It is possible to achieve high levels of health even without high levels of income. Disparities between the wealthiest and poorest nations must be reduced; in the end, each individual is inextricably linked as the world quickly becomes a global community. Maintaining communities and honoring cultural norms and traditions can only help populations become more self-sufficient. It is inherently necessary for health planners to understand this basic fact.

In case 2, what are some of the social and economic factors that may influence the health of the elderly 95-year-old man? Consider the relative affluence of the country in which he lives. What social and economic factors would best contribute to keeping him healthy in the community? How can nurses intervene in improving the conditions of aging persons, particularly in countries where increased aging of the population is a relatively new phenomenon.

Factors Associated with Healthcare Systems

Healthcare systems differ in terms of the degree to which they can adequately serve the population and the degree to which they are centralized in the government. They range from national healthcare systems, such as those in the United Kingdom or Spain, to pluralistic free-market systems, such as those in the United States. National healthcare systems are highly regulated, tend to have salaried physicians and other providers, are funded by governments, and involve relatively high taxes. Free-market healthcare systems depend more on individual or employer and employee contributions than on taxes. In between these two extremes are the systems of various countries whose citizens have access to universal health insurance and pay higher taxes for these services, such as the Scandinavian countries of Denmark, Norway, and Sweden. Other health insurance funding methods include national health insurance programs with single-payer systems, such as those in Canada, and programs with multipayer health insurance systems that offer universal health insurance via sickness funds, such as those in Germany and France.

The U.S. system, which is often characterized as highly fragmented and segmented, depending on the individual's insurance status or level of wealth, spends far more per capita on health than any other country in the world. Although the United States spends the most on healthcare per capita, it has the worst rating in preventable deaths (treatable cancer, diabetes, childhood infections/disease, and complications from surgery); it ranked last among 16 industrialized nations. From 1997–1998 to 2006–2007, the United States lowered its preventable mortality rate by only 20% compared to an average decrease of 31% in other nations (Nolte & McKee, 2011). See Figure 4.4 for comparisons with other countries of the world on various measures (Davis, Sremikas, Squires, & Schoen, 2014).

The United States passed the Patient Protection and Affordable Care Act in March 2010, a landmark national healthcare reform law that was expected to allow 94% of all Americans to obtain health insurance, reduce the growth in healthcare costs, and decrease the federal budget deficit by $143 billion over the next 10 years (Congressional Budget Office, 2010). This legislation has had many hurdles to overcome since its passage but is gradually increasing the number of insured individuals in spite of opposition by

Exhibit ES-1. Overall Ranking

COUNTRY RANKINGS

Top 2
Middle
Bottom 2

	AUS	CAN	FRA	GER	NETH	NZ	NOR	SWE	SWIZ	UK	USA
OVERALL RANKING (2013)	4	10	9	5	5	7	7	3	2	1	11
Quality Care	2	9	8	7	5	4	11	10	3	1	5
Effective Care	4	7	9	6	5	2	11	10	8	1	3
Safe Care	3	10	2	6	7	9	11	5	4	1	7
Coordinated Care	4	8	9	10	5	2	7	11	3	1	6
Patient-Centered Care	5	8	10	7	3	6	11	9	2	1	4
Access	8	9	11	2	4	7	6	4	2	1	9
Cost-Related Problem	9	5	10	4	8	6	3	1	7	1	11
Timeliness of Care	6	11	10	4	2	7	8	9	1	3	5
Efficiency	4	10	8	9	7	3	4	2	6	1	11
Equity	5	9	7	4	8	10	6	1	2	2	11
Healthy Lives	4	8	1	7	5	9	6	2	3	10	11
Health Expenditures/Capita, 2011	$3,800	$4,522	$4,118	$4,495	$5,099	$3,182	$5,669	$3,925	$5,643	$3,405	$8,508

figure 4.4 Overall ranking of countries on health outcomes. (From Davis, K, Sremikas, K. Squires, D, Schoen, C. (2014). *Mirror, mirror on the wall, 2014 update: How the U.S. health care system compares internationally Commonwealth Fund*. Retrieved from http://www.commonwealthfund.org/publications/fund-reports/2014/jun/mirror-mirror)

many Americans and various states. So how does this translate to poorer countries, with less wealth than the United States or Europe? Lessons learned from decades of work focusing on a specific disease of a population have provided data to suggest that focusing on the system may garner better health indexes for global health delivery (Kim, Farmer, & Porter, 2013). Care delivery value chains (CDVCs) targeted at a specific problem can create a system that engages all aspects of care toward one outcome. Creating a value-based delivery system which is focused on the value it achieves for the patient and society, and which emphasizes best practice and includes the need to understand the combined effect of interventions over a cycle of care, is an important aspect of CDVCs (Kim et al., 2013). The cycle includes the patient value that includes performing and engaging, measuring or diagnostics, and accessing care. The elements of the chain to achieve these values include the following:

- Monitoring and prevention
- Diagnosing
- Preparing
- Intervening
- Recovering and rehabilitation
- Monitoring and managing overall outcomes

Integrating this model into health systems may move health indexes to the next level.

Strong healthcare systems are vital, yet they also need sustainable financial support. Some countries are turning to insurance mechanisms. Smith and Sulzbach (2008) describe voluntary, nonprofit health insurance schemes, organized and managed at the community levels, that they call "community-based health insurance" (p. 2461). This concept is based on the principle of risk pooling and involves regular payments of a small premium in exchange for reducing direct payments at the point of service. These types of financing are also referred to as prepayment schemes, private prepaid programs, microinsurance, and mutual health organizations (Smith & Sulzbach, 2008). Although care in these poorer countries involves a completely different paradigm than in developed countries, lack of the greatest resource—healthcare providers—is one of the most compelling problems. Lack of financing either from the government or from the population served further exacerbates this problem.

Extreme shortages of healthcare workers are an endemic problem in developing countries, and yet again, these countries share the greatest burden of disease, spend the least on healthcare expenditures, and have the lowest number of healthcare workers. Fifty-seven countries, most of them in Africa and Asia, face a severe health workforce crisis. With most recent data available, the WHO (2006) estimated that at least 2,360,000 health service providers and 1,890,000 management support workers, or a total of 4,250,000 health workers, are needed to fill the gap. Without prompt action, the shortage will worsen, especially in the poorest countries. Sub-Saharan Africa, for example, had 11% of the world's population and 24% of the GBD, and it manages with only 3% of the world's health workers (WHO, 2006). The number of health workers is directly related to the health of global populations. Further, country-specific data can be found at the website of Global Atlas of the Health Workforce, WHO, Geneva: http://www.who.int/hrh/statistics/hwfstats/.

To add to this problem, many factors that affect the health of global populations are often beyond the control of individual people. Wars, political instability, famine, ecological factors such as global warming and subsequent environmental disasters, and economic trends may lead members of the local health workforce (such as nurses and physicians) to move to highly developed countries where they can work in more favorable conditions.

What has occurred is a global shortage of nurses and physicians in areas of need, and workforce migration leading to a "brain drain" of workers moving from lesser-developed countries to more developed countries. In 2010, the WHO introduced the *Global Code of Practice of the Recruitment of Health Personnel* (WHO, 2010). The code promotes the ethical recruitment of personnel and provides a focus on health work force development and health systems sustainability, and strengthening local health systems. Table 4.2 lists the key facts related to nurse migration. The WHO (2011) assembly on strengthening nursing and midwifery supported a continued focus on including nursing and midwifery in health system planning and employment, and transforming education systems to meet the needs of each country. Gostin (2008) states that the factors contributing to a shortage of healthcare workers are globalization, which has increased over the past 20 to 30 years, and a decreased supply of healthcare workers along with an increased demand for well-trained workers. He says that this leads to a "push–pull" situation, in which healthcare workers are "pushed" from developing countries and "pulled" to developed countries with the promise of a brighter future. Factors leading to this problem include low wages, unsafe environments, the need for better living conditions and facilities, lack of opportunity to be promoted, and unusually heavy workloads and long working hours (Gostin, 2008). The WHO (2010) suggests that in-source countries need to consider better health workforce retention by focusing on maldistribution of nurses and quality of life. Health systems need to provide protection and better treatment of workers in general, as often there are poor working conditions and poor pay. Lastly, in accordance with the WHO goal of improving nursing education, countries need to invest in improving the initial education and training of midwives so that they are better prepared as professional healthcare workers (WHO, 2009). Because migration is a human right, the WHO supports destination or receiving countries to act as responsible global citizens in recruiting migrant workers. This includes building capacity in their own countries as well as treating expatriate workers with the same dignity and respect as all healthcare workers.

Gostin does suggest an upside to migration for the worker and the community: workers who migrate also gain new skills in the receiving countries and can return to their native countries revitalized with education and new outlooks on solving the problems—in other words, "brain gain." Those who leave may also come back with the skills to educate other workers. For example, nurses may return with advanced practice nursing skills and become educators in their respective countries.

The WHO (2006) considers the following to be important requirements for the effective management of health workforce shortages (p. 2):

- Increased investment in education and training: Initial funds are necessary to increase the capacity and diversity of the cadre of healthcare workers. This will be followed by the continued need to pay their salaries. It is estimated that to increase the workforce by 4 million in 57 countries and make it sustainable by 2025, there needs to be an investment of $10 per person.

table 4.2 **Key Facts on Health Workforce Migration**

- There are about 60 million health workers worldwide.
- Many health workers migrate to high-income countries for greater income, job satisfaction, career opportunities, and management quality.
- Demand for health workers is increasing in high-income countries, where health systems can depend heavily on doctors, nurses, and other health workers who have been trained abroad.
- Migration of health workers may result in financial loss and weakens health systems in the countries of origin.
- WHO has developed a Global Code of Practice on the International Recruitment of Health Personnel to achieve an equitable balance of the interests of health workers, source countries and destination countries.

Source: World Health Organization. (2010). *Migration of health workers fact sheet.* Retrieved from http://www.who.int/mediacentre/factsheets/fs301/en/index.html

- National health workforce plans (political leadership and commitment of the necessary funds): Investment in the business of healthcare, to create support systems, and improved management to effectively monitor and implement countrywide road maps are essential for sustainability.
- More efficient use of existing human resources (including redelegation of some of the tasks to less-qualified but well-supervised workers): Evaluating the talent within the existing workforce and creating new programs where services are piggybacked, such as immunizations and vitamin supplements, will create a larger return on investment in health.
- Protection and fairer treatment of health workers: Many healthcare workers are faced with violence within the workplace and are often not paid on a routine basis.
- Access to HIV prevention and treatment for health workers in affected countries: HIV has disproportionately affected healthcare workers, and due to stigma, many workers do not seek or receive adequate treatment.
- Attracting women to health professions and addressing retirement: It is necessary to create flexible opportunities to attract women to all segments of the health sector, provide incentives to those who have retired to return to work, and adjust incentives linked to retirement.
- Comprehensive preparedness for a workforce response to outbreaks and emergencies in every country: Healthcare workers need to be included in planning for emergency preparedness so that there can be a cohesive collaborative process in the event of a catastrophic event.
- Career incentives to attract health workers to rural and disadvantaged areas: Healthcare workers are mostly in rural communities in the countries with the greatest need. Providing incentives for administering quality care in a rural setting could improve healthcare in these areas.
- Health promotion and prevention strategies to reduce demand for health services: Healthcare workers are mostly needed in rural communities in the countries with the greatest need.

When a country invests in its healthcare workers through improved training, improved working conditions, career ladders, and allocation of financial resources toward improving salaries and systems, workers are more likely to remain in that country. HIV protection and treatment, as well as plans for emergency preparedness, are paramount if workers are to feel safe in their environments. The "pull" to other countries is great, and healthcare workers must feel that their contribution is valued and that their future will be improved if they resist the perceived benefits of moving to more developed countries to live out their lives and careers.

ROLE OF NURSES

The world is now a global village. Problems that affect people in other countries also affect people in their own countries. Nurses and community healthcare providers need to be knowledgeable about the needs of all people, as well as of their patients, in the global society. Knowledge of the goals for worldwide health can lead to new cooperative ventures and unique solutions using technology and knowledge transfer techniques. Do all citizens of the world deserve access to good health and a sense of well-being? It is expected that the answer to this question will be "yes," but such a goal can be accomplished only through international cooperation, regardless of national boundaries. Larger questions of inequalities in wealth and resources must be addressed, and as a new generation of providers emerges, they may have the answers that have eluded societies before them.

Nurses are a major part of the solution to world health problems, and if conditions become more favorable and nations more supportive of their role, different and more realistic solutions can be crafted. All nurses and nursing students need to be enlightened about global health issues so that this valuable profession can be part of the solution toward a more healthy global population in the years to come.

key concepts

- Global health encompasses the behavioral and environmental risk factors of a community, which are influenced by politics, economics, and culture.
- Monitoring health indicators and ensuring the inclusion of vulnerable and invisible populations will improve packaged interventions to affect health outcomes.
- Global burden of disease is a term that reflects the health of a nation and the level of opportunity to improve health.
- The Millennium Development Goals are a framework for achieving the right to health. Nurses should participate in forming future goals for countries.
- The road map to achieving health relies on the participation of all individuals and nations to address the basic needs of clean drinking water, sanitation, and alleviating poverty.
- Education is the key to improving the community environment, which, in turn, will improve health.
- Health worker migration increases the burden of care for a society and results in the need to shift tasks primarily to nurses and community health workers.

critical thinking questions

1. Imagine the role that nurses can play in a more egalitarian world where all healthcare providers can contribute equally to the pressing global problems presented here. What are some of your proposed solutions?
2. How can nurses work within communities of interest to determine how the burden of disease is affected by poverty?
3. How can nurses influence the major risk factors related to maternal mortality and HIV?
4. What health factors can nurses address to work with young males of a community to improve overall health?

community resources

- World Health Organization
- International Council of Nurses

references

Alleyne, G., Binagwaho, A., Haines, A., Jahan, S., Nugent, R., Rojhani, A., & Stuckler, D.; Lancet NCD Action Group. (2013). Embedding non-communicable diseases in the post-2015 development agenda. *The Lancet, 381*(9866), 566–574.

Backman, G., Hunt, P., Khosla, R., Jaramillo-Strouss, C., Fikre, B. M., Rumble, C.,…Vladescu, C. (2008). Health systems and the right to health: An assessment of 194 countries. *The Lancet, 372*, 2047–2085.

Benatar, S. (2005). Moral imagination: The missing component in global health. *PLoS Medicine, 2*(12), e400. doi:10.1371/journal.pmed.0020400

Bhutta, Z. A., Das, J. K., Walker, N., Rizvi, A., Campbell, H., Rudan, I., & Black, R. E.; Lancet Diarrhoea and Pneumonia Interventions Study Group. (2013). Interventions to address deaths from childhood pneumonia and diarrhoea equitably: What works and at what cost? *The Lancet, 381*(9875), 1417–1429.

Bhutta, Z., Ali, S., Cousens, S., Ali, T. M., Haider, B. A., Rizvi, A., … Black, R. E. (2008). Alma-Ata: Rebirth and Revision 6 Interventions to address maternal, newborn, and child survival: What difference can integrated primary health care strategies make. *The Lancet, 372*, 972–989.

Bradley, S. E., Prata, N., Young-Lin, N., & Bishai, D. M. (2007). Cost-effectiveness of misoprostol to control postpartum hemorrhage in low-resource settings. *International Journal of Gynaecology & Obstetrics, 97*(1), 52–56.

British Medical Journal. (1999). The champagne glass of world poverty. *British Medical Journal, 318*, 7189.

Cairncross, S., Hunt, C., Boisson, S., Bostoen, K., Curtis, V., Fung, I. C., Schmidt, W.-P. (2010). Water, sanitation and hygiene for the prevention of diarrhoea. *International Journal of Epidemiology, 39*(Suppl 1), i193–i205. doi:10.1093/ije/dyq035

Cancer Research UK. (2014). *Cancer stats: Cancer statistics for the UK*. Retrieved from http://www.cruk.org/cancerstats

Cohen, R. L., Bishai, D. M., Alfonso, Y. N., Kuruvilla, S., & Schweitzer, J. (2014). Post-2015 health goals: Could country-specific targets supplement global ones? *The Lancet Global Health, 2*(7), e373–e374. doi:10.1016/S2214-109X(14)70193-7

Congressional Budget Office. (2010). Retrieved from http://www.cbo.gov/ftpdocs/113xx/doc11379/Manager'sAmendmenttoReconciliationProposal.pdf

Davis, K., Sremikas, K., Squires, D., & Schoen, C. (2014). Mirror, mirror on the wall, 2014 update: How the U.S. health care system compares internationally Commonwealth Fund. Retrieved from http://www.commonwealthfund.org/publications/fund-reports/2014/jun/mirror-mirror

Disease Control Priorities Project. (2008). Retrieved from http://www.dcp2.org/main/Home.html

Dunn, H. (1959). High-level wellness for man and society. *American Journal of Public Health, 49*(6), 786–792.

Ezzati, M., Hoorn, S. V., Rodgiers, A., Lopez, A., Mathers, C., & Murray, C. (2003). Estimates of global and regional potential health gains from reducing multiple major risk factors. *The Lancet, 363*, 271–280.

Farmer, P., Furin, J., & Katz, J. (2004). Global health equity. *The Lancet, 363*, 182.

Fisher, I. (1909). *Report on national vitality, its wastes and conservation. Prepared for the National Conservation Commission*. Washington, DC: Government Printing Office.

Gostin, L. (2008). The international migration and recruitment of nurses: Human rights and global justice. *JAMA, 299*(15), 1827–1829.

Hawkes, S., & Buse, K. (2013). Gender and global health: Evidence, policy, and inconvenient truths. *The Lancet, 381*(9879), 1783–1787.

Horton, R. (2013). Non-communicable diseases: 2015 to 2025. *The Lancet, 381*(9866), 509–510. doi:10.1016/S0140-6736(13)60100-2

Houweling, T. A. J., Morrison, J., Azad, K., Manandhar, D. S., Alcock, G., Shende, S.,…Costello, A. (2014). How to reach every newborn: Three key messages. *The Lancet Global Health, 2*(8), e436–e437. doi:10.1016/S2214-109X(14)70271

Hunter, D. J., & Reddy, K. S. (2013). Noncommunicable diseases. *New England Journal of Medicine, 369*(14), 1336–1343. doi:10.1056/NEJMra1109345

Institute of Health Metrics and Evaluation. (2014). *Global burden of disease* Retrieved from http://www.healthmetricsandevaluation.org/gbd

Institute of Medicine. (1997). *America's vital interest in global health: Protecting our people, enhancing our economy, and advancing our international interests*. Washington, DC: National Academies Press. Retrieved from http://books.nap.edu/openbook.php?record_id=5717&page=11

Jamison, D. T., & Jardel, J.-P. (1994). Comparative health data and analyses. In C. J. L. Murray & A. D. Lopez (Eds.), *Global comparative assessments in the health sector: Disease burden, expenditures, and intervention packages* (pp. v–vii). Geneva: World Health Organization.

Kim, J. Y., Farmer, P., & Porter, M. E. (2013). Redefining global health-care delivery. *The Lancet, 382*(9897), 1060–1069. doi:10.1016/S0140-6736(13)61047-8

Lamberti, L., Walker, C. F., Noiman, A., Victora, C., & Black, R. E. (2011). Breastfeeding and the risk for diarrhea morbidity and mortality. *BMC Public Health, 11*(Suppl 3), S15.

Lawn, J. E., Rohde, J., Rifkin, S., Were, M., Paul V. K., & Chopra, M. (2008). Alma-Alta 30 years on: Revolutionary, relevant, and time to revitalize. *The Lancet, 372*, 917–927.

Lopez, A., Mathers, C., Ezzati, M., Jamison, D., & Murray, C. (Eds.). (2006). *Global burden of disease and risk factors* (2nd ed.). New York, NY: Oxford University Press. Retrieved from http://www.dcp2.org/pubs/GBD/1/Section/27

Lozano, R., Naghavi, M., Foreman. K., Lim, S., Shibuya, K., Aboyans, V., . . . Murray, C. J. L. (2012). Global and regional mortality from 235 causes of death for 20 age groups in 1990 and 2010: A systematic analysis for the Global Burden of Disease Study 2010. *The Lancet, 380*, 2095–128.

Marks, S. (2006). *Health and human rights: Basic international documents* (2nd ed.). Cambridge, MA: François-Xavier Bagnoud Center for Health and Human Rights, Harvard School of Public Health.

Murray, C., & Lopez, A. (Eds.). (1996). *The global burden of disease*. New York, NY: Oxford University Press.

Murray, C. J., Vos, T., Lozano, R., Naghavi, M., Flaxman, A. D., Michaud, C., . . . Memish, Z. A. (2012). Disability-adjusted life years (DALYs) for 291 diseases and injuries in 21 regions, 1990–2010: A systematic analysis for the Global Burden of Disease Study 2010. *The Lancet, 380*(9859), 2197–2223.

Nolte, E., & McKee, M. (2011). Variations in amenable mortality—Trends in 16 high-income nations. *Health Policy, 103*(1), 47–52. doi:10.1016/j.healthpol.2011.1008.1002

Potter, D., Goldenberg, R., Chao, A., Sinkala, M., Degroot, A., Stringer, J. S. A., . . . Vermund, S. H. (2008). Do targeted HIV programs improve overall care for pregnant women? *Journal of AIDS, 47*, 79–85.

Prata, N., Passano, P., Sreenivas, A., & Gerdts, C. E. (2010). Maternal mortality in developing countries: Challenges in scaling-up priority interventions. *Women's health, 6*(2), 311–327.

Ross, C., & Wu, C. (1995). Links between education and health. *American Sociological Review, 60*, 719–745.

Sachs, J. (2005). *The end of poverty*. London: Penguin.

Sachs, J. (2010). The MDG decade: Looking and conditional optimisim for 2015. *The Lancet, 376*, 950–951.

Sepúlveda, M. (2003). *The nature of the obligations under the International Covenant on Economic, Social and Cultural Rights*. Utrecht, The Netherlands: Intersentia.

Setel, P., Macfarlane, S., Szreter, S., Mikkelsen, L., Jha, P., Stout, S., Abouzahr, C.; Monitoring of Vital Events. (2007). The scandal of invisibility: Making everyone count by counting everyone. *The Lancet, 370*(9598), 1569–1577.

Skolnik, R. (2008). *Essentials of global health*. Boston, MA: Jones and Bartlett.

Smith, J. A. (1981). The idea of health: A philosophical inquiry. *Advances in Nursing Science, 3*(3), 43.

Smith, K. V., & Sulzbach, S. (2008). Community-based health insurance and access to maternal health services: Evidence from three West African countries. *Social Science and Medicine, 66*, 2460–2473.

Smith, J. M., Gubin, R., Holston, M., Fullerton, J., & Prata, N. (2013). Misoprostol for postpartum hemorrhage prevention at home birth: An integrative review of global implementation experience to date. *BMC Pregnancy and Childbirth, 13*(1), 44.

Thompson, J. (2007). Poverty, development and women: Why should we care? *Journal of Obstetrics, Gynecology and Neonatal Nursing, 36*, 523–530.

United Nations AIDS. (2013). Women, girls, gender equality and HIV. New York, NY: United Nations. Retrieved from http://www.unaids.org/en/media/unaids/contentassets/documents/factsheet/2012/20120217_FS_WomenGirls_en.pdf

United Nations. (1989). *Convention on the rights of the child (CRC)*. New York, NY: United Nations.

United Nations. (2000). *The Millennium Summit*. New York, NY: United Nations. Retrieved from http://www.un.org/millenniumgoals/

United Nations. (2012a). *The Millennium Development Goals Report 2012*. New York, NY: United Nations. Retrieved from http://www.undp.org/content/dam/undp/library/MDG/english/The_MDG_Report_2012.pdf

United Nations. (2012b). *UNAIDS report on the AIDS epidemic*. New York, NY: United Nations. Retrieved from http://www.unaids.org/en/media/unaids/contentassets/documents/epidemiology/2012/gr2012/20121120_FactSheet_Global_en.pdf

United Nations. (2013a). *The Millennium Development Goals 2013 Report*. New York, NY: United Nations. Retrieved from http://www.un.org/millenniumgoals/pdf/report-2013/mdg-report-2013-english.pdf

United Nations. (2013b). *Countdown to 2015. Maternal, newborn, and chlild health survival*. New York, NY: United Nations. Retrieved from http://www.countdown2015mnch.org/documents/2013Report/Countdown_2013-Update_noprofiles.pdf

United Nations. (2014). *Every women every child*. New York, NY: United Nations. Retrieved from http://www.everywomaneverychild.org/about

Van Lerberghe, W., Matthews, Z., Achadi, E., Ancona, C., Campbell, J., Channon, A., . . . Turkmani, S. (2014). Country experience with strengthening of health systems and deployment of midwives in countries with high maternal mortality. *The Lancet*. doi:10.1016/S0140-6736(14)60919-3

Venro. (2009). *Re-thinking biomass energy for sub-Saharan Africa*. Retrieved from http://www.venro.org/fileadmin/redaktion_afrikas_perspektive/publikationen/Projekt-Publikationen/091124_Arfikas-Perspektive_Bioenergiestudie_Final.pdf

United Nations Economic and Social Council (ECOSOC). (2014). *Millenneum Development Goals and the post development agenda*. Retrieved from http://www.un.org/en/ecosoc/about/mdg.shtml

United States Agency for International Development. (2014). *Demographic and Health Survey Program*. Retrieved from http://www.dhsprogram.com/

Walker, C. L. F., Rudan, I., Liu, L., Nair, H., Theodoratou, E., Bhutta, Z. A., . . . Black, R. E. (2013). Global burden of childhood pneumonia and diarrhoea. *The Lancet, 381*(9875), 1405–1416. doi:10.1016/S0140-6736(13)60222-6

Winslow, C. E. A. (1920). The untilled fields of public health. *Science, 51*(1306), 23–33.

World Bank. (1993). *Investing in health: World development report*. New York, NY: Oxford University Press.

World Bank. (2014). *Poverty overview*. Retrieved from http://www.worldbank.org/en/topic/poverty/overview.

World Health Organization. (1947). *Constitution of the World Health Organization* (p. 1). Retrieved from http://whqlibdoc.who.int/hist/official_records/constitution.pdf

World Health Organization. (1978, September 6–12). *Declaration of Alma-Ata*. Adopted at the International Conference on Primary Health Care, Alma-Ata, USSR.

World Health Organization. (2000). *World health report: Health systems improving performance*. Geneva, Switzerland: World Health Organization. Retrieved from http://www.who.int/whr/2000/en/

references (continued)

World Health Organization. (2004). *World development report 2004: Making services work for poor people*. Washington, DC: The World Bank.

World Health Organization. (2006). *The global shortage of health workers and its impact*. Fact sheet No. 302. Retrieved from http://www.who.int/mediacentre/factsheets/fs302/en/

World Health Organization. (2008). *Definition of the sector wide approach in glossary of globalization trade and health terms*. Retrieved from http://www.who.int/trade/glossary/story081/en/

World Health Organization. (2009). *Global standards for the initial education of professional nurses and midwives* (WHO/HRH/HPN/08.6) (pp. 40). Geneva, Switzerland: World Health Organization. Retrieved from http://www.who.int/hrh/nursing_midwifery/hrh_global_standards_education.pdf

World Health Organization. (2009). Injuries: The neglected burden in developing countries. *Bulletin of the World Health Organization, 87*, 246–246. doi:10.2471/BLT.08.052290

World Health Organization. (2010). *Global code of practice on the International Recruitment of Health Personnel*. Retrieved from http://www.who.int/hrh/migration/code/code_en.pdf

World Health Organization. (2011). *Global status report on non-communicable diseases*. Geneva, Switzerland: World Health Organization.

World Health Organization (2012a). *Born too soon: The global action report on preterm birth*. Retrieved from http://www.who.int/pmnch/media/news/2012/preterm_birth_report/en/index2.html

World Health Organization. (2012b). *Countdown 2015. Partnership for maternal child health*. Geneva, Switzerland: World Health Organization. Retrieved from http://www.countdown2015mnch.org/documents/2012Report/2012-part-2.pdf

World Health Organization. (2013a). *Achieving health-related MDGs*. Retrieved from http://www.who.int/hrh/workforce_mdgs/en/index.html

World Health Organization. (2013b). *Roll back malaria program*. Retrieved from http://www.rollbackmalaria.org/keyfacts.html

World Health Organization. (2013c). *World health statistics report*. Geneva: WHO. Retrieved from http://www.who.int/gho/publications/world_health_statistics/EN_WHS2013_Full.pdf

World Health Organization. (2014a). *Global health observatory*. Retrieved from http://www.who.int/gho/en/

World Health Organization. (2014b). *Maternal mortality: Fact sheet*. Retrieved from http://www.who.int/mediacentre/factsheets/fs348/en/

World Health Organization. (2014c). *Infant and young children: Fact sheet*. Retrieved from http://www.who.int/mediacentre/factsheets/fs342/en/

Yakoob, M. Y., Theodoratou, E., Jabeen, A., Imdad, A., Eisele, T., Ferguson, J., Bhutta, Z. A. (2011). Preventive zinc supplementation in developing countries: Impact on mortality and morbidity due to diarrhea, pneumonia and malaria. *BMC Public Health, 11*(Suppl 3), S23.

web resources

Please visit thePoint® for up-to-date web resources on this topic.

Evidence-Based Practice and Population Health

PART

two

CHAPTER 5

Frameworks for Health Promotion, Disease Prevention, and Risk Reduction

Rosanna F. DeMarco and Mary Margaret Segraves

Perplexity is the beginning of knowledge.

Khalil Gibran

In theory there's no difference between theory and practice. In practice there is.

Yogi Berra

If the facts don't fit the theory, change the facts.

Albert Einstein

chapter highlights

- Influences on health and well-being
- Role of the nurse as an interdisciplinary team member in health promotion and prevention
- Health promotion programs
- Epidemiologic models of health promotion and public health science
- Levels of prevention and pathogenesis
- Immunizations
- Screening
- Behavior change theories
- Ecologic model and women living with HIV/AIDS

objectives

- Discuss the contribution of the Centers for Disease Control and Prevention to the health and well-being of people in the United States.
- Explain three levels of prevention in relation to levels of pathogenesis.
- Identify and define health behavior change models and their practical use in altering behavior to enhance health and well-being.
- Identify a multisystem prevention approach to people, families, and communities.
- Describe epidemiologic models of health promotion and modifiable risk reduction.

key terms

Behavior change models: Models that assist clients, groups, and communities to redirect activities toward health and wellness.

Ecologic model: Models that consider intrapersonal attributes, interpersonal dynamics, person/environment interactions, cultural beliefs, and attitudes.

Health: A quality, an ability to adapt to change, or a resource to help cope with challenges and processes of daily living.

Health belief model: A behavior change model that considers the severity of the potential illness or physical challenge, the level of conceivable susceptibility, the benefits of taking preventive action, and the challenges that may be faced in taking action toward the goal of health promotion.

Learning model: A behavior change model emphasizing reinforcement of social competence, problem-solving, autonomy, and sense of purpose.

Modifiable risk: Susceptibility to disease or injury that can be controlled by individual people, families, or communities.

Motivational interviewing: Client-centered communication style for eliciting behavior change by helping clients and groups explore and resolve ambivalence to change.

Primary prevention: Maximizing health and wellness through strategies that are set in place before illness or injury is present.

Relapse prevention model: A change model that is used primarily to assist people struggling with relapse and recovery from substance use.

Risk reduction: Decreasing the chance of developing an illness, experiencing an injury, or being faced with chronic consequences of both.

Secondary prevention: Maximizing health and wellness through strategies set in place at the early and active chronic stages of illness and injury.

Social learning: A behavior change model that considers environmental influences, personal factors, and behavior as key components to change.

Social support: A component of change in which community members, friends, neighbors, and adjacent communities influence change by offering instrumental assistance, informational support, emotional support, and appraising support.

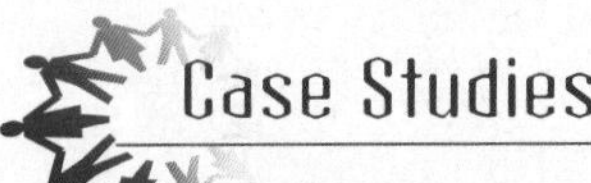

Case Studies

References to case studies are found throughout this chapter (look for the case study icon). Readers should keep the case studies in mind as they read the chapter.

The following three case studies are examples of prevention research by the Centers for Disease Control and Prevention (CDC) to address community health **risk reduction** and health promotion initiatives in people of various ages. They illustrate how healthy behaviors and risk reduction can be addressed through culturally relevant avenues using both epidemiologic evidence and the behavior change models presented in this chapter. The key to success in promoting health and reducing risk in these cases is the thoughtful, planned building of coalitions among individuals, communities, and health professionals. For example, nurses who address a particular healthcare concern need to involve members of communities in identifying goals, objectives, and solutions that can affect lifelong health promotion. It is critical that the risk be modifiable (sometimes referred to as a "modifiable risk"), which means that individual people or groups can actually do something about the problem using social competence, problem-solving, autonomy, and purpose.

CASE 1

At the CDC Prevention Research Centers (PRCs) annual program meeting, 300 participants received a bag that was a product of community prevention research. The PRC program purchased the bags from Threads of HOPE, a small business developed by community partners and the Center for Health Promotion and Disease Prevention of the University of North Carolina at Chapel Hill, one of 33 CDC-funded PRCs. Threads of HOPE is a spin-off of the center's core research project, HOPE Works, which trains community facilitators to run support groups enabling women to help each other make health and lifestyle changes. The women—who are African-American, Native American (Coharie tribe), Latina, or white—live in Sampson and Duplin Counties in eastern North Carolina, where unemployment has been high since the mid-1990s, when tobacco and textile production ceased in the area. In 2000, the poverty rate was close to 20%.

Fifteen years of researcher–community collaboration in the area has indicated that income, education, occupation, and community factors are playing a greater role in health than individual health behaviors or access to healthcare. The economic depression contributed to a sense of hopelessness that made some women less motivated to address health behaviors. The women who participate in this community-owned business receive a living wage, training in textile production and business management, health insurance, a chance to pursue higher education, and access to health promotion interventions primarily concerning nutrition and physical activity (Centers for Disease Control and Prevention [CDC], 2013a).

CASE 2

An organization known as Program to Encourage Active, Rewarding Lives for Seniors (PEARLS) was developed at the Health Promotion Research Center of the University of Washington to help combat depression in seniors. The CDC provided funding for this program, which lasts for 6 months and consists of eight in-home visits by a counselor.

Minor depression is characterized by loss of interest or pleasure in activities, and feelings of sadness or hopelessness. It strikes about 14% of seniors, many of whom are dealing with isolation, loss of friends and family, and debilitating chronic diseases. For example, seniors who have diabetes are more than twice as likely as other people of the same age to have depression. One client who had limited vision said, "I just can't contribute any more." Another woman spent weeks lying hopelessly in bed after recovering from pneumonia. Counselors help clients identify and write down the factors contributing to their depression as well as develop and evaluate solutions. One counselor said, "...just like the cold or the flu has symptoms, so does depression.... There is a close connection between depression and unsolved problems. If the problem is, 'I can't do anything worthwhile,' the goal can be, 'Find something I can do on a small scale that will be beneficial to other people.'" Both the client with limited vision and the one recovering from pneumonia found help in PEARLS, which uses structured behavioral therapy and positive events to resolve depression. A counselor helped the woman with limited sight find ways to help others, such as knitting baby blankets and calling isolated people, which were activities suited to her skills, interests, and personality. Other components of PEARLS include scheduling social and physical activities and planning simple pleasures, such as taking a walk, calling a friend, or soaking in a hot bath.

In its 3-year study phase, PEARLS eliminated depression completely for more than a third of participants. Of seniors in a comparison group, who received usual care, only 12% reportedly eliminated depression completely. PEARLS also reduced depressive symptoms by half for 43% of participants—with almost three times as many people achieving that result as in the comparison group. Investigators have also found that PEARLS reduces hospitalizations, for any reason, in participants. Researchers attribute the success of PEARLS to the behavioral therapy, which affects the same parts of the brain as some antidepressant drugs. Behavioral therapy can be more permanent than drugs, is less expensive, and can be used outside a clinical setting. Because the clients come up with solutions of their own, they feel capable of following through on them (CDC, 2013e).

CASE 3

A project called Planet Health, developed by the Prevention Resource Center on Nutrition and Physical Activity at Harvard University, combines important messages on nutrition and physical activity with four academic subjects in public schools: social studies, math, science, and language arts. Even though obesity affects many American children, officials still find they must eliminate health classes, nurses, and physical education from public schools because of tight budgets.

The Planet Health curriculum meets Massachusetts academic standards and includes lessons designed to fit into a teacher's busy schedule. The programs consists of 24 lessons a year, 6 in each of the 4 main subjects—language arts, math, science, and social studies—plus special activities for physical education classes. Planet Health also challenges students to turn off televisions. Harvard researchers have shown that television viewing is directly related to obesity. The curriculum encourages children to spend less time watching television, playing video games, or using the computer—to reduce their "screen time" to 2 hours or less per day. The curriculum also includes innovative exercises to learn more about food and the properties of food, and styles of eating that make kids healthy.

In a 2-year study at 10 middle schools, Planet Health reduced the amount of time boys and girls watched television and also lowered the prevalence of obesity among girls. According to another study, the program will save money for children later in life; for every dollar spent on the program in middle school, $1.20 in medical costs and lost wages will be saved by the time the children reach middle age. Blue Cross Blue Shield of Massachusetts picked up Planet Health in 2004 as part of an overall school wellness program, and it is now used in more than 120 schools across the state. The YMCA has also started offering a version of Planet Health during after-school programs in Massachusetts. Since 2001, when the curriculum was put into book form, more than 4,000 copies have sold. Researchers are working on a new edition that will add and update information about sugar-sweetened beverages, the different types of fats, and whole grains.

Researchers and administrators say Planet Health's greatest success can be seen in the lifestyle changes it inspires—not just in the classroom, but in the community. Schools that use Planet Health have begun to hold fitness days for families, and teachers have started yoga classes for themselves (CDC, 2013f).

key terms (continued)

Tertiary prevention: Maximizing health and wellness through strategies that are set in place at the palliation and end stage of disease and injury trajectories.

Theory of reasoned action: A behavior model emphasizing that individual performance of a given behavior is primarily determined by a person's intention to perform that behavior.

Transtheoretical model: Sequential approach to behavior change on the basis of process across stages and timely readiness of the learner.

Well-being: A subjective perception of full functional ability as a human being.

According to Glanz, Rimer, and Viswanath (2008), health is a quality, an ability to adapt to change, or a resource to cope with challenges and processes of daily living. Whether **health** is defined as an attribute that helps individuals, families, and communities navigate the stormy sea of life, or as an ideal state of physical, social, and mental **well-being**, the notion of health being the absence of disease is superseded by a complex relationship between health and a person's sense of wellness. For example, it is true that people who make up neighborhoods, communities, and populations can die from lack of health, but they can die well (i.e., with a sense of well-being and at a high level of human functioning). This chapter explores models of health promotion through public health science, with specific emphasis on models of risk prevention and behavior change as vehicles to well-being. In this chapter, "disease" refers not just to illness or injury at the individual level, but also from the perspective of the larger community of people in neighborhoods, cities, states, countries, and the world. An important underpinning to every effort described in this chapter is the ethical imperative to address health as a proactive approach to wellness. The chapter ends with the discussion of an inclusive and integrative behavior change model that describes the need to consider multiple influences on positive health outcomes. This is in contrast to single-focused measures that have been used in the past to develop health promotion interventions and healthcare policy. The issue of African-American women living with human immunodeficiency virus/acquired immunodeficiency syndrome (HIV/AIDS) in the United States is used as an example of how a formidable infectious and communicable disease can be addressed using this model to identify key components that influence behavior change. It also illustrates how interdisciplinary teams that include nurses identify and foster health promotion and policy change.

Every human being is the author of his own health or disease.

Buddha

HEALTH PROMOTION, DISEASE PREVENTION, AND RISK REDUCTION AS CORE ACTIVITIES OF PUBLIC HEALTH

Health has different meanings to individuals, families, and communities. Nurses working with clients in communities with a focus on population-based health gain knowledge about subjective well-being by observing individuals, families, and communities who are directly participating in improving their health. Individuals and groups interact in partnership with public health professionals to enhance their well-being and maximize their progress toward health, rather than just avoid illness, such as in the case studies at the beginning of this chapter.

Improving health is a journey of discovery among health professionals, the science of public health (epidemiology), and people who are motivated to effect change across varied and complex influences on well-being. Ten key components of public health practice are central to keeping populations healthy and safe. Nurses promote health through prevention efforts by belonging to interdisciplinary teams that address the following core activities (American Public Health Association, 2013):

1. Providing essential input to interdisciplinary programs that monitor, anticipate, and respond to public health problems in population groups, regardless of which disease or public health threat is identified
2. Evaluating health trends and risk factors of population groups and helping to determine priorities for targeted interventions
3. Working with communities or specific population groups within the community to develop public policy and targeted health promotion and disease prevention activities
4. Participating in assessing and evaluating healthcare services to ensure that people are informed of available programs and services and are assisted in the utilization of available services

It is important to understand that promoting health and wellness behaviors in individuals as members of a group or population depends on addressing all 10 core activities of public health simultaneously as an integrated whole. Each of these areas is addressed throughout this chapter in more detail. In this chapter, health promotion is presented through frameworks or models that can direct nursing practice to (1) focus on how to approach this complex and almost overwhelming concept of health at the population level; (2) become knowledgeable about how and why behavior change needs to be addressed, related to disease prevention and health promotion, depending on levels of control over an outcome; and (3) devise creative, cost-effective interventions and policy changes related to levels of prevention.

HEALTHY PEOPLE INITIATIVES

The *Healthy People* initiatives and *Healthy People 2000, 2010,* and *2020* (HP 2000, HP 2010, and HP 2020) are a set of health objectives established nationally to address keeping individuals, families, and populations safe and healthy (Brown, 2009). Chapter 4 discusses international approaches to public health issues on the global scale. In the United States, the CDC promotes health at the global level by promoting the sharing of knowledge, tools, and other resources as a global responsibility, as well as creating partnerships throughout the world through health promotion, health protection, and health diplomacy (CDC, 2013b). From a national perspective, HP 2020 is a guidepost for nurses and interdisciplinary teams in community and public health. HP 2020 has historic roots in efforts by the U.S. Surgeon General to establish a definitive plan for state and community organizations to address the health of citizens.

box 5.1 Healthy People 2020 New Focal Areas

1. Adolescent health
2. Blood disorders and blood safety
3. Dementias, including Alzheimer disease
4. Early and middle childhood
5. Genomics
6. Global health
7. Healthcare-associated infections
8. Health-related quality of life and well-being
9. Lesbian, gay, bisexual, and transgender health
10. Older adults
11. Preparedness
12. Sleep health
13. Social determinants of health

Source: http://www.healthypeople.gov/2020/about/new2020.aspx

The effort to establish measurable objectives was developed through a planned process that involves consulting healthcare experts locally and nationally, collecting data obtained from studies of population illness (morbidity, natural progression of disease and injury, and mortality patterns over time), engaging businesses in the process, and listening to the needs and barriers identified by citizens in the United States (Trossman, 2008). HP 2020 is designed to achieve two primary goals: (1) to increase quality and years of healthy life and (2) to eliminate any barriers to accessing care, specifically through health disparities. Currently, 42 topic areas with congruent objectives and data are available for consideration. Of this current grouping, new seminal areas have been identified that include genomics, global health, healthcare-associated infections, LGBT (lesbian, gay, bisexual, and transgender) health, preparedness, and social determinants of health (HP 2020, 2013). Box 5.1 lists all of the new areas of interest in HP 2020.

Where would the first case study, about Threads of HOPE, fit in terms of addressing HP 2020 indicators and focal areas? Identifying specific indicators and focal areas that support health promotion means very little unless professionals in community or public health practice, such as nurses, consider partnerships to be necessary in the promotion of community health. Do you think that Threads of HOPE addresses a particular focal point that is missing from the HP 2020 project?

Knowing how to address the need for change and the actual change at a personal, family, and community level must be based on science—evidence based on rigorous understanding of a problem. Specific actions that can best achieve positive health outcomes can then be determined. Consideration must be given to realistic availability of solutions, cost and benefits, and the degree to which individual people will accept these approaches. It seems too simple to assume that promoting identified HP 2020 goals and objectives in tandem with known scientific methods will promote the health of the nation. Many complicated factors affect the process of educating the public about health, such as people's knowledge of their risk of disease, subsequent health outcomes, and the personal or communal choice to be healthy. It is necessary to consider individual and family perspectives about health and wellness, as well as community definitions of these concepts.

STUDENT REFLECTION

I will never forget giving a presentation to a group of men and women in a senior center as my first effort in trying to convince them that cholesterol was a silent killer. After sharing age- and education-specific information from the American Heart Association and the CDC demonstrating dietary and exercise choices to promote health, one man got up and said, "What difference does it make; we all are going to die from something and I would rather eat fried foods than not eat them." Many people around him nodded their heads, and I realized that until people are convinced that scientific evidence applies to them and that their choices affect their personal well-being, family, and increasing costs in healthcare, we are stuck with lofty goals by tradition rather than through transformation into something new.

The role of the community and the public health nurse in promoting health is challenged by the way health information is shared (cultural relevance), the choices people make (behaviors), the places where people live (social conditions and environment), and the access to care (healthcare insurance coverage, availability of healthcare, and quality of care received) (Andersen et al., 2008). Thus, it is critical to seek out health promotion and behavior change models to use to provide direction in making health promotion, disease prevention, and risk reduction efforts real.

ROAD MAPS TO HEALTH PROMOTION

Epidemiologic Model and Prevention

Although illness care is a primary component of the art and science of nursing, health promotion and disease prevention are important, closely related public health efforts in achieving the goals of nursing care. By definition, health promotion is an action or effort that supports the well-being of individuals, groups, and communities by reducing risk of illness and injury (Markle-Reid et al., 2006). In this chapter, the word "disability" is replaced with the words "physical challenges" or "injury," to emphasize that there is always "ability" to deal with structural and functional problems (Mahoney, Bevers, Linos, & Willett, 2008).

Community health nurses are focused specifically on **modifiable risks** of acquiring disease. This requires nurses to analyze trends in risk surveillance data and consider the physical, emotional, and psychosocial challenges people face when confronting disease, physical stressors, and the possibility of premature death. Public health science uses in-depth processes of data collection across the natural history of disease to define trends, and in this way assists nurses and other public health officials in prioritizing the steps they need to take to minimize risk and improve the quality of care in populations.

PRACTICE POINT

The *Morbidity and Mortality Weekly Report* (MMWR), published weekly by the CDC and available online, contains useful public health information and guidelines that address trends in illness and disease. MMWR readership predominately consists of physicians, nurses, public health practitioners, epidemiologists and other scientists, researchers, educators, and laboratory-oriented professionals. The data provided in the MMWR come from state health departments and compare morbidity and mortality rates annually. These records are very helpful to public health clinicians because they supply information that promotes a proactive approach to resource planning when the rates are increasing. Public health nurses should consider a free subscription to the MMWR reports (CDC, 2013c).

Although the morbidity and mortality data reports are quantitative, it is important to understand that in most cases, perceptions of health or well-being on the part of individuals, families, and communities are subjective. The science of diagnosis and healthcare follow-up may be present, but it is the subjective perceptions of others that often determine a person's willingness to participate in health promotion initiatives. For example, if people perceive that health or "low risk" means the absence of acute symptoms or the absence of disease, many of them may consider themselves healthy and in no need of making an effort toward health promotion. In fact, they could actually be living with real, chronic morbid or comorbid conditions such as diabetes, hypertension, congestive heart failure, or hepatitis C, or they may be at risk for acquiring these conditions.

Keeping in mind the subjectivity of wellness, how would you develop outreach in the PEARLS program to elderly members of the community who are isolated and may want to preserve their privacy? What would be a convincing argument to make to women who are not involved in making bags with Threads of HOPE? How could you convince them that doing so would actually be an act of health promotion and would have a positive effect on their well-being?

Health promotion is a strategy that is used in partnership with health professionals, individuals, and communities. It includes all three levels of disease prevention and has the potential to, or can directly, change health and well-being. Healthcare professionals or people in communities can institute these strategies. In reality, disease and physical challenges can occur at any time. In many cases, predictions made from statistical conclusions (probabilities) through the science of epidemiology are the basis for determining the possibility of getting a disease or becoming physically or emotionally challenged (see Chapters 6 and 7). Analysis of epidemiologic data occurs while health professionals consider what happens at the prepathogenic, early pathogenic, and late pathogenic phases of diseases and physical or emotional disorders. The basis of this scientific approach is the study of causal relationships that yield pathology. Epidemiologists make conclusions about the direction of further study by considering (1) relative risk of an agent causing a problem (e.g., smoking and lung cancer); (2) consistency (i.e., similar results across other studies); (3) exposure (i.e., correlation with a certain distinct pathologic condition such as asbestos and mesothelioma); (4) timing (i.e., cause and resulting condition both occurring within a short period of time, such as inhaled fumes and an asthma attack); and (5) plausibility (i.e., existence of a biologic process) (Escoto Ponce de Leon, Mancilla Diaz, & Camacho Ruiz, 2008).

The central idea here is to prevent illness and physical or emotional challenges from occurring. Or, if they do occur, the goal is to lessen their effects and enhance clients' quality of life. The science of epidemiology helps health professionals such as nurses, and coalitions of interested citizens, develop interventions for the stages of illness or physical or emotional challenges, which enhance the quality of life of individuals and communities. In Figure 5.1, health and wellness change along a developmental timeline. After a disease or physical challenge is identified, it progresses and eventually becomes life-threatening. Although this pattern appears to be linear, in reality the linearity is theoretical. Illness occurs erratically; there are times of stability and times of acute and stressful exacerbation (Ross, Mathis, & Brockopp, 2008). At each pathogenic level, health promotion is intimately linked to prevention.

Levels of Prevention

Activities classified as "preventive" are directed at eradicating, eliminating, or reducing the impact of disease and injury on individuals and populations, thus promoting health instead of disease (Gasink & Lautenbach, 2008). *Disease* in this context refers to communicable and noncommunicable conditions. Examples of noncommunicable diseases (noninfectious diseases or physical or emotional challenges) are substance abuse, obesity, depression, or workplace injuries. Physical or emotional challenges, as well as genetic disorders, are conditions that are generally noncommunicable in nature but cause structural and functional changes that are not statistically normal in the general population. Some examples include glaucoma, scoliosis, Down syndrome, neurofibromatosis, hearing loss, and learning disabilities. Communicable diseases are caused by pathogens (e.g., viruses and bacteria) that multiply and enter hosts through a variety of mechanisms and influences. These diseases have the capacity to cause infections across living organisms, with life-threatening and potentially chronic effects. Examples include HIV, malaria, swine flu, and smallpox (Kieny, Excler, & Girard, 2004).

What type of diseases (communicable or noncommunicable) do the programs in each case study address? Could addressing noncommunicable diseases or physical or emotional challenges through these programs influence vulnerability or resistance to communicable diseases in these populations?

To understand specific health promotion approaches, nurses should think in terms of three levels: primary, secondary, and tertiary prevention. The individual person's or the community's state of health and well-being, as studied within the science of identification, description, and prediction of illness, serve as the basis for the levels.

Primary Prevention

When an individual or a group is considered in good health and shows no signs or symptoms of disease or physical challenges, nurses in interdisciplinary teams and community partnerships are involved in primary prevention. They seek to maximize health and wellness, using a variety of strategies, at a time when they or the clients have some level of control over the trajectory of health and wellness. Examples of primary prevention include the use of seat belts, hand washing, proper preparation of food, exercise, and balanced nutrition (Box 5.2).

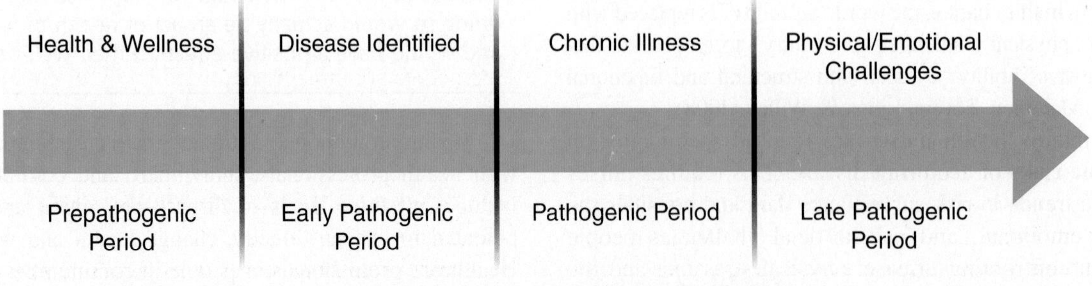

figure 5.1 Natural history of disease and levels of wellness/illness continuum.

box 5.2 Examples of Primary Prevention

Immunizations
Driver's safety classes
Healthy water quality
Healthy air quality
Health education classes
Improving safety designs of equipment
Fire safety
Decreasing exposure to sun
Use of environmentally safe products
Using seat belts
Using earplugs and safety glasses

Surveillance of healthy populations is a continual, dynamic method of gathering data about the health of the general public for the purpose of primary prevention of illness. The CDC and individual states monitor emerging and endemic health hazards that occur in community settings on an ongoing basis. Data are systematically collected, analyzed, interpreted, and disseminated so that they can be used to develop activities and programs that will reduce morbidity and mortality and improve health. The functions of public health surveillance are described in Box 5.3. In addition, local surveillance of community populations can be obtained by using various records—from clinics, community health and visiting nurses, worker's compensation settlements, personnel files, and the like.

It is critical to understand that there are situations in which primary prevention is difficult to achieve at the individual or community level. Sometimes, even with professional support and healthcare information, clients are unable to avoid experiencing disease or physical challenges because the causative agents are "not modifiable," for example, genetic conditions, unexpected tragedies (natural disasters such as floods or tornados), and situations in which there is no developmental control, such as the effect of secondhand smoke. These would be considered conditions where primary prevention strategies are difficult to implement and not modifiable.

Great things are done by a series of small things brought together.

Vincent Van Gogh

An important example of primary prevention is the availability and dispensing of vaccines developed to enhance the body's ability to create antibodies to either live or attenuated antigens. This approach protects individuals and populations from getting communicable diseases, or lessens the severity of the disease. Immunization with vaccines is an effective way to promote primary prevention. Nurses who actively participate in the immunization of children in well-child clinics, young adults in university health clinics, and adults in international travel clinics are promoting primary prevention of measles, human papillomavirus (American Cancer Society, 2013), and yellow fever, respectively. See Box 5.4 for a list of vaccine-preventable diseases (CDC, 2013g).

box 5.3 Functions of Public Health Surveillance

Estimating the impact of a disease or injury
Portraying the natural history of a health condition
Determining the distribution and spread of illness
Generating hypotheses and stimulating research
Evaluating prevention and control measures
Facilitating planning for program activities
Detecting outbreaks

Source: Centers for Disease Control and Prevention. (2004). Framework for evaluating public health surveillance systems for early detection of outbreaks. *Morbidity and Mortality Weekly Report, 53*(RR-05), 1–11.

box 5.4 Vaccine-Preventable Diseases

Anthrax
Cervical cancer
Diphtheria
Hepatitis A
Hepatitis B
Haemophilus influenzae type b (Hib)
Human papillomavirus (HPV)
Influenza (flu)
Japanese encephalitis
Lyme disease
Measles
Meningococcal disease
Monkeypox
Mumps
Pertussis (whooping cough)
Pneumococcal Pneumonia
Poliomyelitis (polio)
Rabies
Rotavirus
Rubella (German measles)
Shingles (herpes zoster)
Smallpox
Tetanus (lockjaw)
Tuberculosis
Typhoid fever
Varicella (chickenpox)
Yellow fever

According to the CDC (2013g), immunity to a disease results from the presence of antibodies to that disease. Antibodies are proteins produced by the body to neutralize or destroy toxins or disease-carrying organisms, and they are disease specific. For example, antibodies to measles protect a person who is exposed to measles but have no effect if the person is exposed to mumps. There are two types of immunity: active and passive.

Active immunity results when exposure to a disease organism triggers the immune system to produce antibodies to that disease. Exposure to the disease organism can occur through infection with the actual live organism (resulting in natural immunity), or introduction of a dead or weakened form of the disease organism through vaccination (vaccine-induced immunity). Either way, if an immune person comes into contact with a disease, his or her immune system will recognize it and immediately produce the antibodies needed to fight it. Active immunity is long-lasting, sometimes lifelong.

PRACTICE POINT

It may be important for nurses working with clients older than 60, or in communities where chronic illnesses abound, to consider the use of the vaccine against shingles. Shingles is a painful localized skin rash, often accompanied by blisters, caused by the varicella zoster virus (VZV), the same virus that causes chickenpox. Any person who has had chickenpox can develop shingles because VZV remains in the nerve cells of the body after the chickenpox infection clears and can reappear many years later. Shingles most commonly occurs in people 50 years of age or older, in those who have medical conditions that keep the immune system from working properly, or in those who receive immunosuppressive drugs. The vaccine against shingles is recommended by the Advisory Committee on Immunization Practices (ACIP) to reduce the risk of this condition and its associated pain in people 60 years of age or older. See http://www.cdc.gov/vaccines/vpd-vac/shingles/default.htm for further information.

Passive immunity results when a person is given antibodies to a disease rather than producing them through his or her own immune system. A newborn infant acquires passive immunity from its mother through the placenta. This type of immunity can also occur with the use of antibody-containing blood products such as immune globulin, which may be given when immediate protection from a specific disease is needed. This is the major advantage to passive immunity; protection is immediate, whereas active immunity takes time (usually several weeks) to develop. However, passive immunity lasts only for a few weeks or months. Only active immunity is long-lasting. *Herd immunity* is a type of passive immunity; the presence of a large proportion of immune individuals in a community decreases the chances of contact between any infected people and susceptible individuals. An entire population need not be immune to prevent an epidemic of a disease. Herd immunity is often attributed to either antibody formation, which occurs when populations acquire an illness in a non–life-threatening form due to medical care interventions or reduced virulence, or to vaccination programs.

Secondary Prevention

Secondary prevention is a planned effort to minimize the impact of disease or injury once it is in effect. Secondary prevention is used at an early stage of pathogenesis or physical or emotional challenges. It includes, through the science of screening, initial recognition of the stage of an illness or physical challenge, which can progress to greater or lesser severity over time. The types of screening procedures and examples are found in Box 5.5.

box 5.5 Types and Examples of Screening Procedures

Mass screening: applied to entire populations
Blood lead level screening
Papanicolaou (Pap) smears
Phenylketonuria of newborns
Selective screening: performed for specific high-risk populations
Mammographies for young women at high risk for cancer
Tuberculin tests for hospital employees
Occupational diseases
Exposure to radiation
Multiphasic screening: a variety of screening tests applied to the same population on the same occasion. Data can be used for establishing baseline data in a healthcare facility and for risk factor appraisal
Series of tests performed on a single blood sample
Periodic surveillance of drug therapy
Monitoring the stage of an illness
Case finding: clinician's search for illness as a part of a client's periodic health examination
Monitoring the health of individuals in a case load

Source: US Preventive Services Task Force. (2002). *Guide to Clinical Preventive Services* (3rd ed.). McLean, VA: International Medical Publishing.

Women diagnosed with HIV/AIDS and children who are identified as having scoliosis are examples of the need for secondary prevention. To screen effectively for the presence of these conditions, a test should be (1) cost-effective, meaning that the cost of producing and distributing the screening tool is justified by the positive effect on protecting the public; (2) easy to use; (3) available to large sectors of the population at risk; (4) sensitive and specific enough to identify true positives and true negatives; (5) backed by a healthcare infrastructure that can implement programs of care for people who have a verified risk of disease or physical challenge; and (6) acceptable to clients. Sensitivity and specificity are criteria used to measure how valid and reliable a screening test can be. Sensitivity measures the strength of a screening test's ability to correctly identify people who have a disease or physical challenge. Specificity measures the strength of a screening test's ability to correctly identify people who do not have a disease or physical challenge. In an ideal world, all screen tests should have both high sensitivity (100%) and high specificity (100%). The 100% level is approached but not met. Thus, confirmatory studies need to be undertaken to verify the presence of the disease. In the case of diseases that could be fatal, sensitivity is crucial (Box 5.6). For nurses participating in

box 5.6 Sensitivity and Specificity

Sensitivity = testing correctly to identify persons who have the disease/physical challenge
High sensitivity: True positive (people who have the disease and test positive)
Low sensitivity: False negative (people who have the disease but test negative [normal])
Specificity = testing to identify persons who do not have the disease
High specificity: True negative (people who do not have the disease and test negative)
Low specificity: False positive (people who do not have the disease but test positive [abnormal])

screening and delivering results of screening, it is most important to be aware of the test's limitations of validity and reliability, and to remember that serious economic costs to communities and health systems can be incurred when testing is not accurate. Nurses should also be aware of the psychological costs when a false-positive result occurs, which can create debilitating fear and anxiety. Calculation of sensitivity and specificity is discussed in Chapter 7.

STUDENT REFLECTION

I recently participated in an immersion trip to Central America as a nursing student. I kept asking questions of our guides about disease screening and secondary prevention related to breast cancer, HIV, human papillomavirus, cholesterol, and high blood pressure. In several instances, it was clear that no screening was being performed in some of the areas. I was upset that screening, which has been established as reputable and accurate, was not occurring—especially in population groups that suffered from poverty and nonoptimal living situations (lack of running water, outdoor ditches for latrines, garbage dumps as housing, unavailable barrier protection with sexual intimacy). After discussions with local health officials, it was clear that the lack of health personnel to offer the screening, the cost of the necessary materials, and the severe lack of infrastructure to follow-up if people tested "positive" meant that there could be no screening at all. This stunned me and allowed me to understand the economic and ethical considerations related to screening and secondary prevention.

For example, when a client is tested initially for HIV with the OraQuick HIV test for oral fluid, a test supported by the CDC based on many years of serum testing (CDC, 2013d), the healthcare team has a responsibility to verify these findings despite the high sensitivity and specificity of this test (99.3% and 99.8%, respectively). If a person tests positive for HIV, the initial result is confirmed by using an HIV antibody test known as the enzyme-linked immunosorbent assay (ELISA), which was developed in the 1980s (Homsy, Thomson-Honnebier, Cheng-Mayer, & Levy, 1988). After all confirmatory HIV testing has been completed and infectious disease experts, including physicians and nurses specializing in infectious disease, have reviewed the findings, these professionals may consider the client to be at the stage of illness early in the trajectory of pathogenesis. For example, the client may have a low viral load or absent viral load with a CD4 count greater than 200 cells/μL. This would mean that the client has ability to fight infection and that replication of the virus is not high. Involving this client in medical care, with the support of infectious disease services such as housing, nutrition services, counseling, addiction recovery, financial support, and primary care services, offers him or her the potential to maintain health and wellness.

Some may question the use of the word "prevention" here, when indeed the person already has a confirmed diagnosis of HIV. In this context, secondary prevention means that efforts are being made to minimize (1) any further extension of the HIV illness to "full-blown" AIDS (CD4 count less than 200 cells/μL, with detectable viral loads); (2) the need to use antiretroviral medications, which have severe and debilitating side effects; (3) any exacerbation of other comorbidities that could affect HIV status, such as intravenous drug use; and (4) any possibility of communicating the virus to others. People living with HIV/AIDS need to have support to counter perceptions of stigma and discrimination that can lead to depression. Depression can be linked with decreased healthcare adherence, which can cause HIV to worsen and AIDS to develop. If these clients are sexually active and not using safe sex practices, which include not maintaining recovery from substance abuse and not using barrier protection, the virus will be spread to others and they, in turn, may become infected with another strain of the virus.

Is it possible to screen for the problems identified in the three case studies (depression, nutrition, and physical activity)? How would this screening occur? What resources would be used?

In a school screening program for idiopathic scoliosis, a school nurse may find that a child has an anatomical abnormality. Depending on the stage of the abnormality, the school nurse makes appropriate referrals on the basis of orthopedic and neurologic screening standards (Scoliosis Screening, 2013). Generally, scoliosis screening is conducted because of evidence-based predictions of development at a cross-section of time when identification of the problem is critical to timely interventions.

Sometimes, when screening is completed, the client's level of disease or injury is found to be at a more advanced stage and is not considered to have been "caught early." This is true for many women of color who are tested for HIV. History of intimate partner violence may inhibit personal motivation to receive care, or may create situations where the client may not be free to get care. Lack of healthcare insurance, mental health challenges, and active substance addictions can also cause women to delay testing for HIV. Subsequently, when they are diagnosed, they may be very ill, experiencing the life-threatening chronic and/or end stage of the illness called AIDS (Earnshaw, Smith, Chaudoir, Lee, & Copenhaver, 2012).

The U.S. government requires screenings for some conditions and not others. Some screenings are mandatory because of the physical and economic costs that may result if they are not performed (e.g., newborn screenings). On the other hand, some people see screenings as stigmatizing and may experience feeling of vulnerability or discrimination in a variety of ways (interpersonally, with regard to health insurance, and at work). Although there are efforts to make HIV screening mandatory and the usual practice, for instance, there has been strong resistance to this (Mahajan, Stemple, Shapiro, King, & Cunningham, 2009). HIV testing continues to be voluntary, no matter the stage of disease at which the client presents. Thus, HIV diagnosis can lead to different prevention plans (secondary or tertiary) based on the staging.

Tertiary Prevention

Tertiary prevention is the long-term management and treatment of clients with chronic conditions, such as HIV/AIDS and cancer, so that quality of life is maintained, despite the fact that the condition will not improve and will most likely worsen. Tertiary prevention includes rehabilitation and palliative care. AIDS-related cancers such as lymphoma are not uncommon. In general, cancer is a life-threatening illness that may occur along with other conditions. Cardiovascular disease, diabetes, and pulmonary disease may be present as well, and require clinicians such as nurses to plan clients' cancer treatment, continue to assess HIV/AIDS disease progression, watch for opportunistic infections, and control pain or other side effects of the treatment. Care also includes supporting life choices that bring emotional comfort to clients such as family involvement, decreased isolation, supportive spiritual development, and organized help from communities.

PRACTICE POINT

Public health nurses should become familiar with those resources available to communities that can help address prevention at all levels. Local and state health departments have directories of both publically and privately funded prevention support programs and services, and many hospital systems provide directories for clients to consider in their time of need. Finally, Internet-based directories are being created to help citizens find a network of services in their community or region.

For example, nurses involved in cardiac care might do the following: rather than envisioning end-stage cardiac rehabilitation as the focus of prevention after a cardiovascular event, or when cardiovascular disease is prominent in a community, they could think about approaches to prevention that are inclusive of all stages of health promotion and prevention. Many cardiovascular centers provide unique, prevention-as-treatment approaches for communities with high incidence and prevalence rates for heart disease, or an unusual number of people who are at risk for developing heart disease. Interdisciplinary teams of clinicians, including nurses, offer clients and communities the strategies and tools necessary to reduce their risks. For example:

- Primary prevention programs: Clients and families who are at risk for heart disease because of family history are treated. This level of prevention focuses on evaluation of personal risks in light of family history to help clients reach their heart health goals.
- Rehabilitation: Cardiac rehabilitation programs assist clients and families in recovery from heart attacks, angioplasty, and cardiac surgery and provide them with important information to make lifestyle changes to prevent recurrence.
- Associated comorbidities programs: Clients and families at risk for, or who already have, diabetes are assisted in weight loss and in managing other cardiac risk factors such as hypertension and high cholesterol. In addition, they are assisted in managing the combination of effects the illnesses have on daily life.

Therapies can include monitored exercise, stress management, yoga and meditation, nutrition counseling, smoking cessation, weight management, and stress testing.

In summary, prevention efforts are intended to decrease the physical, psychological, and economic costs of chronic, serious illness as well as physical and emotional challenges. Efforts to address these potential costs use an epidemiologic model of levels of prevention throughout the natural history of disease (prepathogenesis, early pathogenesis, and pathogenesis across time). These efforts include the use of immunizations, screening, and rehabilitation (see Figs. 5.1 and 5.2). Health promotion using this model is based on public health science and surveillance of trends related to diagnoses that are identified through sensitive and specific screening tests and the natural history of particular diseases. Nurses in public and community health practice, being advocates of decreasing risk in populations, use this model to care for individuals, groups, and communities through instrumental care or through health policy.

BEHAVIOR MODELS

The focus of prevention efforts is the development of culturally relevant and gender-sensitive interventions which demonstrate positive outcomes in health and well-being. To promote health and well-being, one of the key approaches of primary, secondary, and tertiary prevention is a focused effort to change behaviors that have a negative impact on the natural history of disease and to promote behaviors that have a positive impact on the natural history of disease. Approaching

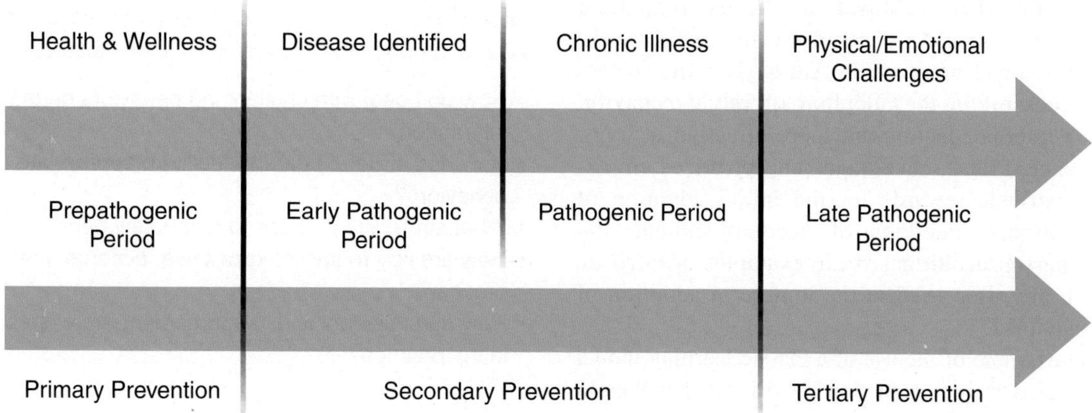

figure 5.2 Natural history of disease, levels of wellness/illness and levels of prevention continuum.

individuals and groups about behavior change must incorporate knowledge of diverse client perspectives, and include the use of counseling skills and motivational interviewing.

Motivational interviewing, which was developed by Rollnick and Miller (1995), is defined as a "directive, client-centered communication style for eliciting behavior change by helping clients/[groups] to explore and resolve ambivalence" (Motivational Interviewing, 2009). It is a focused, goal-directed approach (Box 5.7). It originated with experiences of problem drinkers who presented themselves to clinicians; the drinkers needed help to change a behavior, although they wanted to continue it (ambivalence). To address behavior change using this method, the motivation comes from the client and is not imposed by a clinician. The client needs to resolve ambivalence to change a behavior with autonomy. Persuasion on the part of the clinician only intensifies resistance. The communication style is therefore one of directing the client to examine and resolve ambivalence. This method does not (1) argue with a group or community by insisting it has a problem that needs to change, (2) offer advice without actively encouraging group-identified choices, (3) give advice while the group is put in a passive role, (4) impose diagnostic labels, or (5) use coercive tactics. Motivational interviewing teaches all clinicians

box 5.7 Actions Involved in Motivational Interviewing Behaviors for Clinicians

Seek to understand the person's frame of reference through reflective listening.
Express acceptance and affirmation.
Elicit and select reinforcing motivational statements of problem recognition, concern, desire, intention, and ability to change.
Monitor the degree of readiness to change and ensure that resistance is not generated by clinician control.
Affirm freedom of choice and direction.

Source: www.motivationalinterview.org/clinical/whatismi.html

that making efforts to change behavior is based on a clinician–client exchange. Whether individuals or groups represent specific interests in communities, participation in decision-making, informed consent, advocacy, and health literacy must be considered in using models of behavior change.

The quality of health at the individual, family, and community level is influenced by many factors. As discussed earlier, decreasing health disparities was an objective of HP 2010, and was identified as a key component in addressing barriers for some community dwellers who may desire to keep healthy and are ready to do so. So, despite the desire to change a behavior, there may be social, economic, or biologic nonmodifiable influences that prevent change. Behavior health models describe, explain, or predict prevention health behaviors. The models discussed here are available to help nurses consider creative methods of implementing the preventive measures identified earlier in this chapter. Although they appear to stand alone as unique and unrelated frameworks of behavior change, consideration of multiple influences cannot help but foster health, as in a "perfect world" (ie, one in which nurses understand this concept and use all these methods together). The following section describes the theoretical frameworks of behavior change and many of the **behavior change models** that have been used to address health promotion and risk reduction (Behavior Change Theories and Models, 2009). This section ends by describing the ecologic model. The ecologic model is a model that considers multiple influences as a way to address complex behaviors to promote health at the individual, environmental, and policy level.

Learning Theories

According to Skinner (1953), health behaviors are seen as incremental steps toward a final goal. In the so-called **learning model**, a goal is established and reinforced by the nurse, with rewards given for partial accomplishment, if necessary. Incremental increases are then made as the pattern of behavior is shaped toward a specific goal.

Reinforcement is used as motivation to either continue or discontinue a behavior. This model uses extrinsic, or external, factors for reinforcement. Although extrinsic factors are successful in the adoption of initial behavior, intrinsic, or internal, factors are more effective in long-term adherence. Praise, encouragement, or prizes are examples of extrinsic rewards for the initial adoption of healthy behaviors. Feelings of accomplishment and changes in person health habits are examples of intrinsic rewards that are often used in the long-term adoption of healthy behaviors.

A good example of the use of a classic learning model is the syndicated weight reduction program called Weight Watchers. Through the use of group encouragement, incremental weight loss is rewarded with public recognition and even a presented "ribbon" or "star" to indicate success. Intrinsic rewards, including the ability to show successful weight loss, as well as leadership opportunities within the program, can be helpful to people just beginning Weight Watchers, and have been documented within the past 10 years (Mitchell, Ellison, Hill, & Tsai, 2013).

Nurses in home care situations who work with clients with chronic illnesses, such as diabetes, congestive heart failure, and hypertension, have used the learning approach successfully while being actively involved in teaching and surveillance of client care. The difficulty with this approach is that there is a high level of expectation that intrinsic rewards will last over time, despite the influence of social norms and economic conditions. For example, in inner city communities, it is not uncommon to find a dearth of grocery stores, fresh fruit and vegetable stands, and farmer's markets as options for purchasing low-calorie, low-fat, and low-cost healthy foods. Instead, small stores sell high-calorie, high-fat processed foods (Baker, Schootman, Barnidge, & Kelly, 2006). Thus, clients with diabetes may have received intrinsic and extrinsic rewards for glycemic control but have little opportunity for continuity given the economic and social choices available in their communities.

Anything that changes your values changes your behavior.

George A. Sheehan

EVIDENCE FOR PRACTICE

Watling and Schwartz (2004) describe the application of positive reinforcement in occupational therapy by reviewing the efficacy of positive reinforcement in child behavior, which is well established in literature. Positive reinforcement has been used successfully in research studies to increase social behavior, improve cognitive and language skills, increase functional skills, and improve play skills. For example, the authors suggest that as the incidence of autism increases, all clinicians could benefit by examining their usual practice and including the use of positive reinforcement when applying learning theory. The questions that should be asked in reference to practices related to clients, groups, and communities are as follows:

- How do I deal with challenging behaviors during an interaction?
- How do I structure care to facilitate appropriate behaviors?
- What strategies do I use to teach new behaviors?
- How am I currently using positive reinforcement in my practice?
- How can I use positive reinforcement more effectively in my practice?

Health Belief Model

The **health belief model**, developed by Hochbaum (1956) and Rosenstock (1974), specifies that individual, family, or community health-related behavior depends on (1) the severity of the potential illness or physical challenge, (2) the level of conceivable susceptibility, (3) the benefits of taking preventive action, and (4) what stands in the way of taking action toward the goal of health promotion. This model uses cues as an important way to remind people of healthy behaviors and to promote these actions. Examples of this model include posting a note stating, "Don't overdo it at dinner" (individual) or "Let's try to do one thing tonight that is not related to a television set" (family), and placing a "Got Milk?" billboard in the neighborhood (community/population). Critical to this approach is the belief that the cue messages can be accomplished. If a community group does not believe that they can sustain a "walking" club in a safe section of a neighborhood, cues will not successfully encourage community members to follow a walking program. At the individual level, age-specific considerations are important. If people think they are healthy, they will not adhere to a preventive health program. Older people, who more readily see chronic illness and death as imminent, may become frightened with the prospect of susceptibility, while younger people often believe that they are invincible and impervious to illness and physical challenges.

EVIDENCE FOR PRACTICE

Spector (2007), a nurse, used the health belief model to undertake a descriptive research study. This qualitative study explored the relationships between lifestyle behaviors and risk-reduction strategies in women with the BRCA1 or BRCA2 gene mutation. These two human gene mutations are associated with a significant increase in the risk of breast cancer, as well as some other cancers. Spector interviewed women about their perceptions regarding the benefits and risks of engaging in healthy lifestyle behaviors. Barriers to these behaviors were also a topic of discussion. Five of the women had prophylactic surgery (removal of breasts and/or ovaries), which subsequently decreased their belief that they were at risk. After genetic testing revealed that they had an elevated risk, most women changed their behavior in some way to take better care of themselves. Reported benefits of these healthier lifestyles included increased energy and improved mood. Perceived barriers were related to economics and time (e.g., more healthful eating habits are more costly, and exercise takes time). These findings suggest that there is a need for nursing interventions to improve education and enhance motivation for lifestyle reduction of risk in women with a genetic predisposition for breast and ovarian cancer.

STUDENT REFLECTION

My instructor in community health asked us to use the health belief model in caring for clients who were receiving care in a sexually transmitted infection (STI) clinic. He suggested that I show the clients some of the consequences of syphilis in particular (graphic pictures), because there had been a large increase in the incidence of the disease in the section of town where the clinic was situated. After I interviewed 10 different clients and really tried to increase their fear about the consequences of their actions, more than 50% stated that they never thought they would get an STI despite not using any precautions to reduce the chances of becoming infected. In fact, 30% of the clients revealed during assessment that this was their second or third diagnosis of syphilis. So, despite the severity of the results of the disease, other factors affected choices of risk about acquiring an STI. Some of those factors were alcohol abuse; inability to practice safe sex effectively; and trading unprotected sex for money, housing, and food (Anisha, Senior, Community Health).

Transtheoretical Model

The **transtheoretical model**, developed by Prochaska and DiClemente (1983), is a sequential approach to behavior change that involves timely readiness of the learner. This model promotes change using a five-stage process; the stages are (1) precontemplation, (2) contemplation, (3) preparation, (4) action, and (5) maintenance. Experts believe that individuals, families, and communities progress through these stages in a back-and-forth manner, not in a linear fashion. For nurses, the key to this approach is developing interventions tailored to clients' levels of readiness. For example, using this model to establish a twice-yearly blood pressure screening program in a community setting would require the following stages:

1. Precontemplation (no screening programs scheduled and no intention to schedule screening),
2. Contemplation (no screening programs scheduled but intent to start a program soon),
3. Preparation (no definite screening program but have taken steps to develop a program),
4. Action (a developed screening program and intent to sustain the program),
5. Maintenance (have had the program for some time and intend to continue), and
6. Relapse (had a program, does not have a program currently but intends to be active with a program soon).

EVIDENCE FOR PRACTICE

Herzog (2008) assessed the transtheoretical model in relation to smoking cessation using a "stage model" for health behavior as a criterion. This researcher made a systematic review of the literature, choosing studies that used the transtheoretical model in smoking cessation. To make reasonable comparisons and validity claims, Herzog stipulated that the following criteria needed to be part of the change mechanism: (1) each stage should consist of qualitatively different and mutually exclusive categories of change; (2) there is a specified ordering of the categories; (3) barriers to change for individuals should be similar within each stage; and (4) barriers to stage transitions should be different between people in the different stages. Using the stage model, the investigator concluded that smoking cessation interventions did not meet the validity test, and thus, the stages of change were not distinct enough to be helpful in intervention research.

Theory of Reasoned Action

The **theory of reasoned action** states that a person's given behavior is primarily determined by his or her *intention* to perform that behavior (Fishbein & Ajzen, 1975). This intention is determined by the person's attitude toward the behavior (beliefs about the outcomes of the behavior and value of these outcomes), and the influence of the person's societal environment or subjective norm (beliefs about what others think the person should do). The ability to perform the behavior (a belief that it can be done) is the critical aspect of the change process. Social or subjective norms are significant, and the importance of abiding by these norms is reflected in what people expect of individuals, families, and communities. For example, healthcare practitioners may use this model in smoking cessation. If a client believes that he or she cannot give up the addiction, no social norm will influence the behavior change. Smokers may isolate themselves from others, or from circumstances which might influence their belief in their ability to change. Thus, the notion of addictive behaviors being hidden to decrease social pressure is a formidable challenge when trying to encourage healthy behaviors. The theory of planned behavior (a theory that links attitudes with behavior) is aligned with the theory of reasoned action, which states that perceived control over skills is needed to perform a behavior. This is similar to Bandura's concept of self-efficacy (the belief that one is capable of achieving a certain goal which may be a behavior).

EVIDENCE FOR PRACTICE

Shepard and Towler (2007) used questionnaires to obtain information from 538 participants about their understanding of relationships between nutrition knowledge and attitudes about fat intake from meat, meat products, dairy products, and fried foods. Correlations between the sums of belief evaluations, attitudes, intention, and self-reported behavior were high (ranging from 0.40 to 0.77), with similar correlations for a subgroup of men (35 to 54 years of age). Nutrition knowledge showed some statistically significant (but small) negative correlations to attitudes. Women had higher nutrition knowledge scores and more negative views of the foods than men. The researchers concluded that nutrition knowledge is less clearly related to consumption of certain foods than to specific beliefs and attitudes.

Social Learning (Social Cognitive) Theory

Social learning, or social cognitive, theory is a behavior change approach in which environmental influences, personal factors, and attributes of the behavior itself have an effect. Most importantly, a person must believe in his or her capability to perform the behavior (self-efficacy) as well as perceive an incentive to do so (positive expectations outweigh negative). The immediate or long-term benefits must be valued. Providing skill development by modeling desired behavior can increase self-efficacy (Bandura, 1986).

EVIDENCE FOR PRACTICE

Nowakowski Sims, Noland Dodd, and Tejeda (2008) conducted a study using social learning theory to explore the influence that child maltreatment, witnessing parental violence during childhood, sibling violence, and gender have on the perpetration of dating violence. A weighted scoring method was used to determine how the severity of violence in the home affects the perpetration of dating violence. Bivariate correlations and linear regression models indicate the presence of significant associations between child maltreatment, witnessing parental violence, sibling violence, gender, and subsequent dating violence. Multiple regression analyses indicate that for men, a history of severe violence or victimization (child maltreatment and childhood witnessing of parental violence) and severe violence by siblings are strong indicators of potential dating violence perpetration.

Theories of Social Support

Family members, friends, neighbors, and adjacent communities can influence change by offering **social support**—instrumental assistance, informational support, emotional support, and/or appraising support. An example of instrumental assistance is providing transportation to buy groceries or building a safe place to walk in a community. An example of informational support would be providing a community board with information on how to obtain assistance to clean a polluted pond. An example of emotional support is calling an isolated family that has lost a child to assist them in their bereavement. An example of appraising support is giving positive feedback about a new health skill (Berkman & Glass, 2000). Although the literature suggests that social support is not equivalent to professional support, professionals can assist interested community members in organizing and developing social support opportunities that promote health in the community.

EVIDENCE FOR PRACTICE

Daly, Shin, Thakral, Selders, and Vera (2008) examined the effects of risk factors (e.g., perceived neighborhood crime) and protective factors (e.g., teacher, family, and peer support) on the level of engagement in school (n = 123 adolescents of color, varying ages, and both male and female students). Results indicated that perceived neighborhood crime and violence were uniquely predictive of school engagement. Different levels of social support (protective factors) did not modify the effects of risky neighborhood conditions on adolescents' school engagement. Age modified the relationship between perceived family social support and perceived neighborhood crime on adolescents' levels of school engagement. These results indicate that prevention and intervention programs addressing school engagement among early adolescents of color should be considered.

The Relapse Prevention Model

The **relapse prevention model** has been used specifically with issues that relate to adherence. Relapse often occurs because of (1) negative emotional states; (2) lack of, or limited coping skills; (3) decreased motivation; (4) stress; and (5) high-risk experiences. Taylor (2013) supports the idea that there are differences between a relapse and short lapse from healthy behavior, and suggests that planning a strategy related to high-risk situations is critical for success, especially in the realm of harm reduction efforts. For example, communities interested in crime prevention and harm reduction may be aware that in certain months of the year, there is an increase in violent crime. They would then create a community campaign to promote nonviolence by increasing law enforcement presence and improving faith-based, school system, elder health, and neighborhood watch supports.

EVIDENCE FOR PRACTICE

Godley, Dennis, Godley, and Funk (2004) identified and tracked relapse time after discharge from an outpatient substance abuse treatment program. The participants were teens, that is, 12 to 18 years of age (n = 563), who were randomly selected for one of five interventions. Follow-up occurred every 3 months for 1 year, and then at 30 months. The findings show that the participants could be grouped into five different categories of relapse after treatment: (1) low use of substance with limited number of days in a controlled environment, (2) low use of substance with a high number of days in a controlled environment, (3) moderate/decreasing use of substance, (4) increasing use of substance, and (5) consistently high use of substance. What this means is that there are considerable differences in the motivational needs of the participants depending on the initial response to treatment, the stability (versus increase/decrease) of the response, and the length of time spent in a controlled environment. Cannabis and alcohol were the two main substances involved, although the two groups with the poorest trajectories had increasing levels of cocaine, opiate, and other substance use at the 30-month follow-up. This study demonstrates the chronic nature of substance use, even in a subgroup of teens, and the importance of studying the complex patterns of recovery and relapse.

The Ecologic Model

The **ecologic model** stems from the original work of Bronfenbrenner (1979, 2004). This model is based on the belief that all processes occurring within individuals and their environment should be viewed as interdependent. It suggests that behavior change in individuals needs to be considered in a broader social context, including developmental history, psychological characteristics, interpersonal relationships, physical environment, and culture.

According to this model, behavior is a result of the knowledge, values, and beliefs of people, as well as numerous social influences. These social influences include relationships, social support networks, and community structure. According to the ecologic model, there are four levels of reciprocal influence, and it is necessary to consider all of these levels in order to change behavior. The four levels of influence, which may either promote risk or support protective factors, are (1) ontogenetic, (2) microsystem, (3) exosystem, and (4) macrocultural (El-Bassel et al., 2003) (Fig. 5.3). The influences represent biologic, environmental, and social influences as a dynamic and collective group of variables that need to be considered as a whole.

This model has been successfully used in health promotion and prevention research as a way to decrease barriers to mammography screening and safer sex practices (Eddy, Donahue, Webster, & Bjournstad, 2002; McLeroy, Bibeau, Steckler, & Glanz, 1988; Richards, Viadro, & Earp, 1998; Schaalma, Abraham, Gillmore, & Kok, 2004). Burke (2003) used the ecologic model to provide a better understanding of intrapersonal, interpersonal, and environmental factors associated with intimate partner violence in low-income communities. Others have used this model to identify individual and community resources, such as trust and partnership, to develop effective interventions for health access (Bhattacharya, 2003).

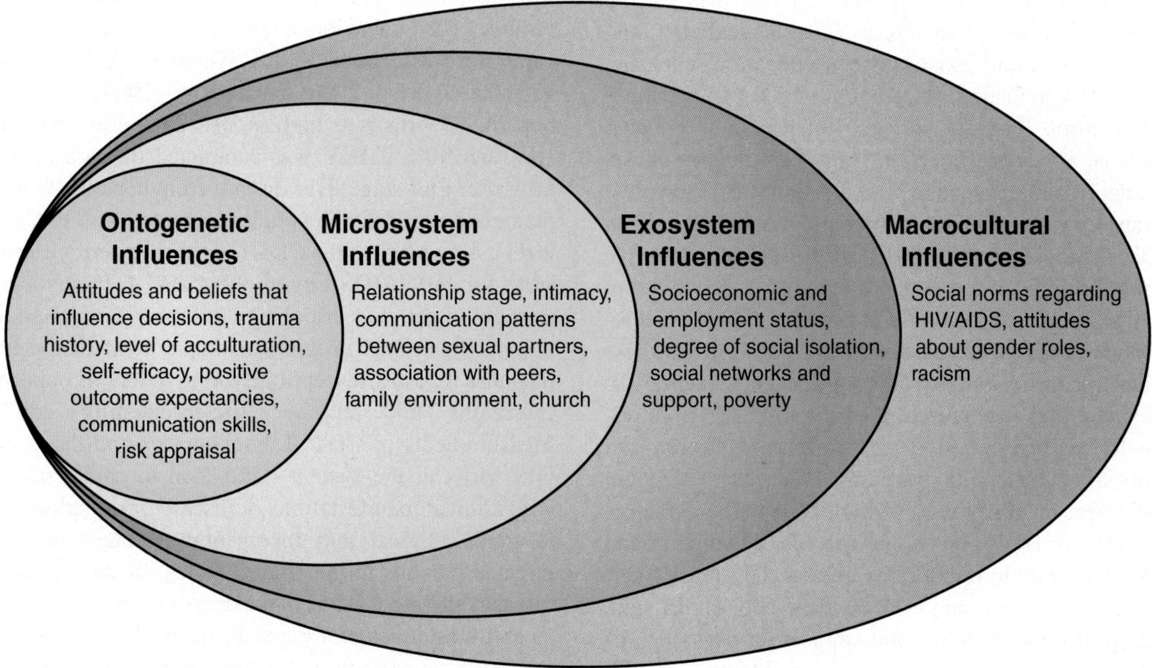

figure 5.3 Ecologic model.

El-Bassel et al. (2003) used the ecologic model to study communication strategies for preventing HIV infection in African-American and Latino heterosexual couples ($n = 217$).

USE OF THE ECOLOGIC MODEL: EVIDENCE FOR HEALTH PROMOTION INTERVENTION

The ecologic model is an appropriate framework to help identify and measure complex processes at a variety of levels for women living with HIV/AIDS. It allows public health interdisciplinary teams to (1) emphasize the unique developmental nature of variables that influence behaviors; (2) use a multilayered understanding of influence on behaviors; and (3) test variables from each of the identified systems in the model to guide the assessment, development, implementation, and evaluation of targeted interventions. The following is an example of how public healthcare providers implement each of the systems in the model in order to develop appropriate health promotion interventions. The ecologic model is more inclusive than many of the theories of behavior change previously discussed. The references used include publications that are more than 5 years old, which indicates the historical development of evidence since the 1980s, when HIV was first identified in gay men in San Francisco, California.

Ontogenic System: Personal Factors

Characteristics such as race, marital status, and level of education are predictors of effective HIV prevention strategies (Hodder et al., 2013). Three trends emerging from these studies are as follows: (1) black women with lower levels of education are less likely to use HIV prevention measures than other groups surveyed; (2) older women and women of color are less likely to use condoms; and (3) strong correlations exist between education level and AIDS-related knowledge. In research which explores sexual risk factors, intimate partner violence, and selected psychosocial illnesses (injection drug use, alcohol abuse, anxiety, depression, psychosis, and dementia), HIV-positive menopausal women without childbearing issues have been overlooked (Stockman et al., 2013). High rates of depressive symptoms, and major depression diagnoses with addiction/recovery histories, are common in persons of color receiving HIV care (Berger-Greenstein et al., 2007). Regardless of gender, race, or ethnicity, traumatic events, mental illness, distrust, and stigma have all been linked to poor adherence to health promotion and prevention efforts, and behaviors associated with increased HIV risk. (Whetten, Reif, Whetten, & Murphy-McMillan, 2008). These factors are barriers to HIV prevention for black women, and the lack of economic opportunity means they must focus on immediate survival, and restricts their choices. In spite of the help of public funding and support services, lack of adequate and sustaining income is formidable (Rice & Wicks, 2007).

The relationship between trauma and HIV in African-American–seropositive women and the contexts in which these risks occur are critical areas in need of understanding and successful intervention. Trauma such as child sexual abuse, intimate partner violence, adult sexual abuse, and victimization from exposure to violent environments, contribute to behaviors associated with increased HIV risk and disease sequelae (Myers, Wyatt, Loeb, & Carmona, 2006; Glover et al., 2010). "Research has shown that histories of physical and sexual trauma can affect the decisions women make with regard to risks for STIs and HIV, including the choice of partners and the ability to negotiate the use of barrier methods of protection" (Myers et al., 2006, p. 401). In African-American women, being a victim of violence increases depressive symptoms, decreases safe sex behaviors, and increases the chance of becoming HIV seropositive, increases the chances of acquiring and being treated for an STI within a year's time (Laughon et al., 2007). Post-traumatic stress disorder (PTSD) in African-American women and also in Latina women has been shown to be an outcome of interfamilial and extrafamilial sexual abuse as children and adults (Myers et al., 2006). Severe child sexual abuse is associated with substance use and lower self-esteem (Liu et al., 2006).

In the health histories of aging African-American women with no history of HIV, comorbid chronic conditions challenge self-care, especially when there is little or no social support (Warren-Findlow & Prohaska, 2008). Risk-taking behaviors, such as having multiple sexual partners, unprotected sex, and drug and alcohol abuse greatly complicate HIV risk, HIV infection, and STIs, when these behaviors are superimposed on chronic conditions such as hypertension, obesity, lupus, diabetes, and congestive heart failure. These behaviors continue to be major issues in prevention efforts (Buzi, Smith, Weinman, & Novello, 2013; Trzynka & Erlen, 2004; Wyatt et al., 2004). Prevalence of hepatitis C virus is as high as 30% among those living with HIV and 90% if HIV was contracted through intravenous drug use. End-stage liver disease from hepatitis C virus is a major cause of death in people coinfected with HIV (HRSA, 2011). According to the CDC (2013c), the retrovirus responsible for HIV/AIDS targets the $CD4^+$ T lymphocyte as a primary target, thus crippling a number of important immunologic functions. Progressive impairment of the immune response leads to susceptibility in a variety of opportunistic infections and chronic life-threatening conditions. Measurements of $CD4^+$ T lymphocytes and the amount of HIV virus in the system (viral load in copies/mL), along with clinical manifestations of disease or infection, are used to guide clinical and therapeutic management of HIV-infected persons in the United States. Results of viral load assessments are used to make decisions regarding initiation of antiretroviral therapy and to determine whether current antiretroviral therapy is effective. These measures are critical in decreasing mortality and morbidity rates.

Microsystem: Relationship between Women and the Environment

Disclosing one's HIV status has been reported to increase feelings of shame and stigma, partner violence, rejection, depression, and high-risk sexual behavior (Herek, Gillis, & Cogan, 2009). Stigma is highly correlated with low self-image, depression, lack of social support, a lack of subjective social integration, and social conflict (Berger, Ferrans, & Lashley, 2001; Bunn, Solomon, Millar, & Forehand, 2007; Kalichman et al., 2009). Withdrawal from personal interaction as a way to reduce tension is part of stigmatization, and for persons living with HIV/AIDS who have strong histories of substance abuse, the temptation to fall out of recovery is profound (Logie & Gadalla, 2009). Poor self-image is linked to increased risk behaviors for HIV infection (Mahajan et al., 2008) and decreased disease adjustment, health promotion, self-advocacy, self-efficacy for negotiating safe sex and safe sex practices (Herek et al., 2009). When women are empowered by HIV prevention efforts, they experience increased self-image, control over healthcare treatment decisions, self-efficacy, increased knowledge, and a positive sense of self as individuals and in relationships (Norris & DeMarco, 2005).

In non-HIV studies, such as breast cancer survivorship, self-image is related to relationship satisfaction and a positive feminine identity (Zimmermann, Scott, & Heinrichs, 2010). Self-image is a factor which affects risk behavior and perceptions of risk for unplanned pregnancies, and is a predictor of the ability to negotiate safe sex behaviors (Sheeran et al., 1999). In women, there is a relationship between poor self-image, depression, and lack of self-advocacy in sexual relationships (DeMarco, Johnsen, Fukuda, & Deffenbaugh, 2001). From a treatment perspective, depressive symptoms are underdiagnosed and are associated with lower medication adherence, risky behaviors, and poor health outcomes (Lennon, Huedo-Medina, Gerwien, & Johnson, 2012). Lack of adherence to antiretroviral medication schedules has an effect on CD4 and viral load counts (i.e., adherence slows the progression of HIV, thereby maintaining health and survivorship). Substance abuse (drugs and alcohol) in HIV-infected persons decreases the use of appropriate and needed healthcare interventions, and in addition, it decreases HIV prevention by increasing the likelihood of risky sexual behavior (Liebschutz, Geier, Horton, Chuang, & Samet, 2005).

Exosystem: Formal and Informal Social Structures

Simoni, Walters, and Nero (2000) found that in women of African descent (Black Hispanics, non-Hispanic Blacks) living in New York City, disclosure of their HIV status to adult family members, friends, and coworkers was related to greater frequency of HIV-related social support but was not directly related to a decrease in depression or mood disturbance. During and after disclosure, social support was found to help with coping and improve psychological distress. Isolation, stigma, managing their medical care, and being a mother caused women to be unwilling to talk about their illness with their children, family, friends, and partners (DeMarco et al., 2001).

There is a strong connection between highly active antiretroviral therapy (HAART) and health. For poor women of color, adherence to medical protocols, which include HAART, and medical follow-up, as well as less high-risk behavior, is compromised by (1) believing that other people in their lives, specifically family and friends (children and sexual partners), come first; (2) subsisting on a low income, which affects resource allocation; (3) experiencing race discrimination, which magnifies the seropositive stigma; and (4) choosing to enter high-risk situations to obtain money (sex work) to change their circumstances. Many strategies are used to improve medication adherence, including counseling, support groups, educational information, telephone/computer-based feedback, improving motivation and self-efficacy, and directly observed therapy. Adherence may be improved with these strategies, but much needs to be understood within a particular group to determine their best use in a cost-effective manner (Haynes, Ackloo, & Sahota, 2008; Wolitski, Janssen, Onorato, Purcell, & Crepaz, 2005). However, despite the use of these methods, a proven method for implementing long-term behavior change remains unknown.

Social support includes relationships with family, friends, and community members. This is usually thought of as perceived social support; it represents the degree to which needs for relevant (or important) support are fulfilled by a person's social network. High levels of depressive symptoms are related to lack of HIV social support from friends, relatives, partners, groups, and organizations. In contrast, increased social support improves self-esteem and mastery. Thus, interventions that include group support can benefit psychological health (Simoni, Huang, Goodry, & Montoya, 2005).

Psychosocial factors contribute to disease progression, which can be measured by CD4 and viral load levels. These levels are indirect measures of adherence to HIV medications (Ironson et al., 2005). Factors that support adherence to HIV treatment protocols include supportive family members and other emotional support, whereas barriers to adherence include stigma, feeling unloved, and relationship turbulence (Edwards, 2006).

Macroculture: Values and Beliefs of Culture

To reduce the spread of HIV/AIDS, women who are seropositive must reduce the number of instances when reinfection by other HIV strains may occur, and protect partners from the virus by increasing safe sex behaviors. Safer sex strategies, from adolescence and onward in sexual development, include assertiveness, self-advocacy to negotiate protection during intercourse, verbal strategies, avoidance of drugs and/or alcohol consumption before or during sex, and avoidance of contact with potentially infected body fluids (Buzi et al., 2013). Negotiated safer sex in adults has almost exclusively been associated with condom use (Widman, Carol, & Noar, 2013). Because of the belief that partners are not sexually active with others, heterosexual adults use condoms less often with primary or regular partners than with casual sexual partners (Widman et al., 2013). In addition, as mentioned earlier, many social and situational factors contribute to decreases in behavior that may prevent HIV in women, such as feeling intense stigma, victimization, substance abuse, mental health problems, and contracting other STIs (Crepaz et al., 2007; Mize, Robinson, Bockting, & Scheltema, 2002).

Gender roles in women and, in particular, the need to maintain connection in relationships at the cost of one's own health are major issues for all women living with chronic diseases, but particularly for those who are HIV positive (DeMarco, Miller, Patsdaughter, Grindel, & Chisholm, 1998; DeMarco & Johnsen, 2002, 2003; DeMarco, Lynch, & Board, 2002). Jack (1991, 1999) discussed the concept of silencing in the context of women's experiences with relationships. Jack's work is relevant today, since the experiences women have in relationships continue to be oriented toward understanding and defining themselves in the context of others. Jack supports the position that women's relationships are influenced not only by biologic factors but also by psychosocial factors (Bancroft, 2002) and asserts "women's orientation to relationships is the central component of female identity and emotional activity" (Jack, 1991, p. 3). This researcher's extensive exploratory and longitudinal studies with diverse groups of women resulted in the development of the concept of "silencing the self" and the Silencing the Self Scale. This concept of "silencing the self" has been used to explain how gender roles negatively influence self-advocacy behaviors in women. Women tend to silence their voice in relationships in order to maintain connections with others, even if that means they will subsequently suffer physically, psychologically, or socially. According to Jack (1991), women are reinforced culturally to (1) care for others' needs before their own, (2) abide by designated societal rules of behavior, (3) refrain from directly expressing their feelings and needs, and (4) outwardly maintain compliance, while feeling hostility inwardly because of their silencing behaviors. Silencing the self is relevant to the proposed study because it is a concept that is identified and understood in the context of relationships with others (i.e., a relational concept). The nature of intimate heterosexual relationships where seropositive safe sex occurs is an example of this relational context. Women living with HIV continue to be sexually active with men. Being quiet during times of sexual intimacy, rather than making direct requests and taking care of themselves, will not protect them against further strains of HIV and other STIs, and will infect others (DeMarco et al., 1998, 2001, 2002; DeMarco & Johnsen, 2002, 2003; DeMarco & Norris, 2004a, 2004b; Norris & DeMarco, 2004, 2005).

HEALTH PROMOTION AND SECONDARY/TERTIARY PREVENTION FOR WOMEN LIVING WITH HIV/AIDS

Using the ecologic model, the aim of any intervention to promote health and minimize the spread of HIV/AIDS requires the creative inclusion of a prevention initiative that is community-based, peer-led, and interdisciplinary. Advancing the scientific understanding of secondary HIV prevention (what is called *positive prevention*) and exploring ways to reduce behavioral risk in African-American women may prevent further transmission of HIV and the serious negative psychological consequences of living with HIV disease. African-American women experience disproportionate levels of (1) interpersonal mistrust and fear of disclosure because of the fear of stigma, (2) poor adherence to treatment and other health promotion and disease prevention efforts, (3) delay in seeking care related to mental health comorbidities and addiction recovery issues, and (4) compromised self-advocacy in sexual relationships. An innovative, culturally relevant, and gender-sensitive intervention that would address these barriers for women who are already disproportionately saddled with HIV/AIDS, racism, ageism, and poverty would be beneficial not only to them but also to their families and the communities in which they live. Ultimately, public health nurses would be trying to improve health outcomes for this underserved population of women.

Within the context of HIV physical care, and efforts to decrease communicability using the ecologic model, consideration should be given to mental health symptoms, severity/frequency of the effects from significant trauma (PTSD), substance use, abuse and addiction. In Table 5.1, the sectors of the model and areas that need to be considered to address prevention are shown as a process of collaboration between interdisciplinary teams, evidence, and real, population-based needs.

ROLE OF NURSES

This chapter addresses real examples of how nurses, as part of an interdisciplinary team, can be involved in fundamental prevention and health promotion efforts. After using public health science and evidence to identify risk, the focus of prevention and health promotion can proceed using culturally relevant, sensitive, ethical, and creative ways to motivate others to consider health and wellness as individuals, groups, and communities. Historical behavior change theories are examples of how health science has developed in using psychology, sociology, anthropology, and ethical perspectives to advance efforts at the national level and beyond. Although primary prevention, in particular, is often overlooked as a critical component to health and wellness when it comes to resource allocation in the U.S. health system, in truth it is one of the most influential areas where nurses as teachers can make a difference in people's lives.

table 5.1 **Ecologic Model with Health Promotion and Disease Prevention Considerations for African-American Women Living with HIV**

Ontogenetic system: *Personal factors*	**Microsystem: *Relationship between the individual and the environment***	**Exosystem: *Formal and informal social structures***	**Macroculture: *Values and beliefs of culture***
Health history Physiologic indicators Comorbidities Mental health Age, education, marital status, income, pregnancies, health history, sexual history, mental health symptoms Effect of trauma CD4 count/viral load Sexually transmitted infections	Relationships and influences in interactions in relationships Stigma related to disclosure Substance abuse/recovery Healthcare adherence Self-advocacy in sexual relationships	Stressors or buffers that influence risky behaviors Relationships with family, friends, community members Healthcare adherence, substance use, self-advocacy in sexual relationships Stigma	Culture of women Culture of African-American women Self-advocacy in sexual relationships Stigma

key concepts

- National goals and directives to maintain the health of individuals, families, and communities are important road maps for healthcare professionals.
- Three levels of prevention assist health professionals to advance quality of life and health through the natural history of disease and disability.
- Identifying modifiable risk and using health promotion models to address change in behaviors, beliefs, attitudes, and intentions can significantly increase the health of individuals, families, and communities.

critical thinking questions

1. What does it mean to be healthy and well when diagnosed with multiple sclerosis?
2. Name community indicators that would demonstrate health and wellness for a particular geographic area.
3. What are the responsibilities of community and public health nurses in promoting health and decreasing illness and injury in populations, families, and individuals?
4. Identify five key influences on health and wellness in the United States.
5. If national health policies are identified but cannot be funded because of national fiscal deficits, how would community/public health nurses initiate support for these policies?
6. Choose a data-based publication that represents each level of prevention and take a position about which level is the most complex to put into action for advancing health and wellness.
7. Critique behavior change from the perspective of measuring the change after a health promotion intervention has been implemented (e.g., teaching communities to decrease saturated fat in their diet and to exercise more).

community resources

- State and local departments of health (divisions of maternal and child health, communicable disease, occupational health, addictions, gerontology)
- YMCA/YWCA programs
- Gyms/athletic complexes
- State and local police departments
- Parks and recreation departments
- Places where blood pressure equipment is sold or screenings are available (local retail stores)
- School systems (school nurse associations)
- Local restaurants
- Air and water control areas
- Primary care physician and advanced nurse practices
- Dentists
- Elder services

references

American Cancer Society. (2013). Retrieved from http://www.cancer.org/cancer/cancercauses/othercarcinogens/infectiousagents/hpv/acs-recommendations-for-hpv-vaccine-use

American Public Health Association. (2013). *The role of public health nurses*. Retrieved from http://www.apha.org/membergroups/sections/aphasections/phn/about/phnroles.htm

Andersen, E.T. & McFarlane, J. (2008). *Community as Partner: Theory and Practice in Nursing*. Philadelphia, PA: Lippincott, Williams, & Wilkins.

Baker, E. A., Schootman, M., Barnidge, E., & Kelly, C. (2006). The role of race and poverty in access to foods that enable individuals to adhere to dietary guidelines. *Preventing Chronic Disease*, *3*(3), A76.

Bandura, A. (1986). *Social foundations of thought and action: A social cognitive theory*. Englewood Cliffs, NJ: Prentice-Hall.

Bancroft, J. (2002). Biological factors in human sexuality. *The Journal of Sex Research*, *39*(1), 15–21.

Behavior change theories and models. (2009). Retrieved from http://www.csupomona.edu/~jvgrizzell/best_practices/bctheory.html

Berger, B. E., Ferrans, C. E., & Lashley, F. R. (2001). Measuring stigma in people with HIV: Psychometric assessment of the HIV stigma scale. *Research in Nursing and Health*, *24*, 518–529.

Berger-Greenstein, J., Cuevas, C. A., Brady, S. M., Trezza, G., Richardson, M. A., & Keane, T. M. (2007). Major depression in patients with HIV/AIDS and substance abuse. *AIDS Patient Care and STDs*, *21*(12), 942–955.

Berkman, L. F., & Glass, T. (2000). Social intergration, social networks, social support, and health. In L. F. Berman & I. Kawachi (Eds.), *Social epidemiology*. New York, NY: Oxford University Press.

Bhattacharya, G. (2003). Social-environmental influences on HIV risks: Implications for HIV prevention. *Journal of HIV/AIDS & Social Services*, *2*(3), 11–31.

Bronfenbrenner, U. (1979). *The ecology of human development: Experiments by nature and design*. Cambridge, MA: Harvard University.

Bronfenbrenner, U. (2004). *Making human beings human: Bioecological perspectives on human development*. Thousand Oaks, CA: Sage Publications.

Brown, D. W. (2009). The dawn of Healthy People 2020: A brief look back at its beginnings. *Preventive Medicine*, *48*(1), 94–95.

Bunn, J. Y., Solomon, S. E., Millar, C., & Forehand, R. (2007). Measurement of stigma in people with HIV: A re-examination of the HIV stigma scale . *AIDS Education and Prevention*, *19*, 198–208.

Burke, J. G. (2003). Intimate partner violence among low income women: Associated individual and contextual risk factors (Doctoral dissertation, Johns Hopkins University). *Dissertation Abstracts International*, *64*(O2), 659B University Microfilms No. 3080630.

Buzi, R. S., Smith, P. B., Weinman, M. L., & Novello, G. (2013). HIV risk perceptions among adolescents attending family planning clinics: An integrated perspective. *AIDS Care,* 25(1), 20–27.

Centers for Disease Control and Prevention. (2013b). *Global health promotion*. Retrieved from http://www.cdc.gov/osi/goals/global/promotion.html

Centers for Disease Control and Prevention. (2013c). *Morbidity mortality weekly report*. Retrieved from http://www.cdc.gov/mmwr/index.html

Centers for Disease Control and Prevention. (2013d). *OraQuick rapid HIV test for oral fluid-frequently asked questions*. Retrieved from http://www.cdc.gov/HIV/topics/testing/resources/qa/pdf/oralfluidqandafin1_1.pdf

Centers for Disease Control and Prevention. (2013e). *PEARLS gives seniors with minor depression new hope*. Retrieved from http://www.cdc.gov/prc/stories-prevention-research/stories/pearls.htm

Centers for Disease Control and Prevention. (2013f). *Reading writing and reducing obesity*. Retrieved from http://www.cdc.gov/prc/stories-prevention-research/stories/planet_health.htm

Centers for Disease Control and Prevention. (2013g). *Why immunize?* Retrieved from http://www.cdc.gov/vaccines/vac-gen/why.htm

Crepaz, N., Horn, A. K., Rama, S. M., Griffin, T., DeLuca, J. B., Mullins, M. M., & Aral, S. O. (2007). The efficacy of behavioral interventions in reducing HIV risk sex behaviors and incident sexually transmitted disease in Black and Hispanic sexually transmitted disease clinic patients in the United States: A meta-analytic review. *Sexually Transmitted Diseases*, *34*, 319–332.

Daly, B. P., Shin, R. Q., Thakral, C., Selders, M., & Vera, E. (2009). School engagement among urban adolescents of color: Does perception of social support and neighborhood safety really matter? *Journal of Youth Adolescence*, *38*, 63–74.

DeMarco, R., & Johnsen, C. (2002). Vulnerable populations: Women living with HIV/AIDS. In E. A. Mahoney & J. K. Shaw (Eds.), *HIV/AIDS nursing secrets* (pp. 135–142). Philadelphia, PA: Hanely & Belfus, Inc.

DeMarco, R., & Johnsen, C. (2003). Taking action in communities: Women living with HIV lead the way. *Journal of Community Health Nursing*, *20*(1), 51–62.

DeMarco, R., Johnsen, C., Fukuda, D., & Deffenbaugh, O. (2001). Content validity of a scale to measure silencing and affectivity among women living with HIV/AIDs. *Journal of Association of Nurses in AIDS Care*, *12*(4), 49–60.

DeMarco, R., Lynch, M. M., & Board, R. (2002). Mothers who silence themselves: Clinical implications for women living with HIV/AIDS and their children. *Journal of Pediatric Nursing*, *17*(2), 89–95.

DeMarco, R. F., Miller, K., Patsdaughter, C., Grindel, C., & Chisholm, M. (1998). From silencing the self to action: Experiences of women living with HIV/AIDS. *Women's Health Care International*, *19*(6), 539–552.

DeMarco, R., & Norris, A. E. (2004a). Women's voices women's lives: A Web-based HIV prevention film project. In J. V. M. Welie & J. Lee (Eds.), *Jesuit health sciences and the promotion of justice: An invitation to a discussion* (pp. 203–209). Milwaukee, WI: Marquette University Press.

DeMarco, R., & Norris, A. E. (2004b). Culturally relevant HIV interventions: Transcending ethnicity. *Journal of Cultural Diversity*, *11*(2), 65–68.

Eddy, J. M., Donahue, R. E., Webster, R. D., & Bjournstad, E. D. (2002). Application of an ecological perspective in worksite health promotion: A review. *American Journal of Health Studies*, *17*(4), 197–202.

Edwards, L. V. (2006). Perceived social support and HIV/AIDS medication adherence among African American women. *Qualitative Health Research*, *16*(5), 679–691.

El-Bassel, N., Witte, S. S., Gilbert, L., Wu, E., Chang, M., Hill, J., & Steinglass, P. (2003). The efficacy of a relationship-based HIV/STD prevention program for heterosexual couples. *American Journal of Public Health*, *93*(6), 963–969.

Earnshaw, V. A., Smith, L., Chaudoir, S. R., Lee, I., & Copenhaver, M. M. (2012). Stereotypes about people living with HIV: Implications for perceptions of HIV risk and testing frequency among at-risk populations. *AIDS Education & Prevention, 24*(6), 574–581.

Escoto Ponce de Leon, M. C., Mancilla Diaz, J. M., & Camacho Ruiz, E. J. (2008). A pilot study of the clinical and statistical significance of a program to reduce eating disorder risk factors in children. *Eating & Weight Disorders*, *13*(3), 111–118.

Fishbein, M., & Ajzen, I. (1975). *Belief, attitude, intention, and behavior: An introduction to theory and research*. Reading, MA: Addison-Wesley.

Gasink, L. B., & Lautenbach, E. (2008). Prevention and treatment of health care-acquired infections. *Medical Clinics of North America, 92*(2), 295–313.

Glanz, K., Rimer, B. K., & Viswanath, K. (2008). *Health behavior and health education: Theory, research and practice* (4th ed.). San Francisco: Jossey-Bass.

Glover, D. A., Loeb, T. B., Carmona, J. V., Sciolla, A., Zhang, M., Myer, H. F., & Wyatt, G. E. (2010). Childhood sexual abuse severity and disclosure predict posttraumatic stress symptoms and biomarkers in ethnic minority women. *Journal of Trauma & Dissociation*, 11(2), 152–173.

Godley, S. H., Dennis, M. L., Godley, M. D., & Funk, R. R. (2004). Thirty-month relapse trajectory cluster groups among adolescents discharged from out-patient treatment. *Addiction, 99*(Suppl 2), 129–139.

Haynes, R. B., Ackloo, E., & Sahota, N. (2008). Interventions for enhancing medication adherence. *Cochrane Database of Systematic Reviews, 2*, CD000011.

Healthy People, 2020. (2013). *2020 Topics and Objectives.* Retrieved from http://www.healthypeople.gov/2020/topicsobjectives2020/default.aspx

Herek, G., Gillis, J. R., & Cogan, J. C. (2009). Internalized stigma among sexual minority adults: Insights from a social psychological perspective. *Journal of Counseling Psychology, 56*, 32–43.

Herzog, T. A. (2008). Analyzing the transtheoretical model using the framework of Weinstein, Rothman, and Sutton (1998): The example of smoking cessation. *Health Psychology, 27*(5), 548–556.

Hochbaum, G. (1956). Why people seek diagnostic x-rays. *Public Health Reports, 71*, 377–380.

Hodder, S. L., Justman, J., Hughes, J. P., Wang, J., Haley, D. F., Adimora, A. A., . . . El-Sadr, W. M. (2013). HIV acquisition among women from selected areas of the United States: A cohort study. *Annals of Internal Medicine,* 158(1), 10–18.

Homsy, J., Thomson-Honnebier, G. A., Cheng-Mayer, C., & Levy, J. A. (1988). Detection of human immunodeficiency virus (HIV) in serum and body fluids by sequential competition ELISA. *Journal of Virological Methods, 19*(1), 43–56.

HRSA (2011). A guide for evaluation and treatment of Hepatitis C in adult co-infected with HIV. Retrieved from http://hab.hrsa.gov/deliverhivaidscare/files/hepccoinfectguide2011.pdf

Ironson, G., O'Cleirigh, C., Fletcher, M. A., Laurenceau, J. P., Balbin, E., Klimas, N., . . . Solomon, G. (2005). Psychosocial factors predict CD4 and viral load change in men and women with human immunodeficiency virus in the era of highly active antiretroviral treatment. *Psychosomatic Medicine, 67*(6), 1013–1021.

Jack, D. C. (1991). *Silencing the self.* Cambridge, MA: Harvard University Press.

Jack, D. C. (1999). *Behind the mask.* Cambridge, MA: Harvard University Press.

Kalichman, S. C., Simbayi, L. C., Cloete, A., Mthembu, P. P., Mkhonta, R. N., & Ginindza, T. (2009). Measuring AIDS stigmas in people living with HIV/AIDS: The internalized AIDS-related stigma scale. *AIDS Care, 21*(1), 87–93.

Kieny, M. P., Excler, J. L., & Girard, M. (2004). Research and development of new vaccines against infectious diseases. *American Journal of Public Health, 94*(11), 1931–1935.

Laughon, K., Gielen, A. C., Campbell, J. C., Burke, J., McDonnell, K., & O'Campo, P. (2007). The relationships among sexually transmitted infection, depression, and lifetime violence in a sample of predominantly African American women. *Research in Nursing and Health, 30*, 413–428.

Lennon, C. A., Huedo-Medina, T. B., Gerwien, D., P., & Johnson, B. T. (2012). A role for depression in sexual risk reduction for women? A meta-analysis of HIV prevention trials with depression outcomes. *Social Science & Medicine,* 75(4), 688–698.

Liebschutz, J. M., Geier, J. L., Horton, N. J., Chuang, C. H., & Samet, J. H. (2005). Physical and sexual violence and health care utilization in HIV-infected persons with alcohol problems. *AIDS Care, 17*(5), 566–578.

Liu, H., Longshore, D., Williams, J. K., Rivkin, I., Loeb, T., Warda, U. S., . . . Wyatt, G. (2006). Substance abuse and medication adherence among HIV-positive women with histories of child sexual abuse. *AIDS and Behavior, 10*(3), 279–286.

Logie, C., & Gadalla, T. M. (2009). Meta-analysis of health and demographic correlates of stigma towards people living with HIV. *AIDS Care, 21*(6), 742–753.

Mahajan, A. P., Sayles, J. N., Patel, V. A., Remien, R. H., Sawires, S. R., Ortiz, D. J., . . . Coates, T. J. (2008). Stigma in the HIV/AIDS epidemic: A review of the literature and recommendations for the way forward. *AIDS, 22*(Suppl. 2), S67–S79.

Mahajan, A. P., Stemple, L., Shapiro, M. F., King, J. B., & Cunningham, W. E. (2009). Consistency of state statutes with the Centers for Disease Control and Prevention HIV testing recommendations for health care settings. *Annals of Internal Medicine, 150*(4), 263–269.

Mahoney, M. C., Bevers, T., Linos, E., & Willett, W. C. (2008). Risk is a statistical concept based on mathematical probabilities: Opportunities and strategies for breast cancer prevention through risk reduction. *Cancer: A Cancer Journal for Clinicians, 58*(6), 347–371.

Markle-Reid, M., Browne, G., Weir, R., Gafni, A., Roberts, J., & Henderson, S. R. (2006). The effectiveness and efficiency of home-based nursing health promotion for older people: A review of the literature. *Medical Care Research & Review, 63*(5), 531–569.

McLeroy, K. R., Bibeau, D., Steckler, A., & Glanz, K. (1988). An ecological perspective on health promotion programs. *Health Education Quarterly, 15*(4), 351–374.

Mitchell, N. S., Ellison, M. C., Hill, J. O., & Tsai, A. G. (2013). Evaluation of the effectiveness of making weight watchers available to Tennessee Medicaid (TennCare) recipients. *Journal of General Internal Medicine, 28*(1), 12–17.

Mize, S. J., Robinson, B. E., Bockting, W. O., & Scheltema, K. E. (2002). Meta-analysis of the effectiveness of HIV prevention interventions for women. *AIDS Care, 14*(2), 163–180.

Motivational Inteviewing (2009). Retrieved from http://www.motivationalinterview.org/Documents/1%20A%20MI%20Definition%20Principles%20&%20Approach%20V4%2001291l.pdf

Myers, H. F., Wyatt, G. E., Loeb, T. B., & Carmona, J. (2006). Severity of child sexual abuse, post-traumatic stress and risky sexual behaviors among HIV-positive women. *AIDS and Behavior, 10*(2), 191–199.

Norris, A. E., & DeMarco, R. (2004). The mechanics of conducting culturally relevant HIV prevention research with Haitian American adolescents: Lessons learned. *Journal of Multicultural Nursing and Health, 11*(1), 69–76.

Norris, A. E., & DeMarco, R. (2005). The experience of African American women living with HIV creating a prevention film for teens. *Journal of the Association of Nurses in AIDS Care, 16*(2), 32–39.

Sims, E. N., Dodd, V. J., & Tejeda, M. J. (2008). The relationship between severity of violence in the home and dating violence. *Journal of Forensic Nursing, 4*(4), 166–173. doi:10.1111/j.1939-3938.2008.00028.

Prochaska, J. O., & DiClemente, R. (1983). Stages and processes of self-change of smoking: Toward an integrative model of change. *Journal of Consulting and Clinical Psychology, 5*(3), 390–395.

Rice, M. C., & Wicks, M. N. (2007). The importance of nursing advocacy for the health promotion of female welfare recipients. *Nursing Outlook, 55*, 220–223.

Richards, C. L., Viadro, C. I., & Earp, J. A. (1998). Bringing down the barriers to mammography: A review of current research and interventions. *Breast Disease, 10*(4), 33–44.

Rollnick, S., & Miller, W. R. (1995). What is motivational interviewing? *Behavioral and Cognitive Psychotherapy, 23*, 325–334.

Rosenstock, I. (1974). The health belief model and preventive health behavior. *Health Education Monographs, 2*, 354–385.

references (continued)

Ross, K., Mathis, S., & Brockopp, D. (2008). Developing a successful palliative care service in an acute care setting. *Journal of Nursing Administration, 38*(6), 282–286.

Schaalma, H. P., Abraham, C., Gillmore, M. R., & Kok, G. (2004). Sex education as health promotion: What does it take? *Archives of Sexual Behavior, 33*(3), 259–269.

Scoliosis screening. (2013). Retrieved from http://iscoliosis.com/symptoms-screening.html

Sheeran, P., Abraham, C., & Orbell, S. (1999). Psychosocial correlates of heterosexual condom use: A meta-analysis. *Psychological Bulletin, 125*(1), 90-132.HYPERLINK "http://psycnet.apa.org/doi/10.1037/0033-2909.125.1.90" \t"_blank"http://dx.doi.org/10.1037/0033-2909.125.1.90

Shepard, R., & Towler, G. (2007). Nutrition knowledge, attitudes and fat intake: Application of the theory of reasoned action. *Journal of Human Nutrition & Dietetics, 20*(3), 159–169.

Simoni, J. M., Walters, K. L., & Nero, D. K. (2000). Safer sex among HIV-positive women: The role of relationships. *Sex Roles, 42*, 691–708.

Simoni, J. M., Huang, B., Goodry, E. J., & Montoya, H. D. (2005). Social support and depressive symptomatology among HIV-Positive women: The mediating role of self-esteem and mastery. *Women and Health, 42*(4), 1–15.

Skinner, B. F. (1953). *Science and human behavior.* New York, NY: Macmillan.

Spector, D. (2007). Lifestyle behaviors in women with a BRCA1 or BRACA2 genetic mutation. *Cancer Nursing, 29*(6), E1–E10.

Stockman, J. K., Lucea, M., Draughon, J. E., Sabri, B., Anderson, J. C. Bertrand, D., . . . Campbell, J. C. (2013). Intimate partner violence and HIV risk factors among African-American and African-Caribbean women in clinic-based settings. *AIDS Care,* 25(4), 472–480.

Taylor, M. (2013). Exploring practices of harm reduction. *Alberta Association of Registered Nurses,* 68(4), 17–19.

Trossman, S. (2008). On the road to Healthy People 2020. ANA, other nursing groups offer their input as nation's health agenda begins to form. *American Nurse, 40*(6), 1–8.

Trzynka, S. L., & Erlen, J. A. (2004). HIV disease susceptibility in women and the barriers to adherence. *Medsurg Nursing, 13*(2), 97–104.

Watling, R., & Schwartz, I. S. (2004). Understanding and implementing positive reinforcement as an intervention strategy for children with disabilities. *American Journal of Occupational Therapy, 58*(1), 113–116.

Warren-Findlow, J., & Porhaska, T. R. (2008). Families, social support, and self-care among older African-American women with chronic illness. *American Journal of Health Promotion, 22*(5), 342–349.

Whetten, K., Reif, S., Whetten, R., & Murphy-McMillan, L. K. (2008). Trauma mental health, distrust and stigma among HIV positive persons: Implications for effective care. *Psychosomatic Medicine, 70*, 531–538.

Widman, L., Golin, C. E., & Noar, S. M. (2013). When do condom use intentions lead to actions? Examining the role of sexual communication on safer sexual behavior among people living with HIV. *Journal of Health Psychology, 18*(4), 507–517.

Wolitski, R. J., Janssen, R. S., Onorato, I. M., Purcell, D. W., & Crepaz, N. (2005). An overview of prevention with people living with HIV. In S. C. Kalichman (Ed.), *Positive prevention: Reducing HIV transmission among people living with HIV/AIDS.* New York, NY: Kluwer.

Zimmermann, T., Scott, J. L., & Heinrichs, N. (2010). Individual and dyadic predictors of body image in women with breast cancer. *Psycho-Oncology, 19*(10), 1061–1068.

web resources

Please visit thePoint thePoint for up-to-date web resources on this topic.

CHAPTER 6

Epidemiology: The Science of Prevention

Gail A. Harkness

There are in fact two things, science and opinion, the former begets knowledge, the latter ignorance.

Hippocrates

Science is organized common sense, where many a beautiful theory was killed by an ugly fact.

Thomas Huxley

Get your facts first, then you can distort them as you please.

Mark Twain

chapter highlights

- Defining epidemiology
- Development of epidemiology as a science
- Epidemiologic conceptual frameworks
- Applying epidemiologic principles in practice
- Assessment of health needs and assets
- Using assessment data for planning and implementing interventions
- Promoting healthy lifestyles
- Preventing and controlling outbreaks
- Contributing to a safe and healthy environment
- Evaluating the effectiveness of health services

objectives

- Trace the origins of epidemiology.
- Comprehend the basic principles and scope of epidemiology.
- Contrast three epidemiologic conceptual models.
- Relate the problem-solving process to both the epidemiologic process and the nursing process.
- Apply epidemiologic principles to the practice of public health nursing.

key terms

Epidemic: An outbreak that occurs when there is an increased incidence of a disease beyond that which is normally found in the population.

Epidemiologic triad: Model based on the belief that health status is determined by the interaction of the characteristics of the host, agent, and environment.

Epidemiology: Study of the distribution and determinants of states of health and illness in human populations; used both as a research methodology to study states of health and illness, and as a body of knowledge that results from the study of a specific state of health or illness.

Natural history: Course of a disease or condition from the onset to resolution.

Outbreak: Epidemic usually limited to a localized increase in the incidence of the illness.

Rate: Primary measurement used to describe either the occurrence or the existence of a specific state of health or illness.

Risk: Probability or likelihood that a disease or illness will occur in a group of people who presently do not have the problem.

Risk factor: Characteristics or events that have been shown to increase the probability that a specific disease or illness will develop.

Web of causation: Epidemiologic model that strongly emphasizes the concept of multiple causation while de-emphasizing the role of agents in explaining illness.

Wheel of causation: Epidemiologic model that de-emphasizes the agent as the sole cause of disease while emphasizing the interplay of physical, biologic, and social environments.

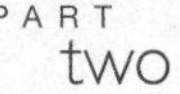

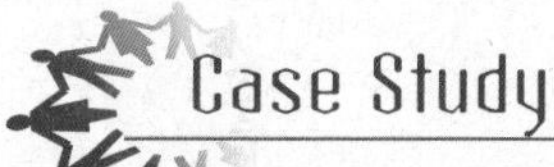

Case Study

References to the case study are found throughout this chapter (look for the case study icon). Readers should keep the case study in mind as they read the chapter.

More than 750,000 youths are active members of gangs in the United States. They often come from socially and economically disadvantaged communities, and they commit a disproportionate amount of violence and crime compared with youths not involved in gangs. Gang members are also more likely to use drugs and alcohol as well as engage in unsafe sex. As a result, youths who belong to gangs can be considered a vulnerable population at increased risk for negative health outcomes. Public health nurses in large cities have developed programs that target youths in gangs. These nurses represent local healthcare facilities, community service agencies, churches, schools, businesses, and other neighborhood groups. Goals are to increase access to expanded community health services, promote healthy living behaviors, and foster a positive community environment.

Katie, a public health nurse in Los Angeles, has developed a partnership with a local police department juvenile diversion program that offers a delinquency prevention program to young people from 13 to 18 years of age. These young people have been arrested for nonviolent offenses, such as possession of drugs, burglary, theft, joy riding, and vandalism. Some of these young people are gang members, and others are at risk for joining gangs because they come from neighborhoods with long histories of gang activity. Katie's responsibilities are to lead interactive 3-hour sessions that primarily focus on health-related issues for the youths. She identifies three topics for discussion: (1) major causes of morbidity and mortality in youth, (2) major health issues common in a particular age group, and (3) risk prevention and health promotion (adapted from Sanders, Schneiderman, Loken, Lankenau, & Bloom, 2009).

Like other types of modern science, epidemiology arose from building blocks constructed by ancient civilizations. Humans have experienced disease for as long as they have existed, and in the early days, attempts that people made to understand the onset of disease and to prevent its occurrence were crude. People perceived health as something holy, and healers looked to the spiritual world to protect health and prolong life. People often considered disease and disability as a great curse and a divine punishment, and they believed that amulets, totems, charms, and rituals prevented all sorts of evils. However, early cave dwellers experimented with medicinal plants and became adept at treating some illnesses. These discoveries were primarily a direct result of trial-and-error observations, enhanced by doses of curiosity, common sense, and chance.

For thousands of years, the practice of healing slowly developed as humans observed that more and more herbal remedies and therapeutic treatments had beneficial results. Some cultures, such as in Egypt, had an extensive repertoire of treatments. More than 700 remedies existed for ailments resulting from crocodile bites to infections following childbirth. Practitioners at that time reduced dislocations, aligned and immobilized fractures, and applied hot and cold treatments to reduce inflammation. People recognized and understood differences in individual constitutions and observed that many diseases were contagious in nature. Interestingly, they conceptualized the influence of the environment on the occurrence of disease. However, priests and religious healers kept most of this knowledge secret.

Hippocrates of Cos (460 to 370 BC), considered the father of modern medicine, was the first person to record these secrets in writing. In a textbook of medicine that was used for centuries, he recorded the belief that external factors in the environment were a cause of illness in humans. He wrote of the effects of seasons, winds, and water, as well as the characteristics of the ground. He encouraged healers to observe what are known today as lifestyle patterns: "what are their pursuits, whether they are fond of drinking and eating to excess, and given to indolence, or are fond of exercise and labor" (Hippocrates, 1938). Hippocrates also wrote *On Air, Waters and Places*, a book that provided details on the relationship between humans and the environment. Experts now consider this book as a milestone in the development of the science of epidemiology, illustrating the connection between human life and the environment. However, people overlooked this concept for centuries, and it was not seriously considered again until investigators in the late 19th century developed the science of bacteriology.

Men and women today still search for reasons for their illnesses, and many still perceive illness as a punishment for sins. However, the wealth of scientific knowledge developed within the last 160 years has permitted the understanding of the complexities of the human body and the effects of internal and external stressors. This knowledge has provided the means for preventing and modifying illness and repairing disabilities. Much of this knowledge has been gained through the extension of the observations of the past to the rigorous study of specific illnesses or disabilities in large groups of people.

DEFINING EPIDEMIOLOGY

Early attempts to understand illness and disease focused on studying the experiences of individual people. Today, clinicians consider these case reports or case studies. Studying individual experiences is invaluable for forming ideas, or hypotheses, about possible causes of specific diseases. However, studying individual people may not provide accurate information about the characteristics of the disease being investigated, because individual experiences with a disease may vary. Also, examining the experiences of individual persons does not provide evidence of causality (see Chapter 8). To gather more accurate information about disease, studying groups of people is essential.

An example is the relationship between smoking and lung cancer that experts statistically determined in the 20th century. Without studying the experiences of groups of people, they may never have identified this relationship. Some smokers never develop lung cancer, and some nonsmokers do develop lung cancer. However, epidemiologists Doll and Hill, in the 1950s, demonstrated the relationship between lung cancer and smoking by comparing a group of people with lung cancer to a group of people without lung cancer. They discovered that the people with lung cancer had smoked significantly more cigarettes than those without lung cancer (Doll & Hill, 1950). Further epidemiologic research studies provided more evidence of a causal link between smoking cigarettes and lung cancer. Unfortunately, after 50 years, smoking is still a cause of significant illness and death throughout the world.

Epidemiology as the science of prevention emerged from the rigorous study of disease and illness in groups of people. **Epidemiology** is defined as the study of the distribution and determinants of states of health and illness in human populations. States of health and illness include health, disease, morbidity, injuries, disability, and mortality. The goals of epidemiology are to prevent or limit the consequences of illness and disability in humans, as well as to maximize their state of health (Harkness, 1995). The word *epidemiology* is derived from the word **epidemic** in the Greek language: *epi*—upon, *demo*—people, and *logos*—thought. In epidemiology, the community replaces the individual client as the primary focus of concern (Mausner & Kramer, 1985).

The science of epidemiology has been traditionally associated with infectious disease. Many of the techniques used in epidemiologic investigations were developed when cholera was killing much of the population of Europe. Therefore, early epidemiologic attempts to control and prevent infectious disease involved altering the characteristics of the agent, the host, and the environment (see Chapter 14).

The scope of epidemiology has expanded and shifted substantially. Primarily as a result of improved public health practices in the early 20th century, life expectancy in the United States, the United Kingdom, and European countries, as well as in other developed countries, rose. With it, a change in the patterns of disease occurred. No longer are infectious diseases the leading causes of death; the morbidity and mortality from noninfectious diseases and chronic degenerative conditions have increased (Table 6.1). Advancing technology in the 20th century made everyday life increasingly complex. There were unparalleled changes in diagnostic practices and therapeutic methods, resulting in expanded strategies for the prevention and control of disease. A focus on maintenance of wellness evolved.

All truths are easy to understand once they are discovered—the point is to discover them.

Galileo Galilei

Investigators now use epidemiologic techniques to study all aspects of health, including factors that keep people well. Chronic disease, psychosocial problems, occupational

table 6.1 **Comparison of the Leading Causes of Death in the United States, 1900 and 2010**

1900[a]	2010[b]
1. Major cardiovascular–renal disease	1. Heart disease
2. Influenza and pneumonia	2. Malignant neoplasms (cancer)
3. Tuberculosis	3. Chronic lower respiratory diseases
4. Gastritis, duodenitis, enteritis, and colitis	4. Cerebrovascular diseases (stroke)
5. Accidents	5. Unintentional injuries
6. Malignant neoplasms	6. Alzheimer disease
7. Diphtheria	7. Diabetes mellitus
8. Typhoid and paratyphoid fever	8. Nephritis, nephritic syndrome, and nephrosis
9. Measles	9. Influenza and pneumonia
10. Cirrhosis of the liver	10. Suicide

[a]U.S. Bureau of the Census. (1975). *Historical statistics of the United States, colonial times to 1970,* bicentennial edition, Part 2, Washington, D.C.
[b]Centers for Disease Control and Prevention. *Health, United States, 2013*. Retrieved from http://www.cdc.gov/nchs/hus.htm

injuries, environmental effects, and the planning and evaluation of health services are but a few of the disciplines that have been enhanced by using principles of epidemiology. Today, epidemiology is both a *research methodology* used to study states of health and illness and a *body of knowledge* that results from the study of a specific state of health or illness. When using epidemiology as a research methodology, the calculation of **rates** is the primary measurement used to describe either the occurrence or the existence of a specific state of health or illness (see Chapter 7).

How can Katie use these principles of epidemiology, both as a research method and as a body of knowledge, in her preparation for the 3-hour sessions?

DEVELOPMENT OF EPIDEMIOLOGY AS A SCIENCE

John Graunt and the Bills of Mortality

The study of illness in groups of people developed gradually. One of the first people to study patterns of disease in populations was a London haberdasher, John Graunt. In 1662, he analyzed the weekly reports of births and deaths in London; his analyses were the precursor of modern vital statistics. Graunt found that more male infants were born than female infants and that more men died than women. He also observed that infant mortality was high, and he noted that seasonal variations occurred in deaths.

Through his analysis of the Bills of Mortality, Graunt developed a better understanding of diseases and conditions that led to death. He published his observations and findings in *Natural and Political Observations Made upon the Bills of Mortality.* Graunt added an essential step in the development of epidemiology as a science. He developed a new logic of statistical inference, demonstrating that examining routinely collected data from groups of people would yield clues to human illness. His publication can be found online.

Two centuries passed before William Farr expanded Graunt's work. In the meantime, James Lind instituted the precursor of the clinical trial when he compared responses to dietary treatments for scurvy, and Percival Pott observed cancer of the scrotum in English chimney sweeps, hypothesizing that soot was the cause. Edward Jenner performed the first successful vaccination against smallpox with the liquid from a cowpox pustule, resulting in the vaccination of more than 100,000 people in England within 3 years. These accomplishments in the 18th century linked specific diseases with the characteristics of groups of people and documented the effects of various treatments. Table 6.2 summarizes the milestones in the evolution of epidemiology from 460 BC through the 20th century.

William Farr, Registrar General

In 1839, William Farr was appointed to the new Office of the Registrar General for England and Wales. Farr set up a system for the consistent collection of the numbers and causes of deaths. With these data, he was able to compare the death rates of workers in various occupations, the differences in mortality according to gender, and the effect of imprisonment on mortality. He also discovered an inverse relationship: deaths from cholera decreased with an increase in elevation above sea level (Farr, 1852).

Farr and his predecessors contributed significantly to the understanding of the distribution of illness and death. As one of the first epidemiologists, he recognized (1) the value of a precise definition of both the illness and the population at risk for the illness, (2) the importance of using appropriate comparison groups, and (3) that factors such as age, health status, and environmental exposure can confound statistical results.

John Snow and the Broad Street Pump

Perhaps the best known epidemiologist of the 19th century was John Snow, a contemporary of William Farr. He was a British physician who used population data and his own observations to investigate the epidemic of cholera that occurred from 1848 through 1854. He observed that deaths from cholera were particularly high in the parts of London supplied by two water companies the Lambeth Company and the Southward and Vauxhall Company.

Sewage heavily polluted a section of the Thames River, and interwoven water mains piped untreated water into the homes of two-thirds of London's residents. Houses on the same street received water from different companies. Sometime between 1849 and 1854, the Lambeth Company changed its water source to a less-contaminated location upstream. During a particularly bad cholera outbreak from 1853 to 1854, Snow demonstrated through calculation of death rates from cholera that the disease decreased in those areas supplied by the Lambeth Company but remained the same in those areas supplied by the Southward and Vauxhall Company (Table 6.3).

The most severe outbreak during this time was in the area of Broad Street, Golden Square, where people obtained their water from a local pump. More than 500 people died from cholera within 10 days. Believing that the water delivered by the pump was responsible for the cases of cholera, Snow removed the handle, and the number of cases immediately declined. However, there also were a number of other factors that contributed to this event, for example, an exodus of the population to other locations. Nonetheless, he is credited for "staying the epidemic," and a pump now has been erected in his honor on the corner of Broad Street in Soho.

Snow, during his investigations, mapped the areas where cholera occurred, developed rates as an objective measure to compare populations, made use of the natural experiment provided by the unusual pattern of water mains, and found evidence for the cause of cholera. These were

table 6.2 **Selected Milestones in the Evolution of Epidemiology**

Time	Person	Accomplishment or Event
460–377 BC	Hippocrates of Cos	First to record the relationship of the external environment to the health of individuals. Considered the first epidemiologist.
ca. 81 AD	Aretaeus the Cappadocian	Described pulmonary tuberculosis in detail.
129	Claudius Galen	Described the four humors and introduced many drugs derived from plants. First to describe smallpox.
500	Susruta	Brahmin physician who associated malaria with the mosquito.
850	Rhazes	Arab physician who wrote *al-Hawi*, papers that incorporated all known medical, anatomical, and pharmacologic knowledge of the time. Differentiated smallpox from measles.
1347		Italian 40-day ban on travel and trade was established to control bubonic plague. Quarantine comes from the Italian word *quarentina*, meaning 40 days.
1589	Thomas Moffet	First description of living organisms causing disease: lice, fleas, and scabies mites.
1662	John Graunt	London haberdasher who analyzed weekly reports of births and deaths. Found infant mortality was high and deaths varied according to seasons.
1683	Anton van Leeuwenhoek	Used a microscope to observe and describe "animalcules" from pond water and human saliva.
1701	Nicholas Andry	French surgeon who proposed that infection by germs was a cause of disease.
1747	James Lind	Observed and compared responses to dietary treatments for scurvy—the first evidence of a clinical trial. Recommended preventive techniques for typhus.
1760	Daniel Bernoulli	Demonstrated that smallpox conferred lifelong immunity through the use of the first life table techniques.
1775	Percival Pott	Observed that many English chimney sweeps developed cancer of the scrotum; hypothesized that exposure to soot was the cause.
1779	Johann Peter Frank	German who wrote *System of Medical Policing*, the first book about public health.
1798	Edward Jenner	Discovered the first vaccination against smallpox with cowpox pustule liquid. Within 3 years, 100,000 people in England were vaccinated.
1800	William Cruikshank	Scottish surgeon who used chlorine to purify water.
1836	Pierre Charles–Alexandre Louis	Conducted observational studies demonstrating the ineffectiveness of bloodletting. Emphasized statistics.
1840s–1860s	William Farr	First Registrar General in England. Considered father of modern statistics. Developed mortality surveillance systems and addressed basic epidemiologic concepts. Pioneered public health reforms.
1846	Peter Ludwig Panum	Danish physician who described the epidemiology of measles and the mechanism for spread of disease.
1847	Ignaz Semmelweis	Hungarian obstetrician who demonstrated that mortality from puerperal fever could be dramatically reduced if doctors washed their hands.
ca. 1850	Jean Baptiste Emile Vidal	French dermatologist responsible for the introduction of an efficient sewage system in Paris.
ca. 1854	John Snow	Performed epidemiologic research on transmission of cholera using natural experiments, mapping, and rates. Removed London's Broad Street drinking water pump handle to stop the spread of cholera.
1854	Florence Nightingale	Initiated sanitary reforms in the Crimean War and demonstrated that preventable or contagious diseases were the primary cause of mortality. Later used statistics to improve public health in England. Considered the founder of the nursing profession.
ca. 1860	John Parkin	English surgeon who used charcoal filters to purify water in an attempt to prevent the spread of cholera.
1860–1880s	Louis Pasteur	Developed pasteurization. Suggested that living organisms called "germs" caused infectious diseases.
1864		Contagious Diseases Act passed in England to combat the spread of venereal disease.
1865–1880s	Robert Koch	German who discovered the causal agents for anthrax, cholera, and tuberculosis. Developed criteria for identifying cause. Won Nobel Prize for bacteriology in 1905.
1866	Joseph Lister	Developed a carbolic acid spray for surgical disinfections.
1921		Johns Hopkins University established the first academic program in epidemiology.
1927	Wade Hampton Frost	Developed cohort analysis of mortality data and developed life tables. Credited for moving epidemiology from a descriptive to an analytical discipline.

(continued on page 110)

table 6.2 **Selected Milestones in the Evolution of Epidemiology** (continued)

Time	Person	Accomplishment or Event
1930		National Institutes of Health established in the United States.
1946		U.S. Communicable Disease Center was established. Now Centers for Disease Control and Prevention (CDC).
1948		Framingham cohort study of cardiovascular disease initiated.
1950s	Richard Doll and A. Bradford Hill	English researchers who conducted the landmark studies on the relationship between smoking and lung cancer.
Second half of 20th century		Chronic degenerative diseases replaced infectious diseases as leading causes of death worldwide.

Sources: Lee, H. S. J. (2002). *Dates in infectious diseases: A chronological record of progress in infectious diseases over the last millennium*. New York, NY: Parthenon Publishing Group; Timmreck, T. C. (2002). *An introduction to epidemiology*. Boston, MA: Jones and Bartlett; Lilienfeld, D. E., & Stolley, P. D. (1994). *Foundations of epidemiology*. New York, NY: Oxford University Press.

table 6.3 **Death Rates from Cholera by Water Company, London, 1853 to 1854**

Water Company	Population, 1851	Cholera Deaths	Deaths/100,000
Southwark and Vauxhall	167,654	192	114
Both companies	301,149	182	60
Lambeth	14,632	0	0

Source: Snow, J. (1855). *On the mode of communication of cholera.* London: John Churchill. http://www.ph.ucla.edu/epi/snow/snowbook.html

outstanding accomplishments in an era that preceded bacteriology. He published his findings in *On the Mode of Communication of Cholera* (Snow, 1855). The entire document is available online.

Florence Nightingale, Nurse and Epidemiologist

Florence Nightingale, the daughter of a wealthy Englishman, was also a contemporary of William Farr and John Snow. She devoted her life to the prevention of needless illness and death. She used compelling statistics to bring about healthcare reforms, both during the Crimean War and later in her English homeland. Also, she is credited with founding the profession of nursing.

Prior to leading a group of nurses to aid the British soldiers in the Crimean War, Nightingale was superintendent of a London hospital. There she supervised nurses, the operation of the physical plant, and the purity of the medicines. In 1854, she and a group of carefully chosen nurses and servants joined the troops in Scutari, in the Crimea. She was appalled by the conditions of the hospital barracks. Rats and fleas infested buildings, facilities were overcrowded, linen was filthy, essential supplies were missing, and an open sewer ran underneath the barracks. The soldiers suffered not only from wounds, but also from dysentery, malnutrition, frostbite, cholera, typhus, and scurvy. The mortality rate for the soldiers was 42.7% (Cohen, 1984).

Using carefully gathered data that were unique at the time, Nightingale documented the results of her sanitary reforms. The polar-area diagram she designed (Fig. 6.1) illustrates the needless deaths in the military hospitals during the Crimean War. Deaths peaked in January 1855. During that month, 83 soldiers died from wounds, but 2,700 died from infectious diseases. If the dead soldiers had not been replaced, infectious diseases would have wiped out the entire army. By the end of the war, the death rate in British soldiers in the Crimea was less than that of the troops at home (Cohen, 1984).

With the help of William Farr, Nightingale continued documenting events after the war that were associated with poor sanitary conditions. She compared mortality in civilians with that in soldiers and found that in peacetime, the soldiers in England had a mortality rate nearly twice that of civilian males. Nightingale asked for and received a formal investigation of military healthcare, and eventually, the government implemented her sanitary reforms. She studied the health of soldiers in India, the mortality in British hospitals, and the mortality following surgery. Throughout her career, she experimented with graphs and diagrams that everyone could understand and tried to introduce statistics into higher education. As a pioneering epidemiologist, she effectively demonstrated that statistics provide an organized way of learning from experience.

EPIDEMIOLOGIC MODELS

Epidemiologic Triad

The **epidemiologic triad** is the classic model based on the belief that health status is determined by the interaction of

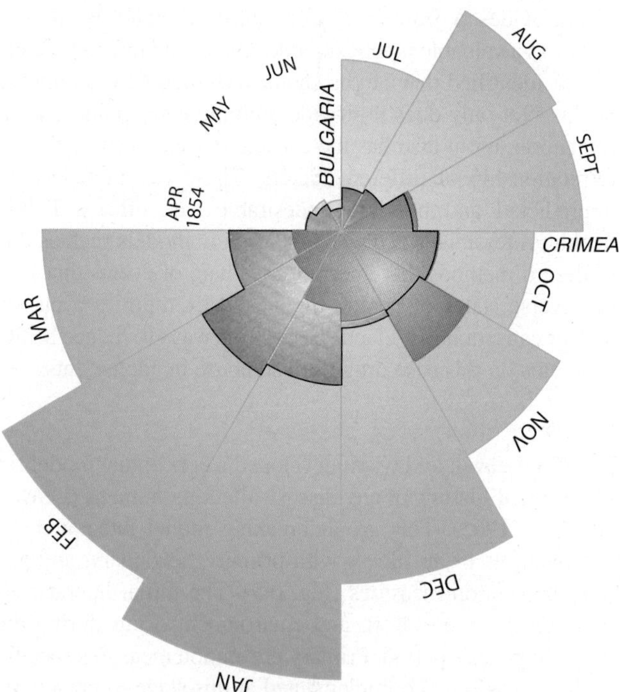

figure 6.1 Florence Nightingale's polar-area diagram illustrating the extent of needless deaths in British military hospitals during the Crimean War, April 1854 to March 1855. The blue wedges measured from the center of the circle represent area for area the deaths from preventable zymotic diseases, the red wedges measured from the center the deaths from wounds, and the black wedges measured from the center the deaths from all other causes. The black lines across the red triangles in September and November 1854 mark the boundaries of the deaths from all other causes during those months. In October 1854, the black area coincides with the red. The entire areas may be compared by following the blue, the red, and the black lines enclosing them. (From Aiken, L. [1988]. *Assuring the delivery of quality patient care.* State of the Science Invitational Conference, Nursing resources and the delivery of patient care [NIH Publication No. 89–3008, pp. 3–10]. Washington, DC: U.S. Department of Health and Human Services, Public Health Service; and Cohen, B. [1984]. Florence Nightingale. *Scientific America, 250*[3], 129.)

the characteristics of the host, agent, and environment, not by any single factor. The host is the client whose health status is the concern, whether it is a person, a family, a group of high-risk people, or the community as a whole. Agents are an element or force that under proper conditions can initiate or perpetuate a health problem. Environment refers to the context within which the agent and host interact (Fig. 6.2).

Host factors, sometimes called intrinsic factors, include both variable (modifiable) and absolute (nonmodifiable) factors. Age, race, and genetic makeup are examples of absolute, or nonmodifiable, factors. Lifestyle, exercise level, nutrition, health knowledge, and motivation for achieving optimal wellness are examples of host factors that are variable, or modifiable.

Agents can be classified into five groups. These agents may be *physical*, such as heat and trauma; *chemical*, such as

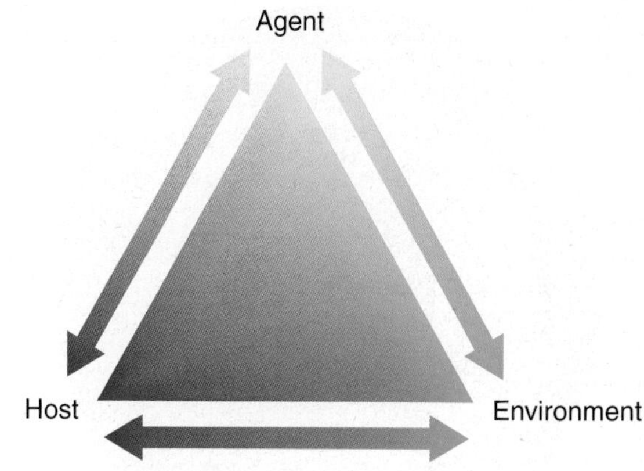

figure 6.2 The epidemiologic triad.

pollutants, medications, and drugs; *nutritional*, such as the absence or excess of water, vitamins, fats, proteins, and carbohydrates; *psychosocial*, such as stress, social isolation, and social support; and *biologic*, such as bacteria, viruses, arthropods, toxins, and conditions that interfere with the normal function of the body.

Environmental factors are frequently divided into three categories: biologic, physical, and social. The biologic environment is composed of plants, animals, and the toxins they produce; this includes pathogenic microorganisms, vectors that carry the infectious agents, and the reservoirs where infectious agents are normally found. The physical environment includes light, heat, air, atmospheric pressure, radiation, geologic factors, and the structures in the environment. The social environment includes culture, technology, educational opportunities, political systems, demographic characteristics, sociologic factors, and economic and legal systems.

The Wheel of Causation

Many diseases, illnesses, and conditions have multiple or no discernible agents, or the agent may be a part of the environment. An alternate model is conceptualized as a wheel, with a circle as the genetic core of the host, surrounded by a larger, segmented wheel representing the biologic, physical, and social environments (Fig. 6.3). The **wheel of causation** de-emphasizes the agent as the sole cause of disease, whereas it emphasizes the interplay of physical, biologic, and social environments. Interaction between the host and environment, with or without an identifiable agent, remains the major determinant of health status in all epidemiologic models.

The Web of Causation

The **web of causation** is an epidemiologic model that strongly emphasizes the concept of multiple causation while de-emphasizing the role of agents in explaining illness. At the time of development, there was a need to create a model that would help describe the multiple factors underlying chronic illnesses. These causal webs are more focused and realistic, and they may be as intricate and complex as needed. In this model, it is necessary to identify all possible antecedent

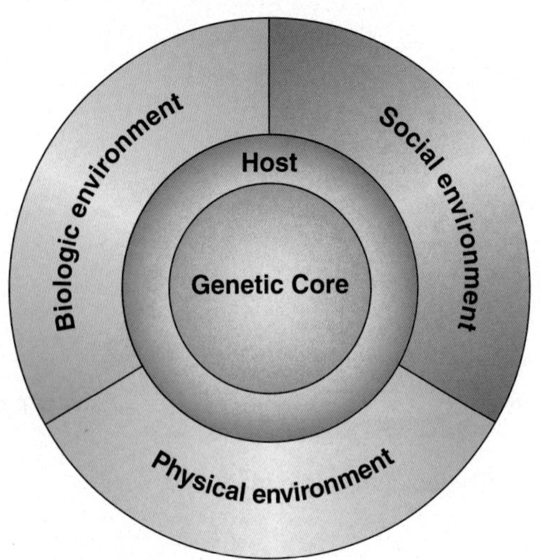

figure 6.3 The wheel of causation.

factors that could influence the development or prevention of a particular health condition. Each factor is perceived as a link in multiple interrelated chains. By making the pathways explicit in a web of causation, a diagram deepens understanding and provides a framework for statistical analysis. It also serves as a valuable practical guide. Direct and indirect factors can be identified that can be changed or modified to improve health. Not only does it provide multiple entry points for intervention, but it also has the capacity to demonstrate the interrelationship of different factors. These can include both unpredicted and possibly undesirable side effects. Public health professionals use web of causation models such as this to design methods that interrupt the chain of events that lead to adverse states of health. Figure 6.4 exemplifies a classic web of causation that identifies multiple ways to reduce health problems, in this case drug use and abuse in adolescents.

Natural History of Disease

In 1958, Leavell and Clark developed a conceptual model for the **natural history** of any disease affecting humans (Leavell & Clark, 1965). This groundbreaking model integrated the pathogenesis of an illness with primary, secondary, and tertiary prevention measures (Fig. 6.5). The initial interactions between the agent, host, and environment occur during the prepathogenesis period. Primary prevention measures specific to the disease can be implemented at this stage to prevent its

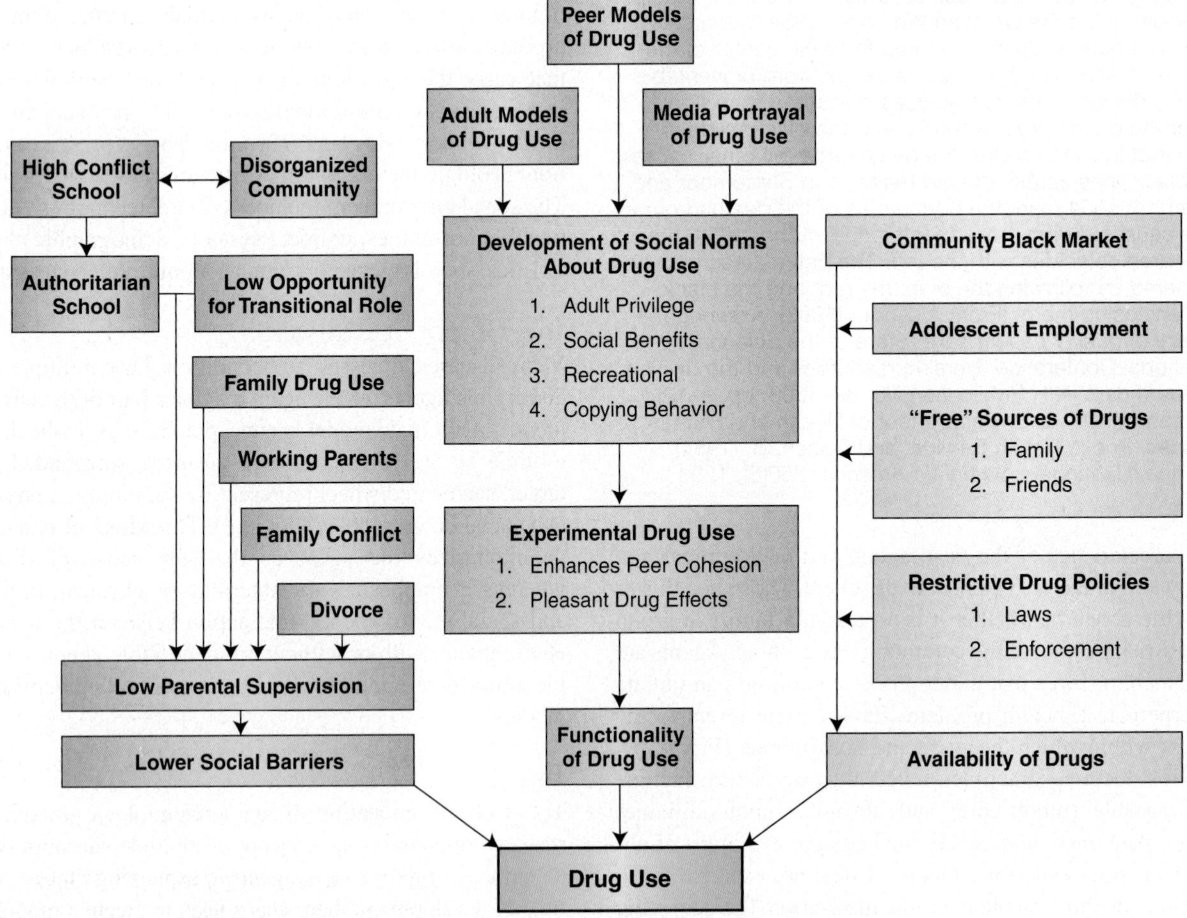

figure 6.4 The web of causation for drug use. (Used with permission from Duncan, D. F., & Petrosa, R. (1999). Social and community factors associated with drug use and abuse among adolescents. In T. P. Gullotta, G. R. Adams, & R. Montemayor (Eds.), Substance Misuse in Adolescence (pp. 56-91). Thousand Oaks, CA: Sage Publications.)

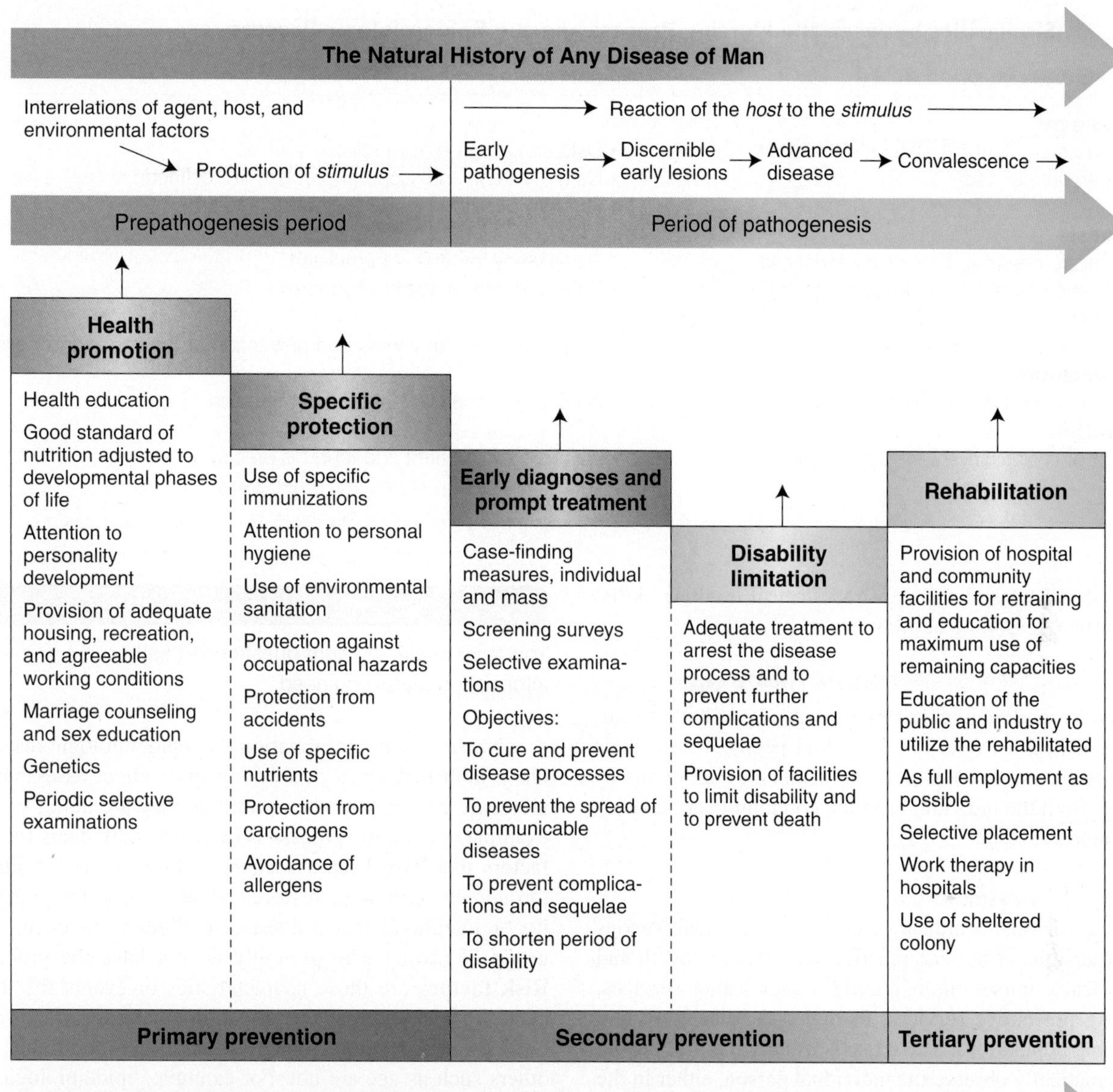

The Natural History of Any Disease of Man
Interrelations of agent, host, and environmental factors
Production of *stimulus*
Reaction of the *host* to the *stimulus*
Early pathogenesis
Discernible early lesions
Advanced disease
Convalescence
Prepathogenesis period
Period of pathogenesis
Health promotion
Health education
Good standard of nutrition adjusted to developmental phases of life
Attention to personality development
Provision of adequate housing, recreation, and agreeable working conditions
Marriage counseling and sex education
Genetics
Periodic selective examinations
Specific protection
Use of specific immunizations
Attention to personal hygiene
Use of environmental sanitation
Protection against occupational hazards
Protection from accidents
Use of specific nutrients
Protection from carcinogens
Avoidance of allergens
Early diagnoses and prompt treatment
Case-finding measures, individual and mass
Screening surveys
Selective examina-tions
Objectives:
To cure and prevent disease processes
To prevent the spread of communicable diseases
To prevent complica-tions and sequelae
To shorten period of disability
Disability limitation
Adequate treatment to arrest the disease process and to prevent further complications and sequelae
Provision of facilities to limit disability and to prevent death
Rehabilitation
Provision of hospital and community facilities for retraining and education for maximum use of remaining capacities
Education of the public and industry to utilize the rehabilitated
As full employment as possible
Selective placement
Work therapy in hospitals
Use of sheltered colony
Primary prevention
Secondary prevention
Tertiary prevention
Levels of application of preventive measures

figure 6.5 Leavell and Clark's natural history of any disease affecting humans. (Reprinted with permission from Leavell, H. F., & Clark, E. G. [1965]. *Preventive medicine for the doctor in his community, an epidemiologic approach*. New York, NY: McGraw-Hill.)

onset in a population of well people. The period of pathogenesis begins when there are biologic, psychological, or other responses within the host. Secondary prevention measures focus on early diagnosis and prompt treatment. This can limit resulting disabilities when implemented during the early stages of the disease. Tertiary prevention follows with rehabilitation measures that enable the individual to function at his or her maximum capability. This model, used widely in practice, is discussed in more detail in Chapter 5 (see Fig. 5.5).

Every human being is the author of his own health or disease.

Buddha

APPLYING EPIDEMIOLOGIC PRINCIPLES IN PRACTICE

The epidemiologic process and the nursing process are both derived from the problem-solving process that provides a framework for gathering data about health problems, analyzing the information, generating diagnoses or hypotheses, planning for resolution, implementing plans of action, and evaluating results (Table 6.4). The focus of the nursing process is on caring for the client within his or her family, whereas the focus of the epidemiologic process is on caring for the population of the community as a whole. Whether caring for the individual or the members of a community,

table 6.4 **Similarities between the Nursing Process and the Epidemiologic Process**

Nursing Process, Client Based	Epidemiologic Process, Population Based
Assessment	
• An individual client database is established • Data are interpreted	• Data are gathered from reliable sources • Nature, extent, and scope of problem are defined • Problem described by person, place, and time
Diagnosis	
• Healthcare needs and assets are identified • Goals and objectives for care are established	• Tentative hypothesis is formulated • Data analyzed to test the hypothesis
Planning	
• Processes for achieving goals are selected	• Plans are made for control and prevention of the condition or event
Implementation	
• Actions initiated to achieve goals	• Actions are initiated to implement the plan
Evaluation	
• Extent of goal achievement is determined	• Actions are evaluated and report is prepared • Further research is conducted if necessary

nurses need access to data, abstract critical thinking skills, and complex reasoning abilities.

Assessment of Health Needs and Assets

Community and public health nurses assess both health needs and health assets for individual people within their environment and for the population within the community as a whole. Both the individual and the community are considered clients.

Individual Assessment

Providing personal healthcare services to individual persons is a cornerstone of nursing practice. Community health and public health nurses often provide direct health services, including preventive services, to high-risk, displaced, and vulnerable populations. The nurse is usually the first person to systematically observe the individual person, either in the home, clinic, parish, or healthcare facility. The public health nurse takes a nursing history, performs a physical assessment, and makes both objective and subjective observations about the condition of the person. He or she establishes where the person is in relation to the full spectrum of health and identifies the person's assets as well as needs. Assets include strengths and resources of the client such as general state of health, prior use of healthcare services, health behaviors, lifestyle, motivation, and other factors. This information establishes the database about the client. The planning process and the interventions that are subsequently implemented are based on this assessment. Also, the database becomes a baseline for measuring the outcomes of care.

Considering the goals of the delinquency prevention program, what information does Katie need to gather from her group of young people? How could she access this information?

PRACTICE POINT

You have to ask the right questions to gather the information (data) you need.

Nurses use the information that epidemiologic research has established when performing most client assessments, although they may not be aware that they are doing so. For example, a common process is to assess individuals for risk factors that have been associated with a disease or illness through epidemiologic research. **Risk** refers to the probability or likelihood that a disease or illness will occur in a group of people who presently do not have the problem. **Risk factors** are those characteristics or events that have been shown to increase the probability that a specific disease or illness will develop. Some risk factors are modifiable, and others such as age are not. For example, epidemiologic research has established that certain risk factors, such as a sedentary lifestyle, obesity, increased cholesterol, hypertension, and smoking, are associated with cardiovascular disease. These risk factors are now a part of the epidemiologic body of knowledge, or the epidemiology, of heart disease. As a result, several health appraisal approaches are now commonly used to profile client risk.

What factors increase the risk of negative health outcomes for youths in gangs?

Epidemiologic research has also established the natural history of most illnesses. This refers to the course of a disease or condition from onset to resolution. It includes (1) pathologic onset stage, (2) the presymptomatic stage, and (3) the manifestation of clinical disease (Leavell & Clark, 1965). Through the individual assessment process, the nurse can begin to determine the stage of the illness in question.

Cues identified at the initial assessment may indicate whether primary, secondary, or tertiary prevention interventions would be most appropriate.

EVIDENCE FOR PRACTICE

Decline in the physical functioning of the elderly is of concern worldwide. Chen, Chang, and Lan (2014) conducted a study that evaluated the association between changes in physical functioning and a variety of other factors in an older population in Taiwan. The data of 907 participants were derived from the Functioning and Aging Study conducted in Taipei between 2005 and 2009.

Functional status was assessed using activities of daily living, instrumental activities of daily living and mobility tasks, and classification as being normal, with mild disability, moderate disability, and severe disability.

The proportion of elderly participants with normal function decreased with time throughout the study period. Risk factors, both modifiable and nonmodifiable, that were associated with changes in physical functioning included the following:

- Age
- Living arrangements, social support
- Self-rated health
- Stroke
- Diabetes
- Parkinson disease
- Osteoporosis
- Depression
- Cognition
- Vision
- History of fracture and falls
- Incontinence of urine and feces
- Physical activity
- Body mass index, short physical performance

Researchers conclude that older persons with stroke, Parkinson disease, diabetes, osteoporosis, geriatric conditions, and poor short physical performance would benefit the most from prevention measures for functional decline. Older people not living with spouses, with poor self-rated health, with low social support, who are malnourished and live a sedentary lifestyle might also benefit from interventions protecting against functional decline. All public health nurses can assess their elderly clients and plan interventions that will protect them from excessive decline in the ability to function well in their daily lives.

Community Assessment

Conceptualizing the community as a client is difficult for the individual-oriented nurse. Assessing the health needs and assets of a community involves creating a comprehensive community profile or database. The individual nurse may be solely responsible for the assessment, but usually he or she contributes to the assessment as a member of a team. Epidemiologic statistical methods, such as calculation of rates, are used in this process (see Chapter 7). A detailed discussion of community assessment is found in Chapter 11.

Epidemiologists gather available demographic data that provide information about the age and sex distribution, socioeconomic characteristics, and cultural and ethnic distributions. They access vital statistics, including applicable epidemiologic morbidity and mortality rates. Additional data can be obtained from community members or community groups. Information about the accessibility and availability of healthcare services, such as health manpower, may or may not be community assets. To obtain information about health beliefs, norms, values, goals, perceived needs, and health practices, healthcare workers may use focus groups, interviews or observation, or surveys. Nurses may participate in field-testing new tools for data collection.

After epidemiologists collect the data, they synthesize and analyze the information and generate a list of community health needs and assets. Identifying patterns of disease, illness, and injuries detects trends that form the rationale for program development. Critical thinking skills are essential for the appropriate analysis of this information. Finally, it is necessary to set goals and objectives to address high-priority problems.

PRACTICE POINT

A thorough and accurate client database, whether that of individuals, groups, or the community, provides the evidence and rationale for your interventions.

To understand the scope of the health problems facing the young people who were enrolled in the delinquency prevention program, a community assessment should be considered. What information does Katie need to gather, and where would she find that information?

STUDENT REFLECTION

Although my nursing program focused a lot on research findings, particularly in writing assignments, I did not fully understand the impact that statistics can make in nursing until I had my community practicum in a local women's health center. When I arrived there, the staff was talking about a violent episode that had occurred the previous week. Everyone seemed to think that there was more violence in the community than there should be, and that we needed to know more about it.

My preceptor was a program developer, and the women at the center asked her if they needed a violence prevention program. One of my first assignments was to find out just how much and what types of violence had occurred in the last year. The first thing my preceptor suggested was to go online and look at websites for various states and towns. I was amazed at how much information was available. For example, I found out that the rates of homicide, assaults, and rapes in our town were greater than the average for both the state and the nation. Also, I found out that 45% of the poor, young males from minority groups were in jail for crimes of violence! I learned that most violence occurs between people who know each other, and that violence is related to substance abuse. I presented my information to the staff, and they all decided to have my preceptor contact other community agencies and the local college to form a coalition to address violence. I attended the first meeting, and people tossed around lots of ideas. They decided to look into a 24/7 free telephone line to give people support in a crisis, increase housing for women suffering from domestic violence, and consider a number of initiatives for youth in the town.

This experience taught me several things.

- Lots of information is available about health problems in a community.
- New ideas require presentation of supportive data.
- Involving other interested communities can enhance whatever is planned to reduce health problems.
- One person's efforts can really make a difference.

Using Assessment Data for Planning and Implementing Interventions

The individual or community client database, much of which has been gathered using epidemiologic methods, provides the rationale for planning and implementing interventions. It is possible to use the epidemiologic body of knowledge that describes the natural progression of specific diseases or illnesses to target ways to break the problem cycle once it has been identified. An intervention plan outlines the goals, objectives, and strategies for achieving the interventions and provides completion dates for their accomplishment. The type of health problem, the readiness of the individual or community to address the problem, the availability of health services, the nurse's role, the characteristics of social change, and other related factors influence successful implementation.

Three goals for the delinquency prevention program are presented at the beginning of this chapter.
Write an objective for each goal.

Promoting Healthy Lifestyles

Every phase of public health nursing involves the provision of health education whenever the opportunity arises. Lifestyle patterns are modifiable, and nurses can help make the public aware of the benefits of preventive health through use of the media and meeting with individuals and community groups.

Following the landmark epidemiologic studies of smoking and lung cancer in the 1950s, the general public gradually recognized that personal behaviors such as smoking were risk factors for the leading conditions causing morbidity and mortality in the United States and other countries. In 1984, the Centers for Disease Control and Prevention (CDC) and the U.S. state health departments collaboratively established the Behavioral Risk Factor Surveillance System (BRFSS). The goal of this surveillance system is to collect, analyze, and interpret specific behavioral risk factor data that can be used to plan, implement, and monitor health promotion and disease prevention programs.

The BRFSS gathers information about health behaviors, such as lack of physical activity, obesity, and safety belt use, primarily by telephone calls. It also gathers data about preventive health services, such as screening for breast and cervical cancer and elevated blood cholesterol. The BRFSS used these epidemiologic statistics when national objectives were established for *Healthy People 2000*, *Healthy People 2010*, and *Healthy People 2020*. *Healthy People 2020*, developed by the U.S. Department of Health and Human Services, sets behavioral objectives to be achieved over the second decade of the 21st century. Experts developed these objectives through a broad consultation process, built on the best scientific knowledge and designed to measure programs over time. Along with the BRFSS data, *Healthy People 2020* serves as the basis for the development of state and community plans to improve the health of their populations. Each state collects statistics for the BRFSS, and thus these data are available for nurses to access when planning educational programs for primary prevention.

Dietary factors are associated with four out of the 10 leading causes of death: heart disease, some types of cancer, stroke, and type 2 diabetes. Obesity rates have doubled in adults and tripled in children and adolescents over the last two decades. The data are alarming (CDC, 2014b):

- 35.9% of adults aged 20 years and older are obese.
- 62.2% of adults aged 20 years and older are overweight, including obesity.
- 18.4% of adolescents aged 12 to 19 years are obese.
- 18% of children aged 6 to 11 years are obese.
- 12.1% of children aged 2 to 5 years are obese.

The estimated cost of these diet-related conditions is more than $123 billion annually in medical expenses. Including lost productivity in these statistics adds billions more (CDC, 2010). The BRFSS data dramatically demonstrate the significant increase in the prevalence of overweight people in the United States (Fig. 6.6). Using these data, *Healthy People 2020* identified overweight and obesity as a major health issue in the United States. Sex and ethnicity are also important factors in the development of obesity (Fig. 6.7). Overweight is most prevalent in African-American and Hispanic females. If nurses find that such statistics

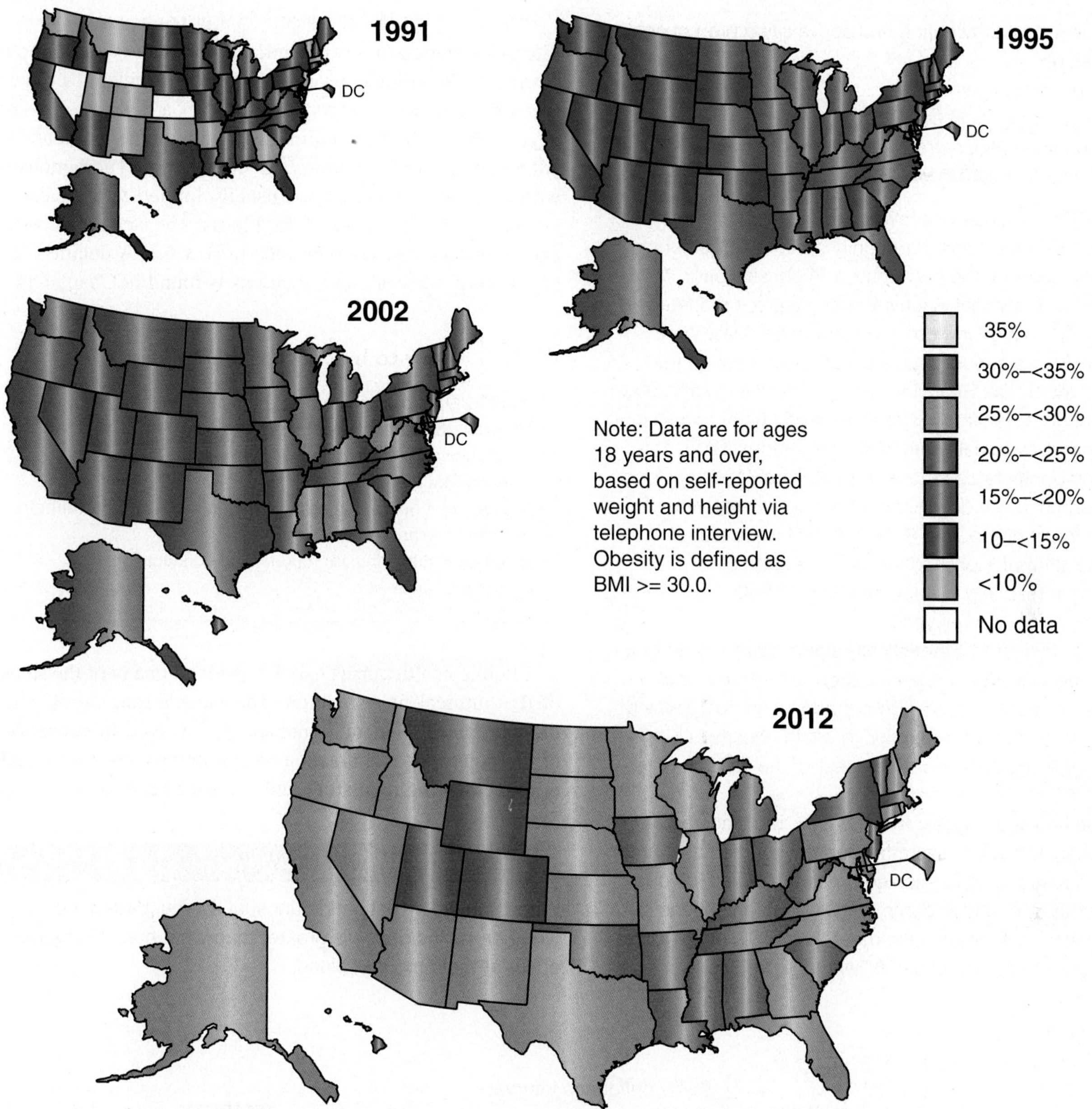

figure 6.6 Changes in prevalence of obesity among U.S. adults. Note that the data are for ages 18 years and over, based on self-reported weight and height via telephone interview. Obesity is defined as body mass index ≥30. (From National Health and Nutrition Examination Survey, NCHS, CDC; BRFSS, 2012.)

apply to the members of their own community, they can initiate programs to address the problem.

The burden of food-related ill health measured in terms of mortality and morbidity is similar to that attributable to smoking. The cost is twice the amount attributable to car, train, and other accidents, and more than twice that attributable to smoking. The vast majority of the burden is attributable to unhealthy diets rather than to food-borne diseases.

PRACTICE POINT

Use statistics to demonstrate the need for program development and community interventions.

EVIDENCE FOR PRACTICE

Healthier food access in schools is a major objective of *Healthy People 2020*. To accomplish this goal, the United States has invested heavily in actions to prevent youth obesity by promoting healthy eating and physical activity. With support from CDC, a Putting Prevention to Work (CPPW) obesity prevention program was initiated in King County, Washington, during 2010 and 2012 (CDC, 2014a). Components of the robust obesity prevention program included the following:

- Implementation of nutrition standards for school meals

- Student-led healthy eating and active living promotional campaigns
- Farm to school initiatives
- High-quality physical education
- Nutrition and culinary training for school cafeteria staff
- Participation in community health coalitions

The CPPW focused on low-income school districts and communities, since community health assessment data indicated that the prevalences of obesity, poor nutrition, and physical inactivity were disproportionately high relative to higher-income communities. Data were obtained from a school-based survey analogous to the national Youth Risk Behavior Survey. The Washington State Department of Health used self-reported height and weight from the survey to calculate body mass index (BMI). The survey response rates ranged from 63% to 71%, resulting in approximately 34,000 respondents per survey year, for the project group, and 61% to 67% for the rest of the population of Kings County and the state of Washington resulting in approximately 18,500 respondents per survey year.

Results indicated a statistically significant 17% decline in youth obesity after implementation of CPPW school districts, but not in non-CPPW districts. Also, there was a statistically significant reduction in youth obesity in Kings County when compared with the rest of the state of Washington.

These findings suggest that focused, multifaceted, and comprehensive policy, systems, and environmental change interventions located in each community can reduce obesity in youth. Continued community level interventions such as these have the potential to meet the CDC's obesity prevention priority as one of its 10 "winnable battles."

Preventing and Controlling Outbreaks

The investigation of an epidemic or **outbreak** is an example of the epidemiologic process in action. Epidemics occur when there is an increased incidence of a disease or event beyond that which is normally found in the population. Although the term *outbreak* is often used synonymously with epidemic, outbreaks are usually limited to a localized increase in the incidence of the illness. The steps of investigating an outbreak are presented in Box 6.1. A detailed description of outbreak investigations is found in Chapter 14.

box 6.1 How to Investigate an Outbreak

- Establish the existence of the outbreak.
- Describe the outbreak according to person, place, and time.
- Formulate and test hypotheses as to the most probable causative factors.
- Implement a plan for control of the outbreak and prevention of further outbreaks.
- Evaluate results, prepare reports, and conduct further research if necessary.

Public health nurses may be involved in any of the steps of the outbreak investigation. The nurse's role varies with the workplace. Generally, nurses are involved in education of the public, in mobilization of community resources, and in implementing regulatory and control measures.

PRACTICE POINT

When you are investigating unusual events, determine whether the incidence is greater than what normally would occur at that time and place.

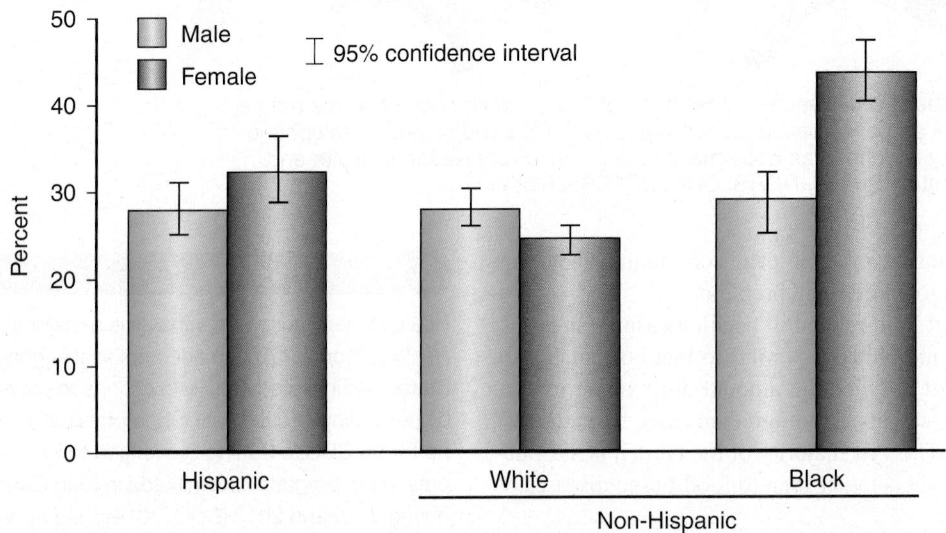

figure 6.7 Age-adjusted prevalence of obesity among adults aged 20 and over, by race/ethnicity: United States, January to June 2013. Note that data are age adjusted to the 2000 standard population. Obesity is defined as body mass index ≥30. (Retrieved from www.cdc.gov/nchs/data/nhis/earlyrelease/earlyrelease201312_06.pdf)

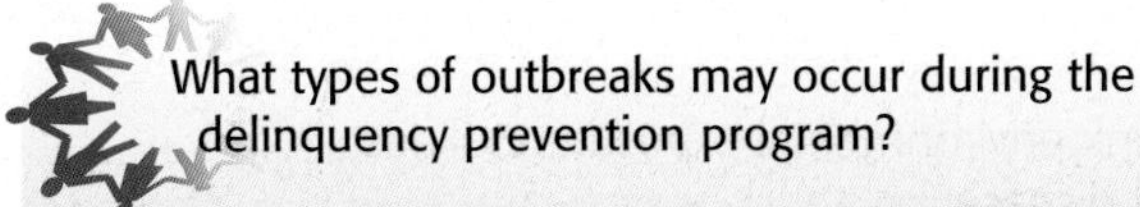

What types of outbreaks may occur during the delinquency prevention program?

Contributing to a Safe and Healthy Environment

Individual and community risk assessments should include detection of real or potential threats from the environment. Environment includes physical, biologic, social, cultural, or any other external factors that can influence the health status of individuals or populations. The principles of epidemiology, normally used in investigating disease and illness, can be applied to the human effects of natural disasters such as hurricanes and earthquakes, as well as to industrial disasters such as injuries, air pollution, nuclear accidents, and release of toxic chemicals.

PRACTICE POINT

Evaluate your community, and subsets of the community, for potential environmental hazards.

When healthcare professionals gather demographic data, vital statistics, and epidemiologic morbidity and mortality statistics, they should also consult environmental health sources. Using detailed individual or community client databases, nurses then have the potential to link environmental exposure to illness and disease. Nurses often provide case management for both communicable and chronic illnesses that result from environmental exposure. Nurses also may be risk consultants, communicators, and educators, working with community groups, agencies, and industry to protect the health of their workers.

What are the environmental risks for the group of delinquent youth? How would Katie address these in her sessions with the youth?

The World Health Organization (WHO), the National Institute for Occupational Safety and Health (NIOSH) in the United States, and other international and national agencies review existing knowledge about chemicals, radiation, and other environmental hazards that have immediate and long-term effects on health, and issue reports concerning environmental health criteria. See Chapter 21 for detailed information regarding environmental assessment.

Evaluating the Effectiveness of Health Services

Public health professionals who collect epidemiologic data during assessments and use them for establishing the need for health programs can also use them to evaluate those services. Evaluation requires a systematic and objective process that determines the relevance, effectiveness, and impact of the health service. Creating objectives that are measurable assists in this process. Nurses should continuously monitor the health status indicators in the community, especially for vulnerable populations. Age-specific mortality rates, low birth rates, infant mortality rates, health services utilization, and other indexes specific to the characteristics of the community are examples (see Chapter 7). This information assists in identifying gaps and detecting emerging problems early so that appropriate responses can be facilitated. In addition, nurses and other healthcare professionals can also use epidemiologic principles to develop surveys to gather specific information from targeted populations such as child care centers or the population of census tracts that may be at high risk.

The primary way to demonstrate prevention or control of a health problem is to compare epidemiologic statistics before and after the implementation of the health service. Planning and evaluation are continuous processes. As new data become available, modification in health services may be necessary, and those modifications require evaluation.

PRACTICE POINT

Use your program objectives to evaluate your interventions.

Outline an evaluation program for the delinquent youth prevention program discussed in the case at the beginning of this chapter.

key concepts

- Early attempts at understanding the reasons for disease were primarily a direct result of trial-and-error observations of individual people.
- Study of illness and causes of death in groups of people began in the 17th century. Founders of epidemiology as the science of preventive medicine included John Graunt, William Farr, John Snow, and Florence Nightingale.
- Epidemiology is defined as the study of the distribution and determinants of the states of health and illness in human populations, with the goal of preventing or limiting consequences and maximizing states of health.
- Individual and community assessments, using epidemiologic principles, form the database that provides the evidence and rationale for interventions.

key concepts (continued)

- Promoting healthy lifestyles uses epidemiologic data such as that found in the BRFSS. The U.S. publication *Healthy People 2020* defines measurable objectives to be achieved over the second decade of the 21st century.
- Nurses, in their care of individual and community clients, have the potential to link environmental exposure to illness and disease.
- Epidemiologic data, collected during assessments that establish the need for health programs, are also used to evaluate those services.

critical thinking questions

1. Jeff is 11 years old and slightly overweight. His father is a truck driver who was recently diagnosed with type 2 diabetes. His mother is a licensed practical nurse at the local hospital. At a recent health science fair at his school, a student-led screening clinic documented Jeff's blood pressure at 140/92 mm Hg.
   a. Is Jeff at risk? If so, for what?
   b. What other data do you need?
   c. How does epidemiologic data define hypertension in a child Jeff's age?
   d. What recommendations would you make?
   e. Are there health promotion activities that you would recommend?
2. Look through several major newspapers for articles containing health statistics.
   a. What are the implications of these statistics for your community?
   b. What further data would you obtain to document the problem in your community?
3. Go to the CDC website: www.cdc.gov. Pick a topic to explore. Show how epidemiologic information has been used to describe the topic.
4. Explore the website "Violence Prevention" (http://www.cdc.gov/ViolencePrevention/pub/PreventingYV.html). Identify at least one activity that Katie could use to meet each of the goals of her program.

references

Centers for Disease Control and Prevention. (2010). *National health priorities, reducing obesity, heart disease, cancer, diabetes and other diet and inactivity related diseases, costs, and disabilities*. Retrieved from http://www.cdc.gov/nccdphp/dnpao/index.html

Centers for Disease Control and Prevention. (2014a). Declines in student obesity prevalence associated with a prevention initiative—King County, Washington, 2012. *Morbidity and Mortality Weekly Reports*, *63*(07), 155–157.

Centers for Disease Control and Prevention. (2014b). *FASTSTATS: Obesity and overweight*. Retrieved from http://www.cdc.gov/nchs/fastats/overwt.htm

Centers for Disease Control. (2013) *Health, United States, 2012*, Retrieved from http://www.cdc.gov/nchs/hus.htm

Chen, C. M., Chang, W. C., & Lan, T. Y. (2014). Identifying factors associated with changes in physical functioning in an older population. *Geriatrics Gerontology International*. doi:10.1111/ggi.12243. Retrieved from http://www.ncbi.nlm.nih.gov/pubmed/24506482

Cohen, I. B. (1984). Florence Nightingale. *Scientific American*, *250*(3), 128–137.

Doll, R., & Hill, A. B. (1950). Smoking and carcinoma of the lung. *British Medical Journal*, 2(4682), 739–748.

Farr, W. (1852). Influence of elevation on the fatality of cholera. *Journal of the Statistical Society of London*, *15*, 155–183.

Harkness, G. A. (1995). *Epidemiology in nursing practice*. St. Louis, MO: Mosby.

Hippocrates. (1938). On airs, waters, and places [400 BC]: Translated and republished. *Medical Classics*, *3*, 19–42.

Leavell, H. F., & Clark, E. G. (1965). *Preventive medicine for the doctor in his community: An epidemiologic approach* (p. 21). New York, NY: McGraw-Hill.

Lee, H. S. J. (2002). *Dates in infectious diseases: A chronological record of progress in infectious diseases over the last millennium*. New York, NY: Parthenon Publishing Group.

Mausner, J. S., & Kramer, S. (1985). *Epidemiology—An introductory text* (2nd ed.). Philadelphia, PA: W. B. Saunders.

Sanders, B., Schneiderman, J. U., Loken, A., Lankenau, S. E., & Bloom, J. J. (2009). Gang youth as a vulnerable population for nursing intervention. *Public Health Nursing*, *26*(4), 346–352.

Snow, J. (1855). *On the mode of communication of cholera*. London: John Churchill. Retrieved from http://www.ph.ucla.edu/epi/snow/snowbook.html

web resources

Please visit thePoint® for up-to-date web resources on this topic.

CHAPTER 7

Describing Health Conditions: Understanding and Using Rates

Gail A. Harkness

Perplexity is the beginning of knowledge.

Khalil Gibran

There are three kinds of epidemiologists: those who can count and those who can't.

Anonymous

Prejudice is a great time saver. You can form opinions without having to get the facts.

E.B. White, author

chapter highlights

- Concept and calculation of rates
- Crude, specific, and adjusted rates
- Incidence and prevalence rates
- Sensitivity and specificity calculations

objectives

- Describe the primary method used to measure the existence of states of health or illness in a population during a given time period.
- Explain the formula and rules for calculation of a rate.
- Differentiate between crude and adjusted rates.
- Contrast incidence rates and prevalence rates.
- Discuss the use of specific rates when describing characteristics of person, place, and time.
- Differentiate between incidence density, incidence rates, and relative risk ratio.
- Discuss differences between the sensitivity and specificity of tests.
- Using examples, interpret the relevance of the use of rates in nursing practice.

key terms

Adjusted rate: Statistical procedure that removes the effects of differences in the composition of a population, such as age, when comparing one to another.

Attack rate: An incidence or occurrence rate.

Attributable risk: The difference between the incidence rates in an exposed and an unexposed group of people.

Case fatality rate: Calculated by dividing the number of deaths from a specific disease by the number of people living with that disease during the year, and multiplying by 100.

Cause-specific mortality rate: The probability of death from a specific cause.

Crude rate: Measurement of the occurrence of the health problem or condition being investigated in the entire population.

Demographic data: The study of the size, distribution, and characteristics of human populations.

Epidemic curve: A graph that plots the distribution of cases by the time of onset of the disease.

Epidemiologic descriptive studies: Research studies designed to acquire more information about the occurrence and distribution of states of health, such as characteristics of person, place, and time.

Incidence density: Use of a person-time denominator in the calculation of rates; a person-day reflects one person at risk for 1 day, and a person-year represents one person at risk for 1 year.

Incidence rate: Measure of the probability that people without a certain condition will develop that condition over a period of time.

Long-term change: Fluctuations in time surrounding health problems that extend over decades, reflecting gradual changes.

Morbidity: A departure from a state of physiologic or psychological well-being.

Mortality rate: The probability of death from any cause among the entire population within a given time frame.

Period prevalence: A prevalence rate that indicates the existence of a condition during an interval of time, often a year.

Periodic change: Seasonal or cyclic fluctuations in time surrounding health problems.

Point prevalence: A prevalence rate that indicates the existence of a condition at a specific point in time.

Population at risk: Groups of people who have specific characteristics, or risk factors, that increase the probability of developing health problems.

Prevalence rate: Measures the number of people in a given population who have an existing condition at a given point in time.

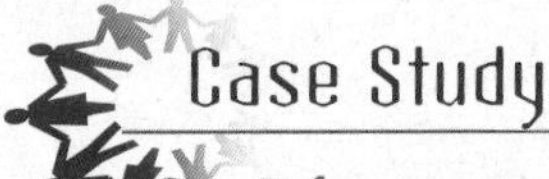

Case Study

References to the case study are found throughout this chapter (look for the case study icon). Readers should keep the case study in mind as they read the chapter.

The Visiting Nurse Association serving two rural counties in Florida has received a grant from the United States Office of Minority Health for a human immunodeficiency virus/acquired immunodeficiency syndrome (HIV/AIDS) prevention outreach program targeted toward the two counties' large African-American population. The counties are adjacent to each other and have a combined population of 312,838 people. The number of African-American people in the two counties is 57,875, or 18.5% of the population.

Lindsay is on the team that developed the program grant, and she is now the program director. She and the team members develop a HIV/AIDS outreach survey, a yes-or-no checklist that serves as a data collection form. Demographic information will be collected at the end of the interview. Outreach workers from the African-American community are hired to interview people, on the street and in their homes, following a week-long training session on HIV/AIDS and methods of establishing rapport (adapted and updated from Brown & Brown, 2003).

HIV/AIDS Outreach Survey Form

1. Do you know about HIV/AIDS?
2. Are you doing anything to protect yourself from HIV?
3. Have you used drugs?
4. Have you been tested for HIV?
5. Modes of HIV transmission reviewed?
6. Risk factors reviewed?
7. Discussed HIV risk reduction?
   a. Correct condom use
   b. Monogamous partners
   c. Reduce number of partners
   d. Cleanliness of equipment
8. Literature given?
9. Condoms given?
10. Is subject male or female?

Comments: ________________

key terms (continued)

Proportion: A type of ratio that includes the quantity in the numerator as a part of the denominator.

Proportional mortality ratio: A ratio that compares deaths from a specific illness with deaths from all other causes.

Rate: The primary measurement used to describe the occurrence (quantity) of a state of health in a specific group of people in a given time period.

Ratio: A fraction that represents the relationship between two numbers.

Relative risk ratio: The ratio of the incidence rate in the exposed group and the incidence rate in the nonexposed group.

Sensitivity: Ability of a test to correctly identify people who have a health problem; the probability of testing positive if the health problem is truly present.

Short-term change: Variations measured in hours, days, weeks, or months; commonly found in outbreaks of infectious disease.

Specific rates: Detailed rates that are calculated using the number of people in the smaller subgroups of the population in the denominator. Often, people are divided into subgroups by age and sex, although any characteristic can be used.

Specificity: Ability of a test to correctly identify people who do not have a health problem; the probability of testing negative if the health problem is truly absent.

To understand the extent of a state of health, whether it is a disease, disability, or factors that keep people well, it is necessary to describe the magnitude or frequency of the condition. Since people differ in terms of health, it is important to know how they differ. By looking at the frequency of the condition in groups of people who either have or do not have the problem under investigation, it can be determined who is at risk or not at risk for that condition. Using this technique, descriptive epidemiology can demonstrate the seriousness of the problem, determine the characteristics of the people it affects, and identify where and when it occurs. It can also provide data, or clues, that suggest how the condition evolves and why the condition exists. This information can indicate which people are likely to develop certain health problems; what diseases, disabilities, or needs they have; how these health problems are distributed within the community; and what kind of health services are needed. The use of existing resources in a community can then be determined and programs planned to address the needs.

Using the information about the frequency and distribution of a condition, nurses and other healthcare professionals can examine the characteristics of groups of people in the community, or within institutions, who are most likely to develop health problems. These groups are considered to be **populations at risk**. Knowledge about the population at risk and risk factors can be also used to set priorities for the development of strategies to meet emerging health needs and for expansion or change in programs or services that are directed toward secondary or tertiary prevention.

The process of using epidemiologic techniques to generate a knowledge base about a specific health problem, and plan for its control and prevention, is best illustrated by cardiovascular disease. The knowledge gained from the study of populations at risk and identification of predisposing risk factors has been the foundation for the primary, secondary, and tertiary prevention strategies used widely today. Since the initial development of objectives in *Healthy People 2000* in the United States, there has been a focus on health promotion activities, such as exercise, good nutrition, smoking cessation, and weight control (primary prevention). Cholesterol and blood pressure screening (secondary prevention) have become a high priority in primary care practices. Also, treatment for people who have cardiovascular disease includes rehabilitation programs with a primary focus on increasing cardiovascular health (tertiary prevention).

Although most epidemiologic studies have focused on disease and disability, it should be emphasized that this process can also be used to study states of wellness. For example, studies of the factors that are associated with healthy, community-dwelling elderly people can lead to the implementation of strategies to enhance wellness in the elderly population.

To demonstrate that African-American people are a population at risk, Lindsay examines Florida statistics. She finds that since the epidemic began, a cumulative total of 107,980 cases of HIV/AIDS have been diagnosed in Florida. Nearly half (48.7%) of these cases have occurred in African-American people. Make a list of other information that Lindsay needs to understand the scope of the HIV/AIDS problem in the two counties.

UNDERSTANDING AND USING RATES

Although the most basic measure of frequency involves counting the number of affected people, this may result in misleading impressions and usually is of limited use. A higher number of cases in one group of people versus another may mean that the number of susceptible people in that group is greater or that the counting took place over a longer period of time. To provide more valid descriptions of the frequency of various states of health, it is necessary to use ratios, proportions, and rates.

However, there are some statistics that are impressive even if they involve counting (or estimating) just the number of affected people. For example, Figure 7.1 illustrates the 10 leading causes of death in the world in 2011. The figure shows that chronic diseases are causing increased number of deaths worldwide. Ischemic heart disease caused 7 million deaths, lung cancers caused 1.5 million deaths, and diabetes caused 1.4 million deaths in 2011 (World Health Organization, 2011).

A **ratio** is a fraction that represents the relationship between two numbers. It is the value obtained by dividing one quantity by another quantity. People (or things) counted in the numerator are not counted in the denominator. For example, the number of boys (160) in an elementary school could be contrasted with the number of girls (80) in that school using a ratio (160/80 = 2/1 = twice as many boys as girls).

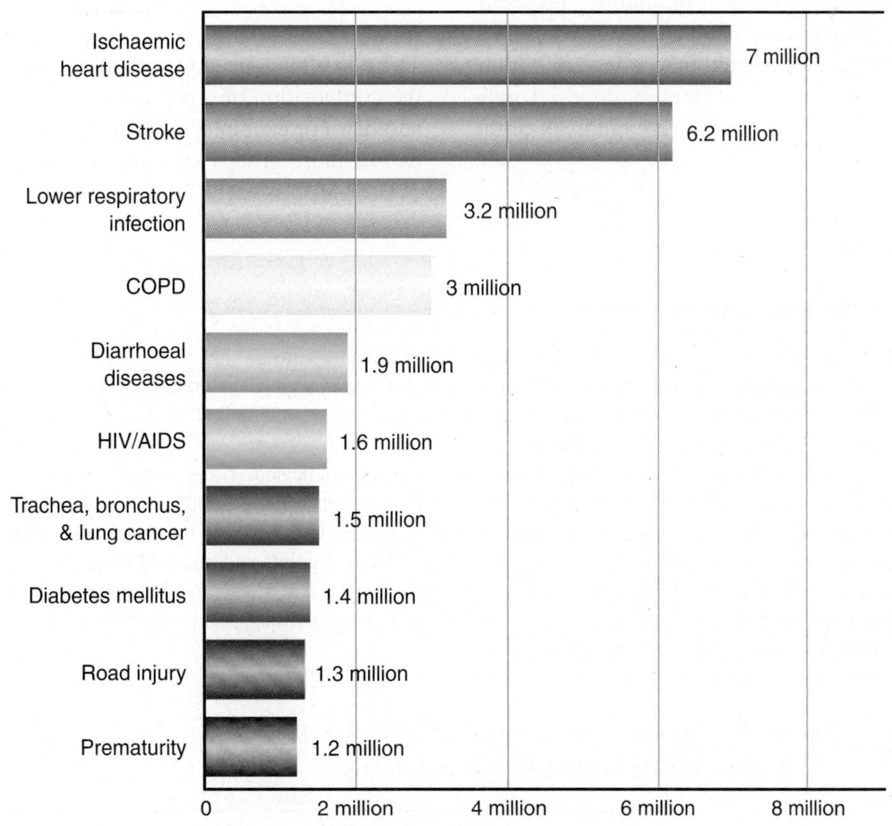

figure 7.1 The 10 leading causes of death in the world, WHO, 2011. (Available from http://www.who.int/mediacentre/factsheets/fs310/en/).

A **proportion** is a type of ratio that includes the quantity in the numerator as a part of the denominator; it is the relationship of a part to the whole. Dividing the number of boys by the total number of children in the school results in a proportion (160 divided by 240 = 0.67; 67% of the students are boys).

The **rate** is the primary measurement used to describe the occurrence (frequency or quantity) of a state of health in a specific group of people in a given time period. It is a proportion that includes the factor of time. Therefore, rates are the best indicators of the risk (probability) that a specific disease, condition, or event will occur. The rules for calculation of rates are outlined in Box 7.1. Rates are used to quantify either the occurrence (incidence) or the existence (prevalence) of states of health or illness. Using rates rather than counting cases takes both the size of the population at risk and the time frame into account.

Not everything that counts can be counted, and not everything that can be counted counts.

Albert Einstein

For example, suppose it is necessary to compare 2,250 cases of H1N1 influenza diagnosed in February in Lake County having a population of 104,000 with 10,500 cases of H1N1 influenza diagnosed in February in Barnes County having a population of 950,000. If only the frequency count is examined, Barnes County has the greatest number of people with the flu, and therefore, it could be concluded that Barnes County has the greater community problem. However, it is not appropriate to compare the raw numbers alone; more cases would be expected in a county with more residents. Indeed, the calculation of rates in Table 7.1 indicates that Lake County had the most severe outbreak of the illness in February.

PRACTICE POINT

When assessing the extent of a health problem in a community at a given time, the number of cases should be counted, the number of people in the population should be obtained, and a rate should be calculated.

Crude Rates

Crude rates are general or summary rates that measure the occurrence of the condition being investigated in the entire population. Calculation of these rates usually involves averaging the population numbers at the beginning and end of the year, and that number is used in the denominator. However, smaller groups within the entire population (subgroups) may differ significantly with regard to their risk of developing the condition, and thus, calculating only crude rates may obscure important information. For example, the formula for a crude birth rate has the entire population in its denominator. Births can occur only to females who are of childbearing age; therefore, the total population may not be an ideal denominator.

There are 2,150 people living with HIV/AIDS this year in two Florida counties. What is the crude rate of the HIV/AIDS burden in these two counties?

Adjusted Rates

There is often a need to remove the effects of differences in the composition of a population when comparing one with another. For example, an investigator may want to compare two or more groups knowing that they differ in terms of a

box 7.1 How to Calculate Rates

1. All of the events being measured should be included in the numerator.
2. Everyone included in the denominator should be at risk for the event in the numerator. For example, it would be inappropriate to include males in the denominator when calculating a rate for ovarian cancer because no males are at risk for the illness.
3. A specific period of time for the observations must be clearly indicated. This can range from a single point in time to several years, depending on the type of rate that is being calculated.
4. A rate is a fraction or a proportion; therefore, it is necessary to multiply by a base, usually a multiple of 10, to make the rates understandable. This removes the decimal points and makes the comparison of rates easier to interpret. Any base multiple of 10 may be chosen that results in a rate above the value of 1. For large populations, 100,000 is often used. For smaller populations, 100 is often used, and the rate can then be expressed as a percentage.
5. Formula for calculation:

$$\text{Rate} = \frac{\text{Number of conditions or events within a designated period of time}}{\text{Population at risk during the same period of time}} \times \text{Base multiple of 10}$$

table 7.1 **Calculation of Rates of H1N1 Influenza in Lake and Barnes Counties**

Lake County	Barnes County
Influenza rate = $\frac{2,250}{104,000} \times 100,000$	Influenza rate = $\frac{10,500}{950,000} \times 100,000$
Influenza rate = 0.0216346 × 100,000	Influenza rate = 0.0110526 × 100,000
Influenza rate = 2,163.5 cases per 100,000 people	Influenza rate = 1,105.3 cases per 100,000 people

Note: A base multiplier of 10,000 would result in a rate of approximately 216 cases per 10,000 people in Lake County and 111 cases per 10,000 in Barnes County.

characteristic, such as age, that may influence the results. The process of adjusting rates controls for these differences. Although age adjustment and other types of **adjusted rates** are artificial, they provide a valid way to compare two populations without the confounding variable (such as age) affecting the results.

As an example, Figure 7.2 shows age-adjusted death rates for selected causes of death for all ages, by sex, in the United States between 2000 and 2010. During this 10-year period, the age-adjusted death rate (where age was removed as a confounding factor) decreased 16% among males and 13% among females. While most causes of death declined in both males and females, Alzheimer disease increased in both sexes (Centers for Disease Control and Prevention, 2012a).

Age-adjusted rates are meaningful only as a comparison and should not be used if an accurate description of a population is desired and not a comparison of populations. It is also possible to adjust rates to remove other variables, such as race or occupation, that are confounding an investigation.

Incidence Rates

An **incidence rate** (also an occurrence or **attack rate**) is a measure of the probability that people without a certain condition will develop the condition over a period of time, often a year. It measures the pace at which new illnesses, such as H1N1 influenza, occur in a previously disease-free group of people. The general rules that apply to rates also apply to calculation of incidence rates (see Box 7.1). However, only the *new* cases that have occurred in the designated time period are counted and placed in the numerator. Common incidence rates and ratios that provide indexes of the health of a community are presented in Table 7.2.

Determination of the date of onset is required for studies of incidence. For acute conditions, this can be quickly

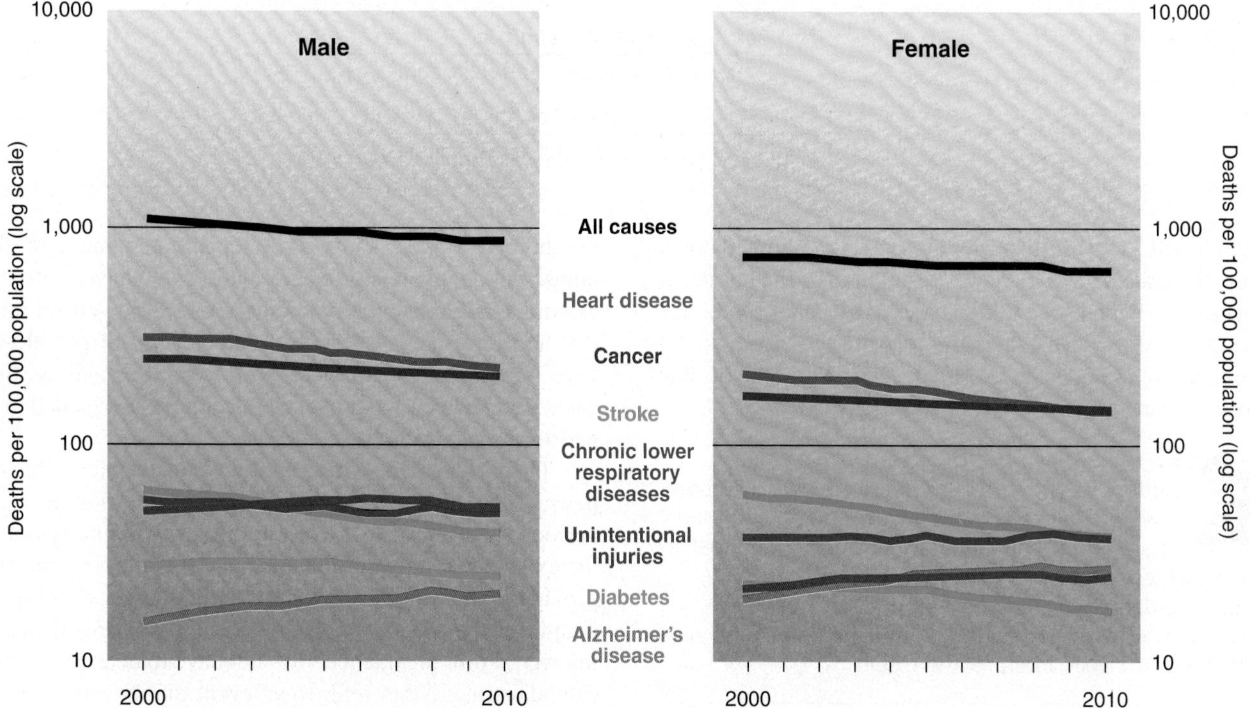

figure 7.2 Age-adjusted death rates for selected causes of death for all ages, by sex, in the United States between 2000 and 2010. (Available from http://www.cdc.gov/nchs/hus.htm)

table 7.2 **Incidence Rates and Ratios That Provide Indexes of the Health of a Community**

Indexes of Health	Calculation
General Mortality Rates	
Crude mortality rate	$\frac{\text{Number of deaths occuring in 1 year}}{\text{Midyear population}} \times 100{,}000$
Cause-specific mortality rate	$\frac{\text{Number of deaths from a stated cause in 1 year}}{\text{Midyear population}} \times 100{,}000$
Age-specific mortality rate	$\frac{\text{Number of people in a specific age group dying in 1 year}}{\text{Midyear population of the specific age group}} \times 100{,}000$
Case fatality rate	$\frac{\text{Number of deaths from a specific disease}}{\text{Number of cases of the same disease}} \times 100$
Proportional mortality ratio	$\frac{\text{Number of deaths from a specific cause within a time period}}{\text{Total deaths in the same time period}} \times 100$
Maternal and Infant Rates	
Crude birth rate	$\frac{\text{Number of live births in 1 year}}{\text{Midyear population}} \times 1{,}000$
General fertility rate	$\frac{\text{Number of live births in 1 year}}{\text{Number of females 15–44 years of age at midyear}} \times 1{,}000$
Maternal mortality rate	$\frac{\text{Number of deaths from puerperal causes in 1 year}}{\text{Number of live births in the same year}} \times 100{,}000$
Infant mortality rate	$\frac{\text{Number of deaths of children 1 year of age in 1 year}}{\text{Number of live births in the same year}} \times 1{,}000$
Perinatal mortality rate	$\frac{\text{Number of fetal deaths plus infant deaths 7 days of age in 1 year}}{\text{Number of live births plus fetal deaths in same year}} \times 1{,}000$
Neonatal mortality rate	$\frac{\text{Number of deaths of children under 28 days of age in 1 year}}{\text{Number of live births in the same year}} \times 1{,}000$
Fetal mortality rate	$\frac{\text{Number of fetal deaths in 1 year}}{\text{Number of live births plus fetal deaths in the same year}} \times 1{,}000$

established. H1N1 influenza is an acute, time-limited condition; thus, the data in Table 7.1 result in incidence or occurrence rates. For other conditions such as cancer or depression, it may be difficult to determine the time of onset. In this case, an event that can be verified, such as the date of diagnosis, is considered as the time of onset.

Lindsay finds that 384 new cases of HIV infection were diagnosed in the two counties within the past year. What is the incidence rate? Contrast this incidence rate with (1) the crude rate of the HIV/AIDS burden calculated above and (2) the incidence rate in the United States of 83.7 new HIV infections per 100,000 in 1 year. Interpret the results.

Prevalence Rates

Both incidence rates and **prevalence rates** can be measures of **morbidity**—a departure from a state of physiologic or psychological well-being. Prevalence rates measure the number of people in a given population who have a specific existing condition at a given point in time. The general rules that apply to rates also apply to calculation of prevalence rates (see Box 7.1). However, both new cases and existing cases (old and new cases) are counted in the designated time period and placed in the numerator.

There are two types of prevalence rates. **Period prevalence** indicates the existence of a condition during a period or an interval of time. **Point prevalence** refers to the existence of a condition at a specific point in time and provides a picture of an existing situation for a group of people. If the time frame is not given, point prevalence is inferred. Point prevalence does not have to be expressed in calendar time; it can refer to an event that happens to different people at different times. For example, it could refer to the day of discharge from an institution for a group of people or a specific day of attendance at a screening clinic.

Prevalence is influenced by two factors: the number of people who have developed the condition in the past and the duration of their illness. The longer the duration of a condition, the higher the prevalence rate. This is best illustrated with chronic diseases. Even if the incidence rate is low, the prevalence rate may be high. For instance, there are many more existing cases of cancer in a community than are indicated by examining the number of new cases of cancer.

Prevalence statistics are very important in identifying public health problems that exist in a community. They are particularly useful to health planning professionals because they measure the burden of a condition or illness in a community. This information documents the need for developing programs such as the initiation of primary, secondary, or tertiary prevention strategies for people at risk. Also, these data provide the rationale for modification of facilities and hiring staff to meet the requirements of the community.

EVIDENCE FOR PRACTICE

Researchers at the Centers for Disease Control and Prevention (CDC, 2010a) used the results of the Oregon Healthy Teens Survey, which had questioned eighth-grade students to determine the demographic characteristics and risk factors for participation in the "choking game." This is an activity where youths become "high" by cutting off blood and oxygen to the brain with a belt, towel, rope, or other item. Evaluation of earlier studies had indicated that youths experiencing peer rejection or other disruptive factors are more likely to participate in strangulation activities.

This investigation (CDC, 2010a) reported prevalence rates as percentages because the base multiplier for calculation of the rates was 100. A total of 36.2% of the youths had heard of the choking game, 30.4% had heard of someone participating, and 5.7% had taken part themselves. Risk factors included substance use and mental health factors such as depression. Youths with these factors had the highest participation rate (15.8%) and were approximately nine times more likely to participate. Of those who reported only substance use and no mental health factors, the participation rate was 7.9%, and of those who reported only mental health factors and no substance use, the participation rate was 4%. In students with no reported risk factors, the participation rate was 1.7%.

Public health surveillance of these strangulation activities in youths should be expanded to understand the frequency of the risk and the motives and circumstances surrounding participation. Along with parents and educators, nurses, counselors, and others who work with youths should be aware of strangulation activities and their serious health effects. They should watch for signs of participation in strangulation activities, especially in youths with suspected substance use or mental health risk factors. The association between participation in strangulation activities and other sensation-seeking behaviors or mental health risk factors suggests that effective methods for substance use prevention might serve as models for effective prevention strategies. However, prevention methods for this activity should be tested before being incorporated into general use. For example, an unintended consequence of prevention methods may be increased youth participation in the choking game. Effective prevention methods could be incorporated into existing substance use and mental health screening instruments, curricula, or related public health tools (CDC, 2010a).

SPECIFIC RATES: DESCRIBING BY PERSON, PLACE, AND TIME

Specific rates are more detailed rates and are calculated using the number of people in the smaller subgroups of the population in the denominator. Often, people are divided into subgroups by age and sex, although any characteristic can be used. The frequency and severity of most illnesses vary according to age more than any other personal characteristic.

When investigating the distribution and the determinants of a health condition, one of the first steps is to use statistics to find out who is experiencing the condition (person), where it is occurring (place), and when it appears (time). This information about the distribution of the condition is an essential step in the identification of high-risk groups and in the search for possible solutions.

There are three ways of examining descriptive information that can be helpful in developing plausible explanations (hypotheses) for the occurrence of the condition under study. First, look for *differences* in frequency of characteristics between groups; second, look for *areas of agreement* where factors are identified that are occurring frequently; and third, look for *variations* in the data that may present clues for control and prevention of the condition. Rates are usually used in this process, and it is often helpful to use graphs or charts to depict the results.

If you can't explain it simply, you don't understand it well enough.

Albert Einstein

Person: Who

Within any general population, whether it consists of members of a neighborhood, the clients in a community clinic, or the residents in an assisted living facility, there are differences among the individual people. These differences are genetic, biologic, behavioral, and socioeconomic. Because of these variations, specific incidence and prevalence rates should be calculated according to these specific characteristics. Statistics of this type that are gathered to describe populations are referred to as **demographic data**, or the study of the size, distribution, and characteristics of human populations.

Two characteristics are considered routine descriptors of a person: age and sex. Most health problems vary in both frequency and severity by age, and many are sex specific. Therefore, morbidity and mortality rates for almost all health conditions vary by age or sex. Because of this, age- and sex-specific incidence and prevalence rates should be calculated whenever describing a problem.

PRACTICE POINT

Age is the most important characteristic to address when describing the state of people's health; it is directly associated with risk for illness or disability.

The CDC has used specific incidence rates in its surveillance of injuries in the United States (CDC 2014a). Figure 7.3 shows the percentage distribution of injury episodes by place of occurrence in 2010. As can be expected, 47% of the nonfatal, medically attended injury episodes took place in or around the home. Nearly 40% of these injuries occurred while a person was engaged in leisure activities, including sports (CDC, 2012b). Figure 7.3 shows percentages; however, these are also rates with a multiplier of 100. Knowing what an injured person was doing and where his or her injury occurred is very important for designing prevention programs.

Figure 7.4 presents an example of specific prevalence rates for adults aged more than 45 years who need help with routine activities, by age-group and selected race or ethnicity. Again, this example shows rates expressed as percentages; examining this figure shows that needing help with routine activities increased steadily with age for all racial/ethnic groups. Non-Hispanic Blacks were more likely to need help with routine activities compared with Hispanics and non-Hispanic Whites for those aged 45 to 74 years. Among adults aged 45 to 54, Hispanics were least likely to need help with routine activities. However, the pattern changes among adults aged 75 years and over. Hispanics and non-Hispanic Blacks were both more likely to need help with routine activities than non-Hispanic Whites. Studying figures such as this one can give public health practitioners data that is needed to institute primary, secondary, and tertiary interventions to enhance the health of these groups (CDC, 2013).

Facts are stubborn, but statistics are more pliable.

Mark Twain

Place: Where

Examining the differences in the rates of illness or disability and determining where they are highest or lowest assists in determining health needs, planning prevention and control measures, and allocating resources. Natural boundaries, political boundaries, and environmental characteristics are taken into consideration in this process.

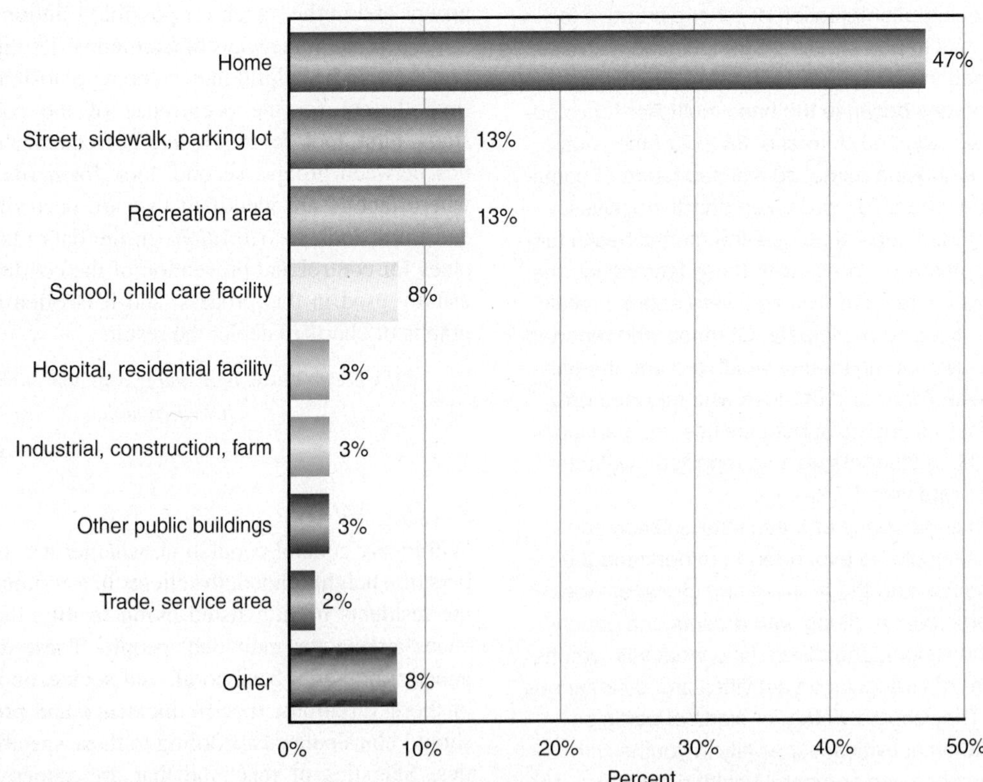

figure 7.3 Percentage distribution of injury episodes, by place of occurrence: United States, 2010. (Source: National Health Interview Survey, 2010. Available from http://www.cdc.gov/nchs/data/factsheets/factsheet_injury.htm)

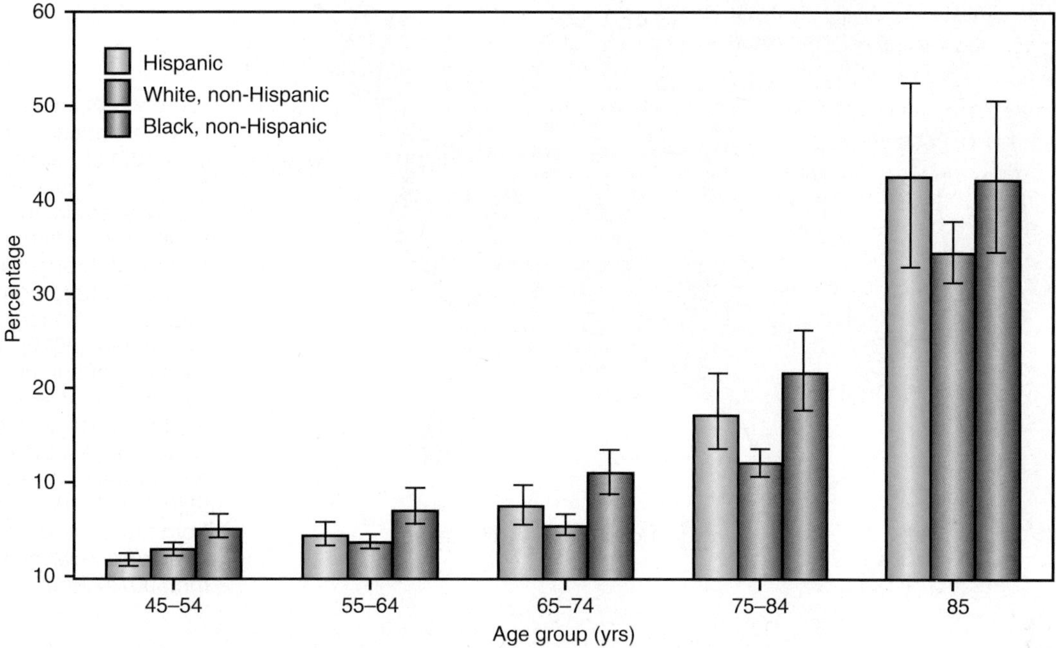

figure 7.4 QuickStats: Percentage of adults aged greater than or equal to 45 years who need help with routine activities by age-group and selected race/ethnicity—National Health Interview Survey, United States, 2011. (Available from http://www.ced.gov/mmwr/preview/mmwrhtml/mm6233a7.htm?s)

Variations in incidence and prevalence rates can be examined by continent, nation, states, city, census tract, city block, or other geographic area. Differences between urban and rural areas or among smaller localities may be helpful in investigating specific health needs for communities. Place of occurrence is almost always examined when investigating outbreaks, both in the community and within institutions. Rates can be compared among institutions, among units in a single institution, or among different groups within any healthcare facility. This information indicates where prevention and control measures and health resources should be concentrated to decrease incidence and prevalence of a particular problem.

EVIDENCE FOR PRACTICE

The CDC monitored the 2008 multistate outbreak of salmonella related to exposure to pet turtles, the third such outbreak since 2006 (CDC, 2010b). A total of 135 cases occurred in 25 states and the District of Columbia, but many more unreported illnesses likely occurred. Figure 7.5 shows the distribution of the confirmed cases by state. The first known (index) case was a 2-year-old girl who was brought to a physician's office in Philadelphia after 3 days of diarrhea and fever. *Salmonella typhimurium* was isolated from her stool specimen. Three weeks earlier, the family had purchased two pet turtles with shell lengths less than 4 inches from a street vendor. Within weeks, more clients in Pennsylvania were diagnosed with the same strain of the organism, and matching isolates had been found in cases from 10 states. Most ill people reported exposure to turtles with shell lengths less than 4 inches that had been acquired from flea markets, street vendors, and souvenir shops. (Small turtles pose a greater risk to young children because they are perceived as safe pets but are small enough to be placed in the mouth or handled inappropriately.)

Investigation of this outbreak documented that young children without direct turtle exposure are at risk for turtle-associated salmonellosis through person-to-person transmission in child care settings. This investigation reinforced the need for continuing the existing prevention and control measures. Increasing enforcement of the existing local, state, and federal regulations against the sale of small turtles, increasing penalties for illegal sales, and enacting more state and local laws regulating the sale of small turtles could enhance federal prevention efforts and facilitate a more rapid public health response.

Time: When

Variations in time can be short term, periodic, or long term. **Short-term changes** are measured in hours, days, weeks, or months. They are commonly found in outbreaks of infectious disease. Figure 7.6 illustrates an **epidemic curve** created from study of an outbreak of mumps that occurred from June 2009 to January 2010 in New York and New Jersey. Cases of reported confirmed or probable mumps (n = 1,494) are shown by week of illness onset and age-group during the outbreak. At the time of the report, local transmission continued to occur (CDC, 2010c).

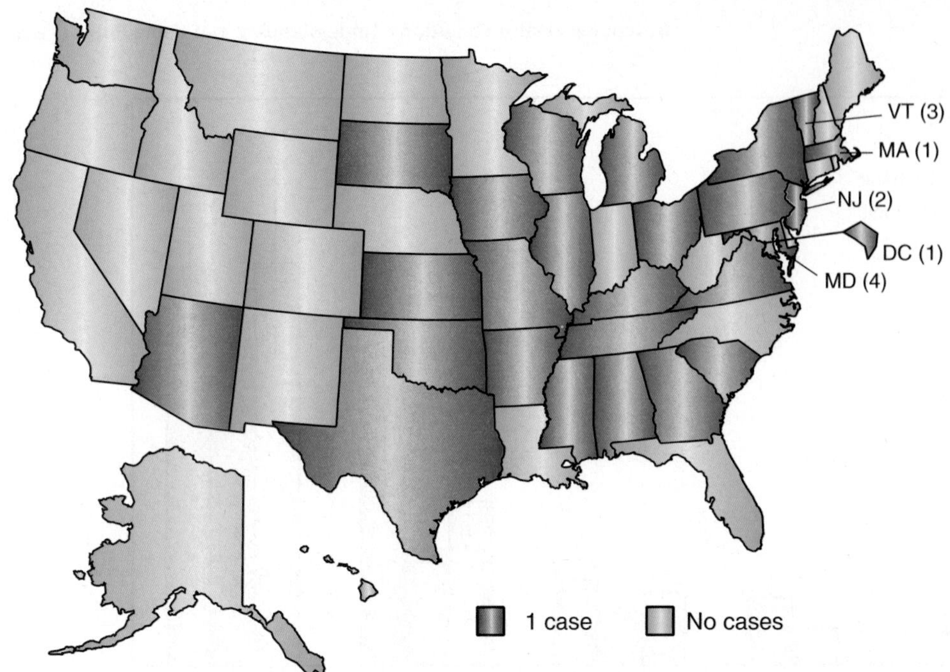

figure 7.5 Number of laboratory-confirmed cases ($n = 135$) of *Salmonella typhimurium* infection with the outbreak strain, involving pet turtles in the United States, March 13 through November 17, 2008. (Data from Centers for Disease Control and Prevention. [2010]. Multistate outbreak of human *Salmonella typhimurium* infections associated with pet turtle exposure—United States, 2008. *Morbidity and Mortality Weekly Report*, *59*[07], 191–196. Retrieved from http://www.cdc.gov/mmwr/preview/mmwrhtml/mm5907a2.htm)

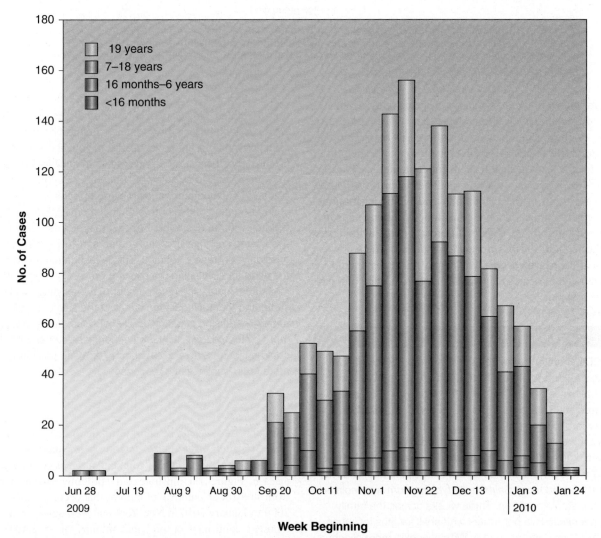

19 years
7–18 years
16 months–6 years
<16 months

No. of Cases

180
160
140
120
100
80
60
40
20
0

Jun 28 2009 | Jul 19 | Aug 9 | Aug 30 | Sep 20 | Oct 11 | Nov 1 | Nov 22 | Dec 13 | Jan 3 2010 | Jan 24

Week Beginning

figure 7.6 Number ($n = 1,494$) of reported confirmed or probable mumps cases, by week of illness onset and age-group in New York and New Jersey, June 2009 through January 2010. (Data from Centers for Disease Control and Prevention. [2010]. Update: Mumps outbreak—New York and New Jersey, June 2009–January 2010. *Morbidity and Mortality Weekly Report*, *59*[05], 125–129. Retrieved from http://www.cdc.gov/mmwr/preview/mmwrhtml/mm5905a1.htm)

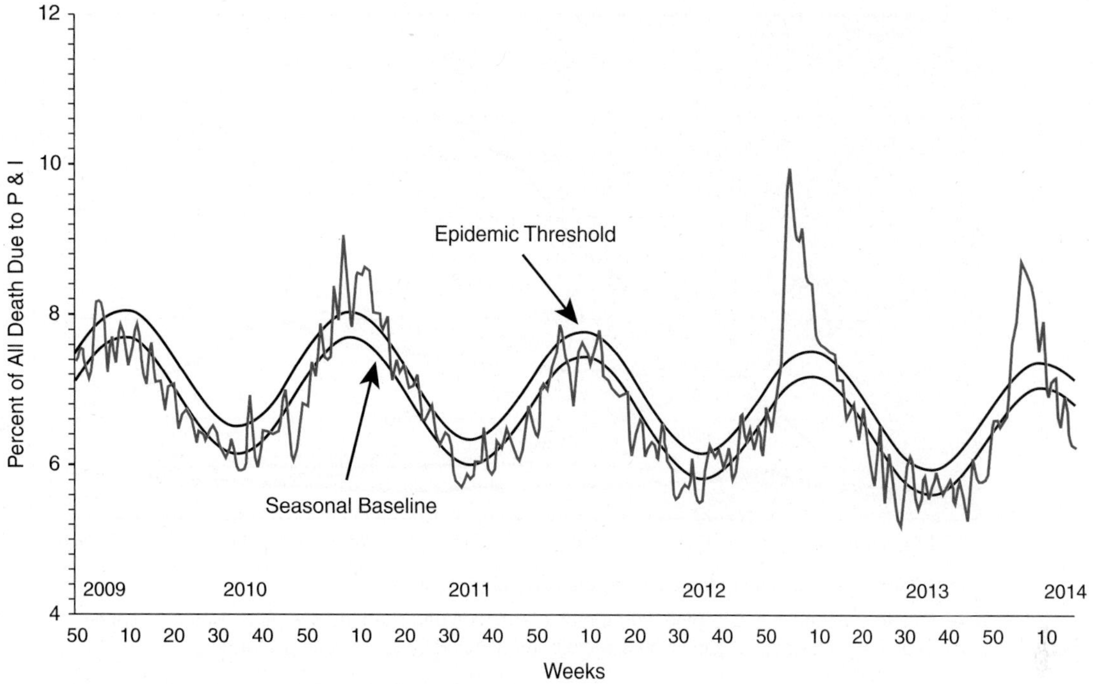

figure 7.7 Pneumonia and influenza mortality for 122 U.S. cities: Week ending March 8, 2014. (Available at http://www.cdc.gov/flu/weekly/)

Periodic changes may be seasonal or cyclic. For example, respiratory diseases are more common in winter and spring, and infectious hepatitis increases in incidence every 7 to 9 years. Figure 7.7 shows the percentage of all deaths attributed to pneumonia and influenza for 122 cities in the United States between 2009 and 2013. The seasonal variation in death rates reflects the seasonal variation in respiratory infections. When studying these mortality statistics, it is possible to compare the percentage of all deaths attributable to pneumonia and influenza with a seasonal baseline and epidemic threshold value calculated for each week. An increase of 1.645 standard deviations above the seasonal baseline deaths is the "epidemic threshold." This is the point at which the observed proportion of deaths attributed to pneumonia or influenza is significantly higher than would be expected at that time of the year. **Long-term changes** extend over decades and reflect gradual changes. An interesting example follows the tracking of West Nile virus infection, a disease that is transmitted by a mosquito vector. Figure 7.8 follows the progression of the illness from one state to another after it was first reported in New York in 1999. This figure combines variation in both place and time over a period of 15 years (CDC, 2014b).

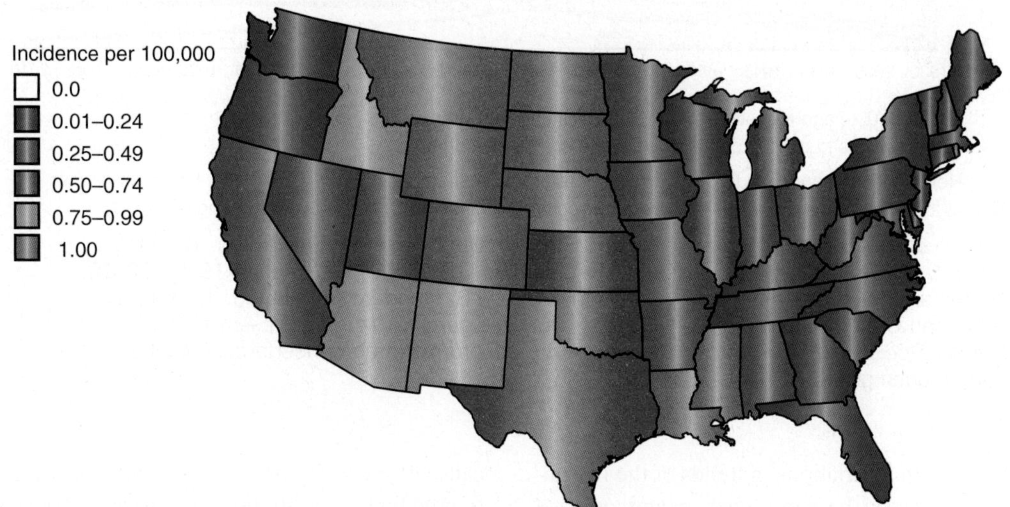

figure 7.8 Average annual incidence of West Nile virus neuroinvasive disease reported to CDC by state, 1999 to 2012. (Source: ArboNET, Arboviral Diseases Branch, Centers for Disease Control and Prevention. Retrieved from http://www.cdc.gov/westnile/statsMaps/cumMapsData.html)

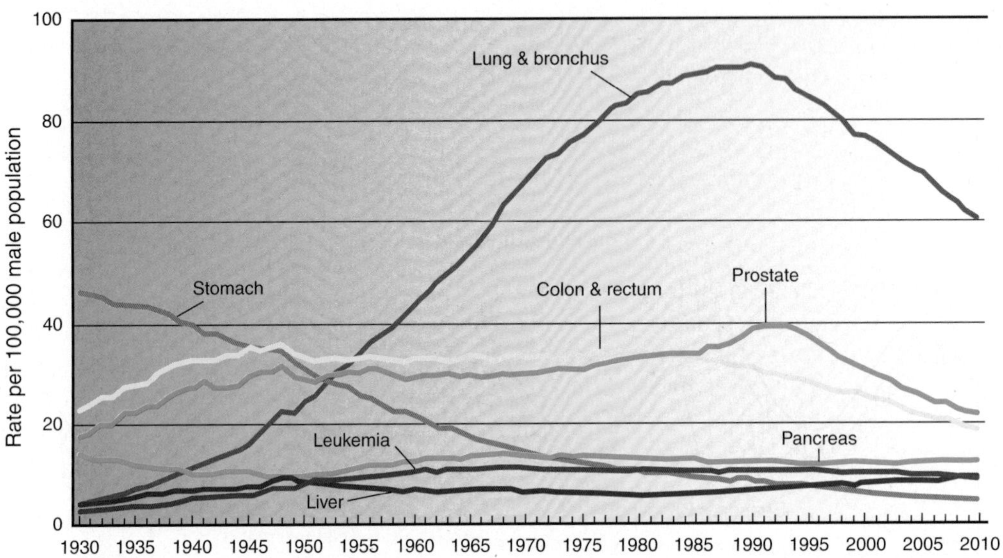

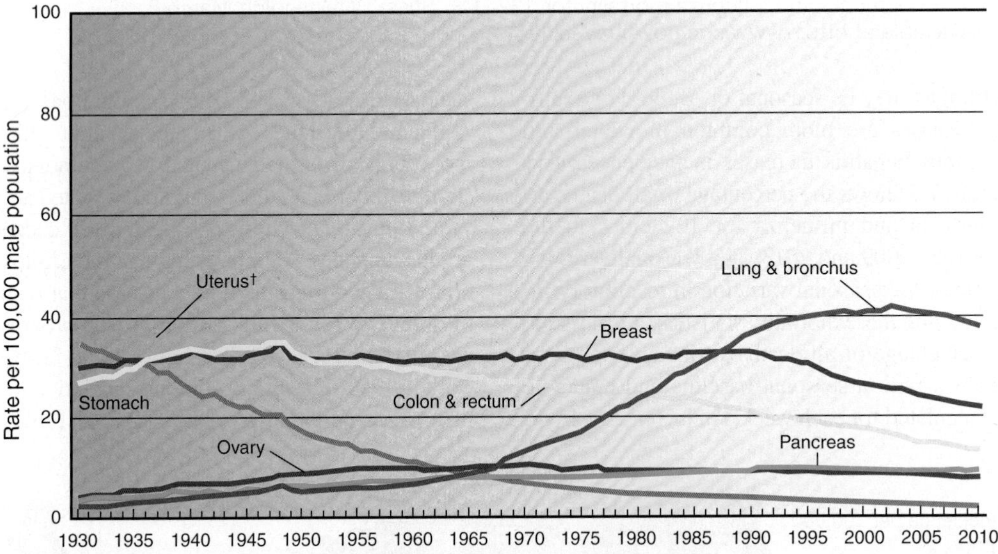

figure 7.9 **A:** Age-adjusted cancer death rates,* males by site, United States, 1930 to 2010. **B:** Age-adjusted cancer death rates,* females by site, United States, 1930 to 2010. *Rates are per 100,000 age-adjusted to the 2000 U.S. standard population. (Data from American Cancer Society. [2014]. *Cancer Facts & Figures 2014*. Atlanta: American Cancer Society. Retrieved from http://www.cancer.org/research/cancerfactsstatistics/cancerfactsfigures2014/)

Figure 7.9 shows that variations in trends of the mortality of various cancers can be seen when examined over many years. Overall, the age-adjusted cancer rates between 1930 and 2010 have fluctuated but are decreasing slowly. Cancer of the lung and bronchus leads all cancers as the cause of mortality in both men and women. It is interesting to note that the mortality rate for cancer of the stomach has decreased steadily since 1930, that cancer of the lung rose steadily until the 1990s, and that cancer of the colon and rectum continues to decrease (American Cancer Society,

2014). This is likely a result of primary prevention measures such as education and increased awareness as well as secondary prevention measures such as colonoscopy screening.

TYPES OF INCIDENCE RATES

Mortality Rates

Mortality rates or death rates are common incidence rates that are calculated for public health purposes. **Crude mortality rates** indicate the probability of death from any cause among the entire population in a designated geographic area. **Cause-specific** (disease-specific) **mortality rates** indicate the probability of death from a specific cause; the number of deaths from a specific disease is divided by the number of people in the population at midyear and multiplied by 100,000. In calculating the **case fatality rate**, the number of people with a specific disease such as lung cancer becomes the subgroup being studied out of the entire population in a designated geographic area. For example, the case fatality rate is calculated by dividing the number of deaths from lung cancer by the number of people living with lung cancer during the year, and multiplying by 100. Further breakdown into specific subgroups might involve age, sex, occupation, tobacco use, or other characteristics for calculation of mortality rates.

It is possible to confuse the **proportional mortality ratio** (PMR) with the cause-specific mortality rate. The PMR compares deaths from a specific illness to deaths from all other causes; it reflects the proportion of deaths due to a specific cause. The PMR is not a rate. The denominator includes all deaths within a given time period rather than the entire population under study. In contrast, the **cause-specific mortality rates** indicate the risk of death from a specific disease for a given living population. Both the PMR and cause-specific mortality rates should be calculated when death statistics are being examined for public health purposes.

Incidence Density

When there are unequal periods of observation for study subjects, it may be necessary to use a person-time denominator in the calculation of incidence rates. This technique provides a measure of **incidence density**. In healthcare, people often enter a study period at different times and therefore contribute unequal periods of time to the study. To identify the precise period of observation for each person and weigh that period of observation properly in calculating rates, a person-time unit, such as person-day or person-year, can be constructed. A person-day represents one person at risk for 1 day, and a person-year represents one person at risk for 1 year. Incidence density can be calculated as:

$$\text{Incidence Density} = \frac{\text{New cases occurring during the study peroid}}{\text{Person-time units accumulated by subjects during the study period}} \times \text{Base multiple of 10}$$

Table 7.3 demonstrates the difference between the calculation of crude incidence rates and incidence density in a study that examined the development of hospital- and institution-associated pneumonia in both an acute care facility and a long-term care facility. These incidence data illustrate the need to calculate and compare both crude incidence and incidence density rates when comparing different settings with varying lengths of stay. In this example, the incidence rate in long-term care was almost five times that of the acute care setting. However, when the researchers included client days in the denominator, the acute care setting reflected twice the incidence density of the long-term care setting. More clients contributed shorter periods of time in the acute care setting, whereas there was relatively little turnover in residents in the long-term care setting.

Measures of incidence density can account for those persons who die, those who are lost to follow-up, or those who have acquired the illness and are therefore not at risk for the entire study period. Normally, it is assumed that the risk of acquiring the illness is constant throughout the entire period of the study.

Attributable Risk

Attributable risk is the difference between the incidence rates in an exposed group of people and an unexposed group of people. It measures the risk of a condition occurring in an exposed group that is attributable to a specific exposure but not to other factors. In almost any health-related event, some risk occurs normally in a population without a specific exposure. In calculating attributable risk, the risk of the event that would have occurred under normal circumstances is subtracted from the risk of the event in the exposed group:

Attributable Risk = Incidence rate in the exposed − The incidence rate in the nonexposed

table 7.3 **Incidence Rates of Institution-Associated Pneumonia in an Acute and Long-Term Care Setting**

Setting	No. of Cases	No. at Risk	Client or Patient Days	Crude Incidence (%)	Incidence (Density/ 100 Patient Days)
Acute care	33	2,249	19,102	1.5	1.75
Long-term care	27	366	37,064	7.4	0.73

Source: Data from Harkness, G. A., Bentley, D. W., & Roghmann, K. (1990). Nosocomial pneumonia in the elderly. *American Journal of Medicine*, *89*, 459.

Relative Risk Ratio

Incidence rates indicate the occurrence of a health-related event in a population in a given period of time. It is an indicator of the probability that people without a specific condition will develop the condition within a designated period of time. Therefore, it is a measure of the risk of developing the condition. Often, incidence rates for groups exposed to a certain risk factor are compared with the incidence rates for people who are not exposed. This procedure results in a **relative risk ratio**. It is a ratio of the incidence rate in the exposed group and the incidence rate in the nonexposed group.

$$\text{Relative Risk} = \frac{\text{Incidence rate in the exposed group}}{\text{Incidence rate in the nonexposed group}}$$

A relative risk of 1.0 indicates that the risk is equal for both groups, and conversely, a relative risk greater than 1.0 indicates that the risk is greater in the exposed group. For example, a relative risk of 6.0 can be interpreted to mean that people who are exposed to a disease are six times more likely to develop it. The CDC used this technique to develop an educational chart for use in HIV prevention programs (Fig.7.10). This chart shows how the relative risk for transmission from a person living with HIV to a person without the infection varies according to sexual activity and condom use. For example, it is possible to contrast insertive oral sex while using a condom, which has a low risk for HIV transmission, with receptive anal sex without a condom, which is 2,000 times more risky. This kind of information regarding HIV transmission can influence decisions about sexual activity and condom use (CDC, 2007).

A relative risk less than 1.0 indicates that the risk is less in the exposed group; the factor in question may possibly protect against the condition under study. Although this finding is not very common, it may signify that further study is warranted. Statistical tests, such as the calculation of the chi-square statistic, are used to determine whether the relative risk ratios are different from those that would be expected by chance. In this way, the statistical significance of the findings can be established.

SENSITIVITY AND SPECIFICITY

Sensitivity and specificity are statistical measures that evaluate the validity and reliability of a test. **Sensitivity** is the ability of the test to identify correctly people who have the health problem under study. It is the probability of testing positive if the health problem is truly present. **Specificity** is the ability of the test to identify correctly people who do not have the health problem. It is the probability of testing negative if the health problem is truly absent. Increasing the sensitivity of a test causes a decrease in specificity, and conversely, increasing the specificity of a test decreases sensitivity. The formulas for calculation of sensitivity and specificity are found in Box 7.2. To obtain sensitivity and specificity values, it is necessary to perform research studies that obtain the values of screening tests and then determine whether the health problem truly exists in each subject.

In an ideal situation, a screening test is able to identify the presence or absence of a health problem correctly in every person screened with a sensitivity and specificity of 100%. However, this is almost impossible to achieve in

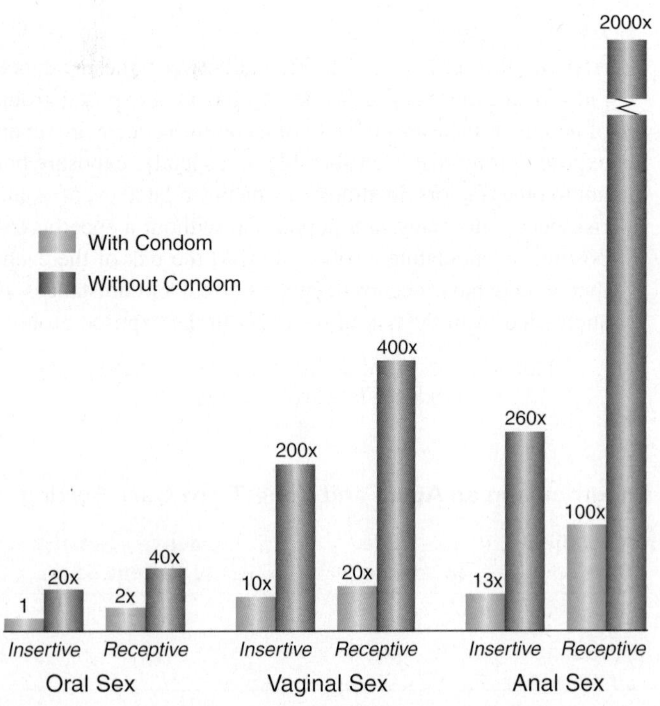

figure 7.10 Relative risk for transmission from a person living with HIV. (Data from CDC. *Relative risk for transmission from a person living with HIV*. Retrieved from http://www.cdc.gov/hiv/topics/treatment/PIC/pdf/chart.pdf)

box 7.2 How to Calculate Sensitivity and Specificity

$$\text{Sensitivity} = \frac{\text{Number of true positives}}{\text{Number of true positives} + \text{Number of false negatives}}$$

$$\text{Sensitivity} = \frac{\text{Number of true positives}}{\text{Number of true negatives} + \text{Number of false positives}}$$

Note: A test with a high sensitivity has a low type II error rate. A test with a high specificity has a low type I error rate.

actual practice. One way to address this problem is to use several screening tests to make health decisions.

Before screening projects are undertaken, it is important to determine carefully the screening levels or test values. Much depends on the consequences of leaving some cases undetected (false negatives) or classifying healthy people as having a health problem (false positives). When the disease being studied is rare, the specificity of a test is rarely high enough to give an adequate positive predictive value. Only the sensitivity of a test is useful in the case of a rare disease. The choice of screening levels is subjective and based on the severity of the disease, cost, time factors, advantages of early treatment, and other screening criteria.

The outreach program promotes HIV testing in the African-American population. Lindsay examines the types of tests available and finds that rapid, same-day testing has a sensitivity between 88.9% and 99.7% and a specificity between 99.6% and 100%. What does this information mean? If a positive test is found, what is the best recommendation?

USE OF RATES IN DESCRIPTIVE RESEARCH STUDIES

Epidemiologic descriptive studies include the descriptions of health conditions, case reports, and correlational studies. Descriptive studies are very useful in describing the characteristics of disease occurrence and in generating hypotheses for further study. They are the first studies to be performed in investigating the determinants of a health problem and are essential in determining the rationale for an experimental or intervention study.

Researchers design descriptive studies to acquire more information about the occurrence of health problems or, alternatively, the factors that keep people well. The specific rates calculated in these studies describe people who have or do not have the health problem in terms of person, place, and time. These studies provide a picture of the events as they naturally occur. Therefore, this type of data is very helpful for nurses involved in health planning or administration in both community and institutional settings. Knowledge of people who are the most or least susceptible to a health problem can help when deciding to implement programs for prevention or control of health problems and to allocate resources.

Lindsay develops a plan to evaluate the effectiveness of the outreach program. Using the HIV/AIDS Outreach Survey, decide what statistics should be calculated for each of the 10 questions. Include the calculation of both general (crude) rates and specific rates where appropriate.

key concepts

- Measuring the magnitude or frequency of a state of health determines the characteristics of those who are at high risk.
- Epidemiologic descriptive studies have determined measurable risk factors for major illnesses.
- Calculation of rates provides the best indicators of the probability that a specific state of health will occur.
- Indexes of the health of a community, region, or country include comparisons of general mortality rates and maternal infant rates.
- A variety of rates can be calculated according to need, including incidence, prevalence, adjusted, and specific rates.
- Specific rates calculated by person, place, and time provide the best description of a health condition.
- Prevalence is influenced by the number of people who have developed the condition in the past and the duration of their illness. Prevalence rates provide essential data for implementing prevention measures.
- Before screening projects are undertaken, the sensitivity and specificity of screening levels or test values should be carefully reviewed.

critical thinking questions

1. Between January 1 and December 31, 35 new cases of tuberculosis were diagnosed in a city. There were a total of 300 active cases among the population of 400,000 on December 31 of that year. Twenty deaths from tuberculosis were recorded during the 1-year period.
   a. What was the incidence rate per 100,000 people for tuberculosis during the year?
   b. What was the prevalence rate of tuberculosis per 100,000 on December 31?
   c. What is the cause-specific death rate per 100,000 for tuberculosis during the year?
2. A recent report from a state health department included a map indicating the distribution and number of rabid animals for each of the 167 towns in the state between January 1 and October 31. What type of information about the occurrence of rabies does this report include? Why were rates not calculated? How might this information be used to control rabies?
3. A community nurse uncovers the following statistics regarding HIV infection in African-Americans in two rural counties in the United States:

	New HIV Infection	Living with HIV	Population Total
Males	150	838	29,560
Females	234	1,312	28,315
African-American population	384	2,150	57,875

   a. What is the incidence rate in black males and black females per 10,000 people in the 1-year period?
   b. What is the prevalence rate in black males and black females per 10,000 people in the 1-year period?
   c. Interpret the incidence and prevalence rates. Which statistics provide the best information to use for program planning?
   d. What population group should be targeted for the HIV/AIDS outreach program? Why?

references

American Cancer Society. (2014). *Cancer facts & figures 2014*. Atlanta: American Cancer Society. Retrieved from http://www.cancer.org/research/cancerfactsstatistics/cancerfactsfigures2014/index

Brown, E. J., & Brown, J. S. (2003). HIV prevention outreach in black communities of three rural North Florida counties. *Public Health Nursing, 20*(3), 204–210.

Centers for Disease Control and Prevention. (2007). *Relative risk for transmission from a person living with HIV*. Retrieved from http://www.cdc.gov/hiv/topics/treatment/PIC/pdf/chart.pdf

Centers for Disease Control and Prevention. (2010a). "Choking game" awareness and participation among 8th graders—Oregon, 2008. *Morbidity and Mortality Weekly Report, 59*(1), 1–5.

Centers for Disease Control and Prevention. (2010b). Multistate outbreak of human *Salmonella typhimurium* infections associated with pet turtle exposure—United States, 2008. *Morbidity and Mortality Weekly Report, 59*(7), 191–196.

Centers for Disease Control and Prevention. (2010c). Update: Mumps outbreak—New York and New Jersey, June 2009–January 2010. *Morbidity and Mortality Weekly Report, 59*(5), 125–129. Retrieved from http://www.cdc.gov/mmwr/preview/mmwrhtml/mm5905a1.htm

Centers for Disease Control and Prevention. (2012a). *Health, United States, 2012*. Retrieved from http://www.cdc.gov/nchs/hus.htm

Centers for Disease Control and Prevention. (2012b). *NCHS fact sheet: NCHS data on injuries*. Retrieved from http://www.cdc.gov/nchs/data/factsheets/factsheet_injury.htm

Centers for Disease Control and Prevention. (2013). QuickStats: Percentage of adults aged ≥45 years who need help with routine activities by age group and selected race/ethnicity—National Health Interview Survey, United States, 2011. *Morbidity and Mortality Weekly Report, 62*(33), 683. Retrieved from http://www.cdc.gov/mmwr/preview/mmwrhtml/mm6233a7.htm?s

Centers for Disease Control and Prevention. (2014a). *NCHS data on injuries: NCHS fact sheet*. Retrieved from http://www.cdc.gov/nchs/data/factsheets/factsheet_injury.htm

Centers for Disease Control and Prevention. (2014b). *West Nile virus disease cases and deaths reported to CDC by year and clinical presentation, 1999–2012. Final cumulative maps & data for 1999–2012*. Retrieved from http://www.cdc.gov/westnile/statsMaps/cumMapsData.html

World Health Organization. (2011). *The top 10 causes of death*. Retrieved from http://www.who.int/mediacentre/factsheets/fs310/en/

web resources

Please visit thePoint® for up-to-date Web resources on this topic.

CHAPTER 8

Gathering Evidence for Public Health Practice

Barbara A. Goldrick

Of course we don't know what we're doing, that's why it's called research.

Albert Einstein

1. Statistical significance is not the same thing as practical importance.

2. The more complex the test required to show statistical significance, the less important to an individual the association is likely to be.

3. The word "significant" without the prefix "statistical" is usually a coward's way of implying "important" without mathematical evidence.

Cowden's Three Rules of Statistics; John M. Cowden, English epidemiologist

People commonly use statistics like a drunk uses a lamppost: for support rather than for illumination.

Mark Twain

chapter highlights

- Epidemiologic/public health research defined
- Observational studies: Descriptive versus analytical research
- Strengths and limitations of epidemiologic research methodology
- Applying epidemiologic research to public health nursing practice

objectives

- Describe the difference between descriptive and analytical research.
- Discuss the strengths and weaknesses of retrospective, prospective, case–control, and experimental designs.
- Generate research questions related to problems identified in community and public health nursing practice.

key terms

Analytical study: Investigation that uses comparisons between groups to determine the role of various risk factors in causing the problem.

Association: Statistical relationship between two or more events, characteristics, or other variables.

Case–control study: Observational analytic study that enrolls one group of persons with a certain health problem (case patients) and a group of persons without the health problem (control subjects). It compares differences in exposures, behaviors, and other characteristics to identify and quantify associations, test hypotheses, and identify causes.

Case study: Research method that involves an in-depth analysis of an individual, group, or institution.

Causality: Relationship between two variables in which the presence or absence of one variable (the "cause") determines the presence or absence of the other (the "effect").

Clinical trial: Experimental study in which the investigator specifies the type of exposure for each study participant and then follows each person's health status to determine the effects of the exposure.

Cohort study: Observational analytic study in which enrollment is based on status of exposure to a certain factor or membership in a certain group.

Controls: Subjects in an experiment who do not receive the "treatment" and provide baseline data against which the effects of the treatment can be measured.

Cross-sectional study: Study in which a sample of persons from a population is enrolled and their exposures and health outcomes are measured simultaneously.

Descriptive study: Study in which information is collected to characterize and summarize a health event or problem.

Epidemiologic research: The study of the distribution and determinants of health conditions or events among populations. The studies may be descriptive or analytic.

Evidence-based nursing practice: Defined as "a problem-solving approach to practice that involves the conscientious use of current best evidence in making decisions about patient care" (Melnyk & Fineout-Overholt, 2005).

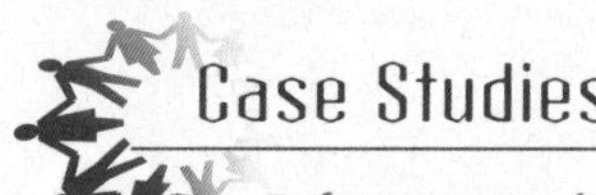

Case Studies

References to the case studies are found throughout this chapter (look for the case study icon). Readers should keep the case studies in mind as they read the chapter.

CASE 1

A *Healthy People 2020* goal, retained from *Healthy People 2010*, is to increase the proportion of adults aged 65 years and older who are vaccinated against pneumococcal disease, which is caused by *Streptococcus pneumoniae*, to at least 90% (U.S. Department of Health and Human Services [USDHHS], 2010). However, data from the Centers for Disease Control and Prevention (CDC)/National Center for Health Statistics (NCHS) National Health Interview Survey estimate that in 2012 only 63% of persons aged 65 years or older had ever received pneumococcal polysaccharide vaccine (CDC, NCHS, 2013).

A group of community health nurses learn that their state is not on target to meet the *Healthy People 2020* objective to increase the proportion of persons aged 65 years or older vaccinated against pneumococcal disease to 90% (USDHHS, 2010). In addition, the state health department has reported the occurrence of four cases of multidrug-resistant *S. pneumoniae* in the state within the past several months.

CASE 2

The first World Health Organization (WHO) *Global Status Report on Noncommunicable diseases* (NCDs), *2010*, launched in 2011, confirmed that NCDs are now the leading cause of mortality worldwide and are on the increase. Cardiovascular diseases account for most NCD deaths at 17 million people annually, followed by cancer (7.6 million), respiratory disease (4.2 million), and diabetes (1.3 million). These four groups of diseases account for about 80% of all NCD deaths and share four common risk factors:

- Physical inactivity
- Tobacco use
- Poor diets
- Harmful use of alcohol

Nearly 80% of NCD deaths in 2008 occurred in low- and middle-income countries, which dismisses the myth that these conditions occur mainly in affluent societies. Without action, the NCD epidemic is projected to kill 52 million people annually by 2030 (WHO, 2011).

key terms (continued)

Hypothesis: Statement of the expected outcome between two or more variables in a specific population.
Intervention study: Investigation designed to test a hypothesized relationship by modifying an identified factor in a population. Studies may be therapeutic (clinical) or preventive.
Null hypothesis: Statement that there is no difference between/among the variables under study.
Observational study: Study in which the investigator observes rather than influences exposure and disease among participants.
Odds ratio (OR): Measure of association used in comparative studies, particularly case–control studies, which quantifies the association between an exposure and a health outcome.
***p* value:** In statistical testing, the probability that the obtained results are not due to chance alone.
Preventive trial: Study in which the investigator provides a specific preventive measure to the group under study and follows the group to determine the effects of the intervention.
Prospective study: Analytic study in which participants are enrolled before the health outcome of interest has occurred.
Relationship: See **association**; the two terms are often used interchangeably.
Relative risk (RR): Ratio of the risk of disease or death among those exposed to the risk among the unexposed; synonymous with risk ratio.
Retrospective study: Analytic study in which participants are enrolled after the health outcome of interest has occurred.
Sample: Selected subset of a population; a sample can be random or nonrandom and representative or nonrepresentative.
Survey research: Systematic canvassing of persons to collect information, often from a representative sample of the population.
Therapeutic trial: Clinical trial in which the investigator provides a specific intervention/treatment (therapy) to the group under study and follows the group to determine the effects of the treatment.
Type I error: An error created by rejecting the null hypothesis when it is true; that is, a difference is seen to exist when in fact it does not.
Type II error: An error created by accepting the null hypothesis when it is false; that is, it is concluded that no difference exists when in fact it does.
Variables: Qualities or characteristics of persons, things, or situations that change and can be manipulated or measured in research. Extraneous variables can affect the measurement and relationship among study variables.

In Chapter 6, epidemiology was defined as the study of the distribution and determinants of states of health and illness in human populations. This information provides the data necessary to justify the establishment of health services designed to maintain and improve health. Epidemiologic surveillance is then conducted to monitor and evaluate these health services. The purposes of **epidemiologic research**, on the other hand, are to (1) identify community/public health problems and (2) describe natural history and etiology of diseases. Community/public health nurses use a variety of epidemiologic research methods to generate new knowledge and provide evidence for best practice. As can be seen in Figure 8.1, the epidemiologic research cycle includes both experimental or intervention studies and observational studies.

OBSERVATIONAL STUDIES

Observational studies may be either descriptive or analytical. In **descriptive studies**, the researcher collects information to characterize and summarize the health event or problem when little is known about the phenomenon. Descriptive studies provide the foundation for the development and testing of **hypotheses.**

In **analytical studies**, the researcher relies on comparisons between groups to determine the role of various risk factors in causing the problem. Descriptive studies, the most basic of these categories, are fundamental to public health research (CDC, 2010).

Descriptive Studies

Descriptive research identifies the characteristics of individuals, situations, or groups and the frequency with which certain phenomena occur (Burns, Grove, & Gray, 2013). In Chapter 6, it was pointed out that quantifying disease (or any unusual occurrence) requires the description of a case, which is rigorously standardized and unambiguous. For epidemiologic purposes, the cases must be related to a population at risk. The concept of risk also was defined in Chapter 6 as it relates to person, place, and time. Therefore, descriptive epidemiologic studies, which are frequently used in public health, are designed to acquire more information about characteristics of health (or disease) as they pertain to person, place, and time. People in the study population will all have some characteristics in common; therefore, some restrictions to this broad definition must be made. For example, research is limited to considering people of the same age range, sex, or geographic location. Most epidemiologic studies are observational; that is, no intervention or treatment is included. Observational studies are divided into hypothesis-generating and hypothesis-testing studies (see Fig. 8.1). Hypothesis-generating research includes case studies and cross-sectional studies. Hypothesis-testing studies, on the other hand, include analytical studies that test the relationship between two or more **variables** in a specified population (see further discussion later).

If it looks like a duck, and quacks like a duck, we have at least to consider the possibility that we have a small aquatic bird of the family Anatidae on our hands.

Douglas Adams, science fiction writer

Case Studies

Case studies involve an in-depth analysis of an individual, group, or social institution (Burns et al., 2013). In epidemiologic and public health research, the case study often is the first clue that a problem may exist. A **case series** is a group of people with the same, or similar, illness or injury and with the same, or similar, factors that may be importantly related to the disease or injury. A historic example of a case series was the first cases of young men who presented with Kaposi sarcoma and *Pneumocystis carinii* pneumonia in California and New York in the early 1980s. What these young men had in common was having sex with other men. In June 1981, the CDC published the first report about AIDS in the United States, which alerted the medical and public health communities 4 months before the first peer-reviewed article on the subject of AIDS was published. For more information on the history of HIV/AIDS, see the CDC website at www.cdc.gov/hiv/topics/basic/#origin and AVERT website at http://www.avert.org/history-aids-1986.htm.

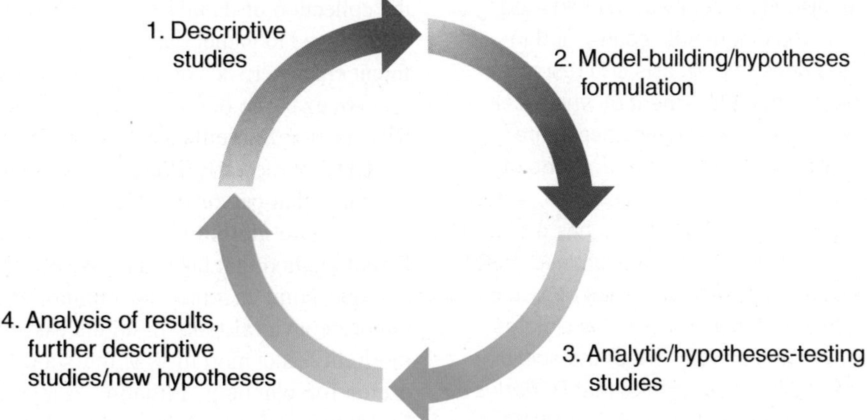

figure 8.1 Epidemiologic study cycle.

EVIDENCE FOR PRACTICE

Pertussis, also known as whooping cough, is a highly contagious respiratory disease caused by the bacterium *Bordetella pertussis*. According to public health officials, pertussis is on a historic resurgence in the United States, returning to record numbers of reported cases not seen since the 1950s. In 2012, the CDC reported a total of 48,277 cases of pertussis, at an incidence rate of 15.2/100,000 population. This is the highest number of cases reported in the United States since 1955, when 62,786 cases were reported. However, many more infections go undiagnosed and unreported.

The number of cases in 2012 had increased from 18,719 cases in 2011. The highest rates were among 11- to 19-year-olds and those aged 20+ years, at 29.9 and 21.6/100,000, respectively. However, 80% of the deaths (16/20) due to pertussis were among infants less than 1 year old; 75% of the deaths (15/20) occurred in infants less than 3 months old (CDC, 2013a). Trends by age group in the United States from 1990 to 2012 indicate that infants aged less than 1 year old, who are at greatest risk for severe disease and death, continue to have the highest reported rate of pertussis. School-aged children (7 to 10 years) continue to contribute a significant proportion of reported pertussis cases. However, 2012 data indicate that pertussis is increasing among adolescents (CDC, 2013b).

Although pertussis tends to have cycles over time with peaks every 3 to 5 years, the increase in cases has been greater and more prolonged in the past several years. A number of states, including Utah, Washington, Ohio, and Wisconsin, had substantial increases in the disease in 2013. For example, the state of Texas reported that it had not seen the number of pertussis cases in 2013 that high since 1959. In addition, Ohio had seen a 20% increase in reported pertussis cases, compared to that in 2012. Pertussis also has been circulating at epidemic levels in Colorado for the past couple of years. Outbreaks of whooping cough continued to be reported in late 2013 (ProMED-mail, 2013a, 2013b, 2013c).

Factors underlying increased incidence of whooping cough may include diminished immunity from childhood pertussis vaccines, improved diagnostic testing, and increased reporting. Rising rates of pertussis and response to vaccination could be due to replacement of whole-cell killed *B. pertussis* vaccines by acellular vaccines in the 1990s. The latter vaccines use only selected portions of pertussis bacteria to stimulate an immune response. A new study from the CDC suggests that *B. pertussis* has mutated in response to vaccine immunity. The team examined 1,300 samples taken from whooping cough outbreaks between 1935 and 2012 in the United States. *B. pertussis* isolates lacking pertactin, a key antigen component of the acellular pertussis vaccine, were observed, indicating that *B. pertussis* is losing its ability to produce pertactin. Before 2010, the researchers saw only one pertussis infection, in 1994, in which the bacteria did not make pertactin. However, by 2012, the majority of pertussis infections the researchers studied were caused by non–pertactin-making *B. pertussis* (Pawloski et al., 2013).

According to the researchers, it may be possible that changes in *B. pertussis* affect the vaccine's ability to protect. The CDC is examining this question and was expected to have data to do so by 2014. However, the mutated bacteria are no more dangerous than the original, and vaccines against the illness are still effective. Also, there is no evidence yet that current pertussis vaccines are less effective against the new strains of *B. pertussis*.

Therefore, as of 2013, the Advisory Committee on Immunization Practices (ACIP) recommendations are to increase vaccination among those aged 0 to 18 years, and for adults older than 18 years, including those older than 65 who have not yet received a dose of Tdap (a combination vaccine with tetanus and diphtheria), to receive a single dose of the vaccine (CDC, 2012a, 2012b, 2013c). To reduce transmission to susceptible infants, the 2013 ACIP recommendations also included revaccination for pregnant women in the second or third trimester for each pregnancy (CDC, 2013c).

Cross-Sectional Studies

One method used in public health to collect observational data is **survey research**. Survey research focuses on the collection of information regarding the status quo of some situation(s) by questionnaire or by interviews with a sample of respondents (Burns et al., 2013). The main principle of survey research is that the **sample** of respondents must represent the population from which it was drawn. **Cross-sectional studies** (prevalence studies) are an example of public health survey research. In this type of study, the population to be studied is defined and data are collected from members of the group about their disease and exposure status. The data represent a point in time; therefore, they provide a "snapshot" of the population. Cross-sectional studies are good for examining the **relationship** between a variable and a disease/condition but not for determining cause and effect, which requires the collection of data over time. Cross-sectional studies may be designed to gather data from two or more groups with different characteristics or with different exposure risk.

An example of cross-sectional studies is the Behavioral Risk Factor Surveillance System (BRFSS) established by the CDC in the early 1980s when scientific research clearly indicated that personal health behaviors played a major role in premature morbidity and mortality. The BRFSS is an efficient method that takes a cross section of the population at a single point in time and monitors the prevalence of the major behavioral risks in adults associated with premature morbidity and mortality at the state level. These data are useful for planning, initiating, supporting, and evaluating health promotion and disease prevention programs. Several states used the data to determine progress toward achievement of *Healthy People 2010* objectives (USDHHS, 2000).

table 8.1 **Assessment of the *Healthy People 2020* Objectives, 2012**

Objective	Year 2012 (%)	Target 2020 (%)
Reduce the proportion of adults (aged ≥20 years) who are obese	28.9	30
Reduce the proportion of adults (aged ≥18 years) who engage in no leisure-time physical activity	49.5	47.9
Reduce cigarette smoking by adults (aged ≥18 years)	18.0	12
Increase the proportion of adults (aged ≥65 years) who are vaccinated annually against influenza	63.4	90
Increase the proportion of adults (aged ≥65 years) who are vaccinated against pneumococcal disease	59.9	90

Sources: Center for Disease Control, National Center for Health Statistics. (2013). *Health, United States, 2012*. Retrieved from http://www.cdc.gov/nchs/data/hus/hus12.pdf; U.S. Department of Health and Human Services. (2010). *Healthy People 2020*. Retrieved from http://www.healthypeople.gov/2020/topicsobjectives2020/default.aspx

For more information on the BRFSS, see the CDC's BRFSS website at http://www.cdc.gov/brfss/.

Table 8.1 outlines an assessment of how progress was being made on selective objectives of *Healthy People 2020* in 2012 on the basis of the survey questions asked in the CDC NCHS questionnaire (CDC, 2013). As can be seen, the prevalence of obesity among U.S. adults aged 20 and older was lower than the 30% targeted 2020 objective for obesity in this age group. Also, the percentage of adults (20 years and older) who had participated in federal guidelines for physical activity in 2012 was higher than the 2020 target of 47.9%. However, the percentage of adults who were current smokers in 2012 was more than the targeted 12% by 2020 (USDHHS, 2010).

Healthy People 2020 targets to increase influenza and pneumococcal vaccination in adults, which had been retained from *Healthy People 2010*, still had not been met as of 2012 (CDC, 2013c). The percentage of adults aged 65 and older who had received influenza and pneumococcal vaccination in 2012 remained well below the targets of 90%, respectively. It will be interesting to see how many of the objectives proposed for *Healthy People 2020* are met by the target date (USDHHS, 2010).

Another example of survey research for public health information is the CDC's Youth Risk Behavior Survey, which assesses risk behaviors such as youth violence. Information is available at the CDC's website at http://www.cdc.gov/HealthyYouth/yrbs/index.htm. An example of outcomes from survey research is the National High Blood Pressure Education Program coordinated by the National Heart, Lung and Blood Institute (NHLBI) of the National Institutes of Health. Established in 1972, the program is succeeding in its mission of increasing awareness, prevention, treatment, and control of hypertension. Considerable success has been achieved in the National High Blood Pressure Education Program. The latest hypertension guidelines published by NHLBI Joint National Committee (JNC) on Blood Pressure in Adults was in 2013 (James et al., 2013). These latest NHLBI recommendations, presented in Table 8.2, are an age-adjusted **evidence-based approach** to the management of hypertension in adults. The JNC 8 used data from randomized controlled trials, the "gold standard" for determining efficacy and effectiveness, and graded the quality of the evidence on the basis of their effect on key outcomes. Table 8.3 outlines the 2014 American Heart Association/American College of Cardiologists recommendations for lifestyle management to lower blood pressure (BP) and cardiovascular risk (Eckel et al., 2013).

table 8.2 **2013 Guidelines for the Management of Blood Pressure in Adults**

Age	SBP (mm Hg)	DBP (mm Hg)
<60 years	<140	<90
>60 years	<150	<90
All ages with diabetes, but no chronic kidney disease (CKD).	<140	<90
All ages with or without diabetes and with CKD.	<140	<90

SBP, systolic blood pressure; DBP, diastolic blood pressure.
Source: James, P. A., Oparil, S., Carter, B. L., et al. (2013). 2014 evidence-based guideline for the management of high blood pressure in adults: Report from the panel members appointed to the eighth joint national committee (JNC 8). JAMA. Published online first: December 18, 2013. doi:10.1001/jama.2013.284427. Retrieved December 19, 2013 from http://jama.jamanetwork.com/article.aspx?articleid=1791497.

Case 1: In an attempt to increase the number of people aged 65 years or older who are vaccinated against pneumococcal disease, the community health nurses in Case 1 decide to conduct the following:

- An assessment of baseline knowledge, attitudes, and practices among healthcare providers in the community regarding pneumococcal vaccination to identify barriers to providing pneumococcal vaccination
- An assessment of baseline knowledge, attitudes, and beliefs among community residents aged 65 years or older to determine barriers to receiving pneumococcal vaccination

1. What research method could the nurses use to perform these assessments?
2. How would you go about gathering the data for these assessments?

table 8.3 **Recommendations for Lifestyle Management to Lower Blood Pressure**

Recommendations		NHLB Strength of Evidence
Diet	1. Consume a dietary pattern that emphasizes intake of vegetables, fruits, and whole grains.	Strong
	2. Include low-fat dairy products, poultry, fish, legumes, nontropical vegetable oils and nuts.	Strong
	3. Limit intake of sweets, sugar-sweetened beverages, and red meats.	Strong
	4. Achieve this by following the USDA food pattern or the AHA diet.	Strong
	5. Lower sodium intake to 1,500 mg/day.	Moderate
	6. Combine the DASH dietary pattern with lower sodium intake.	Strong
Physical activity	Engage in aerobic physical activity 3–4 times a week, lasting on average 40 minutes, and involving moderate-to-vigorous physical activity.	Moderate

Sources: Adapted from Eckel, R. H., Jakicic, J. M., Ard, J. D., Hubbard, V. S., de Jesus, J. M., Lee, I-M.,... Yanovski, S. Z. (2013). 2013 AHA/ACC guideline on lifestyle management to reduce cardiovascular risk: A report of the American College of Cardiology/American Heart Association task force on practice guidelines. *Circulation*. Advance online publication. Retrieved from http://circ.ahajournals.org/content/early/2013/11/11/01.cir.0000437740.48606.d1.long

Analytical Studies

As can be seen in Figure 8.2, analytical research study designs are on a continuum, ranging from strongest to weakest designs. Two analytical designs—the prospective correlational design and the retrospective correlational design—are "weaker" designs on the continuum; however, these studies lead to hypothesis testing based on established **associations** (correlations). There are two general types of analytical epidemiologic studies: cohort studies and case–control studies.

Cohort Studies

Cohort studies, sometimes referred to as longitudinal studies, are **prospective studies** that monitor subjects over time to find associations between risk factors and health outcomes (Porta, 2008). Although they are stronger in design methodology than are case–control studies when well executed (see later discussion), cohort studies also are more expensive. In their simplest form, a sample (cohort) of subjects who are exposed to the risk factor(s) is matched with a sample of subjects not exposed to the risk factor. Some prospective studies, such as the Framingham Heart Study, which were designed to estimate the lifetime risk of coronary heart disease, lasted for decades. Many recommended public health guidelines for BP, total cholesterol, and low-density lipoprotein cholesterol resulted from the Framingham Heart Study (Shortreed, Peeters, & Forbes, 2013).

PRACTICE POINT

A biased sample will result in a biased study with biased results. Randomization is crucial to obtaining a representative sample. The larger the sample, the greater the chances of a true representation of the population.

The advantages of cohort studies are that they minimize selection bias, a threat to internal validity, and provide preliminary evidence of the incidence of a risk factor with which the **relative risk** (RR) can be established. **Internal validity** is the degree to which the effects detected in a study are real rather than from confounding or extraneous variables (Burns et al., 2013). See Box 8.1 for threats to internal validity.

Relative risk is defined as the ratio of disease incidence (or death) in an exposed population to that in an unexposed population. The assumption is that the underlying risk without the exposure is the same in both groups:

$$RR = \frac{\text{Incidence rate in people exposed}}{\text{Incidence rate in people not exposed}}$$

Relative risk is a ratio ranging from zero to infinity that indicates the strength of the association between the risk factor and the outcome. It is calculated by dividing the risk in the group exposed to a risk factor by the risk in the unexposed group.

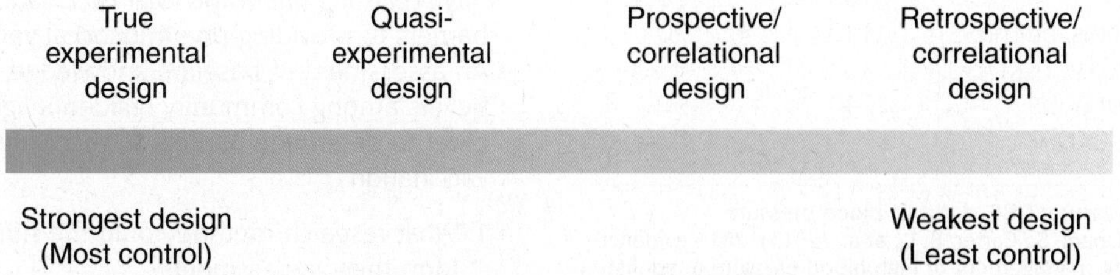

figure 8.2 Research design continuum. (Adapted from Polit, D. F., & Hungler, B. P. [1995]. *Nursing research* (5ed.). Philadelphia, PA: J.B. Lippincott.)

box 8.1 Threats to Internal Validity

History: Refers to events that are occurring during the study, which could influence participants' responses to the intervention.

Maturation: Refers to unplanned and unrecognized changes in the participants that could affect the findings of the study (e.g., fatigue, hunger, or increased knowledge).

Testing: Refers to the effect of multiple measurements of participants' responses that could influence the participants' responses, thereby altering the outcome of the study.

Selection: Refers to the process by which participants are selected and grouped for a study. This threat is more likely to occur when randomization is not possible.

Instrumentation: Refers to changes in the measurement instrument used in the study, which result in inconsistent data collection.

Mortality: Refers to loss of subjects from the study. When those who drop out of the study differ significantly from those who remain in the study, and if there is a difference in those who remain in experimental and control groups, the outcome of the study would be affected.

Source: Burns, N., Grove, S. K., & Gray J. R. (2013). *The practice of nursing research* (7th ed.). St. Louis, MO: Elsevier.

An RR significantly greater than 1 (statistically) indicates that the exposure is associated with increased risk of disease. An RR significantly less than 1 (statistically) indicates that the exposure is associated with decreased risk of disease; that is, the exposure is protective. An RR not significantly different from 1 (statistically) indicates that there is no association between the exposure and the risk of disease (Washington State University, n.d.).

Epidemiologic cohort studies are developed to examine **causality** among variables in illnesses. Causal associations found in this manner are known as inferred causality. Repeated, multiple studies strengthen the causal link. This strategy may not be as powerful as experimental designs; however, in many epidemiologic studies, a true experimental study would not be ethical. For example, a researcher would not deliberately expose one group to an infectious microorganism to study its effect. An important finding of inferred causality came from the well-known **cohort study**, the Harvard Nurses' Health Study, which has followed female registered nurses from 14 states since 1976. A 1994 landmark study established an association between breast cancer and long-time use of hormone replacement therapy (Colditz et al., 1995). The Nurses' Health Study, considered the "grandmother" of women's health studies, is the world's largest, longest-running study of women's health. The study, which is now in its third phase (Nurses' Health Study 3, n.d.), has also provided other valuable information on women's health (e.g., increased dietary calcium intake does not protect against fractures of the hip and wrist among postmenopausal women; birth control pills do not increase the risk of heart disease among nonsmoking women).

box 8.2 Criteria for Causality

The relationship must be clear (*strength of association*).
Observation of the association must be repeatable in different populations at different times (*consistency*).
The cause must precede the effect (*temporality*).
The explanation must make sense biologically (*plausibility*).
There must be a dose–response relationship (*biological gradient*).

Source: Adapted from Hill, A. B. (1965). The environment and disease: Association or causation. *Proceedings of the Royal Society of Medicine. 58*(5), 295-300. [PMC free article] [PubMed].

More information on the Harvard Nurses' Health Study can be found at http://www.channing.harvard.edu/nhs/.

Cohort studies attempt to find cause-and-effect relationships; however, to find statistically meaningful data (i.e., causality), a large number of cases are needed. There may also be threats to internal validity due to loss of subjects from the study (mortality). Nonetheless, data from cohort studies may be used as the basis for hypotheses generation for stronger experimental studies, such as randomized controlled trials (CDC, 2010). In general, the five criteria listed in Box 8.2 must be met to establish a cause-and-effect relationship.

To every complex question there is a simple answer…and it is wrong.

H. L. Mencken, writer and wit

Case–Control Studies

Case–control studies, also known as **retrospective studies**, work backward from the effect to the suspected cause (Porta, 2008). Subjects are selected on the basis of the presence or absence of the disease or outcome in question: one group of people (case subjects) with the health problem and another group without the health problem **(controls)**. The two groups are then compared to determine the presence of specific exposures or risk factors.

For example, diethylstilbestrol (DES) was thought to be a safe and effective way to prevent miscarriages or premature deliveries. It has been estimated that between 5 and 10 million people were exposed to DES in the United States between 1938 and 1971. However, landmark case-controlled epidemiologic studies have found health risks associated with DES in women for whom it was prescribed during pregnancy and the offspring born of those pregnancies (DES sons and daughters). DES daughters and sons are defined as women or men who were exposed to DES in utero. Research has confirmed that daughters of mothers who took DES are at risk for clear cell adenocarcinoma, a rare kind of vaginal and cervical cancer that may affect females from their early teens to their forties. Studies have also demonstrated that sons of mothers who took DES are at risk for epididymal cysts and other genital abnormalities, including testicular hypoplasia, cryptorchidism, and microphallus (CDC, 2012).

In addition, research is underway to determine whether the offspring of sons and daughters of mothers who took DES might have health effects related to DES exposure. These grandchildren of women prescribed DES during pregnancy are sometimes called the "third generation" (CDC, 2012c). More detailed information about DES can be found at the CDC website DES Update Home at http://www.cdc.gov/des/hcp/nurses/index.html.

The relationship between exposure and outcome in a **case–control study** is quantified by calculating the **odds ratio** (OR). The OR is an estimate of RR that is interpreted in the same manner as RR. When a disease is relatively rare (e.g., a cumulative annual incidence of less than 5% in the unexposed population), the OR is similar to the RR. Otherwise, the OR overestimates RR. An OR significantly greater than 1 (statistically) indicates that the exposure is associated with increased risk of disease, and an OR not significantly different from 1 statistically indicates there is no association between the exposure and the risk of disease (CDC, 2010).

Case–control studies have several advantages: they (1) allow for the examination of multiple exposures for a single outcome; (2) are suitable for studying rare diseases and those with long latency periods; (3) require fewer case subjects; and (4) generally are quicker and less expensive to conduct than cohort studies, making them well suited for an outbreak investigation (see Chapter 14). They have several disadvantages: (1) they are not appropriate for studying rare exposures, (2) they are subject to bias because of the method used to select controls, and (3) they do not allow the direct measure of the incidence of disease. Also, because they look backward, case–control studies may create uncertainty about the temporal relationship between exposure and disease (CDC, 2010).

INTERVENTION (EXPERIMENTAL) STUDIES

True experiments that control all factors other than the one under investigation are rare when studying human populations. Many studies, although experimental in design, are not able to either randomize selection of subjects or exert the same degree of control of the study variables that would be found in true experimental studies. Manipulation of the independent variable occurs, but it may not be possible to control influencing or confounding factors.

Case 2: Data from the 2011 to 2012 National Health and Nutrition Examination Survey indicate that adults aged 20 years and older in the United States have at least one of the following three preventable cardiovascular disease risk factors: uncontrolled hypertension, uncontrolled high cholesterol, or smoking (CDC, 2013d).

The U.S. Department of Health and Human Services (DHHS) is prioritizing evidence-based policy and program interventions to address the leading causes of death and disability in the United States, including heart disease, cancer, stroke, chronic lower respiratory tract diseases, unintentional injuries, and preventable behaviors such as tobacco use, poor nutrition, physical inactivity, and excessive alcohol use that contribute to those causes (USDHHS, 2012).

- The incidence of heart disease is increased in persons who are overweight or obese (BMI > 25).
- High BP is twice as common in adults who are obese than in those who have a healthy weight.
- Obesity is associated with elevated triglycerides and decreased HDL cholesterol. (USDHHS, 2013).

Data obtained from the Framingham Heart Study have indicated that those with BP levels between 130 and 139/85 and 89 mm Hg were associated with a more-than-twofold increase in RR for cardiovascular disease as compared with those with BP levels below 120/80 mm Hg.

1. What type of epidemiologic study was conducted in the Framingham Heart Study?
2. What does a "more-than-twofold increase in RR for cardiovascular disease" mean?

STUDENT REFLECTION

In a research class, we were all given the challenge to come up with a practical clinical problem that would be feasible for us to study. We had to apply the *who*, *what*, *where*, *when*, *why*, and *how* questions to clinical problems. For about a half hour each class session, we discussed our issues with our classmates. I remember one that really stumped us. My fellow students wanted to measure hair loss before and after chemotherapy. Our challenge was to come up with a way to measure hair loss—easier said than done. Lots of ideas were suggested, from collecting all hair that falls out in a jar, to shaving the head, counting the hair, and waiting for it to grow back in, when it would be counted again. Nothing seemed satisfactory. Then the solution dawned on us. We decided to measure a square inch on the scalp with permanent ink, trim the hair to 0.5 inch, and take a photograph. We then would count each hair in the photograph. The neat thing about this measurement was that we could take a series of pictures over time and measure the speed of hair loss. We were all pretty pleased with this, and so was the instructor. It demonstrated how creative we could be while following the rules of research measurement. The experience made me realize that a group is better than an individual in the research design process and that we all had to think "out of the box." It was a great learning experience.

PRACTICE POINT

When gathering evidence for practice, nurses should consider the ***strength*** of the evidence as follows:

High: There are consistent results from good-quality studies. Further research is very unlikely to change the conclusions.

Moderate: Findings supported, but further research could change the conclusions.

Low: There are very few studies, or the existing studies are flawed.

Insufficient: Research is either unavailable or does not permit estimation of a treatment effect.

Source: Agency for Healthcare Research and Quality. Retrieved from http://www.effectivehealthcare.ahrq.gov/ehc/products/160/1048/lbd_clin_fin_to_post.pdf

Intervention studies in public health are categorized as preventive trials and therapeutic trials, and both can be either quasi-experimental studies or true experimental studies. Quasi-experimental study designs are weaker because assignment of subjects into groups is not randomized, the researcher is unable to manipulate the variable under study (see Fig. 8.2), or because of situations where it may be unethical or impractical to randomize subjects. The quasi-experimental design is used in preventive trials that focus on primary prevention (i.e., during the prepathogenesis stage to reduce the incidence of disease).

Preventive Trials

An example of a **preventive trial** using a quasi-experimental design is a study of a school district participating in a smoking prevention program. The sample is divided into two groups: some schools receive a health education program on smoking ("treatment"), and the others receive nothing ("control"). The two groups are then assessed for the incidence of smoking at 3 months, 6 months, and 1 year following the program. In this case, assignment to the treatment and comparison groups was not randomized; therefore, it is considered a quasi-experimental study. The greatest strengths of quasi-experimental studies are their practicality, feasibility, and, to some extent, their generalizability (external validity) to similar groups. External validity is the degree to which the results of a study can be generalized to other settings or samples other than the ones studied (Burns et al., 2013). See Box 8.3 for threats to external validity.

When a quasi-experimental design is used, control over other factors (confounding variables) may result in statistical differences due to competing hypotheses (type I error) or result in no statistical difference when it does exist (type II error). Also, if a quasi-experimental design is used, it cannot be assumed that the treatment and control groups were equal. However, the design can be made stronger by pretesting both groups before the intervention. If both groups respond similarly on the pretest, then information obtained after the intervention can be assumed to be the result of the intervention (Burns et al., 2013).

box 8.3 Common Threats to External Validity

Reactivity: Also known as the "Hawthorne effect"; this threat occurs when participants behave in a certain way because they know they are being studied, affecting the generalizability of the findings.

Novelty: Occurs when a new intervention affects the outcome of the study because of either enthusiasm or skepticism by the researchers or the participants.

Experimenter/participant effect: Occurs when the researcher or subject has preconceived expectations of the intervention, resulting in bias and affecting generalizability of the findings.

Interaction of selection and intervention: Occurs when subjects willing to participate in the study are not representative of the target population, thus limiting the generalizability of the results.

Interaction of setting and intervention: Occurs when the characteristics of the study setting influence the outcome of the study, limiting the generalizability of the findings to other settings.

Interaction of history and intervention: Occurs when the circumstances (history) of the study influence the results of the study, and decrease the generalizability of the findings.

Source: Burns, N., Grove, S. K., & Gray, J. R. (2013). *The practice of nursing research* (7th ed.). St. Louis, MO: Elsevier.

From error to error, one discovers the entire truth.

Sigmund Freud

EVIDENCE FOR PRACTICE

Falling is a significant problem among community-living older adults in the United States. Liu and Frank (2010) examined 19 published longitudinal studies that studied the effects of the Chinese art of Tai Chi on reducing the risk of falling among the elderly through regular exercise. They found that Tai Chi exercise duration of 12 weeks or longer, with frequencies of twice a week or more, and session lengths of at least 45 minutes had the following outcomes: reduced fear of falling, increased single-leg stance, decreased rate of falling, increased flexibility, and improved walking. The authors concluded that Tai Chi could be an economic and effective exercise program for improving balance and balance confidence in older adults.

Properly executed experimental studies provide the strongest empirical evidence. The hallmark of the experimental study is random assignment of subjects to treatment (intervention) and control groups, which controls for potential unknown confounding variables. Randomization also provides a better foundation for statistical procedures to prevent type I and type II errors than do observational and quasi-experimental studies. The research continuum in Figure 8.2 indicates that experimental study designs are the strongest because they control for all factors except that which is under investigation (Harkness, 1995). The "gold standard" for experimental studies is the prospective, double-blind, placebo control group design, also referred to as **clinical trials** or therapeutic trials. In double-blind experimental studies, neither the researchers nor the subjects are aware to which group they are randomly assigned.

PRACTICE POINT

Do not evaluate all research studies at the *p* value of .05. No researcher has a fixed level of significance that accepts or rejects hypotheses from year to year, and in all circumstances. Rather, consider each finding according to its usefulness in clinical situations. Studies may have clinical significance and not be statistically significant.

Therapeutic Trials

Therapeutic trials are based on secondary prevention, which focuses on limiting the spread of disease (see Chapter 14). In therapeutic trials the treatment (independent variable) is manipulated by the researcher to determine its effect on controlling the disease. For example, a 1994 landmark study conducted between 1991 and 1993 enrolled 477 HIV-infected pregnant women between 14 and 34 weeks of gestation. In this double-blind, placebo-controlled, randomized therapeutic trial, the women were stratified according to gestational age (14 to 26 weeks or more than 26 weeks) and were randomly assigned to receive either zidovudine (AZT) or placebo. There were no significant differences between the characteristics of the AZT group and the placebo (control) group (Connor et al., 1994).

The AZT regimen consisted of antepartum AZT (100 mg orally five times daily) plus intrapartum AZT (administered intravenously every hour until delivery), as well as AZT for the newborn beginning 8 to 12 hours after birth (2 mg/kg orally every 6 hours for 6 weeks). During the study period, 409 women gave birth to a total of 415 live infants. The infants were evaluated by cultures and HIV serologic tests both at birth and at several weekly intervals until 78 weeks of age. At the 18-month analysis for AZT efficacy, there was a two-third (67%) reduction in the risk of HIV transmission from mother to infant in the AZT group. Because of these rather marked findings, the study was halted, and all mothers were given AZT (Connor et al., 1994). Recent studies of antiretroviral prophylaxis in the prevention of mother-to-child HIV transmission have found similar results (Sturt, Dokubo, & Sint, 2010; Tudor Car et al., 2013).

The U.S. Public Health Service Task Force recommends the use of antiretroviral therapy to reduce perinatal HIV transmission, universal prenatal HIV counseling, and HIV testing with consent for all pregnant women in the United States. As a result, the number of HIV-infected infants born each year in the United States has decreased from approximately 1,750 (in the mid-1990s) to approximately 143 in 2010 (CDC, 2013e). For more information regarding the prevention of maternal–child transmission of HIV, see CDC, *Eliminating Perinatal HIV Transmission,* at http://www.cdc.gov/primarycare/materials/hivtransmission/.

In both preventive trials and therapeutic trials, planning includes sample selection, protocol methodology, data collection, and data analysis. Sample selection is taken from the target population, the population to which the results of the intervention are applicable. In the Connor et al. (1994) AZT trial described earlier, the target population was HIV-infected pregnant women. The sample consisted of HIV-infected pregnant women who were randomly assigned to the treatment (AZT) group or the placebo (control) group. The study was a double-blind study, in which neither the researchers nor the participants knew who was receiving AZT treatment until the study ended. A double-blind study is one method to prevent observation bias. In a single-blind study, only the investigator knows which participants are receiving the treatment and which are not. In unblinded studies, both the investigator and the participants know who is in the treatment group and the control group. Nonetheless, measures should be taken to prevent observation bias in both single-blind and unblinded studies.

Chance favors the prepared mind.

Harlan Ellison, American author

Although statistical analysis is beyond the scope of this text, it is important to know that the sample size in intervention trials should be large enough for adequate statistical power to prevent a type II error. In addition, the researcher should set the expected statistical ***p* value**, generally at .05, to ensure that the study results are not due to chance alone and to avoid committing a type I error. A **type I error** occurs when the **null hypothesis** (H_0, a theory that has been put forward, either because it is believed to be true or because it is to be used as a basis for argument) is rejected when it is true. A **type II error** occurs when one accepts the null hypothesis when it is false (i.e., the alternative hypothesis [H_a] is true). For example, in a clinical trial of a new drug, the null hypothesis might be that the new drug is no better than the current drug. The null hypothesis and alternative hypothesis, respectively, would be as follows:

H_0: There is no difference between the two drugs.
H_a: There is a difference between the two drugs.

Having a basic understanding of research methods allows nurses to interpret and critically analyze studies described in newspapers, magazines, and scientific journals, as well as on the Internet. It also allows nurses to generate research questions related to problems identified in their practice.

key concepts

- Epidemiologic research identifies community/public health problems and describes the natural history and etiology of diseases.
- Epidemiologic/public health research can be descriptive or analytical. Study designs are based on the problem under study and range in strength on a continuum, with the weakest design being the retrospective design and the strongest being the experimental design.
- Descriptive studies are most frequently used in public health research. They may be observational or analytical.
- Findings from descriptive epidemiologic studies lead to hypotheses for future research.
- The case study provides an in-depth examination of a single unit, such as a person, family, community, or institution.
- Case–control studies retrospectively compare subjects (cases) with a condition (disease) and matched subjects/control without the condition/disease (e.g., those with a foodborne infection compared with those without an infection).
- Cohort studies, also called longitudinal studies, examine phenomena prospectively to observe presumed effects over time (e.g., effects of diet and exercise on heart disease).
- Cross-sectional studies examine the relationship of health-related characteristics and other variables of interest (e.g., age, gender) in a defined population at a particular point in time.
- Quasi-experimental and experimental designs are used to examine causality.
- The "gold standard" for research design is the randomized, control group design.
- Preventive trials focus on primary prevention to reduce the incidence of disease.
- Therapeutic trials are based on secondary prevention, which focuses on limiting the spread of disease.
- Community health nurses are the consumers of health-related research, which is the foundation of evidence-based practice and also is used to inform and educate the public.

critical thinking questions

1. Review the following article: Incident diagnoses of breast cancer, active component service women, U.S. Armed Forces, 2000–2012. (2013, September). *Medical Surveillance Monthly Report, 20*(9). Retrieved from http://www.afhsc.mil/viewMSMR?file=2013/v20_n09.pdf#Page=25
   a. What research design was used in the study?
   b. Are there health promotion and disease prevention activities that you would recommend to patients on the basis of these study findings and those of the Colditz et al. (1995) study described earlier?
2. There is a high increase in teenage smoking in your community, and community leaders are developing a plan to decrease the incidence of smoking.
   a. Develop a research question to address the problem.
   b. What kind of study should be undertaken?
   c. Design a study to decrease the incidence of smoking in teenagers.
3. Read the following report: Agency for Healthcare Research and Quality. (2012). *Treatment to prevent osteoporotic fractures: An update*. Retrieved from http://www.effectivehealthcare.ahrq.gov/ehc/products/160/1048/lbd_clin_fin_to_post.pdf
   a. Is the report evidence based?
   b. Identify the strengths and weaknesses of evidence in the report.
   c. Is the evidence strong enough to influence practice?

references

Agency for Healthcare Research and Quality. (2012). *Treatment to prevent osteoporotic fractures: An update.* Retrieved from http://www.effectivehealthcare.ahrq.gov/ehc/products/160/1048/lbd_clin_fin_to_post.pdf

Burns, N., Grove, S. K., & Gray, J. R. (2013). *The practice of nursing research: Appraisal, synthesis, and generation of evidence* (7th ed.). St. Louis, MO: Saunders Elsevier.

Centers for Disease Control and Prevention. (2010). *An introduction to epidemiology.* Retrieved from http://www.cdc.gov/excite/classroom/intro_epi.htm

Centers for Disease Control and Prevention. (2012a). *Epidemiology and prevention of vaccine-preventable diseases, "Pink Book"* (12th ed.). Atlanta, GA: Author.

Centers for Disease Control and Prevention. (2012b). Updated recommendations for use of tetanus toxoid, reduced diphtheria toxoid, and acellular pertussis (Tdap) vaccine in adults aged 65 years and older—Advisory Committee on Immunization Practices (ACIP), 2012. *Morbidity Mortality Weekly Report, 61*(25), 468–470.

references (continued)

Centers for Disease Control and Prevention. (2012c). *DES update for healthcare providers*. Retrieved from http://www.cdc.gov/des/hcp/index.html

Centers for Disease Control and Prevention. (2013a). *2012 final pertussis surveillance report*. Retrieved from http://www.cdc.gov/pertussis/downloads/pertussis-surveillance-report.pdf

Centers for Disease Control and Prevention. (2013b). *Pertussis: Surveillance & reporting*. Retrieved from http://www.cdc.gov/pertussis/surv-reporting.html#trends

Centers for Disease Control and Prevention. (2013c). Advisory Committee on Immunization Practices (ACIP) recommended immunization schedule—United States, 2013. *Morbidity Mortality Weekly Report*, *62*(Suppl.), 1–19.

Centers for Disease Control and Prevention. (2013d). *National Health and Nutrition Examination Survey*. Retrieved from http://www.cdc.gov/nchs/nhanes/new_nhanes.htm

Centers for Disease Control and Prevention. (2013e). *Eliminating perinatal HIV transmission*. Retrieved from http://www.cdc.gov/primarycare/materials/hivtransmission/

Centers for Disease Control and Prevention, National Center for Health Statistics. (2013). *Health, United States, 2012*. Retrieved from http://www.cdc.gov/nchs/data/hus/hus12.pdf

Colditz, G. A., Hankinson, S. E., Hunter, D. J., Willett, W. C., Manson, J. E., Stampfer, M. J.,… Speizer, F. E. (1995). The use of estrogens and progestins and the risk of breast cancer in postmenopausal women. *New England Journal of Medicine*, *332*(24), 1589–1593.

Connor, E. M., Sperling, R. S., Gelber, R., Kiselev, P., Scott, G., O'Sullivan, M.,… James Balsley for the Pediatric AIDS Clinical Trials Group Protocol 076 Study Group (1994). Reduction of maternal-infant transmission of human immunodeficiency virus type 1 with zidovudine treatment. *New England Journal of Medicine*, *331*, 1173–1180.

Eckel, R. H., Jakicic, J. M., Ard, J. D., Hubbard, V. S., de Jesus, J. M., Lee, I-M.,… Yanovski, S. Z. (2013). AHA/ACC guideline on lifestyle management to reduce cardiovascular risk: A report of the American College of Cardiology/American Heart Association task force on practice guidelines. *Circulation*. Advance online publication. Retrieved from http://circ.ahajournals.org/content/early/2013/11/11/01.cir.0000437740.48606.d1.citation

Harkness, G. (1995). Analytic epidemiology. *Epidemiology in nursing practice* (Chapter 6, pp. 97–111). St. Louis, MO: Mosby.

Incident diagnoses of breast cancer, active component service women, U.S. Armed Forces, 2000–2012. (2013, September). *Medical Surveillance Monthly Report*, *20*(9). Retrieved from http://www.afhsc.mil/viewMSMR?file=2013/v20_n09.pdf#Page=25

James, P. A., Oparil, S., Carter, B. L., Cushman, W. C., Dennison-Himmelfarb C., Handler, J.,… Ortiz, E. (2013). 2014 Evidence-based guideline for the management of high blood pressure in adults. Report from the panel members appointed to the eighth joint national committee (JNC 8). *JAMA*. Advance publication online. Retrieved from http://jama.jamanetwork.com/onlineFirst.aspx

Liu, H., & Frank, A. (2010). Tai chi as a balance improvement exercise for older adults: A systematic review. *Journal of Geriatric Physical Therapy*, *33*(3), 103–109.

Melnyk, B., & Fineout-Overholt, E. (2005). *Evidence-based practice in nursing and healthcare*. Philadelphia, PA: Lippincott, Williams and Wilkins.

Nurses' Health Study 3. (n.d.). Retrieved from http://www.nhs3.org/

Pawloski, L. C., Queenan, A. M., Cassiday, P. K., Lynch, A. S., Harrison, M., Shang, W.,… Tondella, M. L. (2013). Prevalence and molecular characterization of pertactin-deficient *Bordetella pertussis* in the US. *Clinical Vaccine and Immunology* Advance online publication. Retrieved from http://www.asm.org/images/Communications/tips/2013/1213pertussis.pdf

Porta, M. (Ed.). (2008). *A dictionary of epidemiology*, (5th ed.). New York, NY: Oxford University Press.

ProMED-mail. (2013a, September 9). *Pertussis*. Retrieved from http://www.promedmail.org/

ProMED-Mail. (2013c, December 25). *Pertussis–USA*. Retrieved from http://www.promedmail.org

ProMED-Mail. (2013b, December 29). *Pertussis–USA*. Retrieved from http://www.promedmail.org

Shortreed, S. M., Peeters, A., & Forbes, A. B. (2013). Estimating the effect of long-term physical activity on cardiovascular disease and mortality: Evidence from the Framingham Heart Study. *Heart* [Epub ahead of print]. Advance online publication. Retrieved from http://heart.bmj.com/content/early/2013/03/07/heartjnl-2012-303461.long

Sturt, A. S., Dokubo, E. K., & Sint, T. T. (2010). Antiretroviral therapy (ART) for treating HIV infection in ART-eligible pregnant women. *Cochrane Database of Systematic Review*, *17*(3), CD008440.

Tudor Car, L., Brusamento, S., Elmoniry, H., van Velthoven, M.H., Pape, U. J., Welch, V.,… Atun, R. (2013). The uptake of integrated perinatal prevention of mother-to-child HIV transmission programs in low- and middle-income countries: A systematic review. *Public Library of Science*, *8*(3), e56550. Advance online publication. Retrieved from http://www.plosone.org/article/info%3Adoi%2F10.1371%2Fjournal.pone.0056550

U.S. Department of Health and Human Services. (2010). *Healthy people 2020*. Retrieved from http://www.healthypeople.gov/2020/topicsobjectives2020/default.aspx

U.S. Department of Health and Human Services. (2012). *Secretary's strategic initiatives*. Retrieved from http://www.hhs.gov/secretary/about/priorities/strat_initiatives.pdf

U.S. Department of Health and Human Services. (2013). *Overweight and obesity: Health consequences*. Retrieved from http://www.surgeongeneral.gov/library/calls/obesity/fact_consequences.html

Washington State University. (n.d.). *Clinical epidemiology & evidence-based medicine glossary: Terminology specific to epidemiology*. Retrieved from http://www.vetmed.wsu.edu/courses-jmgay/GlossepiTerminology.htm

World Health Organization. (2011). *Global status report on noncommunicable diseases 2010*. Retrieved from http://www.who.int/nmh/publications/ncd_report2010/en/

web resources

Please visit thePoint® for up-to-date Web resources on this topic.

Implementing Nursing Practice in Community Settings

PART

three

CHAPTER 9

Planning for Community Change

Susan L. Hamilton and Stephanie M. Chalupka

Change will not come if we wait for some other person or some other time. We are the ones we've been waiting for. We are the change that we seek.

Barack Obama

If you don't like something, change it. If you can't change it, change your attitude.

Maya Angelou

Few things are harder to put up with than the annoyance of a good example.

Mark Twain

Prejudice is a great time saver. You can form opinions without having to get the facts.

E. B. White

chapter highlights

- Health planning at the state, national, and global level
- Social and environmental determinants of health
- Social ecologic model and multilevel interventions
- Community coalitions
- Health impact pyramid
- Health equity and social justice
- Lewin's change theory, force field analysis, and levers of change
- Logic models
- Role of the community health worker
- Funding community health interventions
- Evaluating community health interventions
- Nurse-managed health centers

objectives

- Explain social determinants of health and how they contribute to the health status of a community.
- Describe social justice and health equity.
- Apply force field analysis as a technique for managing change at the community level.
- Explain the importance of changing the social and environmental context to make healthy choices the default.
- Use a logic model as a planning and communication tool for community programs.
- Develop community program objectives that are specific, measurable, achievable, relevant, and time-bound (SMART).
- Describe the role of the community health worker in providing services for poor, underserved, and diverse populations.
- Explain why multilevel interventions are needed to achieve change in complex community health conditions that have multiple determinants.
- Identify sources of funding for community health intervention programs.
- Describe the contributions made by nurse-managed health centers.

key terms

Coalition: Group of consumers, health professionals, policy-makers, and others working together to improve community health status or to solve a specific community health problem.

Key informant: Person knowledgeable about specific aspects of a problem and the community's current and past attempts to address it.

Logic model: Visual representation of how a program is organized, including activities, resources, short-term and intermediate outcomes, and program goals.

Population aggregate: A defined subset of the population such as people with or at risk for a specific health problem or having specific social or demographic characteristics.

Stakeholder: An individual, organization, or group that has an interest (stake) in a specific community health issue or the outcome of a community-level intervention.

Sustainability: Establishing the conditions for the health improvements achieved by an intervention to continue beyond the period of a formal community health program or for a program to continue after grant funding ends.

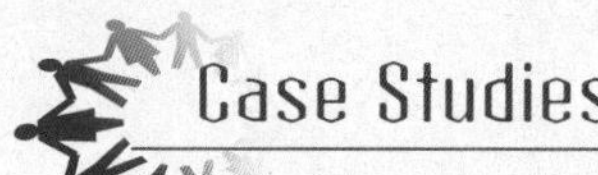

Case Studies

References to case studies are found throughout this chapter (look for the case study icon). Readers should keep the case studies in mind as they read the chapter.

CASE 1

Ellen, a public health nurse, is the program manager for the River City Influenza Immunization Initiative. The program is part of a statewide initiative funded by a 3-year grant from the Massachusetts Department of Public Health. The overall goal of the statewide initiative is to eliminate ethnic and racial disparities in influenza immunization status and to decrease morbidity and mortality from influenza and pneumonia. Ellen's role in the statewide program is to plan and implement a new initiative in River City to increase influenza immunization rates in Hispanic adults aged 50 and older.

CASE 2: WORCESTER: THE HEALTHIEST CITY IN NEW ENGLAND BY 2020

The public health department of the city of Worcester, Massachusetts, is the lead agency for the 2012 Greater Worcester Region Community Health Improvement Plan (CHIP), which has as its vision to make Worcester the healthiest city in New England by 2020. Among the major health priorities identified by the broad coalition of community partners are obesity and associated behaviors, such as nutrition and physical activity. Of particular concern is limited access to healthy foods and environments supporting active living for vulnerable populations and immigrant communities. Limited access to and high cost of healthy foods, inadequate public transportation, fees for recreational facilities and activities, neighborhood safety in parks and outdoor spaces, accessible and walkable spaces, time constraints, and the stress of "living on the edge" were identified as related challenges. Therefore, ensuring equitable resources for active living and healthy eating requires a comprehensive approach, given that multiple sectors—including healthcare, education, public works, transportation, local government, and the business community—need to collaborate to improve current conditions (City of Worcester, 2012).

Gina is a public health nurse in the city of Worcester, Ginny is a nurse program manager at one of Worcester's two federally funded community health centers, and Homero is a school nurse at one of Worcester's elementary schools. Gina, Ginny, and Homero participated in planning through the Community Health Assessment (CHA) and the CHIP. The Worcester public schools and the community health center are being used as intervention sites to (1) implement strategies to enhance and expand mobile farmers' markets in seven low-income/food desert neighborhoods and (2) increase the number of Worcester elementary schools that are partnering with the Massachusetts Safe Routes to Schools program.

HEALTH PLANNING

Health planning is an organized and systematic process in which problems are identified, priorities selected, and objectives set for the development of community health programs on the basis of the findings of CHAs and health surveillance data. Health planning occurs at the global, national, regional, state, county, and local levels. Ideally, health planning is coordinated and consistent among each of these levels.

Health Planning at the Global Level

The World Health Organization (WHO), the United Nations (UN), and many regional organizations engage in global and regional health planning. In 2000, the UN ratified the *Millennium Declaration*, which seeks to build a more equitable world society through a partnership between rich and poor nations with the goals to eliminate extreme poverty and improve the health and well-being of the poorest people in the world by 2015. The Millennium Development Goals include specific health targets to reduce child and maternal mortality; to halt the epidemics of HIV, malaria, and tuberculosis; to increase sustainable access to safe drinking water and sanitation; to reduce violence and injuries; and to decrease tobacco use and chronic disease, including cardiovascular disease (UN, 2012).

In 2008, the WHO Commission on Social Determinants of Health (CSDH) issued their report *Closing the Gap in a Generation*, calling on all nations to address such social issues as poverty, lack of access to education and job opportunities, poor infrastructure, and environmental pollution, which all have a significant impact on health. The three overall recommendations of the CSDH are to (1) improve the conditions under which all people are born, grow, live, work, and age to minimum standards; (2) ensure more equitable distribution of power, money, and resources; and (3) expand knowledge of the social determinants of health and establish a system to measure and monitor health inequity. These national and international health planning documents recognize the need to promote health and prevent disease by addressing their underlying political, economic, and social causes and to ensure health equity.

Health Planning at the National and State Levels

Ongoing health planning occurs within state health departments, the Centers for Disease Control and Prevention (CDC), and the U.S. Department of Health and Human Services (HHS) through initiatives such as *Healthy People 2020* and the National Prevention Strategy (NPS). This ongoing planning is driven by trends in health outcomes and health behavior identified from disease surveillance by the states and the CDC; data produced by the National Center on Health Statistics

(NCHS) from the Behavioral Risk Factor Surveillance System (BRFSS), National Health Interview Survey (NHIS), and other sources; claims data from the Centers for Medicare and Medicaid Services (CMS); and data from the U.S. Census Bureau from the ongoing American Community Survey. Such data are used for the periodic evaluation of progress toward meeting the objectives of *Healthy People 2020* and for identifying trends in the incidence or prevalence of health problems such as diabetes, asthma, or Alzheimer disease; of health behaviors such as binge drinking or smoking; or of communicable diseases such as influenza or chlamydia. Trends identified in these data may lead the CDC, HHS, and other federal agencies or state health departments to develop new initiatives or to change health polices or programs.

Healthy People 2020

Healthy People 2020 are national objectives for improved health outcomes that guide the health promotion and disease prevention efforts in the United States. *Healthy People 2020* objectives are 10-year targets for health improvement that build on four decades of health improvement efforts that began with the publication of *Healthy People: The Surgeon General's Report on Health Promotion and Disease Prevention* in 1979. The overall goals of *Healthy People 2020* are to

- Attain high-quality, longer lives free of preventable disease, disability, injury, and premature death.
- Achieve health equity, eliminate health disparities, and improve health of all groups.
- Create social and physical environments that promote good health for all.
- Promote quality of life, healthy development, and healthy behaviors across all life stages (HHS, 2012, para. 5).

There are 26 leading health indicators (LHIs) that represent strategic opportunities to address high-priority health issues that contribute to preventable death and health disparities across the life span (HHS, 2010). The *Healthy People 2020* objectives are organized into 42 topic areas, including many new topics such as genomics, LGBT health, and healthcare-associated infections. *Healthy People 2020* objectives and resources are available on an interactive website that includes links to data sources, evidence-based practice guidelines, and state-level plans. The *Healthy People 2020* website also includes historical data on progress toward meeting prior Healthy People objectives. *Healthy People 2020* objectives provide a framework for assessing the health status of a community and can serve as the benchmark against which to compare the health status of a **population aggregate** when conducting a CHA. The *Healthy People 2020* objectives can also serve as the long-term goals of a community health intervention.

PRACTICE POINT

When doing a CHA, think of the target level within the *Healthy People 2020* objective as the "normal values" for health indicators. For example, compare the percentage of adults aged 18 and older in your community or population aggregate who currently smoke, with the target of 12% in objective TU-1 and the national rate of 20.6% in 2008 to provide a context for interpreting the rate for your population and for setting health improvement goals.

National Prevention Strategy

The Patient Protection and Affordable Care Act (ACA) of 2010 (Chapter 4) created the National Prevention Council which was charged with developing the NPS, published by the Office of the Surgeon General in 2011. The goal of the NPS and several other initiatives embedded in the ACA is to focus the nation's healthcare system on population health through initiatives and funding to prevent disease and to support health promotion and wellness across the life span (Koh & Sebelius, 2010).

The overall goal of the NPS is to increase the number of Americans who are healthy at every stage of life. The NPS has four strategic directions for national prevention efforts that form the foundation for the plan and its recommendations. These are (1) creating healthy and safe community environments, (2) integrating clinical and community preventive services, (3) empowering people in making healthy choices, and (4) eliminating health disparities. The NPS also makes evidence-based recommendations for actions in seven priorities which have the greatest potential to improve the health of the U.S. population and to reduce the burden of preventable chronic disease, disability, and death. The seven priorities are as follows:

- Tobacco-free living
- Preventing drug abuse and excessive alcohol use
- Healthy eating
- Active living
- Injury- and violence-free living
- Reproductive and sexual health
- Mental and emotional well-being

Detailed recommendations for policies, programs, and system changes at the local, state, and national levels are included for each of the priorities (National Prevention Council, 2011).

We know a great deal about how to improve the health of the nation; decades of research and practice have built the evidence base and identified effective prevention approaches. Improving socioeconomic factors (e.g., poverty, education) and providing healthful environments (e.g., ensuring clean water, air and safe food, designing communities to promote increased physical activity) reinforce prevention across broad segments of society. Broad-based changes that benefit everyone in a community should be supplemented by clinical services that meet individual health needs (e.g., immunization, colonoscopy, tobacco cessation counseling, blood pressure and cholesterol monitoring and control). Through health promotion, education, and counseling, we can provide people with the knowledge, tools, and options they need to make healthy choices.

National Prevention Council, 2011, p. 11

State Departments of Public Health

In the United States, state departments of public health have a central role in health planning. These departments coordinate planning at many levels—with federal agencies, including the CDC, with other agencies of state government, with local or county health departments, and with health providers. Most states have adopted state health plans that build on the national objectives in *Healthy People 2020*. HHS and state departments of public health use state-level data from the BRFSS, Youth Risk Behavior Survey (YRBS), NHIS, and the National Health and Nutrition Examination Survey (NHANES), as well as vital statistics and disease surveillance information, to monitor progress toward meeting the *Healthy People 2020* objectives and other health improvement goals.

PRACTICE POINT

Each state and territory has a healthy people coordinator who is responsible to coordinate with the HHS Office of Disease Prevention and Health Promotion to ensure that the state's health plan is in line with *Healthy People 2020*. To find the healthy people coordinator for your state, go to www.healthypeople.gov and search for state-specific plans.

Community Health Improvement Planning Process

Community health improvement planning is a systematic process that involves all sectors of a community to conduct a comprehensive CHA, identify priorities for action, develop and implement a CHIP, and guide future community decisions and resource allocations. Although similar to several other public health and community organizing models (Box 9.1), the CHIP emphasizes accountability and includes specific performance measures for improvement. Hospitals, community health centers, schools, employers, public officials, housing authorities, faith communities, and many other sectors of a community are included in the planning and implementation process. Nurses working in the community in public health, community health centers, clinics, home care, schools, and occupational settings are often actively involved.

Planning health promotion or prevention interventions at the community level can be a complex process. Several models and frameworks help organize some or all of the steps in the planning process (see Box 9.1). One model developed specifically for public health nursing is the Intervention Wheel that describes 17 public health nursing interventions at the individual, community, and systems levels (see Chapter 1).

box 9.1 Models and Tools for Community Health Planning

MAP-IT is a framework developed by HHS to help communities to implement *Healthy People 2020*. http://www.healthypeople.gov/2020/implement/MapIt.aspx

Mobilizing for Action through Planning and Partnerships (MAPP) is a framework for community health assessment and strategic planning developed by the National Association of County and City Health Officials (NACCHO). MAPP focuses on community engagement to help communities identify and address public health priorities (Lenihan, 2005). http://www.naccho.org/topics/infrastructure/MAPP/index.cfm

Community Toolbox is an online set of tools and practical suggestions for community health assessment, coalition-building, logic models, and the community health improvement process (CHIP) from the University of Kansas. http://ctb.ku.edu/en/default.aspx

Guideline and Template for Community Health Improvement Planning was developed by the Connecticut Department of Public Health to develop comprehensive prevention and control plans for specific diseases or conditions such as HIV, smoking, or lead poisoning. http://www.naccho.org/topics/infrastructure/accreditation/upload/CHIP-Guide.pdf

Precede–Proceed Model was developed for planning health promotion programs to address health behaviors. A toolkit to help use this model in practice is included in the Community Toolkit. http://ctb.ku.edu/en/tablecontents/sub_section_main_1008.aspx

Community Health Assessment and Group Evaluation (CHANGE) is a tool developed by the CDC to help communities focus on changes in policies, systems, and environments to improve population health. Includes a CHANGE tool to track progress. http://www.cdc.gov/healthycommunitiesprogram/tools/change.htm

COMMUNITY ASSESSMENT

Community health assessment is a systematic process that may use several approaches, including **key informant** interviews, analysis of data on health status and health behavior indicators, observation, and community surveys. The goal of a CHA is to identify the community health problems that are the priorities for intervention, as well as community resources available to address each health problem or need. Assessment of a community includes identification of community assets and strengths, as well as specific health problems or health needs. Assessment of community readiness and community capacity to address the identified health problems is also an important part of the process. The process of community assessment is discussed in Chapter 11.

In Case 1, data from the Massachusetts Department of Public Health indicate that of the 256,400 adults aged 50 and older in River City, 43% received flu shots last year, well below the statewide average of 67% and the *Healthy People 2020* objective of 90% for adults aged 65 and older. The proportion of the River City population aged 50 and above who were immunized for influenza was much lower among Hispanic (22%) than White (58%) or Black (45%) residents. Why do you think the influenza immunization rate for the population aggregate of older Hispanics is so much lower than for other older adults in River City?

Ellen has used health status data to identify lower influenza immunization rates among older Hispanics as the community health problem her program will address. What community assets and strengths might be available to address this priority health problem and how might Ellen identify them?

SYSTEMS THEORY

A community is a complex system of human activity conducted within the context of the social and ecologic environment. Every family, neighborhood, workplace, school, and recreational facility is itself a system with its own boundaries, rules, and purpose. These systems overlap to the extent that individual people in each family system participate in the activities or are affected by the decisions made within other systems. Social systems engage in reciprocal exchange or flows of information, energy, resources, and goods or services. Systems within the community are interdependent and interconnected. Change in one system leads to reciprocal changes in interconnected systems (McLeroy, Norton, Kegler, Burdine, & Sumaya, 2003). This interconnectedness means that bringing about change in the community often requires influencing systems at multiple levels because the conditions within one system, such as the family or workplace, are influenced by and reflect the broader social, economic, environmental, or political systems. It also means that changes made within one system, such as the school or workplace, may have an impact on other areas with reciprocal exchange of information or resources such as the family or the broader community.

In Case 2, how might changes in the availability of healthy foods and improved eating habits be expected to result from the expansion and enhancement of farmer's markets sponsored that the Community Health Center and elementary school lead to reciprocal changes in the larger community system? Recognizing the importance of a systems approach, can you think of ways that Ginny and Homero can work together to enhance the impact of this intervention beyond the individual families who participate in other systems in the community?

WORKING WITH THE COMMUNITY

Just as the nurse would engage an individual patient or family in their plan of care, the community health nurse seeks the participation of community members and institutions as partners in planning and implementing programs, or changing policies, to achieve desired health outcomes at the community level. One strategy to enlist the community as a partner in the change process is the formation of a **coalition**, task force, committee, consortium, or community advisory board. (Although each has a distinct meaning, the term coalition is used in this chapter to mean any of these types of community partnership.)

Coalitions bring together consumers, health professionals, policy-makers, and other constituencies to work together to improve community health status. The strategy of using coalitions to bring about change recognizes that (1) population health results from the interaction of social, cultural, economic, and political determinants in the overall community and (2) both the problems and the solutions are embedded in the community system. Systems change and an increase in community capacity are often necessary to improve the health status of the community (Emshoff et al., 2007; McLeroy et al., 2003).

Great things are done by a series of small things brought together.

Vincent Van Gogh

EVIDENCE FOR PRACTICE

The Allies Against Asthma initiative used community coalitions to improve the quality of care and health outcomes of low-income children in seven communities with high prevalence of asthma. These coalitions included diverse groups of stakeholders and focused on systems level changes in homes and schools to help families manage asthma better and to improve the indoor and outdoor air quality. The odds of hospitalizations and emergent treatment for asthma among children under age 18 on Medicaid for the seven communities where these coalitions intervened, was significantly lower than in a matched group of control communities. The evaluation of this program indicated that "...ongoing consumer voices in coalition processes and decisions likely increased the quality of policy and systems changes . . . [because] they reflected the actual needs of families attempting to manage asthma" (Clark et al., 2013, p. e4).

Defining the Population of Interest

To develop a plan for a community program or initiative, first identify the population of interest that will be affected by, benefit from, or participate in the planned change. The population of interest may be an entire nation, state, county, or city on the basis of geographical or political boundaries.

This may be the case, for example, when planning responses to pandemic influenza or programs to reduce carbon emissions at all levels, even global, where the objective is to protect the health of all people. The population of interest may also be a population aggregate such as adults aged 50 and older for an initiative to increase the rate of screening for colon cancer. It is important for the community health nurse who is planning a program to know, for example, whether the population of interest is the population of adults aged 55 to 74 living in Wisconsin; the panel of patients served by a large group medical practice; families of migrant farm workers in Broward County, Florida; or the students in kindergarten through sixth grade in the Chicago public schools.

Coalitions

When forming a coalition, it is important to be clear about the nature and scope of responsibility of the group. A common mistake is to ask people to serve on a coalition to satisfy the requirements of a grant or government agency without providing the coalition with a "real job." The reasons for a coalition's failure may include lack of a clear mission, goals, objectives, and expectations; lack of leadership; and lack of accountability for meeting expectations. Poor management of meetings and lack of consideration for the time and expertise of members can also lead to the failure of a coalition (Zakocs & Edwards, 2006). Organizers should do the following (Box 9.2):

- Make use of the expertise of individual members by asking for their help and input on matters directly related to their field.
- Seek out people with a range of opinions and roles in the community. Find out who has been a valuable member of previous community coalitions or teams.
- Consider how each member of a coalition and the organization or group they represent will benefit from the work of the coalition.
- Understand group dynamics and remember that people agree to serve on coalitions in exchange for more than feeling good about helping address a community issue.
- Try to have a heterogeneous group but one in which members are able to show mutual respect and listen to each other's ideas without criticism of the person.

When we turn to one another for counsel we reduce the number of our enemies.

Khalil Gibran

box 9.2 How to Be a Valuable Member of a Coalition or Program Team

Only say "yes" to invitations to serve when you are really interested and have time to do the work. Do not agree and fail to participate.
Come to meetings on time, stay for the entire meeting.
If you are leading a meeting, start and end on time.
Come to meetings prepared. Read any material sent to you in advance.
Come to meetings undistracted—no "texting" or multitasking.
Practice active listening and ask questions.
Show respect for differing opinions and suggestions—listen without interrupting, look for ways to build on the strengths of all ideas.
Observe group dynamics to learn how group leaders achieve consensus, maintain momentum, and make progress toward goal achievement.
Keep your commitments. Complete your assignments.
Exchange business cards and network with colleagues.

PRACTICE POINT

To run meetings efficiently, it helps to

- Know the purpose of the meeting (to make a decision, generate ideas, communicate something, or to plan).
- Show respect for the time and expertise of coalition members.
- Begin and end on time.
- Send an agenda and background materials in advance.
- Get the right people to attend. Know who your resources are and the role that they play.
- Invite only key stakeholders.
- Stay on topic.
- Communicate results.
- Learn how to resolve conflicts and reach consensus.

Stakeholders and Opinion Leaders

The people and organizations that are **stakeholders** (Box 9.3) are commonly included in coalitions. Factors to consider in forming a coalition include the history of the stakeholders working together (successfully or unsuccessfully); success or failure of prior attempts to resolve the community health problem being addressed, including the

box 9.3 Questions to Help Identify Community Stakeholders

1. Who is most affected by this community health problem or issue? Who is most concerned?
2. Who are the "opinion leaders" in the community who would be interested in this health issue? Who may have different views?
3. Who stands to "gain" or "lose" if this community health problem is addressed? How can they be engaged in finding solutions?
4. Whose help will be needed to address this community health problem?
5. Who needs to be "on board" or "invested" for this intervention to be successful and for the changes to be sustained after the intervention?

reasons for these results; and the degree to which prior improvements were sustained. As part of the community assessment, it is helpful to discuss factors that contribute to the problem, and other issues that may need to be addressed, with community leaders. These community leaders may include formal and informal leaders from faith organizations, schools, and employers. It is important to consider whose opinion counts most with the population group(s) expected to participate in the program. Such "opinion leaders" often make good members of coalitions or may recommend others to participate.

In Case 1, who are the stakeholders in the River City initiative? Who would you suggest Ellen ask to serve on a community coalition to achieve the goals of this program? Why?

SOCIAL ECOLOGIC MODEL

The social ecologic model is based on general systems theory and health promotion theory. Multiple determinants of health interact at different levels to affect the health status of individual people, population aggregates, or communities (Bopp, Kaczynski, & Campbell, 2013; McLeroy et al., 2003; Smedley & Syme, 2002). Planning for change at the community level is often based on a social ecologic approach with interventions at multiple levels. The social ecologic model includes consideration for how social, cultural, economic, political, environmental, organizational, and neighborhood factors influence health behaviors and health status within a community (refer to the discussion of the ecologic model in Chapter 5). Although people may change their health behavior or receive services as part of a community-level program, the concern of public health professionals is primarily the health status of the community as a whole or of a population aggregate. "[T]he goal of community-based interventions is not only to change individual perceptions and behavior but also to embed public health values in our social ecology . . ." (McLeroy et al., 2003, p. 532).

Even small changes in health behavior at the community or population level have the potential to significantly affect health status. The overall impact of interventions implemented at the community level is greater than the sum of the changes made by individuals or families as a result of community-level programs (Smedley & Syme, 2002). Change in health behavior or health status at one level produces changes at other levels of the community system (McLeroy et al., 2003). For example, a community-level intervention that results in 200 people quitting smoking may also lead to changes in community or family norms that affect future levels of smoking initiation or reduce the number of cigarettes smoked each day because of new restrictions at work and public places. A person or family who brings unwanted pharmaceuticals to a community take-back program instead of flushing them down the toilet contributes to environmental health by preventing contamination of drinking water supplies. A city or town that contracts for curbside pickup of recycled materials and charges residents a fee for each bag of trash collected may achieve a greater impact.

Interventions at institutional or societal levels may achieve significant changes in public health without the need for behavior change on the part of individual people. Examples abound. Fluoridation of water and advances in preventive dentistry improved dental health and dramatically reduced the incidence of dental caries in children. Laws banning trans fats in foods served to the public in New York City led to reformulation of foods throughout the fast food and snack food industry. Folic acid supplementation of cereals reduced the incidence of neural tube birth defects.

PRACTICE POINT

Sometimes, the most important action that the community health nurse may take is to advocate for a change in public policy or to collaborate with officials with responsibility for environmental health or elder services. It is important to consider the range of social, cultural, economic, or policy forces that influence the health behavior or health condition of concern and then to work at multiple levels to bring about change.

HEALTH IMPACT PYRAMID

Figure 9.1 presents the health impact pyramid. Developed by Frieden (2010), this is a framework that describes the public health impact of interventions at different levels in the social ecologic model.

At the base of the pyramid are interventions to address socioeconomic conditions such as poverty, lack of education, and lack of access to clean water or sanitation. At the next level are interventions that change the environment or options available so that making the choice for a healthy behavior is the "default" or easy choice while choosing a less healthy option would require a person to spend more time, effort, or money. Examples include food and drug safety, iodization of salt, elimination of trans fats in food, and restrictions on smoking in public places and work sites. Changing food manufacturing to eliminate trans fats, for example, will have a positive impact on the health of the entire population without people having to change their buying or eating habits and would be sustained over time. "Changing the environmental context so that individuals can easily take heart-healthy actions in the normal course of their lives can have a greater population impact than clinical interventions that treat individuals" (Frieden, 2010, p. 592). Interventions to improve socioeconomic conditions and to make the healthy choice the default choice may yield large returns in population health without requiring individuals to change health behaviors, but some may be politically

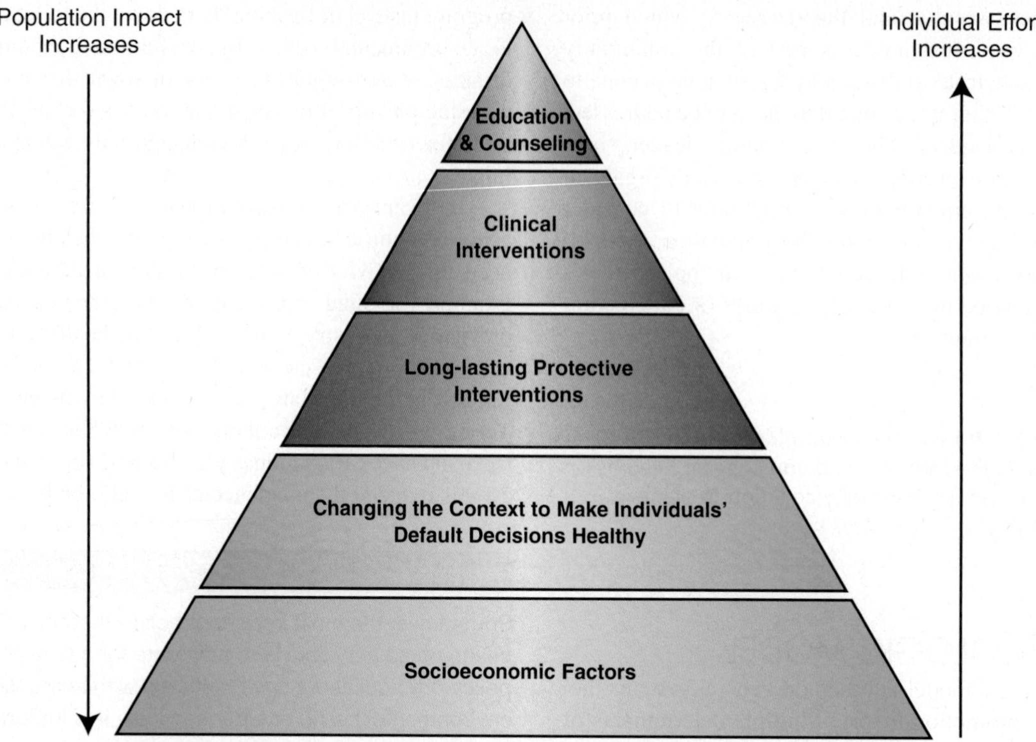

figure 9.1 Health impact pyramid. (From Frieden, T. R. [2010]. A framework for public health action: The health impact pyramid. *American Journal of Public Health*, *100*[4], 590–595. Used with permission.)

difficult to achieve or require significant investment of time, money, or political capital.

At the middle of the pyramid are community health interventions such as immunizations that have a long-term protective effect as well as periodic screenings such as colonoscopy. At the next highest level are clinical interventions such as treatment of hypertension, hyperlipidemia, and diabetes. While clinical interventions can have an important impact on the prevention or control of disease at the individual level, the benefits may be limited because not everyone has access to primary care, people often do not adhere to treatment regimes over the long term, and treatments are not always effective. At the top of the pyramid are counseling and health education. These interventions require the largest effort by individuals, and achieving sustained health behavior change is the exception rather than the rule. In addition, counseling and health education reaches a limited number of people and may have little effect if used as the sole intervention. Health counseling may be helpful in individual and family interventions, but must be repeated with each new client and may have little effect at the population level. "Nevertheless, educational interventions are often the only ones available, and when applied consistently and repeatedly may have considerable impact" (Frieden, 2010, p. 592).

The health impact pyramid is a useful framework for community health nurses when planning health promotion interventions at multiple levels. While we often think about health education and screening interventions, these require the greatest effort on the part of individuals and have the least population impact. In addition to these interventions, we should think about what changes could be made in the environment, in policy, and in programs to make it easier for people to make healthy choices.

MULTILEVEL INTERVENTIONS

Because of the complexity of the problems that most community-level interventions are designed to address and the multiple determinants or causes of such problems, the most successful interventions are those that combine interventions at more than one system level. Even when changes in individual health behaviors such as smoking, exercise, or healthful eating are the desired outcomes of an intervention, it is important to focus efforts on higher levels to change the social and cultural norms or context within which the behavior occurs (Frieden, 2010; McLeroy et al., 2003; Smedley & Syme, 2002). Interventions directed at different system levels can be described as follows:

- Upstream: at the societal, environmental, or policy level
- Mainstream: at the population or community level
- Downstream: at the individual level

Downstream one-on-one interventions do little to address the social or environmental determinants of population health and require continued and repeated efforts as new people continue to experience the relevant health problem. Prevention of disease by intervening upstream at the social or environmental levels or mainstream at the community level amplifies the impact of such interventions on population health (Bekemeier, 2008; Eisen, 2012). "The ways that behavior is institutionalized (organizational-level change), normalized (community-level change), and legally bound (policy-level change) are essential 'social facts,' without which individual behavioral change is not easily sustained" (McLeroy et al., 2003, p. 533).

Bekemeier (2008) points out that practitioners of public health nursing in the early 20th century, including Lillian Wald and visiting nurses, recognized that their most important work was to reform "...the conditions that create and exacerbate disease" (p. 50) and call on nurses to focus their practice and research on primary prevention and the root causes of ill health. "Focusing ...on the underlying causes of poor health and health disparities requires an upstream perspective that brings nursing (back) into the realm of policy analysis, social reform, environmental health, sociology, and international health" (p. 50).

PRACTICE POINT

Remember to always "look upstream" when thinking about where to target interventions. Dr. Richard Jackson at the UCLA School of Public Health explains that "public health needs to look at the cause of the cause." He gives the example of a person struck by a car and killed. That death is recorded as the result of an accident. Dr. Jackson suggests looking upstream: Why was the person hit by the car? Was there a way to walk along the road safely? Was there a sidewalk? Dr. Jackson asks if the cause of death was actually the poor design of the community or the lack of a place to walk in an area without the risk of being hit by a car (Brown, 2012).

How can we apply this same thinking of upstream causes to the primary prevention of chronic disease? What are the "causes of the cause" of diabetes, cancer, or heart disease? How can we better address these upstream determinants of health?

SOCIAL DETERMINANTS OF HEALTH

The circumstances in which people are born, grow up, live, work, and age, and the systems put in place to deal with illness are termed the *social determinants of health*. These circumstances are in turn shaped by the wider context, including economics, social policies, and politics (World Health Organization, 2008).

The social ecologic model recognizes that the determinants of health are complex and multidimensional. The health status of a community, a population aggregate, a group, or an individual person results from a complex interaction of social, economic, environmental, and behavioral factors. Chronic diseases, including cardiovascular disease, diabetes, cancer, and chronic respiratory disease, are among the leading causes of morbidity and mortality in developed nations. These diseases have multiple interactive causes that accrue over the course of the life span, including diet, physical activity levels, smoking, alcohol intake, exposure to toxic environments, genetic and familial factors, socioeconomic status, and demographics (Gostin & Powers, 2006; Smedley & Syme, 2002; Stokols, 1992). Community health nurses may construct a web of causation (Chapter 5) to help identify the multiple factors that contribute to the chronic disease or community problem of interest as part of the planning process.

Obesogenic and Salutogenic Environments

Understanding the impact of the social, economic, and political systems on the factors that contribute to childhood obesity, for example, reframes the problem. Obesity is not just an issue of personal or family responsibility but one created by an *obesogenic* environment—defined as an environment promoting or contributing to obesity (Schwartz & Brownell, 2007; Smedley & Syme, 2002). Rather than directing interventions toward individual behavior change by families whose children are overweight or obese, the goal of community-level interventions is to change the environment to one that creates the conditions where healthy choices are the default or norm. Making school a *salutogenic* environment, where only healthy food choices are available and physical activity is incorporated into school curricula, benefits all children (Schwartz & Brownell, 2007). Salutogenic environments are ones "... that reduce vulnerability to illness and promote enhanced levels of well-being" (Stokols, 1992, p. 12).

Healthy people require healthy environments to live in, work, and play. The *built environment* is broadly defined as human-made surroundings that include buildings, public resources, land-use patterns, the transportation system, and design features. Research is increasingly demonstrating links between the built environment and eating and physical activity behaviors, which in turn affect health outcomes (Prevention Institute, 2008). Environments should be designed in ways that help people access healthy foods and easily incorporate physical activity into their daily routines. The creation of healthy environments is not accomplished by any single group or entity. It requires coordinated and comprehensive efforts by stakeholders, community leaders, multiple sectors, professional organizations, and leaders. Healthy community design integrates evidence-based health strategies into community planning, transportation, and land-use decisions. Healthy community design can improve people's health by increasing physical activity, reducing injury; increasing access to healthy food; improving air and water quality; minimizing the effects of climate change; decreasing mental health stresses; strengthening the social fabric of a community; and providing fair access to livelihood, education, and resources (Centers for Disease Control and Prevention, 2012).

STUDENT REFLECTION

We attended one of the public hearings for "Worcester: The Healthiest City in New England" (Case 2). One of the people that provided testimony was Gina, a public health nurse for the city. She was advocating for the adoption of a Complete Streets policy. She explained that "Complete Streets" are designed and operated to enable safe access for all users. Pedestrians, bicyclists, motorists, and public transportation users of all ages and abilities are able to safely move along and across a complete street. Complete streets make it easy to cross the street, walk to shops, and bicycle to work. It was interesting to see evidence-based practice in action because Gina provided data from research that demonstrated that residents who live in communities with pedestrian- and bicycle-friendly infrastructure are more physically active. She also provided evidence that residents in a highly walkable neighborhood have been shown to engage in about 70 more minutes per week of moderate and vigorous physical activity than residents in a low-walkability neighborhood.

Health Impact Assessment

A health impact assessment (HIA) helps communities make informed choices about improving public health through community design. HIA is a process that helps evaluate the potential health effects of a plan, project, or policy before it is built or implemented. A HIA can provide recommendations to increase positive health outcomes and minimize adverse health outcomes. HIA brings potential public health impacts and considerations to the decision-making process for plans, projects, and policies that fall outside the traditional public health arenas, such as transportation and land use (CDC, 2012).

HIA is usually voluntary, although several local and state laws support the examination of health impacts in decision-making and a few explicitly require the use of the HIA. Outside the United States, HIA is more widely used. Some countries have mandated HIA as part of a regulatory process. In the United States, HIA is a rapidly emerging practice among local, state, and federal jurisdictions, mostly on a voluntary basis.

HIA holds promise for incorporating aspects of health into decision-making because of its applicability to a broad array of policies, programs, plans, and projects; consideration of adverse and beneficial health effects; ability to consider and incorporate various types of evidence; and engagement of communities and stakeholders in a deliberative process (CDC, 2012).

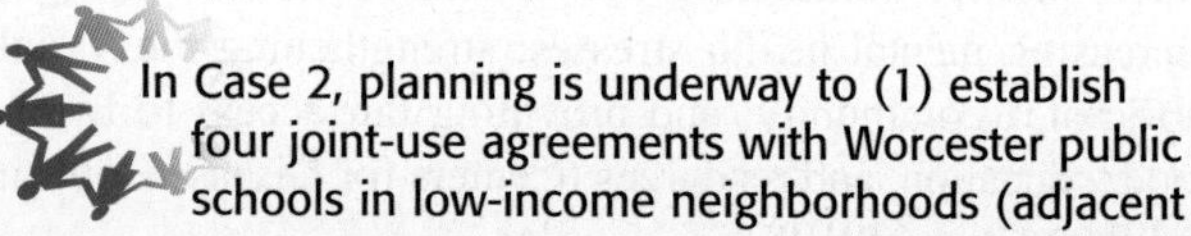

In Case 2, planning is underway to (1) establish four joint-use agreements with Worcester public schools in low-income neighborhoods (adjacent to Housing Authority developments) to allow the use of both indoor and outdoor facilities by the public during nonschool hours on a regular basis; (2) change zoning regulations to promote community gardens and urban agriculture; (3) enhance and expand the Mobile Farmers' Market in seven low-income/food desert communities and on college campuses in Worcester; (4) adopt other evidence-based obesity reduction programs in preschools and elementary schools, including "I am Moving I am Learning" (Head Start) and Hip Hop to Health (City of Worcester, 2012).

Ginny and Homero are both involved in these efforts. If they were using the Public Health Nursing Intervention Wheel (Chapter 1), which types of interventions do these plans represent?

Health Disparities, Health Equity, and Social Justice

The WHO CSDH wrote that the "unequal distribution of health-damaging experiences is not in any sense a 'natural' phenomenon but is the result of a toxic combination of poor social policies and programs, unfair economic arrangements, and bad politics" (WHO, 2008, p. 1). Differences in health status exist at the population level between nations or within nations; the basis of these differences is age, race or ethnicity, gender, socioeconomic status, or other characteristics. "Health disparities become health inequities when they are unnecessary, unfair, and preventable resulting from social injustices that become engrained in the fabric of society through its social, economic, and political structures, laws, policies, and culture so as to become largely invisible" (Falk-Rafael & Betker, 2012, p. 98).

Achieving health equity is the overarching goal established in *Healthy People 2020* as well as the WHO *Millennium Declaration*. Health inequities are *avoidable* inequalities in health between groups of people within countries and between countries. These inequities arise from inequalities within and between societies. Social and economic conditions and their effects on people's lives determine people's risk of illness, and the actions taken to prevent them becoming ill or to treat illness when it occurs (WHO, 2013). There are numerous examples of health inequality within the United States. The United States has the world's highest per capita spending on healthcare, but it ranks 50th in global life expectancy, with a very significant gap in life expectancy between the rich and poor. The gap is as large as 20 years between rich Whites living in Maryland and poor African-Americans living only 20 miles away in Washington, DC (Eisen, 2012). Health equity requires the elimination not only of health disparities, but also of health inequalities resulting from disparities in the living and working conditions that are the social determinants of health. Health equity is based on the principles of fairness and social justice, as well as the belief that all people have an equal value.

Villeneuve (2008) of the Canadian Nurses Association issued a call to action to the world's nurses to rally around a vision of eliminating health disparities and to understand the importance of population health. Nurses need to be informed about the dynamics of economics, global demographics, and access to healthcare and begin to learn to frame health status indicators and health disparities "as examples of *system-level vital signs*" (italics in the original; p. 335). Villeneuve suggests that nurses need to "find policy levers with which to weave these dynamics into their work in order to influence the development of healthy public policy based on broad determinants of health" (2008, p. 339).

Social justice is a value central to the practice of nursing and public health. Social justice refers to an equitable sharing of both the common burdens and the common benefits or advantages in society. The basis of social justice is a value system in which healthcare is a right and achieving health equity and population health are goals. Social justice holds that all individuals are entitled to equal protection from health hazards in the environment produced by the powerful (Beauchamp, 1976). In contrast, in the value system of "market justice," which characterizes modern American society, health is one of personal individual responsibility, and healthcare and other social goods are treated as commodities or economic goods (Beauchamp, 1976; Gostin & Powers, 2006; Kneipp & Snider, 2001). Achieving social justice requires addressing the root causes of ill health, including "poverty, substandard housing, poor education, unhygienic and polluted environments, and social disintegration…[that] lead to systemic disadvantage not only in health, but also in nearly every aspect of social, economic, and political life" (Gostin & Powers, 2006, p. 1054).

The gross inequalities in health that we see within and between countries present a challenge to the world. That there should be a spread of life expectancy of 48 years among countries and 20 years or more within countries is not inevitable. A burgeoning volume of research identifies social factors at the root of much of these inequalities in health…[The Millennium Declaration] goals challenge the world community to tackle poverty in the world's poorest countries. Included in these goals is reduction of child mortality, the health outcome most sensitive to the effects of absolute material deprivation.

Marmot, 2005, p. 1099

PRACTICE POINT

Nurses are in a unique position in society to act as role models, advocates, and champions of community health change. They should identify an issue about which they are passionate and let others know of their interest. They should seek out a mentor and look for opportunities to help bring about changes they want to see in the community. Read the inspirational stories of nurses working in their communities to improve human health and make a difference at the Luminary Project at http://www.theluminaryproject.org.

CHANGE THEORY

Bringing about change in the health status of a community and its members may come through change in health behaviors, as well as through change in the environment, public policy, social or cultural norms, or healthcare delivery. Theories of health-behavior change at the individual, family, and community levels have been discussed in Chapter 5. Such theories of health-behavior change are embedded in many interventions to bring about change at the community level. In addition to changing health behavior, interventions at the community level use theories and techniques designed to bring about change in complex systems, including theories of organizational change.

Lewin's Model of Change

The field theory developed by Karl Lewin, an organizational and social psychologist, in the 1950s is one useful change theory. Lewin envisioned planned organizational change as a three-step process of unfreezing, changing, and refreezing (Schein, 1996; Shirey, 2013). Understanding the three steps of Lewin's theory, the technique of force field analysis, and the levers of change are useful in visualizing and creating change at the community level.

Unfreezing

Unfreezing the status quo is a necessary precursor to change. This may occur either gradually, through generational changes in beliefs, language, and group norms, or rapidly through a paradigm shift (e.g., the terrorist attacks of September 11, 2001). Gradual, incremental change in attitudes and behaviors related to drinking and driving have led to new community norms such as "designated drivers" and the hiring of limousines for prom nights. Rapid unfreezing of a community's indifference about bicycle helmets may occur when a local child riding without a helmet dies or is seriously injured in an accident when a helmet could have prevented injury.

Unfreezing moves a community from the stage of denial or lack of awareness of the need to change a condition or to address an issue, to a stage of preplanning or preparation for change. Education about the extent of the problem or condition and its consequences may begin the process of unfreezing a community's state of denial of a health problem or acceptance of current unhealthy behaviors or norms. Nurses can play a role as change agents during this stage to help mobilize the community by helping to highlight discrepancies between current and desired community health status, or creating a sense of urgency about a health issue (Shirey, 2013). Public policies requiring restaurants and fast food outlets to display the calories and fat grams of menu items or requiring public schools to send parents a periodic "health report card," including a body mass index (BMI) calculation, are examples of interventions intended to begin the process of unfreezing the status quo. Creating dissatisfaction with the current state and raising awareness of a need for change are catalysts for unfreezing (Schein, 1996; Shirey, 2013).

A round man cannot be expected to fit in a square hole right away. He must have time to modify his shape.

Mark Twain

Changing

Once a community has become sufficiently aware of the need for change, or sufficiently dissatisfied with the current conditions through increasing awareness of an issue or as the result of a crisis, the process of changing or transition may begin. Change is a dynamic process that may be more successful when it is actively managed rather than allowed to happen haphazardly. It is seldom a neat, linear process. Change is more often achieved incrementally through repeated cycles or steps than it is by large paradigm shifts. Changing requires an understanding of what needs to be changed, how the change will take place, and an idea of what the change will "look like" when the desired state has been achieved (Schein, 1996).

Refreezing

Refreezing is the process of stabilizing once a change has occurred with the goal of sustaining the change in the community's systems, policies, and customs. Making the new behaviors the community norms helps ensure that the change toward more positive health status will remain in place once the intervention or program is completed. Refreezing establishes a new status quo from which further change may be possible in the future (Schein, 1996; Shirey, 2013).

Sustainability must always be a concern when planning changes in health beliefs, knowledge, behavior, or social conditions. New behaviors are difficult to maintain until they become habitual. Part of the process of planning community health change is to anticipate the support system that must be in place when a program ends so that the positive changes in health are maintained. Involvement of the community as a partner in the change process is a key to such sustainability. Community members and stakeholders must be involved in all stages of the planning process so that they have "ownership" of the process or program and feel empowered by the changes that are accomplished (MacDuffie & DePoy, 2004; Smedley & Syme, 2002). If change is imposed from outside the community or embraced only by the health professional, lasting change is unlikely.

Force Field Analysis

Force field analysis is a change management technique developed by Lewin. Force field analysis involves identifying factors within a community or organization that are driving or reinforcing change in the desired direction, as well as those that are restraining or resisting change. When the driving forces and restraining forces are relatively equal, a state of equilibrium exists. Knowing the direction and strength of each force helps identify which can be increased or decreased to allow the process of unfreezing to occur. It is also important to identify which forces are not possible to change due to political, structural, cultural, organizational, financial, or other constraints so that the plan for change is realistic and achievable. It is not necessary or possible to change every force that is driving or restraining change. Ideally, force field analysis is a participatory process involving the major stakeholders in the community (MacDuffie & DePoy, 2004).

The key is to identify those forces that will require the investment of a reasonable amount of time or resources yet yield the greatest opportunity to effect change in the situation. The primary value of a force field analysis is to help one select the most appropriate targets for intervention(s). Reducing restraining forces and/or strengthening driving forces may create the unfreezing, disequilibrium, and dissatisfaction with the status quo necessary to bring about change in community beliefs, behaviors, social and environmental conditions, and health status.

An example of a force field analysis applied to Case 1 is shown in Figure 9.2. If you were Ellen, which of the restraining forces would you try to decrease and which of the driving forces would you try to increase? Why? What strategies might Ellen use to unfreeze the status quo to create an environment conducive to change?

Levers of Change

The purpose of using levers of change is to increase driving forces and/or to decrease restraining forces—leverage points identified in the force field analysis. Just as physical levers amplify the force applied to move a physical object and allow a person to move a larger object with a smaller expenditure of energy or effort, levers of change are tools or techniques that achieve the largest changes with the least investment of resources. Policy-makers can strategically use these levers in public policy or social marketing to bring about desired change in the health status of the community (Smedley & Syme, 2002; Stokols, 1992).

Examples of public policy levers used to reduce the rates of smoking were laws requiring workplaces, restaurants, and other public places to be smoke-free; ordinances against the sale of cigarettes to minors; and significant taxes on tobacco products. Levers to change social norms about smoking have included social marketing concerning the detrimental effect of secondhand smoke on children and the value of smoke-free homes. These "levers" have helped amplify the impact of health education and smoking cessation programs designed to change individual health behaviors on smoking rates in the United States (Smedley & Syme, 2002).

Community Readiness for Change

Planning programs or interventions to change community health status includes an assessment of the community's readiness to undertake the change process related to a specific health issue. Communities may be at different states of

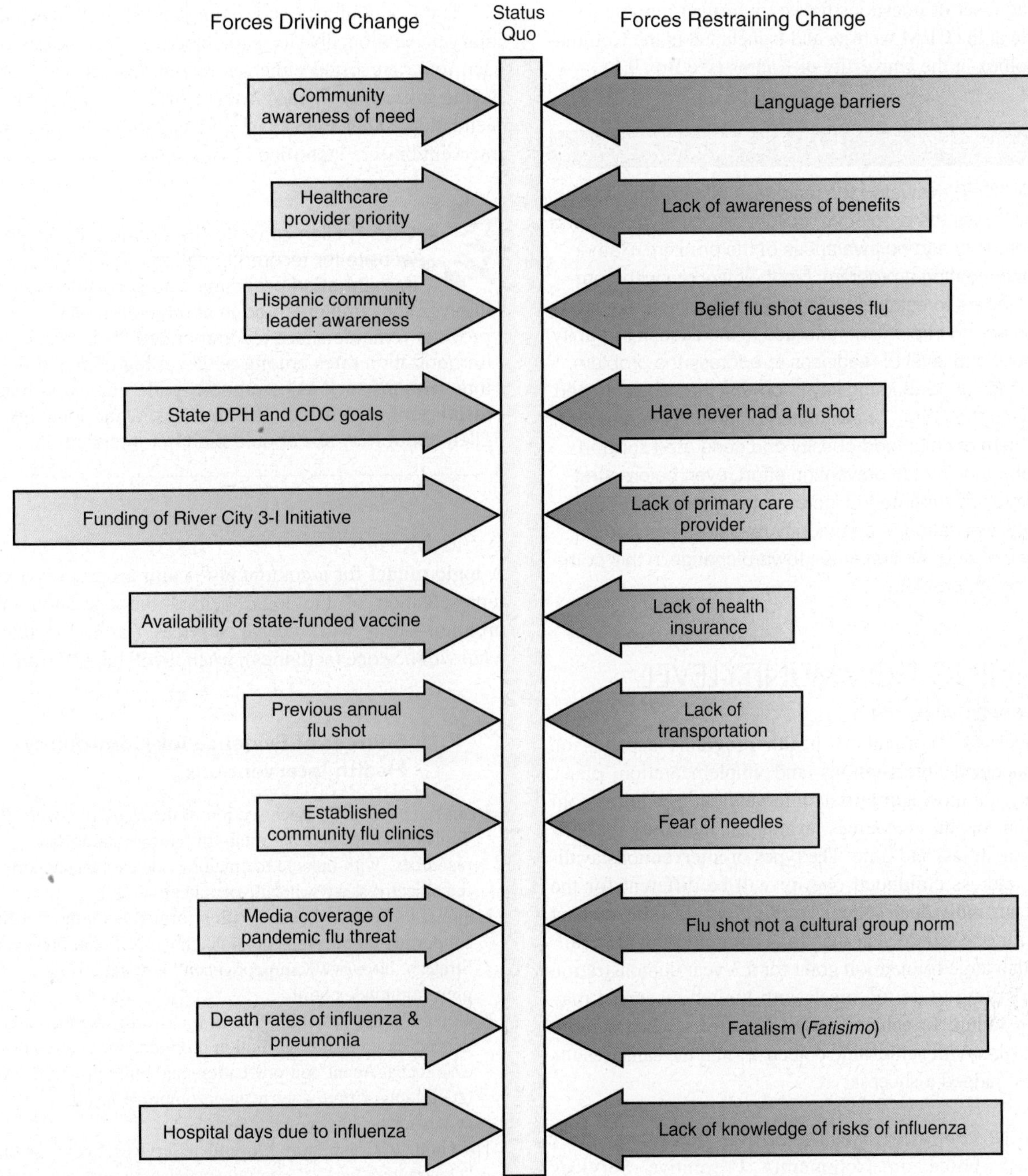

figure 9.2 Force field analysis: influenza immunization in Hispanic adults aged 50 and above. Length of arrow indicates strength of driving or restraining force.

readiness, ranging from not being aware of a problem or denying that a problem exists to having already initiated or undergone changes (Findholt, 2007).

A community's readiness for change is issue specific (Plested, Edwards, & Jumper-Thurman, 2006). The community readiness model (CRM) is a tool used to measure a community's readiness to change in six dimensions through key informant interviews. Developed by the Tri-Ethnic Center for Prevention Research at Colorado State University for drug and alcohol use prevention programs, researchers have shown that the CRM is a useful framework in planning prevention programs addressing such issues as intimate partner violence, HIV/AIDS, breast cancer education, needle exchange programs (York & Hahn, 2007), and childhood obesity (Findholt, 2007). York and Hahn extended the evaluation of the CRM beyond community-based prevention programs to study its usefulness in developing and implementing public policies to limit exposure to smoking. A handbook for using the CRM, including a set of questions for key informant interviews, is available at the CRM website and is included in the Community Toolbox at the University of Kansas (see Box 9.1).

EVIDENCE FOR PRACTICE

Findholt (2007) evaluated the readiness of a county in Oregon to address the problem of childhood obesity and found the community had no awareness of the problem. Rather than implementing a program, Findholt worked with community leaders to establish a childhood obesity prevention coalition and to implement activities to increase community awareness and level of readiness to address the problem. The process of conducting key informant interviews as part of applying the CRM "... stimulated community interest in the problem of childhood obesity and generated support for a community-wide prevention effort, even before strategies were implemented to increase readiness" (p. 570). Findholt's evaluation of community readiness resulted in "unfreezing" and the first steps toward change in this community health problem.

PLANNING COMMUNITY-LEVEL INTERVENTIONS

The success of community health programs depends on well-conceived interventions and implementation plans. Selecting the most appropriate intervention(s) requires consideration of the resources available, including people, money, facilities, and time. The types of interventions available to address childhood obesity will be different for the staff of an individual school working within their current budget for one school year than for a community-wide coalition with a large foundation grant for a 3-year demonstration project. Trying to do too much with limited resources may result in failure to achieve stated objectives when a more realistic plan with achievable objectives and the same results would be judged a success.

Guide to Community Preventive Services

The Task Force on Community Preventive Services (TFCPS) conducts systematic reviews of research for evidence of the effectiveness of community-based prevention and health promotion programs and practices. The goal of the TFCPS is to make recommendations for translation of research into practice. The work of this task force parallels that of the U.S. Preventive Services Task Force, which conducts similar work related to clinical prevention services in primary care. The work of the TFCPS is published online as the Guide to Community Preventive Services, also known simply as The Community Guide. New systematic reviews are published periodically in the *American Journal of Preventive Medicine* and *Morbidity and Mortality Weekly Report (MMWR)* and summarized on the task force website.

The Community Guide is organized by topics such as injury prevention, obesity, and diabetes. Interventions within each topic are listed either as recommended or as not yet having sufficient evidence from research to support a recommendation. Other sources of evidence for community-based interventions are identified in Box 9.4.

In Case 1, Ellen consults The Community Guide website for recommendations on influenza immunization programs. She finds that multiple interventions implemented in combination, and provider reminders, are recommended for increasing immunization rates among adults at high risk. Other interventions such as community-wide education had insufficient evidence of effectiveness. What does this tell Ellen about how she should plan her intervention?

Logic Model

A **logic model** for a community health program is a visual representation of the logic behind the operation of the program—*who* will receive services (target population), *what* will be done (activities), *when* it will happen (timeline),

box 9.4 Sources of Evidence for Community Health Interventions

Healthy People 2020 Each section of the *Healthy People 2020* Topics & Objectives has a tab for "interventions and resources" with links to the major evidence that supports the objectives. www.healthypeople.gov

National Prevention Council with information on the evidence supporting the recommendations in the National Prevention Strategy. http://www.surgeongeneral.gov/initiatives/prevention/index.html

National Council on Aging Center for Healthy Aging—evidenced-based health promotion programs for chronic disease management, fall prevention, and other programs for older adults. http://www.ncoa.org/improve-health/center-for-healthy-aging/

The Guide to Community Preventive Services, known as the "Community Guide." http://www.thecommunityguide.org/index.html

U.S. Preventive Services Task Force (USPSTF) recommendations. http://www.uspreventiveservicestaskforce.org/recommendations.htm

AHRQ Guide to Clinical Preventive Services. http://www.ahrq.gov/professionals/clinicians-providers/guidelines-recommendations/guide/index.html

National Guideline Clearinghouse. http://www.guideline.gov/

The Cochrane Library of systematic reviews. http://www.cochrane.org/cochrane-reviews

Research and systematic reviews published in *Public Health Nursing, American Journal of Public Health, Preventing Chronic Disease,* and other nursing, public health, and health promotion journals.

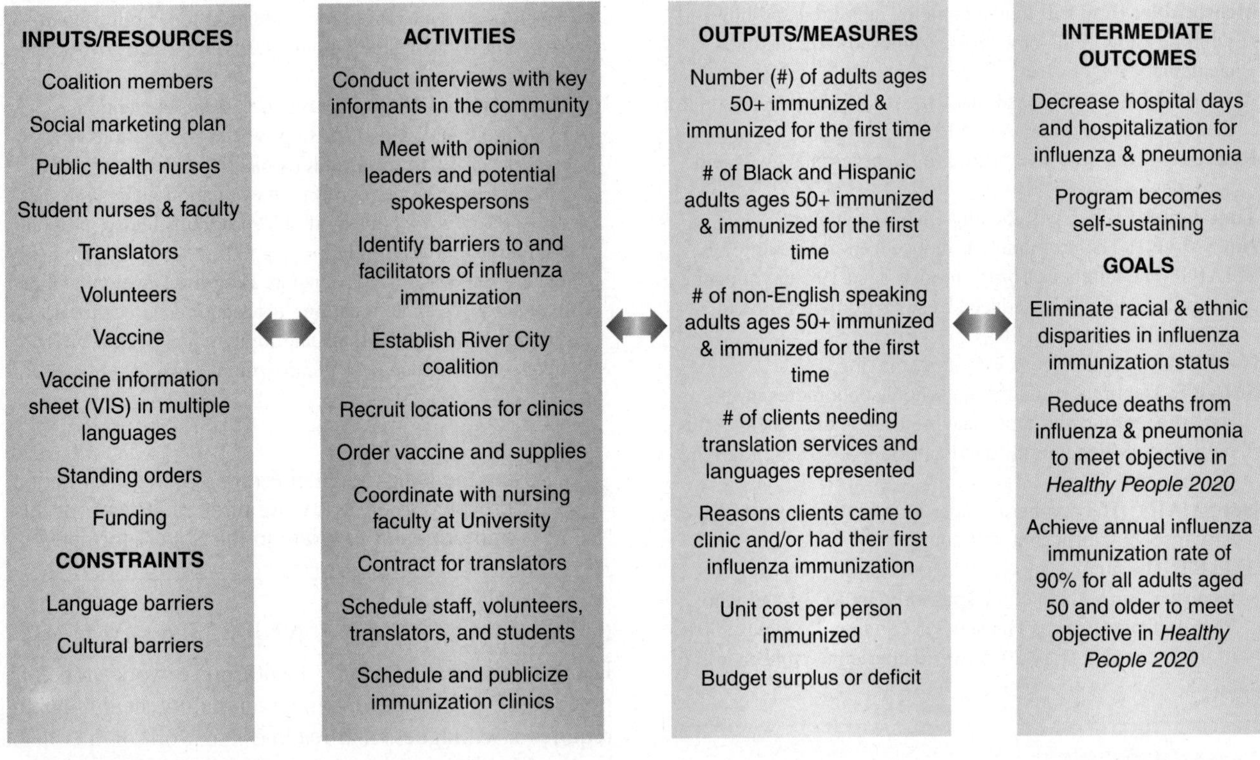

figure 9.3 Logic model for influenza immunization program. (Adapted from Taylor-Powell, E., & Henert, E. [2008]. *Developing a logic model: Teaching and training guide*. Retrieved from http://www.uwex.edu/ces/pdande/evaluation/pdf/lmguidecomplete.pdf. Used with permission.)

where, and *why* (program theory) (Taylor-Powell & Henert, 2008). The model is usually a formal process map or flow diagram (Fig. 9.3) but can be more informal using graphics or pictures. The logic model is a tool for both planning and communication. It helps the community health nurse identify available and needed resources, plan the sequence and timeframe for program implementation, develop a budget, and identify how results will be measured. The logic model also informs community leaders, program staff, stakeholders and decision-makers on the operation of the program and how it will achieve the desired results (Tucker, Liao, & Giles, 2006).

> *Logic will get you from A to B. Imagination will take you everywhere.*
>
> **Albert Einstein**

A program's theory or logic is evidence based and derived from epidemiologic and program research using sources of evidence such as those listed in Box 9.5 and a critical review of relevant literature. The program theory may also be one of those described in Chapter 5, such as the health belief model or the ecologic model. It may be important to adapt or modify the program theory or assumptions to the specific community by using information from the community assessment, such as a community's capacity, resources, results of previous efforts to address the problem, and community readiness to change. Step-by-step guides to developing and using logic models are provided in the Community Toolkit (see Box 9.1) and the resources for program evaluation listed in Box 9.6.

PRACTICE POINT

Logic models are great tools for communicating with decision-makers and grant sources. Proposals that include a well-constructed logic model are more likely to be approved and funded.

box 9.5 Writing SMART Program Objectives

Specific: What behaviors, knowledge, skill, change in health status indicators or outcome will result from the program?
Measurable: How will the outcome be measured and how will one know if the objective is achieved? Are the data available?
Achievable: Is it realistic to reach the desired outcome with the resources and time available to the program?
Relevant: Is the objective related to the program's goals and activities?
Time-bound: When will the objective be achieved?
Not SMART: The program will reduce teen pregnancy.
SMART: The number of births to girls aged 19 and younger in Springfield will be reduced by 20% from 40 births in 2010 to 32 or fewer in 2015.
Not SMART: Fewer teens will start smoking.
SMART: The proportion of high school sophomores in the state of Georgia who report having ever smoked a cigarette on the Youth Behavioral Risk Factor Survey in 2020 will be no more than 7%.
Not SMART: The number of older minority residents of River City receiving a flu shot will double.
SMART: The number of people aged 50 and older who receive a flu shot at a clinic sponsored by RC3-I and who identify themselves as Hispanic or Latino will increase 50% in the fiscal year (FY) 2015 over the baseline number in FY 2012.

In Case 1, Ellen reviews the theory and assumptions underpinning the statewide initiative with the statewide coordinator. She learns that the goals for increasing immunizations in older adults are based on research indicating that (1) the strongest predictor of an older adult's having an influenza immunization this season is having had a flu shot the previous year (Xakellis, 2005), (2) there are significant racial and ethnic disparities among older adults in the rates of influenza immunization and in the rates of hospitalization and death from influenza and pneumonia (Lemon, Rakowski, Clark, Roy, & Friedmann, 2004; O'Malley & Forrest, 2006), (3) older Hispanics who prefer to speak Spanish and who live in areas without established Hispanic populations have lower influenza and pneumonia immunization rates (Haviland, Elliott, Hambersoomian, & Lurie, 2011), and (4) significant reductions in the risks of hospitalization and death from influenza and pneumonia have been documented among older adults who received flu shots (Nichol, Nordin, Nelson, Mullooly, & Hak, 2007).

SMART Objectives

SMART is an acronym for program objectives that are *s*pecific, *m*easurable, *a*chievable, *r*elevant, and *t*ime-bound. Program objectives written in the SMART format help in planning interventions and establishing measurement systems to evaluate programs and outcomes (see Box 9.5).

box 9.6 Resources for Program Evaluation

CDC Framework for Program Evaluation including steps and standards. http://www.cdc.gov/eval/framework/index.htm
CDC Introduction to Program Evaluation for Public Health Programs: A Self-Study Guide. http://www.cdc.gov/eval/guide/index.htm
CDC Division for Heart Disease and Stroke Prevention Evaluation Guides include step-by-step instructions and examples for writing SMART objectives, developing and using a Logic Model, writing an evaluation plan, and other skills. http://www.cdc.gov/dhdSP/programs/nhdsp_program/evaluation_guides/evaluation_plan.htm
University of Wisconsin Extension. Program Development and Evaluation Web site including tools and resources for developing program evaluations and logic models. http://www.uwex.edu/ces/pdande/evaluation/index.html

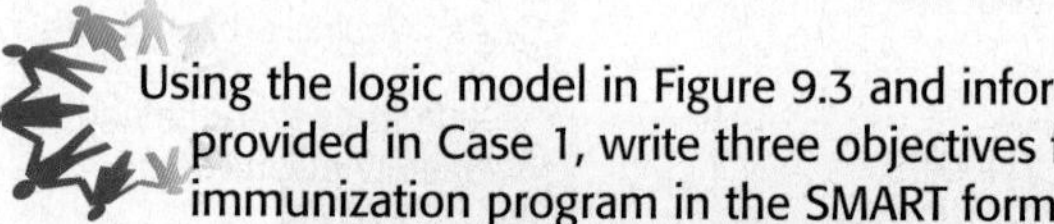

Using the logic model in Figure 9.3 and information provided in Case 1, write three objectives for this immunization program in the SMART format.

COLLABORATION AND TEAMWORK

Rarely does the community health nurse work alone. The practice of public health and community health nursing requires a willingness and readiness to work on a collegial basis with community members from all walks of life and with other professionals from a wide range of fields. Other members of a team may include social workers, policymakers, elected officials, public health professionals, school officials, senior center directors, educators, community health workers (CHWs), and researchers.

Respect for the abilities and appreciation for the contributions of community members and other health and social service professionals are essential to the success of team building and collaboration. Depending on the specific needs and composition of the group, the community health nurse may play many different roles—team leader, team member, consultant, educator, or facilitator. Active listening is just as important a nursing skill when working with community members as it is when caring for an individual person. CHWs and community members have much to teach health professionals about how to provide services that are concordant with the unique social, cultural, and linguistic needs of the community.

One of the tests of leadership is the ability to recognize a problem before it becomes an emergency.

Arnold Glasgow

PRACTICE POINT

Nurses should seek input and feedback from community members using focus groups and key informant interviews to tailor an intervention to the unique needs, culture, and priorities of the community of interest.

Community Health Workers

Community health workers, also called lay health advisors, outreach workers, promotores(as) de salud (promoters of health), peer educators, patient navigators, and community health advocates, are essential to effective and comprehensive health systems globally. CHWs are recognized in the Patient Protection and ACA as important members of the healthcare workforce. They provide a cultural and language bridge to the members of the target population (Health Resources and Services Administration [HRSA], 2007; Pérez & Martinez, 2008). CHWs work with community health nurses and other members of the program team in both urban and rural areas to provide health education, outreach and assistance in accessing services, translation, and specific interventions. Generally recruited from the community of interest and trained by program staff, CHWs make an important contribution to providing patient-centered care and decreasing health inequalities. The evidence shows that they can help improve healthcare access and outcomes; strengthen healthcare teams; and enhance quality of life for people in poor, underserved, and diverse populations and communities (Rosenthal et al., 2010). In addition to connecting patients to existing services, improving outreach, communications and adherence, CHWs can also have an important impact on healthcare costs and on the prevention and control of both chronic and infectious disease. The successes of the CHW model have resulted in more broad use of CHWs into the health delivery system (Sabo et al., 2013).

EVIDENCE FOR PRACTICE

In 2005, community, hospital, and academic leaders in New York City developed the Washington Heights/Inwood Network for Asthma Program to address the burden of asthma in their community in Northern Manhattan, where the rate of pediatric asthma-related emergency department visits was approximately four times the national average. The bilingual CHWs had strong community ties, spoke the same languages as the residents, and were familiar with the obstacles faced by local families. The CHWs were based in community organizations and the local hospital provided culturally appropriate education and support to families who needed help managing asthma. Families participating in the year-long care coordination program received comprehensive asthma education, home environmental assessments, trigger reduction strategies, and clinical and social referrals. Since 2006, 472 families have enrolled in the year-long program. After 12 months, hospitalizations and emergency department visits decreased by more than 50%, and caregiver confidence in controlling the child's asthma increased to nearly 100%. The project leaders attribute the program's success to the consistent commitment and involvement of community partners from its inception (Peretz et al., 2012).

Although CHWs have much to teach healthcare professionals about their communities, the CHWs need a structure within which to work and training to develop skills and to understand the activities and strategies of the specific community health program. Building relationships, mutual respect, and trust between the CHWs, community or public health nurses, and other members of the program team is critical to success. Written job descriptions, step-by-step intervention guidelines, scripts for health education, and ongoing training and supervision for CHWs are required to ensure the fidelity and consistency of interventions as well as to support CHW job satisfaction and job performance (HRSA, 2007; Pérez & Martinez, 2008).

In Case 1, what skills and knowledge might CHWs recruited to work on the River City Influenza Immunization Initiative bring to the program that Ellen may not have? How can Ellen work with the CHWs to make the best use of their talents?

EVALUATING COMMUNITY-LEVEL INTERVENTIONS

Evaluation begins as a program is being planned. The activities and intermediate outcomes identified in the logic model and the SMART program objectives are the start of an evaluation plan. It is critical to make plans for evaluating a program at the time of initial program planning to ensure the development of the necessary tools and methods for collection of data to measure the impact of the program in advance of the intervention. Planning for the evaluation of a program also includes, when possible, measuring preintervention levels of health status or behavior using the same evaluation criteria to establish a baseline for comparison with program results.

The evaluation plan often includes both process and outcome evaluations. Process evaluations focus on how well the program was implemented and looks at processes, activities, and capacity building. Outcome evaluation focuses on the extent to which the intervention achieved its objectives for changes in knowledge, skills, or health behavior and for improvement in community health status. Measures used for evaluation include both quantitative and qualitative data (CDC, n.d.).

Steps in developing the evaluation plan include the following:

1. Develop evaluation questions "focused on what happened, how well it happened, why it happened the way it did, and what the results were" (CDC, n.d., p. 5).
2. Determine indicators or measures you will use to answer your evaluation questions.
3. Identify where you will find the data you need to measure your indicators and answer your questions.
4. Decide what method you will use to collect data.
5. Specify the time frame for when you will collect data.

6. Plan how you will analyze your data based on the type of data you are using.
7. Decide how you will communicate your results (CDC, n.d.).

In addition to evaluation done by the program staff or consultants, foundations or government agencies funding the program may hire outside evaluators to conduct process and outcome evaluations. This often happens with large multisite demonstration projects in which the results of evaluation research are important outcomes used to determine the efficacy and impact of new intervention strategies.

The RE-AIM framework was developed to evaluate health behavior research and has helped to establish the evidence base of many health promotion programs. The RE-AIM framework includes five dimensions that together represent the elements that a health promotion program needs to have an overall impact on population health. The dimensions are *r*each, *e*ffectiveness, *a*doption, *i*mplementation, and *m*aintenance and are measured at both the participant and organizational levels.

- *Reach* is based on how well the intervention reaches its target audience. This includes the number and percent of people in the target population who are served.
- *Effectiveness* is the impact of the intervention on health behaviors, health status, quality of life, and other outcome measures. This includes a consideration of any negative effects or consequences of the intervention.
- *Adoption* looks at the extent to which the community-based organizations or providers who were expected to participate actually implemented the program.
- *Implementation* evaluates intervention fidelity or the extent to which the program was carried out as it was intended and how consistently service delivery was given between providers.
- *Maintenance* evaluates how well the behavior change or health improvements are maintained by the participants as well as the extent to which the program is continued by the participating providers (Belza, Toobert, & Glasgow, n.d.; Gaglio, Shroup, & Glasgow, 2013).

"The overall goal of the RE-AIM framework is to encourage program planners, evaluators, readers of journal articles, funders, and policy-makers to pay more attention to essential program elements that can improve the sustainable adoption and implementation of effective evidence-based health promotion programs" (Belza et al., n.d., p. 2). More information and resources on using the RE-AIM framework are available at www.re-aim.org.

PRACTICE POINT

It is important to include short-term and intermediate objectives and evaluation measures in the logic model and evaluation plan. Most community-level interventions require many years before there are measurable changes in community health status or health outcomes.

In Case 1, the city health departments participating in the statewide influenza immunization initiative each have a representative on the project's steering committee. An evaluation subcommittee has developed process and outcome measures that each health department has agreed to use to facilitate cross-city comparative analysis. In addition, each person attending a flu clinic will be asked to complete a card that asks their reason for having a flu shot, if they ever had a flu shot before, how they heard about the public health clinic, and if they required language assistance. Why did the evaluation committee include these questions?

FUNDING COMMUNITY-LEVEL INTERVENTION PROGRAMS

Planning and implementing community health programs includes finding and securing funding. Funding for a new program may come from the internal budgets of the sponsoring organization and its collaborative partners or may require outside funding from a foundation or government grant. To address a community health problem, some initiatives may not need additional funds but simply the reconfiguration of current programs or creation of a coalition to use existing resources. Additional funding may come from other sources such as community benefit programs of local health providers or insurance companies, in-kind contributions from business enterprises, and sponsorship of specific aspects of a program by a local bank or business.

Accountability

Whether a program is funded by one's own agency or an outside grant, the community health nurse will have to be accountable for how the program was implemented. Accountability includes regular communication about how funds were used, details of program activities, and progress toward achieving program goals. Large foundations and government agencies often expect logic models and formal evaluation plans as part of grant proposals. Performance in meeting the expectations for regular and meaningful progress, outcome, and financial reports is an important factor in decisions about renewal of grant funding.

Sustainability

Sustainability is an important consideration in program planning and a key factor in grant making. Most funding agencies expect programs to give a clear and convincing plan outlining how efforts started with grant funding will be continued after the grant ends. For example, is there a written commitment from the participating agencies that they will maintain changes in the delivery of services brought about by the program if those changes prove effective and produce the desired results? Developing a strategy for how a program will continue after initial funding ends should begin early in the planning process.

In Case 1, Ellen expects the program to increase the number of influenza immunizations, which will generate funds for the health department from insurance payments from Medicare, Medicaid, and other plans. The local School of Nursing has made a commitment to include the immunization clinics in its community health nursing rotation and to provide student nurses and faculty to help with clinic management and administration of vaccines. Students at the local medical translation training program will provide translation at clinics as hourly employees of the health department. Can you think of other possible ways to sustain the program once the 3-year demonstration project funding from the state department of public health ends?

Program Replication

What may have succeeded in one location may reflect how ready the community was to change, not how well a program was designed and/or how well it was implemented. The ability to replicate or reproduce a successful program within a different community or with a new population aggregate is a test of the strength of the design of an intervention. When an intervention has yielded positive results in one community, the next step in establishing evidence for practice is to test the intervention by replication.

STUDENT REFLECTION

The elementary school where I am doing my community health nursing practicum has just begun an "Andrew's Elementary Walking School Bus" program. The program began in the fall, during International Walk to School Month. There is a structured walking route with meeting points, a timetable, and a schedule of trained volunteers. It sounds simple, and it is. It can be as informal as two families taking turns walking their children to school or something larger and more structured such as a route with meeting points, a timetable, and a regularly rotated schedule of trained volunteers. Many other communities have used the "walking school bus" program, and the school was able to take advantage of information available from the CDC and other schools to help the program get off to a good start.

Project Funding

Government Agencies

Funding of community health programs by state or federal government agencies usually involves a formal competitive request for proposal (RFP) process. Most often grants from the NIH, CDC, or HRSA are categorical (e.g., targeted to a specific disease or health behavior such as childhood obesity or smoking initiation by teens), with a limited set of target populations and program models. Grants from federal agencies are usually made to a state's department of health or human services, universities, or large regional service providers with an established track record. Grants from state and local government agencies are often made using a combination of federal funds granted to the state and funds allocated from the state or local government budget.

The ACA has created new opportunities for federal and state funding of health promotion and prevention programs. These opportunities include Community Transformation Grants that will fund programs to improve nutrition, physical activity, and wellness with priority given to strategies to reduce healthcare disparities. Grants will be available to small business to provide comprehensive workplace wellness programs. New funding will be available to expand the services of community health centers and to expand Medicaid. A new Prevention and Public Health Fund was also established by the ACA with funding targeted to be $2 billion in 2015 and beyond to invest in new prevention and wellness initiatives and strengthening the public health infrastructure (Koh & Sebelius, 2010). Some states have also established similar prevention funds. There may be many new opportunities for funding community health nursing programs and interventions as the provisions of the ACA are fully implemented.

Private Foundations

Private foundations of all sizes provide grants for community health services. Most foundations publish guidelines that identify their program interests, proposal guidelines, range of grant amounts, and eligible grantees. It is important to learn as much as possible about a foundation before submitting a proposal, to select a foundation or foundations whose interests align closely with the proposed program, and to follow guidelines carefully. If an applicant is submitting proposals to more than one foundation for the same program, it is important to indicate this fact in the cover letter and proposal budget.

Local Resources

Local banks and other businesses, faith communities, civic groups such as Rotary International or the Junior League, and other local resources may provide seed money, matching funds, or in-kind support for community health programs. In-kind support such as donating items for a silent auction, volunteering hours at a food bank, or printing program materials are valuable contributions that local businesses can make in addition to, or instead of, cash. Even if the amount of funds from local groups is not large, it is important to seek local support. Not only does the support of the program by local groups demonstrate community engagement to larger funding sources, the interest and involvement of local leaders helps ensure program success and increases the likelihood of sustainability.

Community Benefit Programs

Community benefit programs of local or regional hospitals and health maintenance organizations (HMOs) may be valuable partners to the public health department or community health nurse in planning, implementing, and funding programs to improve population health. Each nonprofit hospital is required to provide and document community benefits as the basis for their tax exemption. Community benefits are programs and services designed to improve health in communities and increase access to healthcare (Barnett, 2009). More information and tools for community benefit programs are available on the website of the Association for Community Health Improvement (ACHI).

PRACTICE POINT

Develop long-term relationships with funders by thanking them, providing regular progress reports on the program they have funded, and acknowledging their support in each press release about the program. Foundations and businesses are more likely to fund proposals from organizations that have communicated well and have been accountable for funds previously provided than from organizations that only contact them when funding is needed.

In Case 1, Ellen organized a "kick-off" event at the community health center. The city's mayor and director of the health department spoke, and each received a flu shot in front of cameras from the local media, including the Spanish-language newspaper. Ellen wrote a monthly report of program achievements for the state department of public health. She provided an edited copy to the director of the city's health department to send to the mayor, city council, and local members of the state legislature. Why is this important?

SOCIAL MARKETING

Social marketing is the use of marketing principles and practices to change health behaviors or beliefs, social or cultural norms, or community standards to improve health or benefit society (CDC, 2011). Examples include the use of social marketing to promote health behavior change related to eating fruits and vegetables (five a day), breastfeeding, active play by children, and following guidelines for cancer screenings. It has also been used to change social and cultural norms related to smoking, texting while driving, condom use, and consumption of trans fats. Social marketing is an increasingly important tool in bringing about change in population health. Several resources are available to help the community health nurse learn to use social marketing through the CDCynergy Gateway to Health Communication and Social Marketing Practice (CDC, 2011).

Social marketing is more than just media communication or health education. The goal is to change behavior. All people are exposed to commercial and social marketing each day, and although marketing may look easy and seem intuitive, it is anything but. Most public health programs lack the resources to develop social marketing campaigns; fortunately, it is not necessary to "recreate the wheel." Many social marketing programs and materials that can be adapted for local use are available through the CDC, HHS, and national associations such as the American Heart Association and the National Dairy Council. These programs are available free or for a nominal fee.

STUDENT REFLECTION

When I was in high school, the school nurse showed us an empty soft drink bottle half filled with sugar. She said there are 10 teaspoons of sugar in a 12-ounce (350-mL) bottle. Can you imagine eating that much sugar with a spoon? The nurse said that diet drinks are no better because they change your metabolism and make you crave sweets. I stopped drinking soft drinks that day and started drinking water and diluted fruit juice and lost 10 lb in 6 months without trying. The visual aid that nurse used did more to convince me than anything I had read.

NURSE-MANAGED HEALTH CENTERS

Nurse-managed health centers (NMHCs) are a unique model of community health services led by advanced-practice nurses and providing a wide range of services and programs to vulnerable and underserved populations. The communities served by NMHCs are usually geographically defined and are most often vulnerable and underserved population aggregates such as the rural poor, migrant farm workers, low-income mothers and children, inner-city neighborhoods, and immigrant communities. The NMHC may offer services in subsidized housing projects, homeless shelters, correctional institutions, schools, faith communities, storefronts, and other locations easily accessible to the population aggregate being served. The NMHCs emphasize health promotion, disease prevention, and health education. Many provide specialized programs to meet the needs of specific population aggregates such as pregnant and parenting women, teens, or homeless people. Primary prevention is a core component of the care provided, and the range of services varies from health promotion programs to a full range of primary care and chronic disease management programs (Esperat, Hanson-Turton, Richardson, Debisette, & Rupinta, 2012).

Many NMHCs are academic nursing centers established by colleges of nursing to provide service to the community as well as clinical practice and research opportunities for students and faculty, and to prepare students with skills to work in medically underserved areas. Other NMHCs are federally qualified health centers of federally qualified look-alikes or are clinics within the structure of a hospital or health system. HRSA has funded some NMHCs, particularly those at schools of nursing, and NMHCs are included in provisions for expanded funding of safety-net providers and community health centers under the ACA. NMHCs belong to the National Nursing Centers Consortium, where you can find more information about these community health nursing programs that build on the legacy of Lillian Wald in meeting the needs of vulnerable and underserved communities (Esperat et al., 2012).

key concepts

- Common themes of current national and international health plans include providing health promotion and disease prevention at the population level, addressing social determinants of health, and achieving health equity.
- Social justice and health equity are key values in community health and public health nursing.
- Changing the social and environmental context to make healthy choices the default is an effective strategy for improving the health of a community.
- Even small changes at the community or population level have the potential to create significant change in the health status of a community.
- Logic models provide a visual representation of how a program is organized: what it will do (activities), what resources are needed (inputs), how short-term and intermediate outcomes will be measured, and how the program goals will be achieved.
- The change process can be visualized as three steps of unfreezing the status quo, changing or moving to a new state, and refreezing to sustain the change or changes made.
- Force field analysis is a tool used to identify the forces driving or restraining change.
- The health status of a community and its members is the result of a complex interplay of social, economic, environmental, behavioral, political, and cultural forces.
- Health behavior change, whether at the individual or community level, requires sustained effort, and results may not be evident in the short term.
- Community participation in all steps of the change process helps to increase the potential for program success and sustained change in community health status.
- Community readiness to change needs to be considered in selecting the most appropriate types and levels of interventions.
- Multilevel interventions are needed to achieve change in complex community health conditions that have multiple determinants.
- Public policies such as tax increases on tobacco, alcohol, or soft drinks can serve as policy levers to bring about change in community health status.
- Nurses can play an important role in their professional and personal lives as advocates and champions for health improvement, social justice, and health equity at the local, regional, national, and global levels.
- Community health workers can help bridge the gap between the community health nurse and the community, especially when there are cultural and language differences.
- Nurse-managed health centers provide health promotion and primary care services to vulnerable and underserved population aggregates.

critical thinking questions

1. Think about the factors (social, developmental, environmental, and policy) that contribute to the problem of binge drinking on college campuses. Use a force field analysis to think about how the change process could be applied to reduce binge drinking on your campus.
   a. Which driving force(s) would you want to strengthen? What approach would you use to accomplish this? Why?
   b. Which restraining force(s) would you want to decrease? What approach would you use to accomplish this? Why?
2. Can you think of recent changes in public policy, the environment or social context that have made it easier to make healthy choices in your own health behaviors? How might you apply the concept of making healthy choices the default choice to your nursing practice to support healthier behaviors among your clients?
3. Based on community-level data, you have identified the need to increase immunization rates in the refugee and immigrant population in your community. Who might you enlist as partners in planning and implementing programs to achieve desired health outcomes at the community level? Why did you select these partners?
4. Bekemeier and Villeneuve and Falk-Rafael all suggest that nurses need to actively work to bring about change upstream in the social and environmental determinants of health. How might this vision for the role of nurses in population health manifest itself in your practice?

references

Barnett, K. (2009). *Beyond the numerical tally: Quality and stewardship in community benefit*. Retrieved from http://www.communityhealth.org/communithhlth/files/files_projects/PHI_ASACB_policybriefs_Feb09.pdf

Beauchamp, D. (1976). Public health as social justice. *Inquiry, 12*, 3–14.

Bekemeier, B. (2008). "Upstream" nursing practice and research. *Applied Nursing Research*, 50–52. doi:10.1016/j.apnr.2007.11.002

Belza, B., Toobert, D. J., & Glasgow, R. E. (n.d.). *RE-AIM for program planning: Overview and applications*. Washington, DC: National Council on Aging. Retrieved from http://www.prc-han.org/docs/RE-AIM_issue_brief.pdf

Bopp, M., Kaczynski, A. T., & Campbell, M. E. (2013). Social ecological influences on work-related active commuting among adults. *American Journal of Health Behavior, 37*(4), 543–554. doi:10.5993/AJHB.37.4.12

Brown, J. (2012). Wellness and sustainability. *Greenhealth Magazine*. Retrieved from http://greenhealthmagazine.org/wellness-and-sustainability/

Centers for Disease Control and Prevention. (2011). *CDCynergy: Gateway to health communications and social marketing practice*. Retrieved from http://www.cdc.gov/healthcommunication/CDCynergy/

Centers for Disease Control and Prevention. (2012). *Designing and building healthy places*. Retrieved from http://www.cdc.gov/healthyplaces/default.htm

Centers for Disease Control and Prevention. (n.d.). *Developing an evaluation plan*. Retrieved from http://www.cdc.gov/dhdSP/programs/nhdsp_program/evaluation_guides/docs/evaluation_plan.pdf

City of Worcester. (2012). *Greater Worcester region community health improvement plan*. Retrieved from http://www.worcesterma.gov/uploads/bf/02/bf025dca732a04d5ef3f541cea3113f7/chip-report.pdf

Clark, N. M., Lachance, L. L., Benedict, M. B., Doctor, L. J., Gilmore, L., Kelly, C. W . . . Wilkin, M. (2013). Improvements in health care use associated with community coalitions: Long-term results of the allies against asthma initiative. *American Journal of Public Health, 103*(6), 1124–1127. doi:10.2105/AJPH.2012.300983

Eisen, J. (2012). Sick people or sick societies? *Canadian Dimension, 46*(4), 40–44.

Emshoff, J. G., Darnell, A. J., Darnell, D. D., Erickson, S. W, Schneider, S., & Hudgins, R. (2007). Systems change as an outcome and a process in the work of community collaborative for health. *American Journal of Community Psychology, 39*, 255–267.

Esperat, M. C., Hanson-Turton, T., Richardson, M., Debisette, A. T., & Rupinta, C. (2012). Nurse-managed health centers: Safety-net care through advanced nursing practice. *Journal of the American Academy of Nurse Practioners, 24*, 24–31.

Falk-Rafael, A., & Betker, C. (2012). Witnessing social injustice downstream and advocating for health equity upstream: "The trombone slide" of nursing. *Advances in Nursing Science, 35*(2), 98–112.

Findholt, N. (2007). Application of the community readiness model for childhood obesity prevention. *Public Health Nursing, 24*(6), 565–570.

Frieden, T. R. (2010). A framework for public health action: The health impact pyramid. *American Journal of Public Health, 100*(4), 590–595.

Gaglio, B., Shoup, J. A., & Glasgow, R. E. (2013). The RE-AIM framework: A systematic review of use over time. *American Journal of Public Health, 103*(6), e38–e46. doi:10.2105/AJPH.2013.301299

Gostin, L. O., & Powers, M. (2006). What does social justice require for the public's health? Public health ethics and policy imperatives. *Health Affairs, 25*(4), 1053–1060.

Haviland, A. M., Elliott, M. N., Hambersoomian, K., & Lurie, N. (2011). Immunization disparities by Hispanic ethnicity and language preference. *Archives of Internal Medicine, 171*(2), 158–165.

Health Resources and Services Administration. (2007). *Community health worker national workforce study*. Retrieved from ftp://ftp.hrsa.gov/bhpr/workforce/chw307.pdf

Kneipp, S., & Snider, M. J. (2001). Social justice in a market model world. *Journal of Professional Nursing, 17*(3), 113.

Koh, H. W., & Sebelius, K. G. (2010). Promoting prevention through the Affordable Care Act. *New England Journal of Medicine, 363*(14), 1296–1299.

Lemon, S. C., Rakowski, W., Clark, M. A., Roy, J., & Friedmann, P. D. (2004). Variations in influenza vaccination among the elderly. *American Journal of Health Behavior, 28*(4), 352–360.

Lenihan, P. (2005). MAPP and the evolution of planning in public health practice. *Journal of Public Health Management Practice, 11*(5), 381–386.

MacDuffie, H., & DePoy, E. (2004). Force field analysis: A model for promoting adolescents' involvement in their own health care. *Health Promotion Practice, 5*, 306–313.

Marmot, M. (2005). Social determinants of health inequalities. *Lancet, 365*, 1099–1104.

McLeroy, K. R., Norton, B. L., Kegler, M. C., Burdine, J. N., & Sumaya, C. V. (2003). Community-based interventions [Editorial]. *American Journal of Public Health, 93*(4), 529–533.

National Prevention Council. (2011). *National Prevention Strategy*. Washington, DC: U.S. Department of Health and Human Services, Office of the Surgeon General. Retrieved from http://www.surgeongeneral.gov/initiatives/prevention/strategy/report.pdf

Nichol, K. L., Nordin, J. D., Nelson, D. B., Mullooly, J. P., & Hak, E. (2007). Effectiveness of influenza vaccine in the community-dwelling elderly. *New England Journal of Medicine, 357*(14), 1373–1381.

O'Malley, A. S., & Forrest, C. B. (2006). Immunization disparities in older Americans. *American Journal of Preventive Medicine, 31*(2), 150–158.

Plested, B. A., Edwards, R. W., & Jumper-Thurman, P. (2006). *Community readiness: A handbook for successful change*. Fort Collins, CO: Tri-Ethnic Center for Prevention Research. Retrieved from http://www.triethniccenter.colostate.edu

Pérez, L., & Martinez, J. (2008). Community health workers: Social justice and policy advocates for community health and well-being. *American Journal of Public Health, 98*(1), 11–14.

Peretz, P. J., Matiz, L. A., Findley, S., Lizardo, M., Evans, D., & McCord, M. (2012). Community health workers as drivers of a successful community-based disease management initiative. *American Journal of Public Health, 102*(8), 1443–1446. doi:10.2105/AJPH.2011.300585

Prevention Institute. (2008). *Strategies for enhancing the built environment to support healthy eating and active living*. Retrieved from http://www.calendow.org/uploadedFiles/Publications/Publications_Stories/builtenvironment.pdf

Rosenthal, E. L., Brownstein, J. N., Rush, C. H., Hirsch, G. R., Willaert, A. M., Scott, J. R., . . . Fox, D. J. (2010). Community health workers: Part of the solution. *Health Affairs, 29*(7), 1338–1342. doi:10.1377/hlthaff.2010.0081

Sabo, S., Ingram, M., Reinschmidt, K., Schachter, K., Jacobs, L., Guernsey de Zapien, J., . . . Carvajal, S. (2013). Predictors and a framework for fostering community advocacy as a community health worker core function to eliminate health disparities. *American Journal of Public Health, 103*(7), e67–73. doi:10.2105/AJPH.2012.301108

Schein, E. H. (1996). Kurt Lewin's change theory in the field and in the classroom: Notes toward a model of managed learning. *Systems Practice, 9*(1), 27–47.

Schwartz, M. B., & Brownell, K. D. (2007). Actions necessary to prevent childhood obesity: Creating the climate for change. *Journal of Law, Medicine & Ethics, 35*, 78–89.

Shirey, M. R. (2013). Lewin's theory of planned change as a strategic resource. *The Journal of Nursing Administration, 43*(2), 69–72.

Smedley, B. D., & Syme, S. L. (2002). *Promoting health: Intervention strategies from social and behavioral research*. Institutes of Medicine, Washington, DC: National Academies Press.

Stokols, D. (1992). Establishing and maintaining healthy environments: Toward a social ecology of health promotion. *American Psychologist, 47*(1), 6–20.

Taylor-Powell, E., & Henert, E. (2008). *Developing a logic model: Teaching and training guide*. Retrieved from http://www.uwex.edu/ces/pdande/evaluation/pdf/lmguidecomplete.pdf

Tucker, P., Liao, Y., & Giles, W. H. (2006). The REACH 2010 logic model: An illustration of expected performance. *Preventing Chronic Disease, 3*(1), 1–6. Retrieved from www.cdc.gov/pcd/issues/2006/jan/05_0131.htm

United Nations. (2012). *Millennium Development Goals Report, 2012*. New York, NY: Author. Retrieved from http://www.un.org/millenniumgoals/pdf/MDG%20Report%202012.pdf

U.S. Department of Health and Human Services. (2010). *Healthy People 2020*. Retrieved from http://www.healthypeople.gov/2020/TopicsObjectives2020/pdfs/HP2020_brochure_with_LHI_508.pdf

U.S. Department of Health and Human Services. (2012). *About Healthy People*. Retrieved from http://www.healthypeople.gov/2020/about/default.aspx

Villeneuve, M. J. (2008). Yes we can! Eliminating health disparities as part of the core business of nursing on a global level. *Policy, Politics, & Nursing Practice, 9*(4), 334–341.

World Health Organization. (2008). *Closing the gap in a generation: Health equity through action on the social determinants of health*. Geneva, Switzerland: Author. Retrieved from http://whqlibdoc.who.int/hq/2008/WHO_IER_CSDH_08.1_eng.pdf

World Health Organization. (2013). *Social determinants of health: Key concepts*. Retrieved from http://www.who.int/social_determinants/thecommission/finalreport/key_concepts/en/index.html

Xakellis, G. C. (2005). Predictors of influenza immunization in persons over age 65. *Journal of the American Board of Family Practice, 18*(5), 426–433.

York, N. L., & Hahn, E. J. (2007). The community readiness model: Evaluating local smoke-free policy development. *Policy, Politics, & Nursing Practice, 8*(3), 184–200.

Zakocs, R. C., & Edwards, E. M. (2006). What explains community coalition effectiveness? A review of the literature. *American Journal of Preventive Medicine, 30*(4), 351–361.

web resources

Please visit thePoint® for up-to-date Web resources on this topic.

CHAPTER 10

Cultural Diversity and Values

Teresa Eliot Roberts

I don't think things are moving toward an omega point; I think they're moving toward more diversity.

Clifford Geertz

Preservation of one's own culture does not require contempt or disrespect for other cultures.

Cesar Chavez

I do not want my house to be walled in on all sides and my windows to be stuffed. I want the cultures of all the lands to be blown about my house as freely as possible. But I refuse to be blown off my feet by any.

Mohandas Gandhi

chapter highlights

- Culture in community settings
- Cross-cultural nursing
- Cultural competence and related concepts
- How culture affects health
- Cultural health assessment

objectives

- Define culture and describe ways in which it is propagated.
- Define cross-cultural nursing practice.
- Explain ways in which a nurse can be culturally competent.
- Define subculture and explain how it may come into play in a clinical encounter.
- Describe the limitations and possible pitfalls of cultural competence.
- Explain how culture can affect health.

key terms

Culture: Knowledge, values, practices, customs, and beliefs of a group.

Cross-cultural or transcultural nursing: Any nursing encounter in which the client and nurse are from different cultures.

Cultural competence: Openness to others' ideas and ways of life; respect, curiosity, patience, and self-awareness of one's own culture and culturally mediated ideas.

Cultural safety: Culturally appropriate health services to disadvantaged groups while stressing dignity and avoiding institutional racism, assimilation (forcing people to adopt a dominant culture), and repressive practices.

Ethnocentrism: The assumption that others believe and behave as the dominant culture does, or the belief that the dominant culture is superior to others.

Subculture: A group sharing some practices, language, or other characteristics in common, within a larger society that does not share those characteristics.

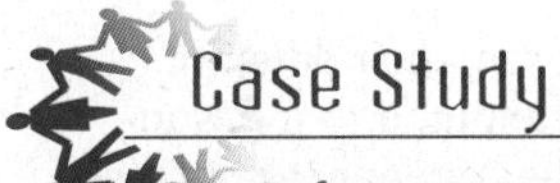

Case Study

References to the case study are found throughout this chapter (look for the case study icon). Readers should keep the case study in mind as they read the chapter.

Susan, who works in a community health clinic, is explaining to her client, Nilda, why she needs a colposcopy. She tells her that her Papanicolaou (Pap) smear shows cell changes that could, if left untreated, develop into cervical cancer. A colposcopy and biopsies are necessary to determine a more exact diagnosis and guide treatment. To Susan's surprise, Nilda looks stricken and begins to cry quietly.

After further conversation, Susan realizes that Nilda, who is from Brazil, believes that she has cancer. Nilda understands English very well; therefore, Susan has not used an interpreter. However, even if she had, her remarks may still have been confusing, because language is not the only difference between people from different countries. Their cultural assumptions may not be the same.

What Susan does not know is that in Brazil serious diagnoses such as cancer are generally not given directly and bluntly; the clinician brings the conversation slowly around to the illness and hints at the serious diagnosis (Roberts, 2004). In Anglo-American culture, clinicians tend to be both direct and blunt. Values such as time efficiency during an appointment and the patient's right to know all the possible differential diagnoses make Anglo-American culture feel impersonal and confusing to many people from other cultures. When Susan explains that cancer is a *possibility*, Nilda assumes that this is a gentle way of saying she probably *has* cancer. So, it is a cultural misunderstanding that makes Susan's first nursing intervention fail.

This chapter introduces the reader to culture as a health mediator, especially as it relates to community health. Aspects of culture that directly affect health and health decision-making are discussed, as well as specific challenges that face nurses and patients when they come from different cultures. Nurses and nursing students face challenges when they consider their cultural origins and assumptions; they need to remain respectful, open, and curious when interacting with patients from cultures different from their own. First, though, an analysis of what culture is will help focus the discussion.

CULTURE AND NURSING

What Is Culture?

Culture has been defined in many different ways, yet it remains hard to describe. A basic definition of culture could be the music, language, economy, fashion, religion, and art of a community. A more thorough analysis reveals, however, that although culture encompasses those phenomena, it also includes intangibles that are even more subtle and sometimes abstract. Culture is a "unique meaning and information system, shared by a group and transmitted across generations, that allows the group to meet basic needs of survival, . . . to transmit successful social behaviors, to pursue happiness and well-being, and to derive meaning from life" (Matsumoto, 2009). Culture has been described as that which occupies the space between people in the world. Anthropologist Renato Rosaldo explains that

> *[c]ulture lends significance to human experience by selecting from and organizing it. It refers broadly to the forms through which people make sense of their lives, rather than more narrowly to the opera or art museums.... All human conduct is culturally mediated. Culture encompasses the every day and the esoteric, the mundane and the elevated, the ridiculous and the sublime. Neither high nor low, culture is all-pervasive.*
>
> **Renato Rosaldo (1993, p. 26)**

Culture includes language, religion, occupation, economics, art, politics, and philosophy. It affects practices of individuals, families, and institutions. Culture is how people approach the world. One difficulty in discussing culture, though, is that because of its nature, people often fail to recognize its influence on themselves. Culture "exist[s] in the heads of human actors who are so thoroughly soaked in culture that it ceases to be something they notice" (Glass, 2006, p. 259).

Nurses and other human service professionals have come to realize what anthropologists have long known, that culture affects how people view health, illness, treatment, regaining and maintaining health, as well as death and dying. For these reasons, culture has become a major nursing concern. It is a fundamental and important issue in evidenced-based practice in community settings.

Properties of Culture

Dynamic, Not Static

Culture is an ever-changing phenomenon. Culture changes over time. For example, the culture of 19th-century Egypt is related to that of present-day Egypt, but it is not the same. The language has lost a few words and gained new ones. Computers have affected Egyptian work and communication. Egyptian religion, language, values, and family dynamics are closely linked to what they used to be but have evolved over time.

Culture also adapts to new circumstances. For example, along the New Jersey shore, the culture changed dramatically after Hurricane Sandy in 2012. Evacuations, damage to infrastructure, housing, and even the landscape radically changed how residents lived and thought about their communities. The cultures of individual people and families also evolve with changes in home life, illness, or migration to a new country, although these changes are usually less dramatic.

All objects, all phases of culture are alive. They have voices. They speak of their history and interrelatedness. And they are all talking at once!

Camille Paglia, author

Shared, Not Private

The definition of culture can vary among anthropologists, but all agree that one characteristic of culture is that it is something that is shared among people. Families and peers are the source of the first cultural sharing for most children. When a parent explicitly explains a value system to his or her children or cooks food for them or even teaches them their primary language, that parent is sharing cultural knowledge. A similar process happens in schools and neighborhoods, on the Internet, or in any place where people interact. Individual people may have cultural values, beliefs, and practices, but the sharing of these among people is the process of culture.

I have always felt that the action most worth watching is not at the center of things but where edges meet.

Anne Fadiman

Learned, Not Inherited

A person is not born *with culture* the way he or she is born *with genes*. Thus, if a Honduran newborn is adopted by an English couple and raised in London, that child will be culturally British. Usually, culture is first "learned" from parents and siblings and then from peers, teachers, neighbors, books, television, and other media. A Hungarian parent may teach a child that rich food is fundamental to a healthy diet and that Christianity is the best religion, for example, whereas a Japanese parent may teach that fish and rice are a healthy diet and that studiousness and selflessness are virtues. These lessons may be explicit, as in when a parent explains his or her own values, or parents or peers may teach cultural norms implicitly, as when they model or reward certain behaviors.

When you learn something from people, or from a culture, you accept it as a gift, and it is your lifelong commitment to preserve it and build on it.

Yo-Yo Ma

Cross-Cultural Nursing

Cross-cultural nursing is any nursing work in which the nurse and patient have different cultures. **Transcultural nursing** is sometimes used as a synonym but can also refer specifically to the work and model of Madeleine Leininger (2002), a nurse-anthropologist who sought to focus nursing attention on culture.

In the case of Nilda and Susan, their different cultural assumptions contributed to a misunderstanding. However, the experiences of cross-cultural clinical encounters are also potentially enriching, showing each participant new ways of looking at the world and providing opportunities for introspection.

How can nurses working in communities develop a non-self-blaming or defensive posture when they make mistakes based on cultural assumptions and misunderstandings? How can mistakes like this be supported and turned into learning experiences?

It is critical that nurses understand that culture is neither static nor deterministic (Carpenter-Song, Schwallie, & Longhofer, 2007). That is, just because a client is Chinese, Sioux, Amish, or Romanian, that person does not necessarily act or believe like most people from the same culture. Moreover, an individual's culture does not necessarily have the same importance to that person at all times or in every situation. Rather than assuming anything, "communicate a recognition that people live their ethnicity differently, that the experience of ethnicity is complicated but important, and that it bears significance in the healthcare setting" (Kleinman & Benson, 2006).

STUDENT REFLECTION

During my first clinical rotation in home care, I was visiting a 50-year-old Vietnamese lady recovering from pneumonia. While I was assessing her respiratory status, I noticed several round brown bruises down her back, bilaterally. I was a little shocked, not knowing what it was. I could not think of anything about her infection that would cause that. But she told me that when she came from the hospital, her sister-in-law had given her a "fire cupping" treatment. I went home and did some research. It turns out that people in many countries treat some respiratory conditions by trapping hot air in little cups on the skin of the back, which can cause bruising. I wrote a paper about it and did a presentation to my community health class. My instructor said that even she had not really known much about cupping until she read my paper!

Cultural Competence

Nurses in an ethnically diverse society, then, should strive to serve their clients in a culturally sensitive, respectful, and effective manner. In other words, they should demonstrate cultural competence. In nursing, **cultural competence** means considering cultural aspects of health, illness, and treatment for each client or community, as well as doing so at each stage of the nursing process. The American Academy of Nursing's Expert Panel on Cultural Competence described cultural competence as *an ongoing process that involves accepting and respecting differences and not letting one's personal beliefs have an undue influence on those whose worldview is different from one's own. Cultural competence includes having general cultural as well as cultural-specific information so the health care provider knows what questions to ask.*

Giger et al. (2007, p. 100)

Institutional Cultural Competence

Nurses and other health professionals should take culture into account in providing client-centered care, but to promote community health and well-being, healthcare organizations must also strive for cultural competence. For community and public health agencies to be culturally competent, they must:

- Have a defined set of values and principles and demonstrate behaviors, attitudes, policies, and structures that enable them to work effectively cross-culturally.
- Have the capacity to (1) value diversity, (2) conduct self-assessment, (3) manage the dynamics of difference, (4) acquire and institutionalize cultural knowledge, and (5) adapt to diversity and the cultural contexts of the communities they serve.
- Incorporate the above in all aspects of policy-making, administration, practice, service delivery, and involve systematically consumers, key stakeholders, and communitites (National Center for Cultural Competence, 2008).

Proponents of cultural competence also conceptualize it as a process, which is to say that as people, groups, and cultures change, nurses will never arrive at one point of mastery but should continue striving for culturally-sensitive care. "Assumptions of knowing can lead to decreased efforts to learn" (Racher & Annis, 2007, p. 265).

In Susan's case, especially if she has many Brazilians in her community service area, it would be good nursing practice to find out more about Brazilian culture. The facility in which Susan works should consider hiring Brazilian staff and/or consultants, find out whether there are health concerns specific to this population (a form of community health assessment; see Chapter 10), have a strong and professional interpretation department, and continuously ask in what ways the facility can improve services to this population, including ongoing self-assessment to consider how the nurses' cultures affect care.

How could nurses organize a descriptive research study that could answer some of these questions? Is there a way to understand how nurses feel about hiring practices and how those who are underrepresented feel?

It is crucial that nurses expand their views beyond the individual practitioner and client. Nurses must be culturally knowledgeable and sensitive, but they should also be critical of the systems and policies in society that perpetuate health disparities among groups. Practitioners who have tolerant nondiscriminatory attitudes will not necessarily be culturally competent if they are not also trained to recognize when behavior unintentionally supports the status quo or a business-as-usual mentality and favors some over others (Kumas-Tan, Beagan, Loppie, MacLeod, & Frank, 2007).

EVIDENCE FOR PRACTICE

Beach et al. (2005) performed a systematic literature review and analysis of 34 studies that evaluated interventions designed to improve the cultural competence of health professionals. A synthesis of the findings indicated that cultural competence training improves the knowledge of health professionals (17 of 19 studies) as well as both the attitudes (14 of 14 studies) and skills (21 of 25 studies) of health professionals. Results also indicated that cultural competence training impacts patient satisfaction (3 of 3 studies demonstrated a beneficial effect). There were no studies that evaluated patient health status outcomes, and evidence that cultural competence training improves patient adherence to therapy, health outcomes, and equity of services across racial and ethnic groups is lacking. It is necessary to increase cultural competence training for nurses and other health professionals in all healthcare settings. Future research should focus on outcomes and should determine which teaching methods and content are most effective.

PRACTICE POINT

Memorizing a list of cultural traits of clients is simplistic: it may facilitate stereotyping and obscure the fact that each client is a multifaceted human for whom culture can play unique roles. It is incumbent that nurses approach their clients as individuals who may be more or less acculturated and should not be prejudged.

Some cross-cultural nursing texts list traits of various cultures, implying that memorizing these will make a person sensitive cross-culturally. However, human beings are complex, and culture is just one of the many factors that influences how they view health and illness. "We cannot 'read off' health status, health beliefs and behaviors from an individual's designated ethnic status" (Culley, 2006, p. 150).

Principles of Cultural Competence

There are thousands of cultures in the world, countless because they are always changing. A nurse cannot have encyclopedic knowledge about every culture a client might come from. But as a nurse is focusing on a certain community, it is advisable to learn what major cultural groups comprise that community and what facets of the community give it its own unique subculture as well. Indeed, nurses should do this while they are doing the general community health assessment. Although the nurses will not be fluent in all cultures at all times, certain principles will make nurses more culturally competent: openness to others' ideas and ways of life; respect, curiosity, patience, and self-awareness of one's own culture and culturally mediated ideas; and the humility to know that one can always learn more about a certain client's culture and that person as an individual. Individual nurses must work toward cultural awareness and competence to help erase health disparities and power imbalances among groups.

In such diffused changes of culture two factors are necessary: contact and understanding.

Hu Shih, Chinese philosopher

Related Concepts

Cultural Safety

Historically, many practices of healthcare institutions and clinicians have been discriminatory and hurtful to minority groups. **Cultural safety** refers to providing culturally appropriate health services to disadvantaged groups while stressing dignity and avoiding institutional racism, assimilation, and repressive practices. Bearskin (2011) explains that cultural safety "involves the recognition of the social, economic, and political position of certain groups. Nurses' responsibility for cultural safety must include paying attention to the disparities in health care, . . . improving health care access for all, . . . exposing the social, political, and historical context of health care, and disrupting unequal power relations" (p. 553).

For the community health nurse, this means ongoing learning about the health beliefs and practices of their clients and never dismissing or disrespecting folk traditions. For instance, communities in the United States that use healing practices of Vodou (or Voodoo), a Haitian religion, often feel that they have to hide their practices because the dominant society considers the religion unacceptable or even evil. A nurse who is not familiar with these practices might at first be shocked or scared by Vodou, but providing culturally safe care means that he or she would need to analyze those feelings and instead approach Vodou with respect and openness, encouraging clients to use Vodou if they see it as beneficial.

EVIDENCE FOR PRACTICE

An interdisciplinary group (Alverson et al., 2007) conducted an ethnographic study to explore cultural differences in discourse about mental illness. Mental health patients belonging to three cultural groups—Puerto Rican Americans, Anglo-Americans, and African-Americans—were interviewed about their illnesses. Ways of discussing mental illness varied among these groups: the researchers noted that the Anglo-Americans more often used jargon and felt at home with the health services, but that the African-American participants often appeared suspicious and saw themselves as "guinea pigs" within the mental healthcare system. This attitude of insecurity is understandable given a history of certain notorious incidents of mistreatment of this group by the medical establishment, such as the Tuskegee Syphilis Study of the mid-20th century and forced sterilization of minority women in the early 20th century.

CULTURAL HUMILITY

Because "competency" implies mastering a finite task, "cultural humility" has been proposed as another, perhaps more appropriate, goal. Cultural humility requires nurses to continually self-evaluate and critique their own cultural assumptions and advocate for their clients in a nonpaternalistic way. To do this, they should:

- Ask open-ended questions about beliefs and practices of the client and family and
- Ask about traditions. What does the client think may have caused an illness, and how has the client already tried to address it?

Rather than trying only to learn tricks or nuggets of cultural knowledge, it is better to have an ongoing, humble attitude and commitment to self-awareness and client-centered care.

For example, a school nurse interacting with students from many cultural groups finds it impossible to be an expert on the health beliefs and practices of all the cultures. However, he or she understands the common health practices of some of the cultures. A teacher complains that a boy is wearing small magnets on his ears, which is against the dress code. After interviewing the child, the school nurse learns that he has been experiencing headaches in class. It turns out that the magnets have been placed on his ears by a traditional Chinese medicine practitioner as treatment for his headaches. The school nurse should explain to the teacher that this is a valid therapeutic technique and that Chinese medicine is a legitimate healthcare system 10 times older than Western allopathic medicine. Also, the therapy is likely to make the child more comfortable in class and better able to learn.

ETHNOCENTRISM

Ethnocentrism refers to two related phenomena. First, ethnocentrism means the tendency of people to assume that everyone else thinks the same way they do, and has the same worldview, logic, and culture. For instance:

- A family that eats a big Christmas dinner of ham and sweet potatoes in the afternoon of Christmas day might assume that everyone celebrates the Christmas holiday that way—even that everyone celebrates the holiday. However, this is a cultural phenomenon that differs significantly across cultural groups, even for those living near each other.

- Nurses often assume that they can reach clients by phone, but if their clients are homeless, they may have neither phones nor addresses.
- A woman drives to work and has an office job, and she forgets that many other people commute on foot, or have an occupation that requires them to be physically active.
- A student nurse asks a client, "What do you usually eat for dinner?" The client answers, "Oh, regular food." The client is assuming that most people eat the same things they do and does not even know how to describe it, perceiving it as the norm.

Ethnocentrism can also refer to the tendency of people to view their way of doing things and their culture as superior to the cultures and ways of others. For instance, someone may feel that a "real" marriage requires a wedding in a certain religious denomination. This may reflect ignorance about or even disdain for hundreds of other ways of creating marriages that occur across our nation and the world. If people think that their own region's fashions or medicines or languages are *better* than those of another region (as opposed to just personally preferring them), they are thinking ethnocentrically.

Perhaps Nilda would like to consult an herbalist about ways to treat her cervical cellular changes. Susan can ethnocentrically reject the idea, telling Nilda that herbalism is primitive and dangerous, or she can find out more about it, offering to work together with Nilda's chosen herbalist to develop a complementary treatment plan.

What would be some concrete first steps in finding an herbalist? How could a nurse build community-collaborative relationships from small-scale relationships with patients in communities?

Subculture

Just as any group of people from a certain place may share a culture, any group of people who share a certain characteristic can share a smaller culture, or **subculture**. For instance, within the United States, Methodists share a subculture of their religion and religious practices. Just as with larger cultures, there is plenty of heterogeneity within Methodism, and not all Methodists are the same or have exactly the same religious beliefs. We can say, however, that it is likely that they share certain beliefs, practices, experiences, and/or religious discourse. Any general culture or ethnic identity "is overlaid with gender, age, socioeconomic and professional identities, each of which may be more or less significant in any specific context, at any specific moment" (Culley, 2006, p. 149).

Subcultures might be grouped by their occupation, age group, sexual orientation, avocation, socioeconomic status, region, or some other characteristic the individuals share. It is reasonable to assume that construction workers from Tampa to Seattle share some experiences, language, and practices. Similarly, motorcycle enthusiasts have interests and knowledge in common that make them a subcultural group, as are nurses, skiers, lesbians, cancer survivors, and café owners. A subculture may be large or small, clustered together or scattered, but its members share some cultural facets such as experience, belief, language (or "lingo"), practices, and values.

It is time for parents to teach young people early on that in diversity there is beauty and there is strength.

Maya Angelou

Nilda's original culture was Brazilian, but the fact that she has had a new experience of migrating to the United States means that she also belongs to a smaller subculture of Brazilians living in the United States. These people have shared certain experiences. She also probably belongs to other subcultures, such as her church, neighborhood, and occupational group. Nilda and Susan also share subcultures; for example, they are both women, they live in the same city, and may be of the same age or love the same television program.

Can common subcultures be shared?

Race

Race can also be thought of as a subculture because people of the same race often share experiences, such as how they are treated by and reflected in a larger society. What is important to understand is that race is a social construct, not a biologic entity. Genetic sciences have shown that there is much more variation *within* traditional racial categories (e.g., Black, White, Hispanic) than there is *between* them (American Anthropological Association, 2007; Braun, 2006). Racism is certainly a reality and can have devastating effects on health (Brondolo, Libretti, Rivera, & Walsemann, 2012), but race itself is based on social ideas and not on biologic determinants. Indeed, there are significant health disparities among races in the United States (United States Department of Health and Human Services, 2013). It is important to know that although a nurse may use a client's appearance to consider what diseases he or she may be susceptible to, appearance may not be a good indicator of genetic propensity, and there are many more factors that are probably more predictive of risk than what apparent race a client might belong to. Similarly, a person's eye shape, skin tone, or hair texture does not tell very much about that person's cultural practices or lifestyle, and not even a great deal about his or her genes.

WESTERN BIOMEDICINE AS "CULTURED"

For many years, anthropologists (scientists who study culture) approached culture in a one-sided way. That is, they studied their subjects, the Maori in New Zealand or the Maasai in Kenya, and did not realize that they themselves were viewing the world from a certain cultural lens. The truth is that no one is "normal" or views the world from a blank slate of neutrality. Every person comes from a certain cultural background. However, people from some cultures, having enjoyed more dominance in the world, may feel more "normal" because their culture is well reflected in world and local media.

Similarly, and importantly, nurses also belong to a cultural subset. The common educational experience, working conditions, such as shift work, and views of health and illness, based on a belief in microbial theory, all contribute to a shared cultural perspective among nurses. In addition, nurses who are from or were educated in the United States share much in common with American national culture and are infused with "Western" values in addition to the values and outlooks shared with medicine and allied health professions. All nurses should recognize and acknowledge this special cultural perspective and the ways in which it influences nursing care of clients.

The first imperative of cultural competence is to be competent in one's own cultural heritage. The nurse should ask himself or herself, "Where are my ancestors and current family from? What traditions and health beliefs did I explicitly inherit and what more subtle assumptions were implicitly handed down to me?" After personal understanding come respect and appreciation for the values and behaviors of others. Knowledge of cultural differences is essential if sensitivity and competence are to occur. Only when self-awareness combines with insight about others can nurses and other healthcare professionals demonstrate true sensitivity (Giger et al., 2007). This concept is important to keep in mind as nurses approach their clients, especially those who come from cultures different from their own. Culture is not a curiosity or a phenomenon that "exotic" clients have, unrelated to the nurses themselves. Indeed, clients from different cultures can just as easily view their clinicians as exotic. In reality, every clinical encounter is a cultural exchange.

ASPECTS OF CULTURE DIRECTLY AFFECTING HEALTH AND HEALTHCARE

Attribution of Illness

Different cultural world views tend to reflect different ideas about what causes disease. Anglo-American culture, for instance, emphasizes infection, genetics, and personal responsibility as factors in disease and health. Illness is seen as something inside or inherent to an individual (Alverson et al., 2007). Other cultures may be "macroreligious," meaning there is more emphasis on divine influence on health and illness. Likewise, luck, fatalism, or disease may be seen as mediated through certain specific organs of the body.

EVIDENCE FOR PRACTICE

A multinational group of scientists conducted an ethnography about birthing practices and beliefs in Awak Ibom, Nigeria (Mboho, Furber, & Waterman, 2013). They found that traditional birth attendants were considered to have supernatural powers. Women often preferred to labor in the homes of traditional birth attendants or even churches, rather than in hospitals, because they felt that there they would be protected from malevolent witchcraft. Additionally, if labor was particularly difficult, it was believed to be an indication of past sin, and a confession of infidelity would be required before traditional birth attendants would intervene.

Diet

What and how people eat vary tremendously among cultures, the understanding of which is crucial to good nursing care. Perhaps a nurse needs to teach a client who is newly diagnosed with diabetes or hyperlipidemia about dietary restrictions. The nurse will be much more effective if he or she chooses examples that resonate with that particular client. For instance, a new immigrant from India is more likely to eat rice and legumes than is a fourth-generation Midwesterner whose staples are red meat and bread. A nurse teaching an anemic client about iron-rich foods would want to use food examples that might appear in the client's own diet. Buddhism, Judaism, Hinduism, Islam, and other religions have dietary restrictions about various meats, for instance, and nursing interventions are more successful if the nurse is sensitive to a client's predilections. Often, various cultures and religions incorporate certain herbs, teas, and honeys into their diets, and the potential medicinal effects should be noted (Fig. 10.1).

EVIDENCE FOR PRACTICE

Reasearchers were interested in finding out more about how Korean immigrants to the United States viewed diabetes, in order to formulate effective strategies to prevent and treat the disease in this group. They held focus groups in a Korean community center, asking adult Korean Americans with type 2 diabetes about the disease. They found that diabetes held a significant social stigma and that, before their own diagnosis, many participants had believed that diabetes happened to "lazy" people and those who "cannot control" themselves (Nam, Song, Park, & Song, 2013).

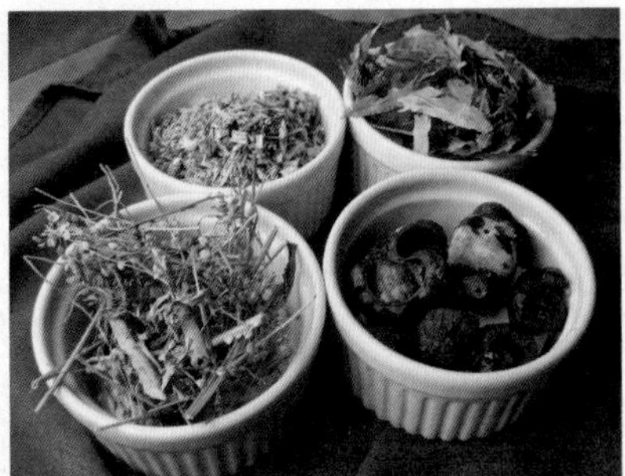
A

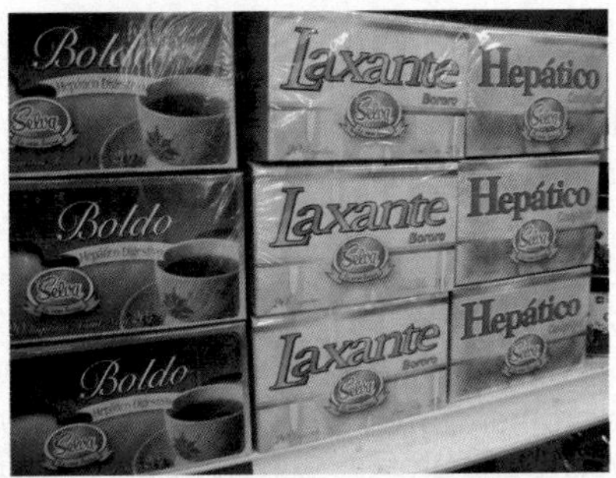

B

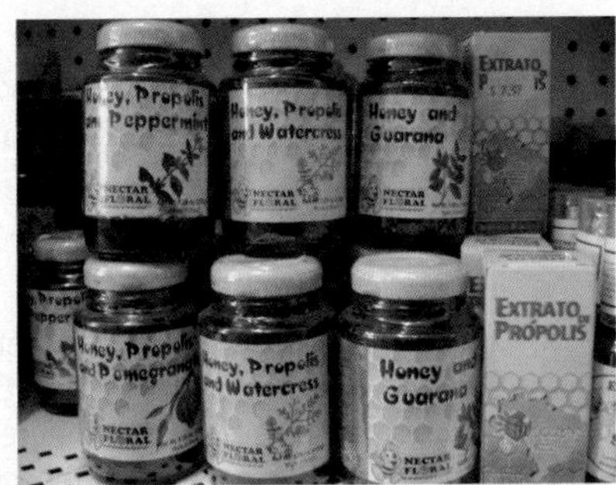

C

figure 10.1 **A:** Examples of herbs used for medicinal purposes, from Dominican botánica. *Clockwise, from bottom left*: mastuerso (vining nasturtium, spitfire, *Tropaeolum majus*)—used as an antimicrobial, source of vitamin C, and to fight coughs and colds; ajenjo (wormwood)—used against intestinal worms and for gallbladder maladies; tilo (linden)—used for anxiety, colds, hypertension, and fevers; guatapanal (divi-divi)—used against infections, especially of the tonsils, for hemorrhoids, and to dress sores. **B:** Medicinal teas for sale in a Brazilian store (Somerville, MA). Boldo (*Peumus boldus*)—for stomach and digestive ailments; Laxante—laxative; Hepatico—liver maladies. **C:** Honeys with medicinal supplements, Brazilian store (Somerville, MA).

Communication

Verbal Communication

Culture also has a significant impact on communication, in terms of verbal as well as nonverbal language, and style of communication. People's "unique cultural backgrounds and orientations have powerful influences on their communication practices that must be carefully accounted for in strategic health communication efforts" (Kreps & Sparks, 2008, p. 329). Clinical encounters should always be held in a language in which the client is fluent, and if interpretation is necessary, a professional interpreter should be used. Interpretation should never be conducted by family or friends of a client, except in emergencies. Use of family or friends as interpreters subverts privacy and confidentiality. Further, professional interpreters are not only fluent in both languages and technical healthcare terms; they are also trained in issues of ethics and cultural brokerage. "Cultural brokerage" means mediating an interaction between people of different cultures. A broker may point out and/or explain cultural differences to the participants, in order for the parties to understand each other better. A professional interpreter knows how and when to carefully add context, as opposed to invisibly translating word for word.

> **PRACTICE POINT**
>
> Lack of fluency in English implies nothing about a client's level of education. Bilingual nurses or those with professional interpreters can aim their teaching at the appropriate educational level for each client, regardless of the client's English language skills.

Nonverbal Communication

Nonverbal language also varies significantly with culture, and misinterpretation of body language can lead to clinical misunderstandings. Some examples are as follows:

- Eye contact: In many cultures (e.g., Native American, Chinese, Haitian), a younger client meeting the gaze of a clinician is a sign of disrespect. However, in other cultures (e.g., White American or German), eye contact is a necessary sign of respect. A clinician from those cultures might misinterpret lack of eye contact as signifying inattention, depression, or noncompliance.
- Personal space: Clients from cultures in which people normally stand close together (e.g., Italian, many Latin-American cultures) may feel that a nurse who sits or stands further away is cold and unfriendly. However, people from a Nordic-influenced culture may be more comfortable with larger spaces between people.

For clinical encounters with refugees and survivors of war or torture, the nurse should conduct interviews gently and pleasantly so that it does not seem like an interrogation. The client should feel in control, and the nurse should explain all procedures. Sometimes, medical devices or procedures reminiscent of healthcare practices are used in torture (shock, acid, excisions, sharps). Gynecologic procedures may invoke memories of rape or sexual assault, especially if the refugee has not had similar gynecologic care in the past. Also, it may be necessary to have interpretation needs more closely regulated by the client if he or she is a refugee of violence or war. The Yugoslav and the Rwandan conflicts of the 1990s, for instance, pitted people who spoke the same languages against each other, and a client may not feel safe with certain groups of people who speak their own language.

Style of Communication

Cultures are often described as communicating either linearly or nonlinearly. People from Western European and U.S. cultures generally favor direct narrations with a beginning, middle, and end (in that order). American medical and nursing cultures may be among the most linear and direct of all, with our emphasis on time efficiency and concise documentation. Many other cultures used nonlinear narratives, communicating ideas in more subtle and, arguably, more sophisticated ways. Interactions between clients from those cultures and U.S.-acculturated care providers can sometimes be jarring for the client and frustrating for the clinician.

Nilda might start explaining her symptoms with a story about her job back in Brazil, only coming slowly around to how this relates to her current condition. Although this could feel frustrating and ambiguous to Susan, Nilda is contextualizing her symptoms, albeit slowly, while also providing quite a bit more detailed information about herself and her illness. If Susan realizes that this style of communication is culturally valid and listens attentively, she may get much more helpful information about her client.

If time constraints on the part of the nurse interfere with giving individuals the culturally relevant time they need to explain their symptoms, what may be some creative options to support this style and use the time of the nurse wisely?

Time Orientation

Cross-cultural studies refer to "past-," "present-," and "future-oriented" cultures. Although this may be somewhat simplistic, it is true that different cultures do view time differently. For instance, northern European and White American-acculturated people tend to plan ahead, are time conscious, and behave in the present with an eye toward the future (Riley-Grimes, 2006). Some cultures, for instance many Native American ones, focus more on the past, consulting history to help make decisions now. Other cultures, such as agricultural-based ones, focus more on the present, meaning that people focus on the activity more than the clock (Galanti, 2006).

Differences in how people view time can create a clash of expectations in clinical encounters. For Anglo-American culture, for instance, time is thought of as linear and perishable. This is especially true in the healthcare world, in which time is considered a scarce commodity. In contrast, a Hispanic immigrant may view 10:00 AM as a suggested time for a clinic appointment and will arrive when other responsibilities are accomplished (Riley-Grimes, 2006). If this patient reports to the appointment at 11:00 AM, an Anglo-American provider is likely to view this negatively (MacDuff, 2006). It is also necessary to consider a client's orientation to time when teaching about medication dosing.

When Susan tells Nilda to "take your medication at the same time every day" she may mean to take it when the clock says 8:00 AM every day, whereas Nilda may infer that anytime between 5:00 and 11:00 AM is OK, because *morning* is the "same time every day."

Can you think of some creative ways to make Susan's message clear to Nilda?

EVIDENCE FOR PRACTICE

Researchers in the United Kingdom examined homelessness using transcultural nursing theory and found several ideas and strategies for nurses caring for homeless patients (Law & John, 2012). The literature indicates that homeless individuals tend to be oriented strongly toward the present. The researchers noted that this group tends to be extremely resourceful, but focuses on survival and not planning for future events. Further, fatalism is common in this group, perhaps related to difficulties in controlling their environments, and can suppress efforts to improve health.

Roles

Cultures around the world have different expectations of the roles of children, young adults, and elderly adults; of men versus women; and of the role of a sick person. For instance, some children speak for themselves, others are taught to remain silent. In some cultures, such as American and British ones, a sick person makes decisions for themselves; in others, such as many Asian and Latin-American ones, the family makes treatment decisions as a group. Some cultures expect difficult prognoses and test results to be discussed with the family first and the patient later, if at all, which explicitly conflicts with the U.S. values of confidentiality and autonomy.

PRACTICE POINT

No matter what culture your clients are from, you want to know what roles they fulfill at home or in their families, because that will affect the significance of their illness and treatment in their lives. For instance, many clients are the primary caregivers in their families, and an illness may have ramifications in their family or community, or in the patient's own sense of self, that might not be immediately apparent to you.

Religion

One central facet of culture is religion, and this also directly affects health, illness, and treatment (Fig. 10.2). Some religions attribute disease to divine forces, for instance. Some cultures are relatively fatalistic, affecting health behaviors (Franklin et al., 2007). *Insha'Allah* ("if God wills") is a common refrain for many Muslims, although they may mean it more or less literally. Some congregations practice faith healing and may reject secular treatment plans. Prayer and other religious practices can also amicably complement nursing interventions. Prayers, especially for a client who believes in a supportive god, may be advantageous to health (Hollywell & Walker, 2009). Indian yoga and Chinese Tai Chi are popular health promotion practices that grew out of ancient religious traditions.

All religions have traditions and rituals around death and dying, and although an individual client and family may or

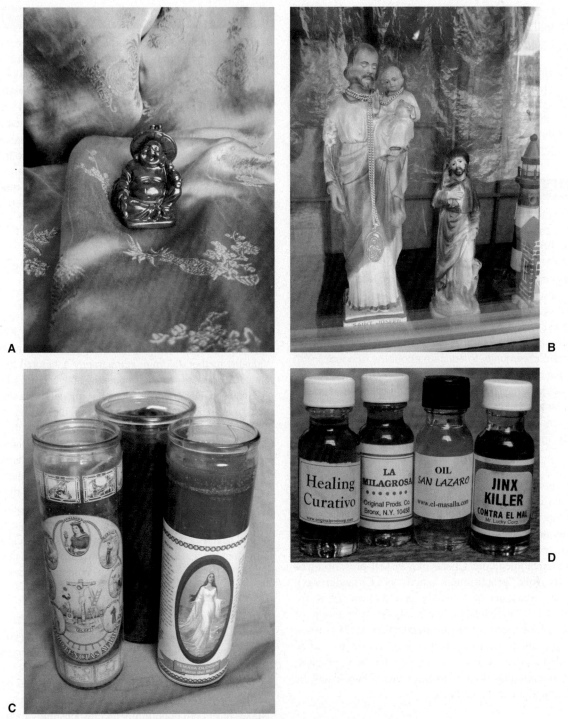

figure 10.2 Religion and spirituality bear directly on health, illness, and treatment. **A:** Buddha statuette, from Puerto Rican botánica (Boston, MA). **B:** Saints, Italian storefront (Somerville, MA). **C:** Candelas from a Boston supermarket. *Left to right:* Siete Potencias Africanas—seven African powers; black candle—against negative spirits; Yamaya Olocun—the ocean goddess Yamaya. **D:** Spiritual remedial oils from a Caribbean botánica (Boston, MA). *Left to right:* Healing Curativo—healing curative; La Milagrosa—the miracle; Oil San Lazaro—Saint Lazarus oil; Jinx Killer Contra El Mal—Jinx killer against evil.

may not desire traditional practices, culture has a tremendous impact on end-of-life issues (Irish, Lundquist, & Nelsen, 2014). The nursing process has a history of acknowledging and incorporating some spiritual interventions, although most nurses could learn more about specific religious beliefs. In a nursing home that serves mostly Jewish clients, for instance, the nurses learn the Jewish death ritual of washing the body after death so that they are ready to do so if the family requests it. Buddhist monks, who come to chant for dying people, may join hospice nurses who serve Burmese clients, or a Hindu family may request that a deceased patient be constantly attended until and after the body leaves the hospital.

If Nilda belongs to a Christian denomination that believes that God regulates health and illness, she may be less likely to make changes in her own health behaviors, such as getting a colposcopy and subsequent Pap smears.

EVIDENCE FOR PRACTICE

To understand how one subculture in New Jersey uses mercury, researchers conducted an ethnographic study, interviewing 22 medical supply store employees and practitioners of Santeria, an Afro-Cuban religion with many adherents in eastern U.S. cities (Newby, Riley, & Leal-Almeraz, 2006). They investigated and described various ways that the religious practitioners used elemental mercury, known as *azogue* in Spanish, which becomes a neurotoxin if inhaled. The authors recommended working closely with the Santero community to educate about the dangers and routes of exposure, especially encouraging the use of closed containers. The researchers emphasize the need to not alienate this community, which has been misunderstood and sometimes vilified by mainstream American authority figures.

Folk Medicine

Herbs and other home remedies are used in every culture around the world (Fig. 10.3). However, some folk healing traditions are currently more robust, whereas others were marginalized in the 20th century with the dominance of professional biomedicine. Clients may be self-prescribing or going to folk practitioners such as Curandero(as), Santero(as), Shamans, or Ayurvedic practitioners. There are myriads of folk remedies a client might be using, some of which can have very powerful effects (Box 10.1). Just as nurses ask about over-the-counter medication use, they should also inquire, respectfully, about what other preparations or nonpharmacologic strategies their clients may be using to maintain or regain health.

box 10.1 **Examples of Folk Remedies and Healing Practices**

Foods	Herbs	Methods
Chicken soup	Comfrey	Coining
Garlic	Ginger	Cupping
Ginger tea	Ginseng	Exorcism
Honey	Lavender	Holy candle burning
Lemon	Rosemary	Massage
Pepper	St. John's wort	Protective jewelry

EVIDENCE FOR PRACTICE

Health researchers conducted a systematic review of the literature to investigate the prevalence of medicinal herbs (or "botanicals") by racial and/or ethnic minorities in the United States (Gardiner et al., 2013). They reviewed 108 studies and found that African-Americans used herbs for health reasons at a rate of 17%, 30% of Hispanics and 30% of Asians used botanicals, although regional and smaller studies tended to find higher rates of use than did national or larger studies. Patients were using herbs for cancer, menopause, diabetes, arthritis, and HIV-related diseases, and many groups rarely disclosed their herb use to their healthcare providers.

CULTURAL HEALTH ASSESSMENT

Individual Clinicians

There are several ways to approach cultural health assessment. Kleinman and Benson (2006) recommend using Kleinman's explanatory models. These researchers prefer using this individualist method (a "mini ethnography"), tailored to each client, as opposed to the concept of generalized cultural competence. Kleinman's explanatory models are a set of questions that explore the clients' view of illness and treatment, including what they think caused it, how serious they think it is, and what they fear about it. These questions can often uncover cultural ideas that the provider would not otherwise have known. They may also show, of course, that the client views his or her illness and treatment much the same way as the provider does. Shellenberger et al. (2007) suggest using a cultural genogram to explore and illustrate how a client's heritage affects his or her health perspectives. Whatever method is chosen, it is important to create an atmosphere that encourages the client to tell his or her own story, with all its cultural nuances.

Healthcare Organizations

As mentioned above, it is also imperative that healthcare organizations such as hospitals and visiting nurses agencies conduct ongoing cultural assessments of their service areas. Racher and Annis (2007) write that "creating spaces for voices to be heard and groups to be represented produces opportunities to break down resistance and facilitate social change. Nurses have both opportunity and responsibility to take action in creating such spaces." The Office of Minority Health (2013) recommends that healthcare organizations "[c]onduct regular assessments of community health assets and needs and use the results to plan and implement services that respond to the cultural and linguistic diversity of populations in the service area."

Cultural competence requires ongoing self-assessment by both individual nurses and by healthcare organizations. "Self-assessment by organizations builds . . . commitment to be inclusive, open, and progressive in meeting the needs of clients from different cultures. Nurses are advocates and resources for this work" (Racher & Annis, 2007, p. 268).

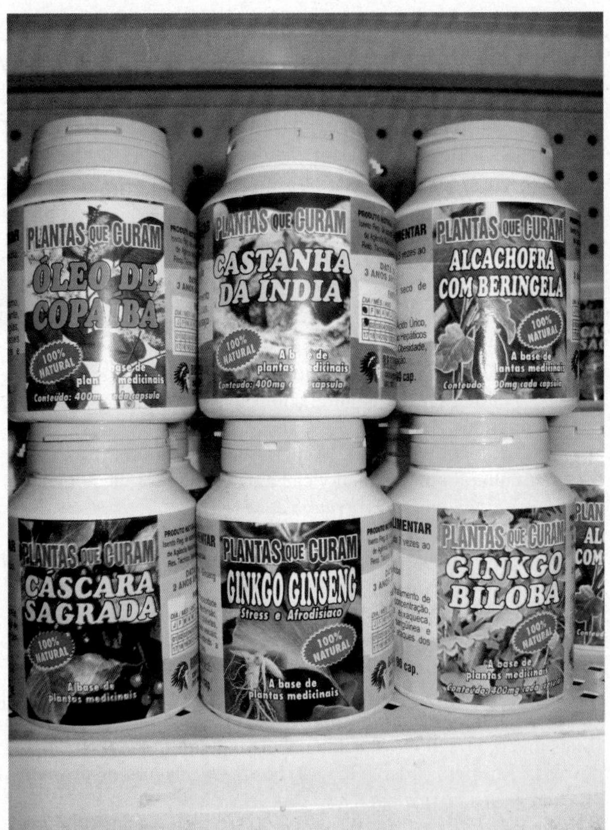

A

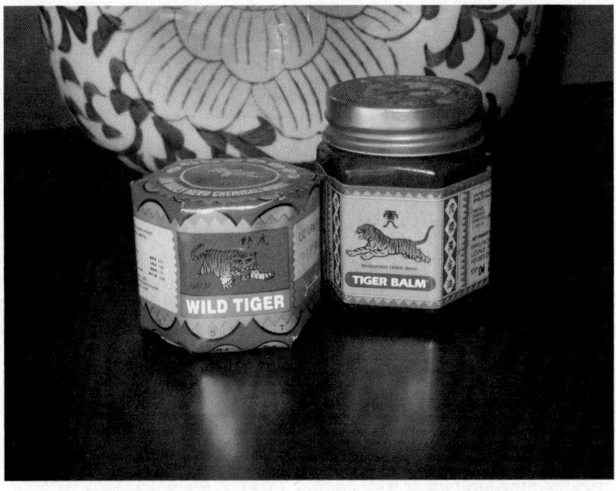

B

figure 10.3 **A:** Supplements for sale in a Brazilian store (Somerville, MA). Óleo de Copa'ba—anti-inflammatory and antimicrobial; Canstanha da India—astringent, analgesic, vasoconstrictor, and anti-inflammatory; Alcachofra com Beringela—problems of the liver and gallbladder as well as diabetes and high cholesterol; Cáscara Sagrada—laxative; Ginkgo Ginseng—(thought to have) numerous beneficial effects; *Ginkgo biloba*—circulation and memory aid. **B:** Tiger balm from Vietnamese store (Boston, MA). Tiger balm, applied topically, is used for muscle strains and soreness as well as for respiratory congestion.

key concepts

- Culture is dynamic, shared, and learned.
- "Cultural competence" is an attitude of openness to, respect for, and curiosity about different cultural values and traditions, and ideally includes a broader critical analysis of power relations affecting health disparities. For community health nurses, it necessitates familiarizing oneself with (and continuing to learn about in an ongoing way) cultures that are represented in the communities they serve. In this way, "culture" could mean a national culture (e.g., Vietnamese or Honduran culture), a religious culture (e.g., Jewish culture), the culture of homelessness, a school's culture, or that of any other subculture. A narrow view of cultural competence risks "not understanding how broader social, economic, political, and environmental variables affect the nurse-client encounter or how situational factors influence health-seeking behaviors. It is often the macrolevel factors that affect health disparities more than the nurse-client encounter does" (Lipson & DeSantis, 2007).
- Advocates for groups that have been sociopolitically marginalized promote "cultural safety," the ideal of considering cultural aspects of groups while working against assimilation and repression.
- "Cultural humility" is an acknowledgment that *everyone's* views are culturally influenced, that our own are not inherently better than those of our clients, and that our clients can teach us.
- Ethnocentrism can be defined as an assumption that everyone shares your cultural values, or an opinion that your culture is superior to others.
- Subcultures, or smaller subgroups of a larger society, have characteristics in common that may impact health beliefs or practices.

critical thinking questions

1. Do you think that the notion of cultural competence risks stereotyping? If so, how, and if not, why not?
2. How can nurses strive for cultural competence without pigeonholing or prejudging clients?
3. What are some of the main cultural groups in the region or city in which you live? What are some of the smaller cultural groups in your city or region?
4. Think for a while about cultural practices and how they affect health or illness in your own family. They may be difficult to identify as such at first, but they do exist. What ideas about illness prevention does your family adhere to? What do you do when someone gets sick? What rituals does your family practice when someone dies?

references

Alverson, H. S., Drake, R. E., Carpenter-Song, E. A., Chu, E., Ritsema, M., & Smith, B. (2007). Ethnocultural variations in mental illness discourse: Some implications for building therapeutic alliances. *Psychiatric Services*, *58*(12), 1541–1546.

American Anthropological Association. (2007). *Race project*. Retrieved from http://www.understandingrace.org/humvar/race_humvar.html

Beach, M. C., Price, E. G., Gary, T. L., Robinson, K. A., Gozu, A., Palacio, A., . . . Cooper, L. A. (2005). Cultural competence: A systematic review of health care provider educational interventions. *Medical Care*, *43*(4), 356–373.

Bearskin, R. L. B. (2011). A critical lens on culture in nursing practice. *Nursing ethics, 18*(4), 548–559.

Braun, L. (2006). Reifying human difference: The debate on genetics, race, and health. *International Journal of Health Services*, *36*(3), 557–573.

Brondolo, E., Libretti, M., Rivera, L., & Walsemann, K. M. (2012). Racism and social capital: The implications for social and physical well-being. *Journal of Social Issues*, *68*(2), 358–384.

Carpenter-Song, E. A., Schwallie, M. N., & Longhofer, J. (2007). Cultural competence reexamined: Critique and directions for the future. *Psychiatric Services*, *58*(10), 1362–1365.

Culley, L. (2006). Transcending transculturalism? Race, ethnicity and health-care. *Nursing Inquiry*, *13*(2), 144–153.

Franklin, M. D., Schlundt, D. G., McClellan, L. H., Kinebrew, T., Sheats, J., Belue, R., . . . Hargreaves, M. (2007). Religious fatalism and its association with health behaviors and outcomes. *American Journal of Health Behaviors*, *31*(6), 563–572.

Galanti, G.-A. (2006). Applying cultural competence to perianesthesia nursing. *Journal of Perianesthesia Nursing*, *21*(2), 97–102.

Gardiner, P., Whelan, J., White, L. F., Filippelli, A. C., Bharmal, N., & Kaptchuk, T. J. (2013). A systematic review of the prevalence of herb usage among racial/ethnic minorities in the United States. *Journal of Immigrant and Minority Health*, *15*(4), 817–828.

Giger, J., Davidhizar, R. E., Purnell, L., Harden, J. T., Phillips, J., & Strickland, O. (2007). American Academy of Nursing Expert Panel report: Developing cultural competence to eliminate health disparities in ethnic minorities and other vulnerable populations. *Journal of Transcultural Nursing*, *18*(2), 95–102.

Glass, T. A. (2006). Commentary: Culture in epidemiology—The 800 pound gorilla? *International Journal of Epidemiology*, *35*(2), 259–261.

Hollywell, C., & Walker, J. (2009). Private prayer as a suitable intervention for hospitalized patients: A critical review of the literature. *Journal of Clinical Nursing*, *18*(5), 637–651.

Irish, D., Lundquist, K. & Nelsen, V., eds. (2014). *Ethnic variations in dying, death and grief: Diversity in universality.* Taylor & Francis.

Kleinman, A., & Benson, P. (2006). Anthropology in the clinic: The problem of cultural competency and how to fix it. *Public Library of Science Medicine*, *3*(10), e294.

Kreps, G. L., & Sparks, L. (2008). Meeting the health literacy needs of immigrant populations. *Patient Education and Counseling*, *71*(3), 328–332.

Kumas-Tan, Z., Beagan, B., Loppie, C., MacLeod, A., & Frank, B. (2007). Measures of cultural competence: Examining hidden assumptions. *Academic Medicine*, *82*(6), 548–557.

Law, K., & John, W. (2012). Homelessness as culture: How transcultural nursing theory can assist caring for the homeless. *Nurse Education in Practice, 12*, 371–374.

Leininger, M. (2002). Culture care theory: A major contribution to advance transcultural nursing knowledge and practices. *Journal of Transcultural Nursing*, *13*(3), 189–192.

Lipson, J. G., & DeSantis, L. A. (2007). Current approaches to integrating elements of cultural competence in nursing education. *Journal of Transcultural Nursing*, *18*(1), 10S–20S.

MacDuff, I. (2006). Your pace or mine? Culture, time, and negotiation. *Negotiation Journal*, *22*(1), 31–45.

Matsumoto, D. (2009). Teaching about culture. In R. A. R. Gurung, & L. R. Prieto (Eds.), *Getting culture: Incorporating diversity across the curriculum*. New York, NY: Stylus.

Mboho, M., Furber, C. & Waterman, H. (2013). Social-cultural practices and beliefs influencing maternal mortality. *African Journal of Midwifery and Women's Health, 7*(1), DOI: http://dx.doi.org/10.12968/ajmw.2013.7.1.26

Nam, S., Song, H.-J., Park, S.-Y., & Song, Y. (2013). Challenges of diabetes management in immigrant Korean Americans. *The Diabetes Educator*, *39*(2), 213–221.

National Center for Cultural Competence. (2008). *Cultural competence: Definition and conceptual framework*. Retrieved from http://nccc.georgetown.edu/foundations/frameworks.html

Newby, C. A., Riley, D. M., & Leal-Almeraz, T. O. (2006). Mercury use and exposure among Santeria practitioners: Religious versus folk practice in northern New Jersey, USA. *Ethnicity and Health*, *11*(3), 287–306.

Racher, F. E., & Annis, R. C. (2007). Respecting culture and honoring diversity in community practice. *Research & Theory for Nursing Practice*, *21*(4), 255–270.

Riley-Grimes, A. (2006). Scheduling havoc? Or time orientation and culture? *AMT Events*, *23*(1), 12–13.

Roberts, T. M. E. (2004). Healthcare experiences of Brazilians residing in Massachusetts: An ethnographic study (Doctoral dissertation, Boston College). *Dissertation Abstracts International*, *65*, 2871.

Rosaldo, R. (1993). *Culture & truth: The remaking of social analysis*. Boston, MA: Beacon Press.

Shellenberger, S., Dent, M. M., Davis-Smith, M., Seale, P. J., Weintraut, R., & Wright, T. (2007). Cultural genogram: A tool for teaching and practice. *Families, Systems, & Health*, *25*(4), 367–381.

United States Department of Health and Human Services. (2013). *National Healthcare Disparities Report, 2010* (AHRQ Publication No. 10-0004). Rockville, MD: Agency for Healthcare Research and Quality. Retrieved from http://www.ahrq.gov/research/findings/nhqrdr/nhdr10/

United States Department of Health and Human Services, Office of Minority Health. (2013). Retrieved from http://minorityhealth.hhs.gov/templates/browse.aspx?lvl=2&lvlID=15

web resources

Please visit thePoint® for up-to-date Web resources on this topic.

CHAPTER 11

Community Assessment

Rosanna DeMarco and Mary M. Segraves

Never doubt that a small group of thoughtful, committed citizens can change the world. Indeed, it is the only thing that ever has.

Margaret Mead

One of the signs of passing youth is the birth of a sense of fellowship with other human beings as we take our place among them.

Virginia Woolf

I don't even know what street Canada is on.

Al Capone

chapter highlights

- Components of a community assessment
- Defining a community
- Frameworks of community assessment
- Different approaches to community assessment

objectives

- Define and describe types of communities.
- Describe the process of a community assessment.
- Identify biologic, psychological, and sociocultural indicators of community health.
- Conduct a systematic community assessment using a specific framework or a combination of frameworks.
- Explain how community health nurses can affect change within a community based on conclusions drawn from assessment.

key terms

Asset-based assessment: Attention is directed to community strengths and resources as a primary approach to community assessment.

Collaborative models: An approach to assessment that begins with planning that includes representative parties of a population, including service organizations, corporations, and government officials.

Community: A group of people sharing common interests, needs, resources, and environment; an interrelating and interacting group of people with shared needs and interests.

Community as partner: Within the process of community assessment, considering the expertise of community dwellers as central to the task of understanding the health and well-being of the community.

Developmental model: A retrospective, historical analysis of system parameters such as the physical environment, education, safety and transportation, politics and government, health and social services, communication, economics, and recreation in a community.

Epidemiologic model: A process used to assess a community using data collected from descriptions and statistical relationships to evaluate the level of health and well-being within a community to address identified healthcare needs.

Framework: A model or a road map that assists the direction toward a goal.

Functional health pattern: A systematic and deliberate approach to community assessment, evaluating patterns of behaviors of community dwellers that occur sequentially across time.

Geopolitical community: Group of people who live within identified boundaries and governing systems.

Phenomenologic community: Group of people who have interpersonal and intrapersonal connections.

Windshield survey: Observation of a community while driving a car or riding public transportation to collect data for a community assessment.

Understanding the interactions between people, health, and environment is a primary concern of nursing practice. Community assessment has been called a critical process for the future which can be used as a means for understanding these interactions, as well as for finding a way to improve both the health status of at-risk populations, and outreach activities. Most recently, we have seen the value of community assessment as a key contributor to advancing humanitarian aid to communities in times of emergency need (Kirsch et al., 2012). In addition to providing information that is essential to understanding the community, community assessment allows for critical thinking about its strengths, weaknesses, assets, and

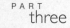

Case Study

References to the case study are found throughout this chapter (look for the case study icon). Readers should keep the case study in mind as they read the chapter.

In many circumstances, communities undertake in-depth assessments to understand what the needs of the community may be and how members of the community who have ways of assisting (health, business, religious, mental health, policing agencies, for example) can be part of a solution for the needs that are uncovered. Some recent examples of this approach include (1) a health foundation using participation of community dwellers to understand the health needs of the community (Williams, Bray, Shapiro-Mendoza, Reisz, & Peranteau, 2009); (2) healthcare providers evaluating barriers to colorectal cancer screening in high-risk populations (Patel et al., 2012); and (3) community leaders against violence evaluating threat assessment related to mental health indicators of potential violence in communities (Interdisciplinary Group on Preventing School and Community Violence, 2013).

Similarly, a classic example of a detailed, step-by-step assessment undertaken more than 10 years ago used a report card approach to assessment. The population of San Diego County is the second largest in California and the fourth largest in the United States. The 2.7 million residents represent diverse racial and ethnic backgrounds, and present many challenges to those providing public health and social services. Many recent social changes, such as welfare reform, managed care, and restructuring of healthcare services, have affected healthcare delivery in the region. The San Diego County Board of Supervisors, along with members of the community, wanted to know what impact these changes might have on the health and well-being of children and families. To address this issue, the board ordered that a monitoring system be developed, and the San Diego County Child and Family Health and Well-Being Report Card was created to monitor community-level outcomes.

The San Diego Health and Human Services Agency (HHSA), which was in the process of creating performance measures for its operations, partnered with Children's Hospital and Health Center in San Diego to develop the components of the community "report card." There were five key stages of development:

- An evaluation of other community report cards
- A literature review
- An extensive community information–gathering process
- Reviews by technical and community advisory groups and a national consultant
- Final approval from the board

The resulting report card reflected a broad definition of health and well-being. Data sources ranged from local health, education, and law enforcement entities to state and federal agencies. Included were 3 to 5 years of historical data, state and national comparative data, and, where available, race/ethnicity data. Compilation of these comprehensive statistics created a population-based, data-driven monitoring system (Simmes, Blaszcak, Kurtin, Bowen, & Ross, 2000).

deficits. Whenever nurses conduct an assessment of a community, they examine biologic, psychological, and sociocultural influences of the environment of a group of people who share specific characteristics. Initially, the idea of conducting a community assessment might seem overwhelming. However, knowledge gained from this endeavor provides valuable insight into the ways that people's health behaviors directly and indirectly influence the overall health and well-being in their community.

A man of a right spirit is not a man of narrow and private views, but is greatly interested and concerned for the good of the community to which he belongs, and particularly of the city or village in which he resides, and for the true welfare of the society of which he is a member.

Edgar Allan Poe

In examining the San Diego case study, we can see that many people representing many groups needed to be identified, be organized with a particular mission, and then be encouraged to work together to establish key indicators that eventually became a report card for health in their community. The information obtained can then be used to design health programs to address the needs that were identified from the assessment data. Thus, the effort has a very practical and important end.

The principles of epidemiology that are described in Chapter 6 provide a valuable framework to begin community assessment. In addition, information about communities can be expanded beyond the context of community health nursing and applied to others areas of nursing practice. This chapter defines communities and identifies a variety of methods and tools that can be used to assess communities. Community assessment is a comprehensive evaluation of the status of a community. It identifies vulnerable populations, determines unmet needs, and documents community resources. The information is then used to set goals, plan programs for intervention, and evaluate outcomes. The approach that is used for community assessment depends on

box 11.1 How to Complete a Community Assessment

1. Establish a working group, including community members.
2. Define the composition of the community.
3. Identify the information that needs to be collected.
4. Identify an organizing framework for collecting data.
5. Use existing data to describe the community's strengths and weakness, assets, and liabilities.
   - Collect demographic data from national, state, county, and city or town from the Internet.
   - Collect local data from libraries, service organizations, municipal records, newspapers, phonebooks, and other local sources.
6. Gather new data as necessary.
   - Community forums
   - Focus groups
   - Key informants
   - Participant observation
   - Surveys
7. Analyze the data, looking for similarities, differences, and inconsistencies.
8. Develop a profile of the community.
9. Identify vulnerable populations, unmet needs, resources, and unique characteristics.
10. Outline a plan for intervention based on findings.
11. Prepare a report and disseminate it to others.
12. Design, implement, and evaluate a project based on findings.

the type and characteristics of community. Most frameworks described will be feasible for the assessment of geopolitical communities, yet using some frameworks with phenomenologic communities or specific aggregates can present challenges. When data are collected, combinations of frameworks can be integrated if it makes sense. The methods of community assessment that will be described are all useful but are not equally appropriate in all settings.

Community assessment is an integral function that supports all aspects of nursing practice. The approaches to assessment that will be described provide a foundation to develop and implement interventions that build and maintain healthy communities. Although community assessment presents some challenges, the information yielded from the assessment is invaluable in accomplishing health-related goals. Within the context of a greater healthcare team, and with the community members as partners, a community assessment assists community health nurses to maintain wellness and prevent illness in a population. An overview of the community assessment process is found in Box 11.1.

DEFINING THE COMMUNITY AND ITS BOUNDARIES

Geopolitical Communities

The word **community** has several meanings that are relevant to the process of assessment. Community can be a group of people who live in the same area, or can be the area in which they live. Types of communities that commonly come to mind are municipalities or townships with identifiable geographic or other designated boundaries. These communities may be cities, towns, neighborhoods, or locales. A community that is described as a specific area, possessing geographic boundaries and sharing the same governing structure, is often called a **geopolitical community**.

The group of people, or an *aggregate* as it is often called in the literature, consists of those who live within the boundary of the geopolitical community. However, these borders are really ambiguous. The aggregate could also include people who work within the community but who do not necessarily live there and could include those living close to community boundaries who visit the communities to purchase goods or use facilities for nonwork activities.

PRACTICE POINT

Seek data about people who funnel in and out of the community. These are often overlooked by students who are trying to understand who constitutes the community. Local town or city employment data may direct you to companies that employ large numbers of people. For example, most of the population from a metropolitan area may work for three or four large corporations. By approaching these corporations, you can find data about employee residence. Interviewing some employees may tell you where they are receiving healthcare. In addition, you may identify these peoples' concerns related to their health and well-being while working for this particular corporation.

EVIDENCE FOR PRACTICE

A community health education center, which was affiliated with an academic institution, recognized that a way to invest in the professional development of students was to develop a project called "Creating Community Connections." This project was designed to characterize the evolving community landscape following Hurricane Katrina while providing opportunities for students to engage in experiential learning. Students in the project gained skills in program planning and community assessment, as well as in leadership and communications. Twenty-three students worked on the project during its 2 years, developing data-collection tools, organizing and conducting key informant interviews, facilitating focus groups and community forums, managing data, and summarizing project findings for community presentations. Participation in this project allowed our students to grow as public health leaders and researchers while gaining a greater appreciation for community collaboration (Martin, Cunningham, & Magnus 2011).

Phenomenologic Communities

Another way to understand or describe a community is to think of it as a group of persons who share common interests or beliefs. For example, neighbors interested in enhancing their property to maintain the unique qualities of a neighborhood have a common interest but not necessarily a formal organizational structure, whereas members of a church congregation do have a formal structure and interests that bind them together. The term **phenomenologic community** (Smith & Maurer, 2009) refers to members of a community with common interests who have interpersonal and intrapersonal connections. Community members share common interests, beliefs, or goals, and together they identify what activities, structures, and outcomes are meaningful specifically to them. Phenomenologic communities frequently exist within a geopolitical community, although their borders are often less well defined. Examples of phenomenologic communities include groups such as the homeless or persons with disabilities.

Phenomenologic communities also include groups that are referred to as "communities of solution" (Smith & Maurer, 2009). A community of solution is formed by an aggregate specifically to address health concerns within a particular area. Communities of solution are not only composed of persons from the area of need, but also include members of neighboring communities who have a vested interest in a challenge the community faces. These communities can form in response to a health threat, such as contaminated water or industrial air pollution. Other examples include certain political action groups or the formation of ad hoc task force groups.

Underserved populations can also be regarded as a phenomenologic community. Social connections between members are likely to be loose and not integrated, and without an organized structure. Often, members of these aggregates are disenfranchised in many ways. Also, members of these communities might be included within other larger groups. Examples are undocumented immigrants, women living with HIV/AIDS, or teens at risk for being involved in violent crimes.

I would never belong to a group that would accept someone like me as a member.

Groucho Marx

STUDENT REFLECTION

One of the most rewarding things I have realized is that my dormitory floor could be a community of solution. I was very concerned for a long time about the drinking behavior of some of the students who lived around me. Three students got drunk beyond belief after a hockey game one week and pulled a fire alarm in the dorms to be funny. All of them were suspended. I talked with some of the students on the floor about this, and we began to plan how we could try to address this situation. The first step involved obtaining accurate information about the rate and severity of the drinking behavior on the floor, what was causing the behavior, and how the behavior compared to that on other floors and to the campus as a whole. It was really interesting to see how many of us banded together out of concern and shared the same valued concerns about the well-being of our colleagues and ourselves while attending school.

EVIDENCE FOR PRACTICE

The topic of this research report was the role of promotoras (health promoters in Spanish language) briefly trained in depression care at community health centers. Community assessment revealed the need to understand and develop interventions within the world of those living in the community. The intervention focused on four contextual sources of depression in underserved, low-income communities: underemployment, inadequate housing, food insecurity, and violence. A multimethod design included quantitative and ethnographic techniques to study predictors of depression. A community assessment was completed to evaluate the intervention's impact. On the basis of an intake interview, 120 patients with depression were randomly assigned to enhanced care plus the promotora contextual intervention, or to enhanced care alone. All four contextual problems emerged as strong predictors of depression (χ^2, $p < 0.05$). Logistic regression revealed housing and food insecurity as the most important predictors (odds ratios (ORs) both 2.40, $p < 0.05$). Research that assessed both ethnic and geographic factors demonstrated a predominantly positive response to the intervention among stakeholders, which included patients, promotoras, primary care practioners (PCPs), nonprofessional staff workers, administrators, and community advisory board members (Waitzkin et al., 2011).

EVIDENCE FOR PRACTICE

To understand differences and similarities in demographics, health, and healthcare access in Chinese and Vietnamese adults, this study used a cross-sectional participatory community health assessment in an urban city in Massachusetts. The researchers collected qualitative data from community stakeholders to create a community health assessment tool that addressed information on healthcare access, health status, behavioral health, and chronic disease history and treatment. Areas of concern were issues of healthcare access and poor health status, particularly among Chinese participants, and mental health symptomotology in both groups. These findings revealed important health concerns in two Asian ethnic groups. Studies like this one are needed to better understand these concerns and inform programs and policies to improve health outcomes in these Asian ethnic groups and other groups (Tendulkar et al., 2012).

Societal, National, or International Communities

In its broadest context, community is used to describe society in general, or a nation. For example, U.S. citizens have a common federal government and share ideals, whereas individual communities within the country have different state and local governments and priorities in relation to individual needs and interests. Recently, however, references have been made to the international community or global community, which encompasses nations outside the United States. Although the overall composition of these communities may differ, some have strikingly similar characteristics, with shared interests and goals, including members' health and safety. To continue to advance the goals of health and safety, there must be a thorough way of understanding each of the communities described, especially if nurses are to accurately target ways to address goals for change. The first step in any plan to help a community is to assess the community's needs. These needs should be assessed in multiple ways.

PRACTICE POINT

Different navigational techniques have evolved over the ages in different cultures, but all involve locating one's position compared to known locations. Patterns are derived from multiple perspectives. Triangulation, which comes from navigation methodology, is defined as the process of planning, recording, and controlling the movement of a craft or vehicle from one place to another. Specifically, triangulation involves finding coordinates and distance to a point by calculating the length of one side of a triangle, using measurements of angles and sides of the triangle formed by that point, and two other known reference points. In summary, triangulation is the use of multiple methods or perspectives to collect and interpret data about some phenomenon, and is used to come together for an accurate representation of reality (Grove, Burns, & Gray, 2013). In other words, whenever you are trying to find an accurate answer to a question you may have about a community, consider looking at the question in different ways or finding more than one way to address it.

The amorphous nature of the community can create some challenges to the identification of its members and to the assessment of their immediate needs. In thinking about the nursing process, the initial phase of gathering data to develop a diagnosis, problem statement, or challenge needs to be addressed. Establishing goals, objectives, and key interventions seems formidable if nurses do not consider how they are defining the community that is to be assessed.

What type of community was described **in the case study** about San Diego? Was more than one type of community represented? If so, what kinds? How did the working group define who was and who was not a member of the community?

STUDENT REFLECTION

I was scared to death when trying to figure out how to complete my community assessment assignment. However, after a while I realized how exciting it was to feel like a private investigator on a quest of trying to solve a problem (i.e., figuring out the truth about the health of the community in which I was serving: elders in their homes). After I was able to understand where to look for health information data on the Internet and in city records, what I really liked was interviewing members of the community about what they thought about living in this city, what was good about it, and what was not so good. After a while, I was able to take all sorts of information I had found and merge it together—like finding hidden pieces of a jigsaw puzzle. What really helped me was organizing a plan of how to do this, and what areas I wanted to investigate, into a priority list. It was a really cool assignment.

How community health nurses conduct a community assessment varies depending on the overall purpose of the assessment. Each setting, and those who are part of the setting, defines the context within which a plan can be developed. The plan should include appropriate ways to access and assess data, validate the findings, and develop a plan to address challenges, and include a plan to evaluate interventions that are instituted.

Often, community assessments are related to a specific practice setting. Some examples of an assessment in a school setting might include the following:

- Learning about the outbreak of a specific communicable infectious disease (lice)
- Learning about healthcare practices associated with a specific chronic disease (asthma)
- Learning how best to protect children and adolescents, as well as their families, from the spread of infectious disease in a school setting

Therefore, school health nurses must be familiar with information about the disease, such as the organism that causes it, incubation periods, mode of transmission, symptoms, protective measures, and necessary treatment.

Knowing these parameters helps these nurses devise a plan to assess the numbers of students and family members who may have symptoms of a disease, and to identify those who are at risk for acquiring the infection. The school nurse can then assist them in understanding how they can care for themselves or access resources. The evidence that follows is an example of the principles and processes of gathering health-related information related to obesity, and an intervention to address this issue in children.

EVIDENCE FOR PRACTICE

This study evaluated a school nurse–delivered intervention in improving diet and activity, and in reducing body mass index (BMI) among overweight and obese adolescents. Six high schools were randomly assigned to either a six-session, school nurse–delivered counseling intervention that utilized cognitive–behavioral techniques or contact with a nurse who provided information. Eighty-four overweight or obese adolescents in grades 9 through 11 completed behavioral and physiologic assessments at baseline and at 2- and 6-month follow-ups. At 2 months, participants who received the counseling intervention ate breakfast on more days per week (difference = 1.01 days; 95% CI: 0.11, 1.92) and had a lower intake of total sugar (difference = −45.79 g; 95% CI: −88.34, −3.24) and added sugar (difference = −51.35 g; 95% CI: −92.45, −10.26), compared to control participants. At 6 months, they were more likely to drink soda once a day or less frequently (OR: 4.10; 95% CI: 1.19, 16.93) and eat at fast food restaurants once a week or less frequently (OR: 4.62; 95% CI: 1.10, 23.76) compared to control participants. There were no significant differences in BMI, activity, or caloric intake (Pbert et al., 2013).

EVIDENCE FOR PRACTICE

One study (Wheeler, Merkle, Gerald, & Taggart 2006) involved how school nurses could develop a coalition between clinicians and students to design a true collaborative solution which addresses asthma as a common and proliferating problem in school children. School nurses caring for children with asthma learned five key lessons that are examples of what these nurses need to assess when considering how to plan for the needs of these children in their school community.

- Establish strong links with asthma clinicians. Self-management helps decrease morbidity, but without ongoing follow-up and communication and coordination with clinicians in the community, student care becomes inconsistent.
- Target students who are most affected by asthma and airway disease related to asthma. Addressing poorly controlled asthma is more practical in terms of time and economics than case-finding. School nurses should assess their school community for those children with high absence rates and large numbers of school nurse visits because of asthmas attacks.
- Identify an appropriate mix of resources, which should include an asthma champion at the school, appropriate school nurse staffing, and the involvement of parents.
- Use a collaborative approach, which is critical. Collaboration in this sense means identifying environmental sources or asthma triggers, such as mold, by working with community members who may be contributing to the source of the problem.
- Support evaluating this combination of efforts by measuring outcomes.

This approach allows for adjustment and readjustment of interventions to make the outcomes more successful over time.

Assessments made by community health nurses are often informal. They use the **windshield survey** to learn about the neighborhoods in which their clients live. Many community health providers use this method, but it has its limitations. It is a subjective process which nurses may use to understand the community by viewing surroundings. It is a descriptive way of understanding what appears to be the physical expression of the community as it is viewed on foot or through the windshield of a car. Anderson and McFarlane (2008) suggest that a community assessment can be accomplished this way by observing the level of economic development through physical environment, educational systems, safety and transportation, health and social services, communication, and recreation. Anderson and McFarlane refer to this approach as "Learning About the Community on Foot."

PRACTICE POINT

A windshield survey is a great way to get a subjective idea of what a community is like. When you decide to either walk or ride through a community (keeping safety precautions in mind at all times and being alert to the level of crime or danger), try to plan the experience by first consulting a map. Get a sense of the physical boundaries that define the community, and explore not only residential spaces, but also recreational open space and businesses. Look at all the details and observe closely. Look at the quality of streets, bridges, types of house materials (e.g., wood, brick), people, light, air quality, and stores, especially grocery stores. Make the survey an adventure.

FRAMEWORKS FOR COMMUNITY ASSESSMENT

Community assessment is not unique to community or public health nursing practice. Epidemiologists, genetic counselors, and social workers also conduct assessments to understand which people are at risk of acquiring a specific illness, or to identify those who may need social support as they experience a traumatic event. Understanding and appreciation for community strengths, deficits, resources, and needs through community assessment is the objective that community health nursing shares with other disciplines (Economos & Irish-Hauser, 2007; Fletcher, Slusher, & Whitaker, 2006; Piper, 2011).

There is recent criticism that community assessments have often emphasized what was missing in communities to address health and safety, rather than looking at the strengths and resources the community may have to address these issues (Piper, 2011).

In the examples presented, nurses followed identical underlying principles and processes to gather health-related data about communities. The nurses developed a planned community assessment to determine how people who share social or spatial relationships respond to internal and/or external influences on health. Identifying patterns of response to these influences can help planning interventions to preserve or improve the health of the community. However, it is always difficult to know how to start and the best way to approach this process. Previously defined **frameworks** are examples of successful ways to assess communities. They provide direction for the assessment. The following frameworks serve as methods that can be used to develop assessments. The approach to the assessment will require considerable organization and a sequential plan.

Most nursing perspectives on community assessment incorporate concepts used in **epidemiologic models** to identify areas that affect the health of communities. The scope of nursing assessment also includes identification of communities' assets and capacity to create and implement changes from within the aggregate. There are two main reasons to conduct a community assessment: (1) to gain information and clarify the need for change and (2) to empower those responsible for implementing that change (Piper, 2011). The following section includes several frameworks for community assessment that can be used individually or in combination to identify key strengths and weakness in a community's health and well-being.

Epidemiologic Approach to Community Assessment

Healthy People 2020, the broad-based collaborative effort among federal, state, territorial, and private and nonprofit organizations, has established the leading health indicators and priorities for action in the United States (Box 11.2). These 10 public health indicators are tracked, measured, and reported regularly using epidemiologic methods and a wide variety of data-collection techniques. Although these objectives can be applied to the nation as a whole, or to populations of a state, county, region, city, or town, it is the practical impact at the individual and family level that is most important. For many reasons, communities vary in their ability to reach targeted objectives. Therefore, investigating the community's status in reaching these objectives is a part of any community assessment.

Community report cards provide a snapshot of the overall health and well-being of a community through the use of indicators or measurements of local social and health trends. Such reports are used increasingly across the United States to communicate critical information concerning local issues to community members, service groups, and policy-makers. Developing a community report card helps articulate the community's desired goals—to establish means of measuring the condition of the community in relation to what is desired, and to collect data to measure progress toward goals. Members of the community and professional groups then decide how to create programs to address needs, change the circumstances that exist, or maintain those activities that have created a healthy community.

In developing the San Diego County community report card, indicators were developed to assess the community. Technical, community, and scientific advisory groups were established to firmly ground the development process in local technical and political realities. More than 20 local data experts reviewed and helped refine a list of indicators from secondary sources that would require no primary data collection. In addition, a scientific advisory committee of eight local leaders from the fields of public health, social work, pediatrics, and medicine provided scientific oversight throughout the development process. These two committees reviewed the preliminary list of indicators and made recommendations for refinement of five domains: economics, health, safety, education, and access to services. Twenty-nine scientifically based or consensus-driven indicators are listed according to their domain (Table 11.1).

What are the epidemiologic methods that have been used to develop the community report card? Explain how these indicators relate to (1) describing the *who*, *what*, *where*, and *when* and (2) the descriptions of person, place, and time that are necessary components of a community report card (see Chapter 6).

box 11.2 Leading Health Indicators: 10 High-priority Public Health Issues in the United States

- Physical activity
- Overweight and obesity
- Tobacco use
- Substance abuse
- Responsible sexual behavior
- Mental health
- Injury and violence
- Environmental quality
- Immunization
- Access to healthcare

Source: Healthy People 2020 (From http://www.healthypeople.gov/HP2020/)

Principles of epidemiology are used throughout the development, planning, implementation, and evaluation phases of the community assessment process. Epidemiologic methods can help identify patterns of health and social inequity and can be used to determine trends in three ways: (1) by describing the disease or disability, (2) by determining relationships that can predict health or health disparities, and (3) by developing and testing interventions.

Describing the Disease or Disability

Before engaging in any data collection, the members of the community must be defined. It should be very clear who is a member of the community and who is not. The organizing

table 11.1 **Community Report Card Indicators: San Diego County, California**

Economics
Average percentage unemployed
Percentage of children living in poverty
Rate of public assistance to children
Percentage of parents receiving public assistance who are working or involved in work-related activities
Rate at which children receive food stamps
Rate at which children are identified as homeless
Health
Infant mortality rate
Percentage of infants born with low birth weight
Rate of births to teenagers
Rate of youth suicides
Rate of hospitalization of children and youth for mental illness
Percentages of adolescent health risk behaviors: cigarette use, binge drinking, marijuana use
Access to Services
Number of subsidized child care spaces
Average wait time for publicly funded outpatient alcohol and drug treatment services for adolescents
Average wait time for publicly funded nonemergency outpatient mental health services for children and youth
Percentage of children who are adequately immunized
Percentage of children with health insurance
Safety
Rate of delinquency petitions filed in juvenile court
Rate of child and youth homicides
Rate of children living in out-of-home placement owing to abuse/neglect
Number of domestic violence reports
Rate of unintentional injuries and unintentional injury–related deaths
Rate at which children and youths are killed or injured in alcohol/drug-related motor vehicle crashes
Education
Annual percentage of students who drop out of high school
Percentage of students who attend school daily
School suspension rate
School expulsion rate

framework and resulting plan of action should articulate what information needs to be collected and how it will be obtained. Then, the working group can begin the assessment (see Box 11.1).

Existing (secondary) data can often be used to identify the community's strengths and weakness, to determine assets and liabilities, and to describe, along with available community resources, the amount of disease/disability or health in a population (Box 11.3). Finding data that identify the "who, what, where, and when" related to disease, disability, and exemplars of health must then be systematically organized and analyzed. Plans for collecting new (primary) data may include community forums, focus groups, key informants, participant observation, and surveys. (For more information on developing and using these methods, please refer to a nursing research textbook.)

By exploring data available on the Internet, community health nurses can not only describe trends but can also identify resources that address the trends and determine where gaps may exist. The aggregate data from these resources include local demographics, such as death rates, causes of death, marital status, gender, age, ethnicity, and density of the population. Depending on the purpose of the community assessment, records in health facilities may be examined. This information can provide a sense of what the people living or working in the community face in terms of health problems, and can assess what happens to them over time in terms of follow-up and wellness. The local chamber of commerce can help identify and describe the physical environment, health and social services, economy, transportation/safety, politics and government, communication, education, and recreation facilities available to the population. In addition, census tract data and the perceptions of informants (people who live in the community) about how they experience the physical environment, health and social services, economy transportation/safety, politics and government, communication, education, and recreation can all be considered descriptive data relative to the community and the way it is experienced by those who live in it. Census tract maps are often electronically produced and accessible by state, city, county, and town. These maps include an option to click and zoom in on a specific area of interest.

box 11.3 Resources for Community Assessment

Administration for Children and Families
Agency for Healthcare Research and Quality
Alcoholics Anonymous
Alzheimer's Association
American Association of Retired Persons
American Cancer Society
American Dental Association
American Diabetes Association
American Heart Association
American Public Health Association
American Red Cross
American School Health Association
Association for Children and Adults with Learning Disabilities
Asthma and Allergy Foundation
Centers for Disease Control and Prevention
Healthy People 2010
Indian Health Services
March of Dimes
National Alliance for the Mentally Ill
National Association for Health Care
National Association of Rural Health Clinics
National Center for Farmworker Health
National Council of the Aging
National Hospice & Palliative Care Organization
National Kidney Foundation
National Wellness Institute
Occupational Safety and Health Administration
Planned Parenthood
Real Solutions to Gun Violence
Substance Abuse and Mental Health Administration
World Health Organization
Women's Health (Health and Human Services)
Youth Risk Survey

Embedded in the maps is the capacity to access specific data related to the earlier mentioned areas of interest.

For example, a Massachusetts census tract and statistical site (MassStats, 2013) provides the opportunity to access specific city data, including health data: birth rate, birth weight rate, teen birth rate, birth rate changes by year, lead poisoning rate, cancer incidence, and presence of hospitals. As shown in Figure 11.1, the city of Brockton, Massachusetts, a suburb of the major metropolitan city of Boston, demonstrates higher-than-normal premature mortality. The color legend for Brockton indicates a higher-than-normal premature mortality rate (>400 per 100,000 people), whereas the town of Avon, which borders Brockton, has a less-than-normal rate (<200 per 100,000 people). Similarly, in a more rural setting in the United States, epidemiologic data may reveal high levels of farm machine fatalities, but may also reveal equally high levels of family instability related to intrafamilial conflict and mental health.

Determining Relationships That Can Predict Health Status

Data can be analyzed in such a way that relationships that predict health status (i.e., illness) can be defined. This information can be very helpful to community health nurses in planning programs and/or interventions. In Chapter 7, measures of association are described as statistical measures which are used to investigate the degree of relationship between events and/or circumstance of illness/disability in cases and cohorts of the population. The idea of association means that events or illness/disability may have a strong tendency to occur together rather than just by chance. In more recent years, statistical information has been transferred graphically so that assessment can be seen as concentrations

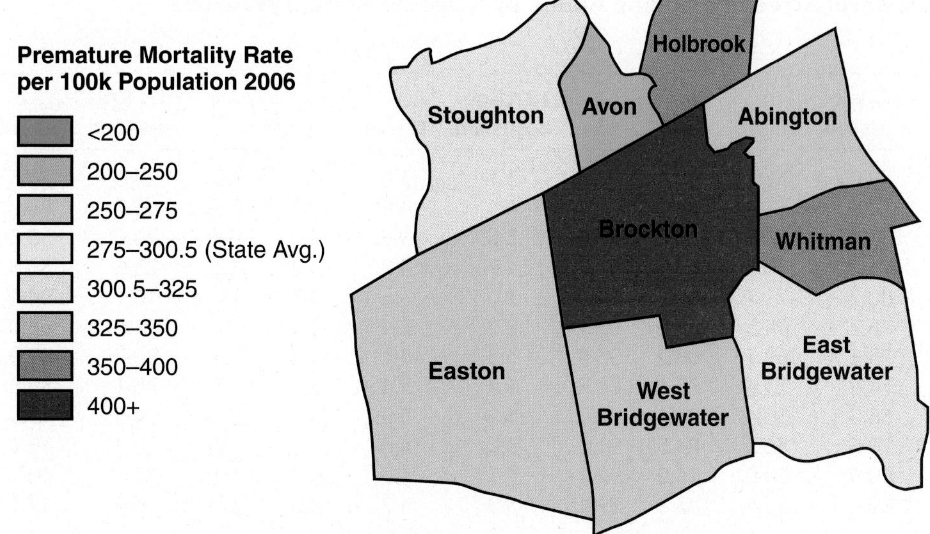

figure 11.1 Premature mortality rate in Brockton, Massachusetts, and surrounding communities (Data from MassStats, 2013. *Premature mortality rate: Brockton, Massachusetts*. Retrieved from http://www.caliper.com/Maptitude/MassStats/Map.aspx)

on maps of cities, towns, counties, and states. The relationships that occur can be vividly portrayed as an association.

CHOLESTEROL AND CARDIOVASCULAR DISEASE

It is known that there is a strong relationship between high levels of cholesterol and cardiovascular disease. The Centers for Disease Control and Prevention (CDC) provide state-by-state information about the rate of screening for cholesterol by providing the percentage of individual responses (Table 11.2). These data, which can be gathered at the state, county, or city level, help to assess the use of prevention in health behaviors of citizens. This helps target education and support programs that can help members of populations obtain the information they need to make decisions that promote health. In addition, it assists healthcare providers in making sure that citizens have access to resources where reasonably inexpensive screening and follow-up are available.

PRACTICE POINT

Scrutinize your data carefully for similarities and differences. For example, using Table 11.2, determine which state has the lowest percentage of cholesterol screening within the past 5 years. If you were going to target an age group for a screening program in this state, what age group would you choose? If you had to choose a state that did the best job of cholesterol screening of its residents within the past 5 years, which state would you choose?

Using the list of San Diego community health indicators, suggest some relationships that could be examined to develop further information about the population.

Geographic Information Systems

Geographic information systems (GISs) are another example of drawing relationships and associations that are important in community assessments. An example of a United States Geological Survey (USGS, 2013) GIS map outlining water deficiencies (hydrologic drought) in the United States is found in Figure 11.2. GIS is a system of hardware and software used for storage, retrieval, mapping, and analysis of geographic data. Spatial features are stored in a coordinate system that refers to a particular place on the earth. Spatial data and associated attributes can be layered together for mapping and analysis. GIS can be used for scientific investigations, resource management, and development planning.

The use of GIS in health sciences is relatively new, but it appears to be expanding faster than any other area of GIS application. Health scientists have long used geographic information conceptually, but the availability of user-friendly GIS tools for community health research is recent. The GIS tools assist in determining locations of disease incidence, characteristics of surrounding environments, location of healthcare facilities, identification of the geographic boundaries of the communities, and other essential community infrastructures (Choi, Afzal, & Sattler, 2006).

Developing and Testing Interventions

Using both descriptive data and relational data, nurses can develop interventions that can empower communities and effect change. These are then evaluated according to the results or outcomes of the interventions. As in the case study, the report card's indicators are now being used as outcome measures for county health and human services programs.

table 11.2 **Cholesterol Screening among Adults by Selected State, 1997–2005**

	≤5 yr				>5 yr				Never			
Location	**18+, Age-adjusted**	**18–44**	**45–64**	**65+**	**18+, Age-adjusted**	**18–44**	**45–64**	**65+**	**18+, Age-adjusted**	**18–44**	**45–64**	**65+**
Alabama	72.0	58.7	85.4	90.2	3.1	3.6	3.2	1.6	24.6	37.3	11.3	8.1
Arkansas	67.7	51.2	83.5	91.5	4.4	4.8	4.8	2.5	27.7	43.8	11.6	5.8
California	71.8	57.5	84.6	94.0	3.6	3.9	4.0	1.9	24.6	38.6	11.4	4.0
Colorado	71.5	56.2	86.5	92.7	4.7	4.8	5.2	3.2	23.6	38.6	8.2	4.0
Washington, DC	80.7	71.7	89.2	94.0	3.0	3.6	2.7	[a]	16.1	24.4	8.1	4.5
Florida	76.2	64.5	88.0	92.1	2.2	2.4	2.4	1.4	21.4	33.0	9.5	6.3
Georgia	75.6	62.7	88.2	93.4	3.5	4.1	3.5	1.9	20.7	32.9	8.2	4.6
Hawaii	71.4	57.4	85.1	90.9	3.2	3.4	3.7	1.7	25.1	38.8	11.1	7.3
Idaho	66.5	50.4	81.4	90.7	5.9	5.9	7.0	3.6	27.5	43.5	11.6	5.7
Illinois	70.6	56.3	84.5	91.0	3.7	4.0	4.2	1.7	25.4	39.3	11.2	7.2
Iowa	69.9	54.8	84.0	92.2	4.7	4.5	6.0	2.9	25.0	40.1	9.9	4.8
Kansas	69.0	53.4	83.8	91.4	3.9	4.2	4.5	2.1	26.9	42.1	11.7	6.4

Other statistics (percentage), gender (all), race/ethnicity (all), year (2003, 2005).
Source: Behavioral Risk Factor Surveillance System (BRFSS); CDC, 2007.
[a]Unreliable data.

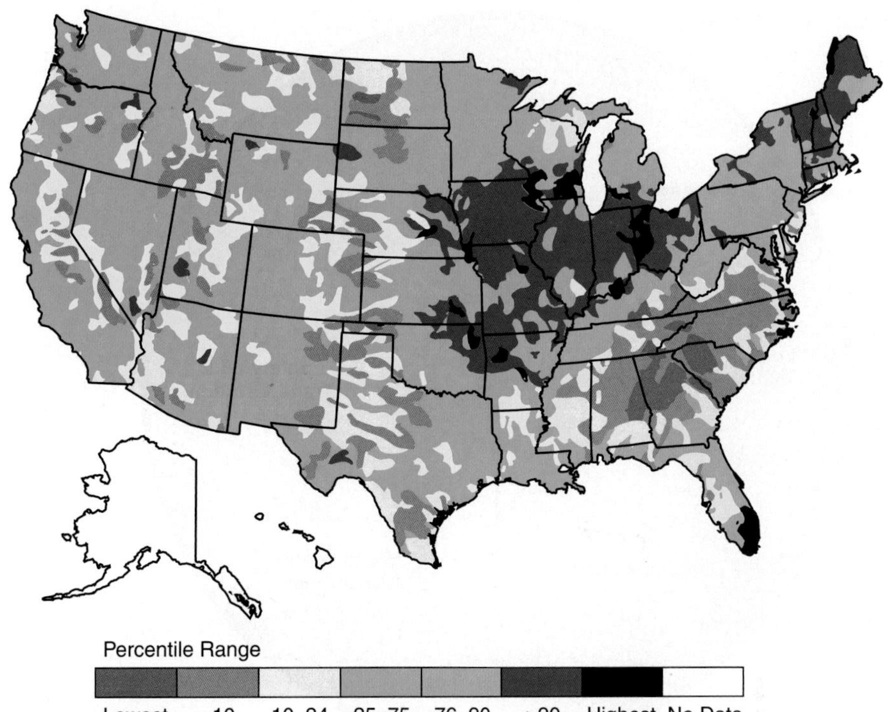

figure 11.2 Hydrologic unit runoff graphs and maps in the United States (Data from United States Geological Survey [USGS], 2008.)

EVIDENCE FOR PRACTICE

Nearly 3,000 children 6 to 12 years of age ($n = 2{,}968$) with *Diagnostic and Statistical Manual of Mental Disorders*, 5th edition (*DSM-5*)–defined attention-deficit/hyperactivity disorder (ADHD) participated in a community assessment study to compare medications that would effectively treat the condition. Protocols included (1) baseline stimulant treatment regimen (Adderall); (2) immediate-release methylphenidate (Concerta), which was converted to an approximately equivalent once-daily dose of 10-, 20-, or 30-mg Adderall extended-release (XR); and (3) mixed amphetamine salts XR (MAS XR), given according to a medication-conversion algorithm. Health-related quality of life was assessed by the Pediatric Quality of Life Inventory 4.0 (PedsQL). Treatment satisfaction and preference were assessed by parent and physician questionnaires. Mean PedsQL total score of baseline treatment was 74.5, compared with 81.0 after 7 weeks of treatment with MAS XR. The 6.4-point improvement was statistically significant ($p < 0.0001$; one-sample *t*-test). Children with ADHD who are being managed in a community practice setting may experience significant clinical benefit, including improved health-related quality of life and parental satisfaction with treatment, after being changed to a treatment regimen which includes MAS XR (Sallee, Ambrosini, Lopez, Shi, & Michaels, 2004).

Community as Partner Framework

Anderson and McFarlane (2008) use a wheel to represent a core surrounded by eight subsystems (Fig. 11.3). The core represents people as central members of the community. The eight parts of the community that interact with the various members of the community are physical environment, health and social service, economy, transportation and safety, politics and government, communication, education, and recreation. Anderson and McFarlane (2008) have proposed that it is necessary to consider the history, demographics, ethnicity, and values and beliefs of the entire community. "Flexible lines of defense" (buffer zones), "normal lines of defense" (health), and "lines of resistance" (strengths) are identified and surround the wheel, as well as separate each subsystem. These lines of defense represent a dynamic level of health after stressors have impinged on the system and can be used as a systems approach by teams to effectively assess a community. The word "partner" and particularly **"community as partner"** is key, because it demonstrates the equity of the nurse's relationship with the community.

The development of the San Diego Community Report Card used a partnership approach. Members of the Child Well-Being Subcommittee, composed of 13 people from diverse professional backgrounds, served as community ambassadors and provided broad policy guidance. To gain the trust and support of the large, diverse San Diego community, the project team solicited extensive feedback from more than 40 community groups. They distributed an information packet and survey in Spanish, English, and Vietnamese. After evaluating the input from the community, the list of indicators was modified to reflect comments made during this process.

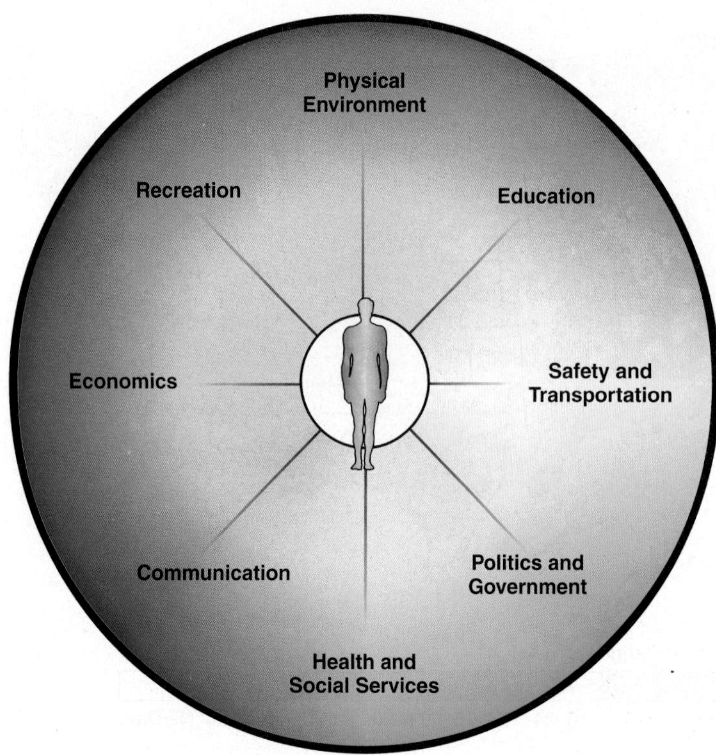

figure 11.3 Communities as interdependent systems.

Functional Health Status Approach

Functional health patterns (FHPs) assessment (Gordon, 1994) is designed to be used for individual, family, or community assessment. FHP assessment involves a systematic and deliberate format. Gordon defines assessment as a form of evaluation. Pattern, according to Gordon, represents "a configuration of behaviors that occur sequentially across time" (p. 70). Understanding community patterns provides insight into how groups respond to problems and take action.

Gordon includes questions that are applicable to community assessment for 11 FHPs (Box 11.4). Because the FHPs were designed for use with nursing diagnoses, clinicians are expected to identify defining characteristics from each pattern and assign relevant diagnoses. Although the FHPs are arranged in numerical order, the assessment format is intended to be used as a guide. Questions for community assessment are open-ended, specifically to elicit responses that provide depth and breadth to inquiries. Gordon acknowledged that because the community encompasses a number of systems, completion of the assessment requires time.

Community and public health nurses will appreciate the format, which is adaptable for use in most communities (Gordon, 1994). Assessment questions are not limited to informants' responses but also include clinicians' descriptions of the community. Novice nurses, especially if they have some familiarity with FHP, might find the model easy to follow as they learn about community assessment. The questions are clear and direct. The FHP community assessment also calls on students to use a variety of means to collect data.

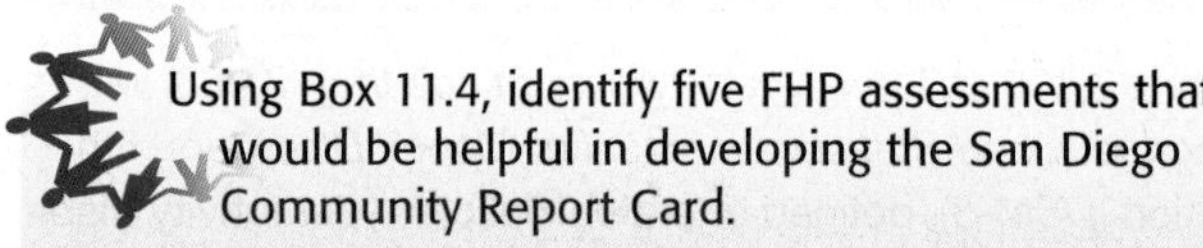

Using Box 11.4, identify five FHP assessments that would be helpful in developing the San Diego Community Report Card.

Developmental Models and Approaches

An effective way to assess a community can be a retrospective, historical approach. Using system parameters, a community health nurse could travel back in history through historical documents, data, figures, and images, and piece together the stages a population or community has experienced. These system parameters can include the physical environment, education, safety and transportation, politics and government, health and social services, communication, economics, and recreation as segments of community life that are shared between those that live and work in a community (see Fig. 11.3). This approach could include gathering historical reports from interviews with community members who could describe their experiences in their own words. Both historical informants and mined data (i.e., data that are examined through extensive and rigorous searches) can help describe the cultural changes within a community or aggregate over time, and help to plan for the future. In this way, developmental data are obtained, and then compared, to determine what variables may have enhanced or detracted from development, and what resources were available at the time.

One generation plants the trees; another gets the shade.

Chinese proverb

box 11.4 Functional Health Patterns

I. Health Perception/Health Management Pattern:
  1. History (community representatives)
    a. In general, what is the health/wellness level of the population on a scale of 1–5, with 5 being the highest level of health/wellness? Any major health problems?
    b. Any strong cultural patterns influencing health practices?
    c. People feel that they have access to health services?
    d. Demand for any particular health services or prevention programs?
    e. People feel that fire, police, safety programs are sufficient?
  2. Examination (community records)
    a. Morbidity, mortality, disability rates (by age group, if appropriate)
    b. Accident rates (by district, if appropriate)
    c. Current operating health facilities (types)
    d. Ongoing health promotion/prevention programs; utilization rates
    e. Ratio of health professionals to population
    f. Laws regarding drinking age
    g. Arrest statistics for drugs, drunk driving by age groups

II. Nutritional/Metabolic Pattern:
  1. History (community representatives)
    a. In general, do most people seem well nourished? Children? Elderly?
    b. Food supplement programs? Food stamps: rate of use?
    c. Foods at a reasonable cost in this area relative to income?
    d. Stores accessible for most? "Meals on Wheels" available?
  2. Examination
    a. General appearance (nutritional appearance; teeth; clothing appropriate to climate)? Children? Adults? Elderly?
    b. Food purchases (observations of food store checkout counters)
    c. "Junk" food machines in schools?
    d. Specific nutritional risk factors: socioeconomic status (SES), culture, gender, and age

III. Elimination Pattern:
  1. History (community representatives)
    a. Major kinds of wastes (industrial, sewage, etc.)? Disposal systems? Recycling programs? Any problems perceived by community?
    b. Pest control (type, method, frequency)? Food service inspection (restaurants, street vendors)?
    c. Water supply source and quality; testing services; water usage costs; drought restrictions?
    d. Concern that community growth will exceed good water supply?
    e. Heating/cooling costs manageable for most? Help programs?
    f. Air pollution sources and control?
  2. Examination
    a. Communicable disease statistics
    b. Air pollution statistics

IV. Activity—Exercise Pattern:
  1. History (community representatives)
    a. How do people find the transportation here? To work? To recreation? To healthcare?
    b. People have/use community centers (seniors, others)? Recreation facilities for children? Adults? Seniors?
    c. Is housing adequate (availability, cost)? Public housing?
  2. Examination
    a. Recreation/cultural programs
    b. Aids for the disabled
    c. Residential centers, nursing homes, and rehabilitation facilities relative to population needs
    d. External maintenance of homes, yards, and apartment houses
    e. General activity level

V. Sleep—Rest Pattern:
  1. History (community representatives)
    a. Generally quiet at night in most neighborhoods?
    b. Usual business hours? Industries round the clock?
  2. Examination
    a. Activity-noise levels in business district? In residential districts?

VI. Cognitive—Perceptual Pattern:
  1. History (community representatives)
    a. Most groups speak English? Bilingual?
    b. Educational level of population?
    c. Schools seen as good/need improving? Adult education desired/available?
    d. Types of problems that require community decisions? Decision-making process? What is the best way to get things done/changed here?
  2. Examination
    a. School facilities (type and condition); dropout rate

VII. Self-Perception/Self-Concept Pattern:
  1. History (community representatives)
    a. Good community to live in? Going up in status, down, about the same?
    b. Old community? Fairly new?
    c. Any age group predominates?
    d. Peoples' moods in general: enjoying life, stressed, feeling "down"?
    e. People generally have the kind of abilities needed in this community?
    f. Community/neighborhood functions?
  2. Examination
    a. Racial, ethnic mix (if appropriate)
    b. Socioeconomic level
    c. General observations of mood

VIII. Role—Relationship Pattern:
  1. History (community representatives)
    a. People seem to get along well together here? Places where people tend to go to socialize?
    b. Type of government? Do people feel they are heard by government? High/low participation in meetings?
    c. Enough work/jobs for everyone? Wages good/fair? Do people seem to like the kind of work available (happy in their jobs/job stress)?

(continued on page 200)

box 11.4 **Functional Health Patterns *(continued)***

d. Any problems with riots, violence in the neighborhoods? Family violence? Problems with child/spouse/elder abuse?
e. Get along with adjacent communities? Collaborate on any community projects?
f. Do neighbors seem to support each other?

2. Examination
a. Observation of interactions (generally or at specific meetings)
b. Statistics on employment, income/poverty
c. Divorce rate

IX. Sexuality—Reproductive Pattern:
1. History (community representatives)
a. Average family size?
b. Do people feel there are any problems with pornography, prostitution? Other?
c. Do people want/support sex education in schools/community?
2. Examination
a. Family size and types of households
b. Male-to-female ratio
c. Average maternal age, maternal mortality rate, infant mortality rate
d. Teen pregnancy rate
e. Abortion rate
f. Sexual violence statistics
g. Laws/regulations regarding information on birth control

X. Coping—Stress Pattern:
1. History (community representative)
a. Any groups that seem to be under stress?
b. Need/availability of phone helplines? Support groups (health related, other)?
2. Examination
a. Delinquency, drug abuse, interpersonal violence, alcoholism, suicide, psychiatric illness statistics
b. Unemployment rate by race/ethnicity/sex

XI. Value—Belief Pattern:
1. History (community representative)
a. Community values: What seem to be the top four things that people living here see as important in their lives (note health-related values, priorities)?
b. Do people tend to get involved in causes/local fund raising campaigns?
c. Religious groups in community? Churches available?
d. Do people tend to tolerate/not tolerate differences/socially deviant behavior?
2. Examination
a. Zoning laws
b. Scan of community health department reports (goals, priorities)
c. Health budget relative to total budget

Source: From Gordon, M. (1994). *Nursing diagnosis: Process and application* (3rd ed.). St. Louis, MO: Mosby. Used with permission.

In the San Diego County case, 3 to 5 years' worth of historical data, as well as comparisons with other areas that were geographically comparable, were used in the development of the report card. What data do you think would be particularly helpful in understanding the historical movement of a community in this particular case, and what do you think would be the strategies to obtain this information?

COMMUNITY ASSESSMENT ASSETS-BASED APPROACH

More than a decade ago, Ammerman and Parks (1998) observed that those who assess communities often approach community assessment with a distinct bias toward traditional deficit-based models. Despite good intentions, the focus of assessment even today is often on numerous problems, grim health statistics, and widening gaps in services. In an effort to build collaboration between a particular university and community, although it could be another institution in another area, an assets model can change the perspective on how one conducts an assessment within a community. When attention is directed to community strengths and resources, better relationships can be developed between all those working on the assessment, especially when the community is part of the process. Working relationships are enhanced when community members realize that the assessment process has the potential to be an empowering experience; the strengths and positive aspects of the community are measured in conjunction with what is needed or not actualized.

Use of the **asset-based assessment** model led to development of the community-based public health initiative (CBPHI) for research, practice, and teaching (Ammerman & Parks, 1998). A key factor of the CBPHI is building coalitions and active partnerships with the community during the assessment phase. Collaboration with community members shifts the focus from dependency on experts to empowerment of all, working together toward a goal. Using an assets model requires taking a different philosophic approach to the assessment process. Interaction with the community is the primary approach.

Using the San Diego Community Report Card indicators as a guideline, create a list of indicators for assessing the strengths and resources of the community.

EVIDENCE FOR PRACTICE

Gerberich, Stearns, and Dowd (1995) supported the idea that overemphasis on statistics and other data resources could divert assessment attention away from opportunities to know a community's "personality." To support a level of understanding, the Community Assessment Instrument for Baccalaureate Learners (CAIBL) was developed, which continues to be used today. Based on Benner's model of skill acquisition, the CAIBL was designed for the novice nurse. The overall purpose of the CAIBL is to allow students to develop observation skills and learn to apply abstract concepts and principles of community health nursing practice. The authors outlined the four-part instrument in detail. Part I of the tool was used to identify and describe the community for assessment. Part II consisted of a windshield assessment. Here, 14 categories for data collection were detailed: housing; zoning; space use; boundaries; common areas; transportation; service centers; stores; street scene; community growth; race, ethnicity and religion; politics; media; and "community personality." Students' task in part III was to review documents and begin to summarize data. Students gathered data by visiting agencies and interviewing key informants. Students were encouraged to share data with other students during post-conference. Part IV is divided into three phases. First, students reviewed the 13 systems to decide whether each was an "important asset," "problem or deficit," or "no effect" in relation to the community (p. 242). Next, to improve community health, students identified goals at a health status, health structure and function, or process level. The final step in this phase included students recommending nursing interventions for each goal on the basis of community assets and resources.

Collaborative Model

A **collaborative model** of assessment is an integral function of community health nursing practice. To develop the skill of collaboration, public health experts can work in partnership in a community assessment model that emphasizes the interdisciplinary nature of the task (Carvalhana & Flak, 2009). Assessment includes nurses as well as social workers in collaboration with community residents. Beyond interdisciplinary expert collaboration, another approach used in community assessment is collaboration between experts and those with health concerns. It is important to ensure that members of a population have an active voice in identifying issues and in making decisions about what is needed. Engaging participants with a "we can do it together" approach is more effective than using a "we/they" approach. For example, Connor, Rainer, Simcox, and Thomisee (2007) worked with migrant workers as partners to increase the availability and accessibility of healthcare services.

The collaboration through mutual group work assists in the development of a community analysis and plan of action. Assessments can be initiated, and analysis is enhanced, in interdisciplinary teams. Interdisciplinary community assessment, with community dwellers offering input, has several advantages: Each professional discipline learns to work interdependently with community leaders (Russell & Hymans, 1999). Disciplines benefit from small group work. Moreover, all those who participate develop mutual understanding and appreciation for each other's viewpoint. This process, however, has distinct drawbacks. This form of assessment is time-consuming, and logistical, systematic approaches must be preestablished to maintain clarity in the process, for all those involved (Russell & Hymans, 1999).

EVIDENCE FOR PRACTICE

Focus groups provide an effective means of incorporating the perspectives of "hidden" populations in assessments of community health needs and assets. In the study reported by Yoshida, Craypo, and Samuels (2011), researchers conducted a series of focus groups with youth in specifically targeted segments of a community to develop a comprehensive picture of community health. Despite differences in age, length of residence, and ethnicity, the focus groups were remarkably similar regarding the issues raised. Leadership capacity was facilitated through teamwork, community assessments, and policy work. Conclusions included that youth gained leadership confidence while successfully advocating for community-level change. Focus group findings have been used to initiate activities which address identified community problems. Focus group participation has the added benefit of increasing community members' participation in other community endeavors.

key concepts

- Community assessment includes examination of biologic, psychological, and sociocultural influences of the environment that surrounds a specific group of people.
- Community can be defined as follows:
  - Geopolitical, sharing geographic boundaries and governing structures
  - Phenomenologic, sharing common interests or beliefs
  - Communities of solution, formed by a group of people to address common interests, beliefs, or needs
  - A society, nation, or international or global communities

key concepts (continued)

- The epidemiologic approach to community assessment includes the following:
  - Describing the health of a population
  - Determining relationships that can predict health and illness
  - Developing and testing interventions to empower communities and affect change
- The community as partner framework uses a systems approach with a focus on partnerships to affect change.
- The functional health status approach evaluates health patterns in the community.
- The developmental approaches use a retrospective historical approach to understand cultural changes over time to provide information for future initiatives.
- The assets-based approach identifies community resources and strengths along with community needs.
- The collaborative model involves assessment by an interdisciplinary term and members of the community.
- The approach used depends on the type of community that is to be assessed. Combinations of frameworks can often be used.

critical thinking questions

Use the following scenario when answering the six questions given below. Use a group format so that sharing can across and between students and faculty.

In conducting a community assessment targeting information about women of color at risk for or living with HIV/AIDS, you gather key collaborative stakeholders together. You want to begin the process by engaging everybody's goodwill for the project. You start the process by having a 2-day retreat where you discuss and educate everybody as to the parameters of this process. You need to consider many things before the retreat. Please answer them as a way of preparing for the retreat by using a critical thinking approach that raises vital questions, offers relevant information, develops well-reasoned conclusions, and fosters open-minded communication by recognizing assumptions. Feel free to use information from websites, such as the Centers of Disease Control and Prevention, which discusses GIS and mapping; the United States Census, which includes expansive census tract data; and local city halls or areas where data are collected statewide describing the community activities and statistics, as resources for answering these questions.

1. What does this assessment involve?
2. How do those in a partnership conduct a community assessment?
3. How can a community assessment engage families and community members?
4. What factors are involved in understanding community assets?
5. How should assessment information be used and by whom?
6. How can a partnership use assessment results to move from planning to action?

references

Ammerman, A., & Parks, C. (1998). Preparing students for more effective community intervention: Assets assessment. *Family and Community Health, 21*(1), 32–45.

Anderson, E. T., & McFarlane, J. (2008). *Community a partner: Theory and practice in nursing* (5th ed.). Philadelphia, PA: Lippincott, Williams, and Wilkins.

Carvalhana, V., & Flak, E. (2009). Role of the pharmacist on a multidisciplinary psychiatry team: Impact on medication adherence in a community setting. *Journal of Pharmacy Technology, 25*(3), 155–158.

Choi, M., Afzal, B., & Sattler, B. (2006). Geographic information systems: A new tool for environmental health assessment. *Public Health Nursing, 23*(5), 381–391.

Connor, A., Rainer, L., Simcox, J., & Thomisee, K. (2007). Increasing the delivery of health services to migrant farm worker families through a community partnership model. *Public Health Nursing, 24*(4), 355–360.

Economos, C. D., & Irish-Hauser, S. A. (2007). Community interventions: A brief overview and their application to the obesity epidemic. *Journal of Law, Medicine & Ethics, 35*(1), 131–137.

Fletcher, C. W., Slusher, I. L., & Whitaker, H. M. (2006). Health care needs: Meeting the health care needs of medically underserved, uninsured, and underinsured Appalachians. *Kentucky Nurse, 54*, 8–9.

Gerberich, S. S., Stearns, S. J., & Dowd, T. (1995). A critical skill for the future: Community assessment. *Journal of Community Health Nursing, 12*, 239–250.

Gordon, M. (1994). *Nursing diagnosis: Process and application* (3rd ed.). St. Louis, MO: Mosby.

Grove, S. K., Burns, N., & Gray, J. R. (2013). *The practice of nursing research: Appraisal, synthesis, and generation of evidence* (7th ed.). St. Louis, MO: Elsevier Saunders.

Interdisciplinary Group on Preventing School and Community Violence. (2013). December 2012 Connecticut school shooting position statement. *Journal of School Violence, 12*(2), 119–133.

Kirsch, T. D., Perrin, P., Burkle, F. M., Canny, W., Purdin, S., Lin, W., & Sauer, L. (2012). Requirements for independent community-based quality assessment and accountability practices in humanitarian assistance and disaster relief activities. *Prehospital & Disaster Medicine, 27*(3), 280–285.

Martin, A. E., Cunningham, S. C., & Magnus, J. H. (2011). Professional development using student-led, community-based activities. *Journal of Public Health Management & Practice*, *17*(4), 354–357.

MassStats. (2013). Massachusetts statistics and maps. Retrieved from http://www.MassStats.com

Patel, K., Hargreaves, M., Liu, J., Kenerson, D., Neal, R., Takizala, Z., . . . Blot, B. (2012). Factors influencing colorectal cancer screening in low-income African Americans in Tennessee. *Journal of Community Health*, *37*(3), 673–679.

Pbert, L., Druker, S., Gapinski, M. A., Gellar, L., Magner, R., Reed, G., . . . Osganian, S. (2013). A school nurse-delivered intervention for overweight and obese adolescents. *Journal of School Health*, *83*(3), 182–193.

Piper, S. M. (2011). Community empowerment for health visiting and other public health nursing. *Community Practitioner*, *84*(8), 28–31.

Russell, K.M. & Hymans, D. (1999). Interprofessional education for undergraduate students. *Public Health Nursing*, *16*(4), 254–262.

Sallee, F. R., Ambrosini, P. J., Lopez, F. A., Shi, L., & Michaels, M. A. (2004). Health-related quality of life and treatment satisfaction and preference in a community assessment study of extended-release mixed amphetamine salts for children with attention-deficit/hyperactivity disorder. *Journal of Drug Assessment*, *7*(3), 145–167.

Simmes, D. R., Blaszcak, M. R., Kurtin, P. S., Bowen, N. L., & Ross, R. K. (2000). Creating a community report card: The San Diego experience. *American Journal of Public Health*, *90*(6), 880–882.

Smith, C. S., & Maurer, F. A. (2009). *Community/public health nursing practice: Health for families and populations* (4th ed.). St. Louis, MO: Saunders Elsevier.

Tendulkar, S., Hamilton, C. R., Chu, C., Arsenault, L., Duffy, K., Huynh, V., . . . Friedman, E. (2012). Investigating the myth of the "Model Minority": A participatory community health assessment of Chinese and Vietnamese adults (includes abstract). *Journal of Immigrant & Minority Health*, *14*(5), 850–857.

United States Geological Survey. (2013). Hydrologic unit runoff graphs and maps in the United States. Retrieved from http://waterwatch.usgs.gov/?m=romap3&r=us&w=real%2Cmap

Waitzkin, H., Getrich, C., Heying, S., Rodríguez, L., Parmar, A., Willging, C., . . . Santos, R. (2011). Promotoras as mental health practitioners in primary care: A multi-method study of an intervention to address contextual sources of depression. *Journal of Community Health*, *36*(2), 316–331.

Wheeler, L. S., Merkle, S. L., Gerald, L. B., & Taggart, V. S. (2006). Managing asthma in schools: Lessons learned and recommendations. *Journal of School Health*, *76*(6), 340–344.

Williams, K. J., Bray, P. G., Shapiro-Mendoza, C. K., Reisz, I., & Peranteau, J. (2009). Modeling the principles of community-based participatory research in a community health assessment conducted by a health foundation. *Health Promotion Practice*, *10*(1), 67–75.

Yoshida, S. C., Craypo, L., & Samuels, S. E. (2011). Engaging youth in improving their food and physical activity environments. *Journal of Adolescent Health*, *48*(6), 641–643.

web resources

Please visit thePoint® for up-to-date Web resources on this topic.

CHAPTER 12

Care Management, Case Management, and Home Healthcare

Rosanna F. DeMarco

Without a sense of caring, there can be no sense of community.

Anthony J. D'Angelo

Never under any circumstances take a sleeping pill and a laxative on the same night.

Dave Barry

Much of your pain is the bitter potion by which the physician within you heals your sick self.

Khalil Gibran

chapter highlights

- Defining care management and case management
- Situating case management as a key component to home visiting
- Historical overview and definition of home care practice
- Description of the home care provision of services
- Examining types of home care agencies, services, and reimbursement
- Exploring role and scope of home care nursing practice during a home visit
- Identifying interdisciplinary roles and use of telehealth
- Describing types of chronic care conditions found in home care patients
- Review of current Health Care Reform and Home Health Care Delivery

objectives

- Identify the relationship between care and case management as a philosophical underpinning to the care given by community health nurses in the home.
- Define home care nursing practice.
- Identify the role of the home care nurse as part of an interdisciplinary team.
- Describe the key components of a home visit.
- Identify common care situations and interventions in home care.

key terms

Assisted living: A model of care for the elderly or disabled that includes services such as home care to maintain the independence of clients.

Balanced Budget Act: Federal act of 1997 that made significant cuts in home care budgets on the basis of the enactment of prospective reimbursement.

Care management: Coordination of a plan or process to bring health services together as a common whole in a cost-effective way.

Case management: Development and coordination of care for a selected client and family.

Client outcomes: Measurable objectives related to specific client (patient) care interventions.

Family caregiver: A member of the client's family, as defined by the client, who has voluntary responsibility to assist with the care of a client.

Homebound: The condition where a client cannot leave his or her home without significant effort.

Home healthcare: A provision of healthcare that occurs in the setting clients consider their home.

Hospital-based agency: A home health agency that is not freestanding in the community, one of many specialty services offered at a hospital setting.

Interdisciplinary collaboration: Sharing of evidence-based practice and skills by several disciplines as an integration strategy with clients and families in homes and other healthcare settings.

Intermittent care: Care that is not required continuously.

Managed care: A framework of fiscal management that emphasizes cost containment.

Necessity: Home care service given by a home care agency is reasonable on the basis of the status of the client.

Official agency: A home health agency that exists at the bequest of local, state, or federal legislation.

Parish nursing: A model of care for members of a faith community that can include wellness care through home visiting.

Plan of care: An agency-generated written document that is guided by a lengthy assessment of client and family needs.

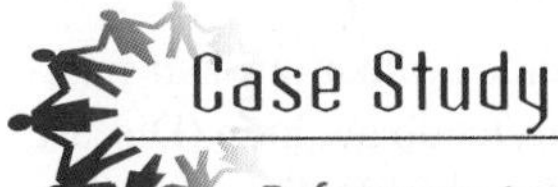

Case Study

References to the case study are found throughout this chapter (look for the case study icon). Readers should keep the case study in mind as they read the chapter.

Eleanor is an 85-year-old woman who lost her husband a year ago. She never learned to drive, and she was dependent on her husband. Now she must rely on her family, both functionally and financially. Eleanor owns a single-family home, and with the support of local family members, she has chosen to live alone there. She has savings of $20,000.

Eleanor is receiving Medicare benefits, including Medicare supplements for prescription drugs at extra cost. On the advice of an internal medicine physician whom she trusts, she takes several prescription drugs and sees a podiatrist. Her blood glucose level has been so high that she requires insulin therapy. She has been unable to leave her home without much effort. A home care nurse who came for 2 months helped find a homemaker and home health aide to provide assistance with bathing, meals, and light housekeeping. (This is a state-funded project for the elderly.)

Even with the help of her family and services, it is becoming less and less safe for Eleanor to live at home alone, and she needs to have more home health aide care for her safety. She has been told that to qualify for more services she would need to become eligible for Medicaid by "spending down" the $20,000 to $2,000. However, before Eleanor could become eligible for Medicaid services, she falls and is admitted to the local hospital with a hairline fracture in her upper humerus.

key terms (continued)

Proprietary agency: A home health agency that is motivated by a for-profit philosophy.
Reimbursement: The form of financial payment offered to home health agencies, among others, for services rendered to clients and families.
Skilled care: The requirement for reimbursement of services in home care (specifically, Medicare, but also Medicaid).
Skilled needs: Refer to the needs of the client that are accomplished through the professional abilities of a registered nurse or his or her supervised designee (e.g., a home health aide).
Telehealth: A form of electronic communication used to deliver healthcare information.
Voluntary agency: A home health agency that is motivated by a not-for-profit philosophy.

Increased longevity and improvements in the ability to care for people with chronic illness have led to an enormous increase in healthcare needs for people older than 65 years, as well as for younger people with chronic or life-threatening conditions. Even though 47 million Americans have no health insurance, the United States spends more on healthcare than other industrialized nations where all citizens are insured (California Health Care Foundation, 2008). Despite the increasing quality of life seen in older people and others who are disabled in some way, experts agree that excessive administrative costs, inflated prices, and inappropriate care are some of the many complicated reasons healthcare costs so much in the United States (Poisal et al., 2007). These are the key demographic factors behind the need to address a multigenerational complex of healthcare management, both globally and locally. Preventing illness and promoting health has often been given a lower priority financially in the United States, as described in Chapter 2. However, on an optimistic note, recent data do suggest that there is (1) a decrease in the prevalence of chronic disability, (2) an earlier diagnosis and treatment of disease, and (3) improved treatment of health problems (National Coalition on Health Care [NCHC], 2013).

Health-related quality of life and well-being is a key objective of *Healthy People 2020* (HP2020, 2014). As such, this chapter emphasizes the need to create, develop, and continue to invest in the evolution of an infrastructure that allows diverse populations to create the best place and circumstances for them to stay well in terms of how they define relevant and sensitive "quality." The following unravels key components of the efforts being made across all three levels of prevention to allow quality of life and well-being to be defined and addressed.

CARE MANAGEMENT

Care management is a term coined to define the evaluation of healthcare interventions, including need and appropriateness of care, and the actions taken to attain effective and efficient outcomes. The Utilization Review Accreditation Commission (URAC) (2008), an independent, not-for-profit organization committed to promoting healthcare quality, identifies utilization management as a key component in the care of clients because of continued rising medical costs. Care management and utilization management are often used as synonyms. In many cases, advances in technology, including the use of predictive modeling and other methods of data analysis, are creating opportunities for utilization management to be targeted to specific disease management areas more precisely.

In the case of Eleanor, care management or utilization management is the process by which her physician's office designates a nurse utilization manager to review client records along with her physician. Eleanor has Medicare coverage and has chosen to be part of a health provider system that offers inpatient and outpatient care directly or by referral. Her care is centralized by electronic record, so the utilization manager or care manager can easily track use of services within the approved system. The tracking is completed not just to keep statistical trends, but to understand the trends and costs associated with them. Once the trends and costs are understood, ways to give quality care at the best cost are offered to Eleanor. Care management and utilization management will inevitably benefit her by helping caregivers anticipate her needs, like home care, as more disability evolves from her advancing chronic comorbid conditions.

CASE MANAGEMENT

The Case Management Society of America (2013) defines **case management** as "a collaborative process of assessment, planning, facilitation and *advocacy* for options and services to meet an individual's health needs through communication and available resources to promote quality cost-effective outcomes." Advocacy in case management is significant, as is the case with all levels of patient care across the lifespan, because it requires health professionals and others to bring private needs to the level of public awareness. Advocacy is always moving the needs of patients, families, and communities to a point of awareness that will advance change and increase quality of a life and experience.

According to the URAC (2008), case management was first practiced by public health service providers early in the last century. The concept has been integrated into other systems over time and has become associated with the care of low-income clients and families who are considered at risk. The chief motivation in this integration is the need for a healthcare professional who advocates for the resources needed by clients. Care management is related to case management; without case management, care management could not be successful. Thus, case management can be considered a building block of care management.

Case management involves an intensive process called disease management. Disease management is a system of coordinated healthcare interventions and communications for groups of people with conditions in which client self-care efforts are significant. Disease management emphasizes prevention at the secondary and tertiary level using evidence-based practice guidelines. Collaborative practice models are a key to the success of disease management programs. These programs include physicians, nurses, and support-service providers, client and family, self-management education, process, and outcomes measurement, evaluation, and management; there is a routine reporting/feedback loop (Disease Management Association of America, 2013). Disease management often focuses on chronic illnesses such as heart disease, heart failure, diabetes, pulmonary disease, urinary incontinence, and asthma.

In disease management programs, in addition to medications, there is strong emphasis on the use of telephone coaching, Internet resources, and intensive client and family teaching to advance self-care and adherence to wellness care. Recently, to help clients and families manage their health problems in an effective and efficient manner, there has been an effort to bundle disease states together in light of many comorbidity patterns.

Eleanor's care and case management takes the form of a home care nurse, who uses a disease management approach to Eleanor's diabetes, congestive heart failure (CHF), and hypertension. This disease management approach involves these three conditions because they are all interrelated.

Other examples of case management approaches may not be disease oriented at all. For example, case management programs may evolve uniquely for pregnancy or postpartum care (Fetterolf, Stanziano, & Istwan, 2008).

EVIDENCE FOR PRACTICE

Fetterolf et al. (2008) address the fact that pregnancy and the care of newborns rank among the top healthcare expenditures. However, disease case management models are not suited for addressing the continuum of care for mothers and babies because the condition of pregnancy is not a disease, is not chronic, and is self-limited. Wellness approaches fail to fully engage the complexities and interventions needed for high-risk pregnancies. Case management alone is too comprehensive and intensive to focus on the large numbers of pregnancies requiring screening before case management is started. The management of a pregnant population through a continuum starting with early prenatal care and transitioning to newborn and maternal postpartum care is ideal. The authors describe a total maternal–newborn solution (TMNS) that considers pregnancy as a unique, high-volume condition with infrequent, but costly, complications that can benefit from primary and secondary preventive efforts to avoid or reduce the impact of complications in a cost-effective manner. A TMNS helps to improve the quality of care delivered, since participants and their healthcare providers are encouraged to follow standardized clinical guidelines and are monitored for compliance (a new way of experiencing case management).

A TMNS is made possible with the use of an information technology platform that provides a common infrastructure to track participant encounters and interventions, and to measure and report on maternal and newborn care delivered. Preliminary outcomes for the TMNS program prove it to be a promising approach for addressing the clinical and cost management of the pregnancy continuum.

To be a case or disease manager, one need not be a nurse. Although the American Nurses Credentialing Center (2013) does certify nurses in this specialty, social workers and public health experts may also serve in this role. The role is complex, and the many responsibilities include addressing the direct and immediate needs of clients and families and achieving quality improvement in the future (Box 12.1).

Care management and case management can be used across the continuum of health from acute care to care within communities. One important area where practices of care management and case management occur is in the home. The rest of this chapter is devoted to discussing home healthcare.

HOME HEALTHCARE

People spend most of their time in their neighborhoods and communities to which they belong. When they are ill and need care, they continue to spend most of their time in those same neighborhoods and communities. Home care nurses are challenged in many ways in caring for clients in their own homes. Home care nurses continue a historical legacy of autonomy, creativity, connection, and talent in advancing nursing practice using research and professional experience as their guides. If there is one thought that comes to mind when one says "home care," it is the place where the faint-hearted need not apply. Home care is a place where nurses practice in the extremes of complexity. It takes a competent and knowledgeable professional to make home care their professional "home."

People facing an acute or chronic illness or a new health-related situation may be candidates for **home healthcare**. This service involves caring for clients and their families wherever they may call "home," regardless of economic and class divisions. Home healthcare is part of a continuum of care to which nurses contribute. It has evolved over time on the basis of three distinct needs: (1) quality healthcare in places and spaces where people live most of their lives (homes and communities), (2) continued development of ways to inform healthcare providers what realities affect health promotion and prevention in the diverse, complex lives of people and families, and (3) cost containment in the healthcare industry. The development of health insurance, rising costs in healthcare in general, and medical and nursing specialization all have played a part in the development of home healthcare as it is today.

History of Home Healthcare

In the United States, home healthcare began in the early 1800s. Key historical points are listed in Box 12.2. The last historical event in this list, the establishment of Medicare, has set a pattern for payment for home services for the next

box 12.1 Case Managers' Role

A case manager's responsibilities include the following functions:

- Advocacy and education—ensuring that the client has a representative who can speak up and represent their needs for needed services and education
- Clinical care coordination/facilitation—coordinating multiple aspects of care to ensure that the client progresses
- Continuity/transition management—transitioning of the client to the appropriate level of care needed
- Utilization/financial management—managing resource utilization and reimbursement for services
- Performance and outcomes management—monitoring and, if needed, intervening to achieve desired goals and outcomes for both the client and the hospital
- Psychosocial management—assessing and addressing psychosocial needs, including individual, familial, and environmental
- Research and practice development—identifying practice improvements and using evidence-based data to influence needed practice changes

Source: Data from Kongstvedt, P. R. (2001). *The managed health care handbook* (4th ed.). New York, NY: Aspen.

box 12.2 History of Home Healthcare

- 1800s—Large wave of immigration to the United States with poverty and poor health facing families and professional caregivers
- 1859—William Rathbone, a wealthy Quaker philanthropist business man, with the help of Florence Nightingale, sent trained nurses into the homes of the sick poor in Liverpool, England.
- 1885—First Visiting Nurse Associations established in Buffalo (NY), Boston (MA), and Philadelphia (PA)
- 1893—Henry Street Settlement established by nurse Lillian Wald in New York City
- 1894—VNAs are established and grow rapidly.
- 1909—Metropolitan Life Insurance Company offers home care services as a benefit.
- 1910—Columbia University offers the first university course in public health nursing.
- 1929—Crash of the stock market occurs, and federal government allocates funds to help those in need of home care.
- 1940s—Hospitals interested in home care because of chronic illness rates
- 1966—Medicare established

Source: Data from Buler-Wilkerson, K. (2001). *No place like home.* Baltimore, MD: The Johns Hopkins University Press.

40 years. The federal government and its fiscal intermediaries at the state level established Medicare's initial payment protocol. This protocol involved fee-for-service (i.e., a set fee for a particular service) charges. Home health agencies such as visiting nurse associations (VNAs) and other agencies established the cost for a particular service and then billed Medicare for that service. Unfortunately, this payment approach left Medicare and clients vulnerable to a blossoming industry where some home care services fraudulently inflated costs and service billing frequency to increase profit margins (National Center for Policy Analysis, 2013).

In the past 20 years, Medicare regulations have served as the basis for Medicaid programs, as well as for other health insurance protocols for payment or **reimbursement**. In this context, payment for healthcare costs was scrutinized because of its inflationary nature. As clients aged and became more seriously ill with chronic illnesses, the system of **managed care** was introduced to encourage healthcare providers to hold costs down through the streamlining of services (Kongstvedt, 2001). Managed care efforts included the idea of prospective reimbursement. Prospective reimbursement is a system in which reimbursement rates are set, for a given period of time, prior to the circumstances giving rise to actual reimbursement claims (Prospective Reimbursement, 2008). In response to this payment approach, hospitals began to reduce the stays of clients and more clients went home earlier and sicker than before. In a continued effort to decrease costs in home health industry, in 1997, Congress passed the **Balanced Budget Act** (DeMarco & O'Brien, 1999). Congress cut $16 billion in payments to the home health industry over 5 years; that is, it slashed reimbursement rates. As a result, home health agencies closed or began to merge because they could not keep up with the costs. In 1997, there were 10,000 home care agencies. After the Balanced Budget Act of 1997, there were 7,000 such agencies (Magee, 2007). Agencies were forced to develop so-called care mixes, where the incentive based on reimbursement encouraged them not to take care of the sickest or the most costly "cases"—clients.

As the previous discussion indicates, many home care agencies depend on reimbursement trends, and trends in payment for home care are beginning to change again. In 2003, the Medicare Modernization and Improvement Act included a provision to eliminate what would have been an inflation increase in home health rates (Centers for Medicare & Medicaid Services [CMS], 2013). Medicare is exploring reimbursement based on performance (i.e., successful outcomes) (Rosenthal & Frank, 2006). However, home care agencies continue to be needed for the aging population of the United States because most people continue to want to be cared for in their own homes, whether they are facing acute or chronic illness or death. The saying "there is no place like home" is truly a reality.

Types of Agencies

Because of the variety of reimbursement mechanisms that have evolved over time in home healthcare, many different forms of services have evolved based on levels of philanthropy; profit-making needs; and federal, state, and city funding. There are four distinct types of home healthcare agencies: private/voluntary (not-for-profit), hospital-based, proprietary (for-profit), and public (Medline Plus, 2013).

Private/Voluntary Agencies

Voluntary agencies are generally established as not-for-profit entities, although they operate with the same fiscal objectives as "for-profit agencies." The difference is that they are often governed by a voluntary board of directors and community-based advisory boards that are interested in fiscally sound, high-quality care for clients they decide will be their service population. Any profit margin that is acquired is reinvested in the operations of the home healthcare service. The advisory and legislative members of the boards direct the chief executive and fiscal officers in how home healthcare should be offered to the service population. A good example is a VNA.

Hospital-Based Agencies

Hospital-based agencies have developed within the past 25 years to save money and maintain control of client care costs. In addition, a key objective is to maintain levels of quality and increase collaboration by establishing home healthcare services as part of a continuum of care offered by the hospital. As a healthcare system, hospitals embraced an approach to care that included prevention and health promotion through divisions that offer primary care, emergency care, acute care, and chronic care in various onsite or offsite facilities. The home is one such site. The principal idea was to establish plans of care that were congruent with a hospital system philosophy. Hospital-based home healthcare agencies are governed by not only the same board that governs the hospital but also an advisory board similar to that of a VNA; this helps match their care initiatives to the realities of the population they serve. Depending on the hospital, hospital-based agencies can be "for-profit" or "not-for-profit."

An example of a home healthcare agency associated with a hospital is the Home Health Care Department of Boston General Hospital. All Boston General Hospital clients who need skilled nursing care at home are referred to the Home Healthcare Department of the hospital and followed over time. People that have been readmitted, and others, may also be referred to this group.

Eleanor receives all of her home care services, including skilled nursing, physical therapy, and occupational therapy, through a hospital-based hospice program that is part of a hospital system made up of five hospitals. The hospitals are owned by the Catholic diocese of the city in which Eleanor lives.

Proprietary Agencies

Proprietary agencies are private agencies that plan to and want to make a profit. They can be part of a local, national, or international chain of home healthcare agencies directed toward any group of clients with particular healthcare problems or challenges. For example, an agency that has as its goal the provision of home health aides and homemaking services to people in need of personal care and housekeeping services, will provide, for profit, trained home health aides and homemakers to assist people and families with these needs. Their services are often paid for privately by families, and any profit margin is used to benefit the owner of the agency or chain of agencies.

Official Agencies

Official agencies are supported by public monies that often come from taxes. The public monies can come from local, state, or federal governments. Essentially, citizens and legislators identify a need for home health services that are often part of a larger public health approach to certain populations. For example, a county health department may be established with several goals and objectives to promote the health of people in the area for which they are responsible. This may include lead paint screening for children, tuberculosis treatment and follow-up, well-child clinics, water-testing facilities, and a public home care agency. Generally, there is a mandate to serve all people without exception. Thus, public home health programs often care for many clients that may not be admitted to private, voluntary, or proprietary home health programs. However, with the constant rise in public health problems such as obesity, diabetes, human immunodeficiency virus/acquired immunodeficiency syndrome (HIV/AIDS), low-birth-weight births, and infant mortality, many public home health agencies are supported financially for the care they give to citizens who may have little access to any other care.

Financing and Regulation of Home Care

Home healthcare services are reimbursed by local, state, and federal funds; private insurance; and private individuals. Government funding for home healthcare includes Medicare (federal), Medicaid (state) (CMS, 2013) as well as monies from TRICARE (federal funds for military personnel and their dependents) and the Veterans Administration (federal funds for those who are currently serving or have served in the armed services of the United States [TRICARE, 2013]). Insurance companies that pay for home healthcare can be independent (e.g., State Farm Insurance) or can be part of a health maintenance organization (HMO) or a case management organization. Medicare, Medicaid, TRICARE, and Veterans Administration coverage is generated from monies that citizens contribute to the state or federal government through taxes. Insurance companies, HMOs, and case management organizations give coverage based on monies that are paid directly to them in monthly or annual increments for the purpose of giving home healthcare when and if they are needed. What is common in the latter type of insurance is these organizations coordinate with home healthcare agencies from which the clients are able to obtain care.

Home healthcare is regulated by the state and federal government. Insurance companies generally align themselves with the regulations stipulated by these governments, but may have their own rules and regulations. Home health agencies are certified through a process where stipulated conditions must be present for the agency to give services to the public and receive payment for those services. For example, Medicare has the following criteria for eligibility: homebound, a plan of care, skilled needs, intermittent care needs, and necessity.

Homebound refers to a condition based upon how difficult it is for a client to leave the home. To leave home must require a taxing effort and must be related to maintaining health and personal care. This may include attending a medical day care program where they would receive medications and therapy while family members may be at work. It may also include only leaving home when going to an appointment with a healthcare provider. There may be variations in why a client must leave home (church, a family birthday event, to buy a pair of shoes), but the key stipulation is the taxing effort required to do this, and the infrequency of the event. Determining a client's homebound status is primarily a way reimbursement systems qualify the severity level of an illness for which they will pay for services.

Eleanor manages to move from a chair in the kitchen to a chair in the living room and to the bathroom with a walker. She requires great effort in ambulating with a walker. In the past, if she had to leave the house, she used to need two people to descend eight steps. Eventually, her family installed an exterior elevator lift to help her access a car to go to physician appointments or family gatherings. By definition, she is homebound because of the taxing effort required to leave her home.

A **plan of care** is an agency-generated written document that is guided by a lengthy assessment. The assessment that is currently used across the United States is called the Outcome and Assessment Information Set (OASIS, 2013). This assessment tool represents items that help home care professionals assess adult home care clients. The items in OASIS assessment include sociodemographic, environmental, health, functional health, personal support data and the status of adult clients who are in a pre- or postnatal state. The OASIS data are reported to the state where the home health agency exists to create a larger database that can be used for state comparisons across the United States. The accuracy needed to complete this assessment is critical because each assessment item becomes the standard from which **client outcomes** are measured. In addition, the OASIS data are used by Medicare to help determine how home healthcare agencies are paid for their services (CMS, 2014).

EVIDENCE FOR PRACTICE

O'Connor and Davitt (2012) recognized that the OASIS is the patient-specific, standardized assessment used in Medicare home healthcare to plan care, determine reimbursement, and measure quality in home care settings. The authors studied the debate over the reliability and validity of the OASIS as a research tool and outcome measure. They undertook a systematic literature review of English-language articles and identified 12 studies published in the last 10 years examining the validity and reliability of the OASIS. Empirical findings indicated the validity and reliability of the OASIS range from low to moderate but vary depending on the item studied. Limitations in the existing research include nonrepresentative samples; inconsistencies in methods used, items tested, measurement, and statistical procedures; and the changes to the OASIS itself over time. The inconsistencies suggest that additional research is needed to confirm the value of the OASIS for measuring patient outcomes, research, and quality improvement.

The home health nurse completes the assessment and establishes the functional needs of the client and the services required. What is important to understand is that, like many areas of healthcare, home healthcare is progressing toward a system of reimbursement that will be based not just on prospective reimbursement (diagnosis and presumed trajectory of care) but on outcomes of care. Therefore, a plan of care based on an accurate assessment, with identified activities leading to outcomes, will be critical to sustaining all types of home healthcare agencies in the future.

Another very well-known system that assists healthcare providers in organizing clinical data in the context of assessment is called the Omaha System (Omaha System, 2013). This model of organizing data includes three relational components: a problem classification scheme (client assessment); an intervention scheme (care plans and services); and a problem rating scale of outcomes (client change/evaluation). The work on creating this model began in the 1970s by the Visiting Nurse Association of Omaha, Nebraska, while adopting a problem-oriented approach as a guide to practice and documentation and management (Omaha System, 2013). The idea was conceived and developed so that an information system could be used that was standardized (written or now computerized) based on an integrated, valid, reliable clinical approach which was organized for clients who received services, and their specific needs. Over 10 years of nationally funded research yielded consensus on standardized language used in client assessment, care plans, and outcomes. This system currently meets Medicare/Medicaid, Joint Commission, and Children's Health Care Assistance Plan (CHAP) guidelines and regulations. It has been recognized by the American Nurses Association (ANA) since 1992, and passed the Healthcare Information Technology Standards Panel (HITSP) Tier 2 selection criteria for Use Cases in 2007. It is integrated into the National Library of Medicine's Metathesaurus; CINAHL; ABC Codes; NIDSEC; Logical Observation Identifiers, Names, and Codes (LOINC®); and SNOMED CT®. It is registered (recognized) by Health Level Seven (HL7®), and is congruent with the reference terminology model for the International Organization for Standardization (ISO). It is being mapped to the International Classification of Nursing Practice (ICNP®) (Omaha System, 2013). Current users are mostly in the United States and include home care, public health, and school health practice settings, nurse-managed center staff, hospital-based and managed care case managers, educators and students, occupational health nurses, faith community staff, acute care and rehabilitation hospital/long-term care staff, researchers, members of various disciplines, and computer software vendors (Omaha System, 2013). In each instance, the focus of care is **skilled needs** provided by these professionals and directed to patients, families, and communities. See Box 12.3 for domains, intervention schemes, and outcome rating scales of the Omaha System.

Skilled needs refer to the needs of the client that are accomplished through the professional abilities of registered nurses or their supervised designees (e.g., home health aides). This includes skilled observation, assessment, teaching, management, and evaluation of a variety of conditions and situations. Examples of skilled nursing needs versus nonskilled nursing needs are presented in Table 12.1.

Eleanor has had several admissions for home care. Each admission stopped after a 60-day period (required by Medicare guidelines), when her **skilled care** condition stabilized. For example, one admission occurred after a hospitalization for CHF. When her weight, breathing patterns, medication adherence, and blood pressure stabilized, she was discharged to the care of her daughters, and the local elder services provided her with home health aides to help with meals, bathing, and housekeeping needs.

Intermittent care refers to a situation in which skilled care is usually provided over several hours during the day, several days during the week, for a specified time period. Medicare requires the specified time period to be 60 days with appropriate renewals if skilled needs continue to exist.

Necessity means that the service given by a home care agency is reasonable based on the status of the client. For example, it would be unreasonable to schedule daily visits to the home of clients who have learned to use a glucometer to test their blood glucose levels effectively. It would be reasonable to visit twice a week for 2 weeks to see if the client is conducting the blood glucose test correctly and accurately.

box 12.3 **Omaha System (Domains, Intervention Schemes, and Outcome Rating Scale) (Omaha System, 2013)**

Domains and Problems of the Problem Classification Scheme

Environmental domain: Material resources and physical surroundings both inside and outside the living area, neighborhood, and broader community
- Income
- Sanitation
- Residence
- Neighborhood/workplace safety

Psychosocial domain: Patterns of behavior, emotion, communication, relationships, and development
- Communication with community resources
- Social contact
- Role change
- Interpersonal relationship
- Spirituality
- Grief
- Mental health
- Sexuality
- Caretaking/parenting
- Neglect
- Abuse
- Growth and development

Physiological domain: Functions and processes that maintain life.
- Hearing
- Vision
- Speech and language
- Oral health
- Cognition
- Pain
- Consciousness
- Skin
- Neuromusculoskeletal function
- Respiration
- Circulation
- Digestion–hydration
- Bowel function
- Urinary function
- Reproductive function
- Pregnancy
- Postpartum
- Communicable/infectious condition

Health-related behaviors domain: Patterns of activity that maintain or promote wellness, promote recovery, and decrease the risk of disease
- Nutrition
- Sleep and rest patterns
- Physical activity
- Personal care
- Substance use
- Family planning
- Healthcare supervision
- Medication regimen

Intervention Categories

Teaching, guidance, and counseling: Activities designed to provide information and materials, encourage action and responsibility for self-care and coping, and assist the individual/family/community to make decisions and solve problems

Treatments and procedures: Technical activities such as wound care, specimen collection, resistive exercises, and medication prescriptions that are designed to prevent, decrease, or alleviate signs and symptoms of the individual/family/community

Case management: Activities such as coordination, advocacy, and referral that facilitate service delivery, improve communication among health and human service providers, promote assertiveness, and guide the individual/family/community toward use of appropriate resources.

Surveillance: Activities such as detection, measurement, critical analysis, and monitoring intended to identify the individual/family/community's status in relation to a given condition or phenomenon.

Targets

- Anatomy/physiology
- Anger management
- Behavior modification
- Bladder care
- Bonding/attachment
- Bowel care
- Cardiac care
- Caretaking/parenting skills
- Cast care
- Communication
- Community outreach worker services
- Continuity of care
- Coping skills
- Day care/respite
- Dietary management
- Discipline
- Dressing change/wound care
- Durable medical equipment use
- Education
- Employment
- End-of-life care
- Environment
- Exercises
- Family planning care
- Feeding procedures
- Finances
- Gait training
- Genetics
- Growth/development care
- Home
- Homemaking/housekeeping
- Infection precautions
- Interaction
- Interpreter/translator services
- Laboratory findings
- Legal system
- Medical/dental care
- Medication action/side effects
- Medication administration

(continued on page 212)

box 12.3 **Omaha System (Domains, Intervention Schemes, and Outcome Rating Scale) (Omaha System, 2013) *(continued)***

Medication coordination/ordering
Medication prescription
Medication setup
Mobility/transfers
Nursing care
Nutritionist care
Occupational therapy care
Ostomy care
Other community resources
Paraprofessional/aide care
Personal hygiene
Physical therapy care
Positioning
Recreational therapy care
Relaxation/breathing techniques
Respiratory care
Respiratory therapy care
Rest/sleep
Safety
Screening procedures
Sickness/injury care
Signs/symptoms—mental/emotional
Signs/symptoms—physical
Skin care
Social work/counseling care
Specimen collection
Speech and language pathology care
Spiritual care
Stimulation/nurturance
Stress management
Substance use cessation
Supplies
Support group
Support system
Transportation
Wellness
Other

Concepts and Ratings of the Problem Rating Scale for Outcomes

Concept	1	2	3	4	5
Knowledge: Ability of the client to remember and interpret information	No knowledge	Minimal knowledge	Basic knowledge	Adequate knowledge	Superior knowledge
Behavior: Observable responses, actions, or activities of the client fitting the occasion or purpose	Not appropriate behavior	Rarely appropriate behavior	Inconsistently appropriate behavior	Usually appropriate behavior	Consistently appropriate behavior
Status: Condition of the client in relation to objective and subjective defining characteristics	Extreme signs/ symptoms	Severe signs/ symptoms	Moderate signs/ symptoms	Minimal signs/ symptoms	No signs/ symptoms

table 12.1 **Comparison of Skilled and Nonskilled Nursing Care**

Skilled	Nonskilled
Assessment of lungs and weight of a client diagnosed with congestive heart failure	Changing a dry dressing
Teaching a newly diagnosed diabetic client how to fill insulin syringes or use an insulin pen	Teaching the client's significant other/spouse how to pay healthcare bills
Management of care given to a client postcerebrovascular accident by speech therapy, physical therapy, and home health aide services	Managing care of a home health aide after all healthcare skilled needs have been stabilized
Changing a complicated wet to dry dressing on a client's abdomen	Pouring medications in plastic labeled container
Monitoring the fluctuating blood pressure of an elderly man who has just started taking antihypertensive medication	Visiting the client to decrease loneliness

Role and Scope of Home Health Practice

The ANA has provided nurses in home health practice with an official document called the *Scope and Standards of Home Health Nursing Practice* (American Nurses Association, 2007). It provides guidelines for nurses involved in home healthcare practice, including standards of care and standards of professional practice. The standards of care include the key elements of the nursing process:

1. Assessment by collecting data about home care clients
2. Diagnosis through the analysis of data
3. Outcome identification that helps home care nurses identify nurse-sensitive measures
4. Planning in the form of nurse-sensitive interventions directed to the identified outcomes
5. Implementation-identified, nurse-centered actions in collaboration with clients and families
6. Evaluation outcome accomplishment through nurse-sensitive interventions

Although this may sound familiar in view of the standards of care in many areas of the continuum of nursing practice, Medicare, Medicaid, and private insurance agencies are moving in the direction of using these standards of practice as reimbursement strategies for agencies based on successful outcome management. Thus, fiscal rewards in the future may be related to identifying nurse-sensitive outcomes as described in this process.

Standards of professional performance described in the ANA document are areas that home care nurses must address in the context of their practice. They include the following:

- Evaluating quality of care
- Evaluating their performance in the agency or home care work in which they are involved, maintaining current competency
- Helping develop nursing students and other colleagues who aspire to become home care nurses, as well as collaborating with others in the care of home care clients
- Being ethical in their practice, as well as using evidence-based practice in their encounters with clients and families

One of the most powerful professional performance standards, unique to home care because of client and family engagement in clients' own world (their home), is the emphasis on helping clients and families to be consumers of healthcare. This may take the form of helping clients and families receive information about their health conditions, health promotion, and disease prevention, as well as the risks and benefits of receiving healthcare in the home.

How can I be useful, of what service can I be? There is something inside me, what can it be?

Vincent van Gogh

STUDENT REFLECTION

I absolutely loved my clinical rotation in home care. One of my clients was an older man. I really liked traveling to his home and meeting him in his own living space. I could really teach and apply principles of medical surgical care by adapting them to his world. For example, I needed to figure out where the cleanest and most optimal place for him to sit and bend over to change a small dressing on his leg would be, and I managed to do this successfully by observing the cleanest and safest place during the home visit. We together decided that the first floor bathroom would work because he could sit on the elevated toilet, reach the sink to wash his hands, and bend effectively without becoming hypotensive.

I have to admit that, despite having a cell phone and easy access for help and advice, when I was allowed to visit my client without my instructor for the first time, I was nervous. There is a lot of autonomy in this role, and many people say that before you take a job in home care, you should have 2 years of hospital experience. If I really wanted to concentrate in home care, I would need to figure out how to be mentored as a new graduate so my confidence would be supported by a system that would help me learn to think critically while being a solitary practitioner of nursing care in the community.

Interdisciplinary Care

Home care, like many areas of healthcare, is an area where **interdisciplinary collaboration** occurs. Various members of the healthcare team, not just nurses, contribute their expertise to client management in the home. Generally, the following groups receive care from home health agencies: adults with acute or chronic illnesses, older adults, mothers and newborns, and children and their parents. Nurses are often the clinical leaders who manage the necessary care. Often, this care is highly specialized and requires the expertise of other members of the healthcare team. Often, physical therapists, occupational therapists, speech therapists, recreational therapists, social workers, nutritionists, and home health aides assist the nurse in meeting client-centered outcomes. Home health aide assistants and home care nurses follow through with delegated tasks that are legally appropriate in terms of the standards of practice designated by the ANA and the local board of registration of nursing. Other members of the home health team are members of different disciplines—professionals who have a special and unique knowledge about an area of clinical science, such as physicians or nurse practitioners in specific fields. It is not uncommon for clinicians on these teams to work together on particular outcomes that benefit the client and family as a whole (Lehning & Austin, 2011).

The challenge of interdisciplinary work and teams is to be able to work together in a complementary way to help clients and families on the basis of their assessed needs. This is not always easy because many members of various healthcare disciplines see only the unique contribution they make as an isolated involvement with clients and families (Chatfield, Christos, & McGregor, 2012). In reality, all healthcare professionals, regardless of discipline, must work together and find common outcomes so that clients and families can achieve wellness. For example, a woman diagnosed with a cerebrovascular accident may be a client of a home health agency. In this case, she may have speech difficulties and restricted use of her upper and lower extremities. Together with coping with the loss of control, she also needs to make healthier food choices directly related to the pre-existing condition that is thought to have caused the "stroke" (hypertension). The nurse who makes the home visit would immediately consult with a speech and language expert, physical therapist, occupational therapist, and a nutritionist in conjunction with a physician as a team. The home care nurse, acting as a clinical leader, would talk together formally at case conferences, or informally with a group of experts, about the need to change or to maintain the plan of care to meet identified outcomes.

Some healthcare authorities believe that the word "interdisciplinary" is a misnomer. They say that a better term is perhaps "transdisciplinary" (Cartmill, Soklaridis, & Cassidy, 2011). This term means that in the context of working together, home care experts are not just contributing specialty knowledge in the care of clients and families in homes, they are also learning from each other and creating a whole, connected disciplinary approach.

Telehealth

Telehealth is a form of electronic communication used to deliver (1) acute care and specialty consultations, (2) home telenursing, and (3) electronic referrals to specialists in expert health facilities. According to Thede, it involves "using electronic communications for transmitting healthcare information such as health promotion, disease prevention, professional or lay education, diagnosis, or actual treatment to people located at a different geographical area" (2003, p. 129). Telehealth relates to two kinds of approaches that are applicable in home care. The first involves electronically stored information that can be shared with others using technology, and the second involves a real interaction between a client and a healthcare provider. The latter telehealth approach is called real-time technology (Thede, 2003), which can include the use of diagnostic instruments that can transmit images or sounds to professionals in other areas. For example, an otoscope can be used in a client's home to send images electronically to an otolaryngologic expert for evaluation. In another instance, monitoring devices can be installed in homes to record the blood pressure, pulse, and weight of a client who has been diagnosed with CHF. Telecommunication of this information to home health agencies allows them to enhance their responsiveness related to subtle changes in client's conditions (Omboni, Gazzola, Carabelli, & Parati, 2013). The goal is for the clients to be stable and well at home.

EVIDENCE FOR PRACTICE

Antonicelli, Mazzanti, Abbatecola, and Parati (2010) undertook a research study addressing the needs of the elderly diagnosed with CHF. Despite evidence showing that administration of β-blockers (β-adrenoceptor antagonists) can improve the clinical status of CHF patients, use of these agents in adequate dosages is not routine at home because of the possible risk of bradyarrhythmia. Telecardiology has recently been investigated as a means of constantly monitoring the heart rate of CHF patients in their homes, and may be a solution to increase use of β-blockers (β-adrenoceptor antagonists) while decreasing the risk of bradyarrhythmia. Antonicelli and colleagues assessed the impact of telemonitoring on patients' adherence to prescribed therapeutic regimens, particularly β-blockers, and whether use of home telemonitoring reduced mortality and rate of readmission to hospital in elderly CHF patients compared with normal specialized CHF team care. A total of 57 patients with CHF (31 New York Heart Association [NYHA] class II, 23 NYHA class III, and 3 NYHA class IV), with a mean ± SD age of 78.2 ± 7.3 years, were randomized to a control group who received standard care, or to a home telemonitoring (TM) group. Patients were followed up over 12 months. Compared with the control group, the TM group had a significant increase in the use of β-blockers, HMG-CoA reductase inhibitors (statins) and aldosterone-receptor antagonists. A reduction in nitrate administration compared with baseline was also seen in the TM group. The 12-month occurrence of the primary combined endpoint of mortality and hospital readmission for CHF was significantly lower in the TM group than in the control group ($p < 0.01$). This study showed that a home care model, including telemonitoring of relevant clinical parameters, may provide useful support in the management of patients with CHF.

Telehealth can also be used in other ways. Information that is stored electronically and shared with others using electronic devices is another way home care providers can keep records of client and family progress, but it can also be a way to share client education information (Thede, 2003). For example, slide presentations can be transferred to help clients and families learn about an intervention that may help with their care or help them learn more about a chronic illness and the usual care practices offered to help their situation. Other examples are programs that allow downloadable information with dynamic pictures and multimedia effects to help clients understand their illness, or transition to a new role (new mothers), or adjust to changes in mobility (Thede, 2003).

Home Care Models

Assisted Living

Long-term supportive services have evolved and currently include assisted living and continuing care communities, as well as nursing homes.

Assisted living is a type of community-based care that combines quasi-independent living with the availability of nursing care onsite and through home care visits (Stefanacci & Podrazik, 2005). It generally is a level of care for people who cannot live on their own, but are not yet ready for a nursing home. This type of living arrangement is different from living independently in one's own apartment, such as living in a senior living facility, in that many activities are provided communally (e.g., eating, recreation). There is an organized effort to create a "caring community" where residents are supervised and help is available for day-to-day living tasks. Many older community dwellers find assisted living or continuing care communities to be places where gradual changes in physical, cognitive, and emotional abilities can be addressed with centralized services. In many cases, this choice is made on the basis of financial ability to support such an option. Many people may want to stay in their own home as a way to protect a long-term investment financially and emotionally.

Eleanor does not want to leave her home. She is willing to "spend down" her $20,000 in the bank to become eligible for Medicaid so that she can receive more services in her home and not have to move to an assisted living or retirement community. But this decision to live alone, despite having family nearby, puts her in jeopardy for falls and other possible emergencies. The decision is an autonomous one because she has no cognitive deficits. Once she was "admitted" to home care for a skilled need, a social worker came to visit her and tried to convince her to think about a safer way to live, but she adamantly refused.

Home health nurses see many clients in assisted living communities. The care they give is congruent with the standards of care described previously, but often the other members of the assisted living community become the client's "family"—and rightfully so. Retirement community dwellers consistently live an ethic of caring for each other and are involved with each other's care. Interdisciplinary teams from home care agencies have developed, with great success, extensive resources to support community elders in assisted living units (Flatt, Agimi, & Albert, 2012). There is a growing belief that not only do patients (particularly elders experience chronic care issues), families, and communities benefit from the contributions of the many healthcare professionals (physicians, nurses, midwives, dietitians, pharmacists, podiatrists, mental health and addiction professionals, physiotherapists occupational therapists, and chiropractors among others), but these professions themselves benefit in the context of case and care management. Interdisciplinary collaboration improves patient care and outcomes, access to care, recruitment and retention of health providers, and improved satisfaction among patients and health providers. Family health teams are evolving in effectively providing comprehensive primary healthcare as well as long-term care for elders for improved health-related quality of life (Zubritsky et al., 2012). The opportunity to be part of an interdisciplinary team can expand the scope of services by allowing teams to evolve with unique cultures and skill sets.

The patient-centered medical home (PCMH) is an evolving model that improves access to care by increasing coordination between patients, families, and their interdisciplinary team. Emerging data show that an integrated approach from a professional team to care of the whole person improves management of chronic illnesses wherever the patient lives (National Committee for Quality Assurance, 2014).

EVIDENCE FOR PRACTICE

Masotti, Fick, Johnson-Masotti, and MacLeod (2006) used the determinants of a health model to hypothesize that environmental determinants have a different impact on people at different ages. These researchers refer to retirement or assisted living communities as naturally occurring retirement communities (NORCs). Health benefits to living within NORCs have been observed and likely vary depending on where the specific NORC exists on the healthy NORC spectrum. Some NORC environments are healthier than others for seniors. Health benefits within healthy NORCs are higher where physical and social environments facilitate greater activity and promote feelings of well-being. Compared with the provision of additional medical or social services, healthy NORCs are a low-cost, community-level approach to facilitating healthy aging. Municipal governments should pursue policies that stimulate and support the development of healthy NORCs.

Home Visits to the Homeless

The thought of making a home visit to a person who may not have a home seems counterintuitive, but home care nurses do visit many homeless people (Pijl-Zieber & Kalischuk, 2011). There are unique challenges related to timing, location, and clean conditions in making a visit and providing care to someone who is homeless, but it is possible and quite rewarding. Many facilities provide shelter to homeless clients, including shelters devoted to posthospitalization care, until the clients are strong enough to return to their usual way of surviving in the community. These shelters may be where the home visit occurs. "Home" care for stasis ulcer care or follow-up related to tuberculosis or HIV is not unusual. There are also groups of interdisciplinary caregivers who make visits to clients throughout the streets of the community, especially at times when many homeless people are at great risk for injury and may need care. This includes during very cold or hot weather, natural disasters, and during unstable conditions related to violence in communities. The comorbidities that are often present pose challenges

(Wong, 2008). Many homeless people have two or more medical and/or surgical conditions, along with mental health problems or addiction histories, including smoking (Okuyemi et al., 2013). For example, people may have mental health problems as well as alcoholism and other addictions. Special skills are required to understand how to assist these people while trying to obtain affordable and safe housing for them.

Other underserved adults and older adults, including uninsured, underinsured, and racially and ethnically diverse populations, are being treated in hospitals, or are receiving extended care in long-term care facilities because they face serious, chronic illness that require palliative care. Many clinical management issues are pertinent to caring for seriously ill clients and their families, including the need to integrate *Healthy People 2020* objectives, such as those that specifically address the epidemic of HIV, cancer, kidney disease, diabetes, chronic and disabling health conditions, respiratory illness, heart disease and stroke, dementia, drug safety, mental health, nutrition, and preventive services. Home care nurses who specialize in the area of palliative care may visit these areas specifically because they offer the client and staff expertise in comfort care as a client's condition deteriorates. Hospice home care is one example of a "home visit" made to facilities that care for the serious and chronically ill who are choosing to stop all curative interventions. Hospice home care is discussed in more detail in Chapter 23.

Parish/Faith Community Nursing

According to Carson and Koenig (2011), **parish nursing** is an approach to holistic care for clients and families in the community. The seminal work of Westberg (1999) identified seven key roles of the parish or faith community nurse: (1) health educator, (2) personal health counselor, (3) referral agent, (4) coordinator of volunteers, (5) developer of supportive groups, (6) integrator of faith and health, and (7) health advocate. Faith community nursing can be delivered in several ways in communities. One aspect of faith community nursing is that of home visiting. The home visits are focused on care given in the context of the seven roles identified by Westberg (1999) and are often negotiated with a faith leader in a community parish, congregation, or synagogue. In many cases, these roles are not reimbursed by insurance, but serve as ways to coordinate care to families as needed.

Tis not enough to help the feeble up, but to support them after.

William Shakespeare

The Home Visit

There are five phases to a home visit: (1) initiating the visit, (2) preparation, (3) the actual visit, (4) termination of the visit, and (5) postvisit planning. In the context of each of these phases, attention must be paid to safety for the nurse as well as for the client.

Initiating the Visit

Community health nurses initiate home visits for a variety of reasons. Many home care agencies receive referrals from physicians or their designees (discharge planners from other healthcare institutions). Referrals can be sent to home health agencies at any time (24/7). Generally, home care agencies make sure that an initial visit is made within 24 hours after receiving a referral. The client's situation must satisfy the reimbursement criteria mentioned earlier if Medicare funding is to be used. Often, these conditions are validated during the first home visit, and plans or alternatives are discussed if these are not met. When receiving a referral, it is particularly important to make sure that the orders and directions for care are clear and accurate. If necessary, a clarifying phone call should be made, prior to the visit, to the person who has referred the client to the agency.

Preparation

Documentation is critical. All appropriate paperwork required for the assessment of the client and family must be available, in electronic format if the nurse plans to use a laptop computer for charting, or as hard copy.

EQUIPMENT

The home care nurse must bring supplies and equipment that may be needed for the visit, depending on the client's diagnosis and specific skilled need. Examples include sterile or clean dressings, urinary catheters, a walker, sterile saline solution, and distilled water, as well as antimicrobial agents and paper towels that can be used for handwashing. A home care nurse does not use client sink areas to wash his or her hands, in order to decrease the chance of cross-contamination. Many nurses use alcohol-based cleansers as a reasonable and aseptic way to cleanse their hands in home situations. In addition, the nurse must keep equipment that is often used, and may be needed unexpectedly (e.g., dressings, sterile solutions if weather permitting, catheters) in his or her vehicle. These articles should be secured in the trunk or hatch of the car so that they are not visible; this decreases the potential for theft and damage to the vehicle used for the home visit.

DIRECTIONS

Getting directions for the home visit is very important. Portable or installed global positioning systems (GPSs) are available, which work via a satellite, or generic maps can help home care nurses locate clients (Wikipedia, 2013). However, becoming familiar with the directions of routes (north, south, east, west), using landmarks, and making sure that unusual locations are explained before one leaves for a visit are important.

PERSONAL SAFETY

Safety prevention for home care nurses is part of preparing for a home visit. Many issues need to be considered. Some key advice is given in Box 12.4. Home care nurses must think about questions such as, "When and where will I go to

box 12.4 Safety Tips for Home Care Nurses

- Be alert and aware of your surroundings.
- Act like you know where you are going.
- Do not let your guard down.
- Trust your gut; if you feel unsafe, *leave* the area.
- Go to high-risk areas early in the day.
- Carry a whistle.
- Keep car doors locked at all times.
- Vary your parking spot or route.
- Keep your keys in your hand en route to and from your car.
- Dress comfortably and conservatively, and wear comfortable and sturdy shoes.
- Make connections in the community.
- Do not carry large amounts of cash or valuables.

the bathroom? When and where will I eat? What will I do if I get lost? What will I do if I am involved in an automobile accident?" Generally, home care nurses locate public restrooms in the community where they can stop for a bathroom break safely. Stopping in the community for eating breaks is also a decision that requires familiarity and safety as part of a process during the average work day, although many nurses bring their own break food from home. In both cases, this not only allows the nurse privacy but also does not expose them to conditions where they could contaminate clients and their families and vice versa. Carrying a functioning cell phone and having a list of emergency numbers to call is critical. A cell phone can also help if directions are lost or if an accident occurs.

The In-home Visit

The actual home visit includes introducing home care services to the client and family, as well as the process of obtaining help from the home care agency when a planned home visit is not occurring. Details are given orally and in writing about when, whom, and how to call in an emergency or nonemergency. It also includes the application of the standards of care for home care practice, which includes the use of the nursing process with defined initial outcomes. The key component of the first in-home visit is assessment. The home care nurse is a guest in the client's home, and must obtain the client's permission and ask for the client's guidance about how to carry out the initial assessment in the context of the home. It is necessary to carry out an overall assessment of the client's and family's strengths, weaknesses, and challenges. In addition, it is also essential to assess home safety risks—medication errors, falls, and abuse and neglect.

ASSESSING FOR RISK OF MEDICATION ERRORS

The risk of errors associated with medications is inherently high. Medications may be taken incorrectly (wrong medication, wrong route, wrong dose) and may have adverse effects or interactions. These negative side effects include hypotension/bradycardia/syncope, dizziness, ataxia, adverse bleeding, confusion/sedation, and urinary urgency (Romagnoli, Handler, Ligons, & Hochheiser, 2013). Taking the wrong medication/wrong dose/wrong route can occur because of errors in prescribing, errors in transcribing during the referral phase of the home care visit process, and errors in hearing the medication order; client and family confusion; pharmacy errors; and cultural beliefs (Setter et al., 2009). Although all of the various kinds of medication errors can occur in hospitals as well as homes, there are some unique circumstances that make home care medication safety particularly challenging. Sometimes, in the freedom of their own home, clients refuse to take medications, forget to take medications, do not fill prescriptions because of cost, or need a renewal of a prescription and do not know how to proceed, or do not have access to a pharmacy. Sometimes, medication errors occur because of multiple physician involvement in care, transitions from hospital to home, client or family error, or the use of over-the-counter (OTC) drugs in addition to prescribed medication that may cause adverse reactions.

On average, community-dwelling elders use 4.5 prescription medications, at any giving time, in addition to OTC drugs. Corbett, Setter, Daratha, Neumiller, and Wood (2010) found a mean of 10.4 medications prescribed to patients at time of hospital discharge, supporting the frequency with which polypharmacy is occurring at time of hospital discharge (Box 12.5). Adverse reactions included death, falls/confusion/sedation, adverse bleeding, inappropriate/ineffective treatment, disease exacerbation, emergency department visits and/or rehospitalizations, and ineffective pain control (Romagnoli et al., 2013). At the initial home visit, it is important for the home care nurse to develop a medication profile that is accurate and will be reviewed at each visit. It is critical to talk about the use of prescribed medications with OTCs and herbal supplements, and develop a plan that includes the client and family being vigilant about medication safety (Box 12.6).

ASSESSING FOR RISK OF FALLS

Falls are a major health problem in home care. One-third of older adults fall every year with serious consequences that include death, fractures, and head injuries. For the elderly, there are even more consequences when a fall is sustained. These include an ongoing fear of falling, loss of function and mobility, disability, restriction of activity, decreased independence,

box 12.5 Interventions Related to Medication Safety at Home

- Teach clients and/or families to always check prescription label when filling or refilling prescriptions.
- Use medication prefill systems.
- Have the client and/or family repeat back medication instructions given over the phone.
- Focus on tricyclic antidepressants, benzodiazepines, and antipsychotic medications, since they are prone to medication errors.

box | 12.6 **Herbal Medications and Adverse Interactions**

Ginkgo biloba
Used as an antioxidant and natural blood thinner
Adverse interactions with anticoagulants, OTC pain relievers (causes adverse bleeding), anticonvulsants, and antidepressants

Ginseng
Decreases stress and effects of aging
Adverse interactions with digoxin, anticoagulants, antidepressants, and analgesics

St. John's wort
Used as antidepressant
Adverse interactions with chemotherapy, indinavir, cyclosporine, digoxin, and theophylline

Source: Data from Salmond, S. (2002). Polypharmacy and phytotherapy: Issues of herb/drug interactions in the elderly. *Australian Journal of Medical Herbalism, 14*(1), 12–14.

increased social isolation, depression, and nursing home placement (Wong, Masters, Maxwell, & Abernethy, 2008).

Fifty-five percent of fall-related injuries occur inside the home (Greene, Sample, & Fruhauf, 2009). The most common rooms where people fall include the living room (31%), bedroom (30%), kitchen (19%), bathroom (13%), and hallway (10%). Fall rates for the elderly are related to intrinsic and extrinsic factors (Table 12.2). In the context of the first home visit, many of these factors are modifiable. For example, the home care nurse can make plans with the family or home care agency to make environmental modifications that can decrease the chance of a fall. For example, this may involve having handrails installed in the bathroom and removing scatter rugs or putting nonskid pads under them. The initiation of an exercise program, medication adjustments, and the management of pain, orthostatic hypotension, and corrected vision all can begin at this first visit (multimodal exercise programs for older adults [Baker, Atlantis, & Fiatarone-Singh, 2007]).

Eleanor and her family obtain a "fall alert" bracelet from their local hospital. This encourages them. The technology works very much like other wireless systems, alerting emergency services and the police if needed. This alert system is connected electronically to Eleanor's home phone with a special piece of equipment that always allows a person to converse with her if she pushes the alert bracelet and needs help. During two occasions in the early evening, Eleanor uses the alert bracelet when she slips off the side of her bed and cannot get up. This effectively allows her to stay at home and have the psychological feeling of being connected to someone who could help her in an emergency when her children are not available.

ASSESSING FOR RISK OF ABUSE AND NEGLECT

Unfortunately, in community settings, there can be instances when clients and family members can be victims of abuse and neglect. This is often hidden until home care nurses or other home care personnel enter the home and observe the potential, or actual, abuse or neglect. In thinking about the difference between abuse and neglect, there are not only subtle differences between the two conditions but also differences in motivating factors behind the situations. Some authors define *abuse* as blatant disregard for the safety and welfare of a client versus neglect as a chronic, eroding lack of physical, psychosocial, and spiritual support of another (Stark, 2011). Abuse can be physical, emotional (often in the form of verbal abuse), and, especially with the elderly, financial. This is often true when caregivers are responsible for the financial management of the household. Neglect is not always the responsibility of others. Some clients, for a variety of reasons that include diagnosed and undiagnosed depression, can be victims of self-neglect (Underwood et al., 2013). Self-neglect can take the form of not taking care of personal hygiene, refusing to take medications that may improve their physical or mental condition(s), and refusing to eat.

table | 12.2 **Intrinsic and Extrinsic Factors Related to Falls in the Home**

Intrinsic	Extrinsic
Age	Poor or inadequate lighting
Previous history of falls	Changes in floor surface or slippery surface
Cognitive impairment	High-gloss floors
Muscle weakness, decreased lower extremity strength	Lack of handrails on stairs
Female	Inappropriate chair height
Taking four or more medications a day	Clutter, throw rugs, electrical cords, loose carpeting
Taking psychotropic medications	Poor sidewalk and pavement conditions, snow and ice
Vision impairment	Pets
Peripheral neuropathy	
Parkinson disease	
History of a stroke (cerebrovascular accident)	
Arthritis	

Abuse and neglect are sometimes motivated intentionally, but more often they can be unintentionally present as issues for clients. This is the case particularly with neglect and self-neglect. Extenuating circumstances may involve a lack of knowledge (not being aware of the resources in the community that are available to help with a situation) (Truglio-Londrigan & Gallagher, 2003).

One important cautionary note is that home care nurses need to be careful about making judgments related to identifying abuse and neglect involving clients and families. Consideration must be given to cultural beliefs, lack of caregiver knowledge and/or skill, caregiver burden or lack of support, well-intended but misguided care, and client autonomy and the right to self-determination (Killick & Taylor, 2009).

Termination

In terminating the initial visit, it is critical to make sure that clients and families know how to reach the home care nurse at any time of the day, and that an emergency plan is understood by the client and the family. This understanding may involve the neighbors. It is equally important to establish an initial plan of care, and to make a plan for the next scheduled visit. If there are any circumstances that would impede future visits, it is important to address these at this time. For example, if the client or family members smoke, and the home care nurse is allergic to smoke or cannot tolerate smoking, the home care nurse should make a contract related to a "no smoking" visit policy. If there are pets that disrupt the visit, the home care nurse needs to make a contract that the pet will be put in another area during future home visits.

STUDENT REFLECTION

I have to admit, with the short length of stay in hospital settings, caring for clients in the community over many months, depending on their skilled needs, and recertification of care by members of a physician team, makes it difficult to discharge the client. It is not just the client but the family that is missed because they are often caregivers that make the care a possibility. So the goodbye is doubly hard sometimes. As a student, I became much more aware of the realities facing clients when they left the hospital and now often wonder why there is such a separation in practice from the hospital to the home. Wouldn't it be great if nurses in the hospital could visit or check in on clients at home after they left!

Postvisit Planning

After the initial visit, the home care nurse establishes, through the nursing process and the use of the initial assessment protocol, a specific plan of care that may include other healthcare disciplines and home health aide services. Outcome goals are established, and a schedule of planned visits is organized. The most crucial postvisit activity is the establishment of outcome measures, so that the home health team can plan an intervention approach that allows reasonable time and effort for healthcare providers and the client and family to achieve these measures. This is accomplished through the expert judgment of the home care nurse, who manages the home care effort, and consideration of the constraints of Medicare, Medicaid, and other health insurance policies.

Nurse–Family Interactions in Home Care

Professional boundaries in the home care setting are an important consideration because home care nurses are guests in a client's home (Rowem & Kellam, 2011). Home care nurses are very aware that dealing with the three Cs—culture, contracts, and confidentiality—is important and that they have unique applications in nonhospital settings.

Culture

In Chapter 10, culture and cultural competency are addressed extensively. However, it is important to reiterate that in home visiting, it is important to converse with clients and families about cultural patterns with which the home care nurse may not be familiar. This includes assessing the degree of acculturation, religious or spiritual needs, the client and family understanding of the health problem that brought the home care nurse to the home, etiquette, and social customs and rituals and practices.

Contracting

In many home care client and family situations, one of the roles of the home care nurse is to develop a plan of care that is mutually accepted so that health outcomes can be met, and at a variety of levels of prevention (primary, secondary, and tertiary; see Chapter 5). In many instances, a client- or family-centered approach leads to differences in levels of motivation to meet outcomes. For example, the home care nurse established positive glycemic control as an outcome for a client who is living with type 2 diabetes at the age of 85. There are instances when the client and family find it difficult to accomplish this mutually agreed-upon activity, related to exercise, food portion control, types of food selections, and medication scheduling. On the surface, it may seem as though a client or family is "fighting against" needed lifestyle changes that are highly connected with health outcomes. On the other hand, a client may say that he wants to get well and be healthy, which results in two conflicting and ambivalent positions. Thus, finding a way to make a contract that is mutually binding between the client, family, and nurse is crucial.

Motivation to change behaviors may be related to ambivalence. Motivational interviewing is a client-centered, directive method for enhancing intrinsic motivation to change by exploring and resolving ambivalence (Motivational Interviewing, 2013). There are four principal approaches used in motivational interviewing: express empathy, support self-efficacy, roll with resistance, and find a discrepancy (Motivational Interviewing, 2013).

An empathetic approach involves identifying with the emotional aspects of the client's experiences, attempting to understand those experiences from the client's perspective. When clients perceive empathy on a counselor's part, they become more open to gentle challenges about lifestyle issues and beliefs about substance use. Clients become more comfortable fully examining their ambivalence about change and less likely to defend unhelpful attitudes, such as the denial of problems (Motivational Interviewing, 2013).

Self-efficacy is the belief on the part of the client that change is possible. Self-efficacy by definition is a critical motivator to operational change in health behaviors. A person who has a high sense of self-efficacy regarding a particular behavior is more likely to engage in that behavior. For example, people with stronger perceived self-efficacy for carrying out safer healthcare behaviors will be more likely to persist with these behaviors in the face of interpersonal pressure to behave otherwise (Bandura, 1997). Home care nurses can help clients believe that they can make a change by asking about other changes they have made in their lives in the past and how they were particularly successful. This approach emphasizes the ability of the client to accomplish a goal successfully.

In motivational interviewing, the home care nurse does not fight client resistance but "rolls with it." Statements demonstrating resistance are not challenged. Instead the home care nurse lets the client take the lead. Using this approach, resistance tends to be decreased rather than increased. Client's argumentative resistance to suggestions is not reinforced and the "devil's advocate" role is minimized.

Home care nurses also work to develop opportunities for clients to discover discrepancies between their current behavior and what they want to accomplish through changed behaviors. When clients perceive that their current behaviors are not leading toward some important future goal, they become more motivated to make important life changes. This approach is accomplished gently and gradually to help clients see that the way they approach health issues may be leading them away from accomplishing their stated goals.

Privacy, Confidentiality, and Security

In 1997, the Health Insurance Portability and Accountability Act (HIPAA) was passed in the United States (United States Department of Labor, 2013). The law assures that personal healthcare information will be kept private and secure. Home care as an industry has strived to maintain privacy of clients and families since its inception. However, new challenges arise related to longitudinal medical records and the numerous healthcare professionals who will have access to healthcare information over a continuum of care. In recent years, the increased use of portable Internet systems to document client and family information brings new challenges to the rights of clients and confidentiality (Thede, 2003). Protecting client and family privacy is a nursing responsibility. Home care nurses must be careful to do the following:

1. Conduct assessment interviews in environments that protect privacy (i.e., a place where conversation may not be overheard, if applicable).
2. When using a computer to access or document data, be mindful that no one else can view the screen.

In addition, home care computerized records must be maintained with an organizational commitment to allow only those with an appropriate identification and password to "log in." This approach is associated with ethical responsibility. Confidentiality also is an issue when healthcare data are transmitted. Much data is transferred electronically through facsimiles (faxes) or computer transfers. Encryption is often used as a way of protecting information so that only persons with special "keys" can decrypt messages that are sent (Thede, 2003). The best way to enhance a commitment to confidentiality in a home care agency is to maintain written policies about the use of client and family data. This includes an orientation and annual updates with staff to ensure that the policies are understood.

Finally, it is the responsibility of all home health agencies to keep all the data they collect secure. Data must be checked for accuracy. Decisions must be made at the organizational level as to (1) who are the personnel that absolutely need access to the information, (2) what type of firewalls will be established on computerized documents to protect client data from outside intruders, and (3) when and how data will be backed up to prevent loss of information.

Key Chronic Conditions and Quality Improvement in Home Care

In many healthcare situations, there are several chronic diseases and conditions that are often managed in the home by nurses in collaboration with other healthcare providers. Because of the management of this care by nurses, they often are involved with quality improvement related to these key conditions. Quality improvement simply means that nurses are interested in developing and managing healthcare interventions of a home health team that can improve or stabilize chronic conditions in the home. Common diseases and conditions include diabetes (Hartman, Litchman, Reed, & Burr, 2009), incontinence (Flanagan et al., 2012), pain (Duke, Botti, & Hunter, 2012), hypertension, and CHF (Taylor & Campbell, 2007). It is important to understand that, although these conditions are studied by nursing students in adult healthcare or medical–surgical nursing class and clinical settings, they take on a new complexity when clients leave a controlled environment such as an acute care hospital or rehabilitation facility.

During in-home care, complexity of care may include such issues as (1) family, (2) environment, and (3) even the home care nurse's capacity to attend consistently to assessment and intervention criteria. Complexity of care also arises from the fact that many clients cared for in homes live with multiple healthcare problems and conditions (comorbidities). For example, a client living with diabetes at home who has a problem with chronic incontinence needs a **family caregiver** to be informed of nutritional needs from the "grocery store to the stove" (Dalton, Garvey, & Samia, 2006). If a family caregiver does not collaborate or participate, the interactive effects of glycemic and incontinence control through diet will be defeated. Although incontinence may have many complex etiologies in and of itself, often the bundling of interventions can help clients have positive outcomes in several areas of concern as long as a principal caregiver participates in the plan of care.

In the same way, if the household environment is not safe, the client with diabetes or dyspnea from CHF may suffer falls and unexpected injuries that could lead to nonhealing wounds, further dyspnea, and unnecessary pain. Careful analysis of safety within the home, and interventions directed toward making the home environment safer through physical adjustments or through the assistance of ambulation strengthening, are key in keeping clients healthy at home.

Finally, home care nurses must be exacting and consistent in their assessment and follow-up with clients and their family caregivers. Because clients are in their own homes, many times home care nurses are faced with trying to balance the need to expeditiously care for clients when they are often fully dressed. This is different than in the hospital setting where clients are often in hospital gowns. In caring for clients living with diabetes, it is critical for home care nurses to ask clients to take off their socks and shoes so that full neurovascular assessments can be completed consistently over time. Symptoms such as subtle changes in sensation may be ignored or overlooked in the context of a chronic health condition, although these same symptoms would warrant immediate care in a more acute illness (Hartman et al., 2009; Centers for Disease Control and Prevention [CDC], 2012).

CASE MANAGEMENT, HOME HEALTHCARE, AND CURRENT HEALTHCARE REFORM

According to the Medicare Payment Advisory Committee (MedPAC), in 2011 about 3.4 million Medicare beneficiaries received home care, and the Medicare program spent about $18.4 billion on home health services (MedPAC, 2013). The number of agencies participating in Medicare reached 12,199 in 2011 where indicators of payment adequacy for home healthcare were seen as generally positive (MedPAC, 2013). However, almost one in five Medicare patients will be readmitted to the hospital within 30 days of discharge, at a cost of $15 billion and which does not include the heavy emotional and health toll on the patients and their families (Jenks, William, & Coleman, 2009; MedPAC, 2013). Avoidable hospital readmissions are typically caused by insufficient posthospitalization care, failure to adhere to recommended medication or therapy regimens, and lack of physical support for the discharged patient.

The federal government's Medicare program has created initiatives and incentive programs in a broad effort to lower the costs of avoidable utilization and to improve the quality of care that is delivered and received at healthcare institutions nationwide (MedPAC, 2013). The healthcare home model is an evolving, comprehensive and cost saving model that includes home care and case management. This model was introduced originally in the late 1960s as a model of healthcare delivery for children with special needs, and was a way to coordinate multiple services to children with complex developmental and physical challenges. Outcomes of the model, beyond family-centered comprehensive care, included a way to coordinate care effectively while being culturally relevant and sensitive (Sia, Tonniges, Osterhus, & Taba, 2004). This model is currently referred to as the PCMH and includes a chronic care model congruent with home care services described in this chapter. The distribution of services was originally introduced as a way to address those populations who were underserved and at high risk who needed coordinated care when they could not access primary care easily. The current terminology referring to this model is "healthcare home" versus "medical home" so that the true nature of the coordination is interdisciplinary with nursing as a central role (American Nursing Association, 2008). The healthcare home model intends to reduce barriers to access by providing services such as enrollment into healthcare services, transportation, and coordination with service providers that include home care services.

Currently pilot projects and efficacy and efficiency studies are underway that use this approach to develop a reimbursement structure. Projects are particularly looking at care coordination for patients with chronic conditions where decreased emergency room and hospital use, in terms of rehospitalization, brought notable savings per year (National Partnership for Women and Families, Side-by-Side Summary of State Medical Home Programs, 2013).

Challenges related to adopting and implementing healthcare home approaches continue to be formidable because current reimbursement rates do not cover the larger scope of services that are meant to be provided. The Accountable Care Organization (ACO) model now utilized by hospital systems was created to coordinate care with an emphasis on prevention, and provide incentive structures in the context of the provisions of the Affordable Care Act (ACA) where the healthcare home model would be seen as a key component in partnership with those hospital systems utilizing the ACO approaches (McClellan, McKethan, Lewis, Roski, & Fisher, 2010). For many, the need to reform the current primary care model in partnership with case management and home care is critical, so that collaborations between ACOs and healthcare home models can truly coordinate care for individuals, families, and communities (Child and Adolescent Health Initiative, 2013).

EVIDENCE FOR PRACTICE

The National Partnership for Women and Families (2011) last updated a list of all those states that have used medical home programs. Factors include organizational leadership, populations served, provider requirements, payment policies, and outcome measures of success. Please refer to http://www.nationalpartnership.org/site/DocServer/HC_Summary_StateMedicalHomePrograms_081028.pdf?docID=4262.

Look up your state or regional location for ongoing information/evidence of success.

In the final analysis, it is the home care nurse who has a significant role in reducing acute care emergency department and hospital use. As healthcare reform continues, the home care nurse will play a significant role in reducing emergency department and hospital use by improving outcomes in chronic care. In a recent study of all home healthcare agencies, Medicare-certified agencies offered training in outcome-based quality improvement to their professional staff, particularly nursing, as a way to ensure outcomes that did not involve expensive and unnecessary interventions (Pace & Johnson, 2006). Those that addressed (1) pain interfering with activity, (2) improvement in transferring, (3) improvement in managing oral medications, and (4) improvement in ambulation and locomotion, demonstrated improved outcomes in comparison with national rates. Improvement continues to be needed in (1) emergent care needs, (2) dyspnea, (3) acute care hospitalization, (4) care of surgical wounds, (5) bathing, and (6) incontinence, as home care progresses in its scope and standards of care to the public.

Healing is a matter of time, but it is sometimes also a matter of opportunity.

Hippocrates

key concepts

- Home care is part of a continuum of care where clients have the opportunity to live and move through the experiences of subacute, chronic, and end-of-life care.
- The care given in home care settings is often managed and directed by a registered nurse.
- Many aspects of the care in both generic and hospice home care are part of a larger care management plan that is individualized using a case management approach.
- The care given in home care settings is interdisciplinary in nature.
- Caregivers are often family members and friends. They must be considered members of the home care team and offered appropriate support if their commitment to care for a loved one at home is to be successful.

critical thinking questions

1. You are caring for a home care client with a large venous stasis wound on her left calf. She is obese and also suffers from CHF and osteoarthritis. She has trouble transferring out of her recliner chair due to pain and shortness of breath. Her physician has recommended daily cleansing of her venous ulcer in the shower. Her bathroom is fully handicapped-accessible with grab bars, a handheld shower head, and a transfer bench, but her pain and shortness of breath prevent her from using the shower. What would you do first?
   a. Explain to the physician that given the client's limitations, showering is not a possibility.
   b. Order a Hoyer lift for the client to assist with transfers.
   c. Consult with a physical therapist about getting the client an electric scooter to facilitate transfers.
   d. Consult with the physician about a better regimen to manage the client's arthritis pain and add a home health aide to her home care services.
2. Look through several major newspapers for articles that discuss care of the elderly in the community or care of those at the end stage of a life-threatening illness.
   a. What is the role of a community health nurse in assisting families in the care of these citizens in their homes?
   b. What are some of the barriers related to the initiation of home care services in communities?
   c. How does living in an urban area versus a rural area affect home care services?
3. According to Cooney & Pascuzzi (2009), the increased use of drugs with elderly populations raises concerns related to adverse outcomes, falls, and hospitalizations. The following list of references represent published manuscripts that may be of interest to nurses interested in addressing this serious and complex situation facing healthcare practice in the home and other locations of care. Choose three articles of interest from the list, and share your insights with your class.
4. Go to the National Association for Home Care and Hospice website (http://www.nahc.org/) and choose a legislative issue that affects home care. What are the key issues related to the political efforts made by promoters of home care? What are the political barriers that affect home care?

community resources

- Local hospitals that have hospital-based generic or hospice home care programs
- Visiting nurse associations
- Elder affairs organizations
- Local and state health departments
- State offices of Medicare and Medicaid

references

American Nurses Credentialing Center. (2013). Retrieved from http://www.nursecredentialing.org/NurseSpecialties/CaseManagement.aspx

American Nurses Association. (2007). *Scope and Standards of Home Health Nursing Practice.* Washington, DC: American Nurses Association.

American Nursing Association. (2008). *Urge committee to include nurse practitioners in the definition of medical homes*. Retrieved from http://www.nursingworld.org/HomepageCategory/NursingInsider/Archive_1/2008NI/Apr08NI/NursePractionersinMedical HomesDefinition.aspx

Antonicelli, R., Mazzanti, I., Abbatecola, A. M., & Parati, G. (2010). Impact of home patient telemonitoring on use of β-blockers in congestive heart failure. *Drugs & Aging*, *27*(10), 801–805.

Baker, M. K., Atlantis, E., & Fiatarone-Singh, M. A. (2007). Multimodal exercise programs for older adults. *Age-and-Ageing*, *36*(4), 375–381.

Bandura, A. (1997). *Self-efficacy: The exercise of control*. New York, NY: W. H. Freeman.

California Health Care Foundation. (2013). Retrieved from http://www.chcf.org

Carson, V. B., & Koenig, H. G. (2011). *Parish nursing: Stories of service and care*. West Conshohocken, PA: Templeton Press.

Cartmill, C., Soklaridis, S., & David Cassidy, J. (2011). Transdisciplinary teamwork: The experience of clinicians at a functional restoration program. *Journal of Occupational Rehabilitation*, *21*(1), 1–8.

Case Management Society of America. (2013). Retrieved from http://www.CMSA.org

Centers for Disease Control and Prevention. (2012). *Diabetes complications*. Retrieved from http://www.cdc.gov/diabetes/statistics/complications_national.htm

Centers for Medicare & Medicaid Services. (2013). Retrieved from http://www.cms.gov/Medicare/Quality-Initiatives-Patient-Assessment-Instruments/HomeHealthQualityInits/index.html?redirect=/homehealthqualityinits/

Centers for Medicare and Medicaid Services. (2014). *OASIS data set*. Retrieved from http://www.cms.gov/Medicare/Quality-Initiatives-Patient-Assessment-Instruments/HomeHealthQualityInits/HHQIOASISDataSet.html

Chatfield, L., Christos, S., & McGregor, M. (2012). Interdisciplinary therapy assessments for the older adult. *Perspectives on Gerontology*, *17*(1), 11–16.

Child and Adolescent Health Measurement Initiative. (2013). *2005–2006 National survey of children with special health care needs. Data Resource Center for Child and Adolescent Health.* Retrieved from http://www.cshcndata.org/DataQuery/DataQueryResults.aspx

Cooney, D., & Pascuzzi, K. Polypharmacy in the elderly: focus on drug interactions and adherence in hypertension. *Clin Geriatr Med*. 2009;*25*(2):221–33.

Corbett, C., Setter, S., Daratha, K., Neumiller, J., & Wood, L. (2010). Nurse identified hospital to home medication discrepancies implications for improving transitional care. *Geriatric Nursing*, *31*(3), 188–196.

Dalton, J., Garvey, J., & Samia, L. W. (2006). Evaluation of a diabetes disease management home care program. *Home Health Care Management & Practice*, *18*(4), 272–285.

DeMarco, R., & O'Brien, L. (1999). Home health care in Massachusetts: The impact of reductions in medicare spending on lay caregivers. *Massachusetts Nurse*, *69*(6), 12.

Disease Management Association of America. (2013). Retrieved from http://www.onemedplace.com/network/list/cid/1892/

Duke, M., Botti, M., & Hunter, S. (2012). Effectiveness of pain management in hospital in the home programs. *Clinical Journal of Pain*, *28*(3), 187–194.

21. Fetterolf, D. E., Stanziano, G., & Istwan, N. (2008). Application of disease management principles to pregnancy and the postpartum period. *Disease Management*, *11*(3), 161–168.

Flanagan, L., Roe, B., Jack, B., Barrett, J., Chung, A., Shaw, C., & Williams, K. S. (2012). Systematic review of care intervention studies for the management of incontinence and promotion of continence in older people in care homes with urinary incontinence as the primary focus (1966–2010). *Geriatrics & Gerontology International*, *12*(4), 600–611.

Flatt, J. D., Agimi, Y., & Albert, S. M. (2012). Homophily and health behavior in social networks of older adults. *Family & Community Health*, *35*(4), 312–321.

Greene, D., Sample, P., & Fruhauf, C. (2009). Fall-prevention pilot: Hazard survey and responses to recommendations. *Occupational Therapy in Health Care*, *23*(1), 24–39.

Hartman, A., Litchman, M. L., Reed, P., & Burr, R. E. (2009). In-home chronic disease management in diabetes: A collaborative practice model for home health care and endocrinology providers. *Home Health Care Management & Practice*, *21*(4), 246–254.

Healthy People 2020. (2014). *2020 Topics and objectives*. Retrieved from http://www.healthypeople.gov/2020/topicsobjectives2020/default.aspx

Jenks, S., William, M., & Coleman, E. (2009). Rehospitalizations among patient in the Medicare fee-for-service program. *New England Journal of Medicine*, *360*(14), 1418–1428.

Killick, C., & Taylor, B. J. (2009). Professional decision making on elder abuse: Systematic narrative review. *Journal of Elder Abuse & Neglect, 21*(3), 211–238.

Kongstvedt, P. R. (2001). *The managed health care handbook* (4th ed.). New York, NY: Aspen.

Lehning, A. J., & Austin, M. J. (2011). On Lok: A pioneering long-term care organization for the elderly (1971–2008). *Journal of Evidence-Based Social Work*, *8*(1/2), 218–234.

Magee, M. (2007). *Home-centered health care*. New York, NY: Spencer.

Masotti, P. J., Fick, R., Johnson-Masotti, A., & MacLeod, S. (2006). Healthy naturally occurring retirement communities: A low-cost approach to facilitating healthy aging. *American Journal of Public Health*, *96*(7), 1164–1170.

McClellan, M., McKethan, A. N., Lewis, J. L., Roski, J., & Fisher, E. S. (2010). A national strategy to put accountable care into practice. *Health Affairs, 29*(5), 982–990. doi:10.1377/hlthaff.2010.0194

Medline Plus. (2013). Retrieved from http://www.medicare.gov/publications/pubs/pdf/10969.pdf

references (continued)

Medicare Payment Advisory Committee. (2013). Retrieved from http://www.medpac.gov/documents/Mar13_EntireReport.pdf

Motivational Interviewing. (2013). Retrieved from http://www.motivationalinterview.org

National Coalition on Health Care. (2008). Retrieved from http://nchc.org/blog/nchc-white-paper

National Partnership for Women and Families. (2013). *Side by side summary of state medical home programs*. Retrieved from http://www.nationalpartnership.org/site/DocServer/HC_Summary_StateMedicalHomePrograms_081028.pdf?docD=4262

National Center for Policy Analysis. (2013). Retrieved from http://www.ncpa.org/sub/dpd/index.php?Article_ID=18680

National Committee for Quality Assurance. (2014). *Patient-centered medical homes*. Retrieved from http://www.ncqa.org/Programs/Recognition/PatientCenteredMedicalHomePCMH.aspx

Outcome and Assessment Information Set. (2013). Retrieved from http://www.cms.hhs.gov/oasis/hhoview.asp

O'Connor, M., & Davitt, J. K. (2012). The Outcome and Assessment Information Set (OASIS): A review of validity and reliability. *Home Health Care Services Quarterly*, *31*(4), 267–301.

Okuyemi, K. S., Goldade, K., Whembolua, G. L., Thomas J. L., Eischen, S., Guo, H., … Des Jarlais, D. (2013). Smoking characteristics and comorbidities in the power to quit randomized clinical trial for homeless smokers. *Nicotine & Tobacco Research*, *15*(1), 22–28.

Omaha System. (2013). Retrieved from http://www.omahasystem.org/overview.html

Omboni, S., Gazzola, T., Carabelli, G., & Parati, G. (2013). Clinical usefulness and cost effectiveness of home blood pressure telemonitoring: Meta-analysis of randomized controlled studies. *Journal of Hypertension*, *31*(3), 455–468.

Pace, K. B., & Johnson, K. E. (2006). Nursing counts. *American Journal of Nursing*, *106*(1), 38.

Pijl-Zieber, E. M., & Kalischuk, R. G. (2011). Community health nursing practice education: Preparing the next generation. *International Journal of Nursing Education Scholarship*, *8*(1), 1–13.

Poisal, J. A., Truffer, C., Smith, S., Sisko, A., Cowan, C., Keehan, S., & Dickensheets, B. (2007). Health spending projections through 2016: Modest changes obscure Part D's impact. *Health Affairs*, *26*(2), W242–W253.

Prospective Reimbursement. (2008). Retrieved from http://www.online-medicaldictionary.org/Prospective+Reimbursement.asp?q=Prospective+Reimbursement

Romagnoli, K. M., Handler, S. M., Ligons, F. M., & Hochheiser, H. (2013). Home-care nurses' perceptions of unmet information needs and communication difficulties of older patients in the immediate post-hospital discharge period. *BMJ Quality & Safety*, *22*(4), 324–332.

Rosenthal, M. B., & Frank, R. G. (2006). What is the empirical basis for paying for quality in health care? *Medical Care Research and Review*, *63*(2), 135–157.

Rowem, J., & Kellam, C. (2011). Ethics and moral development: Core ingredients of a compliance culture. *Home Health Care Management & Practice*, *23*(1), 55–59.

Setter, S. M., Corbett, C. F., Neumiller, J. J., Gates, B. J., Sclar, D. A., & Sonnett, T. E. (2009). Effectiveness of a pharmacist—Nurse intervention on resolving medication discrepancies for patients transitioning from hospital to home health care. *American Journal of Health-System Pharmacy*, *66*(22), 2027–2031.

Sewell, J., & Thede, L. (2012) *Informatics and nursing: Opportunities and challenges* (4th ed.). Philadelphia, PA: Lippincott, Williams, & Wilkins.

Sia, C., Tonniges, T. F., Osterhus, E., & Taba, S. (2004). History of the medical home concept. *Pediatrics*, *113*(Suppl. 5), 1473–1478.

Stark, S.W. (2011). Blind, deaf, and dumb: Why elder abuse goes unidentified. *Nursing Clinics of North American*, *46*(4), 431–436.

Stefanacci, R. G., & Podrazik, P. M. (2005). Assisted living facilities: Optimizing outcomes. *Journal of the American Geriatrics Society*, *53*(3), 538–540.

Taylor, J. R., & Campbell, K. M. (2007). Home monitoring of glucose and blood pressure. *American Family Physician*, *76*(2), 255–262, 187–189, 298.

TRICARE. (2013). Retrieved from http://www.tricare.mil/Welcome/SpecialPrograms/ECHO/Benefits.aspx?sc_database=web

Truglio-Londrigan, M., & Gallagher, L. P. (2003). Using the seven A's to determine older adults community resource needs. *Home Healthcare Nurse*, *21*(12), 827–831.

Underwood, M., Lamb, S., Eldridge, S., Sheehan, B., Slowther, A., Spencer, A., … Taylor, S. (2013). Exercise for depression in care home residents: A randomised controlled trial with cost-effectiveness analysis (OPERA). *Health Technology Assessment*, *17*(18), 1–281.

United States Department of Labor. (2013). *Health plans & benefits: Portability of health coverage (HIPAA)*. Retrieved from http://www.dol.gov/dol/topic/health-plans/portability.htm

Utilization Review Accreditation Commission. (2008). Retrieved from http://www.urac.org/resources/careManagement.aspx

Westberg, G. (1999). A personal historical perspective of whole person health and the congregation. In P. A. Solari-Twadell & M. A. McDermott (Eds.), *Parish nursing: Promoting whole person health within faith communities*. Thousand Oaks, CA: Sage.

Wikipedia. (2013). *Global positioning systems*. Retrieved from http://en.wikipedia.org/wiki/GPS

Wong, B. (2008). Nursing the homeless: Lessons learned. *Alberta Association of Registered Nurses*, *64*(7), 18.

Wong, W. L., Masters, R. S. W., Maxwell, J. P., & Abernethy, A. B. (2008). Reinvestment and falls in community-dwelling older adults. *Neurorehabilitation and Neural Repair*, *22*(4), 410–414.

Zubritsky, C., Abbott, K., Hirschman, K., Bowles, K., Foust, J., & Naylor, M. (2012). Health-related quality of life: Expanding a conceptual framework to include older adults who receive long-term services and support. *The Gerontologist*. doi:10.1093/geront/gns093

web resources

Please visit thePoint® (http://thepoint.lww.com/Harkness) for up-to-date Web resources on this topic.

CHAPTER 13

Family Assessment

Mary Margaret Segraves

Your children are not your children. They are the sons and daughters of Life's longing for itself. They came through you but not from you and though they are with you yet they belong not to you.

Khalil Gibran

My mother had a great deal of trouble with me, but I think she enjoyed it.

Mark Twain

He that raises a large family does, indeed, while he lives to observe them, stand a broader mark for sorrow; but then he stands a broader mark for pleasure too.

Benjamin Franklin

So live that you wouldn't be ashamed to sell the family parrot to the town gossip.

Will Rogers

chapter highlights

- Definitions of family
- Descriptions of the components of family
- Nursing theory in relation to nursing care of families
- Influence of diversity on family health patterns
- Indicators of family health
- Family dynamics and coping styles
- Vulnerable families

objectives

- Define family and examples of family systems.
- Describe the key components of family assessment.
- Identify situations that make families vulnerable.
- Apply recommendations from *Healthy People 2020* to meet family health needs.
- Identify indicators of family health across the life span and risks to family health.

key terms

Caregiver burden: Fatigue or frustration expressed by persons who care for convalescing or chronically ill persons on a daily basis.

Ecomap: A diagram used to identify the direction and intensity of family relationships between members and/or community institutions of importance to the family (e.g., schools, workplaces, places of worship).

Family: Two or more persons who share emotional closeness and identify themselves as members of a family.

Family assessment: The process community health nurses make to appraise family healthcare needs. An assessment is holistic, and includes examination of cultural, spiritual, and developmental needs with biopsychosocial needs.

Family risk reduction: Family health protection and promotion behaviors directed to health risks that family members can or cannot control directly.

Framework: A loose organization of concepts used to explain a phenomenon in nursing.

Genogram: A diagram of family relationships between blood relatives that can span two or more generations. Life events such as marriages, divorces, births, and deaths are included in the diagram. The genogram is used to identify relationships as well as possible patterns of disease.

Grand nursing theory: A nursing theory that is used as a broad explanation of human experience or environment.

Health appraisal: The process families use to perceive the health status of its members, for example, the use of selected measures of specific dimensions of health.

Health disparities: Differences or inconsistencies in healthcare delivery that frequently occur with families with low socioeconomic status.

Informant: Person who provides information for either himself or herself, or for someone who is unable to do so, as in the case with a parent with an infant, or an adult child for a parent with dementia.

Intergenerational diversity: The differences expressed between people of different generations. The differences, which include individual work and lifestyles, affect relationships between family members.

Intrafamily strain: The effect of stressors on families that make members less sensitive and loving to each other.

Marital strain: The effect of stressors on a couple in a relationship that make them less sensitive and loving to each other.

Odds ratio: The number of persons likely to have an identified disorder in a defined group versus the number of persons likely to have the identified disorder in a control group. The odds ratio would be the number found in the first group divided by the number found in the second group.

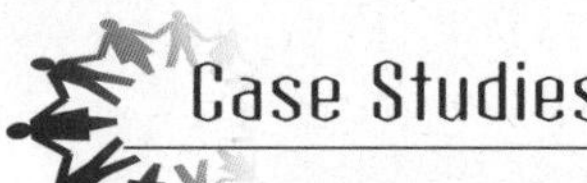

Case Studies

References to case studies are found throughout this chapter (look for the case study icon). Readers should keep the case studies in mind as they read the chapter.

CASE 1

Lucy, a public health nurse in a mid-sized city, has been following the Barnes family for 2 years. Eight-year-old Tanya and her 6-year-old brother Luke have asthma, and Lucy has been helping the family control asthma triggers at home. Tanya and Luke's 51-year-old grandmother, Elsa Morris, is their guardian. The children's mother is in the military and is now overseas. She sends e-mails, with photos, to the children almost daily. The children's father, who never married their mother, has had no contact with the children for more than 4 years.

At Lucy's most recent home visit, Elsa tells Lucy that Tanya has been unable to sleep through the night. Lucy also learns that the children have "too many treats" between meals and after dinner. Mrs. Morris tries to get the children to go to bed around 8 pm, but they like to watch television. Elsa says that she knows she needs to be stricter, but the children miss their mother and she wants to avoid upsetting them.

Elsa's husband has been unemployed for several months. Although he received a generous severance payment from his company, he has had to apply for unemployment. He is generous and caring to the children and to their mother. Elsa works part-time and only makes enough money to cover expenses. She tells Lucy that the cost of the children's medications is "adding up." She also wants to enroll the children in extracurricular activities, but they are "too expensive."

- What three priorities for this family can you identify?
- What additional information would you want from Mrs. Morris?
- What types of community resources to support this family would you recommend?

CASE 2

Agnes and Mark Thomas are 83 and 84 years of age, respectively. They have four adult children and eight grandchildren; all live within 25 miles of the couple. Mrs. Thomas likes the family to have dinner together at least twice a month at her home. Over the past 6 months, her children have noticed that their mother often forgets her grandchildren's names. Mr. Thomas, a retired firefighter and once avid swimmer, has arthritis in his spine, which has decreased his mobility.

Mr. Thomas's elder daughter, 58-year-old Arlene, is developmentally delayed and has lived in various state-run residential facilities since she was 5 years old. Arlene's siblings had little contact with her when she was growing up except on birthdays and holidays. Recently, the director of the facility sent the Thomases a letter to inform that the state is closing the facility and that they need to find housing for Arlene.

Laura, a nurse from the residential facility where Arlene lives, phones Agnes to arrange a home visit. Agnes tells Laura that Arlene cannot live with her and Mark, and she asks Laura to talk to her youngest son Jim, 47 years old. Although Jim has had minimal contact with his sister, he agrees to meet with Laura. He tells her that his parents' health is declining, especially his mother's, and proposes that Arlene might be able to move into the in-law apartment in his home. Jim and Laura arrange another meeting that includes Arlene, as well as Jim's wife and their adolescent twin daughters.

- What potential conflicts can arise in this family?
- What information about the family's resources could help to offset their anxiety about Arlene's change in housing?
- Who else should be included in any plans?

key terms (continued)

Spillover: Permeability between two boundaries (work and home).

System: A group that works on the principle that each part contributes to the way the whole functions.

Theory: A system of interrelated statements that is used to explain, predict, control, or understand a phenomenon.

Working with families is an inevitable aspect of nursing practice. Much emphasis in clinical practice is on individual problems and needs. Family care is frequently the focus of concern in particular clinical situations, such as nursing sick children, family-centered maternity care, and home nursing care, especially hospice care. Learning about the complex nature of family life can provide insight into the ways that family life and practices influence individual health. In many cases, family connections play a vital role in providing support to members. Yet, at other times, family influences can be perceived less positively, and can cause challenges to both family members and the healthcare providers who care for them. This chapter includes a discussion of the expanded definition of family and assessment of family health using an evidence-based approach. Nursing perspectives in family assessment are provided with examples of clinical applications. The case studies at the beginning of the chapter illustrate how complex issues can affect families and their health management.

FAMILIES IN COMMUNITIES

Nurses Working with Families

Contact with families is a significant aspect of nursing practice. Although such assessments may be rare, nurses' assessment of a family's history and relationships can provide insight into how family members interact and make decisions regarding health practices. The process of conducting a **family assessment** might not be deliberate. Typically, nurses ask questions about family members only to obtain emergency contact information or to make arrangements for discharge. In-depth family assessments are rarely routine in adult nursing practice and are usually reserved for crisis situations. Family health is frequently identified as a goal of clinical practice, with the family defined as the unit of care. Overcoming contemporary public health issues, such as heart disease, rising rates of childhood obesity, and poor sleep habits, are challenges that require family lifestyle modifications. A nursing perspective on family in community health nursing practice can help ensure healthy communities.

Yet composition of families can vary, which can lead to some inconsistencies in what comprises a family. The assessment and clinical approach to families and family health, now and in the future, require expanding the traditional notions of family. Looking at different definitions of family is a good place to begin exploring this concept.

The Essence of Family

Families today assume a variety of forms. A nurse's own family of origin is usually a frame of reference for what comprises **family** and how its members relate to one another. The concept of family has broadened and become more inclusive, and extends beyond blood relatives. Families share common traits. Often, groups of close friends form bonds that can be stronger than those with their families of origin. Cohabiting couples or gay/lesbian partners form close connections that communities now acknowledge as families. The following two definitions of family serve as a basis for consideration of family assessment.

One broad definition of family is "two or more persons who are joined together by bonds of sharing and emotional closeness . . . who identify themselves as being part of the family" (Friedman, Bowden, & Jones, 2003, p. 10). This definition characterizes the range of families in 21st-century America and covers a wide range of relationships, including those outside the genetic and legal definitions of family. Another definition is that families decide who they are, and family boundaries are not limited to traditional definitions (Wright & Leahey, 1999, 2009). Although this definition might seem simplistic, it draws attention to individual group needs to affirm identity as family and establish connection to others within that group.

In nursing practice, the word *system* is often used to describe families. A **system** works on the principle that each part contributes to the functioning of the whole. Its structure, personal history, and patterns of communication affect how well the system operates. Family systems are groups of individual people whose functioning depends on one another (Wright & Leahey, 1999, 2009). Family members spend time together to strengthen these bonds. Specific caregiver functions include protecting and nourishing family members, as well as socializing with them. A grandparent or older sibling might care for children in the parent's absence in an attempt to ensure normalcy in the children's home life.

Overall, both definitions of family have characteristics of living in a diverse society that includes groups of different ethnic, religious, or political backgrounds. Both definitions clearly indicate that individual people determine their status as family. An advantage to this definition is that the ideal of what constitutes family includes groups that 50 years ago would not be recognized as such (e.g., gay and lesbian families, cohabiting partners, and single-parent families). However, sociologic trends make describing families based solely on their attributes difficult (Wright & Leahey, 1999, 2009).

The family can also have a profound influence on health and illness (Friedman et al., 2003; Wright & Leahey, 1999, 2009). Members share a common history that can affect their individual behaviors as well as provide a context for their individual actions and health-related actions. Learning about preventive health begins at home, for example, parents taking their children for dental screening every 6 months. Cultural practices also affect families' health decisions, for example, first- or second-generation Americans are more receptive to health education about infant feeding practices than their parents. They have already assimilated into the culture and become more accepting about learning new skills.

Typically, people describe families in terms of members' relationships to each other, with the degree of kinship identified as being either a nuclear or an extended family. Nuclear families consist of first-degree relatives—that is, two generations who live together. Commonly, the two generations include parents and children. Extended families include both first- and second-degree relatives and can include grandparents, aunts, uncles, and cousins. Traditional definitions of extended family indicate that the family shares a dwelling, but members can live in the same neighborhood or in relatively close proximity to one another. The time that an extended family spends together depends not only on geographic closeness to one another but also on family customs. Extended family can also include persons who are not blood relatives, but who share a common locale of origin or culture. This situation is common in immigrants or in persons whose own families live elsewhere.

Happiness is having a large, loving, caring, close-knit family in another city.

George Burns

Nontraditional Families

Blended families form when two partners either cohabit or bring children into the relationship. This type of family has become widespread as more divorced or widowed people marry, and more gay and lesbian relationships become recognized.

Cohabiting Couples and Families

Marriage is a valued institution in most cultures. In American culture, the decision to marry or not is regarded as individual and personal. Still, some unmarried adults can feel marginalized because they have never married. Other couples might choose to cohabit either before they marry, or instead of marrying. According to U.S. Census Bureau (2012b) figures, 7.7 million unmarried couples comprise households. This figure represents a 41% increase of unmarried couples over the past 10 years.

Families often form when couples in a group of people cohabit. They consider themselves to be a family. They have formed committed emotional bonds and share possessions and home ownership.

Gay and Lesbian Families

Marriage between people of the same sex is a relatively recent phenomenon. In 2013, 11 states recognized same-sex marriages, and 12 other states issued laws to protect domestic partnerships (National Conference of State Legislatures, 2013). The 2010 decennial census was the first to include the number of same-sex marriages in the United States. Current figures show that nearly 600,000 married or unmarried same-sex couples live in the United States (U.S. Census Bureau, 2012b).

The number of children with same-sex parents is growing. Almost 20% of households include children whose parents have nontraditional relationships (American Fact Finder, 2010). Some couples decide to have a child together through adoption or artificial insemination.

PRACTICE POINT

Families form when a group of persons has strong emotional bonds, and they may simply proclaim themselves to be families. Members might not have blood or legal relationships, such as marriage. Cohabiting couples and gay and lesbian couples consider themselves to be a family regardless of legal relationships.

Tools That Help Identify Families and Their Relationships

Identifying relationships with families can be complicated. Diagrams are a useful visual aid to identify these relationships. Two diagrams used frequently to supplement family assessments are genograms and ecomaps. Although they are similar, each highlights different aspects of family connections and relationships.

Genograms are diagrams that show relationships across two or more generations. Primarily, they depict traditional family relationships such as marriage, divorce, birth, and death across generations (Tavernier, 2009) (Fig. 13.1). Genograms show how interdependent family members are related to each other. Nurses can use genograms to help families identify common traits as well as unique attributes of various members, recognize patterns of intergenerational conflict, and demonstrate relationships to prevent "scapegoating" a particular family member, especially when discussing hereditary medical conditions.

Sister is probably the most competitive relationship within the family, but once the sisters are grown, it becomes the strongest relationship.

Margaret Mead

Family genograms are usually superimposed on a pedigree, or graphic illustration of a person's medical and biologic history. Pedigrees are tools for learning about patterns of inheritance and isolating genetic or other risk factors. They also make invaluable teaching aids for nurses to use with families who need to make decisions about surveillance for genetic medical diseases, such as hemophilia or Huntington disease.

Ecomaps outline the influence that other systems or groups have on families (Fig. 13.2). They illustrate family relationships and show vital connections, which can include religious, work, cultural, or social groups. Solid or hatched lines plot the strength of family connections. Community health nurses often find that ecomaps are especially helpful to show families whether resources are available to assist them (Rempel, Neufeld, & Kushner, 2007).

PRACTICE POINT

Genograms and ecomaps are graphic representations of family relationships. Nurses can use genograms to identify key events and relationships within families, and ecomaps can be used to identify interactions between families and the communities in which they live.

NURSING PERSPECTIVES ON THE FAMILY AND APPLICATIONS FOR ASSESSMENT

Nurses who can fully appreciate family relationships promote mutual understanding and provide a rich context for care. Families are not simply static groups of individual people who have close physical and emotional bonds, but are a complex evolving network of people.

- Joyful events, such as births, marriages, or partnerships, as well as tragic ones such as natural disasters or catastrophic or chronic illness, add new dimensions to family interactions.
- Children who live apart from their parents might love their caregivers, yet feel their mother's absence acutely.
- Family members separated from the nexus of family interaction (e.g., the "black sheep") retain some connections to the family, albeit loosely. The same holds true for disenfranchised family members who have lived apart from their families for extended periods.
- Deceased family members leave an impression long after their deaths.

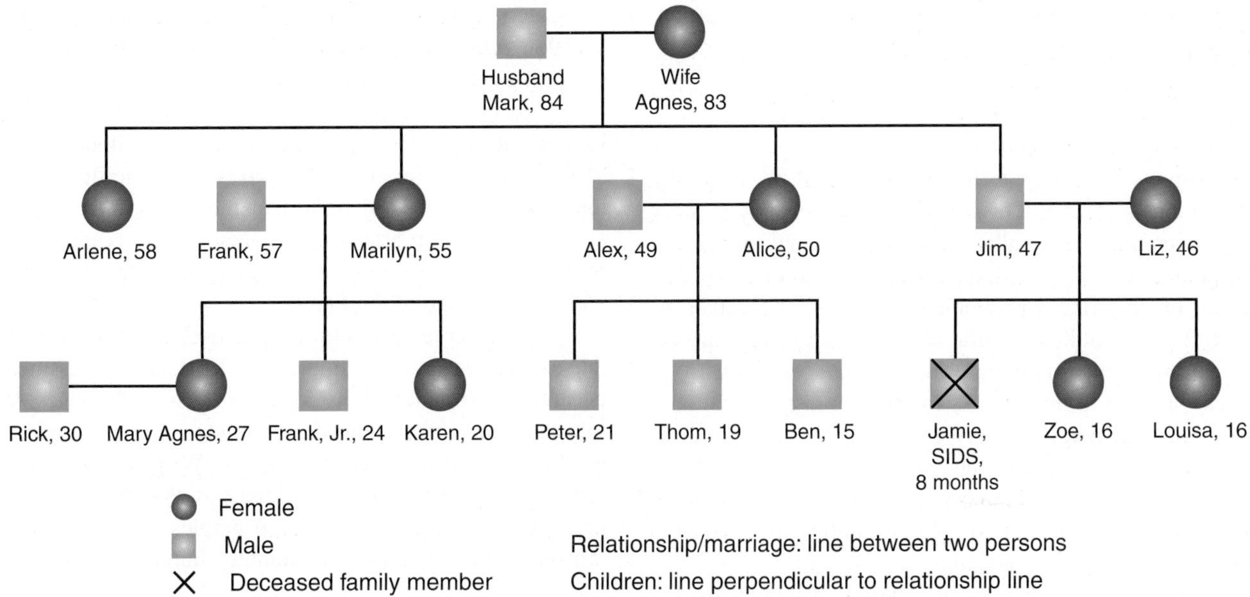

figure 13.1. Example of the Thomas family's genogram. SIDS, sudden infant death syndrome.

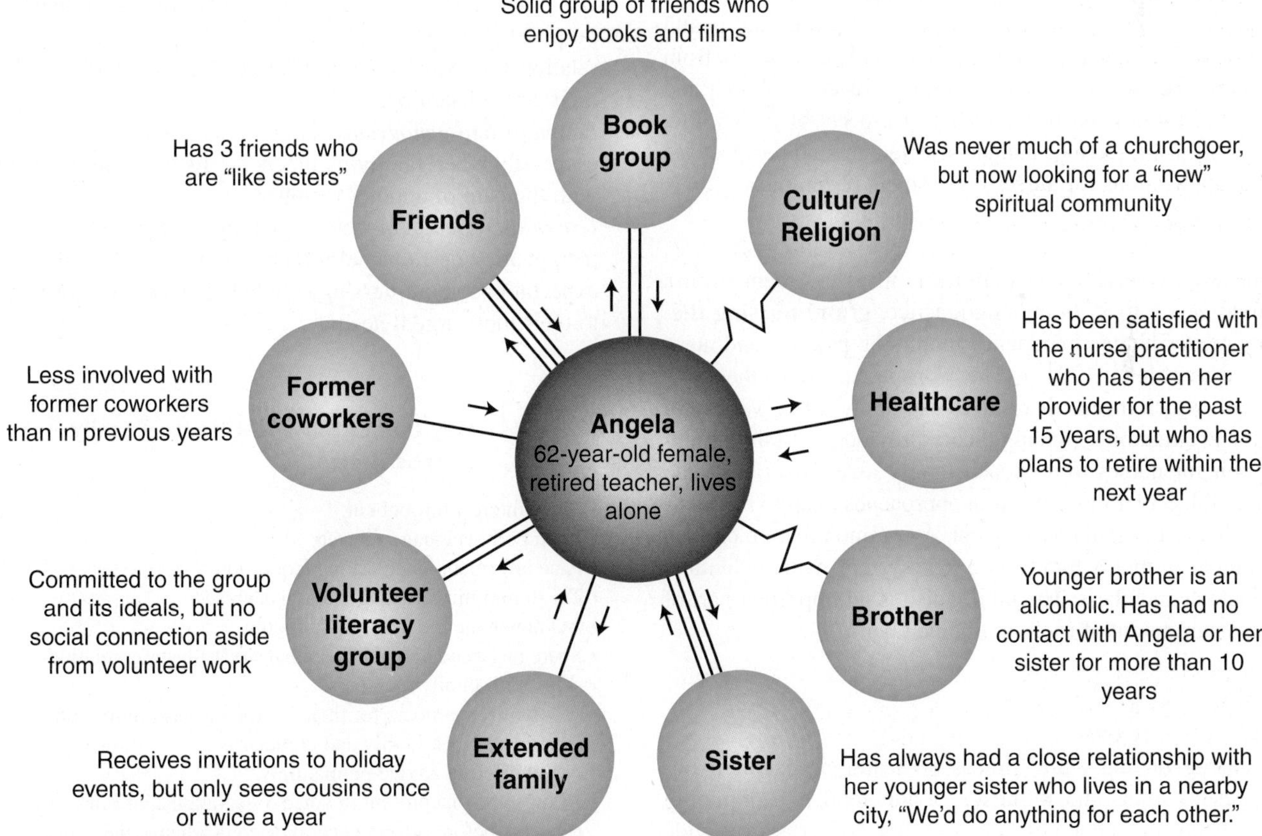

figure 13.2. Ecograph. The circles represent both persons and institutions or organizations to which a person or family is connected. The number of lines indicates the strength of the relationship, the *jagged line* indicates a negative relationship, and *arrows* indicate the direction or reciprocity of the relationship.

The following section includes an overview of different nursing perspectives and their application to family assessment.

Theoretical Approaches to Family in Community Health Nursing

The word *theory* brings to mind ideas based on scientific observations and results from controlled laboratory experiments over time. Generally speaking, a **theory** presents a systematic view of related statements to describe, explain, predict, or prescribe a phenomenon of interest (Walker & Avant, 2010). Unlike the basic sciences (e.g., chemistry or physics), theoretical nursing principles are generated from clinical practice in nursing. As in theories in the basic and social sciences, nursing theory can be used to explain how nurses interact with people, the environment, and the health-care establishment. Community health and family nursing provide nurses with numerous opportunities to observe a wide range of these interactions.

Allowing adequate time for a thorough family assessment can be overwhelming because families are complex groups. Families are not only a group of people but also an environment that reflects its relationships. Families also provide an opportunity to learn about social mores and health practices. The nurse who approaches family assessment from a particular perspective might find it easier to absorb and process information that pertains to aspects of family life. The following sections include selected nursing perspectives with applications for nurses' assessment of families.

Perspectives on Family: Grand Nursing Theory

One way to learn about families is to assess them from a broad perspective. In nursing practice, **grand nursing theory** relates human experience to nursing practice and nursing care (Meleis, 2011). The wording in grand theory is broad, which means that nurses can apply it to a variety of clinical situations. Nursing theory provides a possible foundation for nurses to approach family assessment and plan care. Table 13.1 describes four approaches to applying nursing theory to family assessment. A common feature of each example is that a family is a key system, with individual people as members. The family also is an important part of the environment of each family member.

Family Assessment

Family Interview

Focusing on individual illness or health needs often obscures or omits the influence of the family. Community health nurses encounter family health concerns in a wide range of circumstances. Attention to the dimensions and influence of family helps identify ways to support everyone involved. Identifying key relationships, both within and outside the family, is a good starting point. Genograms and ecomaps can be valuable visual aids when helping families work through areas of concern. Nurses can ask questions about families' routines to keep the assessment focused, as well as deepen understanding about factors that influence families' responses to health and illness (Denham, 2002). In addition, when nurses develop assessment skills in a variety of settings, it becomes easier for them to distinguish the family as both a functional unit and one of care. When an **informant** (person who provides information either for himself or herself or for someone who is unable to do so [e.g., unconscious]) is the only family member or significant other available for the assessment, nurses' observations and broad, open-ended questions about family life help gain a wider perspective of the family.

As in other areas of clinical practice, community health nurses frequently have limited time for family assessments because of demanding caseloads or staffing shortages. Yet focused family interviews of 15 minutes or less can yield a wealth of information (Box 13.1). Wright and Leahey (1999, 2005, 2009; Duhamel, Dupuis, & Wright, 2009) suggest the following five leading principles which maximize information gleaned in a "15-minute" family interview:

- *Manners*: Common courtesies, such as the nurse introducing himself or herself to the family, indicate a desire to connect with the family and to instill trust in family members.
- *Use of therapeutic conversation*: When time is limited, purposeful and focused conversation helps build a relationship. Nurses validate family concerns with their active listening.
- *Ecomaps and genograms*: These tools are invaluable, especially when family members are likely to be involved with the care of another member.
- *Use of therapeutic questions*: Asking family members therapeutic questions helps them not only identify their expectations about nursing care but also assign priorities to their most urgent needs.

box 13.1 Key Points for a 15-Minute Family Assessment

- Show interest throughout.
- Keep body language relaxed.
- Face informant when asking a question.
- Try to minimize writing while listening.
- Acknowledge the family's strengths.
- Share any genograms and ecomaps that illustrate relationships with family members.
- Ask family members for their interpretations/impressions (shared between family and clinician).
- Avoid offering advice prematurely.
- Allow everyone present to voice observations, insights, or concerns before offering how they could change the situation.
- Ask family if they see an area that could be changed.
- Plan goals and outcomes with family.
- Forge a partnership with the family's full participation.
- Collaborate with family to set priorities, plan care, and evaluate goals.

Source: Adapted from Wright, L., & Leahey, M. (2005). The three most common errors in family nursing: How to avoid or sidestep. *Journal of Family Nursing*, *11*(2), 90–101.

table 13.1 **Grand Nursing Theory That Guides Establishment of Assessment Goals for Families**

Theory	Perspective	Nursing Goals for Assessment	Example
Science of unitary beings (Rogers, 1970)	Family represents a group energy field. Family is part of an individual's environment. Individual and family patterns are part of this environment.	To identify family patterns, which enables nurses to gain understanding and appreciation for the family To help family partners to make changes and define outcomes	Two boys, aged 6 and 9 years, have asthma. The younger boy's asthma has worsened over the past 2 months, and he uses his inhaler three times a day. His teacher notes that he is more agitated in class. A public health nurse visits the home and notices two cats. The boys' mother states that she has a new job and that she no longer has time to clean her house "like she used to do." The boys' grandfather, who visits daily, smokes a cigar indoors.
Health as expanding consciousness (Newman, 1994)	Families and environments that are active, constantly interacting, and evolving.	To develop a therapeutic relationship with the family that helps them identify areas for change To build a story with the family as a means to change pattern	Linda, aged 45 years, has multiple sclerosis. Over the past year, her ability to walk has decreased, and she needs the assistance of another person to leave home. She can no longer drive. Both she and her husband are frustrated. They have no children. Both their families live out of state.
Roy Adaptation Model (Roy, 2008)	Role and relationships within the family are part of family functioning and adaptation. External influences also influence the family environment.	To identify basic health needs and the key roles and relationships within the family To determine how different stimuli affect the family's ability to adapt to change	A public health nurse makes a home visit to a Chinese family. The 3-month-old daughter was born prematurely at 32 weeks' gestation and had mild respiratory distress syndrome. Her mother reports that she has not been sleeping because the baby is "fussy." She has deep circles under her eyes. She reports that her husband, who speaks little English, has been sleeping at his parents' home.
Self-care agency (Orem, 2000)	Family is the foundation for self-care and a setting for care. Family members are an integral part of each other's lives.	To identify roles and relationships within the family To determine the family's ability to respond to critical situations and support each other	An older woman, who fell at home and broke her hip, was recently discharged to home after 3 months in a rehabilitation center. She has three adult daughters who are at home for the nursing visit. Two daughters live within 30 minutes of her home; the other daughter, who is a single parent, has a 2-hour drive. The unmarried daughter is helpful, but says that she would like her sisters to share the responsibility for their mother's care.

- *Acknowledgment of family strengths*: Informing families about the assets and resources they already possess leads them to view their situation differently and makes them more likely to move toward more effective problem-solving.

EVIDENCE FOR PRACTICE

Nurses might question that family assessments truly yield information that can help with planning care. Several investigators demonstrated how family interviews could benefit both the person needing care and the family as a supportive group (Eggenberger & Nelms, 2007). The purpose of this study was to describe interviewing families as a group to understand their experience of a member who is critically ill. In this study, the investigators interviewed 41 people from 11 families who had a family member hospitalized in the critical care unit. All families except two had their interviews at the hospital.

The findings showed that families found that the group interview was therapeutic early in the illness cycle. Families said they learned how to manage the experience from telling their stories. Although many family members described that the process is draining, they thought their connectedness to one another strengthened in a way they found rewarding. The family interview also gave members the opportunity to hear mutual concerns and issues, as well as identify their own strengths and weaknesses. Nurses also had the opportunity to observe the family and note nonverbal responses. The authors also noted that families might feel more comfortable being interviewed either at home or in a more familiar setting.

Findings from this study can be applied to community health nursing practice. Illness within a family, whether the person is hospitalized or not, affects all its members. Family interviews allowed nurses the opportunity to hear individual stories and facilitate resolution of problems or concerns. The interview as an assessment not only is important to identify the needs related to a person's illness, but is also vital to determine how the illness affects interpersonal relationships within the family.

Using Conceptual Models of Family Assessment

Other approaches to family assessment use particular concepts that nurses typically encounter in practice. Selected perspectives are described in Table 13.2. Unlike the broader perspectives discussed earlier, these models provide an organized **framework** with which to conduct a family assessment. Although each example has a basic format, nurses can be flexible using them and adapt them, if necessary, to combine with other models. Most nurses select an approach based on familiarity or preference. Some agencies use one particular approach. The key to selecting a certain model is to consider the situation, health concerns, and cultural background of the family.

Similarities between these models underscore the need to integrate informants' reports with objective information about the location of the interview, as well as verbal and nonverbal interactions between family members. Maintaining flexibility during the assessment is essential to help establish rapport with the family. Providing family members with opportunities to ask questions opens dialogue. Sometimes, more than one meeting is necessary to complete the assessment. The guidelines for the "15-minute" assessment (Wright & Leahey, 2005, 2009) are useful to help keep the interview focused and family-centered (Box 13.2).

FAMILY HEALTH ROUTINES AND RITUALS

A thorough family assessment involves in-depth examination of a complex system. One approach to gaining perspective on family health is to observe and inquire about the family's routines and rituals. Routines are observable, repetitive patterns that involve two or more family members. These patterns are repetitive and predictable. Rituals, on the other hand, are more formal, repetitive patterns that strengthen family self-image or identity. Denham (2002) identified six categories of family health routines: self-care; safety and precaution; mental health behaviors; family care; illness care; and member caregiving (see Table 13.2). This "routines and rituals" approach can be used as a guide to integrate with other models for family assessment. The assessment is flexible, which allows family members and informants to validate behavior patterns that affect family health. Data can also be collected over time, as with other models.

table 13.2 **Examples of Approaches to Family Assessment Using Selected Nursing Models**

Approach	Aim of Family Assessment	Key Considerations	Example of Clinical Application
Rituals and routines (Clausson & Berg, 2008)	To identify family routines and rituals that could influence family health	Family members learn and develop health behaviors from family rituals. Family routines are likely to be enduring. Acute illness or life transitions can alter routines.	A young mother from Mexico performs certain postpartum massages on her body daily and ties a shawl around her hips to help her body return to its pre-delivery state.
Life span development (Rankin, 2000)	To identify family health practices within a social and historical context	Social history provides a background in which to frame particular health behaviors or events within a broader perspective. Application to diverse groups could be difficult without knowledge of their history. This model can be used either alone or to complement another model for family assessment.	An 82-year-old World War II veteran with lung cancer explains that he started smoking when he joined the army because soldiers were given free cigarettes.
Functional health patterns (FHPs) (Gordon, 1994)	To assess health patterns in 11 areas of family health: Health perception/health management; nutritional/metabolic; elimination; activity/exercise; sleep/rest; cognitive/perceptual; self-perception/self-concept; role/relationship; sexuality/reproductive; coping/stress tolerance; and value/belief	The questions in the format are a guide for focused inquiry. Questions are direct and include probes to explore particular areas in depth.	A 59-year-old woman who has always lived alone must move in with her older sister and her husband, both in their 60s after she is diagnosed with end-stage renal failure.
Family systems (Anderson, 2000)	To engage the family as a way to identify its strengths, with attention to family dynamics and concerns related to health and illness	Identification of patterns of family relationships is key. Genograms and ecomaps are important tools to identify key relationships that will enable the nurse–family partnership to develop a family care plan.	A family from south Asia whose teenaged son was treated for substance abuse worries that he will resume socializing with his old friends and "fall off the wagon."

There was never a child so lovely but his mother was glad to get him to sleep.

Ralph Waldo Emerson

Transitions and life events affect family routines. For example, a young mother may alter her self-care practices after the birth of her first child. Questions about her diet, activity and exercise, and hygiene serve to open discussion about cultural childbirth practices. A discussion about self-care could also reveal information about family caregiving and expectations about the level to which her partner and/or immediate family support self-care.

FUNCTIONAL HEALTH PATTERNS

The functional health patterns (FHPs) scheme is a systematic, structured approach to family assessment (Gordon, 1994). Patterns are groups of behaviors that occur over time, and these help identify sequences of events as opposed to isolated incidents. The interview format for the assessment includes a specific set of questions for each assessment (see Table 13.2). The format structure is sequential yet can also be a guide for the interview. Questions are open-ended, which allows for additional probing.

In the FHP model in Table 13.2, the example involves a 59-year-old woman with renal failure who is leaving her home to live with her older sister and her family. At the initial home visit, the community nurse observes that the woman's sister has deep circles under her eyes, and she tells you that she is exhausted. Questions about the sleep–rest pattern such as "Has it been difficult to get a good night's sleep?" might be a good opening for the interview. Related questions might include asking about sleep aids, time for relaxation, and obstacles to sleeping soundly at night. Objective observations related to the pattern include looking at sleeping arrangements. If the woman's sister mentions how her interrupted sleep might have had an effect on her ability to cope, the assessment questions can naturally progress to those for the coping–stress tolerance pattern, which can lead to asking how other family members are similarly affected.

box 13.2 Overview: Questions and Considerations for Family Assessment

Who is Part of the Family?

- Who comprises the individual's or group's family?
- What is the nature of individuals' connections to one another?
- Does the individual live alone or have no living family members?
- What influences from the family of origin are present in daily life?
- Is the individual part of a communal living arrangement, for example, a religious community?

Who is the Informant?

- How many informants are present?
- How do they interact with one another?
- Do informants talk about their relationships with other members or support persons who are not present?
- Do members speak independently or is an interpreter present?
- What observations can be made about the interpersonal dynamics between members?
- Does illness or disability, for example, expressive aphasia, psychiatric illness, or amyotrophic lateral sclerosis, affect anyone's ability to speak for himself or herself?

Where is the Interview Located?

- Is the setting comfortable and conducive for the interview?
- If the assessment is part of a home visit, what observations provide insight into family life?
- What community institutions or resources influence family life?

Where Do Family Members Live?

- Do family members live in close proximity to each other?
- Are there reasons why family members are unavailable?
- If the individual lives alone, is there a reliable support person or network available?

How Much Time is Available for the Assessment?

- Can the assessment extend beyond one encounter?
- Does anyone in the family have a special concern or issue of urgency?

How Community Health Nurses Can Support Families

The demand for community health nursing has grown. This need will continue to expand as social, economic, and political trends continue to shift. People living with chronic illnesses or disabilities, the elderly, the poor, and the less educated, frequently remain in their own homes, which has increased the need for home health nurses. As many as 43.5 million adult family members are caregivers for someone 50 years or older (Family Caregiving Alliance, 2012). For example, a home care nurse can help an adult child manage a parent's congestive heart failure and arrange respite care following a hospitalization. Home care nurses note caregivers' needs on initial assessment, using the Outcomes Assessment Information Set (OASIS). OASIS includes questions about the type and frequency of caregiver involvement; characteristics which are used to determine reimbursement for Medicare home care services. Questions about caregiver functional status and psychological or cognitive limitations are also vital with initial family assessments, especially if families might need referrals to outside agencies.

Public health nurses, including school nurses, maintain a high profile with families and communities, primarily regarding health promotion and disease prevention. Their roles have gained additional significance with the recent threats of bioterrorism and outbreaks of new communicable diseases, such as sudden acute respiratory syndrome (see Chapter 14). Given that many health behaviors are learned within the family (Denham, 2012; Sterrett et al., 2013), public health nurses can sponsor events for families, such as health fairs within the community, as a way to build partnership and address family health needs.

Case Study 1—Both Tanya and Luke Barnes have been sleeping poorly at night. They have not received any e-mails or phone calls from their mother for 10 days. Lately, they show little interest in school or other activities they usually enjoy. They constantly ask Elsa and her husband when they will hear from their mother. One afternoon before the children returned from school, an army chaplain visits the home to inform the family that Elaine has been severely wounded in a mortar attack. Elsa phones Lucy immediately and asks, "What do I do now?"

- In what ways could a nurse support Tanya and Luke after they hear about their mother's injury?
- What other professionals would need to know about the current situation?

Case Study 2—Laura arranged a meeting at Jim's home with his family, Arlene, and Nancy, the social worker assigned to the case. Jim took everyone to see the new facility. Arlene would eat breakfast and lunch at a day program from 7:30 to 4:00 on weekdays and have dinner with the family. Arlene was unhappy with the plan because she does not want to leave her "home." Jim's daughters were also upset about their aunt moving into their home and said their life will not be "normal" anymore.

Later that week, Laura phoned Jim and Liz to tell them that several vacancies have opened in a residential community. Several of Arlene's friends are moving there. Although Arlene would receive a small subsidy to move into the facility, the family would have to pay approximately $2000 a month for expenses.

Jim wants to talk to his sisters, especially because their parents' health is declining. The elder Thomases receive homemaker services through their town's council on aging. Mrs. Thomas's dementia is advancing, and she might need placement in an Alzheimer care facility. Mr. Thomas receives a monthly pension, and his savings are limited.

The three Thomas siblings have had difficulty trying to agree on care arrangements for both their parents and older sister. The elder of the two, Marilyn, 55 years old, strongly opposes placement. Their sister Alice, 50 years old, is relatively indifferent.

- Identify the factors that will affect the Thomas siblings' decisions about placement for their mother and sister.
- What type of community resources could help the Thomas family, especially to help allay their anxieties about finances?
- How would you support Alice during the decision-making process?

DIVERSITY AND FAMILY

Issues related to diversity and the family are multifaceted, which can pose challenges in many areas of community nursing practice. Chapter 10, on cultural diversity and values in communities, contains a more detailed discussion of cultural diversity. The focus of discussion in this chapter is on issues community health nurses frequently encounter that relate to diversity and family care.

The Relationship between Culture, Diversity, and Family

Culture and diversity are issues that affect all families, whether or not clients openly express it. The terms *culture* and *diversity* also have several meanings. In a wider context, culture refers to a particular civilization or manner of living. A culture is a social group that shares ethnic origins, language, and characteristic features of everyday life. Culture also refers to a group of people who share attitudes, values, goals, and practices. Diversity is a range or variety of differences. More recently, the term *cultural diversity* has come into use to describe people of different racial or ethnic backgrounds in society. Yet, a more expanded meaning can also include different levels of education, socioeconomic status, belief systems, and practices. Working with families requires nurses to consider cultural diversity so that they can appreciate and understand its influence on families.

Diversity: An Evolving Concept in Families

Diversity is hardly a new concept in community nursing practice. All families have diverse qualities; nurses can look within their own communities to find diversity. Perhaps the age distribution of the community has shifted from young families to older residents. Middle-class families of different ethnic or racial origins might now populate neighborhoods that were formerly composed of white working-class residents. Chances are that changes have occurred so gradually within the community that they were barely noticeable.

Conversely, other changes might be more readily apparent. According to a local school nurse, the number of single mothers or same-sex couples has increased steadily over the past 5 years. Relatives, such as grandparents, are raising children because a parent is ill, deployed in the armed forces, incarcerated, or deceased. New immigrants move into communities and open shops and other businesses, thus making the commercial enterprises more diverse. The existence of public notices in two or three languages other than English indicates that staff in municipal offices are available to help them with inquiries about services. Events such as gay pride parades or Cinco de Mayo celebrations signify that different cultures coexist happily and embrace community diversity.

Diverse Families Living in a Diverse Culture

Patterns of immigration have shaped the cultural complexion of family in the United States. Between the end of the 19th century and the mid-20th century, more than 12 million persons immigrated to the United States. The U.S. Department of Homeland Security publishes an annual Yearbook of Immigration Statistics available as an online resource that includes a section on patterns of immigration, which outlines the different groups that have come to the United States (United States Department of Homeland

Security, 2013). Most striking is that almost every group that came to the United States experienced some form of discrimination before completely assimilating into American culture. Assimilation is the process of adopting the cultural mores and practices unique to an individual culture. Immigrant groups strove to assimilate to life in the United States; however, many families chose to retain customs and practices from their countries of origin. New immigrants settled in communities that were primarily composed of other persons from their homelands, where they retained some familiar aspects of their previous lives (e.g., speaking their native language at home and with friends, celebrating their own holidays, or following time-honored health practices). Families could be comfortable in their new communities because everyone shared a common language and familiar customs.

Changes became more visible over time. Typically, in the first generation of immigrants, many of the "old" ways remained, but families gradually began to assimilate and demonstrated their pride in being American. Yet with subsequent generations, practices once dominant in the family of origin often changed. The new ways, that other family members embraced, could be a source of conflict within the family, and sometimes within the community in which they lived. Change could be especially trying for older members of the family and community. Social scientists who study immigrants and their patterns of assimilation use the term *culture-bound* to describe a family's restricted outlook of character as part of belonging to a particular culture. Culture-bound status is not necessarily restricted to conflicts related to language or ethnicity but can extend to regional, racial, or lifestyle choices. The following sections will examine how each affects family relationships and interpersonal dynamics.

EVIDENCE FOR PRACTICE

Nearly 40% of school-aged children in North America are either overweight or clinically obese. This study noted that the trend has also affected Chinese-American children, particularly second- and third-generation Chinese-Americans. Long-term health sequelae associated with children who are overweight include type 2 diabetes, cardiovascular disease, sleep disorders, and psychosocial problems (bullying, depression, anxiety). Little is known about factors that make Chinese-American children overweight. The authors of this study sought to describe factors that influence being overweight in children (Chen & Kennedy, 2005). They examined relationships between family functioning, parenting style, dietary intake, and physical activity. They also looked at the relationships between these factors and the children's body mass index (BMI) and factors that relate to BMI, such as gender, age, maternal acculturation, and educational level.

The study group included 68 children between the ages of 8 and 10 years who identified themselves as either Chinese or of Chinese origin. To learn about family life patterns, the authors used several instruments to measure acculturation, family communication and functioning, and parenting style. They found that children of highly acculturated parents, including those who were more authoritative, were less likely to be overweight. Children from families that showed poor communication, or whose parents tended to be more democratic, were more likely to be overweight or obese.

Findings from this study demonstrate that family lifestyle and communication can affect individual health choices. The authors explained that in Chinese culture, authoritative parenting differs from strictness in Western culture. The parental role in Chinese families, or "chiao-shun," has a similar meaning to "training," which means to show concern or care for children. In this respect, this type of parenting style actually supports teaching how to make healthy life choices. Close attention to how the families interact can provide insight into resolving health issues. Community health nurses are likely to encounter immigrant and first- and second-generation families from a range of cultural backgrounds. Although the focus of this study is the health issue within Chinese culture, study findings have wider applications for community health nurses who work with immigrant families.

All happy families resemble one another, each unhappy family is unhappy in its own way.

Leo Tolstoy

Disharmony within the Family

At some point, almost every family encounters conflict. Issues that precipitate conflict might relate to a particular event, or they can coincide with a life event, such as a wedding, pregnancy and birth, and illness or death. Other conflicts can be ongoing, such as sibling conflicts, or issues between a parent and an adult child. Family members can also clash over lifestyle choices. To help nurses examine some of these issues more closely, family discord has been divided into two categories: conflicts between people in a formal relationship, such as marriage, and conflicts within families.

Discord When Families Join

Marriage is typically viewed as a joyous occasion that brings people together. Yet, conflict can arise when two people from different, or even similar, backgrounds, are in a relationship or marriage. The number of cohabiting unmarried couples has grown over the past 30 years, but family members might jokingly use terms such as "living in sin," or "haven't made it legal yet," to hide their disapproval of the practice.

INTERRACIAL MARRIAGE

Historically, the purpose of marriage was to unite two families and strengthen combined family wealth and resources. Although this clannish aspect of marriage is less prevalent in American culture today, many cultures still view marriage this way. American culture with its mosaic of many different cultures is no exception. Different cultures can coexist compatibly, but certain culture-bound beliefs persist.

Today, intermarriage between cultures is relatively common. Nonetheless, in some families, if a member chooses to marry someone from a different culture, there is greater potential for conflicts because marriages between people of different religions or races can lead to fundamental and untenable differences which are difficult to resolve with compromise or integration. Interfaith marriages can threaten family integrity, particularly around religious traditions and holidays. Treasured rituals and practices represent a connection to heritage and identity (Walsh, 2010). For example, interfaith families might experience conflict surrounding holiday practices or differences around birth, child rearing, illness, or death.

Accounts of marriage across racial and ethnic lines may have begun as early as Columbus's exploration of the Caribbean, and his arrival at the island known as Hispaniola. From that time onward, interracial marriages began to increase. Early settlers in colonial America married Native Americans or had children with them. Plantation owners and workers, including Thomas Jefferson, fathered children with their African-American slaves. Many states enacted laws that prohibited racial intermarriage, particularly of African-Americans and Whites. Marriage of two persons of different races, or *miscegenation*, was a crime in some states until 1967, when the U.S. Supreme Court ruled the law unconstitutional.

Although interracial unions are more common nowadays than in the past, they can still create conflict within families. Reported interracial marriages and partnerships in the United States have increased 28% between 2000 and 2010. Ten percent of married couples and 18% of unmarried partners are in interracial relationships (U.S. Census Bureau, 2012a). Recent census data show that 45% of married couples are composed of Hispanic and non-Hispanic persons (Kreider, 2012). Despite the numbers of interracial couples, whether married or cohabiting, families might view relationships across racial boundaries as "not right." This response can occur regardless of culture or ethnic origin. Family members might be unwilling to accept the relationship, and this feeling can persist for years.

ARRANGED MARRIAGE

Patterns of communication within families have changed over time. Levels of education, geographic location, and the predominance of the nuclear family have created more insular family arrangements. For the most part, extended families have less influence on the daily practices of individual members. Even within the family, members might frequently disagree on issues such as childbirth and childrearing, religious practices, and other lifestyle choices. A young mother, for example, might perceive her mother-in-law's extended visit to help after the arrival of a new baby as intrusive and meddlesome. A son's decision to pursue a career in education might not be "good enough" when his parents had high expectations that he would choose medicine or law.

Recent immigrants to the United States include people from areas of the world where arranged marriage is the norm. Families might find the transition to American culture difficult and struggle to maintain continuity with long-established customs, such as arranged marriage. Arranged marriage is common in Muslim culture, as well as in the cultures of western Asia and North Africa. Furthermore, about 50% of marriages between people from Iraq, Saudi Arabia, and Pakistan are between either first or second cousins. Parents might choose to sever relationships with a son or daughter who breaks from this tradition and selects his or her own partner, or chooses not to marry at all. In addition, divorce is a difficult option for spouses, especially in arranged marriages, because of the value placed on the union between the two families.

Gay and Lesbian Family Members

Over the past 40 years, nontraditional unions have gradually gained acceptance. In many ways, gay and lesbian life is celebrated and accepted in American life, especially in large cities. Many individuals no longer feel the need to be "in the closet," and are open about their relationships. Television shows and movies include openly gay characters. Regardless of the openness around gay and lesbian issues, the response to someone in a family "coming out" might not be as accepting. The process of accepting that member's lifestyle choice can be painful and cause anger. Some parents might grieve that they will never have grandchildren, or feel shame at being "different."

Intergenerational Diversity

Age is commonly overlooked as a form of diversity; it accounts for **intergenerational diversity**. Intergenerational relationships deserve mention, given that there are four generations of Americans in the workforce today. In the 1960s, the term *generation gap* was frequently used to describe differences between the communication styles and expectations of the postwar *baby boom* generation (1946–1960) and their parents, who lived through the Great Depression and World War II. People of the so-called *war generation* were used to authoritarian leadership and direct personal interaction with superiors and others. "Baby boomers" respected authority but wanted recognition for their individual contributions. People who were born between 1965 and 1983 are known as *generation X* (Gen X) and are likely to want more flexibility in their lifestyles. Although their parents were goal-oriented and focused, people in Gen X are more likely to multitask and may have more than one career in their lifetime. People born between 1984 and 2002 are known as *generation Y,* and also want flexibility in life, like their Gen X counterparts, but with guidance.

Not surprisingly, variations of the generation gap still exist within families, even in "functional" ones. Several generations may live in a single household. For example, adult children might share a home with their parents, who have grown accustomed to empty-nest households, or grandparents with early signs of dementia might live with their children and their families. Observation of interpersonal dynamics in these intergenerational households during family assessment can provide much insight into patterns of coping and communication within the family. Drawing an ecomap can be especially helpful.

Human beings are the only creatures on earth that allow their children to come back home.

Bill Cosby

Diversity embraces every aspect of family life and finds expression in family history, heritage, and language, as well as in the ways that families manifest and maintain health. Understanding diversity in individual families emphasizes the need for community health nurses to pay close attention to various dimensions of family life. Patterns of everyday family life are likely to change if a family member has to assume full-time or part-time responsibility for the care of another family member. Cultural considerations related to ethnicity, religion, and language figure prominently; however, generational difference and lifestyle choices also contribute significantly to diversity among and within families.

In the case of the Thomas family (**Case Study 2**), cultural considerations regarding the care for Arlene are not what people usually think of as "culture." She has grown up in a culture of a special unit of residential care because of her needs, and has not had connection with her older brother, who is now faced with decisions about where she will live, within the context of a mother who is cognitively deteriorating.

- Describe strategies for an open discussion at a family meeting.
- What approaches could help the Thomas family learn about possible placement options?
- Identify social factors that might influence the Thomas family's decision-making.

FAMILIES AND HEALTH RISK

What Is Family Risk Reduction?

Most families tend to express more concern about the possibility that one member might become ill than about overall family wellness (Friedman et al., 2003). A family member who is "at risk" has an increased probability of becoming sick or disabled, or even dying. The five types of risk relate to genetics, age, biological background, personal health habits/lifestyle, and environment (Pender, Murdaugh, & Parsons, 2002). Primary prevention activities cannot reduce or eliminate all risk factors. For example, genetic diseases are unavoidable; however, emphasis on wellness and quality of life can attenuate them (Sullivan-Bolyai, Knafl, Tamborlane, & Grey, 2004).

Predictions underlying probability and risk can affect families directly. Healthcare professionals can alert family members of the possibility of illness, disability, or death. To identify risk, they rely on mathematical formulas (Friedman et al., 2003). An **odds ratio** is the ratio between a risk group and a control group to predict the chance of occurrence of illness. Probabilities related to health or illness are calculated from statistical trends collected and stored in epidemiologic databases that report information about disease and disability trends (Behrens, Taeger, Wellmann, & Keil, 2004; Rosenbaum, 2004; Rothman, Lanes, & Sacks, 2004). The Centers for Disease Control and Prevention (CDC) has several health databases, one of which is the Traumatic Brain Injury Surveillance Program Web site (CDC, 2005). This database holds information that tracks and monitors the incidence of traumatic brain injury. The program holds collected data, which contribute to decision-making about efforts to prevent traumatic brain injury and lists services for people with traumatic brain injury and their families.

PRACTICE POINT

Family risk factors include genetics, age, biological factors, personal health habits, lifestyle, and environmental factors.

Databases themselves do not necessarily include information on the probability or the odds that individual people or family members will develop a disease or sustain an injury, but they do show the relationships between a variety of variables that, when analyzed, help predict the combination of characteristics or factors that yield or cause a result. People with certain genetic backgrounds have an increased likelihood of neurofibromatosis, a more common neurologic disorder, which is often misdiagnosed in childhood (Dylis, 2003). People who were sexually abused as children by an adult could be more susceptible to HIV/AIDS and other sexually transmitted infections (Kalichman, Gore-Felton, Benotsch, Cage, & Rompa, 2004; O'Leary, Purcell, Remien, & Gomez, 2003; Wyatt et al., 2004). Still others may have a greater chance to begin and sustain smoking (Hershey et al., 2005).

As illustrated in the two case studies, illness, disability, and death can affect family structure (the head of the household), function (decision-making), and outcomes (economic stability) both positively and negatively, in a variety of ways, (Mactavish & Schleien, 2004; Maes, Broekman, Dosen, & Nauts, 2003; McIntyre, Blacher, & Baker, 2002; Williams et al., 2002). Families approach the idea of health risk in many different ways depending on (1) what they have learned from their experiences in their family of origin; (2) economic circumstances, especially healthcare insurance coverage; (3) stress and coping styles; and (4) internal and external culture.

Some families who have experienced a life-threatening illness such as cancer may approach that particular health risk with greater vigilance (i.e., becoming concerned that they have cancer whenever they feel ill) (Harmon Hanson, 2001). Other families might overlook times when they actually feel sick because they rationalize that a person has to die eventually.

Forty-one million Americans, many of whom are children, are without health insurance coverage (U.S. Census Bureau, 2005). People without health insurance can find themselves in situations where health risk is less of an issue; instead, they might worry how they might get help when they or other family members are ill (Baker, Sudano, Albert, Borawski, & Dor, 2001; Davis, 2000; Guyer, Broaddus, & Dude, 2002; Lave et al., 1998). In relation to health insurance, some people view families as a structural–functional system, in which members act according to a set of norms and values that they learn through a socialization process within the family (Friedman et al., 2003; Spruijt, DeGoede, & Vandervalk, 2001). So it may be a normative expectation that family take care of what insurance does not address. On the other hand, some people may show little or no concern for family health and wellness, because their socialization toward individual family members is one of detachment. They perceive that other family members' health status has nothing to do with them. Lastly, they have learned through the internal culture of living together that discussion about health or health-related risks at home is unacceptable or "off limits." Other families might consider physical appearance more important than health prevention (Harmon Hanson, 2001).

Healthcare professionals use health and illness factors, and characteristics from the database like the one previously described, to create clinical guidelines specifically related to health promotion at all levels of prevention. Over time, researchers have used epidemiologic data to develop a variety of **health appraisals** or checklists to help family members evaluate individual risk that inevitably affects the family unit as a whole (American Academy of Pediatrics Committee on School Health, 2005; Beach & Dixson, 2001; Ho, Davidson, & Ghea, 2005; Roberts, 1999). Appraisals often include information that identifies a common problem, specific criteria that confirm that the problem exists, tangible examples of the problem, and treatment recommendations. Examples include policy statements from the American Academy of Pediatrics (2010) that promote physical activity in school-aged children to reduce overweight and public health announcements to encourage immunizations against influenza. These references are helpful for teaching families about measures of normative or abnormal conditions for initial screening (secondary prevention). Yet, a critical need exists for public health and community health nurses to help families interpret findings, as well as to provide information on community-based resources that provide further screening and treatment.

Numerous resources are available to help families evaluate risk and make decisions about their priorities with their healthcare providers. *Healthy People 2020* is an example of a public health policy initiative. This document is important because it is oriented to families as consumers of health. Its mission is to identify national health priorities in the United States, and increase public awareness of determinants of health, disease, and disability (CDC, 2011). *Healthy People 2020* tracks nearly 1,200 measurable goals and objectives in 42 topic areas. Each area includes lists of determinants or indicators of health that can help families' direct priorities to address their own health risks. These leading indicators of health relate to physical activity, obesity, tobacco use, substance abuse, responsible sexual behavior, mental health, injury and violence, environmental quality, immunization, and access to healthcare. From a practical perspective, one of the mental health determinants in the *Healthy People 2020* is to increase the proportion of adults with recognized depression who receive treatment. Public health nurses can encourage the family members of an individual with depression to be evaluated by a mental health professional. In communities with few mental health services, families might rally together to lobby for mental health centers that provide care at a reasonable cost within their locality. Table 13.3 briefly summarizes studies that directly relate to the *Healthy People 2020* objectives.

Healthy People 2020 also lists the five leading causes of death in the United States. With information about trends in morbidity and mortality, community health nurses and providers work with families to identify creative interventions that prevent illness or premature death. In recent years, studies have been done which show that racial differences and economic deprivation in families are associated with increased death rates (Bielho, Niccolai, Kershaw, Lin, & Ickovics, 2013; Singh, Azuine, Siahpush, & Kogan, 2013; Sparks, Sparks, & Campbell, 2013). These trends are disturbing, and underscore the need to eliminate **health disparities** on account of race or economic status.

Family risk reduction is the process by which either individual family members or entire families work together toward a goal of reducing the probability of sickness, disability, or death. Through this process, they are making an effort to reduce the probability or occurrence of illness (Harmon Hanson, 2001). The action the family takes is anticipatory, and can occur at any level of prevention (primary, secondary, or tertiary). Family risk reduction before illness is primary prevention. For example,

- If children are fighting with each other to compete for attention, parents might find it helpful to spend time alone with each child individually at a "special time," rather than to ignore the situation, and then have to deal with an emergency department visit for sutures sustained when a child is pushed into a wall (Harrison, 1998).
- Parents might ask their guests to refrain from smoking in the home to reduce the exposure of their children to second-hand smoke that could aggravate their asthma.
- Family members who prepare meals may try to decrease serum cholesterol levels in other members of their family by making healthy food choices at home or by making suggestions for healthy foods in restaurants (secondary prevention).
- Family members caring for an elderly parent may install adaptive devices in their home to help the parent feel more secure when showering or walking (tertiary prevention).

table 13.3 **Studies That Relate to *Healthy People 2020* Objectives**

Objectives Addressed	Significant Findings	Reference
• Modify risk behaviors and improve lifestyle choices. • Decrease chronic illness. • Improve disease prevention and health promotion behaviors.	The Behavioral Risk Factor Surveillance System provides a critical analysis of cholesterol screening to prevent heart disease and stroke. The aim was to meet *Health People 2020* targets for cholesterol screening especially in younger men and the Hispanic population.	Center for Disease Control & Prevention, 2012a
• Decrease risk behaviors that might cause cancer. • Increase number of persons who receive screening. • Provide access for underserved populations.	National Health Interview Survey data are used to assess the use of cancer screening among adults over 18 years. Persons with higher education levels are more likely to seek screening. Targeted cancer screening in immigrants and persons without health insurance should be increased.	Center for Disease Control & Prevention, 2012b
• Decrease alcohol consumption. • Reduce sexually transmitted diseases. • Improve physical activity. • Reduce violence.	Youth Risk Behavior Surveillance System (YRBSS) monitors six categories of priority health-risk behaviors among youth and young adults. Age, gender, race and ethnicity, and geographic location are taken into account. Areas of interest include personal safety, sexual activity, lifestyle, and risk behaviors.	Eaton et al., 2012

Sources of Family Risk Reduction Information

In formal settings, families receive health and wellness information at a ubiquitous and rapid pace. Members of families hear information from a variety of sources that include printed media (e.g., newspapers). Both television and radio have public service announcements and topical news programs. More recently, adults are using the Internet to search for information on health issues. Healthcare providers offer clients health information in clinics, physicians' offices, emergency departments, and urgent care centers. Local public health department clinics and school health offices are also sources of health information in communities.

In informal settings, family members may receive inaccurate information about risk reduction, primarily because people interpret risk reports at their level of understanding (i.e., their own level of education or the level of information given). In fact, family members often hear ambiguous reports or interpretations about how someone became disabled, ill, or died. Family assessment is beneficial to help organize important knowledge across the domains of health, environment, and interpersonal interactions. Information about risk reduction is often difficult to decipher due to unknown factors. For example, when a man learns that his paternal grandfather died from pneumonia at the age of 41 years, the level of risk reduction information changes depending on whether the man died from emphysema related to habitual, heavy smoking of cigars and cigarettes as opposed to a bacterial or viral infection (Daley et al., 1999; Frame, 2000; Keiley et al., 2002; Wimbush & Peters, 2000).

Many pieces of information are written about risk. Health literacy means that language, either written or verbal, has to be understandable. More importantly, nurses in public health practice can observe whether members choose to apply risk information to their lives or ignore it, as a health literacy assessment and as a means of understanding whether family members are actively or passively alerted to health risks (Friedman et al., 2003). Pender (1996) emphasized that prevention requires a defensive approach, with some families (1) being neither ready nor wanting to take preventive action or (2) experiencing stressful life events that complicate such action. Pender et al. (2002) coined the phrase "health protection" to refer to families or individual people who are motivated to avoid illness, detect it early, or preserve function even when ill.

EVIDENCE FOR PRACTICE

The population of Latinos in the United States has been increasing steadily. The authors of one study noted that Latino youth have disproportionately higher rates of mental health issues that include depression, anxiety, suicidal ideation, and suicidal attempts (Garcia, Skay, Sieving, Naughton, & Bearinger, 2008). To understand the underlying risk and protective factors, they used the resiliency framework to determine how family connectedness, communication, and caring affect the mental health of Latino students. The study examined the relationships between family protective factors and emotional distress, suicidal ideation, and suicidal attempts. To obtain information about the students, the researchers used a state survey that they modified for their own purposes. Analysis also included examining relationships involving family connectedness, parental care, and students' perception of their communication with their parents.

Adolescence is a transitional period that can cause emotional upset in vulnerable youth. Minimizing disparities surrounding mental health concerns in persons of color is a priority of *Healthy People 2020*. Study findings show how family relationships can affect the health and well-being of individual members. Although the study group is limited to Latino high school students, findings suggest that students of mixed racial background can have a higher incidence of emotional distress, anxiety, or depression. This risk increases without open communication with parents. The authors also underscore the need for school nurses to ask students who are anxious or have depressed affect about their relationships with parents. The authors suggest that communities provide venues for family events that support and nurture relationships between young adolescents and their parents. Instituting a program like this in elementary schools, and in high schools, might help build relationships over time.

Families with Problems: Stressful Life Events

Life events that most people and their families find stressful are listed in Box 13.3. Stressful family life events may affect physical, cognitive, affective, and social functioning. Descriptions of stressful life events in family literature have evolved from being a single event that brings a family to a crisis with a presumed negative outcome, to one where the crisis becomes a challenge in which families can make positive changes to adapt to the stressor (Hill, 1949; McCubbin & McCubbin, 1993). Several theories address the process of experiencing a stressful life event and how families can move in the direction of wellness through an adaptive process.

box 13.3 Examples of Family Inventory of Life Events

- **Losses**
  A spouse or child dies
- **Family legal violations**
  Domestic violence or child abuse
- **Marital strains**
  Divorce or decreased sexual intimacy
- **Illness and family care strains**
  Filial responsibility for oldest girl sibling, or child of either gender to care for chronically ill parents
- **Intrafamily strains**
  Family feud when two sisters refuse to speak to each other
- **Finance and business strains**
  Filing for bankruptcy
- **Pregnancy and childbearing strains**
  Teen pregnancy
- **Work and family transition strains**
  Retirement or involuntary loss of a job
- **Transitions**
  Child adoption or teen goes to college

Source: Adapted from McCubbin, H. I., & Patterson, M. (1983). The family stress process: Double ABCX model of adjustment and adaptation. In H. I. McCubbin, M. B. Sussman, & J. M. Patterson (Eds.), *Social stress and the family* [Special Issue]. *Marriage and Family Review*, *6*, 7–27.

PRACTICE POINT

A stressful life event that begins as a crisis can lead family members to make changes that enable them to adapt to the stressor.

Resilience is a concept used to describe some families who experience enormous strain from life events and yet continue to live normally, even thriving despite the circumstances (Boerner, Wortman, & Bonanno, 2005; McCubbin & McCubbin, 1993; Pilowsky, Zybert, & Vlahov, 2004; Rossi-Ferrario, Baiardi, & Zotti, 2004). In addition to models of explanation, measures to appraise risk describe types of life events that can cause the greatest strain and therefore may require the most health intervention. The Family Inventory of Life Events and Changes (FILE) is a particular appraisal measure that is useful to identify stressful life events in families (McCubbin & Patterson, 1983) (see Box 13.3). The following section describes examples of stressful events that families might frequently encounter and ways that community health nurses can support family structure, functions, and outcomes during stressful events. The following Evidence for Practice section summarizes a study using the resiliency model as a framework for study.

EVIDENCE FOR PRACTICE

More than 4 million American households are multigenerational, meaning that grandparents reside with their grandchildren. Although this figure accounts for fewer than 5% of all American households, more than one-third of these households have no parent in residence. In nearly all these households, the grandmother usually assumes total responsibility as the head of the household. Considering previous studies of social support and depression in grandmothers raising children, the authors of this study (Musil, Warner, Zauszniewski, & Standing, 2009) examined family life stresses and strains that affect grandmothers. They also tested how resourcefulness and social support affect the relationship between family stresses and strains with grandmothers' depressive symptoms as their grandchildren's primary caregiver. The framework for the study was the resiliency model of family stress, adjustment, and adaptation demands, which could affect grandmother caregivers' mental health to (McCubbin, Thompson, & McCubbin, 1996).

Three groups of grandmothers (n = 486) completed surveys for the study. One group took care of at least one grandchild younger than 16 years and was responsible for raising the child without a parent living in the home. The second group consisted of multigenerational families with at least one grandchild and one parent, and the third group of grandmothers lived within an hour or 50 miles of their grandchildren.

The authors used statistical analyses to compare scores from instruments to measure family life events, resourcefulness, social support, and depression, and attempted to predict depressive symptoms on intrafamily strain and family life stresses. Findings showed that grandmothers raising children reported more depressive symptoms; however, when controlled for demographic variables, being the primary caregiver was not related to depressive symptoms. Reports of higher levels of social support and resourcefulness seemed to minimize the effects of family stresses and strains.

This study is an example of how the resiliency model of family stresses and adjustment and adaptation provides a useful framework to examine any societal variant of family that has relevance for community health nursing practice. The comparisons and predictions help community health nurses anticipate the need for individual and community resources to support grandmothers as primary caregivers. Most importantly, family demands without adequate support and resources can lead to reports of depressive symptoms. Acknowledging the grandmother as primary caregiver and establishing rapport can help build a collaborative relationship. Identifying needs for specific support within the family and referrals to community agencies, as needed, foster good health and well-being for the entire family.

STUDENT REFLECTION

Throughout my nursing program, I have struggled to find a balance between being a student and a nurse. After my community health clinical practice, I am struck by the difficulty families have in making decisions for one another, even if it's in their best interest. Today, I worked with an 84-year-old woman who was discharged from the hospital after treatment for a fall at home. She cannot remember what happened right before she fell, but her doctors suspected that she had a mild seizure or stroke. The nurse at the center let me come along on a visit to the woman's home last week to assess home safety. The woman's children are concerned about her living alone, and until now, they have been reluctant to talk about alternative living arrangements.

At the family meeting, the woman's doctor said that it was in the family's best interest to consider assisted living arrangements because of Mrs. J's impaired mobility and decreased cognitive status. Both her social worker and community health nurse expressed that the family needed more time to make a decision. Her adult children said that they could see the advantages of assisted living. They worry about their mother's safety living alone and want to make sure that she is safe and has some independence, and they would like to visit a local facility.

As a student nurse, I thought this situation was difficult. Clearly, the decision to move a parent into an assisted living facility is complicated, but I observed that the goal of the meeting was to help them make an informed decision and support them through the process. I realized how difficult it was for adult children to make decisions on their parents' behalf. I can't imagine having to do that for my mom or dad. Every family has a different way of dealing with difficult situations. As I develop as a nurse, I have to remember that everyone I care for has someone to call family, and learn how to meet individual and family needs. Experience will help me master this skill.

The Death of a Family Member

The death of a family member, whether expected or sudden, has physical, cognitive, affective, and social consequences for family functioning. Family members describe a sense of disorientation, trouble sleeping, and overwhelming sadness. Some families feel anger, blame, and shame. Community health nurses can be resourceful and help families understand that "feeling" is an important phase in the process of bereavement. Sharing the experience of bereavement with professionals or peers is a way to cope (Chan, O'Neill, McKenzie, Love, & Kissane, 2004; Kaunonen, Aalto, Tarkka, & Paunonen, 2000; Kissane, Bloch, McKenzie, McDowall, & Nitzan, 1998). This is a critical first step to help families explore all potential sources of comfort. Some family members may need or ask for individual counseling, whereas others may choose group therapy. Some families prefer the comfort of close relationships or their faith communities. A primary goal is to identify those sources of comfort for family members and help them avoid isolation while in the process of grieving. Realistically, resources that help families generate new roles, and financial aid to maintain family functioning, are vital.

EVIDENCE FOR PRACTICE

Women's informal caregiving is a long-established societal norm, yet little is known about the dramatic effect it can have on their lives. Typically, women juggle family, work, and social obligations when caring for their sick or dying parents. Read and Wuest (2007) investigated the experiences of adult daughters who cared for dying parents. Using grounded theory, a qualitative method, the authors attempted to understand the daughters' experiences and explain the process of relinquishing. To elicit responses that would help reveal similarities and differences, the authors asked 12 women, who were between 34 and 66 years of age at the time of their parents' death, the question *What's going on here?*

Findings showed that anticipated loss of a parent created emotional, relational, or societal turmoil that disrupts normal patterns of daily life for daughters and their families. The authors used the theory of relinquishing, which they generated from data, to explain the daughters' process of letting go of their relationship with their parents. Daughters observed a sense of obligation to their parents. Family expectations; unresolved conflicts; and differing beliefs, experiences, and information could lead to tensions. Dominant social values led the daughters to raise their expectations about what they could reasonably accomplish in terms of caregiving, and this led to frustration. It is necessary to include respite for caregivers to conserve physical and mental health.

Nurses' attention to coordination of care and resources can lead to improved care overall, which reduces caregiver turmoil. Caring for dying parents disrupts everyday life. Therefore, it is necessary to support adult children as caregivers, and to advocate on their behalf to enhance overall care and well-being for the family.

Divorce

Divorce is a major variation in the family life cycle that can compound the complexity of developmental tasks (Friedman et al., 2003). It affects families at every stage of development (U.S. Census Bureau, 2005). Most importantly, divorce has far-reaching effects for family members at every generational level in both the nuclear and extended family. The sequelae of divorce depend on the family. For example, divorce in a family without children is substantially different from one with children. A child's age and stage of development determines his or her perception of the change in marital relationship, and the resolution of any conflicts. For the married couple, the stage of their relationships helps determine the level of loss and bereavement. For example, divorce that occurs after 25 years of marriage can be devastating and cause "couple identity" crisis as shared financial investments and possessions are dissolved (Friedman et al., 2003). In the same way, divorce that occurs in marriages of shorter duration can be equally upsetting; marital identity is in process and may leave members of the family unit with a sense of unfinished process or a sense of abject failure that may impact other relationships in the future.

Marital/Partner Strain

Conflict management and intimacy are key determinants of marital/partner health and wellness (Bomar, 2004). **Marital strain** is a term that describes how couples manage tensions and promote intimacy as opposed to create negativity (strain) in conflict resolution (Gottman, 1994). Defensiveness, criticism, contempt, and withdrawal erode trust in many relationships. Couples who lack the skills to deal with conflicts and avoid or minimize conflict put pressure not only on their own relationship but also on their relationships with other family members who encounter those conflicts and tensions directly or indirectly (Grych, Raynor, & Fosco, 2004). Community health nurses can observe tensions between spouses and partners, as well as the effects of these tensions on other family members and significant others. A critical point to remember is that in extreme circumstances, conflict erodes the connection between partners. Many couples experience strain from conflicts at various points in their relationships, but show resiliency through connectedness and intimacy because they respect and validate each other at other times (Julien, Chartrand, Simard, Bouthillier, & Begin, 2003).

Legal Issues and Effect on Family Life

Many families experience pain and suffering when a family member receives a legally imposed penalty or is incarcerated. These circumstances can bring embarrassment, financial suffering, physical separation, or stigma. Examples of criminal activity include the following:

1. Failure to provide financial support (heads of households or people, responsible person) for care of children or disabled adults (Rozie-Battle, 2002)
2. Illegal substance possession, use, and trafficking (Houck & Loper, 2002) (see Chapter 16)
3. Prostitution (McClanahan, McClelland, Abram, & Teplin, 1999)
4. Violent actions
5. Theft (Tsang, 2000)

In many of these cases, if a family member is arrested and incarcerated, the separation between individual family members seriously affects developmental relationships. For example, children whose mothers are in prison are separated from them, and they often receive care from foster parents or other family members during the mother's period of incarceration (Houck & Loper, 2002). They may have a court-appointed guardian. Some prison systems have programs that allow children to visit their parents and share activities on scheduled days to lessen the separation between parents and children (Baker, 2005). The program designers take into account the type of criminal infraction and security needs of the incarcerated parent.

Illness, Disability, and Intrafamily Strain

When illness or disability becomes part of a family experience, community health nurses distinguish themselves as facilitators by helping both the family unit and individual family members to find balance. Whether caring for an elder who is homebound or a child with a disability, **caregiver burden** has been well documented in the literature as a significant stressor on the family member who assumes primary responsibility for care (Spurlock, 2005). In most cultures, women (mothers, wives, sisters, daughters, or female "in-laws") have assumed this role, usually by default. Caregiver burden is a significant issue for families because it can cause the development of physical or emotional illness in the caregiver over time. Caregivers might express feeling trapped and isolated with no possible help with care. In addition, caring for a family member can lead to financial strain in some circumstances. An important consideration is that, although caregiver burden does exist, caregivers articulate their desire to provide caregiving in grateful appreciation for what the recipient has done for them in the past. Expression of positive feelings and the privilege connected with caring for another is plentiful in the literature (Lund, 2005). Yet, caregiver burden inevitably affects the dynamic of the entire family unit and is considered **intrafamily strain**.

Illness or disability can alter many family functions. For example, opportunities for recreation can be stifled when someone in the family needs to stay home to assist the person who is ill. The primary caregiver often opts to put the needs of the ill or disabled family member first before taking care of his or her own health needs. Some studies have shown there is a relationship between caregiver burden and elder or child abuse in families (Lachs & Pillemer, 2004). The attention parents give to their child with chronic illness affects healthy siblings. Parental behavior with a child who is chronically ill or disabled can also significantly affect family cohesion, and the sense of connection children feel within the family. Socioeconomic status influences the mood of parents and can indirectly affect other family members. Study findings have shown that a healthy sibling's knowledge about his or her brother's or sister's illness, attitude toward the illness or disability, mood in the household, self-esteem, and feelings of social support are interrelated, and specifically related to the behavior of the ill family member.

Pregnancy and Childbearing

Pregnancy is a developmental event in families. Whether a pregnant woman is an adolescent or an adult, accessible high-quality prenatal care is essential. Infant mortality rates in the United States are considered high for a developed country, and low birth weight continues to be directly related to poverty more than any other variable (Meade & Ickovics, 2005). Prevention initiatives are essential to respond to situations that are threatening to the mother, child, father, and extended family engaged in the prospective birth. Efforts to prevent substance abuse, including alcohol use, during pregnancy are vitally important (Koniak-Griffin, Anderson, Verzemnieks, & Brecht, 2000). Finally, pregnant adolescents need support from their families and schools because teen pregnancy is a distinct predictor of poverty, intrafamily conflict, substance abuse and addiction, and violence (Pickett, Mookherjee, & Wilkinson, 2005).

Infants with fetal alcohol syndrome (FAS), as well as those born to mothers who are drug addicted, face neurological abnormalities, developmental delays, behavior issues, intellectual deficits, and facial abnormalities. As infants reach developmental milestones, the potentially disabling needs of a child with FAS or the sequelae of drug addiction at birth places enormous stress and pressure on the family, as well as on the child who is "different." The special needs of these children require coordination using case management skills, as well as energy and financial resources. Other support may be necessary.

HIV-infected women face unique reproductive decision-making issues. The possibility of transmitting HIV to their infants is the most obvious concern (Mofenson, 2002). Many women may know that they are involved in risk-taking behaviors (intravenous drug use, unprotected sex, multiple sexual partners) and choose not to be tested for HIV because of fear or denial. In fact, many women find out they are seropositive when they receive prenatal care. Many unplanned pregnancies lead to making decisions whether to continue the pregnancy (Ingram & Hutchinson, 1999), but those pregnancies in the context of HIV diagnosis put particular strain on women in knowing that there may be a chance of perinatal transmission of the virus to a neonate. If they decide to have the child, constant worry persists about perinatal transfer of HIV to the infant or seroconversion after birth (Sandelowski & Barroso, 2003). Much progress has been made involving treatment of the mother with zidovudine (AZT) during pregnancy and short-term treatment of the infant after birth. There has also been great success with proactive delivery planning (Mofenson, 2002).

Families of women infected with HIV are deeply concerned because of the continuing uncertainty related to the quality of life of someone in the family living with HIV. These families also often bear a stigma because one member's lifestyle choices might make some family members feel "different." In addition, families might worry about the growth and development of a child with HIV. For the past 15 years, children who were born infected with HIV have responded to current care alternatives.

Work–Family Interface

The effect of family on work has received much less attention than the effect of work on the family. For example, many studies addressed work time and occupational attainment and their relationships to marital solidarity, parent–child affiliations, and choices of hours worked (Aryee, Srinivas, & Hwee, 2005). Kanter questioned the centrality of work in setting economic conditions for family life in 1977, which influenced researchers' interest in exploring the relationship between work and family roles. Despite this critique, the strength and direction of the relationships between family and work have been inconsistent over time (Aryee et al., 2005).

Some researchers have suggested that family and work are separate and independent entities (Aryee et al., 2005), whereas others have found a relationship between job and life satisfaction (Judge, Bono, Erez, & Locke, 2005).

Findings in early studies on family work have recognized that family and work are interdependent. Researchers viewed family factors as influencers of job satisfaction (Hoppock, 1935). Family attitudes predetermined adjustment on the job (Bullock, 1952; Friend & Haggard, 1948). Studies in the 1950s showed that work and family are independent of each other (Parsons & Bales, 1955), whereas later study findings in the 1970s and 1980s showed them as overlapping (Crosby, 1987; Kanter, 1977).

The increasing participation of women in the labor force has catalyzed research efforts on the interaction between family and the workplace and the effects on different aspects of people's life roles. **Spillover** describes the relationship between work and family—that is, requirements in different roles are similar, or fulfillment is sought in one role because of lack of gratification in others (Hammer, Cullen, Neal, Sinclair, & Shafiro, 2005). The boundary between work and home could be more permeable than researchers think. Some research indicates that a person's subjective experience, at work or at home, arouses feelings that are brought into the other context of life, and subsequently affect the processes of the other arena. Past experiences in life may have an effect on the relationship between home or work (Aryee et al., 2005). Most interpretations of how people cope with multiple roles between home and work have been made across genders (Barnett, 1994). Home-to-work spillover might be reduced if full-time hours were reduced, and workers were allowed to adjust their work schedules to accommodate family needs. When one family member is employed full-time, work schedules can impede accommodation, resulting in negative spillover for women as well as men. There is one hypothesis that the high quality of women's marital and parental roles would buffer any negative mental health effects that come with a poor experience in a full-time job (Arnett, 1995). Additional studies to identify specific stressors and stress reducers will help clarify the effect of dual-earner support in marital relationships.

Homeless Mothers and Children and Other Displaced Families

Family homelessness has become a major national problem. Children are born to parents who are homeless, or who have become homeless because of eviction, overcrowding, abuse, conflict, or natural disasters. Homeless families are at greater risk for illness and disability, substance abuse, violence-related injuries, and mental health problems. Living in shelters or temporary facilities is associated with aggressiveness, anxiety, and sadness (Institute of Medicine, 1988).

Forced immigration on an international level, whether permanent or temporary, creates chaos in family and national culture (Committee on Community Health Services, 2005). Many families suffer separation because of economic need. Migrant workers and other types of temporary visiting workers or students often send their earnings back to their families. These disconnected families live impoverished lives and cannot share relationships because of geographic distances (Committee on Community Health Services, 2005). The experience of living in a refugee camp can be unintentionally painful and dangerous. Camps and refugee areas increase the likelihood of physical illness such as dysentery, HIV/AIDS, tuberculosis, and malaria, as well as mental illnesses such as depression and post-traumatic stress disorders (Connolly et al., 2004; Rhodes & Simic, 2005). In addition, families without homes of their own lack a sense of autonomy and are thereby made vulnerable.

COMMUNITY HEALTH NURSES' RESPONSIBILITY TO FAMILIES

Communities have different types of families. Yet they have characteristics that are similar in composition and manner. Individuals who comprise families share emotional bonds that have strengthened or weakened over the course of its history. Yet, even when dealing with individuals' concerns, family influence weighs heavily when meeting specific needs.

Working with families frequently requires community health nurses to be creative when planning interventions. Family assessment provides a good starting point, which enables nurses to explore a family's practices and priorities related to health and wellness. The ultimate goal should be to enable the family to identify its health needs and to help them choose the best way they can meet that need. In this instance, a community health nurse's responsibility is to listen and facilitate building consensus within the family.

Community health nurses are known for being resourceful. Sharing information about available agencies and relevant resources will help families meet their health goals. Actions could be as simple as providing Internet websites or as complex as finding a clinic for a family of refugees.

Often, community health nurses make initial contact with families through referrals that another healthcare facility, or an individual person has made. Acute care facilities and clinics regularly refer people to home care agencies. Community health nurses who work in elder day care centers or day facilities for developmentally disabled individuals frequently require contact with the primary care physicians, nurse practitioners, or others involved directly in the client's care; contact with family members may be necessary. Collaboration with other members of a family's healthcare team ensures continuity of care, and provides perspective from other disciplines that are involved with the family.

Health literacy also is a vital area that requires nurses to advocate on behalf of families within the community. Providing health information available to families in language and content that is clear, concise, and understandable is essential for a well-informed public. Community health nurses can invite families to review with them health-related materials printed for circulation in the community (e.g., reminders about children's immunizations or efforts to curb mosquito breeding to discourage the spread of West Nile virus), to make sure that they fit the community's language and educational levels. Such actions not only promote learning and cooperation but also foster a spirit of partnership and trust between families and nurses.

Most importantly, community health nurses have a responsibility to advocate for families. A primary challenge is to promote health and wellness within the family. The two overarching goals of *Healthy People 2020* are to improve the quality and years of healthy life, and to eliminate health disparities. Community health nurses often intervene on a family's behalf to make sure that families receive access to optimal healthcare. Families often need assistance to navigate the healthcare system, especially when the family is unfamiliar with the setting or trying to cope with illness or crisis that disrupts everyday life.

PRACTICE POINT

The responsibilities of community health nurses to families are to advocate for their health and wellness, to eliminate disparities in healthcare delivery, and to promote health literacy.

key concepts

- Family assessment requires flexibility to include key informants, and in the location and timing of the interview.
- Family health practices, routines, and responses to difficult situations evolve from complex environmental and interpersonal interactions.
- Significant events can put family health at risk.

critical thinking questions

1. Consider a family from your clinical practice that is different in some way from your own. Discuss the challenges of working with the family and describe how you were able to support them. Write a short paragraph about something you learned from that experience. Include an action that you might approach differently if you were in a similar situation again.
2. Draw an ecomap for a family that you recently encountered. Identify what could be an obstacle to that family's health. Discuss how limitations in a family could be made more positive, and how using the ecomap would be helpful.
3. Family assessment can be challenging, often because of time constraints. Describe how you could gather valuable information about a family in the following situations:
    a. A student's aunt who comes to the school health office to take her nephew home because of head lice
    b. A single father who brings his toddler to the clinic because of an earache
    c. The adult daughter of an elderly woman with dementia during a home visit
    d. An elderly man who never married visits the local senior center for a blood pressure check
4. Describe a situation from clinical experience in which a family's culture influenced how they approached healthcare. Include factors that affected interaction, for example, language barriers.
5. Discuss how unexpected life crises or catastrophic illness affects families. Use examples from your clinical experience to illustrate the ways families can support or impede coping with these events.
6. Identify public health events, such as outbreaks of influenza or West Nile virus, in which community health nurses work with groups of families. What practices have you observed in communities? Describe different types of venues that nurses use or could use to provide outreach education.

references

American Academy of Pediatrics. (2010). *Prevention and treatment of Childhood overweight and obesity.* Retrieved November 3, 2010, from http://www.aap.org/obesity/index.html

American Academy of Pediatrics Committee on School Health. (2005). Health appraisal guidelines for day camps and resident camps. *Pediatrics, 115*(6), 1770–1773.

American Fact Finder. (2010). *Family and Households.* Retrieved November 3, 2010, from http://factfinder.census.gov/servlet/STTable?_bm=y&-geo_id=01000US&-qr_name=ACS_2008_3YR_G00_S1101&-ds_name=ACS_2008_3YR_G00_&-redoLog=false

Anderson, K. H. (2000). The family health system approach to family systems nursing. *Journal of Family Nursing, 6,* 103–119.

Arnett, J. J. (1995). Broad and narrow socialization: The family in the context of a cultural theory. *Journal of Marriage and the Family, 57*(3), 617–628.

Aryee, S., Srinivas, E. S., & Hwee, H. T. (2005). Rhythms of life: Antecedents and outcomes of work—Family balance in employed parents. *Journal of Applied Psychology, 90*(1), 132–146.

Baker, D. W., Sudano, J. J., Albert, J. M., Borawski, E. A., & Dor, A. (2001). Lack of health insurance and decline in overall health in late middle age. *New England Journal of Medicine, 345*(15), 1106–1112.

Baker, L. (2005). *Inmates and daughters connect through scout troop.* Retrieved September 21, 2005, from http://www.connectforkids.org/node/3009

references (continued)

Barnett, R. C. (1994). Men's jobs and partner roles: Spillover effects and psychological distress. *Sex Roles*, *27*, 455–472.

Beach, W. A., & Dixson, C. N. (2001). Revealing moments: Formatting understandings of adverse experiences in a health appraisal interview. *Social Science and Medicine*, *52*(1), 25–44.

Behrens, T., Taeger, D., Wellmann, J., & Keil, U. (2004). Different methods to calculate effect estimates in cross-sectional studies. A comparison between prevalence odds ratio and prevalence ratio. *Methods of Information in Medicine*, *43*(5), 505–509.

Biello, K. B., Niccolai, L., Kershaw, T. S., Lin, H., & Ickovics, J. (2013). Residential racial segregation and racial differences in sexual behaviours: An 11-year longitudinal student of sexual risk of adolescents transitioning to adulthood. *Journal of Epidemiology and Community Health*, *67*(1), 28–34.

Boerner, K., Wortman, C. B., & Bonanno, G. A. (2005). Resilient at risk? A 4-year study of older adults who initially showed high or low distress following conjugal loss. *Journal of Gerontology*, *60*(2), P67–P73.

Bomar, P. J. (2004). *Promoting health in families*. Philadelphia, PA: Saunders.

Bullock, R. P. (1952). *Social factors related to job satisfaction: A technique for the measurement of job satisfaction*. Columbia, OH: Ohio State University Press.

Centers for Disease Control and Prevention. (2011). *Healthy People 2020*. Retrieved April 22, 2013, from http://www.cdc.gov/nchs/healthy_people/hp2020.htm

Centers for Disease Control and Prevention. (2012a). Cancer screening—United States, 2010. *Morbidity & Mortality Weekly Report*, *61*(3), 41–45. Retrieved from http://www.cdc.gov/mmwr/preview/mmwrhtml/mm6103a1.htm?s_cid=mm6103a1_w

Centers for Disease Control and Prevention. (2012b). Prevalence of cholesterol screening and high blood cholesterol among adults, United States, 2005, 2007, 2009. *Morbidity & Mortality Weekly Report*, *61*(35), 697–702. Retrieved from http://www.cdc.gov/mmwr/preview/mmwrhtml/mm6135a2.htm?s_cid=mm6135a2_w

Chan, E. K., O'Neill, I., McKenzie, M., Love, A., & Kissane, D. W. (2004). What works for therapists conducting family meetings: Treatment integrity in family-focused grief therapy during palliative care and bereavement. *Journal of Pain and Symptom Management*, *27*(6), 502–512.

Chen, J. Y., & Kennedy, C. (2005). Factors associated with obesity in Chinese American children. *Pediatric Nursing*, *31*(2), 110–115.

Clausson, E., & Berg, A. (2008). Family intervention sessions: One useful way to improve schoolchildren's mental health. *Journal of Family Nursing*, *14*(3), 289–313.

Committee on Community Health Services. (2005). Providing care for immigrant, homeless, and migrant children. *American Academy of Pediatrics*, *115*(4), 1095–1100.

Connolly, M. A., Gayer, M., Ryan, M. J., Salama, P., Spiegel, P., & Heymann, D. L. (2004). Communicable diseases in complex emergencies: Impact and challenges. *Lancet*, *364*, 1974–1983.

Crosby, F. (1987). *Spouse, parent, worker: On gender and multiple roles*. New Haven, CT: Yale University Press.

Daley, M., Farmer, J., Harrop-Stein, C., Montgomery, S., Itzen, M., Costalas, J. W.,... Gillespie, D. (1999). Exploring family relationship in cancer risk counseling using the genogram. *Cancer Epidemiology Biomarkers and Prevention*, *8*(4), 393–398.

Davis, J. B. (2000). Conceptualizing the lack of health insurance coverage. *Health Care Analysis*, *8*(1), 55–64.

Denham, S. A. (2002). Family routines: A structural perspective for viewing family health. *Advances in Nursing Science*, *24*(4), 60–74.

Denham, S. A. (2012). *Diabetes: A family matter*. Retrieved May 28, 2013, from http://www.diabetesfamily.net/family/family-health-model/ecological/

Duhamel, F., Dupuis, F., & Wright, L. (2009). Families' and nurses' responses to the "One question question": Reflections for clinical practice, education and research in family nursing. *Journal of Family Nursing*, *15*(4), 461–485.

Dylis, A. M. (2003). Effects of personal and environmental factors, uncertainty stress, and coping on family functioning in parents of children with Neurofibromatosis 1: A Nursing path analytic study (Doctoral dissertation, Boston College). *Dissertation Abstracts International*, *64*(09B), 4283. (Accession No. AAT 3103302).

Eaton, D. K., Kan, L., Kinchen, S., Shaklin, S., Flint, K. H., Hawkins, J.,... Weschler, H. (2012). Youth risk behavior surveillance—2011. *Morbidity and MortalityWeekly Report, Surveillance Summaries*, *61*(4), 1–162. Retrieved from http://www.cdc.gov/mmwr/preview/mmwrhtml/ss6104a1.htm?s_cid=ss6104a1_w

Eggenberger, S. K., & Nelms, T. P. (2007). Family interviews as a method for family research. *Journal of Advanced Nursing*, *58*(3), 282–292.

Family Caregiving Alliance. (2012). *Selected caregiver statistics*. Retrieved May 10, 2013, from http://www.caregiver.org/caregiver/jsp/content_node.jsp

Frame, M. W. (2000). The spiritual genogram in family therapy. *Journal of Marital and Family Therapy*, *26*(2), 211–216.

Friedman, M. M., Bowden, V. R., & Jones, E. G. (2003). *Family nursing: Research, theory and practice* (5th ed.). Upper Saddle River, NJ: Prentice Hall.

Friend, J. G., & Haggard, E. A. (1948). *Work adjustment is related to family background: A conceptual basis for counseling*. London: Oxford.

Garcia, C., Skay, C., Sieving, R., Naughton, S., & Bearinger, L. H. (2008). Family and racial factors associated with suicide and emotional distress among Latino students. *Journal of School Health*, *78*(9), 487–495.

Gordon, M. (1994). *Nursing diagnosis: Process and application* (3rd ed.). St. Louis, MO: Mosby.

Gottman, J. M. (1994). *What predicts divorce: The relationship between marital processes and marital outcomes*. Hillsdale, NJ: Lawrence Erlbaum Associates.

Grych, J. H., Raynor, S. R., & Fosco, G. M. (2004). Family processes that shape the impact of interparental conflict on adolescents. *Development and Psychopathology*, *16*, 649–665.

Guyer, J., Broaddus, M., & Dude, A. (2002). Millions of mothers lack health insurance coverage in the United States. Most uninsured mothers lack access both to employer-based coverage and to publicly subsidized health insurance. *International Journal of Health Services Planning Administration Evolution*, *32*(1), 89–106.

Hammer, L. B., Cullen, J. C., Neal, M. B., Sinclair, R. R., & Shafiro, M. V. (2005). The longitudinal effects of work-family conflict and positive spillover on depressive symptoms among dual earner couples. *Journal of Occupational Health Psychology*, *10*(2), 138–154.

Harmon Hanson, S. M. (2001). *Family health care nursing: Theory, practice and research* (2nd ed.). Philadelphia, PA: F. A. Davis Press.

Harrison, K. A. (1998). Sibling rivalry in nosing and the role of nurse psychologist. *Perspectives in Psychiatric Care*, *34*(4), 32–39.

Hershey, J. C., Niederdeppe, J., Evans, W. D., Nonnemaker, J., Blahut, S., Holden, D.,... Haviland, M. L. (2005). The theory of truth: How counterindustry campaigns affect smoking behavior among teens. *Health Psychology*, *24*(1), 22–31.

Hill, R. (1949). *Families under stress*. New York, NY: Harper and Brothers.

Ho, R., Davidson, G., & Ghea, V. (2005). Motives for the adoption of protective health behaviors for men and women: An evaluation of the psychosocial appraisal health model. *Journal of Health Psychology*, *10*(3), 373–395.

Hoppock, R. (1935). *Job satisfaction*. New York, NY: Harper & Row.

Houck, K. D., & Loper, A. B. (2002). The relationship of parenting stress to adjustment among mothers in prison. *American Journal of Orthopsychiatry*, *72*(4), 548–558.

Ingram, D., & Hutchinson, S. A. (1999). HIV-positive mothers and stigma. *Health Care for Women International, 20*, 93–103.

Institute of Medicine. (1988). *Homelessness, health, and human needs*. Washington, DC: National Academy Press.

Judge, T. A., Bono, J. E., Erez, A., & Locke, E. A. (2005). Core self-evaluations and job and life satisfaction: The role of self-concordance and goal attainment. *Journal of Applied Psychology, 90*(2), 257–268.

Julien, D., Chartrand, E., Simard, M. C., Bouthillier, D., & Begin, J. (2003). Conflict, social support, and relationship quality: An observational study of heterosexual, gay male, and lesbian couples' communication. *Journal of Family Psychology, 17*(3), 419–428.

Kalichman, S. C., Gore-Felton, C., Benotsch, E., Cage, M., & Rompa, D. (2004). Trauma symptoms, sexual behaviors, and substance abuse: Correlated of childhood sexual abuse and HIV risks among men who have sex with men. *Journal of Child Sexual Abuse, 13*(1), 1–15.

Kanter, R. M. (1977). *Work and the family in the USA: A critical review and agenda for research and policy*. New York, NY: Russell Sage Foundation.

Kaunonen, M., Aalto, P., Tarkka, M. T., & Paunonen, M. (2000). Oncology ward nurses' perspectives of family grief and a supportive telephone call after the death of a significant other. *Cancer Nursing, 23*(4), 314–324.

Keiley, M. K., Dolbin, M., Hill, J., Karuppaswamy, N., Liu, T., Natarajan, R., . . . Robinson, P. (2002). The cultural genogram: Experiences from within a marriage and family therapy training program. *Journal of Marital and Family Therapy, 28*(2), 165–178.

Kissane, D. W., Bloch, S., McKenzie, M., McDowall, A. C., & Nitzan, R. (1998). Family grief therapy: A preliminary account of a new model to promote healthy family functioning during palliative care and bereavement. *Psycho-Oncology, 7*(1), 14–25.

Koniak-Griffin, D., Anderson, N. L., Verzemnieks, I., & Brecht, M. L. (2000). A public health nursing early intervention program for adolescent mothers: Outcomes from pregnancy through 6 weeks postpartum. *Nursing Research, 49*(3), 130–138.

Kreider, R. (2012). *A look at interracial and intraethnic married couple households in the United States in 2012*. Retrieved May 26, 2013, from blog.census.gov./2012/04/26/a-look-at-interracial-and-intraethnic-married-couple-households-in-the-u-s-in-2010

Lachs, M. S., & Pillemer, K. (2004). Elder abuse. *Lancet, 364*, 1263–1272.

Lave, J. R., Keane, C. R., Lin, C. J., Ricci, E. M., Amersbach, G., & LaValle, C. P. (1998). The impact of lack of health insurance on children. *Journal of Health and Social Policy, 10*(2), 57–73.

Lund, M. (2005). Caregiver, take care. *Geriatric Nursing, 26*(3), 152–153.

Mactavish, J. B., & Schleien, S. J. (2004). Re-injecting spontaneity and balance in family life: Parents' perspectives on recreation in families that include children with developmental disability. *Journal of Intellectual Disabilities Research, 48*, 123–141.

Maes, B., Broekman, T. G., Dosen, A., & Nauts, J. (2003). Caregiving burden of families looking after persons with intellectual disability and behavioral or psychiatric problems. *Journal of Intellectual Disabilities Research, 47*, 447–455.

McClanahan, S. F., McClelland, G. M., Abram, K. M., & Teplin, L. A. (1999). Pathways into prostitution among female jail detainees and their implications for mental health services. *Psychiatric Services, 50*(12), 1606–1613.

McCubbin, H. I., & Patterson, M. (1983). The family stress process: Double ABCX model of adjustment and adaptation. In H. I. McCubbin, M. B. Sussman, & J. M. Patterson (Eds.), *Social stress and the family: Advances in family stress theory and research* (pp. 7–38). New York, NY: Haworth Press.

McCubbin, M. A., & McCubbin, H. I. (1993). Family coping with illness: The resiliency model of family stress, adjustment and adaptation. In C. B. Danielson, B. Hamel-Bissell, & P. Winstead-Fry (Eds.), *Families, health and illness* (pp. 21–63). St. Louis, MO: Mosby.

McCubbin, H. I., Thompson, A. I., & McCubbin, M. A. (Eds.). (1996). *Family assessment: Resiliency, coping and adaptation-Inventories for research and practice* (pp. 639–686). Madison, WI: University of Wisconsin System.

McIntyre, L. L., Blacher, J., & Baker, B. L. (2002). Behavior/mental health problems in young adults with intellectual disability: The impact on families. *Journal of Intellectual Disabilities Research, 46*, 239–249.

Meade, C. S., & Ickovics, J. R. (2005). Systemic review of sexual risk among pregnant and mothering teens in the USA: Pregnancy as an opportunity for integrated prevention of STD and repeat pregnancy. *Social Sciences & Medicine, 60*, 661–668.

Meleis, A. (2011). *Theoretical nursing: Development and Progress* (3rd ed.). Philadelphia, PA: Wolters Kluwer; Lippincott Williams & Wilkins.

Mofenson, L. M. (2002, November 22). U.S. Public Health Service Task Force recommendations for use of antiretroviral drugs in pregnant HIV-1–infected women for maternal health and interventions to reduce perinatal HIV-1 transmission in the United States. *MMWR, 51*(RR18), 1–38.

Musil, C., Warner, C., Zauszniewski, M. W., & Standing, T. (2009). Grandmother caregiving, family stress and strain, and depressive symptoms. *Western Journal of Nursing Research, 31*, 389–408.

National Conference of State Legislatures. (2013). *Defining marriage: Defense of marriage acts and same sex marriage laws*. Retrieved May 10, 2013, from http://www.ncsl.org/issues-research/human services/same-sex-marriage-overview.aspx

Newman, M. (1994). *Health as expanding consciousness* (2nd ed.). New York, NY: National League for Nursing.

O'Leary, A., Purcell, D., Remien, R. H., & Gomez, C. (2003). Childhood sexual abuse and sexual transmission risk behavior among HIV-positive men who have sex with men. *AIDS Care, 15*(1), 17–26.

Orem, D. E. (2000). *Nursing: Concepts of practice of practice* (6th ed.). New York, NY: McGraw-Hill.

Parsons, T., & Bales, R. (1955). *Family socialization and interaction process*. Glencoe, IL: Free Press.

Pender, N. J. (1996). *Health promotion in nursing practice* (3rd ed.). Stamford, CT: Appleton & Lange.

Pender, N. J., Murdaugh, C. L., & Parsons, M. A. (2002). *Health promotion in nursing practice* (4th ed.). Upper Saddle River, NJ: Prentice Hall.

Pickett, K. E., Mookherjee, J., & Wilkinson, R. G. (2005). Adolescent birth rates, total homicides, and income inequality in rich countries. *American Journal of Public Health, 95*(7), 1181–1183.

Pilowsky, D. J., Zybert, P. A., & Vlahov, D. (2004). Resilient children of injection drug users. *Journal of the American Academy of Child and Adolescent Psychiatry, 43*(11), 1372–1379.

Rankin, S. H. (2000). Life-span development: Refreshing a theoretical and practice perspective. *Scholarly Inquiry for Nursing Practice, 14*, 379–388.

Read, T., & Wuest, J. (2007). Daughters caring for dying parents: A process of relinquishing. *Qualitative Health Research, 17*, 932–944.

Rempel, G. R., Neufeld, A., & Kushner, K. E. (2007). Interactive use of genograms and ecomaps in family caregiving research. *Journal of Family Nursing, 13*, 403–419.

Rhodes, T., & Simic, M. (2005). Transition and the HIV risk environment. *BMJ, 331*, 220–223.

Roberts, G. (1999). Age effects and health appraisal: A meta-analysis. *Journals of Gerontology: Psychological Science and Social Sciences, 54*(1), S24–S30.

Rogers, M. (1970). *An introduction to the theoretical basis of nursing*. Philadelphia, PA: F. A. Davis.

Rosenbaum, P. R. (2004). The case-only odds ratio as a causal parameter. *Biometrics, 60*(1), 233–240.

Rossi-Ferrario, S., Baiardi, P., & Zotti, A. M. (2004). Update on the family strain questionnaire: a tool for the general screening of

references (continued)

caregiving related problems. *Quality of Life Research, 13*(8), 1425–1434.

Rothman, K. J., Lanes, S., & Sacks, S. T. (2004). The reporting odds ratio and its advantages over the proportional reporting ratio. *Pharmacoepidemiology and Drug Safety, 13*(8), 519–523.

Roy, C. (2008). *The Roy Adaptation Model* (3rd ed.). Upper Saddle River, NJ: Pearson.

Rozie-Battle, J. L. (2002). Child support and African American teen fathers. *The Journal of Health and Social Policy, 15*, 45–58.

Sandelowski, M., & Barroso, J. (2003). Motherhood in the context of maternal HIV infection. *Research in Nursing & Health, 26*, 470–482.

Singh, G. K., Azurine, R. E., Siahpush, M., & Kogan, M. D. (2013). All-cause and cause-specific mortality among US youth: Socioeconomic and rural-urban disparities and international patterns. *Journal of Urban Health 90*(3), 388–405.

Sparks, P. J., Sparks, C. S., & Campbell, J. J. A. (2013). An application of Bayesian spatial statistical methods to the study of racial and poverty segregation and infant mortality rates in the US. *GeoJournal, 78*(2), 389–405.

Spruijt, E., DeGoede, M., & Vandervalk, I. (2001). The well-being of youngsters coming from six different family types. *Patient Education and Counseling, 45*(4), 285–294.

Spurlock, W. R. (2005). Spiritual well-being and caregiver burden in Alzheimer's caregivers. *Geriatric Nursing, 26*(3), 154–161.

Sterrett, E. M., Williams, J., Thompson, K., Johnson, K., Bright, M., Karam, E. & Jones, V. F. (2013). An exploratory study of two parenting styles and family health behaviors. *American Journal of Health Behaviors, 37*(4), 458–468.

Sullivan-Bolyai, S., Knafl, K., Tamborlane, W., & Grey, M. (2004). Parents' reflections on managing their children's diabetes with insulin pumps. *Journal of Nursing Scholarship, 36*(4), 316–323.

Tavernier, D. L. (2009). The genogram: Enhancing student appreciation of family genetics. *Journal of Nursing Education, 48*(4), 222–225.

Tsang, H. (2000). Families of offenders. *Psychiatric Services, 51*, 819–820.

United States Department of Homeland Security. (2013). *Yearbook of immigration statistics*. Retrieved May 28, 2013, from http://www.dhs.gov/yearbook-immigration-statistics

U.S. Census Bureau. (2005). *Health insurance data*. Retrieved from http://www.census.gov./hhes/www/hlthins/hlthins.html

U.S. Census Bureau. (2012a). *2010 Census shows interracial and interethnic married couples grew by 28% over decade*. Retrieved May 26, 2013, from http://www.census.gov/newsroom/releases/achives/2010_census/cb1268.html

U.S. Census Bureau. (2012b). *Households and families: 2010*. Retrieved March 22, 2013, from http://www.census.gov/prod/cen2010/briefs/c2010br-14.pdf

Walker, L. O., & Avant, K. C. (2010). *Strategies for theory construction in nursing* (5th ed.). Upper Saddle River, NJ: Pearson.

Walsh, F. (2010). Spiritual diversity: Multifaith perspectives. *Family Therapy, 49*(3). 330–348.

Williams, P. D., Williams, A. R., Graff, J. C., Hanson, S., Stanton, A., Hafeman, C., . . . Sanders, S. (2002). Interrelationships among variables affecting well siblings and mothers in families of children with a chronic illness or disability. *Journal of Behavioral Medicine*, *25*(5), 411–424.

Wimbush, F. B., & Peters, R. M. (2000). Identification of cardiovascular risk: Use of a cardiovascular specific genogram. *Public Health Nursing*, *17*(3), 148–154.

Wright, L., & Leahey, M. (1999). Maximizing time, minimizing suffering: The 15-minute (or less) family interview. *Journal of Family Nursing*, *5*, 259–274.

Wright, L., & Leahey, M. (2005). The three most common errors in family nursing: How to avoid or sidestep. *Journal of Family Nursing*, *11*(2), 90–101.

Wright, L., & Leahey, M. (2009). *Nurses and families: A guide to family assessment and intervention* (6th ed.). Philadelphia, PA: F. A. Davis Co.

Wyatt, G. E., Longshore, D., Chin, D., Carmona, J. V., Loeb, T. B., Myers, H. F., . . . Rivkin, I. (2004). The efficacy of an integrated risk reduction intervention for HIV-positive women with child sexual abuse stories. *AIDS and Behavior*, *8*(4), 453–462.

suggested readings

Centers for Disease Control and Prevention. (2014). Injury prevention and control: Traumatic brain injury. Retrieved November 1, 2014, from http://www.cdc.gov/traumaticbraininjury.

Centers for Disease Control and Prevention. (2011). Surveillance for Traumatic brain injury-related deaths - United States, 1997-2007. Morbidity & Mortality Weekly Report, 60(SS05); 1-32. Retrieved November 1, 2014, from http://www.cdc.gov/mmwr/preview/mmwrhtml/ss6005a1.htm?s_cid=ss6005a1_w

web resources

Please visit thePoint® for up-to-date web resources on this topic.

Challenges in Community and Public Health Nursing

PART

four

CHAPTER 14

Risk of Infectious and Communicable Diseases

Barbara A. Goldrick

WE ARE LEGEND

We are HIV. Our family is ancient.
Out of Africa,
Monkey to man,
From the trees and forests,
To the towns and cities.
We are here.
For we are HIV, we are legion.
Our children are billions,
Our home, in your defenses,
In your blood, your brain,
Your saliva, your semen.
We are everywhere.
For we are HIV, we are immortal.
We are part of you,
And you of us,
We live with you, but
May not die with you.
We go on.
For we are HIV, we are travelers.
From lover to lover,
Mother to baby,
Donor to blood bank,
Blood bank to patient,
We follow you.
For we are HIV, we evolve.
NRTIs, NNRTIs, PIs, INIs,
New designs, new drugs,
Bring it on, bring it on,
Q151M, K103 N, L90M.
We adapt, we survive.
We are HIV. We consume.
Your resources, your time,
Your hope, your lives,
Your new drugs are easy.
Where are your vaccines?
Can you stop us? We will see.

Julian W. Tang

chapter highlights

- Infectious versus communicable disease
- Outbreak investigation: person, place, time
- Public health surveillance
- Food-borne and waterborne illnesses
- Sexually transmitted diseases

objectives

- Explain the difference between infectious and communicable diseases.
- Examine the agent, host, and environmental characteristics of healthcare-associated infections and common community-acquired infections.
- Describe the major means of transmission of communicable diseases.
- Define an outbreak investigation by person, place, and time.
- Describe public health surveillance.
- Differentiate between food-borne and waterborne illnesses.
- Outline prevention and control measures for sexually transmitted diseases.

key terms

Carrier: A person or animal that harbors an infectious organism and transmits the organism to others, although having no symptoms of the disease.

Colonization: The presence and multiplication of infectious organisms without invading or causing damage to tissue.

Common source outbreak: An outbreak characterized by exposure to a common, harmful substance.

Contagious: Communicable by direct or indirect contact.

Endemic: The constant or usual prevalence of a specific disease or infectious agent within a population or geographic area.

Epidemic: Significant increase in the number of new cases of a disease than past experience would have predicted for that place, time, or

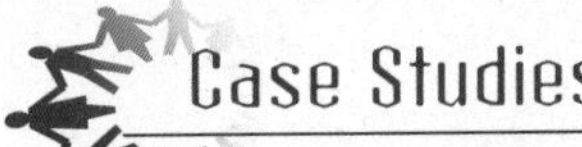

Case Studies

References to case studies are found throughout this chapter (look for the case study icon). Readers should keep the case studies in mind as they read the chapter.

CASE 1

Rob, the nurse at a weekly summer camp for adolescent boys and girls in Wyoming, observed that an excessive number of children were seeking help for diarrhea and/or vomiting during a week in late June. Normally, two or three children per week would report to the health office with these symptoms; however, 22 children sought help during this time, clearly more than what would normally be expected. Rob reported the increased incidence to the camp manager, who immediately notified the Wyoming Department of Health. Suspecting that the well water was contaminated, a sample of the water was analyzed.

In mid-July, the department notified the camp that a water sample from the camp well tested positive for fecal contamination. The camp was closed. Representatives from various state agencies investigated the outbreak (adapted from Centers for Disease Control and Prevention [CDC], 2007).

CASE 2

Megan is a high school sophomore who moved into the community several months ago with her parents and younger brother. She has been sexually active for 2 years. She has had unprotected intercourse with three classmates since her arrival in town. For the past 2 weeks, she has had an urge to urinate frequently. Her vaginal secretions have increased, and the mucus has an unusual odor. She has made an appointment with the school nurse to discuss her symptoms.

key terms (continued)

population; an increase in incidence beyond that which is expected.

Healthcare-associated infection: Originating in a healthcare facility; formerly called nosocomial infection.

Incubation period: Time period between initial contact with the infectious agent and the appearance of the first signs or symptoms of the disease.

Infectious disease: Presence and replication of an infectious agent in the tissues of a host, with manifestation of signs and symptoms.

Pathogenicity: Ability of the agent to produce an infectious disease in a susceptible host.

Propagated outbreak: Outbreak resulting from direct or indirect transmission of an infectious agent from an infected person to a susceptible host; secondary infections can occur.

Reservoir: Location where an infectious agent is normally found, where it lives and reproduces under normal circumstances.

Secondary infection: Infections that occur within the accepted incubation period following exposure to a primary case.

Surveillance: A continual dynamic method for gathering data about the health of the general public for the purpose of primary prevention of illness.

Transmission: The transfer of an infectious agent from one person or place to another.

Infectious disease is universal, and any attempt to imagine how it arose ... will inevitably take us back to the very earliest phases of life.

Frank MacFarlane Burnet and D. O. White

Infectious diseases remain a leading cause of death in developing countries, with approximately half of all deaths caused by infectious diseases each year attributed to just three diseases: tuberculosis (TB), malaria, and HIV/AIDS. Together, these diseases cause over 300 million illnesses and more than 5 million deaths each year. Although deaths due to HIV/AIDS are projected to fall by 2030, it will remain the 10th leading cause of death worldwide. Deaths due to other communicable diseases are projected to decline at a faster rate. For example, TB will fall to number 20 in the list of leading causes of death by 2030 (World Health Organization [WHO], 2008). However, new pathogenic microorganisms have emerged, new strains of known organisms have developed that are more virulent, microorganisms have become resistant to many antibiotics, and infectious diseases have now become a means of terrorism. The characteristics of infectious diseases have changed, but they still are a significant health burden in most of the world.

This is true despite the great advances during the 20th century in the prevention and control of infectious diseases. These advances primarily occurred in developed countries and included purified drinking water, waste control, plentiful foods, immunizations, and drug therapy. This was preceded, however, by the need to prevent and control epidemics of infectious diseases, such as cholera, typhus, and influenza, which killed many people in Europe, America, and much of the rest of the world in the later part of the 19th century. By 1900, infectious diseases were the leading cause of death in the United States. Today, changes in health patterns in the world's more developed countries reflect an increased life span, with associated chronic diseases such as heart disease, cancer, and cardiovascular accidents. Nonetheless, influenza/pneumonia and septicemia remained in the top 15 causes of death in the United States in 2010 (National Center for Health Statistics [NCHS], 2012). As populations age in middle- and low-income countries over the next 20 years, the proportion of deaths due to noncommunicable diseases will also rise significantly. Globally, deaths from cancer will increase from 7.4 million in 2004 to 11.8 million in 2030, and deaths from cardiovascular diseases will rise from 17.1 million to 23.4 million during the same period (WHO, 2008). The *Healthy People 2020* initiative in the United States outlines specific goals and objectives for prevention and control of infectious diseases. These are designed to reduce morbidity, mortality, and costs associated with infectious diseases. Selected objectives from *Healthy People 2020* for immunization and infectious diseases are found in Box 14.1.

box 14.1 *Healthy People 2020* Objectives for Immunization and Infectious Diseases

Reduce, eliminate, or maintain elimination of cases of vaccine-preventable diseases.
Reduce early-onset group B streptococcal disease.
Reduce meningococcal disease.
Reduce invasive pneumococcal infections.
Reduce the number of courses of antibiotics for ear infections for young children.
Reduce the number of courses of antibiotics prescribed for the sole diagnosis of the common cold.
Achieve and maintain effective vaccination coverage levels for universally recommended vaccines among young children.
Increase the percentage of children aged 19 to 35 months who receive the recommended doses of DTaP, polio, MMR, Hib, hepatitis B, varicella and pneumococcal conjugate vaccine (PCV).
Decrease the percentage of children in the United States who receive 0 doses of recommended vaccines by age 19 to 35 months.
Maintain vaccination coverage levels for children in kindergarten.
Increase routine vaccination coverage levels for adolescents.
Increase the percentage of children and adults who are vaccinated annually against seasonal influenza.
Increase the percentage of adults who are vaccinated against pneumococcal disease.
Increase the percentage of adults who are vaccinated against zoster (shingles).
(Developmental) Increase hepatitis B vaccine coverage among high-risk populations.
(Developmental) Increase the scientific knowledge on vaccine safety and adverse events.
Increase the percentage of providers who have had vaccination coverage levels among children in their practice population measured within the past year.
Increase the percentage of children under 6 years of age whose immunization records are in a fully operational, population-based immunization information system (IIS).
Increase the number of states collecting kindergarten vaccination coverage data according to CDC minimum standards.
Increase the number of states that have 80% of adolescents with two or more age-appropriate immunizations recorded in an IIS among adolescents aged 11 to 18 years.
Increase the number of states that use electronic data from rabies animal surveillance to inform public health prevention programs.
Increase the number of public health laboratories monitoring influenza virus resistance to antiviral agents.
Reduce hepatitis A.
Reduce chronic hepatitis B virus infections in infants and young children (perinatal infections).
Reduce hepatitis B.
Reduce new hepatitis C infections.
Increase the proportion of persons aware they have a hepatitis C infection.
(Developmental) Increase the proportion of persons who have been tested for hepatitis B virus within minority communities experiencing health disparities.
Reduce tuberculosis (TB).
Increase treatment completion rate of all tuberculosis patients who are eligible to complete therapy.
Increase the percentage of contact to sputum smear–positive cases who complete treatment after being diagnosed with latent tuberculosis infection.
Reduce the average time for laboratories to confirm and report tuberculosis cases.

Source: U.S. Department of Health and Human Services. Healthy People 2020: *Immunization and infectious diseases objectives.* Retrieved April 29, 2013, from http://healthypeople.gov/2020/topicsobjectives2020/objectiveslist.aspx?topicId=23

Several new infectious diseases were identified in the last 30 years of the 20th century. Some examples are briefly described below.

1. In the 1970s, toxic shock syndrome (TSS) killed several women before it was linked to the use of high-absorbency tampons that provided a moist, warm home where the bacteria could thrive. It was also found to be associated with the contraceptive sponge and diaphragm birth control methods. TSS is caused by a well-known organism, *Staphylococcus aureus*. Streptococcal TSS, a related infection, is caused by *Streptococcus* bacteria.
2. Another new disease that occurred in the last century is acquired immunodeficiency syndrome (AIDS), which was first observed in a few young men in 1981. Infection with HIV, largely transmitted through sexual contact, is now a major cause of morbidity and mortality throughout the world. Today, an estimated 34 million people worldwide live with HIV/AIDS, with more than two-thirds living in developing countries. Nearly three-fourths of the 2.5 million new HIV infections in 2011 occurred in these countries, with sub-Saharan Africa the worst affected region. AIDS is the leading cause of death in sub-Saharan Africa and the fourth leading cause of death worldwide (AVERT, *HIV and AIDS*; CDC, *Global HIV/AIDS at CDC—our story*). The U.S. Centers for Disease Control and Prevention (CDC) provides support to over 75 countries to strengthen their national HIV/AIDS programs and build sustainable public health systems through the U.S. President's Emergency Plan for AIDS Relief (PEPFAR). As of 2012, PEPFAR has supported life-saving antiretroviral treatment for more than 5.1 million people, HIV testing and counseling for more than 11 million pregnant women, and antiretroviral drug prophylaxis to prevent mother-to-child HIV transmission for more than 750,000 HIV-positive pregnant women that allowed approximately 230,000 infants to be born HIV-free (CDC, *Global HIV/AIDS at CDC—our story*).
3. Lyme borreliosis was discovered to be caused by a tick-borne spirochete similar to the organism that causes syphilis. It is focally endemic in North America, Europe, and Asia and is probably the most common tick-borne bacterial disease in the world. Lyme disease is the most commonly reported vector-borne illness in the United States; in 2011, it was the sixth most common nationally notifiable disease. However, this disease is concentrated heavily in the northeast and upper Midwest, and so far it has **not** occurred nationwide (CDC, *Lyme disease*).
4. A new respiratory disease appeared in May 1993, when several healthy young members of the Navajo Nation in New Mexico died within a short period of time from an unexplained respiratory condition. This cluster of strange, unexplained deaths caught the attention of the world, resulting in rapid diagnosis of what was later called hantavirus pulmonary syndrome (HPS).
5. About this same time, a toxic strain of *Escherichia coli* (O157:H7), an organism that normally inhabits the intestines of animals, caused illness and death in children in many parts of the United States. When there are news reports about food-borne outbreaks of "*E. coli*" infections, they are usually talking about *E. coli* O157.
6. Also, a virulent strain of *Streptococcus pyogenes* (Group A strep), known for its ability to evade the normal walling-off process by human immune systems, was named a "flesh-eating bacteria" (necrotizing fasciitis) because of the serious consequences of the infection.
7. In 1996, the possible transmission of mad cow disease (bovine spongiform encephalopathy, or BSE) to humans resulted in the slaughter of thousands of cattle in England. This is a particularly interesting disease, because the infectious agent is a protein (prion) rather than a microorganism.
8. Ebola hemorrhagic fever was initially recognized in 1976, with two simultaneous outbreaks in Nzara, Sudan, and in the Democratic Republic of Congo in Africa. The latter outbreak occurred in a village near the Ebola River, from which the disease takes its name. Ebola hemorrhagic fever outbreaks, with a case-fatality rate of up to 100%, have appeared sporadically since its initial recognition, most recently in the summer of 2014. Researchers believe that the virus is zoonotic (animal-borne) and is normally maintained in an animal host that is native to the African continent. The Ebola virus is transmitted through close contact with the blood, secretions, organs, or other bodily fluids of infected animals.
9. In 2003, newspapers, television, and the Internet were full of frightening articles and images about an outbreak of severe acute respiratory syndrome (SARS), a viral illness, in Asia. At that time, the possibility of a SARS pandemic was worldwide news.
10. Shortly thereafter, also in 2003, fear of a bird flu (avian influenza virus H5N1) outbreak captured the attention of the world. Avian viruses do not usually infect humans, which means that the risk for avian influenza is generally low for most people. However, as of early 2013, the World Health Organization (WHO) had reported a total of 622 human cases of H5N1 avian influenza, with 371 deaths (WHO, 2013). Most cases of H5N1 avian influenza infection in humans have resulted from contact with infected poultry. See Chapter 15 for more on H5N1 avian influenza.
11. In 2009, H1N1 (sometimes called "swine flu"), a new influenza virus, was identified that caused illness in people. This new virus, which was first detected in Mexico and the United States in April 2009, caused the first flu pandemic in more than 40 years. The virus spread from person to person worldwide, in much the

same way that regular seasonal influenza viruses spread. In mid-2009, the WHO had declared a pandemic of 2009 H1N1 influenza. By August 2010, worldwide more than 214 countries and territories had reported laboratory-confirmed cases of pandemic influenza H1N1 2009, including over 18,449 deaths. The CDC estimated that the total number of 2009 H1N1 cases in the United States between April 2009 and April 2010 ranged between 43 and 89 million, with an estimated 12,469 related deaths (CDC, *Updated CDC Estimates of 2009 H1N1 Influenza Cases, 2009–2010;WHO, Pandemic (H1N1) 2010*). For more information on the 2009 H1N1 virus, see Chapter 15, Emerging Infections.

STUDENT REFLECTION

Five years ago, when I was 13, I went to an Outward Bound camp in Connecticut. It was great—we were outdoors hiking or riding almost all day, cooked our own meals over a campfire in the evenings, and slept outside a couple of times. It was one of the most memorable times of my life. The day before we left for home, though, I found a fat tick on my thigh. We were warned about bug bites and used a spray when we remembered to. I went to the camp nurse and she cleaned it out really well, so I forgot about it. After a couple of weeks, I got a nasty headache, had a fever, and felt like I was coming down with the flu. Mom made me go to a doctor when she saw that I had a large red sore at the site of the tick bite. The doctor found several red sores on my legs and said I probably had Lyme disease! I had to be on antibiotics for 3 weeks, and then I felt fine. That experience made me very interested in infectious diseases and nursing as a career.

With the global mobility of humans, animals, food, and feed products greater than ever before, the spread of dangerous pathogens has and will continue to increase. Infectious diseases are a growing threat to all nations, although the burden is greatest in the developing world. To address these issues, the CDC and a network of international public health partnerships have been formed. These partnerships, which include WHO, the United Nations, the World Bank, and the Bill & Melinda Gates Foundation, are contributing to the increased availability of drugs and vaccines, and providing better public health education programs worldwide (CDC, *CDC Global health partnerships*).

EPIDEMIOLOGY OF THE INFECTIOUS PROCESS: THE CHAIN OF INFECTION

According to the germ theory of disease, specific microorganisms cause specific diseases. As described in Chapter 6, the epidemiologic triangle is a model that scientists have developed for studying health problems. It helps us understand infectious diseases and how they spread. The *agent*, or the microbe that causes the disease, is the "what" of the triangle. The *host*, or the organism that is harboring the infectious agent, is the "who" of the triangle. The *environment*, which includes those external factors that cause or allow disease transmission, is the "where" of the triangle.

An **infectious disease** in a human host is one caused by the growth of pathogenic microorganisms in the body. Other necessary elements that add to the epidemiologic triangle are in the so-called chain of infection, which include a portal of exit from the host, environmental reservoirs, transmission, and a portal of entry to a new host (McKenzie, Pringer, & Kotecki, 2005) (Fig. 14.1). For a disease to be

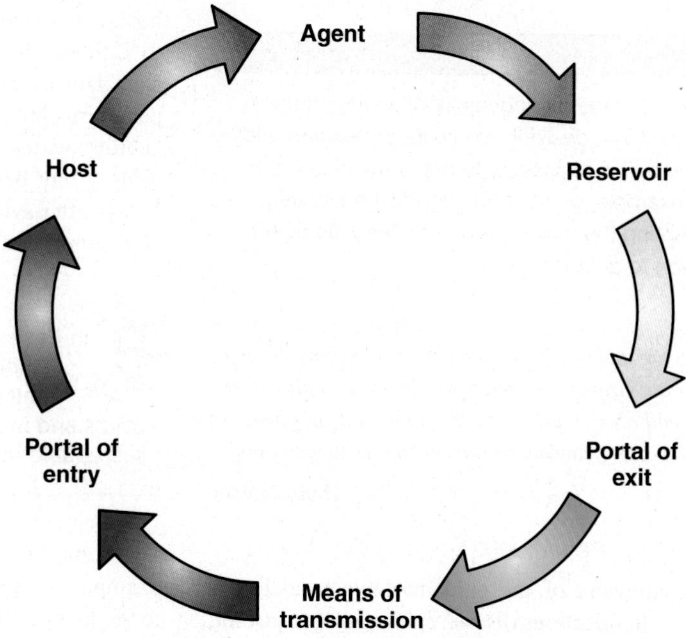

figure 14.1 Chain of infection.

communicable, or **contagious**, there must be a portal of exit from the infected person (or animal), a means of transmission, and a portal of entry to a susceptible host.

Agent

Infectious agents are biological agents capable of producing an infection or infectious disease and include bacteria, viruses, rickettsiae, fungi, protozoa, and helminths (Heymann, 2008). An infectious disease need not be contagious, or communicable.

In the Wyoming summer camp outbreak, 23 stool samples were obtained from symptomatic campers and tested for bacterial and viral pathogens. Fifteen out of the 23 (65.2%) stool samples were positive for norovirus, the bacteria *Campylobacter jejuni*, or both. Well water samples also were positive for these agents. Are these infectious diseases communicable diseases?

In addition to the interaction between the infectious agent, the host, and the environment, the progression of an infectious agent depends on its pathogenicity. **Pathogenicity** is the ability of an infectious agent to cause disease in a susceptible host (Heymann, 2008). It depends on the infectivity of the infectious agent, its ability to invade and destroy body cells (invasiveness), produce toxins (toxicity), and its virulence.

Infectivity varies depending on the route of entry of the infectious agent and the susceptibility of the host. For example, if *Clostridium tetani* (tetanus bacilli) gains entry into the body through a puncture wound, and the person has current tetanus immunization, the person (host) is not susceptible to infectivity by *C. tetani*. Various characteristics of an infectious agent are found in Box 14.2.

PRACTICE POINT

An understanding of the pathogenicity of an infectious agent is important in a decision to initiate prevention and control measures. It is necessary to break the chain of infection. For example, good hand hygiene breaks this chain by preventing the transmission of infectious agent from one person to another.

But however secure and well-regulated civilized life may become, bacteria, Protozoa, viruses, infected fleas, lice, ticks, mosquitoes, and bedbugs will always lurk in the shadows ready to pounce when neglect, poverty, famine, or war lets down the defenses.

Hans Zinsser

Host

The second component of the epidemiologic triad is the susceptible host. In infectious disease epidemiology, just the

box 14.2 Properties of Infectious Agents Influenced by the Host and the Environment

Pathogenicity: Ability of the agent to produce an infectious disease in a susceptible host

Infectivity: Ability of the agent to invade the host and replicate

Virulence: Severity of the infectious disease that results from exposure to the agent

Toxicity: Ability of the agent to produce toxins

Immunogenicity: Ability of the agent to produce specific immunity within the host

Invasiveness: Ability of the agent to destroy body cells

presence of an infectious agent is not sufficient to produce an infectious disease. The process requires a susceptible host. There are several host factors that determine whether a person is at risk for an infection or an infectious disease. These include age, sex, race, physical and emotional health, and immune status.

Portals of Entry and Exit

Infectious agents both enter and leave the body in multiple ways. Portals include the skin, respiratory tract, alimentary tract, genital tract, conjunctiva, and vertical transmission from parent to offspring. An example is the fecal–oral transmission of hepatitis A through indirect contact with infected fecal material.

Incubation Period

If an infectious agent enters the host and begins to multiply, an infection occurs. The time between exposure to an infectious agent and the manifestation of symptoms in the host is called the **incubation period**. Each infectious disease has its own incubation period, but it can also vary in different hosts. For example, the incubation period for influenza is 24 to 72 hours after the virus enters the body, when symptoms start. However, some people can be infected with the influenza virus but have no symptoms. The period of communicability varies. Adults can begin spreading the influenza virus 1 day before they have any symptoms and for 3 to 7 days after symptoms start. Children can transmit the virus after more than 7 days (Heymann, 2008).

In **Case 1**, the incubation periods for the agents responsible for the gastroenteritis in the Wyoming summer camp are 12 to 48 hours for norovirus and usually 2 to 5 days for *C. jejuni*. Who are the susceptible hosts at the camp?

Some diseases have longer incubation periods. For example, hepatitis B has an average incubation period of 60 to 90 days, but it can be as short as 2 weeks and as long as 6 to 9 months. A person infected with hepatitis B virus (HBV) may be asymptomatic but still can transmit the virus to others. Asymptomatic people with chronic hepatitis antigenemia (the presence of HBV antigen in the blood) are **carriers** of the HBV and can transmit the virus to others through percutaneous inoculation, exposure to mucous membranes, and sexual contact (Heymann, 2008). More information about hepatitis can be found in medical–surgical textbooks.

When an infectious agent is present and there are no clinical signs of disease, **colonization** with the infectious agent is said to have occurred, and the infected person is capable of transmitting the agent. An example is methicillin-resistant *S. aureus* (MRSA), which has become increasingly common in many healthcare facilities over the past decade. A person can carry MRSA in his or her nose and throat and can then shed the bacteria. For example, a healthcare worker colonized with MRSA can transmit the organism to neonates or to postoperative patients (surgical wounds), causing severe morbidity and mortality. In recent years, MRSA has become a community-acquired infection (CA-MRSA), with outbreaks in athletes, schoolchildren, military recruits, and prison inmates. Factors that have been associated with the spread of CA-MRSA skin infections include close skin-to-skin contact, openings in the skin such as cuts or abrasions, contaminated items and surfaces, crowded living conditions, and poor hygiene. CA-MRSA most often presents as skin or soft tissue infection such as a boil or abscess (CDC, *MRSA*). Asymptomatic, subclinical, or occult infections are identifiable only by certain laboratory tests, such as serology or skin tests. An example of a skin test to identify infection is the purified protein derivative (PPD) skin test used to identify TB infection. Screening for specific conditions such as TB is also a form of secondary prevention.

Infection with HIV is unapparent in its early stages and may be transmitted from one person to another when infected blood, semen, or vaginal secretions come in contact with an uninfected person's broken skin or mucous membranes. In addition, an infected pregnant woman can transmit HIV to her infant during pregnancy or delivery, as well as through breast-feeding. At the end of 2009, an estimated 1,148,200 persons aged 13 and older were living with HIV infection in the United States, including 207,600 (18.1%) persons whose infections had not been diagnosed. The majority of those living with HIV infection were nonwhite (72%) (CDC, *HIV/AIDS, basic statistics*). In 2009, adolescents and young persons (aged 13–24 years), who represented 21% of the U.S. population, comprised 6.7% of those living with HIV. More than half (60%) were unaware of their infection, the highest for any age group. Nearly 75% of the 12,200 new HIV infections in 2009 among this age group were attributable to male-to-male sexual contact (CDC, 2012a).

Environment: Reservoir

The third component in the epidemiologic triad, the environment, provides reservoirs of infectious agents (microbes); these **reservoirs** can be humans, animals, plants, insects, water, and soil. Microbes live everywhere and their habitats expand as humans alter the environment and extend contact with them. Microbes are adept at adaptation and change under selective pressures for survival and replication. For example, influenza viruses continually evolve, resulting in annual epidemics and an ongoing need to develop new influenza vaccines each year. Another example is antibiotic-resistant strains of microorganisms, such as MRSA.

Infectious disease, then, is not nature's tantrum against humanity. Often it is an argument in what becomes a long marriage.

Arno Karlen

Infections transmitted from animal reservoirs to humans are known as *zoonoses*. Examples of zoonoses are rodent-transmitted plague, hantavirus, and monkeypox. Although rare, zoonotic infections occur in the United States. HPS, a severe, sometimes fatal, respiratory disease in humans, is caused by an infection with a hantavirus. Anyone who comes into contact with rodents or their droppings that carry hantavirus is at risk for HPS (CDC, Hantavirus pulmonary syndrome). In November 2012, the National Park Service announced a total of 10 confirmed cases of hantavirus infection in people who recently visited Yosemite National Park. Three of the confirmed cases were fatal (CDC, *Outbreak of hantavirus infection in Yosemite National Park*).

Changes in the environment tend to have the greatest influence on the transmission of microbial agents that are waterborne, airborne, food-borne, or vector-borne, or those that have an animal reservoir. Transformation of forest to agricultural land in Venezuela led to emergence of a new disease in 1989: Venezuelan hemorrhagic fever. Reforestation of abandoned farmlands in the northeast was a factor in the emergence of Lyme disease in the United States.

In **Case 1**, two untreated wells provided the Wyoming camp with water. The wells were 30 to 50 feet deep and 25 feet apart. An underground metal septic tank that had been installed in the 1950s was approximately 120 feet from the wells. The septic tank was filled to capacity and had not been maintained properly. The leach field was not properly constructed, and the ground immediately downhill from the septic tank was damp with sewage. It was hypothesized that the large number of camp attendees overburdened the septic system and created a heavy demand for well water. This allowed the septic system effluent to contaminate the water that replenished the wells. An ongoing drought in the area was probably an additional contributing factor. What other environmental factors in this rural area might have contributed to this outbreak?

Transmission

Mechanisms of **transmission** of an infectious agent from a reservoir to another host include airborne transmission, direct contact, indirect contact, and droplet transmission.

Airborne Transmission

Airborne transmission occurs when microorganisms are carried in the air in small particles, called droplet nuclei, at distances that exceed a few feet. TB is an example of an airborne infection transmitted by droplet nuclei. A person with active TB disease of the lungs or throat releases TB bacteria into the air when he or she coughs, sneezes, speaks, or sings. People nearby may breathe in these bacteria and become infected. TB bacteria also may spread by droplet nuclei to persons who are not nearby (e.g., through air-conditioning units).

Bacterial spores (e.g., *Aspergillus* spores) can spread by airborne transmission through dust when they are mixed in with dry soil (Heymann, 2008).

Direct Contact

Direct contact occurs through direct body surface-to-body surface contact and physical transfer of microorganisms between a susceptible host and an infected or colonized person (or animal). For example, sexually transmitted diseases (STDs) are transmitted by direct contact with an infected person.

An example of direct contact with an animal reservoir is the transmission of the H5N1 avian influenza virus, which was transmitted from poultry to humans in the "bird flu" epidemic that occurred between 2004 and 2008. Recently published papers indicate that we are only three genetic changes away from a pandemic of H5N1 influenza (Enserink, 2012). See Chapter 15 for more information on H5N1 avian influenza virus.

Indirect Contact

Indirect contact involves contact of a susceptible host with a contaminated intermediate inanimate object, called a vehicle, such as a contaminated surgical instrument, needle, toy, soiled clothing, or bed linen. Vehicles also include food, water, and contaminated hands that are not washed (Heymann, 2008). Indirect contact also includes vector transmission. Vectors are animal or insect carriers of infectious agents. Mechanical vector-borne transmission occurs when an insect carries the microorganisms on its feet or proboscis, or through its gastrointestinal tract. Biologic vector-borne transmission occurs when propagation of the microorganism is required within the insect before it can be transmitted to another host. Malaria is an example of biologic vector-borne infectious disease, which is transmitted by mosquitoes (Heymann, 2008).

EVIDENCE FOR PRACTICE

The CDC has reported an increasing number of outbreaks of enteric disease associated with animals at fairs and petting zoos. Investigators found the route of transmission was usually from direct hand-to-mouth contact with animal feces. Guidelines to reduce the risk of disease are designed to interrupt this route. They include recommendations to wash hands after touching animals, to keep food and drinks outside of animal areas, and to prevent children from putting their hands or objects (such as pacifiers or sippy cups) in their mouths while interacting with animals. Most petting zoos provide hand hygiene facilities, but handwashing compliance varies. See CDC (2011a)—Compendium of measures to prevent disease associated with animals in public settings, 2011 at http://www.cdc.gov/mmwr/pdf/rr/rr6004.pdf.

Droplet Transmission

Although droplet transmission theoretically is a form of contact transmission, the mechanism of transfer of the pathogen to the host is quite distinct from either direct or indirect transmission. Therefore, droplet transmission is considered a separate route of transmission. Droplets are generated from the source person primarily during coughing, sneezing, and talking, and are propelled a short distance (less than 3 feet) through the air and deposited on the conjunctivae, nasal mucosa, or mouth of another person. Measles and influenza are examples of communicable diseases transmitted by droplet spread (Heymann, 2008).

In Case 1, use Figure 14.1 to construct a chain of infections specific to the outbreak of gastroenteritis at the Wyoming camp. What were the reservoirs? What was the method of transmission? Indicate where the chain of infection could be broken and how this could be accomplished.

OUTBREAK INVESTIGATION

An **endemic** disease, infection, or infectious agent occurs when it becomes prevalent within a population or geographic area. For example, chloroquine-resistant malaria is endemic in most of Africa, the Middle East, Asia, and all of the South Pacific islands (CDC, *The yellow book 2012*). An **epidemic** refers to a significant increase in an infection or infectious disease beyond the expected (endemic) level in a certain population and/or geographic area. Epidemics also occur when a new infectious agent emerges or reemerges. A pandemic is an epidemic that generally spreads worldwide. An example of a pandemic is the AH1N1 influenza outbreak that occurred in 2009 to 2010. The use of "outbreak" in this text is synonymous with epidemic (Porta, 2008). The steps of an outbreak investigation are outlined in Box 14.3.

Establishing the Existence of an Outbreak

To establish that an outbreak exists, a comparison of the current incidence of cases with baseline or endemic status is essential. If local data are not available, the incidence of cases should be compared with that in the literature. Observed

box 14.3 **Steps in an Outbreak Investigation**

- Establish and verify diagnosis of reported cases; identify agent.
- Search for additional cases; collect critical data and specimens.
- Characterize cases by person, place, and time.
- Formulate and test tentative hypotheses regarding possible causative factors.
- Implement control measures to control the outbreak.
- Evaluate efficacy of control measures.
- Communicate findings; prepare written report.

Source: Association for Professionals in Infection Control and Epidemiology. (2009). *APIC text of infection control and epidemiology* (3rd ed.). Washington, DC: Author.

rates should be greater than the expected level. In some situations, a single case of a communicable disease long absent from the population, or the first occurrence of an infection not previously recognized in that geographic area, requires immediate reporting and epidemiologic investigation; two such cases associated in time and place may indicate the start of an epidemic (Heymann, 2008). For example, two cases of smallpox in the United States are above the expected level, because smallpox was eradicated worldwide in 1977.

The criteria used for defining a case are important aspects of an outbreak investigation; however, the case definition may change as more data are collected. Once the criteria have been established, the suspected cases are grouped into definite cases, probable cases, and possible cases categories.

In **Case 1**, active case finding and surveillance began after the Wyoming Department of Health was notified of the *E. coli*-positive well water sample on July 19. A case of gastroenteritis was defined as an illness lasting for more than 24 hours that included three or more episodes of diarrhea, vomiting, or both. The attack had to occur in a camper or staff member after arriving at or leaving the camp during the period from June 1 through July 19.

Describing Cases by Person, Place, and Time

As was discussed in Chapter 6, person, place, and time characterize the description of an epidemiologic problem. As data are collected on individual cases in an outbreak investigation, attack rates can be calculated according to demographic variables such as age, sex, and other factors or attributes like occupation or exposure to the suspected agent. These data are helpful in comparing the characteristics of those who develop the infection with the characteristics of those who do not when conducting case-control studies (see Chapter 8). This occurs when epidemiologists test tentative hypotheses to explain the outbreak and identify the population at risk (CDC, *Excite: Epidemiology in the classroom*).

In **Case 1**, lists of camp attendees were obtained from camp managers, and a retrospective cohort study was conducted by administering a telephone questionnaire to 210 out of 277 (75.8%) campers. A total of 141 (67.1%) cases were identified. What was the attack rate among the interviewed campers?

Diarrhea was reported by 102 (72.3%) people, vomiting by 92 (65.2%), and stomach cramps by 89 (63.1%). What were the symptom-specific attack rates (see Chapter 7 for calculating rates)?

When describing an outbreak by place, it may be necessary to use spot maps to identify concentrations of cases within certain areas, and this may show clustering of cases. The use of maps also further defines the population at risk. The use of time in describing an outbreak requires that investigators go back to the first case or indication of outbreak activity. These data graphically provide a histogram of the epidemic curve, which helps determine whether the outbreak is from a common source or from a propagated (continuous) source. The epidemic curve also helps determine the incubation period of the infection and if the problem is ongoing (CDC, *Excite: Epidemiology in the classroom*).

The data in Figure 14.2 illustrate an epidemic curve from the well-known common source outbreak of cholera in London in 1854, which was investigated by John Snow, the "father of epidemiology." Dr. Snow established that cholera was spread by water from the contaminated Broad Street well. When the pump handle was removed and people could no longer obtain water from the well, the epidemic subsided. Note that although the typical incubation period for cholera is 1 to 3 days, the outbreak lasted more than 1 month, because of the contaminated water supply, before the Broad Street pump handle was removed. Figure 14.3 is an example of a propagated epidemic curve of a measles outbreak. The incubation period for measles is typically 10 days, but may be as short as 7 days and as long as 18 days (CDC, *Excite: Epidemiology in the classroom*).The secondary infections, which are spread from person to person, show intervals in the epidemic curve, indicating that the outbreak is not from a common source.

A **common source outbreak** is one that has the same origin (i.e., same person or vehicle as the reservoir or means of transmission). A **propagated** (continuous) **outbreak** is one in which the infection is transmitted from person to person over a longer period of time than with a common source outbreak, and it can generate secondary infections with intervals between peaks that approximate the usual incubation period for the infection. An example of measles cases is outlined in Figure 14.3. **Secondary infections** are those that occur within the accepted incubation period following exposure to a primary case (Porta, 2008). Characterizing an outbreak by person, place, and time is called

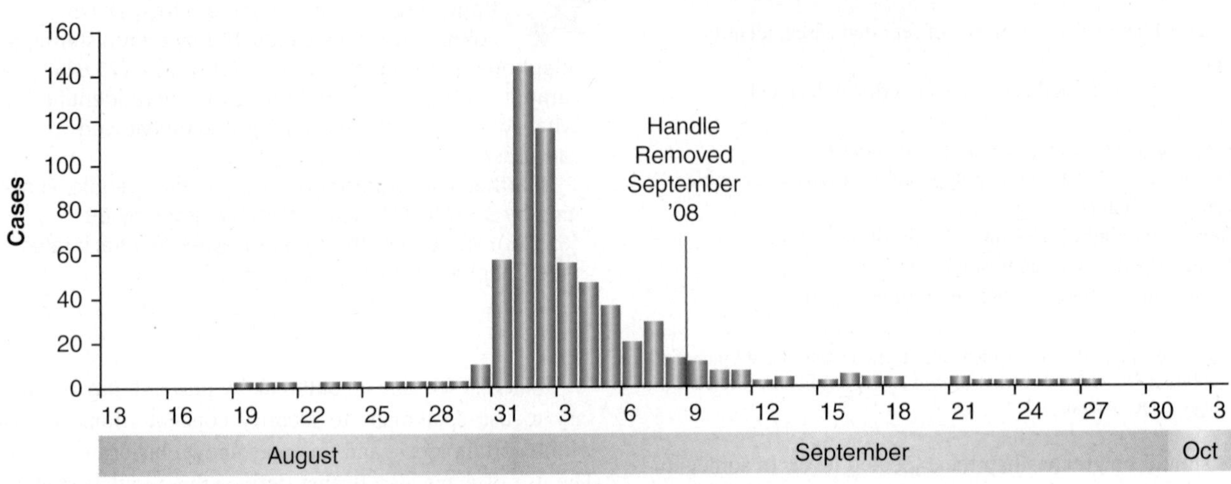

figure 14.2 Common source epidemic curve: Broad Street pump cholera outbreak, London, 1854. (Source: Centers for Disease Control and Prevention).

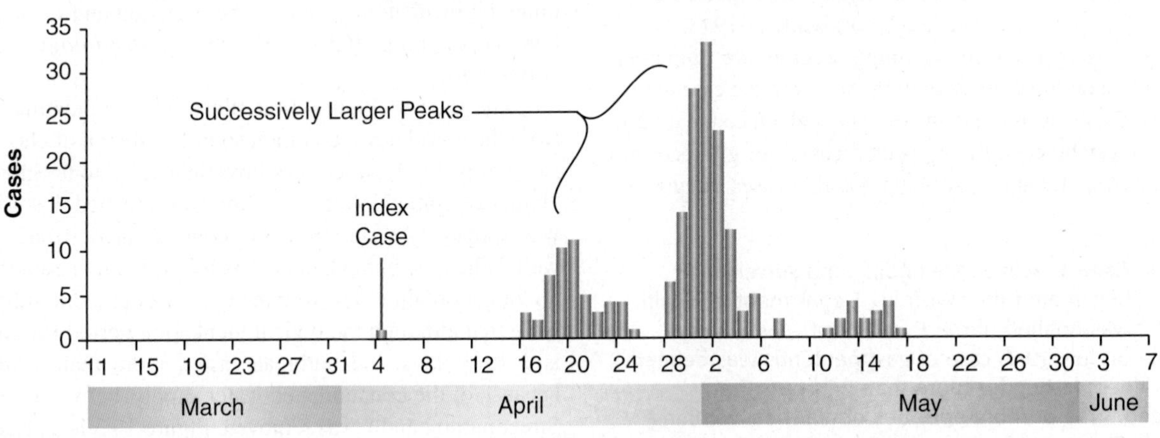

figure 14.3 Propagated epidemic curve: Measles outbreak. (Source: Centers for Disease Control and Prevention. Retrieved from http://www.cdc.gov/epo/dih/Epidemic_Curve/page06.htm)

descriptive epidemiology (see Chapter 7), because it describes the population under study. This step is critical for several reasons. First, by becoming familiar with the data, it is possible to learn what information is reliable and informative (e.g., the same unusual exposure reported by many of the people affected) and what may not be as reliable (e.g., many missing or "don't know" responses to a particular question). Second, a comprehensive description of an outbreak is provided by showing its trend over time, its geographic extent (place), and the populations (people) affected by the disease and the time period in which it occurs. This description lets an epidemiologist begin to assess the outbreak in light of what is known about the disease (e.g., the usual source, mode of transmission, risk factors, and populations affected) and to develop causal hypotheses (CDC, *Excite: Epidemiology in the classroom*). In turn, these hypotheses can be tested using the techniques of analytic epidemiology (see Chapter 8).

HEALTHCARE-ASSOCIATED INFECTIONS

Healthcare-associated infections (HAIs) (previously called nosocomial infections) are a significant cause of morbidity and mortality in the United States. It is estimated that about 1 in every 20 inpatients has an infection related to healthcare. These infections cost the U.S. healthcare system billions of dollars each year and lead to the loss of tens of thousands of lives. In addition, HAIs can have devastating emotional, financial, and medical consequences. The majority of HAIs are urinary tract infections (UTIs), surgical site infections (SSIs), bloodstream infections, and pneumonia (CDC, *Estimates of Healthcare-Associated Infections*). The U.S. Department of Health and Human Services (USDHHS) identified the reduction of hospital-acquired central line-associated bloodstream infections and catheter-associated UTIs as a goal by the end of fiscal year 2013 (USDHHS, *Healthcare-associated infections*).

The CDC's National Healthcare Safety Network (NHSN) is a public health surveillance system that maintains and supports the USDHHS national HAI prevention priorities. Since its inception in 2005, NHSN has been used by healthcare facilities in all 50 states, the District of Columbia (DC), and Puerto Rico. As of December 2012, 30 states and DC required, or have plans to require, use of NHSN for state-specific HAI reporting mandates. NHSN data are reported annually to measure progress toward the HHS goal of HAI prevention. As of the third quarter of 2012, a 41% reduction occurred in central line-associated bloodstream infections since 2008, up from the 32% reduction reported in 2010; a 17% reduction in SSIs since 2008, up from the 7% reduction reported in 2010; and a 7% reduction in catheter-associated UTIs since 2009, which is the same percentage of reduction that was reported in 2010 (Malpiedi et al., 2011).

An estimated 1 to 3 million HAIs occur among residents in long-term care settings each year. In addition to infections that are largely endemic, such as UTIs and lower respiratory tract infections, outbreaks of respiratory and gastrointestinal infections are also common. Pneumonia and other lower respiratory tract infections are the most frequent reasons for transferring residents of long-term care facilities to the hospital (CDC, *Tracking infections in long-term care facilities*). When an outbreak occurs in a healthcare setting, an epidemiologic investigation is conducted, using the same criteria outlined above. Applying the basic principles of infection control, which include hand hygiene, aseptic technique, and isolation precautions, can prevent HAIs. Community/public health nurses also can prevent and control infections in the home by using appropriate aseptic techniques, attention to good hand hygiene, and educating family members in the principles of infection control.

EVIDENCE FOR PRACTICE

In September 2012, an alert clinician notified the Tennessee Department of Health of a patient who had developed culture-confirmed *Aspergillus fumigatus* meningitis after he had received an epidural steroid injection in July at an ambulatory surgical center. The patient was admitted to the hospital in late August. The Tennessee Department of Health notified the CDC, and within days, the CDC had identified the source of the largest multistate healthcare-associated outbreak to be an injectable steroid medication prepared by a compounding center in Massachusetts. At that time, the CDC and the Food and Drug Administration (FDA) recommended that all healthcare professionals discontinue use and remove from their pharmaceutical inventory any product produced by that compounding center. A massive effort to contact nearly 14,000 potentially exposed patients and their physicians was undertaken by the CDC.

As of May 2013, there were 733 cases and 53 deaths reported among patients in 20 states who received injections of the contaminated steroid medication associated with the outbreak. A probable case was defined as a person who received a methylprednisolone acetate (MPA) injection, linked to injectable steroids from three recalled lots of preservative-free MPA distributed by the compounding center in Massachusetts after May 21, 2012, and subsequently developed any of the following: meningitis of unknown etiology; posterior circulation stroke without a cardioembolic source; osteomyelitis, abscess, or other infection of unknown cause at or near the site of injection; osteomyelitis or worsening inflammatory arthritis of a peripheral joint (e.g., knee, shoulder, or ankle) of unknown cause. A confirmed case included identification of a fungal pathogen (by culture, histopathology, or molecular assay) associated with a clinical syndrome listed above.

In the early stages of the outbreak, the majority of patients were diagnosed with meningitis. However, the majority of patients developed a localized infection following exposure to contaminated injections, including epidural abscess, arachnoiditis (a disorder caused by the inflammation of the arachnoid membrane that surrounds and protects the nerves of the spinal cord), discitis (an infection in the intervertebral disc space), or vertebral osteomyelitis.

Most of the cases occurred in Michigan (n = 259), followed by Tennessee (n = 152). The predominant fungus identified in the outbreak was *Exserohilum rostratum*. One patient, the index case from Tennessee, had a laboratory-confirmed *A. fumigatus* infection. These fungi are common in the environment, and fungal infections are not transmitted from person to person. But fungal infections can be slow to develop; therefore, patients and clinicians were advised to remain vigilant for onset of symptoms (CDC, *Multistate fungal meningitis outbreak investigation*).

This is an example of the importance of public health preparedness to identify rare pathogens and implement measures to control them.

PUBLIC HEALTH SURVEILLANCE

At the federal level, the USDHHS is the U.S. public health infrastructure that develops policies to protect the nation's health. The CDC is a major USDHHS agency that protects the nation's health by developing guidelines that promote health and quality of life by preventing and controlling disease, injury, and disability (CDC, *About CDC*).

Surveillance for infectious and/or communicable diseases in the United States consists of a variety of efforts at both the state and federal levels. At the state level, healthcare providers and healthcare facilities are required to report certain infectious diseases to state health departments. State public health departments that monitor disease incidence and identify possible outbreaks within their states report these data to the CDC. Certain infectious and/or communicable diseases must be reported to the CDC. For the current list of notifiable diseases, see the CDC's Nationally Notifiable Diseases website at http://wwwn.cdc.gov/nndss/default.aspx.

The CDC is also a partner with the WHO through the Global Outbreak Alert and Response Network and the WHO Surveillance and Response System, which provide international epidemic alerts and responses (WHO, *CSR and global team*).

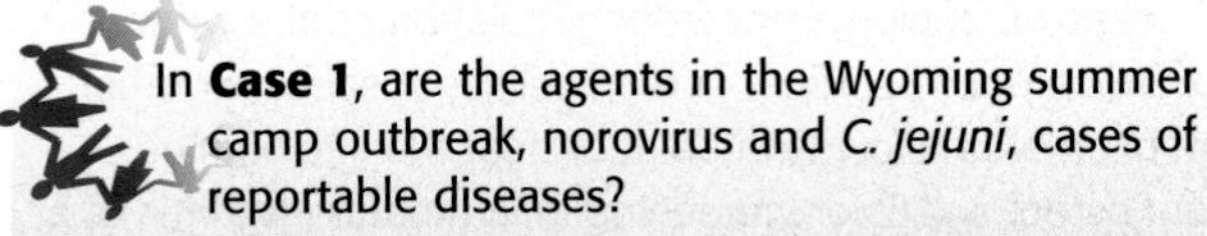
In **Case 1**, are the agents in the Wyoming summer camp outbreak, norovirus and *C. jejuni*, cases of reportable diseases?

At the U.S. federal level, the CDC maintains surveillance systems to analyze data for disease trends and outbreaks. For example, one such surveillance system is FoodNet (Foodborne Disease Active Surveillance Network), which is a collaborative effort among the FDA, the U.S. Department of Agriculture, and the CDC. Specific states, which report cases and outbreaks of food-borne illnesses, are selected to participate in the CDC Emerging Infections Program (CDC, *FoodNet*). The Department of Defense (DoD) also has an electronic surveillance system for the early notification of community-based epidemics (ESSENCE), which has been in operation since 2001 to detect infectious disease outbreaks (DoD, *Global emerging infections system*).

SPECIFIC COMMUNICABLE DISEASES

Food-borne Diseases

Food-borne diseases involve biological and nonbiological agents and can be caused by microorganisms and their toxins, marine organisms and their toxins, fungi and their related toxins, and chemical contaminants. Raw and undercooked foods of animal origin are the most likely to be contaminated. The CDC estimates that each year roughly one in six people in the United States (or 48 million people) get sick, 128,000 are hospitalized, and 3,000 die of food-borne diseases. The top five pathogens contributing to domestically acquired food-borne illnesses in 2011 were noroviruses, *Salmonella*, ***Clostridium perfringens,*** *Campylobacter*, and ***Staphylococcus aureus*** (CDC, *Estimates of foodborne illness in the United States*).

Recent changes in human demographics and food preferences, changes in food production and distribution systems, microbial adaptation, and lack of support for public health resources and infrastructure have led to the emergence of novel as well as traditional food-borne diseases. With increasing travel and trade opportunities, it is not surprising that the risk of contracting and spreading a food-borne disease now exists locally, regionally, and even globally.

Food-borne diseases monitored through the CDC FoodNet include infections caused by bacteria: *Campylobacter, Listeria, Salmonella*, Shiga toxin–producing *Escherichia coli* (STEC) O157 and non-O157, *Shigella, Vibrio, Yersinia*; and parasites: *Cryptosporidium* and *Cyclospora*. FoodNet surveillance data for 2010 indicated a significant decrease in the incidence of STEC O157 infections, which had declined since 2006, and reached the *Healthy People 2010* target of less than 1 case per 100,000. However, the incidence of STEC O157 infection no longer decreased in 2012, and exceeded the previously met target of 1 case per 100,000 persons. The incidence of food-borne diseases in 2012 per 100,000 population, by pathogen, were as follows: *Salmonella* (16.42), *Campylobacter* (14.30), *Shigella* (4.50), *Cryptosporidium* (2.60), STEC non-O157 (1.16), STEC O157 (1.12), *Vibrio* (0.41), *Yersinia* (0.33), *Listeria* (0.25), and *Cyclospora* (0.03). The highest reported incidence was among children less than 5 years of age for *Cryptosporidium* and bacterial pathogens other than *Listeria* and *Vibrio*, for which the highest incidence was among persons aged 65 years and older (CDC, *Trends in Foodborne Illness in the United States, 2012*). *Salmonella* infections have not declined for nearly two decades, and in 2010, the incidence was nearly three times the *Healthy People 2010* target (see Box 14.4 for *Healthy People 2020* objectives for food

box 14.4 *Healthy People 2020* Objectives for Food Safety

Reduce infections caused by key pathogens commonly transmitted through food.

Reduce the number of outbreak-associated infections due to Shiga toxin–producing *E. coli* O157, or *Campylobacter, Listeria,* or *Salmonella* species associated with food commodity groups.

Prevent an increase in the proportion of nontyphoidal *Salmonella* and *Campylobacter jejuni* isolates from humans that are resistant to antimicrobial drugs.

Reduce severe allergic reactions to food among adults with a food allergy diagnosis.

Increase the proportion of consumers who follow key food safety practices.

(Developmental) Improve food safety practices associated with food-borne illness in food-service and retail establishments.

Source: U.S. Department of Health and Human Services. *Healthy People 2020 food safety objectives*. Retrieved July 11, 2013, from http://healthypeople.gov/2020/topicsobjectives2020/objectiveslist.aspx?topicId=14

safety). These findings highlight the need to continue to identify and address food safety gaps that can be targeted for action by the food industry and regulatory authorities. Effective measures include preventing contamination of meat during slaughter and of all foods, including produce, during processing and preparation; cooking meat thoroughly; vigorously detecting and investigating outbreaks; and recalling contaminated food (CDC, 2011b; 2013a). Nurses and other healthcare providers should educate their patients about the hazards of potentially life-threatening food-borne diseases and the preventive measures to reduce them.

Noroviruses

Noroviruses are common food-borne pathogens. Norovirus infections are often called "stomach flu"; however, this is a misnomer, because the norovirus is not an influenza virus. Noroviruses are recognized as the most common cause of acute infectious gastroenteritis in people of all ages. They are responsible for more than 50% of all food-borne gastroenteritis outbreaks in the United States (CDC, *Estimates of foodborne illness in the US*).

Noroviruses are spread primarily from one infected person to another by the fecal–oral route through contaminated hands, contaminated food or water, or by contact with contaminated objects in the environment. In some cases, aerosolized vomitus has been implicated in transmission of noroviruses. The incubation period for norovirus gastroenteritis is 12 to 48 hours; it causes more vomiting than diarrhea, is self-limited, and usually resolves within 48 hours. However, the elderly, children, and those with severe underlying medical conditions are at increased risk due to fluid volume depletion and electrolyte imbalance (CDC, *Norovirus*).

Nearly two-thirds of all norovirus outbreaks reported in the United States occurred in long-term care facilities. Outbreaks of norovirus illness also have occurred in restaurants, cruise ships, schools, banquet halls, summer camps, and even at family dinners. These are all places where people often eat food handled or prepared by others. Outbreaks of noroviruses on cruise ships and continuation of the outbreaks with the same strains on consecutive cruises in new passengers suggest that noroviruses have high infectivity (CDC, *Norovirus*).

Oral hydrating solutions should be given for attacks of norovirus, and in severe cases, intravenous fluid and electrolyte replacement may be necessary. At the first signs of this acute gastroenteritis outbreak, good handwashing, thorough and immediate disinfection with appropriate solutions, and isolation of sick people until 72 hours after they are symptom-free are critical (CDC, *Norovirus*).

Campylobacter Enteritis

Campylobacter is the most common cause of bacterial food-borne illness in the United States, and it is an important cause of diarrheal illness throughout the world regardless of people's age. It is often implicated in traveler's diarrhea. Consumption of contaminated poultry is the most common source of *Campylobacter* infection, although undercooked meats, ground beef, pork, cheese, eggs, shellfish, unpasteurized milk, and direct exposure to pets and farm animals have been implicated. Generally, the incubation period ranges from 2 to 5 days. The resulting diarrheal illness usually lasts no more than a week. Typical symptoms include nausea, vomiting, abdominal pain, fever, headache, and muscle pain. Occasionally, a severe case may last longer, and about 25% of the people affected may experience a relapse (CDC, *Campylobacter*).

Campylobacter infection is usually a self-limited illness, diagnosed by stool culture, and treated by antidiarrheal medications such as loperamide. In more severe cases, antibiotics are prescribed. It is essential that affected people drink plenty of fluids, such as oral rehydration solutions, and wash hands carefully to prevent transmission to others.

Listeria Monocytogenes

Listeria monocytogenes can cause listeriosis, an uncommon but potentially fatal food-borne bacterial disease. The disease primarily affects older adults, pregnant women, newborns, and adults with weakened immune systems, and can result in miscarriage, stillbirth, or severe illness and death in newborn infants. However, rarely, persons without these risk factors can also be affected. The risk may be reduced by recommendations for safe food preparation, consumption, and storage (CDC, *Listeria*).

PRACTICE POINT

Nurses and other healthcare providers should suspect listeriosis in high-risk patients who become ill with diarrhea and/or flu-like symptoms, and have a recent history of eating delicatessen food, soft cheeses, or smoked seafood.

Nontyphoid Salmonella

Nontyphoid *Salmonella* is a bacterial disease transmitted by contaminated food and water, or contact with infected animals and reptiles. Every year, approximately 42,000 cases of salmonellosis are reported in the United States. Because many milder cases are not diagnosed or reported, the actual number of infections may be 30 times greater. There are many kinds of *Salmonella* bacteria. *Salmonella* serotypes Typhimurium and Enteritidis are the most common in the United States. People at risk for severe or complicated illness include infants, the elderly, people with compromised immune systems, and organ transplant recipients. Salmonellosis is characterized by diarrhea, fever, and abdominal cramps 12 to 72 hours following exposure, and generally lasts 4 to 7 days. The majority of those infected recover without treatment. However, approximately 400 persons die each year with acute salmonellosis. A small number of persons with *Salmonella* develop pain in their joints. This is called reactive arthritis, and it can last for months or years. It also can lead to chronic arthritis which is difficult to treat. Treatment of dehydration and electrolyte imbalance is essential. Antibiotics are not usually necessary unless the infection spreads from the intestines. The CDC has identified *Salmonella* bacteria that have become resistant to antibiotics, largely as a result of the use of antibiotics to promote the growth of food animals (CDC, *Salmonella).*

PRACTICE POINT

An efficient and effective homemade oral rehydration solution is to stir one level teaspoon of salt and eight level teaspoons of sugar into one quart or liter of clean drinking water or water that has been boiled and cooled.

Salmonella enteritidis, generally found in shell eggs, has been decreasing as a source of food-borne illness during the past decade, attributed in part to farm-based egg control programs, as well as education of farm worker and consumers. Nonetheless, outbreaks continue to occur. For example, the CDC recently reported a multistate outbreak caused by *Salmonella* Heidelberg, linked to chicken (CDC, *Multistate outbreak of Salmonella* Heidelberg *infections linked to chicken*). Outbreaks of *Salmonella* also have been associated with direct or indirect contact with live poultry, frogs, and turtles (CDC, *Salmonella).* In 2013, three ongoing multistate outbreaks of human *Salmonella* infections linked to live poultry were reported by the CDC (CDC, *Multistate outbreaks of human Salmonella infections*). Since 1990, 45 outbreaks have been associated with live poultry, which included 1,563 cases and five deaths (Fig. 14.4).

Escherichia coli O157:H7

Shiga toxin–producing *Escherichia coli* O157 is a deadly form of *E. coli*, which produces symptoms of severe abdominal cramps, bloody and nonbloody diarrhea, and vomiting that generally resolve within 7 to 10 days. In the very young and the elderly, infection with STEC O157:H7 can cause fatal hemolytic–uremic syndrome and renal failure (CDC, *E. coli*). This severe complication includes temporary anemia, profuse bleeding, and kidney failure.

Several outbreaks of *E. coli O157:H7* have been associated with commercially packaged *foods* and fresh produce (CDC, *Multistate Foodborne Outbreak Investigations*). A recent multistate outbreak of *E. coli O157:H7* involved prepackaged organic spinach and spring mixed blend from a common producer in Massachustetts, but the source of contamination was not identified (CDC, *E. coli*). See Chapter 15 for a further discussion of *E. coli O157:H7*. Food-borne infections should be considered in people with diarrheal illness who are residents of, or travelers to an area where food-borne outbreaks have been reported. A careful history also should consist of contact with animals and reptiles as a source of infection.

Waterborne Diseases

In the United States, Canada, United Kingdom, and much of Europe, the drinking water supply is normally safe. The United States has one of the safest public water supplies in

Since the 1990s,
45 *Salmonella* **outbreaks**
have been linked to **live**
poultry.

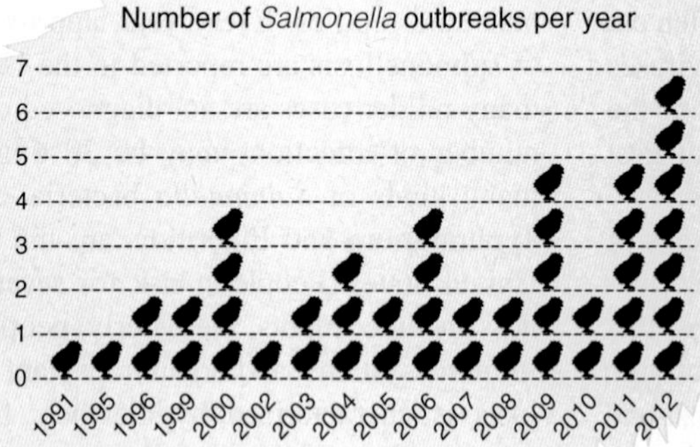

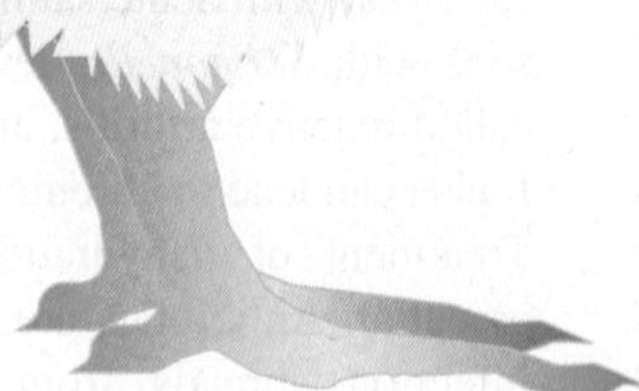

figure 14.4 Salmonella outbreaks linked to live poultry 1990–2012. (Source: Centers for Disease Control and Prevention. Multistate outbreaks of human Salmonella infections linked to live poultry. Retrieved May 2, 2013, from http://www.cdc.gov/salmonella/)

the world. The year 2008 marked the 100th anniversary of one of the most significant public health advances in U.S. history, the disinfection of drinking water. However, 780 million people worldwide do not have access to safe water, and an estimated 2.5 billion people, 50% of the developing world, lack access to adequate sanitation. Diarrheal diseases such as cholera kill more children than AIDS, malaria, and measles combined, making it the second leading cause of death among children less than 5 years of age. Approximately 88% of deaths due to diarrheal illness are attributable to unsafe water, poor sanitation, and inadequate hygiene (CDC, 2013c).

In the United States, state and local governments establish and enforce regulations for protecting recreational water from naturally-occurring and human-made contaminants. No federal regulatory agency has authority over treated recreational water (e.g., pools and interactive fountains), and no minimum federal design, construction, operation, disinfection, or filtration standards exist. The Environmental Protection Agency (EPA) sets water quality guidelines for natural, untreated recreational water (e.g., lakes, rivers, and oceans). Despite drinking water treatment advances, an estimated 4 to 33 million annual diarrheal illness episodes still occur in the United States from exposure to contaminated municipal drinking water. At least 40,000 hospitalizations at a cost of $970 million per year result from just five waterborne pathogens: noroviruses, *Cryptosporidium, E. coli O157:H7*, *Pseudomonas*, and *Legionella*. In addition, we face emerging public health concerns such as chlorine-tolerant pathogens and the increasing complexity of waterborne diseases (CDC, 2011c, 2013c).

In surveillance conducted between 2007 and 2008, the CDC reported a total of 134 waterborne illness outbreaks, of which 116 (86.6%) were associated with treated recreational water (e.g., pools and interactive fountains). *Cryptosporidium* was confirmed as the etiologic agent of 60 (44.8%) of 134 outbreaks. Two outbreaks associated with recreational water were caused by *E. coli O157:H7* and two others were shigellosis outbreaks. Four outbreaks caused by *Pseudomonas* were each linked epidemiologically to hotel/motel pools or spas. An additional 10 outbreaks caused by *Legionella* were linked epidemiologically to pools or spas. Norovirus was identified as the etiologic agent in each of five outbreaks; two were associated with treated water and three with lakes. Nine other outbreaks were associated with chemicals or toxins (CDC, 2011c).

The U.S. EPA and the CDC set national standards to protect drinking water and its sources against naturally occurring or human-made contaminants. In the United States, all public water systems must be monitored for total coliform bacteria (fecal contamination), which is 0 (or no) total coliform per 100 mL of water at a prescribed frequency. State and local governments establish and enforce regulations to protect recreational water against naturally occurring or human contaminants. Standards for operating, disinfecting, and filtering public swimming and wading pools are regulated by state and local health departments and, as a result, vary throughout the United States. Reports of outbreaks in the states and territories are voluntary. However, waterborne diseases associated with recreational activities have been added to the CDC waterborne-disease outbreak surveillance system. Most recreational water outbreaks have been associated with treated water venues such as swimming pools or spas. Box 14.5 presents selected *Healthy People 2020* objectives for environmental health and water quality.

Two criteria must be met for an event to be defined as a water-associated disease outbreak. First, two or more people must be linked epidemiologically by time, location of exposure to water, and illness characteristics. Second, the epidemiologic evidence must implicate recreational water or volatilization of water-associated compounds into the air surrounding the water as the probable source of illness. Multiple etiologic agents should be considered when waterborne disease is suspected and might be related to sewage or septic contamination (CDC, 2011c).

CASE 1: Examine Figure 14.5.

1. Did the outbreak at the Wyoming camp meet the criteria for definition as an outbreak?
2. If so, what type of outbreak was it?
3. Why were the national standards set by the EPA not met?

It was determined that the camp's water system should be regulated as a public water system. A new septic system was installed following a professional site evaluation. In the future, the camp's water system will be subject to periodic EPA testing guidelines and subsequent evaluations. Public health officials, healthcare providers, and water quality regulators should be aware of the potential for septic contamination of well water at rural summer campsites. In addition, parents should inquire about recent water quality testing at camps.

box 14.5 *Healthy People 2020* Environmental Objectives Related to Water Quality

- Increase the proportion of persons served by community water systems who receive a supply of drinking water that meets the regulations of the Safe Drinking Water Act.
- Reduce waterborne-disease outbreaks arising from water intended for drinking among persons served by community water systems.
- Reduce per capita domestic water use.
- Maintain the percentage of days that beaches are open and safe for swimming.
- Reduce the global burden of disease due to poor water quality, sanitation, and insufficient hygiene.

Source: U.S. Department of Health and Human Services. *Healthy People 2020 environmental objectives: Water quality.* Retrieved April 29, 2013, from http://healthypeople.gov/2020/topicsobjectives2020/objectiveslist.aspx?topicId=12#364

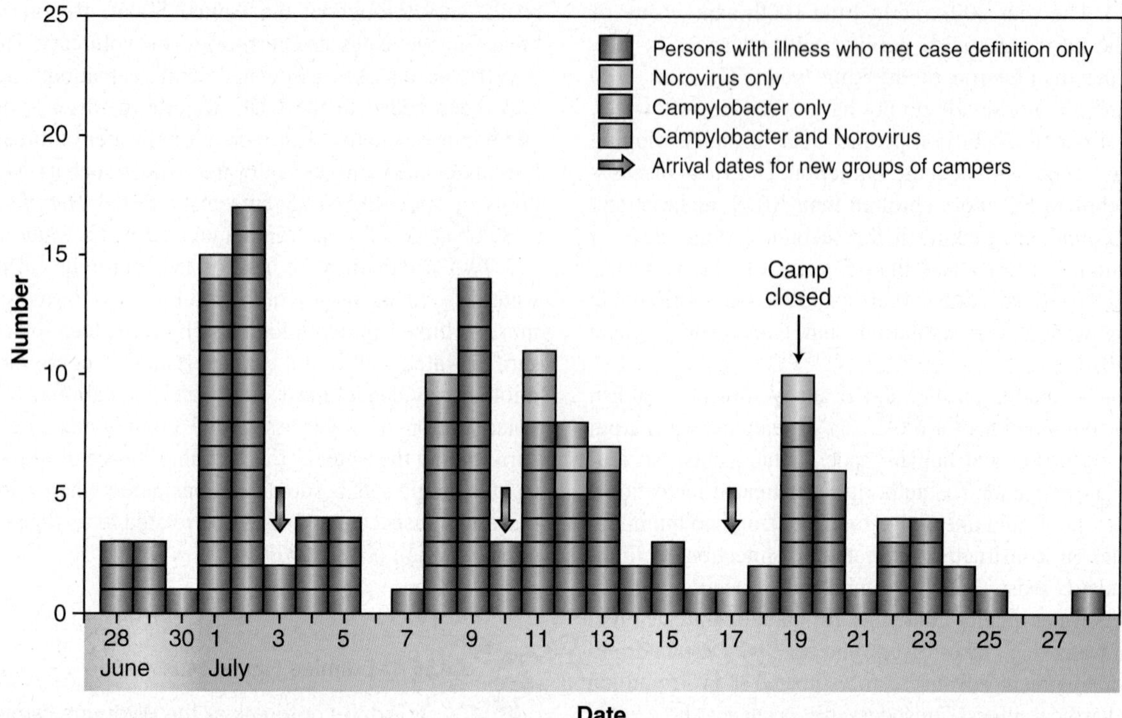

figure 14.5 Epidemic curve for the outbreak of gastroenteritis at the Wyoming camp. (Data from Centers for Disease Control and Prevention. [2007]. Brief report: Gastroenteritis among attendees at a summer camp, Wyoming, June–July 2006. *Morbidity and Mortality Weekly Report, 56*(15), 368–370.)

Legionnaires disease, which is caused by the *Legionella pneumophila* bacterium, was first recognized among hotel guests during an outbreak in Philadelphia in 1976. Between 8,000 and 18,000 people are hospitalized with Legionnaires disease in the United States each year; However, many infections are not diagnosed or reported, so this number may be higher. More illness is usually found in the summer and early fall, but it can happen any time of year. Outbreaks of this disease have been associated with potable water sources, air-conditioning cooling towers, and cruise ships. *Legionella* bacteria are not transmitted from person to person (CDC, *Legionella*).

EVIDENCE FOR PRACTICE

The CDC investigated an outbreak of eight cases (seven confirmed and one possible) of Legionnaires disease among guests at a Maryland hotel. Symptom onset occurred a median of 7.5 days (range: 4–9 days) after leaving the hotel. Underlying medical conditions associated with increased risk of Legionnaires disease included smoking, diabetes, and an immunocompromised condition. Seven patients were hospitalized, but fortunately none died. Although the rooms in which the people with confirmed disease stayed were located in different areas and on different floors of the hotel, all had showered or bathed in their respective rooms, and one had used the whirlpool spa. Six reported exposure to the swimming pool and whirlpool area.

Epidemiologists reported that *L. pneumophila* was recovered from multiple sites in the hotel, including the hot water storage tank; cooling tower; multiple hot water heaters; and showers and faucets in rooms occupied by patients and healthy guests. To kill the bacteria, specialists conducted superheating of the water, hyperchlorination treatment of potable water, and disinfection with a bleach solution. After the remediation interventions, there were no further cases of Legionnaires disease associated with the hotel. However, during postremediation follow-up testing, one low-level isolate of *L. pneumophila* from the cooling tower was identified, and the cooling tower was hyperchlorinated. The recovery of *Legionella* from multiple points in the hotel potable water system suggests that it was the source of the outbreak.

Sexually Transmitted Diseases (Sexually Transmitted Infections)

Sexually transmitted diseases (STDs) or sexually transmitted infections (STIs) affect men and women of all backgrounds and economic levels. Despite the fact that a great deal of progress has been made in STD prevention over the past four decades, the CDC new estimates show that there are about 20 million new STDs in the United States each year, with a cost of nearly $16 billion in direct medical costs alone. Almost half of the new cases occur in young people aged 15 to 24 years. It has been estimated that the actual rate of infection may be twice that of the reported rate, because many cases are undiagnosed and untreated. In addition, the new CDC data suggest that there are more than 110 million total STDs among men and women across the nation. Its analyses included eight common STDs: chlamydia, gonorrhea, hepatitis B, herpes simplex (caused by herpes simplex virus type 2 [HSV-2]), HIV infection, human papillomavirus (HPV) infection, syphilis, and trichomoniasis (CDC, *STI fact sheet*).

Although the consequences of untreated STIs often are worse among young women, new data reveal that the annual number of new infections to be roughly equal among young women and young men (51% among young women vs. 49% among young men). Chlamydia, gonorrhea, syphilis, and trichomoniasis are easily treated and cured if diagnosed early. However, too many of these infections go undetected because they often have no symptoms. But even STIs without symptoms can have serious health consequences. Undiagnosed and untreated chlamydia or gonorrhea, for example, can put a woman at increased risk of chronic pelvic pain, life-threatening ectopic pregnancy, and an increase in infertility (CDC, *STI fact sheet*).

Any genital symptoms such as discharge or burning during urination or unusual sore or rash should be a signal for a person to stop having sex and to see a healthcare provider immediately. Infections caused by bacteria can be treated and usually cured with antibiotics, but those caused by viruses cannot be cured this way. All partners must be notified so that they can be examined and treated, if necessary. Other than abstinence, a long-term mutually monogamous relationship with a partner who has been tested and is known to be uninfected is the best way to avoid STIs. Sexual partners should talk to each other about their STIs so that preventive action can be taken. Prevention of STI transmission does not include washing the genitals, urinating, and/or douching after sex. Latex condoms can reduce the risk of transmission but only when used consistently (every time) and correctly. However, genital ulcer diseases, such as syphilis, can occur anywhere within the male and female genital areas, whether or not they are covered by a latex condom. Correct and consistent use of latex condoms can reduce the risk of STIs *only* when the infected area or site of potential exposure is protected. Condoms lubricated with spermicides (especially nonoxy-nol-9 or N-9) are no more effective than other lubricated condoms in protecting against the transmission of STIs. Based on the findings from several research studies, N-9 may itself cause genital lesions, providing a point of entry for HIV and other STIs. Therefore, the CDC recommends that N-9 not be used as a microbicide or lubricant during vaginal or anal intercourse (CDC, 2010). The *Healthy People 2020* objectives for STDs are presented in Box 14.6.

PRACTICE POINT

Any person is in a high-risk group for STDs if they

- Have multiple sexual partners.
- Do not use a condom during sex.
- Have other STDs.
- Have a sexual partner who has had an STD.

box 14.6 *Healthy People 2020* Objectives for Sexually Transmitted Diseases

Reduce the proportion of females aged 15 to 44 years who have ever required treatment of pelvic inflammatory disease (PID).

Reduce congenital syphilis.

Reduce the proportion of adolescents and young adults with *Chlamydia trachomatis* infections.

Reduce gonorrhea rates.

Reduce sustained domestic transmission of primary and secondary syphilis.

Reduce the proportion of adults with genital herpes infection due to herpes simplex type 2.

Reduce the proportion of females with human papillomavirus (HPV) infection.

Increase the proportion of sexually active females aged 24 years and younger enrolled in commercial health insurance plans who are screened annually for genital *Chlamydia* infections.

Increase the proportion of sexually active females aged 24 years and younger enrolled in Medicaid who are screened annually for genital *Chlamydia* infections.

Increase the proportion of HIV-infected persons who know they are infected.

Source: U.S. Department of Health and Human Services. *Healthy People 2020 sexually transmitted diseases objectives*. Retrieved April 29, 2013, from http://healthypeople.gov/2020/topicsobjectives2020/objectiveslist.aspx?topicId=37

EVIDENCE FOR PRACTICE

The clinical treatment guidelines for STDs typically recommend antibiotic therapy to cover common infections. However, overtreatment and undertreatment of STIs are common during emergency department (ED) visits.

Huppert et al. (2013) examined a quality improvement project that aimed to improve follow-up care for STIs in the ED. They compared the point-of-care (POC) treatment patterns for gonorrhea and trichomoniasis among young women seen in an ED over an 18-month period. Of the 1,877 visits, 8.8% of women had gonorrhea and 16.5% had trichomoniasis. Overtreatment was higher for women with gonorrhea than with trichomoniasis (54% vs. 23%, $p < 0.001$). However, overtreatment for gonorrhea decreased from 58% to 47% ($p < 0.01$) and overtreatment for trichomoniasis decreased from 24% to 18% ($p < 0.01$), which corresponded to improvements in patient follow-up for the QI project. Undertreatment was higher for women with gonorrhea than with trichomoniasis (29% vs. 21%, $p = 0.03$), and did not change over time. An unanticipated benefit of the QI project to improve patient follow-up was the decrease in antibiotic usage in the ED. Given the ability of gonorrhea to develop antibiotic resistance, Hubbert and colleagues recommended that future studies focus on the development of an accurate POC test for gonorrhea.

In **Case 2**, Megan discussed her urinary frequency and abnormal vaginal discharge with the school nurse. What advice might the school nurse have given her?

Chlamydia

Chlamydial infection is the most frequently reported bacterial STD in the United States, with an estimated 3 million new infections occurring annually. The highest rates of chlamydial infection occur in 15- to 19-year-old adolescents, and the infection has nearly three times the prevalence among persons aged 25 to 39 years. Substantial racial/ethnic disparities in chlamydial infection exist, with prevalence among non-Hispanic Blacks approximately five times the prevalence among non-Hispanic Whites. Chlamydia is also common among men who have sex with men (MSM) (CDC, *Chlamydia fact sheet*). Chlamydia is a nationally notifiable disease, and CDC data indicate that nearly all 50 states and territories failed to meet the *Healthy People 2010* (USDHHS, 2000) objective to reduce the proportion of adolescents and young adults with *C. trachomatis* infections to 3% (CDC, 2012b). Chlamydial infection is caused by a bacterium, *Chlamydia trachomatis*, which is transmitted during vaginal, oral, or anal sexual contact with an infected partner.

Chlamydia is known as a "silent" infection because most infected people are asymptomatic and lack abnormal physical examination findings. In women, the bacteria initially infect the cervix, where the infection may cause signs and symptoms of cervicitis (e.g., mucopurulent endocervical discharge, easily induced endocervical bleeding), and sometimes the urethra, which may result in signs and symptoms of urethritis (e.g., pyuria, dysuria, urinary frequency). Infection can spread from the cervix to the upper reproductive tract (i.e., uterus, fallopian tubes), causing pelvic inflammatory disease (PID), which may be asymptomatic and is a major cause of infertility among women of childbearing age. A pregnant woman may pass chlamydial infection to her newborn during delivery, resulting in subsequent neonatal eye infection or pneumonia. Men who are symptomatic typically have urethritis, with a mucoid or watery urethral discharge and dysuria. A minority of infected men develop epididymitis (with or without symptomatic urethritis), presenting with unilateral testicular pain, tenderness, and swelling (CDC, *Chlamydia fact sheet*).

Screening programs have been demonstrated to reduce rates of adverse sequelae in women. There are a number of diagnostic tests for chlamydia, including cell culture (the criterion standard) and nucleic acid amplification tests (NAATs), and others. NAATs are the most sensitive tests and can be performed on easily obtainable specimens such as vaginal swabs (either clinician- or patient-collected) or urine. Urine is the specimen of choice for males. Self-collected vaginal swab specimens perform at least as well as other approved specimens using NAATs. Adolescent girls may be particularly good candidates for self-collected vaginal swab- or urine-based screening because pelvic exams are not indicated if they are asymptomatic. Persons with chlamydia should abstain from sexual activity for 7 days after single-dose antibiotics or until completion of a 7-day course of antibiotics, to prevent spreading the infection to partners. Chlamydia can be easily cured with antibiotics. HIV-positive persons with chlamydia should receive the same treatment as those who are HIV-negative (CDC, Chlamydia fact sheet). A number of antibiotics such as azithromycin (Zithromax), doxycycline, or erythromycin may be prescribed for treatment (CDC, *Chlamydia curriculum*).

EVIDENCE FOR PRACTICE

The CDC and the U.S. Preventive Services Task Force (USPSTF) recommend yearly chlamydia screening of all sexually active women aged 25 or younger and older women with risk factors for chlamydial infections (e.g., women who have a new or more than one sex partner). Pregnant women should be screened during their first prenatal care visit. Pregnant women under 25 or at increased risk for chlamydia (e.g., women who have a new or more than one sex partner) should be screened again in their third trimester. Any woman who is sexually active should discuss her risk factors with a healthcare provider who can then determine if more frequent screening is necessary. Routine screening is not recommended for men. However, the screening of sexually active young men should be considered in clinical settings with a high prevalence of chlamydia (e.g., adolescent clinics, correctional facilities, and STD clinics) when resources permit and will decrease screening programs for women (CDC, *Chlamydia fact sheet*; Agency for Health Research and Quality [AHRQ], 2006).

Gonorrhea

Gonorrhea is second only to chlamydia in number of cases reported to the CDC. Medical cost for treatment of gonorrhea and its complications is estimated at $56 million per year. In 2011, the highest rates were observed among women aged 15 to 19 and 20 to 24 years. Among men, the rate was highest among those aged 20 to 24 years. Approximately 86% of all cases occurred in men and women aged 15 to 29 years. Infection rates for men and women are very similar. However, in the last 10 years, gonorrhea rates among women have been slightly lower than those among men. Infections with *Neisseria gonorrhoeae*, like those resulting from *Chlamydia trachomatis*, cause several clinical syndromes, including urogenital, pharyngeal, and rectal infections in males and females, and conjunctivitis in adults and neonates. If untreated, gonorrhea can cause PID, tubal infertility, ectopic pregnancy, and chronic pelvic pain (CDC, *Gonorrhea fact sheet*).

Following implementation of the national gonorrhea control program in the mid-1970s, the national gonorrhea rate declined significantly despite a small increase in 1998. Like chlamydia, gonorrhea is substantially underdiagnosed and underreported; the number of reported cases is suspected to underestimate incidence by approximately 50%. The decline in new cases of gonorrhea halted for several years; however, in 2009 the gonorrhea rate decreased further to 98.1 cases per 100,000 population. This was the lowest rate since recording of gonorrhea rates began. The rate increased slightly in 2010 to 100.2 and increased again in 2011 to 104.2 per 100,000 population (CDC, 2012b). These data illustrate that the rate of gonorrhea still remains significantly higher than the *Healthy People 2010* targeted objective of 19 cases per 100,000 (USDHHS, 2000) (see Box 14.6 for *Healthy People 2020* objectives).

Patients infected with *N. gonorrhoeae* frequently are coinfected with *C. trachomatis.* Therefore, patients with gonorrhea should be tested for other STIs. Because of findings that chlamydial and gonorrheal infections often coexist led to the recommendation that patients treated for gonococcal infection also be treated routinely with a regimen that is effective against uncomplicated genital *C. trachomatis* infection. In addition, because most gonococci in the United States are susceptible to doxycycline and azithromycin, routine cotreatment might also hinder the development of antimicrobial-resistant *N. gonorrhoeae* (CDC, 2012c).

Drug-resistant strains of gonorrhea are increasing in many areas of the world, including the United States, making successful treatment of gonorrhea more difficult. Antimicrobial susceptibility patterns of *N. gonorrhoeae* have been closely monitored since 1986 through the Gonococcal Isolate Surveillance Project (GISP), and the information has been used to update treatment recommendations. The increased prevalence of fluoroquinolone-resistance in *N. gonorrhoeae* became widespread in the United States in the 1990s and 2000s, when the proportion of *N. gonorrhoeae* isolates in MSM that were resistant to ciprofloxacin (a fluoroquinolone antimicrobial) increased significantly. While the first fluoroquinolone-resistant *N. gonorrhoeae* cases were detected among heterosexuals, fluoroquinolone-resistance became widespread in the continental United States among MSM with gonorrhea before becoming widespread among heterosexuals. The CDC no longer recommends the use of fluoroquinolones for the treatment of gonococcal infections and associated conditions such as PID (CDC, 2011d). In 2010, 27% of all GISP isolates were resistant to penicillin, tetracycline, ciprofloxacin, or some combination of those antimicrobials, and 7% of isolates were resistant to all three antimicrobials. The GISP detected recent increases in minimum inhibitory concentrations (MICs) for cephalosporins among gonococcal isolates in the United States. These increases were most notable in the western United States and among MSM. The epidemiologic pattern of cephalosporin susceptibility in the West and among MSM during 2009 to 2010 was similar to that previously observed during the emergence of fluoroquinolone-resistant *N. gonorrhoeae* in the United States (CDC, 2011d). Therefore, the CDC no longer recommends the routine use of oral cephalosporins for treatment of gonococcal infections. It recommends dual therapy with ceftriaxone (an injectable cephalosporin) 250 mg intramuscularly as a single dose plus either azithromycin 1 gram orally as a single dose or doxycycline 100 mg orally twice a day for 7 days as the most effective treatment for uncomplicated gonorrhea (CDC, 2012c).

The potential emergence of gonococcal cephalosporin resistance is of particular concern because the U.S. gonorrhea control strategy relies upon effective antibiotic therapy. Previously, the emergence and spread of gonococcal antibiotic resistance in the United States was addressed by changing the recommended antibiotics for treatment. No other well-studied and effective antibiotic treatment options or combinations currently are available (Bolan et al., 2012). Therefore, the emergence and spread of cephalosporin-resistant *N. gonorrhoeae* (Ceph-R NG) would severely limit treatment options for gonorrhea in the United States. To prevent the emergence of Ceph-R NG in the United States, the CDC asks that all cases that meet the criteria for suspect or probable Ceph-R NG infection be reported to the state or local health department (CDC, 2012d).

People who have had gonorrhea and have been treated can get the disease again if they have sexual contact with people infected with gonorrhea. Every person who has been diagnosed and treated for gonorrhea should notify all recent sex partners so that they can see a healthcare provider and be treated. This will reduce the development of serious complications from gonorrhea and also reduce the possibility of reinfection. All people involved must avoid sex until they have completed their treatment of gonorrhea.

In **Case 2**, following the suggestion of the school nurse, Megan saw a nurse practitioner at a local women's health clinic. After taking a history, the nurse suspected an STD. A pelvic examination revealed mucopurulent cervicitis, and a tissue culture was taken. A dipstick urine analysis of a urine sample was positive for bacteria. A chlamydial infection was suspected, and a UTI was diagnosed.

1. What other information should the nurse practitioner consider in this case?
2. What treatment is indicated in this case?
3. What additional recommendations would you make?

EVIDENCE FOR PRACTICE

The USPSTF, an independent panel of experts supported by the Agency for Healthcare Research and Quality (AHRQ), recommends that clinicians routinely screen all sexually active women, including pregnant women, for gonorrhea infection if they have a history of previous STDs, new or multiple sexual partners, inconsistent condom use, sex work, and drug use. Currently, the USPSTF recommends against routine screening for gonorrhea infection in men and women at low risk for infection. Also, **the USPSTF recommends prophylactic ocular topical medication for all newborns for the prevention of gonococcal ophthalmia neonatorum** (USPSTF, 2011). (*Note:* The USPSTF has a draft gonorrhea research plan: "Proposed Analytic Framework for Asymptomatic Men and Women, Including Adolescents," which was issued for public input in 2013 [USPSTF, 2013].)

In **Case 2**, within a few days, Megan's tissue culture that was collected before treatment came back positive for *N. gonorrhoeae* in addition to *C. trachomatis*.

Does the nurse practitioner need to report these infections to the local health authorities?

Syphilis

Syphilis has often been called "the great imitator," because many of the signs and symptoms are indistinguishable from those of other diseases. This genital ulcerative disease is caused by the bacterium *Treponema pallidum.* It is transmitted from person to person through direct contact with a syphilitic sore. These sores occur mainly on the external genitals, vagina, anus, or in the rectum, although they can occur on the lips or in the mouth. Transmission occurs during vaginal, anal, or oral sex, and the organism can pass the placental barrier and infect the fetus.

Syphilis causes significant complications if untreated and facilitates the transmission of HIV infection (CDC, Syphilis profiles, 2011). Primary and secondary syphilis are the most infectious stages of the disease, and if not adequately treated, can lead to visual impairment, stroke, and in rare cases, even death. The primary stage of syphilis consists of a single sore or multiple sores. The sore(s) appears at the location where syphilis entered the body. The sore is usually firm, round, and painless. Because the sore is painless, it can easily go unnoticed. The sore lasts 3 to 6 weeks and heals regardless of whether the person is treated. However, if the infected person does not receive adequate treatment, the infection progresses to the secondary stage. Skin rashes and/or sores in the mouth, vagina, or anus (also called mucous membrane lesions) mark the secondary stage of symptoms. This stage usually starts with a rash on one or more areas of the body. Rashes associated with secondary syphilis can appear from the time when the primary sore is healing to several weeks after the sore has healed. The rash usually does not cause itching. This rash may appear as rough, red, or reddish brown spots both on the palms of the hands and/or the bottoms of the feet. However, this rash may look different on other parts of the body and can look like rashes caused by other diseases. The latent (hidden) stage of syphilis begins when primary and secondary symptoms disappear. Without treatment, the infected person can continue to have syphilis in their body, even though there are no signs or symptoms. This latent stage can last for years (CDC, *Fact sheet, syphilis*). Untreated early syphilis in pregnant women results in perinatal death in up to 40% of cases and, if acquired during the 4 years before pregnancy, can lead to infection of the fetus in 80% of cases (CDC, *Syphilis profiles, 2011*).

Syphilis cases had been declining significantly in the United States since reporting began in 1941. For example, the overall rate of primary and secondary syphilis in the United States had declined 90% between 1990 and 2000. However, the syphilis rate in the United States had increased each year from 2001 through 2008. Once again, the overall rate of syphilis infection has been falling since 2008. In 2010, the overall rate decreased for the first time in 10 years, and the rate of primary and secondary syphilis in 2011 remained unchanged from 2010 at 4.5 cases per 100,000 population. Nonetheless, this overall steady trend masks declining infections among women and increases among men, particularly gay and bisexual men. Trend data available for the first time show that MSM now account for nearly three-quarters (72%) of all primary and secondary syphilis cases. During 2010 to 2011, the number of cases of early latent syphilis reported to the CDC decreased 3.4%, and the number of cases of late latent syphilis increased 2.7% (from 18,079 cases to 18,576) (CDC, 2012b). After an 18% increase in the rate of congenital syphilis between 2006 and 2008, the rate of congenital syphilis decreased during 2008 to 2011 (from 10.5 to 8.5 cases per 100,000 live births). In 2011, a total of 360 cases were reported, a decrease from 387 cases in 2010 and 429 cases in 2009. This recent decrease in the rate of congenital syphilis is associated with the decrease in the rate of primary and secondary syphilis among women that has occurred since 2008 (CDC, 2012b), but rates of congenital syphilis remained higher than the *Healthy People 2010* objective of 1/100,000 live births (USDHHS, 2000).

Penicillin G, administered parenterally, is the preferred drug for treatment of all stages of syphilis. The preparation or preparations used (i.e., benzathine, aqueous procaine, or aqueous crystalline), the dosage, and the length of treatment depend on the stage and clinical manifestations of the disease. Selection of the appropriate penicillin preparation is important, because *T. pallidum* can reside in sequestered sites (e.g., the CNS and aqueous humor) that are poorly accessed by some forms of penicillin. Parenteral penicillin G is the only therapy with documented efficacy for syphilis during pregnancy. Pregnant women with syphilis in any stage who report penicillin allergy should be desensitized and treated with penicillin (CDC, 2010).

Doxycycline and tetracycline are recommended alternative therapy for syphilis in nonpregnant patients with a penicillin allergy; however, the U.S. FDA reported that doxycycline was available in limited supply and tetracycline was unavailable (CDC, *Doxycycline and tetracycline shortage update*).

Because effective treatment is available, it is important that people be screened for syphilis on an ongoing basis if their sexual behaviors put them at risk for STDs. People who are diagnosed and treated for syphilis must abstain from sexual contact until the syphilitic sores are completely healed. All persons who have syphilis should be tested for HIV infection. In geographic areas in which the prevalence of HIV is high, persons who have primary syphilis should be retested for HIV after 3 months if the first HIV test result was negative. Reinfection can occur; syphilitic sores may not be detected because they may be hidden in the vagina, rectum, or mouth (CDC, *Syphilis profiles*, 2011).

EVIDENCE FOR PRACTICE

The USPSTF strongly recommends that clinicians screen people at increased risk for syphilis infection; this includes MSM, commercial sex workers, people who exchange sex for drugs, and people in correctional facilities. Also, the USPSTF strongly recommends that all pregnant women be screened for syphilis infection (USPSTF, 2004, 2009).

Human Papillomavirus

Genital HPV infection is one of the most common causes of STDs in the world. It is estimated that 100% of sexually active men and women acquire genital HPV infection at some point in their lives. With an estimated annual incidence of 14.1 million cases, the CDC estimates that HPV accounts for the majority of newly acquired STIs in the United States. There is an estimated $1.7 billion annual cost in direct medical costs to treat conditions associated with genital HPV infection (e.g., warts, cervical dysplasia, cancer). An estimated 79 million women aged 14 to 59 years are infected with HPV, with the highest prevalence in those between the ages of 20 and 24 years. While the vast majority (90%) of HPV infections will go away on their own within 2 years and cause no harm, some of these infections will take hold and potentially lead to serious disease, including cervical cancer. Although rare, genital HPV infection with low-risk types can be transmitted from mother to newborn during delivery and can cause respiratory tract warts in the child, known as juvenile-onset recurrent respiratory papillomatosis (CDC, *CDC curriculum HPV*).

More than 100 types of HPV exist, more than 40 of which can infect the genital area. Genital HPV types are divided into two groups: low-risk types and high-risk types. Low-risk (nononcogenic) types can cause genital warts and benign or low-grade cellular changes (e.g., mild Pap test abnormalities), but are not associated with increased risk of cancer. High-risk (oncogenic) types can cause cervical dysplasia (both low-grade and high-grade cervical cellular changes), moderate to severe Pap test abnormalities, and, in rare cases, cancers of the cervix. In addition, these types of HPV infection have been associated with cancers of the vulva, vagina, anus, penis, and oropharynx. Infection is predominantly associated with sexual activity, including vaginal and anal intercourse, oral sex, and nonpenetrative sexual activity (genital–genital contact); therefore, it requires contact with viable HPV and microtrauma to skin or mucous membranes to establish infection, but transmission can occur from asymptomatic and subclinically infected persons. The natural history of HPV infection is usually benign. Low-risk genital HPV types are associated with mild Pap test abnormalities and genital warts. High-risk types are associated with mild to severe Pap test abnormalities, and rarely, cancers of the cervix, vulva, vagina, anus, penis, and oropharynx. Most women infected with HPV infection do not develop cervical cancer. Recurrence of genital warts within the first several months after treatment is common (CDC, *curriculum HPV*).

A free HPV testing toolkit that can help practicing clinicians effectively implement HPV testing in their practice for patients at risk has been developed by the National Association of Nurse Practitioners in Women's Health (National Association of Nurse Practitioners in Women's Health, *HPV* Toolkit). Also, two HPV vaccines are licensed in the United States. The bivalent vaccine (HPV2), Cervarix, protects against two HPV types (16 and 18), which are responsible for 70% of cervical cancers. The quadrivalent vaccine (HPV4), Gardasil, protects against four HPV types (6, 11, 16, 18), which are responsible for 70% of cervical cancers (16 and 18) and 90% of genital warts (6 and 11). The CDC recommends that all teenage girls and women through age 26 receive HPV vaccines, as well as all teenage boys and men through age 21 (and through age 26 for gay, bisexual, and MSM). Also, immunocompromised persons (including those with HIV infection) should be vaccinated through age 26 years. Neither vaccine is recommended for persons over age 26. Ideally, the vaccines should be administered before onset of sexual activity (CDC, *curriculum HPV*; CDC, *STI fact sheet*).

Treatment of warts or cervical cellular abnormalities may reduce, but likely does not eliminate infectiousness of HPV. Most genital HPV infections, whether caused by low-risk or high-risk types, are transient, asymptomatic, and have no clinical consequences. CDC-recommended patient-applied and provider-administered treatment regimens are available. Choice of treatment should be guided by location of the lesion(s), patient preference, experience of the healthcare provider, available resources, and pregnancy status. Healthcare providers should identify warts for patient-applied treatment and teach patients how to apply substances. Patient-applied treatments consist of podofilox 0.5% solution or gel, imiquimod 5% cream, or sinecatechins 15% ointment. Podofilox, an antimitotic drug that destroys warts, is relatively inexpensive, easy to use, and safe. Imiquimod 5% cream is a topically active immune enhancer that stimulates production of interferon and other cytokines. The safety of podofilox, imiquimod, and sinecatechins during pregnancy has not been established. Also, the safety of sinecatechins has not been established in HIV- or HSV-coinfected individuals. CDC-recommended provider-administered regimens for external genital warts include cryotherapy with liquid nitrogen or cryoprobe, podophyllin resin 10% to 25% in compound tincture of benzoin, trichloroacetic acid (TCA) or bichloroacetic acid (BCA) 80% to 90%, or surgical removal (CDC, *curriculum HPV*).

Human Immunodeficiency Virus

HIV is a retrovirus that infects cells of the human immune system, impairing and destroying their function. Symptoms may be absent in the early stages of infection. However, as the infection progresses, the immune system becomes more compromised, and the person becomes more susceptible to opportunistic infections. In addition, HIV infection increases the risk of reactivation of latent TB (CDC, *HIV and tuberculosis*). The most advanced stage of HIV infection is AIDS (stage 3). It can take 10 to 15 years for an HIV-infected person to develop AIDS, but antiretroviral therapy (ART) can slow down the process even further. Before the highly active ART (HAART) era, the median time from HIV seroconversion to the development of AIDS was 7.7 to 11.0 years, with a median survival rate from 7.5 to 12 years. These effective drug therapies keep HIV-infected persons healthy longer and significantly reduced the death rate in 20 years by 50%. AIDS is now considered a chronic and controlled disease. Therefore, the number of people living with HIV is increasing in countries where HAART treatment is available (Gonzalo, García Goñi, & Muñoz-Fernández, 2009). Still, the global burden of HIV/AIDS remains grim (Table 14.1).

table 14.1 **Estimates of People Affected by Global HIV/AIDS Epidemic, End of 2010**

HIV/AIDS Epidemic 2010	Estimate
People living with HIV/AIDS	34 million
Adults living with HIV/AIDS	30.6 million
Women living with HIV/AIDS	15.3 million
Children living with HIV/AIDS	3.4 million
People newly infected with HIV	2.7 million
Children newly infected with HIV	369,000
AIDS-related deaths in adults and children	1.8 million

More than 30 million people have died of AIDS since 1981.
Africa has more than 15 million AIDS orphans.
At the end of 2010, women accounted for 50% of all adults living with HIV worldwide.
Most countries aspire to expand antiretroviral treatment access to around 80% of those in need. However, this target has not been met, with current global treatment coverage at 54%.
Source: UNAIDS/WHO. *AIDS epidemic statistics 2010*. Retrieved April 30, 2013, from http://www.avert.org/worldstats.htm#.http://www.avert.org/worldstats.htm#

The WHO reports that the number of people living with HIV worldwide has risen from 29.4 million in 2001 to an estimated 34 million (prevalence: 0.8) in 2011, an increase of 16% (Fig. 14.6). These data are beginning to stabilize at this unacceptably high level, and reflect not only the numbers of people newly infected with HIV, but the prevalence of all

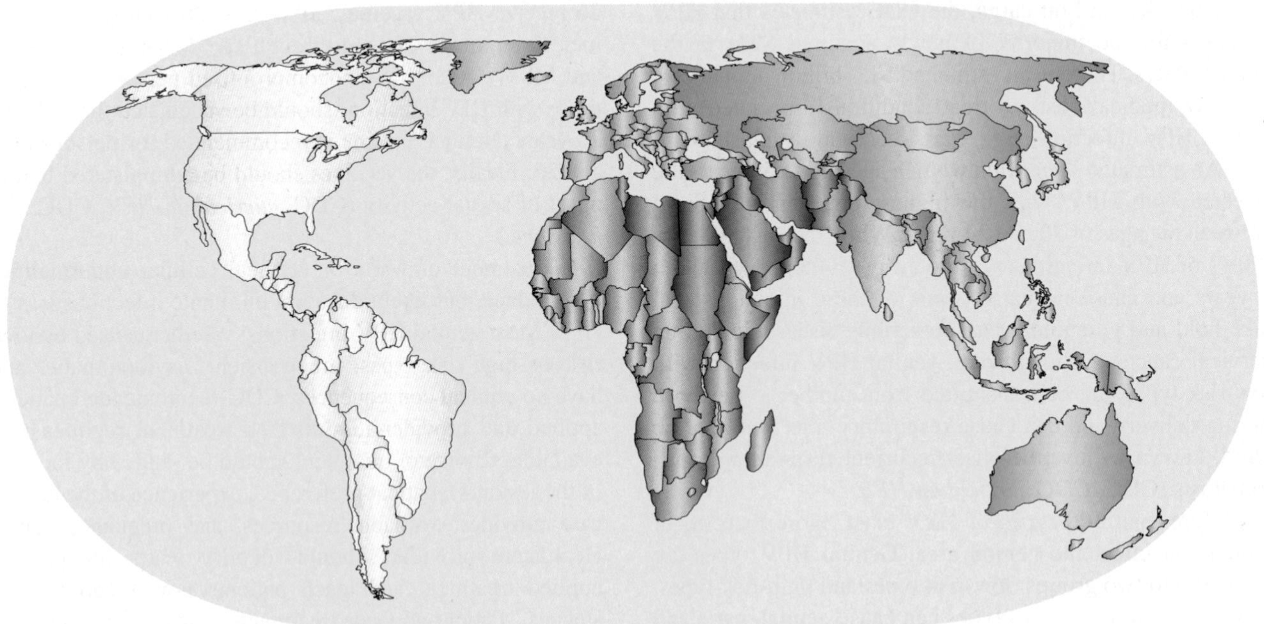

figure 14.6 Adults and children estimated to be living with HIV, 2011, by WHO region. (Data from http://www.who.int/gho/hiv/epidemic_status/cases_all/en/index.html)

cases of HIV due in part to the expanded access to ART, which has helped to reduce the number of people dying from AIDS-related causes. Sub-Saharan Africa still bears a disproportionate share of the global HIV burden. Although the rate of new HIV infections has decreased in this region, the total number of people living with HIV continues to rise. In 2011, that number reached 23.5 million, or 69% of the global total (WHO, *Number of people living with HIV*).

HIV targets predominantly young and middle-aged adults who are the mainstay of the economy and the principal support of their families. As the loss of productive people in a society gradually increases, poverty also increases; there are fewer resources to cope with the situation, and fewer options for change whether at family, community, or national level. Economic growth is compromised, and the very fabric of society can be destroyed (CDC, *Global HIV/AIDS*).

The CDC estimates that more than 1.2 million people in the United States are living with HIV infection, and almost one in five (18.1%) are unaware of their infection. Gay, bisexual, and other MSM are most seriously affected by HIV. The estimated incidence of HIV has remained stable overall in recent years, at about 50,000 new HIV infections per year. Within the overall estimates, however, some groups are affected more than others. MSM continue to bear the greatest burden of HIV infection, and among races/ethnicities, African-Americans continue to be disproportionately affected. In addition, the CDC estimates that one in four new HIV infections in the United States occur in youth at ages 13 to 24 years, and about 60% of all youth with HIV do not know they are infected. The risk for HIV for most young people begins when they start having sex or start injecting drugs (CDC, *Vital signs, HIV among youth in the US*). Those who are infected with HIV and are unaware of their HIV status may unknowingly be transmitting the virus to others, as well as putting themselves at risk for AIDS (CDC, *HIV/AIDS in the United States*).

> *As for AIDS, it's a plague. We are human, we get plagues. They come along every so often, kill off two-thirds of the population; in the next generation it's a quarter; after that it's a childhood disease.*
>
> **Larry Niven**

From 2008 through 2011, the annual estimated rate of diagnoses of HIV infection in the United States remained stable, with the estimated rate in 2011 at 15.8. Although the infection rate among males remained stable, surveillance data from 2008 through 2011 indicate that the rates for persons aged 20 to 29 increased, with males accounting for 79% of all diagnoses of HIV infection among adults and adolescents. The increased number of HIV infections among adult and adolescent males attributed to male-to-male sexual contact (including male-to-male sexual contact *and* injection drug use) and those attributed to heterosexual contact accounted for approximately 92% of diagnosed HIV infections in the United States. The rate of diagnosed HIV infections among adult and adolescent females and for all persons aged 30 to 49 and 55 to 64 years decreased. The numbers of HIV infections attributed to injection drug use and to heterosexual contact among adult and adolescent females also decreased. The rates remained stable for children (aged less than 13 years) and persons aged 13 to 19, 50 to 54, and 65 and older (CDC, 2013b).

From 2008 through 2011, the annual estimated rate of infections classified as AIDS (stage 3) in the United States remained stable, with an estimated rate of 10.3 in 2011. Although the rate of infections classified as AIDS for males remained stable in 2011, adult and adolescent males accounted for 75% of all infections classified as stage 3 among adults and adolescents, with the annual increased number of cases attributed to male-to-male sexual contact. The number of infections classified as stage 3 among adult and adolescent females with HIV infection attributed to injection drug use decreased; however, the number with infection attributed to heterosexual contact remained stable (CDC, 2013b). Healthy People 2020 covers 42 topic areas and has nearly 600 objectives; 18 of these objectives are focused on HIV. A major objective in this category is to increase the *Proportion of Persons Living with HIV Who Know Their Serostatus* (Objective HIV-13) (CDC, *Healthy People 2020 leading health indicators: Objective HIV-13*).

HIV is spread by unprotected sexual contact with an infected person, by sharing needles and/or syringes with someone who is infected, or, very rarely in countries where blood is not screened for HIV antibodies, through transfusions of infected blood or blood clotting factors. Also, infants born to HIV-infected women may become infected before or during birth or through breast-feeding after birth (CDC, *HIV/AIDS Fact Sheets*). There are many misconceptions about HIV transmission. Scientists and medical authorities agree that HIV does not survive well in the environment, making the possibility of environmental transmission remote. HIV is not transmitted through insects or insect bites. There is no known risk of HIV transmission to coworkers, clients, or consumers from incidental contact in industries such as food-service establishments. Although HBV has been transmitted through tattooing or body piercing, HIV has not been transmitted in this manner. Casual contact through closed-mouth or "social" kissing is not a risk factor for transmission of HIV. The CDC recommends against engaging in "French" or open-mouth kissing with a person known to be infected, although the risk of acquiring HIV in this manner is believed to be very low. Contact with saliva, tears, or sweat has never been shown to result in transmission of HIV. Biting is a risk factor only when there is severe trauma with extensive tissue tearing and damage and presence of blood (CDC, *HIV transmission*). Box 14.7 presents guidelines for prevention of exposure to the blood of persons who are HIV infected, at risk for HIV infection, or whose infection and risk status are unknown.

Strategies for preventing infection with HIV emphasize testing to identify infected people and ensuring access to appropriate medical care, treatment, and prevention

box 14.7 Measures for Preventing HIV Exposure and Transmission When Caring for an Infected Person

Wear gloves during contact with blood or other body fluids such as urine, feces, or vomit.
Cover cuts, sores, or breaks on both the caregiver's and the patient's exposed skin with a bandage.
Wash hands and other parts of the body immediately after contact with blood or other body fluids.
Disinfect surfaces soiled with blood with a bleach solution.
Avoid practices that increase the likelihood of blood contact, such as sharing of razors and toothbrushes.
Use and dispose of needles and other sharp instruments appropriately.

services. The only way to know whether someone has HIV infection is to be tested for HIV. To increase awareness of HIV status, the CDC established its Expanded Testing Initiative, which is aimed at (1) significantly increasing the number of persons tested in jurisdictions with a high rate of HIV among disproportionately affected populations, and (2) supporting implementation of the *revised recommendations for HIV testing of adults, adolescents, and pregnant women in healthcare settings* (CDC, *Expanded Testing Program*). The CDC *Revised Recommendations for HIV Testing* advocates routine voluntary HIV screening as a normal part of clinical practice *and are targeted to* subpopulations of persons at higher risk for HIV, typically defined on the basis of behavior, clinical, or demographic characteristics. The revised recommendations *include* HIV screening for persons aged 13 to 64 years in all healthcare settings (e.g., hospitals, acute-care clinics, and STD clinics) after the patient is notified that testing will be performed, unless he/she declines (opt-out screening), HIV screening in the routine panel of prenatal screening for all pregnant women after the patient is notified that testing will be performed, unless she declines (opt-out screening), and patients initiating treatment for TB (CDC, 2006).

HIV infection can be diagnosed by serologic tests that detect antibodies against HIV-1 and HIV-2 and by virologic tests that can detect HIV antigens. Antibody testing begins with a sensitive screening test (e.g., the conventional or rapid enzyme immunoassay [EIA]). Currently available serologic tests are both highly sensitive and specific and can detect all known subtypes of HIV-1. Most also can detect HIV-2 and uncommon variants of HIV-1. The advent of HIV rapid serologic testing has enabled clinicians to make an accurate presumptive diagnosis of HIV infection within half an hour, which could potentially facilitate the identification of the approximately 250,000 persons estimated to be living with undiagnosed HIV in the United States. In addition to screening, prevention counseling should be offered and encouraged in all healthcare facilities that serve patients at high risk (e.g., STD clinics), because these facilities routinely gather information that places persons at high risk for HIV. Prevention counseling need not be explicitly linked to HIV testing. However, some patients might be more likely to think about HIV and consider their risk-related behavior when undergoing an HIV test. HIV testing presents an excellent opportunity to provide prevention counseling to assist with behavior changes to reduce the risk for acquiring HIV infection (CDC, *HIV infection: Detection, counseling, and referral*). In addition to the strategies outlined above, barriers to HIV prevention and screening programs can be eliminated by making these programs culturally sensitive. Box 14.8 presents *Healthy People 2020* objectives for HIV infection.

box 14.8 *Healthy People 2020* Objectives for HIV

Diagnosis of HIV Infection and AIDS

(Developmental) Reduce new HIV diagnoses among adolescents and adults.
(Developmental) Reduce new (incident) HIV infections among adolescents and adults.
Reduce the rate of HIV transmission among adolescents and adults.
Reduce new AIDS cases among adolescents and adults.
Reduce new AIDS cases among adolescent and adult heterosexuals.
Reduce new AIDS cases among adolescent and adult men who have sex with men.
Reduce new AIDS cases among adolescents and adults who inject drugs.
Reduce perinatally acquired HIV and AIDS cases.

Death, Survival, and Medical Healthcare after Diagnosis

(Developmental) Increase the proportion of new HIV infections diagnosed before progression to AIDS.
(Developmental) Increase the proportion of HIV-infected adolescents and adults who receive HIV care and treatment consistent with current standards.
Increase the proportion of persons surviving more than 3 years after a diagnosis with AIDS.
Reduce deaths from HIV infection.

HIV Testing

Increase the proportion of persons living with HIV who know their serostatus.
Increase the proportion of adolescents and adults who have been tested for HIV in the past 12 months.
Increase the proportion of adults with tuberculosis (TB) who have been tested for HIV.

HIV Prevention

Increase the proportion of substance abuse treatment facilities that offer HIV/AIDS education, counseling, and support.
Increase the proportion of sexually active persons who use condoms.
(Developmental) Reduce the proportion of men who have sex with men (MSM) who reported unprotected anal sex in the past 12 months.

Source: U.S. Department of Health and Human Services. *Healthy People 2020 HIV objectives*. Retrieved 29, 2013, from http://healthypeople.gov/2020/topicsobjectives2020/objectiveslist.aspx?topicId=22

HIV does not make people dangerous to know, so you can shake their hands and give them a hug: Heaven knows they need it.

Princess Diana

In **Case 2**, when Megan was seen by the nurse practitioner, a rapid HIV test was performed. The results were negative. What primary prevention measures would you recommend?

Caring for the HIV/AIDS patient in the community is a challenge. Because the disease is chronic and there is no cure, infected people continue to live, work, and socialize as they normally have in the past. However, appropriately timed interventions in HIV-positive persons can reduce risks for clinical progression, complications or death from the disease, and HIV transmission.

EVIDENCE FOR PRACTICE

In 2006, the USPSTF strongly recommended HIV screening for all adolescents and adults at increased risk for HIV infection. This includes MSM; men and women having unprotected sex with multiple partners; past or present injection drug users; men and women who exchange sex for money or drugs; individuals whose sex partners were HIV infected, bisexual, or injection drug users; people being treated for STDs; people who have had a blood transfusion between 1978 and 1985; and those people who request a HIV test despite reporting no individual risk factors. In addition, the USPSTF also recommended that clinicians screen all pregnant women for HIV (AHRQ, 2006).

However, in its 2012 draft revised *Recommendation Statement*, the USPSTF strongly recommends that clinicians screen all people aged 15 to 65 years for HIV infection. It also recommends HIV screening for all pregnant women, including those who present at the time of labor, and for younger adolescents and older adults who are at increased risk (USPSTF, *Screening for HIV: draft recommendation statement)*.

Other Sexually Transmitted Diseases

HERPES SIMPLEX VIRUS

There are two types of herpes simplex virus (HSV), both of which can cause genital herpes. HSV type 1 (HSV-1) most commonly causes sores on the lips (known as fever blisters or cold sores), but it also can cause genital infections. HSV-2 most often causes genital sores, but it also can infect the mouth. The CDC estimates that 16.2% of persons aged 14 to 49 years in the United States have HSV infection, but the overall prevalence is likely higher than 16.2%, because an increasing number of genital herpes infections are caused by HSV-1. HSV-2 infection is more common among women than among men (21% vs. 12%), and is more common among non-Hispanic Blacks (39%) than among non-Hispanic Whites (12%). This disparity remains even among persons with similar numbers of lifetime sexual partners (e.g., two to four partners). Annually, 776,000 people in the United States acquire new herpes infections. While the percentage of persons in the United States who were infected with HSV-2 decreased from 21% in 1994 to 17% by 2004, HSV-2 prevalence has changed very little since 2004, and increases in genital HSV-1 infections have been found in patient populations worldwide (CDC, *Fact sheet: genital herpes*).

Most individuals infected with HSV-1 or HSV-2 are asymptomatic, or have very mild symptoms that are mistaken for another skin condition. As a result, 81% of infected individuals remain unaware of their infection. Generally, HSV-2 infection is transmitted during sexual contact with someone who has a genital HSV-2 infection, and most commonly occurs from an infected partner who does not have a visible sore and may not know that he or she is infected. The average incubation period after exposure is four days (range, 2–12). The vesicles break and leave painful ulcers that may take 2 to 4 weeks to heal. Experiencing these symptoms is referred to as having an "outbreak," or episode. Although the infection can stay in the body indefinitely, the number of outbreaks tends to decrease over time. Recurrences are much less frequent for genital HSV-1 infection than for genital HSV-2 infection. Genital ulcerative disease caused by herpes makes it easier to transmit and acquire HIV infection sexually. There is an estimated two- to fourfold increased risk of acquiring HIV, if exposed to virus when genital herpes is present. Type-specific HSV tests may be useful among persons with HIV infection and MSM at increased risk for HIV acquisition. Healthcare providers should also screen pregnant women if they have a history of genital herpes, as the virus can be passed from mother to child, resulting in a potentially fatal infection (neonatal herpes), one of the most serious complications of genital herpes. However, the CDC does not recommend screening for HSV-1 or HSV-2 in the general population (CDC, *Fact sheet: Genital herpes*).

HEPATITIS VIRUSES

In 2009, an estimated 38,000 persons in the United States were newly infected with HBV, for an estimated incidence of 1.5 cases per 100,000 population, the lowest ever recorded. However, because many HBV infections are either asymptomatic or never reported, the actual number of new infections was estimated to be approximately 10-fold higher. Rates were highest among adults, particularly males aged 25 to 44 years (CDC, *Hepatitis B information for health professionals*).

Hepatitis B viral infection becomes an STD when it is transmitted through mucosal contact with infectious blood or body fluids (e.g., semen, saliva) during sex with an infected partner. Those at increased risk of becoming infected with HBV include sexually active persons who are not in a long-term, mutually monogamous relationship (e.g., more than one sex partner during the previous 6 months) and MSM. Although 95% of adults recover completely from HBV infection and do not become chronically infected, 15% become chronically infected and die prematurely from cirrhosis or liver cancer; the majority remain asymptomatic until onset of cirrhosis or end-stage liver disease. In the United States, chronic HBV infection results in an estimated 2,000 to 4,000 deaths per year. Therefore, the Advisory Committee on Immunization Practices recommends that hepatitis B vaccination also include the following:

- Susceptible sex partners of hepatitis B surface antigen (HBsAg)–positive persons
- Sexually active persons who are not in a long-term, mutually monogamous relationship
- Persons seeking evaluation or treatment for an STD
- Men who have sex with men (CDC, *Hepatitis B information for health professionals*).

In addition to hepatitis B, other types of hepatitis viruses, such as hepatitis C and D, can be transmitted sexually; however, sexual transmission is not the primary means of spread as with HBV.

PREVENTION AND CONTROL OF SPECIFIC INFECTIOUS DISEASES

Nurses can intervene in the infectious process through primary, secondary, and tertiary prevention strategies that address the specific characteristics and transmission patterns of the infectious agents. Methods of prevention make it possible to reduce the risk of exposure. The use of vaccines can reduce the risk of infection before exposure to an infectious agent; this is termed primary prevention. The CDC recommends vaccinations for children, adolescents, and adults. The latest recommendations for vaccination can be found at the CDC website: http://www.cdc.gov/vaccines/schedules/. Postexposure prophylaxis can reduce the risk of an infectious disease after exposure, if the prophylactic treatment is provided shortly after the exposure; this is called secondary prevention. An example of tertiary prevention is treating opportunistic infections among HIV-infected adults and adolescents. The CDC periodically updates its guidelines for treating opportunistic infections. The latest guidelines can be found at the CDC website. Chapters 5 and 6 discuss the natural history of disease and the levels of prevention (primary, secondary, and tertiary) that are appropriate to each stage of the illness.

PRACTICE POINT

Nurses can reduce the risk of infection through primary and secondary prevention measures that are specific to the characteristics of the infectious disease. For example, use of insect repellants and wearing light-colored long pants tucked inside socks is a primary prevention measure for tick-borne Lyme disease. Examining a "bull's eye" lesion, prescribing antibiotics, and performing ELISA testing of serum at a later date are secondary prevention measures.

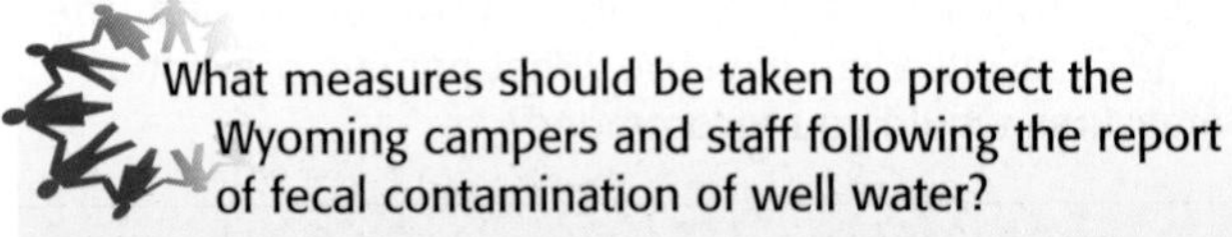

What measures should be taken to protect the Wyoming campers and staff following the report of fecal contamination of well water?

Prevention of Food-borne Diseases

Making food safe is a major undertaking, involving all steps in moving from the farm or fishery to the table. Many different organizations and regulatory agencies are involved in preventing or limiting food contamination. Consumers can do their part by purchasing foods that have been processed for safety, such as juices and ciders that have been pasteurized. *Basics for Handling Food Safely*, guidelines for shopping, storage, preparation, thawing, cooking, serving, handling leftovers, and refreezing food safely can be found at the United States Department of Agriculture Food Safety and Inspection Service website. Other precautions include good handwashing after handling raw eggs, meat and poultry, pets, and farm animals. Also, use soap and hot water to wash utensils and other surfaces that might have come in contact with raw or undercooked meat, poultry, or eggs (CDC, *Food safety*). Consumers should be advised to avoid eating fresh produce irrigated with water of unknown quality. Illnesses that primarily cause diarrhea or vomiting can lead to dehydration if the person loses more electrolytes than he or she takes in. Replacing lost fluids and electrolytes and keeping up with fluid intake are important. Medical treatment is necessary for a diarrheal illness that is accompanied by fever (temperature of more than 101.5°F), prolonged vomiting, bloody stools, or dehydration.

Prevention of Waterborne Diseases

It is important to know where drinking water comes from, how it has been treated, and if it is safe to drink (e.g., a septic tank should not be too close to a private well). Although most community water systems use groundwater for their water supply, more people actually depend on community water systems that use surface water. Community water systems supply water to the same population year-round. Transient noncommunity water systems provide water to 25 or more people for at least 60 days/year, but not to the same people and not on a regular basis (e.g., campgrounds).

The EPA has published guidelines for microbiologic water quality for recreational freshwater (e.g., lakes and rivers) and marine water, which set the monthly water quality indicators for such venues (EPA, *Water quality standards for surface water*). States have latitude regarding their guidelines or regulations and can post warning signs to alert potential bathers until water quality improves. Unlike treated areas, where disinfection can be used to address most problems with the microbiologic quality of water, contaminated freshwater can require weeks or months to improve or return to normal. However, swimming pools might need to be closed until the water has been adequately treated and filtered or the swimming pool drained and refilled to remove contamination. Prompt identification of potential sources of contamination and remedial action are necessary to return bathing water to an appropriate quality for recreational use.

Swallowing, breathing, or having contact with contaminated water from swimming pools, spas, lakes, rivers, or oceans spreads recreational water illnesses. Contamination of recreational water can be avoided when nurses educate the public to remember the following:

- Do not swim if you have diarrhea.
- Do not swallow the pool water.
- Wash hands with soap and water after using the restroom or changing diapers.
- Take children to the bathroom often. Change diapers in the bathroom and not at poolside.
- Wash children thoroughly with soap and water before swimming (CDC, *12 Steps for prevention of recreational water illnesses*).

Prevention of Sexually Transmitted Infections

At the time of the 1997 Institute of Medicine (IOM) report, *The Hidden Epidemic: Confronting Sexually Transmitted Diseases*, an effective national system for STD prevention did not exist in the United States. However, the CDC's efforts to implement the recommendations of the IOM 1997 report resulted in the development of Comprehensive STD Prevention Systems and publication of the STD Program Operation Guidelines. The purpose of the guidelines is to further STD prevention by providing a resource to assist in the design, implementation, and evaluation of STD prevention and control programs. The target audience for the guidelines is public health personnel and other persons involved in managing STD prevention programs (CDC, *Program operations guidelines for STD prevention*).

STDs are among the leading causes of morbidity and mortality in the United States. They affect men and women of all backgrounds and economic levels, and account for substantial healthcare spending. With nearly 19 million new STDs occurring each year, almost half of them among young people aged 15 to 24, prevention of STDs is more important than ever. Anticipated advances in health reform in the United States present opportunities to focus on prevention and wellness and support the development of national strategies to improve the nation's health through evidence-based clinical and community prevention and wellness activities. The updated 2010 CDC *Guidelines for the Treatment of Sexually Transmitted Diseases* (CDC, 2010) integrates recommendations on the most effective treatment regimens, screening procedures, and prevention strategies for STDs. The CDC revised these guidelines in 2012, based on scientific evidence-based review (CDC, 2012c).

key concepts

- The epidemiology of the infectious disease process adds other elements to the epidemiologic triad (agent, host, environment): a portal of exit for the infectious agent, a means of transmission, and a portal of entry to a new host.
- The environment/reservoirs of infectious agents can be humans, animals (zoonotic), plants, insects, water, and soil.
- Mechanisms of transmission of an infectious agent from one host to another include direct contact, indirect contact, droplets, and airborne transmission.
- An infectious disease may or may not be contagious or communicable.
- An epidemic refers to a significant increase in an infection or infectious disease beyond the expected (endemic) level in a certain population and/or geographic area.
- Nurses play an important role in the prevention of healthcare-associated infections and represent the first line of defense for such adverse outcomes.
- The CDC is a major agency that protects the nation's health by developing guidelines that promote health and quality of life by preventing and controlling disease, injury, and disability. It also maintains surveillance systems to analyze data for infectious disease trends and outbreaks.
- Food-borne illnesses include biological and nonbiological agents and can be caused by microorganisms and their toxins.
- Waterborne illnesses are associated with drinking water and recreational water.
- STDs are among the leading causes of morbidity and mortality in the United States.
- The CDC reports indicate that 18% of persons infected with HIV are not aware that they are infected.
- HPV is one of the most common causes of STD in the world and can lead to cancer of the cervix in women.
- The CDC provides an effective system for STD prevention to assist community/public health professionals in the design, implementation, and evaluation of STD prevention and control programs.

critical thinking questions

1. An outbreak of hepatitis A has been reported. As a general rule, the unit of time used in an outbreak investigation is roughly one-fourth (0.25) of the average incubation period for the illness under investigation.
   a. Draw an epidemic curve using the data below.
   b. Given that the incubation period for hepatitis A is 28 to 30 days, what intervals would you use on the *x*-axis?
   c. Was this a common source or propagated outbreak?

Case number	Date of onset
1	12/13
2	1/5
3	1/6
4	1/8
5	1/9
7	1/10
8	1/20

2. A public health nurse is asked to investigate contacts of an identified TB case. Prioritize screening of the following contacts:
   a. Classmates of the case patient
   b. All students in the school the case patient attends
   c. Household/family members of the case patient
3. There is a community project to decrease the incidence of STDs.
   a. What is a target population? Why?
   b. What are some key factors to consider in designing an STD prevention program?

references

Agency for Health Research and Quality, U.S Preventive Services Task Force. (2006). *The guide to clinical preventive services* (AHRQ Publication No. 06-0588, pp. 79–82).

Avert. *HIV and AIDS*. Retrieved April 14, 2013, from http://www.avert.org/worldstats.htm

Bolan, G. A., Sparling, P. F., & Wasserheit, J. N. (2012). The emerging threat of untreatable gonococcal infection. *New England Journal of Medicine*, 366, 485–487.

Burnet, F. M., & White, D. O. (1972). *Natural history of infectious disease* (4th ed.). New York, NY: Cambridge University Press.

Centers for Disease Control and Prevention. (2006). Revised recommendations for HIV testing of adults, adolescents, and pregnant women in health-care settings. *Morbidity and Mortality Weekly Report*, 55(RR14), 1–17.

Centers for Disease Control and Prevention. (2007). Brief report: Gastroenteritis among attendees at a summer camp, Wyoming, June–July 2006. *Morbidity and Mortality Weekly Report*, 56(15), 368–370.

Centers for Disease Control and Prevention. (2010). Sexually transmitted diseases treatment guidelines, 2010. *Morbidity and Mortality Weekly Report*, 59(RR-12), 1–116.

Centers for Disease Control and Prevention. (2011a). Compendium of measures to prevent disease associated with animals in public settings, 2011. *Morbidity and Mortality Weekly Report*, 60(RR04), 1–28.

Centers for Disease Control and Prevention. (2011b). Vital signs: Incidence and trends of infection with pathogens transmitted commonly through food—foodborne diseases active surveillance network, 10 U.S. sites, 1996–2010. *Morbidity and Mortality Weekly Report*, 60(22), 749–755.

Centers for Disease Control and Prevention. (2011c). Surveillance for waterborne disease outbreaks and other health events associated with recreational water—United States, 2007–2008. *Morbidity and Mortality Weekly Report*, 60(SS12), 1–32.

Centers for Disease Control and Prevention. (2011d). Cephalosporin susceptibility among Neisseria gonorrhoeae isolates—United States, 2000–2010. *Morbidity and Mortality Weekly Report*, 60(26), 873–877.

Centers for Disease Control and Prevention. (2012a). Vital signs: HIV infection, testing, and risk behaviors among youths—United States. *Morbidity and Mortality Weekly Report*, 61(47), 971–976.

Centers for Disease Control and Prevention. (2012b). *Sexually transmitted disease surveillance, 2011*. Atlanta, GA: U.S. Department of Health and Human Services.

Centers for Disease Control and Prevention. (2012c). Update to CDC's sexually transmitted diseases treatment guidelines: Oral cephalosporins no longer a recommended treatment for gonococcal infections. *Morbidity and Mortality Weekly Report*, 61(31), 590–594.

Centers for Disease Control and Prevention. (2012d). *Cephalosporin-resistant Neisseria gonorrhoeae public health response plan.* Atlanta, GA: U.S. Department of Health and Human Services.

Centers for Disease Control and Prevention. (2013a). Incidence and trends of infection with pathogens transmitted commonly through food—foodborne diseases active surveillance network, 10 U.S. sites, 1996–2012. *Morbidity and Mortality Weekly Report*, 62(15), 283–287.

Centers for Disease Control and Prevention. (2013b). *HIV surveillance report, 2011*. Atlanta, GA: U.S. Department of Health and Human Services.

Centers for Disease Control and Prevention. (2013c). *National center for emerging and zoonotic infectious diseases: Our work, our stories, 2011–2012*. Atlanta, GA: U.S. Department of Health and Human Services.

Centers for Disease Control and Prevention. *12 Steps for prevention of recreational water illnesses*. Retrieved April 17, 2013, from http://www.cdc.gov/healthywater/swimming/pools/twelve-steps-for-prevention-rwi.html

Centers for Disease Control and Prevention. *About CDC*. Retrieved April 8, 2013, from http://www.cdc.gov/aboutcdc.htm

Centers for Disease Control and Prevention. *Campylobacter*. Retrieved April 9, 2013, from http://www.cdc.gov/nczved/divisions/dfbmd/diseases/campylobacter/

Centers for Disease Control and Prevention. *CDC curriculum HPV*. Retrieved April 15, 2013, from http://www2a.cdc.gov/stdtraining/ready-to-use/hpv.htm

Centers for Disease Control and Prevention. *CDC global health partnerships*. Retrieved April 9, 2013, from http://www.cdc.gov/globalhealth/partnerships.htm

Centers for Disease Control and Prevention. *Chlamydia—CDC fact sheet*. Retrieved April 12, 2013, from http://www.cdc.gov/std/chlamydia/STDFact-chlamydia-detailed.htm

Centers for Disease Control and Prevention. *Chlamydia curriculum*. Retrieved April 12, 2013, from http://www.2a.cdc.gov/stdtraining/ready-to-use/chlamydia.html

Centers for Disease Control and Prevention. *Doxycycline and tetracycline shortage update*. Retrieved April 15, 2013, from http://www.cdc.gov/std/treatment/doxycyclineShortage.htm

Centers for Disease Control and Prevention. *E. coli (Escherichia coli)*. Retrieved April 4, 2013, from http://www.cdc.gov/ecoli/

Centers for Disease Control and Prevention. *Estimates of foodborne illness in the United States*. Retrieved April 8, 2013, from http://www.cdc.gov/foodborneburden/

Centers for Disease Control and Prevention. *Estimates of healthcare-associated infections*. Retrieved April 15, 2013, from http://www.cdc.gov/ncidod/dhqp/hai.html

Centers for Disease Control and Prevention. *Excite: Epidemiology in the classroom*. Retrieved April 5, 2013, from http://www.cdc.gov/excite/classroom/index.htm

Centers for Disease Control and Prevention. *Expanded testing program*. Retrieved April 17, 2013, from http://www.cdc.gov/hiv/resources/factsheets/HIV-ETP.htm

Centers for Disease Control and Prevention. *Fact sheet: Genital herpes* Retrieved April 19, 2013, from http://www.cdc.gov/std/Herpes/STDFact-Herpes.htm

Centers for Disease Control and Prevention. *Fact sheet: Syphilis*. Retrieved April 20, 2013, from http://www.cdc.gov/std/syphilis/STDFact-Syphilis-detailed.htm

Centers for Disease Control and Prevention. *FoodNet*. Retrieved April 17, 2013, from http://www.cdc.gov/foodnet/

Centers for Disease Control and Prevention. *Food safety*. Retrieved April 17, 2013, from http://www.cdc.gov/foodsafety/index.html

Centers for Disease Control and Prevention. *Fact sheet: genital herpes*. Retrieved April 19, 2013, from http://www.cdc.gov/std/Herpes/default.htm

Centers for Disease Control and Prevention.. *Global HIV/AIDS*. Retrieved April 16, 2013, from http://www.cdc.gov/globalaids/default.html

Centers for Disease Control and Prevention. *Global HIV/AIDS at CDC—our story*. Retrieved April 15, 2013, from http://www.cdc.gov/globalaids/Global-HIV-AIDS-at-CDC/default.html

Centers for Disease Control and Prevention. *Gonorrhea fact sheet*. Retrieved April 13, 2013, from http://www.cdc.gov/std/gonorrhea/STDFact-gonorrhea-detailed.htm

Centers for Disease Control and Prevention. *Hantavirus pulmonary syndrome (HPS)*. Retrieved April 4, 2013, from http://www.cdc.gov/hantavirus/hps/

Centers for Disease Control and Prevention. *Healthy people 2020 leading health indicators: Objective HIV-13*. Retrieved from http://www.cdc.gov/hiv/resources/factsheets/PDF/LHI-Factsheet-FINAL-6-26-12.pdf

Centers for Disease Control and Prevention. *Hepatitis B information for health professionals*. Retrieved April 19, 2013, from http://www.cdc.gov/hepatitis/HBV/HBVfaq.htm#overview

Centers for Disease Control and Prevention. *HIV and tuberculosis*. Retrieved April 15, 2013, from http://www.cdc.gov/hiv/resources/factsheets/hivtb.htm

Centers for Disease Control and Prevention. *HIV basic statistics*. Retrieved April 16, 2013, from http://www.cdc.gov/hiv/statistics/basics/ataglance.html

Centers for Disease Control and Prevention. *HIV in the United States: At a glance*. Retrieved April 13, 2013, from http://www.cdc.gov/hiv/statistics/basics/ataglance.html

Centers for Disease Control and Prevention. *HIV infection: Detection, counseling, and referral*. Retrieved April 17, 2013, from http://www.cdc.gov/std/treatment/2010/hiv.htm#detect

Centers for Disease Control and Prevention. *HIV transmission*. Retrieved April 17, 2013, from http://www.cdc.gov/hiv/resources/qa/transmission.htm

Centers for Disease Control and Prevention. *HIV/AIDS fact sheets*. Retrieved April 13, 2013, from http://www.cdc.gov/hiv/topics/surveillance/factsheets.htm

Centers for Disease Control and Prevention.. *HIV/AIDS in the U. S.* Retrieved April 12, 2013, from http://www.cdc.gov/hiv/resources/factsheets/us.htm

Centers for Disease Control and Prevention. *Legionella (Legionnaires' disease and Pontiac fever)*. Retrieved April 10, 2013, from http://www.cdc.gov/legionella/index.html

Centers for Disease Control and Prevention. *Listeria*. Retrieved April 9, 2013, from http://www.cdc.gov/listeria/index.html

Centers for Disease Control and Prevention. *Lyme disease*. Retrieved April 4, 2013, from http://www.cdc.gov/lyme

Centers for Disease Control and Prevention. *MRSA*. Retrieved April 7, 2013, from http://www.cdc.gov/mrsa/

Centers for Disease Control and Prevention. *List of selected multistate foodborne outbreak investigations*. Retrieved October 30, 2014, from http://www.cdc.gov/outbreaknet/outbreaks.html

Centers for Disease Control and Prevention. *Multistate fungal meningitis outbreak investigation*. Retrieved April 9, 2013, from http://www.cdc.gov/HAI/outbreaks/meningitis.html

Centers for Disease Control and Prevention. *Multistate outbreak of Salmonella Heidelberg infections linked to chicken*. Retrieved April 9, 2013, from http://www.cdc.gov/salmonella/heidelberg-02-13/index.html

Centers for Disease Control and Prevention. *Multistate outbreaks of human Salmonella infections linked to live poultry*. Retrieved May 2, 2013, from http://www.cdc.gov/salmonella/live-poultry-04-13/index.html

Centers for Disease Control and Prevention. *National healthcare safety network (NHSN) national HAI reports*. Retrieved April 6, 2013, from http://www.cdc.gov/hai/surveillance/nhsn_nationalreports.html

Centers for Disease Control and Prevention. *Necrotizing fasciitis*. Retrieved April 4, 2013, from http://www.cdc.gov/Features/NecrotizingFasciitis/

Centers for Disease Control and Prevention. *Norovirus*. Retrieved April 9, 2013, from http://www.cdc.gov/norovirus/index.html

Centers for Disease Control and Prevention. *Outbreak of Hantavirsus in Yosemite National Park*. Retrieved April 4, 2013, from http://www.cdc.gov/hantavirus/outbreaks/yosemite-national-park-2012.html

Centers for Disease Control and Prevention. *Program operations guidelines for STD prevention*. Retrieved April 17, 2013, from http://www.cdc.gov/std/program/partners.pdf

Centers for Disease Control and Prevention. *Salmonella*. Retrieved April 9, 2013, http://www.cdc.gov/salmonella/general/index.html

Centers for Disease Control and Prevention. *STI fact sheet*. Retrieved April 11, 2013, from http://www.cdc.gov/std/stats/STI-Estimates-Fact-Sheet-Feb-2013.pdf

Centers for Disease Control and Prevention. Syphilis profiles, 2011. Retrieved April 15, 2013, from http://www.cdc.gov/std/Syphilis2011/default.htm

Centers for Disease Control and Prevention. *The yellow book 2012*. Retrieved April 8, 2013, from http://wwwnc.cdc.gov/travel/page/yellowbook-2012-home.htm

Centers for Disease Control and Prevention. *Tracking infections in long-term care facilities*. Retrieved April 8, 2013, from http://www.cdc.gov/nhsn/LTC/

Centers for Disease Control and Prevention. *Trends in Foodborne Illness in the United States, 2012*. Retrieved April 18, 2013, from http://www.cdc.gov/features/dsFoodNet2012/index.html.

Centers for Disease Control and Prevention. *Updated CDC estimates of 2009 H1N1 influenza cases, hospitalizations and deaths in the*

references (continued)

United States, April 2009–April 10, 2010. Retrieved April 15, 2013, from http://www.cdc.gov/h1n1flu/estimates_2009_h1n1.htm

Centers for Disease Control and Prevention. *Vital signs (2012), HIV among youth in the US*. Retrieved April 17, 2013, from http://www.cdc.gov/vitalsigns/HIVAmongYouth/index.html

Department of Defense. *Global emerging infections system*. Retrieved April 8, 2013, from http://www.afhsc.mil/viewDocument?file=GEIS/GEISAnnRpt2010.pdf

Enserink, M. (2012). Public at last, H5N1 study offers insight into virus's possible path to pandemic. *Science*, 336, 1494–1497.

Environmental Protection Agency. *Water quality standards for surface water*. Retrieved April 30, 2013, from http://water.epa.gov/scitech/swguidance/standards/

Gonzalo, T., García Goñi, M., & Muñoz-Fernández, M. A. (2009). Socio-economic impact of antiretroviral treatment in HIV patients. An economic review of cost savings after introduction of HAART. *AIDS Reviews*, *11*(2), 79–90.

Heymann, D. L. (2008). *Control of communicable diseases manual* (19th ed.). Washington, DC: American Public Health Association.

Huppert, J. S., Taylor, R. G., St. Cyr, S., Hesse, E. A., & Reed, J. L. (2013). Point-of-care testing improves accuracy of STI care in an emergency department. Sexually Transmitted Infections, 89(6), 489–494.

Karlen, A. (1996). *Man and microbes: Disease and plagues in history and modern times*. New York, NY: Simon & Schuster.

Malpiedi, P. J., Peterson, K. D., Soe, M. M., Edwards, J. R., Scott, R. D., Wise, M. E., . . . McDonald, L. C. (2011). *National and state healthcare-associated infection standardized infection ratio report*. Retrieved April 6, 2013, from http://www.cdc.gov/hai/national-annual-sir/index.html

McKenzie, J. F., Pringer, R. R., & Kotecki, J. E. (2005). *An introduction to community health* (5th ed.). Boston, MA: Jones & Bartlett.

National Association of Nurse Practitioners in Women's Health. *HPV toolkit*. Retrieved April 15, 2013, from http://www.npwh.org/

National Center for Health Statistics. (2013). Births: Preliminary data for 2012. *National vital statistics reports*, 60(4). Atlanta, GA: U.S. Department of Health and Human Services.

Niven, L. *Quotes from Larry Niven*. Retrieved April 30, 2013, from http://www.brainyquote.com/quotes/authors/l/larry_niven.html

Porta, M. (Ed.). (2008). *A dictionary of epidemiology* (5th ed.). New York, NY: Oxford University Press.

Tang, J.W. (2008). We are legend. *Emerging Infectious Diseases*, 14(9). Retrieved from http://www.cdc.gov/EID/content/14/9/1420.htm

U.S. Department of Health and Human Services. (2000). *Healthy people 2010* (2nd ed.). With understanding and improving health and objectives for improving health. 2 Vols. Washington, DC: U.S. Government Printing Office.

U.S. Preventive Services Task Force. (2004). *Screening for syphilis infection*. Retrieved April 15, 2013, from http://www.uspreventiveservicestaskforce.org/3rduspstf/syphilis/syphilrs.htm

U.S. Preventive Services Task Force. (2009). *Screening for syphilis infection in pregnancy*. Retrieved April 15, 2013, from http://www.uspreventiveservicestaskforce.org/uspstf/uspssyphpg.htm

U.S. Preventive Services Task Force. (2011). *Ocular prophylaxis for gonococcal ophthalmia neonatorum*. Retrieved April 23, 2013, from http://www.uspreventiveservicestaskforce.org/uspstf/usps-gononew.htm

U.S. Preventive Services Task Force. (2013). *Screening for gonorrhea and chlamydia: Draft research plan*. (AHRQ Publication No. 13-05184-EF-5).

U.S. Department of Health and Human Services. *Healthcare-associated infections*. Retrieved April 6, 2013, from http://www.hhs.gov/ash/initiatives/hai/index.html

U.S. Preventive Services Task Force. *Screening for HIV: Draft recommendation statement* (AHRQ Publication No. 12-05173-EF-3). Retrieved April 20, 2013, from http://www.uspreventiveservicestaskforce.org/uspstf13/hiv/hivdraftrec.htm

World Health Organization. *CSR and global team*. Retrieved April 9, 2013, from http://www.who.int/csr/about/structure/en/

World Health Organization. *Number of people living with HIV*. Retrieved April 22, 2013, from http://www.who.int/gho/hiv/epidemic_status/cases_all_text/en/index.html

World Health Organization. *Pandemic (H1N1) 2009—update 112*. Retrieved April 9, 2013, from http://www.who.int/csr/don/2010_08_06/en/index.html

World Health Organization. (2008). *World health statistics, 2008*. Retrieved April 9, 2013, from http://www.who.int/whosis/whostat/EN_WHS08_Full.pdf

World Health Organization. (2013). *Cumulative number of confirmed human cases of avian influenza A (H5N1) reported to WHO as of March 2013*. Retrieved April 9, 2013, from http://www.who.int/influenza/human_animal_interface/EN_GIP_20130312CumulativeNumberH5N1cases.pdf

Zinsser, H. (1935). Rats, lice and history. *Dictionary of science quotations*. Retrieved April 10, 2013, from http://todayinsci.com/Z/Zinsser_Hans/ZinsserHans-Quotations.htm

suggested readings

Centers for Disease Control and Prevention. *Multistate outbreak of Shiga toxin-producing Escherichia coli O157:H7 infections linked to organic spinach and spring mix blend (final update)*. Retrieved April 10, 2013, from http://www.cdc.gov/ecoli/2012/O157H7-11-12/index.html

Centers for Disease Control and Prevention. *Multistate outbreak of Salmonella enteritidis infections linked to ground beef (finalupdate)*. Retrieved April 9, 2013, from http://www.cdc.gov/salmonella/enteritidis-07-12/index.html

Centers for Disease Control and Prevention. *STD curriculum: Gonorrhea*. Retrieved April 13, 2013, from http://www2a.cdc.gov/stdtraining/ready-to-use/gonorrhea.htm

Centers for Disease Control and Prevention. STDs today. Retrieved April 15, 2013, from http://www.cdcnpin.org/scripts/std/std.asp

Healthy People 2020. Retrieved April 8, 2013, from http://www.healthypeople.gov/2020/

U.S. Department of Health and Human Services. Healthy People 2020. Retrieved April 10, 2013, from http://www.healthypeople.gov/2020/

web resources

Please visit thePoint® for up-to-date Web resources on this topic.

CHAPTER 15

Emerging Infectious Diseases

Barbara A. Goldrick and Gail A. Harkness

FANTASTIC VOYAGE: INFLUENZA

Time to go! Time to go!
An influenza virus,
Hiding in saliva, buried in a cell,
Antibodies and T cells are coming.
Get out! But how?
Induce a sneeze? Kickstart a cough?
Ah yes, here we go...
Aahhh-choo! Freedom at last!
Where are we?
A quick look around
A hospital? I see children,
Very thin, sick children,
Must be the cancer ward.
No B cells or T cells—a virus paradise!
Let's travel, find a breeze and float.
Where's my next victim?
My previous young doctor host
Walking quickly away
Head down, embarrassed
Scolded by a nurse—where was his mask?
Too busy and careless, poor fool
He still serves me well, dragging me into his wake.
Here I go, following and floating
A door nearby opens—negative pressure!
In I go, but on a cancer ward,
This should be positive pressure!
To keep bugs out, not draw them in.
I cannot complain
All good for me, for now I can see
A young girl with leukemia
Sitting in bed, watching TV
Laughing, inhaling, bringing me close.
But wait, what's this? Her mother!
Opening the toilet door,
Even greater negative pressure in there.
And worse, wet surfaces glistening inside,
Cleaned by her mother with chlorhexidine.
No! Not yet! Not now! I'm so close!
Being pulled in. No escape. Falling, falling...
The young girl is laughing. Now her mother is too.

JT Tang, National University Hospital, Singapore

chapter highlights

- Emerging versus reemerging infectious diseases
- Factors that influence the emergence/reemergence of infectious diseases
- Recent emerging/reemerging infectious diseases
- Prevention and control of emerging infectious diseases

objectives

- Identify factors that influence emerging and reemerging infectious diseases.
- Describe recent emerging and reemerging infectious diseases from a global perspective.
- Relate the methods of transmission of emerging and reemerging infectious diseases to methods of control and prevention.

key terms

Antigenic drift: Slow and progressive genetic changes that take place in DNA and RNA as organisms replicate in multiple hosts.
Antigenic shift: Sudden change in the molecular structure of DNA and RNA in microorganisms, resulting in a new strain of the microorganism.
Convergence model: Model illustrating the interaction of 13 factors that contribute to the emergence of infectious diseases.

Directly observed therapy: Observation of clients to ensure that they ingest each dose of anti-TB medication to maximize the likelihood of completion of therapy.
Ecosystem: Natural unit consisting of all living things (plants, animals, bacteria, viruses) interacting with, and dependent on, one another for survival within their nonliving environment.
Emerging infectious disease: Newly identified clinically distinct infectious disease, or the reappearance (reemergence) of a known infectious disease after its decline, with an incidence that is increasing in a certain geographic area or among a specific population.
Herd immunity: Type of immunity in which a large proportion of people in a population are not susceptible to a communicable disease and the few people who are susceptible will not likely be exposed and contract the illness.
Microbial adaptation: Process by which organisms adjust and change to their environment.
Pandemic: Epidemic occurring worldwide.

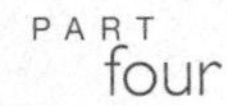

Case Studies

References to case studies are found throughout this chapter (look for the case study icon). Readers should keep the case studies in mind as they read the chapter.

CASE 1

The World Health Organization (WHO) declared an A (H1N1) influenza pandemic in June 2009, the first global pandemic in 40 years and the first in the 21st century. In making the announcement, the WHO reported that 74 countries, including the United States, had provided data for 28,774 cases, including 144 deaths. At that point, the pandemic was in phase 6, the WHO's highest alert level, which meant that a global epidemic was under way. The virus was characterized as unstoppable. By August 2010, more than 214 countries and overseas territories or communities had reported laboratory-confirmed cases of pandemic influenza H1N1 2009, including at least 18,449 deaths (CDC, *2009 H1N1: Overview of a pandemic)*.

Symptoms of influenza A (H1N1) 2009 included fever, cough, sore throat, runny or stuffy nose, body aches, headache, chills, and fatigue. Vomiting and diarrhea also occurred. People may have been infected, and had respiratory symptoms without a fever (CDC, *2009 H1N1: Overview of a pandemic)*.

CASE 2

Occupational groups such as firefighters, healthcare workers, and military personnel may receive periodic tuberculosis (TB) tests because of potential occupational exposure to TB. An estimated 1.1 million firefighters in the United States are at risk for TB exposure while performing first-responder duties such as cardiopulmonary resuscitation. In addition, firefighters and emergency medical technicians (EMTs) live in close quarters while on duty, which might facilitate rapid spread of TB among them. Therefore, in order to comply with the National Fire Protection Association (NFPA) 1582 "Standard on Comprehensive Occupational Medical Programs for Fire Departments," annual tuberculin skin tests should be conducted for firefighters and EMTs (NFPA, 2013).

Infectious organisms have been with humanity since the dawn of civilization; a basic part of life, they are universal. Diseases will continue to emerge and reemerge. Emerging infectious diseases and their basic causes are a global threat, which affect the stability of nations and the entire planet. Developing nations, which have the fewest resources to respond to this emergence and reemergence, bear the greatest burden of this threat. However, infectious diseases, which may spread rapidly and indiscriminately, present a significant risk to the health and development of all nations. No country or population is immune.

In its 1992 report, the Institute of Medicine (IOM) (IOM, 1992) defined an **emerging infectious disease** as either (1) a newly identified clinically distinct infectious disease or (2) the reappearance (or reemergence) of a known infectious disease after its decline with an incidence that is increasing in a certain geographic area or in a specific population. An example of a new infectious disease was made very clear when severe acute respiratory syndrome (SARS) appeared worldwide in 2003. A WHO physician in Hanoi, Vietnam, first recognized SARS early in 2003.

PRACTICE POINT

Astute clinicians can detect a possible emerging infectious disease by taking a careful history that includes travel history, which may reveal travel to an area where an emerging infection has been reported.

FACTORS THAT INFLUENCE EMERGING INFECTIOUS DISEASES

Factors that influence the emergence/reemergence of infectious diseases are complex and interrelated. In *The Coming Plague* (1995), Pulitzer Prize-winning author Laurie Garrett pointed out that by the end of the 20th century, microbes were no longer confined to remote ecosystems but had transformed the planet into a global village. Although a global village provides social and economic opportunities, it also gives emerging infectious diseases a chance to spread.

More than 36 new emerging infectious diseases have been identified worldwide in the past 40 years. Figure 15.1 illustrates recent infectious diseases identified by the WHO and the Centers for Disease Control and Prevention (CDC). An IOM report (2003) illustrated that "health protection and disease prevention among the U.S. population requires global awareness and collaboration with domestic and international partners to prevent the spread of infectious diseases" (Smolinski, Hamburg, & Lederberg, 2003). In *Microbial Threats to Health: Emergence, Detection, and Response*, the IOM (2003) identified 13 factors that affect emerging infections, which are listed in Box 15.1. Its **convergence model** (Fig. 15.2) demonstrates how these 13 factors are grouped. The ability of microbes to adapt and the dynamic interaction between microbes and humans are central to the IOM convergence model. There are four types of interrelated and overlapping microbe–human interactions, which can lead to emerging/reemerging infectious diseases: (1) genetic and biological; (2) physical/environmental;

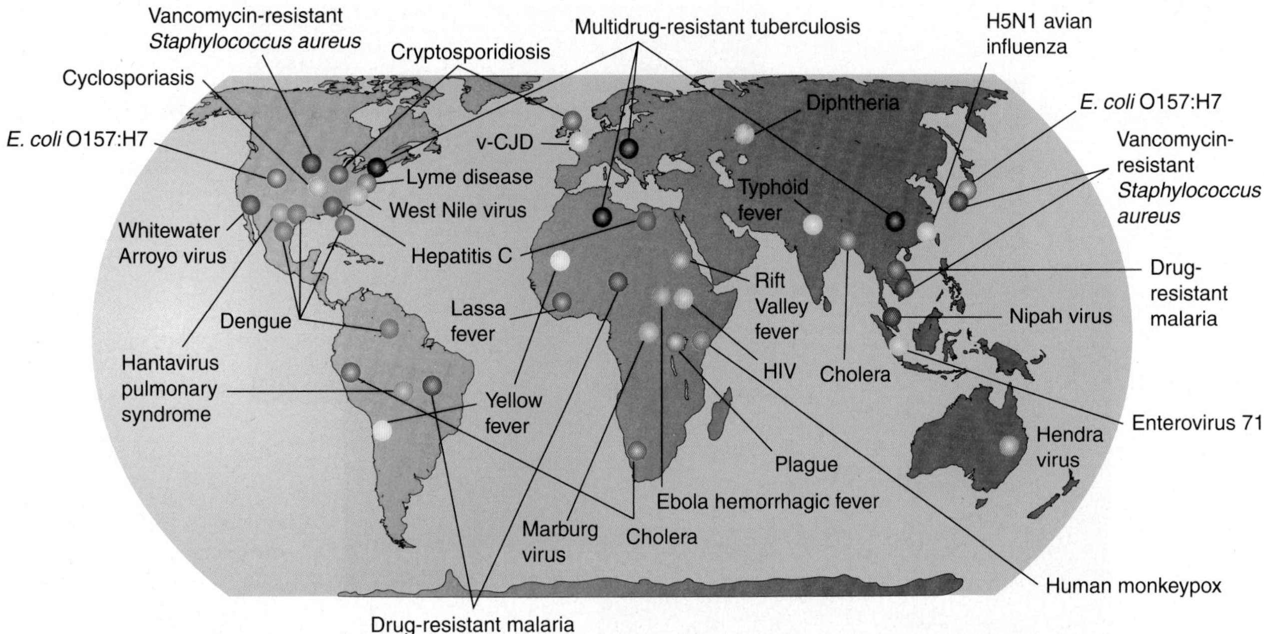

figure 15.1 Examples of recent emerging and reemerging infectious diseases.
(From Smolinski, M. S., Hamburg, M. A., & Lederberg, J. [2003]. *Microbial threats to health: Emergence, detection and response.* Washington, DC: Institute of Medicine. The National Academies Press.)

(3) ecological; and (4) social, political, and economic. Several of these factors are discussed below.

Microbial Adaptation and Change

Microbes live everywhere and are very adept at adaptation. They are constantly interacting with other living organisms and changing in response to their environment. Their habitats expand as humans alter the environment, extending their contact with a wider variety of microbes. As microbes reproduce, genetic changes may result in pathogens that are immunologically distinct from their parental strains. For example, **antigenic drift**, the slow and progressive genetic changes that take place in DNA and RNA as organisms replicate in multiple hosts, causes changes in influenza viruses each year. **Antigenic shift** occurs when there is a sudden change in the DNA and RNA, resulting in a new strain of the microorganism, and people have little or no acquired immunity.

Three stages of **microbial adaptation** and change occur over varying periods of time. During stage I, an epidemic occurs. The microbes enter a "virgin" population where hosts have no prior exposure to the organism and have few defenses. This leads to further spread in the population. Ultimately, survivors are usually left with improved defenses against reinfection. During stage II, the infection becomes endemic or continuously present in a geographic area or population of people. Routine childhood diseases are an example of such infections. During stage III, symbiosis is possible. Further adaptation occurs, resulting in mutual tolerance and sometimes mutual benefit for both the microorganism and the host. This is the preferred outcome.

> *Our relationship to infectious pathogens is part of an evolutionary drama. Here we are. Here are the bugs.*
>
> **Joshua Lederberg, molecular biologist**

As microbes adapt over the centuries, the illnesses they produce become less acute. Symptoms become milder, and fewer organs are involved as immunity develops. Syphilis

box 15.1 Factors That Contribute to the Emergence and Reemergence of Infectious Diseases

- Microbial adaptation and change
- Human susceptibility to infection
- Climate and weather
- Changing ecosystems
- Human demographics and behavior
- Economic development and land use
- International travel and commerce
- Technology and industry
- Breakdown of public health measures
- Poverty and social inequality
- War and famine
- Lack of political will
- Intent to harm (bioterrorism)

Source: Smolinski, M. S., Hamburg, M. A., & Lederberg, J. (2003). *Microbial threats to health: Emergence, detection, and response.* Washington, DC: The National Academies Press.

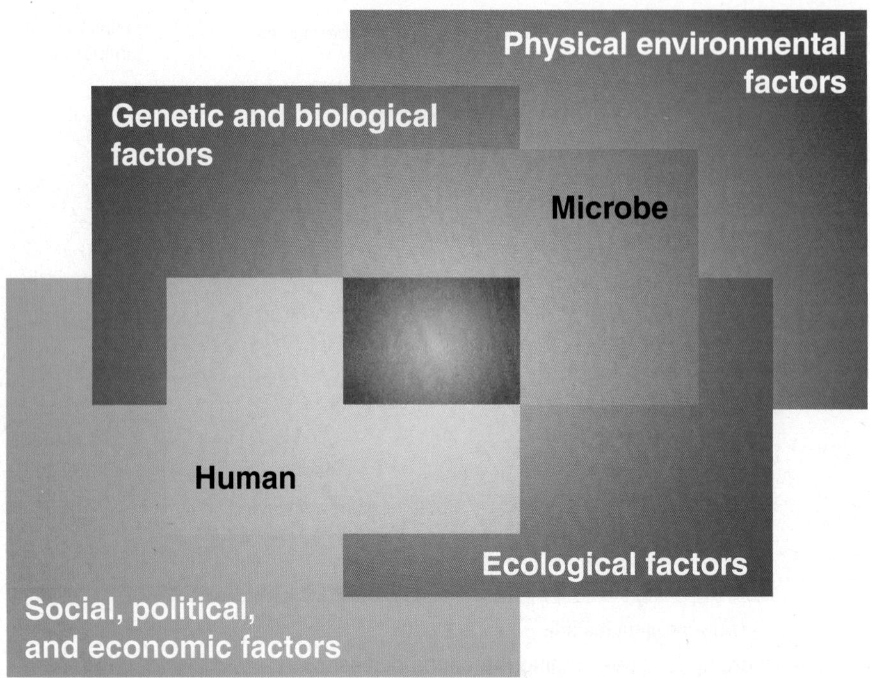

figure 15.2 Institute of Medicine convergence model.
(From Smolinski, M. S., Hamburg, M. A., & Lederberg, J. [2003]. *Microbial threats to health: Emergence, detection, and response*. Washington, DC: Institute of Medicine, The National Academies Press.)

first appeared in the late 15th century in Europe, causing repulsive pustules over the entire body. Many internal organs were involved, and death occurred within a few years. Just 50 years later, symptoms were limited to the genitals, face, and nervous system, and people could live with the disease for decades, thus having an opportunity to transmit it. Even the mode of transmission can change over time. For example, the "black plague," or bubonic plague, that devastated the European population in the 12th and 13th centuries was transmitted through the bites of fleas that lived on rats. Centuries later, a new form of the disease emerged. The organism, normally trapped in the lymph nodes, was released and the lungs became infected. As a result, an even more deadly form of the disease, the pneumonic plague, emerged. Transmission was now airborne, and the disease was transmitted from person to person. Pneumonic plague was fatal in 95% of its victims and remains resistant to antibiotic treatment today.

. . . a flea has smaller fleas that on him prey; And these have smaller still to bite 'em, And so proceed ad infinitum.

Jonathan Swift, On Poetry: A Rhapsody (1733)

Fortunately, a new acute illness is usually the exception rather than the rule. Relatively few potentially pathological microbes enter humans, and few survive. Actually, to cause disease, microbes must beat enormous odds. There is a "parasite's dilemma." If the microbe proliferates rapidly, it may kill the host. If it cannot be transmitted quickly to a new host, the microbe dies. However, if the microbe proliferates slowly, within a week the host's immune system will recognize the microbe as foreign, form antibodies, and destroy the microbe. If microbes survive and cause disease, the reason is usually due to changes illustrated by the epidemiologic triad: (1) a change in the behavior of humans—the host, (2) a change in the behavior of the microbes—the agent, or (3) a change in the environment.

Human Susceptibility to Infection

Many characteristics of the human body and the physical environment determine whether a microbe will cause a disease. For infections to occur, people must be susceptible to infection. If the host has not been exposed to the microbe in the past, there is no acquired immunity to the organism. Immunity can be impaired because of environmental stresses, poor nutrition, medication, or the presence of other illnesses. Normal defense mechanisms can be bypassed through injury or deliberate medical or surgical procedures. Diseases persist only if the population is dense enough to allow continued transmission of germs and large enough to produce a continual supply of susceptible hosts. If a substantial proportion of people in a population are not susceptible to a communicable disease, the few people who are susceptible are not likely to be exposed and contract the illness. This is a process called **herd immunity**.

Infectious diseases introduced with Europeans, like smallpox and measles, spread from one Indian tribe to another, far in advance of Europeans themselves, and killed an estimated 95% of the New World's Indian population.

Jared Diamond, scientist and author

Climate, Changing Ecosystems, and Human Behavior

Many infectious diseases have characteristic geographic distributions and seasonal variations. Probably the most common is the influenza virus that peaks each fall and winter. Factors such as temperature, precipitation, and humidity affect the life cycle of many disease pathogens and their vectors, and consequently they can affect disease outbreaks. Natural changes in climate, such as the effects of El Niño ocean current, global warming, and natural disasters, result in a change in environmental conditions. These changes are not always beneficial to infectious organisms. However, the relationships between climate and infectious disease are a complicated web of causation that includes almost all of the factors that underlie the emergence of these diseases. Dr. Claire Heffernan, a trained veterinarian and a specialist in global health and disease interaction between animals and humans, is concerned that as the climate warms in Arctic regions, more and more diseases from around the world are spreading there, threatening both animal and human populations (ISDA, June 2013).

Ecological changes are one of the most frequently identified factors in the emergence of infectious diseases. **Ecosystems** are groups of interacting living things (e.g., plants, animals, bacteria, and viruses) that depend on each other for survival. Ecosystems become unstable with climate change, and throughout history, humans have contributed to ecological flux. Humans are responsible for land use changes, which are often associated with economic development, with the accompanying dislocation of indigenous animals, plants, and microorganisms. For example, logging and the clearing of timber means that homes and sources of food are lost.

With the death or relocation of indigenous organisms, niches open up for those that thrive under marginal conditions. Also, practices associated with food production can result in the creation of ideal homes for the creatures that carry pathogens (vectors). In developing countries, where ditches may be contaminated by fecal material, irrigation fields can contribute to the contamination of local water supplies.

Changes in the environment cause new interactions between agents and hosts and can potentially lead to new infectious disease threats (IOM, 2010). Human population upheavals caused by war or civil conflicts often result in the forced dislocation of large groups of people, and migration of such groups of people from rural areas to cities can be accompanied by a breakdown of public health measures. These have often been the factors in disease emergence (Fig. 15.3). Although cities have distinct advantages, such as water supplies and transportation, it was only when towns became big cities that massive die-offs became a regular part of human life. Urban life, with malnutrition, overcrowding, and poor sanitation, enhances the major pathways for transmission of infectious disease; plagues and cities have always developed together. For example, cholera outbreaks occurred four times between 1831 and 1854 in England because of the large influx of people into cities and the lack of proper sanitary services. These outbreaks resulted in a total of 10,675 deaths.

EVIDENCE FOR PRACTICE

In 2013, the WHO reported that only three countries (Afghanistan, Nigeria, and Pakistan) remained polio-endemic countries, down from more than 125 in 1988. Most countries have expanded efforts to tackle infectious diseases by building effective surveillance and immunization systems.

As long as a single child remains infected, children in all countries are at risk of contracting polio. Failure to eradicate polio from these last remaining strongholds could result in as many as 200,000 new cases every year, within 10 years, all over the world (WHO, *Poliomyelitis*).

Wild poliovirus type 1 (WPV1) was isolated from sewage samples collected in April 2013 in southern Israel, a non-endemic country. The virus was detected through routine environmental surveillance in Israel that involves regular testing of sewage water. Israel has been free of indigenous WPV transmission since 1988.

Health authorities in Israel conducted a full epidemiological and public health investigation, actively searching for potential cases of paralytic polio, along with any unimmunized persons. Routine immunization levels are estimated at 94%. Outcomes of the investigation determined the need for any additional catch-up immunization activities (WHO, *Poliovirus detected from environmental samples in Israel*).

EVIDENCE FOR PRACTICE

The spirochete *Borrelia burgdorferi* has been identified as being responsible for most human cases of Lyme disease. In the northeastern and midwestern United States, *B. burgdorferi* is transmitted by the vector the *Ixodes scapularis* tick, also known as a deer tick. Global climate change can affect the distribution of vector-borne diseases. Lyme disease is one of the most commonly reported vector-borne illnesses in the United States. In 2012, 95% of Lyme disease cases were reported from 13 states, and it was the seventh most common nationally notifiable disease. However, this disease does **not** occur nationwide and is concentrated heavily in the Northeast and upper Midwest (CDC, *Lyme disease data*).

Travel, Technology, and Industry

International air travel now allows people to reach any destination in the world in an average of 10 to 16 hours. Infected travelers can introduce new microbes into new environments, both while traveling to new places and returning home. An increasing number of travelers increases the chances of contamination. Also, adventure travelers, who venture into new environments with exotic wildlife, increase their chances of coming into contact with microbes that have never before been recognized as human pathogens. In addition, mass food production that processes or uses biological

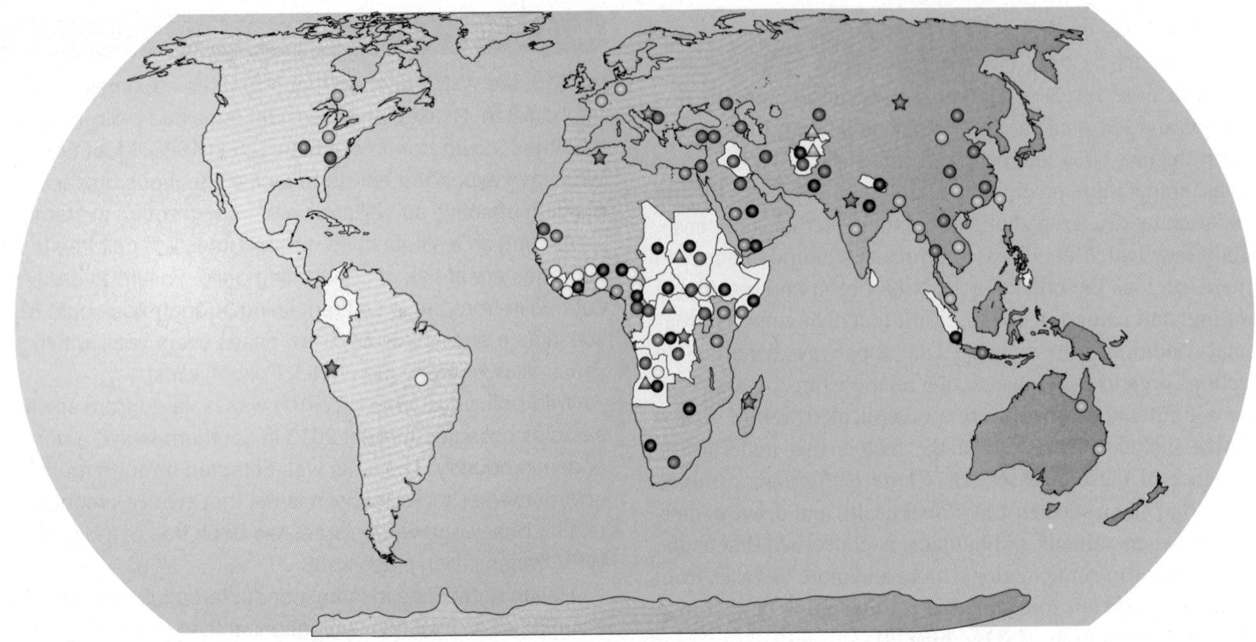

- Ebola, Marburg, and CCHF
- Influenza (H5N1)
- Lassa fever
- Monkeypox
- Nipah and Hendra
- Rift Valley fever
- SARS-CoV
- Yellow fever
- Poliovirus
- Plague
- Tularemia
- Malaria
- Trypanosomiasis

Symbols:	Outbreaks of emerging or reemerging infectious diseases during this period
Circles:	Diseases of viral origin
Stars:	Diseases of bacterial origin
Triangles:	Diseases of parasitic origin
CCHF:	Crimean–Congo hemorrhagic fever
SARS-CoV:	Severe acute respiratory syndrome coronavirus

figure 15.3 Geographic distribution of recent emerging or reemerging infectious disease outbreaks and countries affected by conflict, 1990–2006. Countries in yellow were affected by conflict during this period. Symbols represent outbreaks of emerging or reemerging infectious diseases.
(From Gayer, M., Legros, D., Formenty, P., & Connolly, M. A. [2007, November]. *Conflict and emerging infectious diseases*. [Vol. 13, No. 11]. Geneva, Switzerland: World Health Organization.)

products increases the chance of unknown contamination at every stage. These contaminated food products can be distributed widely, often to grocery shelves or restaurants within a day, and they may be eaten shortly thereafter. A single source of contamination has the potential to affect thousands of people in a large geographic area. The *Escherichia coli* outbreak from spinach grown in contaminated fields in 2006 and the intentional contamination of Chinese milk with melamine in 2009 (food counterfeiting) are just two examples of the types of problems created by mass food production.

There have been profound changes in society within the last 100 years, perhaps few greater than the changes in healthcare technology. Infections acquired in healthcare facilities affect millions of people annually worldwide. The sickest people are at the highest risk. Microbial adaptation and change in response to the overuse of antibiotics and consequent accumulation in the environment have caused the rapid evolution of resistant pathogens. Microorganisms such as methicillin-resistant *Staphylococcus aureus* (MRSA) are now found in the community as well as in healthcare institutions. Antibiotic-resistant pathogens, one of the plagues of the 20th century, continue to be a problem in the 21st century.

Lack of Political Will and Breakdown of Public Health Infrastructures

Unlike the United States, Canada, the United Kingdom, and European countries, most developing nations do not have the public health network and technological advances required to fight against infectious diseases. Many of these countries have to choose between funding economic development initiatives and investing in a national public health infrastructure.

The 1991 outbreak of cholera in Peru is a good case study; this outbreak illustrates the complex web of causation that contributed to the onset and spread of the disease. Historically, there have been seven acknowledged cholera pandemics. The seventh pandemic of cholera commenced in 1961 in Indonesia; by 1991, it had reached Peru. Cholera is a disease transmitted through the fecal–oral route that is associated with poverty. The disease had been absent from Peru for more than 100 years. It has been suggested that human waste contaminated with *Vibrio cholerae* was discharged from a Chinese freighter offshore from infected crew members on board the ship. The microbes then found their way into plankton, which was in turn ingested by fish and shellfish. Consumption of raw shellfish is a delicacy in Peru, and one possible source of the epidemic was contaminated shellfish. Cholera infection in humans occurred because a series of complex factors existed along Peru's shores. The rapid population growth in the coastal cities exceeded the capability of the public health infrastructure to deal with fecal contamination of water supplies. The cholera outbreak in Peru cost the country US$770 million due to food trade embargoes and adverse effects on tourism. The disease subsequently quickly spread to other Latin American countries (Mutreja et al., 2011; WHO, *Global epidemics and impact of cholera*).

PRACTICE POINT

Infectious disease prevention requires global consciousness. Not all countries have the public health infrastructure to combat emerging infectious diseases.

RECENT EMERGING AND REEMERGING INFECTIOUS DISEASES

Severe Acute Respiratory Syndrome, 2002 to 2003

At least 7 of the 13 factors affecting emerging infections, identified in the 2003 IOM Report, occurred during the 2002 to 2003 SARS outbreak. The SARS epidemic, which occurred worldwide between February and July of 2003, began in mainland China in November 2002 but was not reported to the WHO until February 2003, when the Chinese Ministry of Health reported that an outbreak of 305 cases of "atypical pneumonia," including five deaths, had occurred in Guangdong Province. By then, SARS had spread to several countries, including Hong Kong, Taiwan, Singapore, Vietnam, and Canada. Secondary cases of SARS were imported to the respective countries by a "superspreading event" that occurred through exposure to an index case of SARS from mainland China. Although the causative agent for SARS had not been identified early in the outbreak, a case definition for SARS was established, and secondary attack rates of more than 50% were observed in healthcare providers caring for clients with SARS in both Hong Kong and Vietnam (CDC, *Remembering SARS*).

The causative agent for SARS was identified in April 2003 as a variant coronavirus (CoV), with an average incubation period of 4 to 6 days (range, 1 to 14 days) and a maximum of 10 days. Although SARS-CoV was found to be mostly transmitted by close contact with respiratory secretions and aerosols, other body fluids, such as saliva, tears, urine, and feces, also demonstrated presence of the virus. Most cases of SARS among healthcare providers occurred from contacts with clients and visitors who were not identified as having SARS and before infection control and quarantine measures were in place or, when infection control precautions were relaxed (CDC, *Remembering SARS*).

Canada became the first SARS epicenter in the Western Hemisphere, with two clusters of SARS infection epidemiologically linked to two hospital outbreaks. Globally, the WHO received reports of SARS from 29 countries and regions; 8,096 persons with probable SARS, resulting in 774 deaths. In the United States, eight SARS infections were documented by laboratory testing and an additional 19 probable SARS infections were reported (CDC, *Remembering SARS*).

Isolation precautions and quarantine measures to prevent the spread of SARS-CoV were established early in the outbreak, which were effective in containing the epidemic. SARS-CoV was less transmissible than most respiratory infections; therefore, it was highly susceptible to appropriate control measures. About 30% of the early SARS cases in China were in healthcare providers, with the majority of cases occurring before the cause of SARS was identified and before correct infection control measures were in place. By the end of the epidemic, 21% of SARS cases had occurred in healthcare providers, ranging from 3% in the United States to 43% in Canada. Several secondary SARS cases also occurred in household contacts before quarantine measures were instituted.

In 2012, the National Select Agent Registry Program declared SARS-CoV a select agent. A select agent is a bacterium, virus, or toxin that has the potential to pose a severe threat to public health and safety. There have been no known cases of SARS reported anywhere in the world since 2004, when human cases of SARS-CoV infection were reported in China in an outbreak resulting from laboratory-acquired infections (CDC, *Remembering SARS*). However, in June 2014, Chinese scientists discovered a new type of SARS-like CoV in bats in the Yunan Province of China that could be the precursor of the SARS virus or its "relative" (He et al., 2014). There is no evidence that transmission of the new SARS-like CoV to human beings has occurred. Nonetheless, this discovery represents an important clue in the hunt for the source of SARS.

The main lessons learned from SARS, the first new infectious disease to emerge in the 21st century, were that

(1) astute healthcare providers are likely to be the key to early detection and reporting of initial cases of new CoV infections; (2) containment of disease requires the diligent application of enhanced infection control measures at the national and local levels; and (3) control of an emerging infection necessitates swift action by healthcare providers as well as an adequate public health infrastructure.

Middle East Respiratory Syndrome Coronavirus

In late 2012, the WHO received reports of two clusters of human infection with a novel coronavirus (nCoV) in the Middle East. Although this nCoV is distantly related to SARS-CoV, it is different, and this particular strain of CoV has not been previously identified in humans (WHO, *Coronavirus infections*). Nonetheless, the WHO and the CDC recognized that the emergence of a new CoV capable of causing severe disease raised concerns because of the recent experience with SARS.

From September 2012 to July 18, 2014, the WHO reported a global total of 721 laboratory-confirmed cases of human infection with *Middle East respiratory syndrome* coronavirus (MERS-CoV) in 19 countries, including 297 deaths (41% case fatality rate). Cases of MERS-CoV have been reported throughout the Middle East, Africa, Europe, Asia, and the United States (WHO, http://www.moh.gov.sa/en/CCC/PressReleases/Pages/default.aspx). MERS-CoV has been reported in 109 healthcare providers in the Middle East. While the majority (57%) were asymptomatic or with mild symptoms, 32% (n = 35) had moderate symptoms, requiring hospitalization, and another 6% (n = 7) had severe disease, with 4 (4%) being fatal. The recent upsurge of new cases was attributed in part due to breaches in infection prevention and control measures in healthcare settings. The WHO also has reported that MERS-CoV has been found in some camels and in some MERS patients who have had contact with camels. Therefore, in addition to a travel history, patients should be asked if they have visited farms, markets, barns, or other places where animals are present (WHO, *MERS-CoV Summary 11 June, 2014*).

The first two imported cases of MERS-CoV infection in the United States (Indiana, Florida) were reported in May 2014. Both cases were healthcare workers who lived and worked in Saudi Arabia and had traveled to the United States. The two cases were not linked (CDC, 2014). A third asymptomatic Illinois patient, who had contact with the Indiana MERS case, had previously been identified through contact screening. However, further testing by the CDC found that the Illinois resident was not previously infected with MERS-CoV (CDC, *Press release*, May 28, 2014). As of the latest report, all of the cases were transferred from the Middle East to other countries for care of the disease or returned from the Middle East and subsequently became ill. In addition, some healthcare providers have been diagnosed with MERS-CoV infection after exposure to infected patients. Although active surveillance has identified an increase in community-acquired cases, there was no evidence of sustained spreading of MERS-CoV in community settings. Healthcare facilities that provide care for patients with suspected MERS-CoV infection should take appropriate measures to decrease the risk of transmission of the virus to other patients and healthcare providers by systematic implementation of infection prevention and control measures. A probable case of MERS-CoV infection is defined as a person with an acute respiratory infection with clinical, radiological, or histopathological evidence of pulmonary parenchymal disease (e.g., pneumonia or acute respiratory distress syndrome), *and* close contact with a laboratory-confirmed case *or* recent travel to the affected area (WHO, *Coronavirus infections*).

In consultation with the WHO, the definition of a probable case of MERS-CoV infection has been updated by the CDC to also include persons with severe acute respiratory illness with no known etiology with an epidemiologic link to a confirmed case of MERS-CoV infection (CDC, *MERS-CoV*). The CDC continued to work in consultation with the WHO and other partners to better understand the public health risk posed by the new CoV (MERS-CoV). Updated information from the WHO indicated that the period for considering evaluation for MERS-CoV infection in persons who develop severe acute lower respiratory illness days after traveling from the Middle East and other affected countries should be extended to within 14 days of travel (CDC, 2014).

Infection Control for the Prevention of MERS-CoV Transmission

The WHO developed interim guidance to meet the urgent need for up-to-date information and evidence-based recommendations for the safe care of patients with probable or confirmed nCoV (MERS-CoV) infection: *Infection prevention and control during health care for probable or confirmed cases of novel coronavirus (nCoV) infection (WHO, Coronavirus infections)*. Although further studies were needed to better understand the risk of MERS-CoV (nCoV) infection transmission at the time, the WHO interim guidelines were based on clear evidence of limited, unsustainable, human-to-human transmission, possibly involving different modes of transmission such as droplet and contact transmission. These guidelines relate to, and can be used in conjunction with the document entitled, *Avian Influenza, Including Influenza A (H5N1): WHO Interim Infection Control Guidelines for Health-care Facilities*, published by the WHO (2007).

Healthcare-associated outbreaks with transmission to healthcare personnel highlight the importance of infection control procedures. To prevent the transmission of *all* acute respiratory infections, respiratory hygiene/cough etiquette measures should be implemented at the first point of contact with a potentially infected person and should be incorporated into standard precautions. This includes covering the nose and mouth when coughing or sneezing, using tissues to contain respiratory secretions and disposing of them in the nearest waste receptacle after use, and hand hygiene (e.g., hand washing with nonantimicrobial soap and water, alcohol-based hand rub, or antiseptic hand wash) after having contact with respiratory secretions and contaminated objects/materials (CDC, 2004a).

The 2013 WHO guidelines for a suspected or confirmed case of MERS-CoV infection called for placing the patient in a single isolation room with equal or greater than 12 air exchanges per hour (WHO, 2013a). Until the transmission characteristics of MERS-CoV are better understood, patients under investigation, and probable and confirmed cases should be managed according to CDC's infection control recommendations for the CoV that caused SARS (CDC, *Update, Case Definitions, and Guidance MERS*).

The use of personal protective equipment (PPE) should be guided by a risk assessment concerning anticipated contact with blood, body fluids, secretions, and nonintact skin for routine patient care. When procedures include a risk of splash to the face and/or body, PPE should include the use of facial protection by either a surgical mask, and eye visor or goggles, or a face shield; *and* a gown and clean gloves. In addition to standard precautions, all individuals, including visitors and healthcare providers, in contact with patients with acute respiratory tract infection should use droplet precautions, which include wearing a surgical mask when in close contact (i.e., within approximately 3 feet) and upon entering the room of the patient; perform hand hygiene before and after contact with the patient and his or her surroundings, and immediately after removal of a surgical mask (CDC, *MERS*; WHO, 2013a).

Additional precautions should be observed and PPE worn when performing aerosol-generating procedures, which may be associated with an increased risk of infection transmission, in particular, intubation. These include a particulate respirator (e.g., N95 respirator), eye protection (i.e., goggles or a face shield), gown, and gloves (some procedures may require sterile gloves). These guidelines are interim ones to control transmission of the nCoV (MERS-CoV). In addition, not all suspected MERS-CoV patients would be admitted to healthcare facilities. They may prefer to stay in their homes. The CDC and WHO publications are available for MERS-CoV patient care at home and in the community. The CDC website, at http://www.cdc.gov/MERS, and the WHO website, at http://www.who.int/csr/disease/coronavirus_infections/en/index.html, should be consulted for periodic updates regarding MERS-CoV recommendations and guidelines.

Clients in the United States, with a history of MERS-CoV who are hospitalized with a severe febrile respiratory illness, or those who are being evaluated for MERS-CoV, should be managed using isolation precautions identical to those recommended for clients with known avian influenza. These precautions are outlined in Appendix A: "Type and duration of precautions needed for selected infections and conditions" in the CDC *2007 Guideline for Isolation Precautions: Preventing Transmission of Infectious Agents in Healthcare Settings* at http://www.cdc.gov/coronavirus/mers/downloads/Isolation2007.pdf. Clusters of severe acute respiratory illness of unknown etiology in the community also should be thoroughly investigated, and if no etiology is identified, this should prompt immediate notification of local public health officials, and testing for MERS-CoV should be conducted if indicated. In addition, any clusters of severe acute respiratory illness in healthcare personnel in the United States should be thoroughly investigated (CDC, *Update, case definitions, and guidance MERS*).

PRACTICE POINT

Observance of infection control practices can reduce the risk of transmission of an acute respiratory illness, such as MERS-CoV infection, to healthcare providers. Community and public health nurses are educators who provide information to prevent the transmission of all respiratory infections, including MERS-CoV.

Avian Influenza

During the past century, three influenza A pandemics have occurred, and pandemic influenza will inevitably occur in the future. Although the timing and severity of the next pandemic cannot be predicted, the probability that a pandemic will occur has increased based on the recent outbreaks of influenza A (H5N1) in Asia, Europe, and Africa.

Influenza A viruses, which originate in birds, are categorized into subtypes on the basis of their surface antigens. These viruses have 16 hemagglutinin (H) surface antigen subtypes and nine neuraminidase (N) surface antigen subtypes. Only viruses of the H5 and H7 subtypes are known to cause the highly pathogenic form of type A influenza. New influenza virus variants result from frequent antigenic change (i.e., antigenic drift), which is a consequence of point mutations that occur during viral replication. These frequent changes that result from antigenic drift mean that there is a new seasonal influenza vaccine each year (CDC, *How the flu virus changes*).

Knowledge of the history of past influenza A pandemics has increased the awareness of the potential for another pandemic. Three influenza A pandemics have been reported in the past century. The first pandemic occurred in 1918 to 1919. Known as the "Spanish flu" (influenza A [H1N1]), it resulted in 20 to 40 million deaths worldwide and more than 500,000 deaths in the United States. The "Spanish flu" was unique because the causative agent was very deadly, and it spread across the globe within 6 months. Almost half of the people who died were young, healthy adults between 20 and 40 years of age, and many died within the first few days after infection. Others died of complications soon thereafter. The second pandemic, known as the "Asian flu" (influenza A [H2N2]), occurred in 1957 to 1958, and it was first identified in China in late February 1957. In less than 6 months, it spread to the United States, where it caused approximately 70,000 deaths. The highest mortality with Asian flu occurred in the elderly. The H2N2 influenza A virus that caused the pandemic of 1957 disappeared from the human population 10 years later. The third pandemic, known as "Hong Kong flu" (influenza A [H3N2]), occurred in 1968 to 1969. The first cases were detected in Hong Kong in early 1968. Later that year, the virus spread to the United States, where it claimed approximately 34,000 lives (Kilbourne, 2006). Influenza A (H3N2) viruses are still circulating today.

Avian Influenza A (H5N1) Outbreaks, 2003 to 2014

Until 1997, the risk of avian influenza was considered rare in humans. However, confirmed cases of human infection from several subtypes of avian viruses have been reported since then. Most of these human cases have resulted from contact with infected domestic poultry (e.g., chickens and ducks) or surfaces contaminated with blood and secretions/excretions from infected birds. Until 2003, the last epidemic of *human infection with avian influenza A* (H5N1) occurred in Hong Kong in 1997, with 18 confirmed cases and six deaths (WHO, 2011). In 2003, an outbreak of avian influenza A (H5N1), a highly pathogenic virus, spread among millions of birds (mostly chickens) across Southeast Asia. Although the H5N1 virus rarely infects humans, from 2003 to the spring of 2014, the WHO reported 664 laboratory-confirmed human cases of avian influenza A (H5N1) viral infection from 15 countries, of which 391 died (a 59% case fatality rate) (WHO, *Avian influenza*). This was the largest number of documented cases since the virus first emerged in humans in 1997. Nearly all of the infections were the result of people having direct or close contact with infected poultry or contaminated surfaces (WHO, *Avian influenza fact sheet*). In 2012, Russell et al. reported that as few as five amino acid substitutions, or four with reassortment, might be sufficient for mammal-to-mammal transmission of A (H5N1) viruses through respiratory droplets. While the technical aspects of the study by Russell et al. are beyond the scope of this text, their "analyses ..., using current best estimates, indicate that the remaining mutations could evolve within a single mammalian host, making the possibility of a respiratory droplet-transmissible A/H5N1 virus evolving in nature a potentially serious threat" (p. 1547).

The H5N1 virus can improve its transmissibility among humans by two mechanisms. The first is antigenic shift, a "reassortment" event, in which genetic material is exchanged between human and avian viruses during coinfection of a human or an animal such as a pig. Reassortment could result in a fully transmissible pandemic virus, which could rapidly spread throughout the world (Fig. 15.4). The second mechanism is a more gradual process of *antigenic drift*, an adaptive mutation, whereby the capability of the virus to bind to human cells increases during subsequent infections of humans. Adaptive mutation, which is expressed initially as small clusters of human cases with some evidence of human-to-human transmission, would probably give the world some time to take defensive action. If H5N1 viruses gain the ability for efficient and sustained transmission among humans, an influenza **pandemic** (an epidemic occurring worldwide) could result, with potentially high rates of illness and death worldwide. Therefore, the epizootic H5N1 continues to pose an important public health threat (CDC, *Public health threat of highly pathogenic avian influenza A (H5N1) virus*).

PRACTICE POINT

Travel history is an important aspect of assessment for emerging and reemerging infectious diseases such as MERS-CoV and A (H5N1) influenza.

Infection Control for the Prevention of Avian A (H5N1) Influenza Transmission

Clients with a history of travel within 10 days to a country with avian influenza activity and who are hospitalized with a serious febrile respiratory illness, or are otherwise being evaluated for avian influenza, should be managed using isolation precautions. The isolation procedures are the same as those that were used for SARS-CoV and for suspected or confirmed MERS-CoV. In addition to standard precautions, which include careful attention to hand hygiene before and after all client contact or contact with items potentially con-

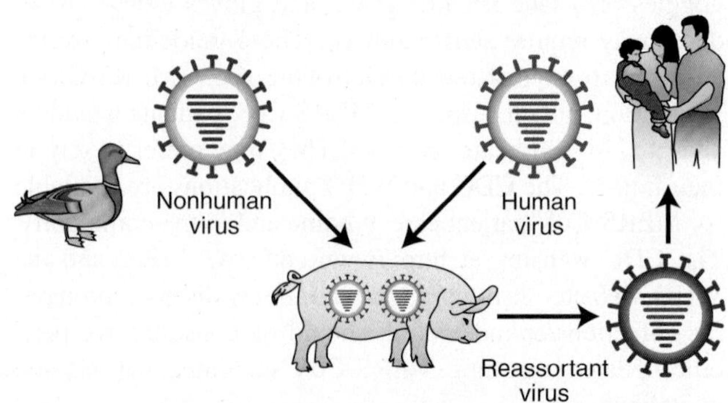

figure 15.4 Reassortment: A mechanism of antigenic shift. (Adapted from National Institute of Allergy and Infectious Diseases, National Institutes of Health. Retrieved from http://www.niaid.nih.gov/topics/flu/research/basic/pages/antigenicshiftillustration.aspx

taminated with respiratory secretions, the CDC recommends the following enhanced isolation precautions when avian influenza is diagnosed or suspected.

- Contact precautions
  - Use gloves and gown for all client contact.
  - Use dedicated equipment such as stethoscopes, as well as disposable blood pressure cuffs and disposable thermometers.
- Eye protection
  - Wear goggles or face shields when within 3 feet of the client.
- Airborne precautions
  - Place the client in an airborne isolation room (AIR). Such rooms should have monitored negative air pressure in relation to corridor, with 6 to 12 air changes per hour (ACH), and exhaust air directly outside, or have recirculated air filtered by a high-efficiency particulate air (HEPA) filter. If an AIR is unavailable, a portable HEPA filter should be used to augment the number of ACH.
  - Use a fit-tested respirator, at least as protective as a National Institute of Occupational Safety and Health (NIOSH)-approved disposable N95 filtering face piece respirator, when entering the room (DHHS, 2006).

The CDC also has recommended nonpharmaceutical community interventions that use social distancing strategies to reduce contact between people (Box 15.2). The Department of Health and Human Services (DHHS, 2006) and the CDC have developed a checklist that identifies important, specific activities that each state and local community can implement to prepare for a possible pandemic. Nurses practicing in the community should be aware of what some of these guidelines are. Many of these activities are specific to pandemic influenza, but many also pertain to any public health emergency. The DHHS website will have the latest guidelines to follow in the event of an outbreak.

PRACTICE POINT

Stress the personal steps that everyone can take to reduce the spread of infection:

- Recognize symptoms of the flu and see a healthcare provider immediately if you have
  - A temperature of greater than 100°F
  - A cough
  - A sore throat
  - An underlying condition that increases risk
- Cover your cough or sneeze
- Wash hands often and keep hands away from your face
- Stay home and do not travel if you are ill
- Be prepared for increased illness in your schools and community

box 15.2 Nonpharmaceutical Strategies to Contain a Community-wide Epidemic

- Closing schools
- Canceling public gatherings
- Planning for liberal work leave policies
- Telecommuting strategies
- Voluntary isolation of cases
- Voluntary quarantine of household contacts

Source: CDC. (2007b). *Interim pre-pandemic planning guidance: Community strategy for pandemic influenza mitigation in the United States.* Retrieved from http://www.flu.gov/planning-preparedness/community/community_mitigation.pdf

H1N1 Influenza (Swine Flu) Pandemic, 2009 to 2010

In June 2009, the WHO declared that the moderately severe global influenza A H1N1 (swine flu) represented a pandemic. This declaration was based on the sustained worldwide spread of H1N1 from person to person, not the severity of illness caused by the virus. By no means was infection with H1N1 as severe as the 1918 pandemic. However, it was expected that cases would continue to increase because of the onset of the influenza season in the Southern Hemisphere. The influenza A H1N1 virus can cause very different patterns in different countries. It may result in more severe illness in people who have limited access to health facilities and services. Key WHO goals were to determine where the virus was spreading in the global community and to reduce its impact, particularly on people who are most vulnerable (CDC, 2009 H1N1: *Overview of a pandemic*).

In **Case 1**, the WHO declared that H1N1 influenza had reached a stage 6 pandemic, with 74 countries reporting 28,774 cases of influenza A (H1N1) infection, including 144 deaths. By December 2009, more than 208 countries and overseas territories had reported laboratory-confirmed cases of pandemic influenza H1N1 2009, including at least 12,220 deaths. Pandemics have two characteristics. First, they affect younger people disproportionately, and second, they may be caused by a new virus that occurs in addition to an influenza virus that circulates every year. Both were characteristics of the new H1N1 virus. About half of the people who died from the new H1N1 virus were young and healthy, and cases of the new infection quickly outpaced the virus that was circulating prior to this time (CDC, *2009 H1N1: Overview of a pandemic*).

- What were the factors that contributed to the development of a pandemic with the 2009 H1N1 influenza virus?
- What process had occurred that resulted in the development of this new H1N1 virus?
- How was the H1N1 influenza different from the regular seasonal influenza virus that occurs every year?

- What had happened that allowed the new H1N1 virus to outpace the regular influenza virus that was already in circulation?
- Why were so many people susceptible to this influenza strain?
- What helpful lessons have been learned through the study of prior epidemics, such as outbreaks of avian influenza?

Novel Avian Influenza A (H7N9) Virus, 2013 to 2014

Influenza A (H7N9) is one of a subgroup of influenza viruses that normally circulate among birds. This virus has not been previously seen in humans; however, human infections with the H7N9 virus have now been detected in China (WHO, *WHO risk assessment: Human infections with avian influenza A (H7N9) virus*). During the first wave from February to May of 2013, a total of 133 human cases and 43 deaths occurred. The second wave, which occurred from October 2013 through early June 2014, had many more cases than the first wave, with 313 cases. The total number of human cases of A (H7N9) influenza as of early June 2014 was 448, including at least 157 deaths (35% case fatality rate) (Centre for Health Protection, *Communicable disease watch*). Reports of family clusters of H7N9 have been rare, providing evidence that the virus is not easily spread from person to person. Although most cases had contact with live poultry or had visited live-animal markets before the onset of illness, the source of infection remained unclear. While the second wave of H7N9 infections had tapered off by June 2014, experts felt that cases would continue to emerge since the virus appears to be present in poultry and their environments. Findings from this latest emerging influenza virus highlight the importance of zoonotic viruses on global health (University of Minnesota Center for Infectious Disease Research and Policy) (WHO [2013a], *Influenza at the human–animal interface*).

Li et al. (2014) conducted an epidemiologic study of A (H7N9) influenza using the 2006 WHO case definition for human infections with A (H5N1) virus (WHO, 2006) and identified through the Chinese surveillance system for pneumonia of unknown origin. A total of 139 cases with confirmed H7N9 infection had a median age of 61 years (range: 2 to 91 years), 71% were male, 73% were urban residents, and 9 were poultry workers. Except for four case clusters among family members who had provided care to case patients, most of the cases were epidemiologically unrelated. Of the data available among 131 patients, 82% had a history of exposure to live animals, including chickens. Ninety-nine percent ($n = 137$) were hospitalized with pneumonia or respiratory failure, with a 34% fatality rate. Analysis of 2,675 close contacts of case patients, 28 (1%) developed respiratory symptoms. However, all 28 close contacts tested negative for the H7N9 virus. Using available data and identifying the date of exposure to live poultry among 111 early cases of A (H7N9) influenza, Gao and colleagues (2013) estimated the incubation period of A (H7N9) to be 5 days.

Early in the outbreak of novel A (H7N9) bird flu, Hu et al. (2013) found an emergence of antiviral resistance to oseltamivir (Tamiflu) in 3 of the 14 patients studied. While early treatment of suspected or confirmed cases of A (H7N9) with oseltamivir was advised, Wang et al. (2014) developed an assay to help clinicians monitor emergence of oseltamivir resistance in the A (H7N9) virus. Hu and colleagues warned: "The apparent ease with which antiviral resistance emerges in A/H7N9 viruses is concerning; it needs to be closely monitored and considered in future pandemic response plans" (p. 6).

Pure bird flu strains, such as the new H7N9 strain and the H5N1 virus, where the latter virus killed 59% of people it infected since 2003, are generally more deadly for humans. All of the reported cases of A (H7N9) up to mid-2014 had been from China (WHO [2013a], *Influenza at the human-animal interface*; *WHO risk assessment: human infections with avian influenza A [H7N9]*). However, ongoing surveillance can identify reassortment of zoonotic viruses that can spread human-to-human transmission, leading to a pandemic. While there may be limited person-to-person spread of the A (H7N9) virus, many people travel between China and the United States; therefore, the CDC has issued a public health alert for healthcare providers to be aware of patients who present with acute respiratory illness and a travel history to countries where the A (H7N9) virus has been confirmed (CDC, *Influenza: H7N9*). Recommendations for infection control may be found at the CDC website www.cdc.gov/flu/h7n9-virus.htm.

West Nile Virus

Human cases of West Nile virus (WNV) infection appeared for the first time in the Western Hemisphere in New York in 1999, and by 2003, an epidemic of WNV had expanded across the United States. WNV has now become endemic in the United States. The virus moved from eastern United States to the west coast within a 3-year period, and the continued expansion of WNV indicates that it is permanently established in the Western Hemisphere. Although the incidence of WNV outside North America is low, the virus has been found in Central America, parts of South America, and the Caribbean. Recent reports have found WNV in the Artic (ISDA, June 2013).

Transmission of WNV involves animals. The most common route of transmission is from the bite of an infected mosquito. Mosquitoes become infected when they feed on infected birds and then spread the disease to humans and other animals when they bite them. Symptoms typically develop between 3 and 14 days after the infected mosquito bites someone. The majority of WNV cases occur among males, with the date of onset ranging from late March to early October. However, in warmer climates, WNV infections can occur year round.

Symptoms of WNV vary. Approximately 80% of infected people (about four out of five) do not have any symptoms. Another 20% of those who become infected have symptoms such as fever, headache, body aches, nausea, vomiting, and sometimes swollen lymph glands or a skin rash on the chest, stomach, and back. Symptoms can last for as short a period as a few days; however, some *healthy people* have become sick for several weeks. About 1 in 150 people infected with WNV develops severe illness, with severe symptoms that can include high fever, headache, neck stiffness, stupor, disorientation, coma, tremors, convulsions, muscle weakness, vision loss, numbness, and paralysis. These symptoms may last for several weeks, and neurological effects may be permanent. People older than 50 years are more likely to develop serious symptoms of WNV if they do become sick; therefore, they should take special care to avoid mosquito bites (CDC, *West Nile virus*).

In the 2002 WNV outbreak, nonvector routes of transmission were identified, including blood transfusions, organ transplantation, and vertical transmission in utero. Nonvector WNV transmission has also been reported in laboratory workers and poultry farm workers. Because of the transfusion-related cases of WNV in 2002, the CDC has established a mechanism through state and local health departments for reporting WNV infection occurring in people who have received blood component transfusions within 4 weeks prior to onset of illness. Therefore, WNV disease should be considered in any person with a febrile or acute neurologic illness who has had recent exposure to mosquitoes, blood transfusion, or organ transplantation, especially during the summer months in areas where virus activity has been reported. The diagnosis should also be considered in any infant born to a mother infected with WNV during pregnancy or while breast-feeding (CDC, *West Nile virus*).

Prevention of WNV Infection

West Nile virus is not transmitted from person to person. No isolation precautions are indicated other than standard precautions. The CDC guidelines emphasize avian, animal, mosquito, and human WNV surveillance, along with control and elimination of mosquito breeding sites such as standing water in flowerpots, buckets, and old tires.

There are no medications to treat, or vaccines to prevent WNV infection. The CDC recommends using an insect repellent such as DEET (*N*, *N*-diethyl-m-toluamide) or picaridin when outdoors, following the directions on the package. Because mosquitoes are most active at dusk and dawn, in addition to an insect repellent, long sleeves and pants should be worn when outdoors during these hours. Screens on windows and doors will keep mosquitoes out (CDC, *West Nile virus*).

WNV disease is a nationally notifiable condition. All cases should be reported to local public health authorities. Reporting can assist local, state, and national authorities to recognize outbreaks and to implement control measures to reduce future infections. More information on WNV is available at the CDC website at http://www.cdc.gov/westnile/index.html.

PRACTICE POINT

Community and public health nurses should educate the public about how to prevent WNV infection:

- **Use of Food and Drug Administration (FDA)-approved repellents for skin and/or clothing for protection from mosquito-borne diseases**
- **When weather permits, wear long-sleeved shirts and long pants outdoors.**
- **Place mosquito netting over infant carriers when outdoors with infants.**
- **Consider staying indoors at dawn, dusk, and early evening, which are peak mosquito biting times.**
- **Install or repair window and door screens so that mosquitoes cannot come indoors.**

Lyme Disease

Epidemiology of Lyme Disease

Lyme disease was described nearly 40 years ago by Steere, who recognized it as an important emerging infection when it appeared in a cluster of children in the Lyme, Connecticut, area, who were thought to have juvenile rheumatoid arthritis. However, it became apparent that Lyme arthritis was a late manifestation of a multisystem disease, of which some symptoms had been recognized previously in Europe and America (Steere, Coburn, & Glickstein, 2004).

Lyme disease, which is caused by a bacterium and transmitted by ticks, is the most commonly reported vector-borne disease in the United States. In 1981, Burgdorfer and colleagues discovered a previously unidentified spirochetal bacterium, subsequently named *B. burgdorferi* (as noted in a previous Evidence for Practice feature). The spread of Lyme disease and its vectors have developed from the recent proliferation of deer and the process of reforestation now taking place. As a result, increasingly large numbers of people live where risk of Lyme disease is increased. The agents of these infections, which once were transmitted by an exclusively rodent-feeding vector, have now become zoonotic. The deer tick (*I. scapularis* in the northeastern and north central United States; *I. pacificus* in the western United States) is an important vector in human Lyme borreliosis along with the white-tailed deer, the preferred host of the adult deer tick. The white-tailed deer populations seem to be critical for the survival of the ticks. However, the deer is not involved in the life cycle of the spirochete (Steere et al., 2004). The life cycle of the *Ixodes* tick takes 2 years (Fig. 15.5). Once a tick becomes infected with *B. burgdorferi*, it remains infected for life and can transmit the organism to new hosts.

In 2012, the CDC reported 22,014 confirmed cases and 8,817 probable cases of Lyme disease in the United States, at an incidence rate of 7.0 per 100,000 population, and it was the seventh most common nationally notifiable disease that year. The majority of Lyme disease cases in 2011 and 2012

Proper tick removal

Wear protective gloves if available. Grasp the tick with a pair of tweezers as close to the skin as possible. Gently but firmly pull it straight out. If tweezers and gloves are unavailable, use a tissue or piece of cloth as a barrier to protect your hands.

Do *not* apply a lit match, petroleum jelly, nail polish remover, or other solvents.

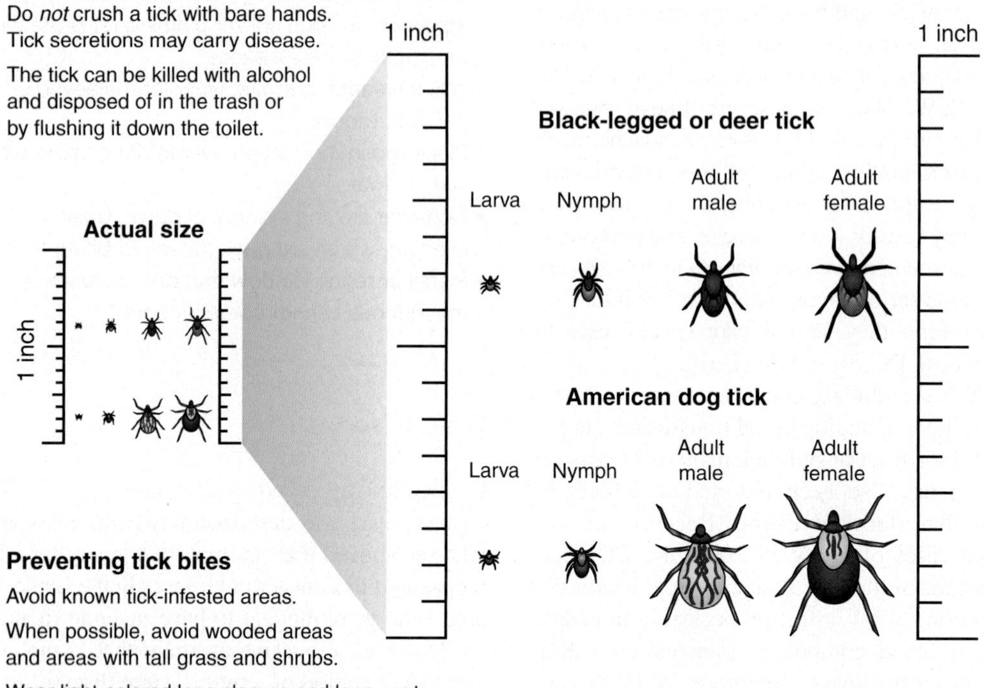
Do *not* crush a tick with bare hands. Tick secretions may carry disease.
The tick can be killed with alcohol and disposed of in the trash or by flushing it down the toilet.
1 inch
1 inch
Black-legged or deer tick
Larva
Nymph
Adult male
Adult female
Actual size
1 inch
American dog tick
Larva
Nymph
Adult male
Adult female
Preventing tick bites
Avoid known tick-infested areas.
When possible, avoid wooded areas and areas with tall grass and shrubs.

Wear light-colored long sleeves and long pants.

Tuck long pants into socks or boots.

Walk in the center of trails to avoid brushing against tall grass, shrubs, or brush.

Apply DEET-containing repellants primarily to clothes and sparingly to exposed skin. Follow product directions carefully and supervise children when using repellants.

Treat pets with repellants that are specifically formulated for pets.

figure 15.5 Tick ID card.

(96% and 95%, respectively) were reported from 13 states in New England, the mid-Atlantic states, and the upper Midwest. Note the difference among the incidence rates over years10 and 11 in Table 15.1. Lyme disease does **not** occur nationwide and is concentrated heavily in the Northeast and upper Midwest (CDC, *Lyme disease data*). The 2011and 2012 incidence rates of Lyme disease in the United States were up to six times the *Healthy People 2010* targeted rate of 9.7 new cases per 100,000 population where the disease is endemic (DHHS, 2000). Although the incidence of human Lyme disease in the northeastern United States is more than twice that in the Midwest, the prevalence of *B. burgdorferi* in the tick vector is nearly identical in the two regions (Brisson, Vandermause, Meece, et al., 2010). Lyme disease is spreading throughout the world. Cases have been found on all continents except Antarctica.

A recent study by Hersh and colleagues (2014) found that humans in the northeastern and midwestern United States are at increasing risk of not only Lyme disease, but also coinfection with two emerging pathogens *Anaplasma phagocytophilium* and *Babesia microti*. *B. burgdorferi*, *B. microti*, and *A. phagocytophilium* are transmitted by the same tick vector, *I. scapularis*. Although coinfection with the gram-negative bacterium *A. phagocytophilium* was found to be less common in the ticks they studied, 83% were found to be coinfected with *B. burgdorferi* and *B. microti*. Human babesiosis, caused by *B. microti*, a protozoan blood parasite, has been increasing in prevalence, especially in the Northeast. Babesiosis can be asymptomatic or present with flu-like symptoms (e.g., fever, chills, body aches, weakness, and fatigue) that may not appear for weeks or months after exposure to *B. microti*. In addition, Krause et al. (2014) found that *B. miyamoti* is prevalent in southern New England. Therefore, healthcare providers should be aware that acute *B. miyamoti* infection may be misdiagnosed as Lyme disease. They also should keep in mind an increased risk of coinfection with *B. burgdorferi* and *B. microti* when diagnosing and treating tick-borne illness. Babesiosis became a notifiable disease in 2011 (CDC, *Babesiosis*).

table 15.1 **Lyme Disease Incidence Rates among 13 States with Highest Incidence, United States, 2011, 2012, and 2002**

State	Incidence Rate, 2011[a]	Incidence Rate, 2012[a]	Incidence Rate, 2002[a]
Delaware	84.6	55.3	24.0
Vermont	76.0	61.7	6.0
New Hampshire	67.3	75.9	20.5
Maine	60.3	66.6	16.9
Connecticut	56.0	46.0	133.8
Wisconsin	42.2	23.9	20.0
New Jersey	38.5	30.8	27.4
Pennsylvania	37.2	32.5	32.3
Massachusetts	27.3	51.1	28.1
Minnesota	22.2	16.9	17.3
Maryland	16.1	18.9	13.5
New York	16.0	10.4	28.9
Virginia	9.3	9.8	3.6
U.S. Incidence	7.8	7.0	8.2

[a] Incidence rate: confirmed cases per 100,000 persons.
Source: CDC. *Lyme disease incidence rates by state, 2002–2011*; CDC. *Lyme disease incidence rates by state, 2003–2012.* Retrived from http://www.cdc.gov/lyme/stats/chartstables/incidencebystate.html

Symptoms and Signs of Lyme Disease

Lyme disease is diagnosed based on symptoms, physical findings (e.g., a "bull's-eye rash," which is the hallmark symptom of Lyme disease), and the possibility of exposure to infected ticks; laboratory testing is helpful if used correctly and performed with validated methods.

Exposure to Lyme disease is defined as having spent time (less than or equal to 30 days before onset of the initial skin lesion) in wooded, brushy, or grassy areas (i.e., potential tick habitats) in a county in which Lyme disease is endemic. A history of tick bite is not required. A county in which the disease is endemic is one in which at least two confirmed cases have been previously acquired or in which established populations of a known tick vector are infected with *B. burgdorferi* (CDC, *Lyme disease*).

The best clinical marker of Lyme disease is the initial skin lesion (i.e., erythema migrans), which occurs in 60% to 80% of people with the disease. For purposes of surveillance, erythema migrans is defined as a skin lesion that typically begins as a red macule or papule and expands over a period of days to weeks to form a large round lesion, often with partial central clearing. Within 1 to 2 weeks of being infected with *B. burgdorferi*, people may have the bull's-eye rash with fever, headache, and muscle or joint pain. Some people have Lyme disease and do not have any early symptoms. Other people have fever and other flu-like symptoms without a rash (CDC, *Lyme disease*).

After several days or weeks, the bacteria may spread throughout the body of an infected person. Symptoms such as rashes in other parts of the body, pain that seems to move from joint to joint, and signs of inflammation of the heart or nerves may occur. If the disease is not treated, additional symptoms, such as swelling and pain in major joints or mental changes, months after becoming infected, may occur in a few cases (CDC, *Lyme disease*). People who are treated with antibiotics early in the infection generally recover quickly and completely, as do those in the later stages of the infection. However, clients with persistent and recurring symptoms may require a second 4-week course of antibiotics (CDC, *Lyme disease*).

STUDENT REFLECTION

When I was in middle school, I attended a Boy Scout camp with my best friend Mark. The camp was near my home in eastern Connecticut. We hiked in the hills almost every day. I loved it, but we often came home with lots of insect bites. One time, I actually counted over a hundred of them—it was sort of a badge of honor! I started to think differently, though, when Mark found an engorged tick behind his knee in the crease of his leg. The nurse at the camp removed it with tweezers and cleaned it, and at the time we didn't think much about it. It was almost time to start school when Mark started to complain about aching everywhere. When he got a fever, his Mom took him to the clinic and they found a large, sore, red lesion where the tick had bitten him. It looked infected. The sore was almost 6 inches long, and the doctor found secondary lesions on both of his legs. I think Mark was scared at this point. After a few days of antibiotics, he felt better, but he had to take the pills for 3 weeks. What surprised me at the time was that he had to be followed for a year to be sure that complications were not present. He got over it, but the two of us talk about it once in a while.

Prevention of Lyme Disease

Steps to prevent Lyme disease include using insect repellent, identification and removal of deer ticks promptly, applying pesticides, and reducing tick habitat. Nymphal deer ticks are the size of poppy seeds, and adult deer ticks are the size of apple seeds (Fig. 15.5). Although interventions are inexpensive, are unlikely to be harmful, and have probably slowed the increase in Lyme disease in the United States, the epidemic continues to gain momentum.

According to the American Lyme Disease Foundation, the best precaution against Lyme disease in tick-infested areas is to avoid contact with soil, leaf litter, and vegetation as much as possible. People who garden, hike, camp, hunt, work outdoors, or otherwise spend time in brush, overgrown fields, or the woods should use the precautions listed in Box 15.3 to reduce their risk of getting Lyme disease (American Lyme Disease Foundation, *Lyme disease*).

PRACTICE POINT

Community and public health nurses must be prepared to educate the public about the signs and symptoms of Lyme disease and other tick-borne diseases, as well as the prevention of these diseases. Because the population density and percentage of infected ticks that may transmit Lyme disease and other tick-borne infections vary markedly from one region of the country to another, people should know whether infected deer ticks are active in their area or in places they may visit. There is even great variation from county to county within a state and from area to area within a county. For example, less than 5% of adult ticks south of Maryland are infected with *B. burgdorferi*, whereas up to 50% are infected in areas with a high tick infection rate in the Northeast. The tick infection rate in Pacific coastal states is between 2% and 4% (American Lyme Disease Foundation). As noted above, healthcare providers should also be aware of an increased risk of coinfection with *B. burgdorferi*, *B. microti*, and *B. miyamoti*.

box 15.3 Lyme Disease Combined Prevention Techniques

- Know how to identify deer ticks.
- Wear enclosed shoes and light-colored clothing with a tight weave to make it easier to spot ticks.
- Scan clothes and any exposed skin frequently for ticks while outdoors.
- Stay on cleared, well-traveled trails.
- Use insect repellant containing diethyl-meta-toluamide (DEET) on skin or insect repellant for clothes.
- Avoid sitting directly on the ground or on stone walls since they are havens for ticks and their hosts.
- Keep long hair tied back, especially when gardening.
- Do a final, full-body tick check at the end of the day for adults, children, and pets.
- Ticks tend to climb to warm, hidden areas of the head and neck if not intercepted first.
- Performed consistently, this is the most effective current prevention technique.
- Shower and shampoo on returning home; crawling ticks may be removed, but not attached ticks.
- Spin clothes in a dryer for 20 minutes to kill any unseen ticks.

Source: Adapted from American Lyme Disease Foundation. *Lyme disease*. Retrieved from http://www.aldf.com/lyme.shtml

E. coli O157:H7

Escherichia coli O157:H7, a Shiga toxin-producing *E. coli* (STEC), may also be referred to as verocytotoxin-producing *E. coli* (VTEC) or enterohemorrhagic *E. coli* (EHEC). This deadly toxin-producing bacterium is the one most commonly heard about in the news in association with foodborne outbreaks in the United States, and have led to national recalls of several food products (CDC, *E. coli*). It produces symptoms of severe abdominal cramps, bloody and nonbloody diarrhea, and vomiting, which generally resolve within 7 to 10 days.

Most people recover fully from an *E. coli* infection in 2 or 3 days; however, *E. coli* O157:H7 can cause fatal hemolytic-uremic syndrome (HUS) and renal failure in the very young and the elderly, and clients may require dialysis. HUS generally occurs up to a week after a gastrointestinal infection with *E. coli*. In these cases, HUS develops when the bacterial toxins enter the bloodstream and destroy red blood cells (CDC, *E. coli*).

PRACTICE POINT

E. coli O157:H7 infections can also be caused by zoonotic transmission through contact with animals that carry the organism.

Recent cases of HUS have been associated with outbreaks of *E. coli* O157:H7 infections, which were apparently caused by contact with animals in public settings, including fairs, farm tours, and petting zoos. Experience from these and previous outbreaks underscores the necessity for adequate control measures to reduce zoonotic transmission. The CDC has developed standardized recommendations for public health officials, veterinarians, animal exhibitors, and visitors to animal exhibits; it established that hand washing is the single most important prevention step for reducing the risk for disease transmission. Other critical recommendations for venues with animals are the inclusion of transition areas between animal and nonanimal areas (e.g., where food is sold) and proper care and management of animals in public settings. In addition, the CDC recommends educating the operators and staff of animal venues, as well as visitors, about the risk of disease transmission if animal contact is possible (CDC, 2005a). More information about zoonotic transmission of *E. coli* O157:H7 can be found in Chapter 14.

Tuberculosis

Epidemiology of TB

Tuberculosis (TB) is a disease caused by *Mycobacterium tuberculosis* that is spread from person to person through the air when a person with TB disease of the lungs or throat coughs, sneezes, speaks, or sings. The TB bacteria (droplet nuclei) can stay suspended in the air for several hours, depending on the environment. Persons who breathe in the air containing these TB bacteria can become infected. The bacteria usually attack the lungs, but they can attack any part of the body such as the kidney, spine, and brain. If not treated properly, TB disease can be fatal (CDC, *Tuberculosis*).

Tuberculosis is one of the most common infectious diseases worldwide. The WHO reports that there were an estimated 8.6 million new cases of TB worldwide in 2012. Thirteen percent of these cases were coinfected with HIV, and 1.3 million people died from TB. Nearly 1 million TB deaths occurred among HIV-negative individuals and 430,000 among people who were HIV-positive. TB is one of the top killers of women, with 250,000 deaths among HIV-negative women and 160,000 deaths among HIV-positive women in 2012. The TB mortality rate has decreased by 45% since 1990, and the world is on track to achieve the global target of a 50% reduction by 2015. Nevertheless, in 2013 only 7 of the 22 WHO "high-burden" countries, which account for over 80% of the world's TB cases, had met all 2015 targets for TB reduction in incidence, prevalence, and mortality rates. The burden of TB is highest in Southeast Asia (29%) and Africa (27%). India and China together account for almost 40% of the world's total TB cases, at 29% and 12%, respectively. Nearly 75% of TB cases among people living with HIV reside in Africa (WHO, 2013b).

Tuberculosis was once the leading cause of death in the United States. After approximately 30 years of decline, the number of reported cases of TB increased 20% between 1985 and 1992. This led to a renewed emphasis on TB control and prevention in the 1990s and actions that reversed the increase in cases.

A total of 9,945 TB cases (a rate of 3.2 cases/100,000 population) were reported in the United States in 2012, the lowest recorded since national reporting began in 1953. However, a total of 63% of the 2012 reported TB cases in the United States occurred in foreign-born persons. The case rate among foreign-born persons (15.9 cases/100,000) in 2012 was approximately 11 times higher than among U.S.-born persons (1.4 cases/100,000). Racial and ethnic minorities and foreign-born persons continue to be disproportionately affected by TB. In 2012, the highest TB rates in the United States occurred among persons who were Asian (18.9 cases/1000,000 population), Black or African-American (5.8 cases/1000,000), Hispanic/Latino (5.3 cases/1000,000), American Indian or Alaskan Native (6.3 cases/1000,000), or Native Hawaiian and other Pacific Islanders (12.3 cases/1000,000). In addition, multidrug-resistant TB (MDR-TB) remains a threat among foreign-born people. Of the total number of reported primary MDR-TB cases, the proportion occurring in foreign-born persons increased from 25.3% (103 of 407) in 1993 to 86.1% (62 of 72) in 2012 (CDC, *TB Facts*).

Despite successful declines in TB cases and case rates over the past 60 years, it is unlikely that current TB control and prevention efforts will result in TB elimination (<1 case per 1,000,000 population) in this century. The improvement of TB control among racial/ethnic minorities and foreign-born persons is essential as the United States strives to prevent TB transmission and meet TB elimination goals (CDC, 2012).

In Case 2, first responders, such as EMTs and firefighters, are now scheduled to have annual tuberculin testing. What are the factors that have contributed to this change? How do these factors differ from those associated with seasonal influenza?

PRACTICE POINT

M. tuberculosis is an example of an infectious agent that can cause an infection in an individual, but not be contagious at all times.

M. tuberculosis infection occurs when a susceptible person inhales airborne droplet nuclei containing the TB bacilli, which pass through the upper respiratory tract and bronchi. When the bacilli reach the alveoli of the lungs, they are taken up by macrophages and spread throughout the body. Generally, 2 to 10 weeks after initial infection with *M. tuberculosis*, an immune response limits additional multiplication and spread of the bacilli. *M. tuberculosis* generally affects the lungs but can attack any part of the body such as the kidney, spine, and brain. If not treated properly, TB can be fatal (CDC, *Tuberculosis*).

However, some of the TB bacilli remain dormant and viable for many years and are defined as latent TB infection. People with latent TB infection usually have a positive purified protein derivative (PPD) tuberculin skin test but no symptoms of active TB and therefore are not contagious. In many people who have latent TB infection, the *M. tuberculosis* bacteria remain inactive for a lifetime without causing active TB disease. But in other people, especially those who have weak immune systems, the bacteria become active and cause TB disease (CDC, *Tuberculosis fact sheets*). See Table 15.2 for the difference between latent TB infection and active TB disease.

Symptoms and Signs of TB

Active TB infection is characterized by a chronic productive cough, low-grade fever, night sweats, and weight loss, along with a positive PPD-tuberculin skin test. People with active TB are contagious. However, certain people who are anergic (lack an immune response to an antigen) may not have a positive PPD (e.g., persons with HIV).

table 15.2 **Symptomatic Differences between Latent Tuberculosis (TB) Infection and Active TB Disease**

A Person with Latent TB Infection	A Person with Active TB Disease
• Has no symptoms • Does not feel sick • Cannot spread TB to others • Usually has a positive skin test or QuantiFERON-TB Gold In-Tube test (QFT-GIT) • Has a normal chest X-ray and sputum test	• Has symptoms that may include the following: A bad cough that lasts 3 weeks or longer Pain in the chest Coughing up blood or sputum Weakness or fatigue Weight loss No appetite Chills Fever Sweating at night • May spread TB to others • Usually has a positive skin test or QFT-GIT • May have an abnormal chest X-ray or positive sputum smear or culture

Notes: QuantiFERON-TB Gold In-Tube test (QFT-GIT) is an FDA-approved indirect blood test for *M. tuberculosis infection (including infection resulting in active disease) when used in conjunction with risk assessment, radiography, and other medical and diagnostic evaluations.*

Sources: CDC, *Tuberculosis fact sheets.* Retrieved from http://www.cdc.gov/tb/topics/testing.htm; CDC. (2010). Updated guidelines for using interferon gamma release assays to detect *Mycobacterium tuberculosis* infection—United States, 2010. *Morbidity and Mortality Weekly Report, 59*(RR05), 1–25.

EVIDENCE FOR PRACTICE

A nurse case-managed intervention, with incentives and tracking procedures to increase adherence to treatment of latent TB infection, was evaluated to determine the efficacy of the program. Twelve homeless subgroups were chosen that had characteristics previously identified in the literature as predictive of nonadherence to treatment. These characteristics included female gender, African-American ethnicity, a history of military service, lifetime injection drug use, daily alcohol and drug use, poor physical health, and a history of poor mental health. Five hundred twenty homeless adults in homeless shelters in Los Angeles were followed prospectively over a period of 5 years. The intervention achieved a 91% completion rate for homeless shelter residents, and there was significantly improved latent TB infection treatment adherence in 9 of the 12 subgroups. However, daily drug users, participants with a history of injection drug use, daily alcohol users, and people who were not African-American had particularly poor completion rates. It was concluded that nurse case management with incentives appears to be a good foundation for improving adherence to treatment for latent TB infection, especially for sheltered homeless populations (Nyamathi et al., 2008).

Latent TB and HIV Infections

People infected with HIV, especially those with low CD4$^+$ cell counts, develop TB disease rapidly after becoming infected with *M. tuberculosis.* Because HIV infection weakens the immune system, people with prior untreated latent TB infection and HIV infection are at very high risk of developing active TB disease (American Thoracic Society, CDC, & Infectious Disease Society of America, 2000a). Therefore, all people with HIV infection should be tested to find out if they have latent TB infection. If they have latent TB infection, they need treatment as soon as possible to prevent them from developing active TB disease. If they have active TB disease, they must take medicine to cure the disease (American Thoracic Society, CDC, & Infectious Disease Society of America, 2000a, 2003; CDC, 2005e).

Prevention and Control of TB

TARGETED TUBERCULIN TESTING AND TREATMENT OF LATENT TB INFECTION

In the United States and other countries with a low incidence of TB, most new, active cases have occurred in people with latent TB infection who later developed active TB. Targeted identification and treatment of infected people at highest risk for developing disease benefits both infected people and susceptible people. Because health departments often lack access to high-risk populations and the resources necessary to undertake targeted testing programs, the participation of other healthcare providers is essential to ensure the successful implementation of community efforts to prevent TB in high-risk groups. Community sites where healthcare professionals may find people at high risk for TB and where targeted testing programs have been evaluated include neighborhood health centers, jails, homeless shelters, inner-city areas, methadone clinics, syringe/needle-exchange programs, and other community-based social service facilities (American Thoracic Society, CDC, & Infectious Disease Society of America, 2000b). The WHO recommends directly observed therapy (DOT), using the most effective standardized, short-course regimens, and of fixed-dose TB drug combinations as an approach to TB control (WHO, *The five elements of DOT*).

Treating latent *M. tuberculosis* infection (LTBI) is a cornerstone of the U.S. strategy for TB elimination. Randomized controlled studies have shown that a new combination regimen of isoniazid (INH) and rifapentine administered weekly for 12 weeks as DOT is as effective for preventing TB as other regimens and is more likely to be completed than the U.S. standard regimen of 9 months of INH daily without DOT. These "first-line" treatment drugs are highly effective against nonresistant TB but much less so against MDR-TB. The new regimen is recommended as an equal alternative to the 9-month INH regimen for otherwise healthy patients aged 12 years or older who have LTBI and factors that are predictive of TB developing (e.g., recent exposure to contagious TB) (CDC, 2012). See Box 15.4 for people at high risk for progressing from latent TB infection to active TB disease.

TREATMENT OF ACTIVE TB

Active TB can be treated even in people with HIV infection. Because of the relatively high proportion of adults with TB caused by organisms that are resistant to INH, four drugs are necessary in the initial phase to be maximally effective. Thus, in most circumstances, the treatment regimen for all adults with previously untreated TB should consist of a 2-month initial phase of INH, rifampin (RIF), pyrazinamide (PZA), and ethambutol (EMB), followed by a choice of several options for the continuation phase of either 4 or 7 months. However, if the organisms are fully susceptible, EMB need not be included. For children whose visual acuity cannot be monitored, EMB is usually not recommended. Management of HIV-related TB is complex and requires expertise in the management of both HIV disease and TB. However, with a few exceptions, recommendations for the treatment of TB in HIV-infected adults are the same as adults without HIV infection. People with latent TB infection should be treated with INH for 9 months, RIF (with or without INH) for 4 months, or RIF and PZA for 2 months (for those who are unlikely to complete a longer course and who can be monitored closely) (American Thoracic Society, CDC, & Infectious Diseases Society of America, 2003).

Drug susceptibility tests should be performed on initial isolates from all clients to identify what should be an effective anti-TB regimen. In addition, drug susceptibility tests should be repeated if the client continues to produce culture-positive sputum after 3 months of treatment or develops positive cultures after a period of negative cultures (American Thoracic Society et al., 2003).

Directly observed therapy (DOT) is one in which healthcare professionals observe clients to ensure that they ingest each dose of anti-TB medication to maximize the likelihood of completion of therapy. Programs using DOT as the central element in a comprehensive, client-centered approach to case management (enhanced DOT) have higher rates of treatment completion than less intensive strategies. Each client's management plan should be individualized to incorporate measures that facilitate adherence to the drug regimen. Such measures may include, for example, social service support, treatment incentives and enablers, housing assistance, referral for treatment of substance abuse, and coordination of TB services with those of other providers (American Thoracic Society et al., 2003; WHO *The five elements of DOT*). There is no need to hospitalize a person solely because they are infectious. Outpatients should be instructed to remain at home, without visitors, until they are no longer thought to be infectious. Also, people who are particularly susceptible to developing TB disease if they become infected (small children, immunocompromised people) should not visit or live with an infected client while he or she can transmit the TB bacterium (American Thoracic Society et al., 2000a, 2000b, 2003; CDC, 2005e).

box 15.4 Factors That Influence Progression from Latent Tuberculosis (TB) Infection to Active TB Disease

People infected with HIV
People infected with *Mycobacterium tuberculosis* within the previous 2 years
Infants and children aged <4 years
People with any of the following clinical conditions or other immunocompromising conditions:

- Silicosis
- Diabetes mellitus
- Chronic renal failure
- Certain hematologic disorders (leukemias and lymphomas)
- Other specific malignancies (e.g., carcinoma of the head, neck, or lung)
- Body weight >10% below ideal body weight
- Prolonged corticosteroid use
- Other immunosuppressive treatments
- Organ transplant
- End-stage renal disease
- Intestinal bypass or gastrectomy

Source: People with a history of untreated or inadequately treated TB disease, including people with chest radiograph findings consistent with previous TB (CDC, *Tuberculosis*).

DIAGNOSTIC AND PUBLIC HEALTH EVALUATION OF TB CONTACTS

By law and regulation, cases of active TB in the United States must be reported to the local health department. Reporting is essential for action by TB control programs at local, state, and national levels. TB case finding is important for understanding the magnitude and the distribution of the disease in the United States. Therefore, reporting of TB suspects promptly (prior to bacteriologic confirmation) is important. Public health services are available for epidemiologic evaluation, including the identification and examination of source cases and contacts (American Thoracic Society et al., 2000a).

The probability that a person who is exposed to *M. tuberculosis* will become infected depends primarily on the concentration of infectious droplet nuclei in the air and the duration of exposure to a person with infectious TB disease. The closer the proximity and the longer the duration of exposure, the higher the risk of becoming infected. Close contacts are people who share the same air space in a household or other enclosed environment for a prolonged period (days or weeks, not minutes or hours) with a person with pulmonary TB disease. A suspect TB client is a person in whom a diagnosis of TB disease is being considered, whether or not anti-TB treatment has been started. People generally should not continue to be suspected of having TB for more than 3 months (American Thoracic Society et al., 2000a).

Initial assessment of contacts should be accomplished within 3 days of reported exposure to a person who has active TB disease. During that initial assessment, a history of previous *M. tuberculosis* infection or disease and treatment should be taken along with any current symptoms of TB illness and medical conditions that increase the risk of TB infection. The type, duration, and intensity of exposure should be documented to provide data for high- and medium-priority contact follow-up with diagnostic tests and possible treatment. All high- and medium-priority contacts who do not have a documented previous positive tuberculin skin test or previous TB disease should receive a baseline PPD tuberculin skin test (CDC, CDC, 2005b). The reaction to the intracutaneously injected PPD-tuberculin skin test is the classic example of a delayed (cellular) hypersensitivity reaction, which induces induration. Induration of 5 mm or more is considered a positive result in people who have an initial induration of 0 mm. See Figure 15.6 (CDC, 2005b).

PRACTICE POINT

Nurses in health departments and in community and public health settings may be responsible for conducting TB contact investigations. By taking a careful contact history, nurses are able to determine which contacts are at greatest risk for TB exposure. Nurses also administer PPD-tuberculin skin tests during evaluation of exposure.

Questions often arise about the interpretation of tuberculin skin test results in people with a history of bacillus Calmette–Guérin (BCG) vaccine, HIV infection, and recent contacts with an infectious case of TB. History of BCG vaccine administration is not a contraindication for tuberculin testing. If more than 5 years have elapsed since administration of BCG vaccine, a positive tuberculin test reaction is most likely a result of *M. tuberculosis* infection (CDC, *Tuberculosis*).

TB DIAGNOSTIC TESTS

The majority of experience with diagnosing *M. tuberculosis* infection, primarily in contacts, has been with the PPD skin test. In 2005, the CDC issued guidelines for using the FDA-approved QuantiFERON-Gold (QFT-G) test for diagnosing *M. tuberculosis* infection, including both active TB disease and latent TB infection. The 2005 guidelines indicated that

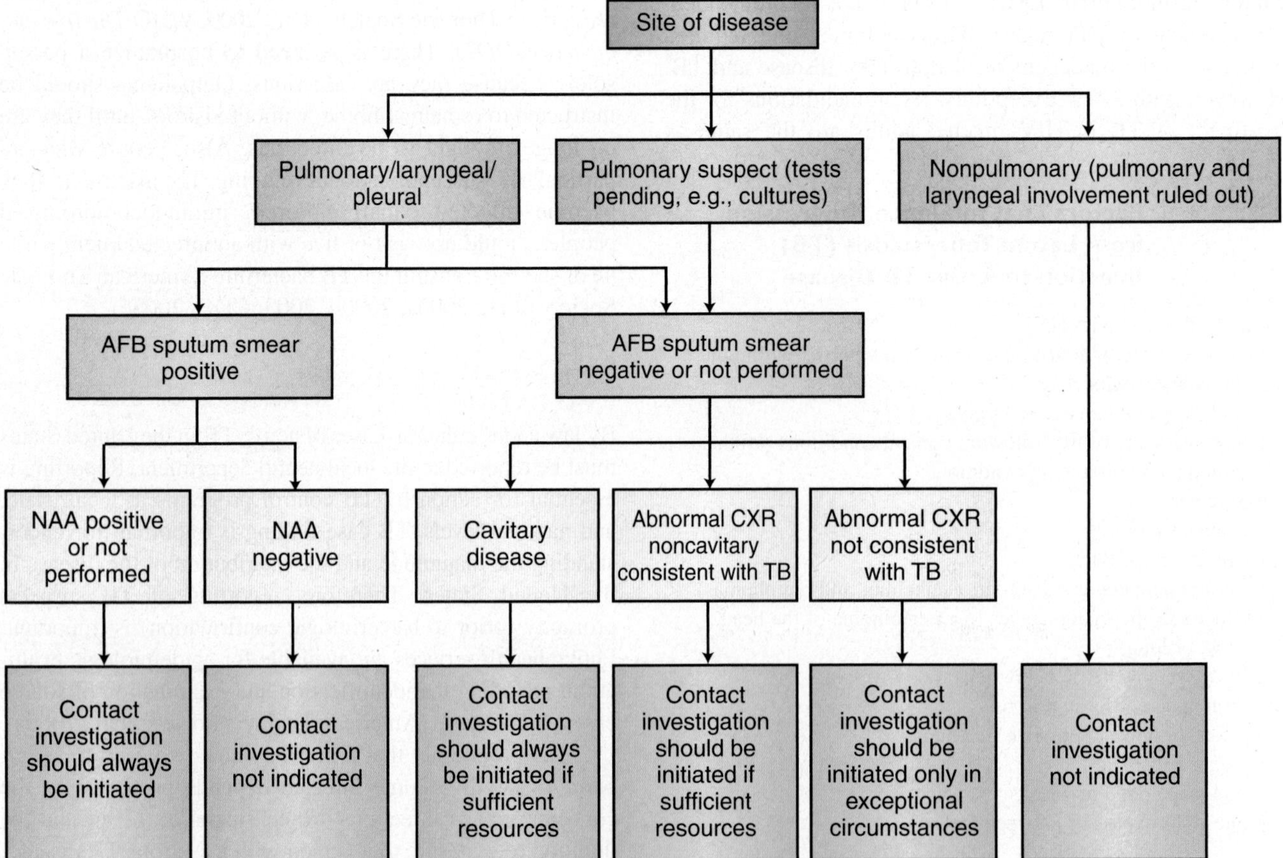

figure 15.6 Decision-making factors when initiating a tuberculosis (TB) contact investigation. AFB, acid-fast bacilli; NAA, nucleic acid assay; CXR, chest radiograph; Approved indication for NAA.

(From CDC [2005]. Guidelines for the investigation of contacts of persons with infectious tuberculosis. *Morbidity and Mortality Weekly Report, 54*(RR15), 1–37.

QFT-G may be used in all circumstances in which a PPD test was recommended, including contact investigations, evaluation of recent immigrants, and serial-testing surveillance programs for infection control (e.g., those for healthcare workers). However, the guidelines provided cautions for testing persons from selected populations, including persons at increased risk for progression to active disease if infected (CDC, 2005c).

Subsequently, two new interferon gamma (IFN-γ) release assays (IGRAs) were approved by the FDA as aids in diagnosing both latent and active *M. tuberculosis* infection. These tests are the QuantiFERON-TB Gold In-Tube test (QFT-GIT) (Cellestis Limited, Carnegie, VIC, Australia) and the T-SPOT TB test (T-Spot) (Oxford Immunotec Limited, Abingdon, United Kingdom). The antigens, methods, and interpretation criteria for these assays differ from those for IGRAs previously approved by the FDA. In 2007, QFT-GIT became the third IGRA approved by the FDA as an aid for diagnosing *M. tuberculosis* infection. The T-Spot became the fourth IGRA to be approved by the FDA in 2008.

In 2010, the CDC, the American Academy of Pediatrics, the American Thoracic Society, and the Infectious Disease Society of America coordinated development of updated guidelines for using IFN-γ assays for U.S. public health officials, healthcare providers, and laboratory workers to detect TB infection. Control materials and antigens for QFT-GIT and T-Spot are contained in special tubes used to collect blood for the test, thus allowing more direct testing of fresh blood. Both tests are approved as indirect tests for *M. tuberculosis* infection (including infection resulting in active disease) when used in conjunction with risk assessment, radiography, and other medical and diagnostic evaluations. The FDA-approved indications for QFT-GIT and T-Spot are similar to indications for QFT-G and TST. Because of administrative and logistic difficulties associated with the PPD skin test, IGRAs are attractive diagnostic aids for detecting *M. tuberculosis* infection. Unlike PPD, IGRA results can be available within 24 hours without the need for a second visit. As laboratory-based assays, IGRAs are not subject to the biases and errors associated with PPD placement and reading. However, the cost for an IGRA is substantially greater than that for a PPD skin test. Nonetheless, this additional cost might be offset by decreasing the number of persons testing positive and the associated costs of evaluating and treating persons with positive test results (CDC, 2010).

Persons at increased risk for *M. tuberculosis* infection include the following:

- Close contacts of persons known or suspected to have active TB
- Foreign-born persons from areas that have a high incidence of active TB (e.g., Africa, Asia, Eastern Europe, Latin America, and Russia)
- Persons who visit areas with a high prevalence of active TB, especially if visits are frequent or prolonged
- Residents and employees of congregate settings whose clients are at increased risk for active TB (e.g., correctional facilities, long-term care facilities, and homeless shelters)
- Healthcare personnel who serve clients who are at increased risk for active TB
- Populations defined locally as having an increased incidence of latent *M. tuberculosis* infection or active TB, possibly including medically underserved, low-income populations, or persons who abuse drugs or alcohol
- Infants, children, and adolescents exposed to adults who are at increased risk for LTBI or active TB (CDC, 2010)

In **Case 2**, the health department is notified to investigate the local fire department concerning a potential TB problem. Six months earlier, the fire department had administered two-step tuberculin skin tests and determined that nine firefighters tested positive for TB infection. A community/public health nurse is sent to the fire department to evaluate the situation.

How should the community/public health nurse proceed?

PRACTICE POINT

Best-practice nursing interventions must be tied into the role of community and public health nurses in the care and supportive aspects of TB case management. The American Thoracic Society, the CDC, and the Infectious Diseases Society of America support client-centered case management with an emphasis on evidence-based DOT options.

Multidrug-Resistant TB

Although effective drugs exist, a major reason for the failure to stem the spread of TB lies in the rise of drug-resistant strains of *M. tuberculosis*. Some strains are resistant to several drugs. Multidrug-resistant TB is defined as resistance to the two most potent "first-line" anti-TB agents. MDR-TB is difficult and expensive to treat and fails to respond to the two most potent anti-TB agents (INH and RIF). In addition, extensively drug-resistant TB (XDR-TB), another emerging threat, is a rare type of multidrug-resistant tuberculosis (MDR-TB) that is resistant to the first-line TB drugs, plus resistance to any fluoroquinolone and at least one of three injectable second-line drugs (CDC, *Tuberculosis fact sheets*).

The WHO estimates that there were about 0.5 million new MDR-TB cases in the world in 2011. About 60% of these cases occurred in Brazil, China, India, the Russian Federation and South Africa alone ("BRICS" countries) (WHO, *MDR-TB [2013b] update*). The development of drug-resistant strains occurs when healthcare providers do not follow treatment guidelines or fail to ensure that clients complete the entire treatment course.

TB Infection Control Guidelines for Healthcare Settings

The CDC updated the TB infection control guidelines for healthcare settings in 2005 (CDC, 2005d). These recommendations reflect shifts in the epidemiology of TB, advances in scientific understanding, and changes in healthcare practice that have occurred in the United States during the preceding decade. The updated TB infection control guidelines emphasize actions to maintain momentum and expertise needed to avert another TB resurgence and to eliminate the lingering threat to healthcare personnel, which is mainly from clients or others with unsuspected and undiagnosed infectious TB disease. A sample recommendation is that the term "tuberculin skin tests" be used rather than PPD. The scope of settings in which the guidelines apply has been broadened to include laboratories and additional outpatient and nontraditional healthcare settings.

These recommendations also apply to an entire healthcare setting rather than to areas within a setting. New terms such as "airborne infection precautions" (airborne precautions) and "airborne infection isolation (AII) room" have been introduced. One of the most critical risks for healthcare-associated transmission of *M. tuberculosis* in healthcare settings is from clients with unrecognized TB disease who are not promptly handled with appropriate airborne precautions or who are moved out of an AII room too soon (e.g., clients with unrecognized TB and MDR-TB). The CDC *Guidelines for Preventing the Transmission of Mycobacterium tuberculosis in Health-Care Settings* can be found online at http://www.cdc.gov/mmwr/PDF/rr/rr5417.pdf.

Ebola Virus Disease

Ebola first appeared in 1976 during two simultaneous outbreaks in Nzara, Sudan, and in Yambuku, Democratic Republic of Congo. It was named from the Ebola River, which is located in Yambuku. The Ebola virus is a member of the *Filoviridae* family (filovirus), and has five distinct species:

- *Bundibugyo ebolavirus* (BDBV)
- *Reston ebolavirus* (RESTV)
- *Sudan ebolavirus* (SUDV)
- *Taï Forest ebolavirus* (TAFV)
- *Zaire ebolavirus* (EBOV) (WHO, *Ebola virus disease*)

Ebola virus disease (EVD), previously called Ebola hemorrhagic fever, is a severe, often fatal illness with a reported case fatality rate as high as 100%. The virus can be brought into human populations through close contact with blood, secretions, or other body fluids and organs of infected animals such as chimpanzees, gorillas, fruit bats, monkeys, forest antelope, and porcupines. It can be spread from person-to-person through direct contact (through broken skin or mucous membranes) with blood, secretions, excretions, or other body fluids of an infected person. Ebola virus has been found in semen up to 61 days. The virus can also be spread by indirect contact through medical equipment and the contaminated environment in contact with these fluids. Large outbreaks of EVD in Africa have been associated with BDVD, EBOV, and SUDV since 1976, but not RESTV and TAFV. Although RESTV has been reported in China and the Philippines, it has not caused illness or death in humans to date (WHO, *Ebola virus disease*).

The last reported outbreak of EVD, which was caused by BDBV, occurred in the Democratic Republic of Congo in 2012. However, in the spring of 2014, an outbreak of EVD was reported in the forested areas of southeast Guinea and quickly spread to several districts. This was the first time EBV had been detected in West Africa. Confirmed cases have been reported in Guinea, Liberia, and Sierra Leone. The WHO confirmed that this outbreak was caused by the EBOV. The Ebola virus was introduced into Nigeria on July 20, 2014 by a Liberian traveler, resulting in a total of 20 cases and 8 deaths. However, by late October 2014, WHO had declared that Nigeria was free of Ebola virus transmission (WHO, *Nigeria ends Ebola*).

Intense transmission continued in Guinea, Liberia, and Sierra Leone. By the end of October 2014, the reported cases in the four West African countries (Guinea, Liberia, Sierra Leone, and Nigeria) had totaled 13,560 with 4,949 deaths (37% fatality rate), making it the worst EVD outbreak in history. Most of the EVD cases reported as of October 2014 had occurred in Liberia, with 2,413 deaths among 6,535 cases (37% fatality rate). However, Guinea reported the highest death rate (61%) at 1,018 among 1,667 cases (WHO, *Ebola Roadmap Apps*). A small number of cases of Ebola infection had been reported in the Democratic Republic of the Congo, but was not related to the ongoing outbreaks in Guinea, Liberia, and Sierra Leone (CDC, *Ebola in Democratic Republic of the Congo*).

The first imported case of Ebola infection in the United States occurred in Dallas, Texas, in September 2014 in a man who had traveled from Liberia. Two healthcare providers who had cared for that patient, who died, became ill with the Ebola virus and have since recovered. A third U.S. case of Ebola infection occurred in October 2014 in a doctor who had worked treating Ebola patients with Doctors without Borders in Guinea. He was hospitalized in New York City, and was recovering (CDC, *Cases of Ebola diagnosed in the United States*).

Although the Ebola virus posed little to no risk to the U.S. general population, on July 31, 2014, the CDC issued a level 3 travel alert (Avoid Nonessential Travel) for Sierra Leone, Guinea, and Liberia and reminded all healthcare providers to (1) take a good travel history to identify patients who had traveled to/from West Africa in the past 3 weeks, (2) know the signs and symptoms of EVD, and (3) follow infection control precautions for suspected and symptomatic cases of EVD to prevent the spread of the Ebola virus (CDC, *Travel Health Notices* at: wwwnc.cdc.gov/travel/notices). The CDC also posted and updated protocols for managing ill passengers and crewmembers on airlines and notification of CDC regarding ill passengers/crew on a plane from the affected countries before arrival in the United States (CDC, *Airline Guidance*).

In late October 2014, the CDC announced that state and local public health departments would begin daily active post-arrival monitoring of travelers from Sierra Leone, Guinea, and Liberia for 21 days from the date of their departure from West Africa. Postarrival monitoring was an additional safeguard to exit screening of all travelers from the affected countries. Travelers were provided information and guidance at the airport and were required to provide their temperature and the presence or absence of Ebola symptoms during the 21-day period. They also were to report their intent to travel in- or out-of-state (CDC, *Media Release*). The CDC also provided epidemiologic risk factors, ranging from "High Risk" to "No Identifiable Risk," to consider when evaluating people for EVD, classifying contacts, and public health actions needed based on exposure (CDC, *Epidemiologic Risk Factors...for Exposure to Ebola*).

Signs, Symptoms, and Diagnosis of EVD

Ebola virus disease has an incubation period from 2 to 21 days, but the average is 8 to 10 days. Early symptoms include sudden onset of fever, muscle pain and weakness, headache, and sore throat. These symptoms are followed by vomiting, diarrhea, rash, compromised liver and kidney function, and, in some cases, internal and external bleeding (CDC, *EVD Signs and Symptoms*). Before the diagnosis of EVD is made, other diseases should be ruled out, such as malaria, influenza, and typhoid fever, since these diseases may have similar signs and symptoms. Laboratory tests for a definitive diagnosis of EVD include ELISA, antigen detection tests, PCR assay, and culture isolation of the virus (CDC, *EVD Diagnosis*).

Infection Prevention and Control of EVD

In the absence of a human vaccine and lack of effective treatment for EVD, public health measures should focus on risk reduction, which include the following:

- Reduction of animal-to-human transmission from contact with infected wildlife and consumption of their raw meat. Animal workers should wear gloves and PPE when handling animals. Hand hygiene should be employed after handling animals. Animal products should be thoroughly cooked before consumption.
- Reduction of person-to-person transmission from direct/close contact with infected patients and their body fluids. Gloves and PPE should be worn when caring for infected patients in the home, and good hand hygiene should be practiced to prevent contamination and cross-infection (WHO, *Ebola virus disease*).
- Use of standard contact and droplet precautions and other infection control measures in healthcare settings to prevent exposure to blood and body fluids and the potentially contaminated environment when caring for patients with suspected or confirmed EBV
- When caring for a hospitalized patient with confirmed or suspected EVD, specific infection control guidance has been provided by the CDC, including patient placement and PPE to be used by healthcare providers, including donning and removing PPE.
- When entering the room of a patient with suspected or known EBV, *all* healthcare providers should wear PPE, including fluid-resistant gown, gloves, mask, and face shield/goggles (CDC, *Infection prevention and control recommendations for hospitalized patients with known or suspected Ebola in U.S. hospitals*).

PRACTICE POINT

For better or for worse, invisible invasive organisms have been a part of life since life began. Their life cycles are so short in comparison with ours that they have multiple generations to react to obstacles in their environment, adapt to adverse conditions, and increase their strength and capacity to reproduce. Therefore, the public health system must continue to be vigilant.

CONCLUSIONS

By the middle of the 20th century, many researchers regarded the threat of infectious diseases to be significantly diminished. However, in the globally interconnected world of the 21st century, it has become clear that the threat of epidemics and pandemics remains a current and pressing possibility. Recent publicity associated with the potential for the Influenza A (H5N1) virus to mutate so that it is both easily transmitted from person to person while maintaining extreme virulence has highlighted the broader problem: Conditions around the globe are set for the possible development of epidemics of zoonotic diseases that have the potential to become pandemic. Unlike other public health threats such as TB and malaria, the emergence of these zoonotic diseases represents the potential of rare events with catastrophic consequences, as seen in the 1918 influenza pandemic and the more recent HIV epidemic. To date, scientists and public health advocates have focused on surveillance as the critical tool for detecting and monitoring outbreaks of zoonotic diseases in human and animal populations, but questions remain as to how to make zoonotic disease surveillance more comprehensive and timely in human and animal populations in order to prevent or minimize the potential for outbreaks to occur in human populations. Scientists have been concerned for some time about climate change and its effect on zoonotic diseases in human and animal populations.

To address this problem, in 2010, the IOM and the National Research Council convened an expert committee. The committee's task was to provide consensus advice on the challenge of achieving sustainable global capacity for surveillance and response to emerging diseases of zoonotic origin such as avian influenza, and ways to protect the public from them. The 2-day workshop by the Committee can be summarized by the following statement: "Because it would be impossible to test every species ..., the strategy must be to focus on so-called hotspots—areas with high biodiversity as well as high human population density—where zoonoses are most likely to be found." Several options are available to monitor and track emerging zoonotic diseases in humans. By conducting "smart surveillance," scientists will be able to target their resources and efforts in areas where human–animal interaction is most likely to provide conditions favorable to zoonoses (IOM, 2010).

Most of the world, including the United States, lacks a skilled workforce to combat emerging diseases. There is a call to increase educational programs in applied epidemiology and infectious disease prevention and control. Nurses are the largest group of healthcare professionals; therefore, they are in a position to take leadership initiatives. Hands-on experience, such as those obtained through the CDC Epidemic Intelligence Service (EIS) 2-year postgraduate program, can equip nurses with surveillance skills.

key concepts

- Factors that influence the emergence or reemergence of infectious diseases are multiple, complex, and interrelated.
- Epidemics and pandemics can place sudden and intense demands on healthcare systems.
- In addition to morbidity and mortality, outbreaks of emerging and reemerging infections can disrupt economic activity and development.
- Certain zoonotic diseases can be transmitted to humans through contact with animals and birds.
- There is a worldwide need for a skilled public health workforce to combat emerging diseases.
- Nurses must be able to recognize new and reemerging infectious diseases, identify the conditions that foster their development, and act to protect the health of the public.

critical thinking questions

1. You spent last weekend hiking in the woods but forgot to bring insect repellant. Two days ago, a circular flat rash with a white center appears high on the back of your calf. It does not hurt; therefore, you decide to forget about it. Today, you develop a fever, are fatigued, and have a headache along with muscle and joint pain.
   a. Explain what may have happened.
   b. Outline your plan of action.
   c. How would you prevent similar occurrences?
2. Your neighbor, Millie, asks to talk to you because she has felt tired for the last 2 days, has a headache, a rash, and does not feel like eating. You take her vital signs and find that she has a low-grade fever. Millie has just returned from a visit with her mother in New Jersey, where she was helping her clean up hurricane damage. It had been unusually dry there until the recent hurricanes hit, resulting in extensive flooding. Millie tells you that she was appalled at the number of birds that had died or were dying while she was there. She says that she helped pick up and dispose of the dead birds and received several mosquito bites on her arms in the process. The lymph glands in her arm pits are swollen.
   a. What could Millie have been exposed to, and how would the exposure have occurred?
   b. What advice would you give to Millie?
3. Outline the factors that have contributed to the emergence or reemergence of each of the following infectious diseases. Explain how these factors differ with each disease.
   a. Lyme disease
   b. West Nile virus
   c. *E. coli* O157:H7
4. Identify at least two changes that have occurred in your local community within the last few years that may contribute to emerging infectious diseases.

references

American Lyme Disease Foundation. *Lyme disease*. Retrieved June 30, 2014, from http://www.aldf.com/lyme.shtml

American Thoracic Society, Centers for Disease Control and Prevention, & Infectious Disease Society of America. (2000a). Diagnostic standards and classification of tuberculosis in adults and children. *American Journal of Respiratory and Critical Care Medicine, 161*,1376–1395.

American Thoracic Society, Centers for Disease Control and Prevention, & Infectious Diseases Society of America. (2000b). Targeted tuberculin testing and treatment of latent tuberculosis infection. *American Journal of Respiratory and Critical Care Medicine, 161*(4), S221–S247.

American Thoracic Society, Centers for Disease Control and Prevention, & Infectious Diseases Society of America. (2003). Treatment of tuberculosis. *Morbidity Mortality Weekly Report, 52*(RR11), 1–77.

Brisson, D., Vandermause, M. F., Meece, J. K., Reed, K. D., & Dykhuizen, D. E. (2010). Evolution of northeastern and midwestern *Borrelia burgdorferi,* United States. *Emerging Infectious Diseases, 16*(6), 911–917.

Centers for Disease Control and Prevention, National Institute of Occupational Safety, & Health. (2007a). *Health hazard evaluation report 2007-0012-3046*. Atlanta, GA: Department of Health and Human Services Centers for Disease Control and Prevention.

Centers for Disease Control and Prevention. (2003). Update: Outbreak of severe acute respiratory syndrome—worldwide, 2003. *Morbidity and Mortality Weekly Report, 52*(12), 241–248.

Centers for Disease Control and Prevention. (2004). *Interim recommendations for infection control in health-care facilities caring for patients with known or suspected avian influenza.* Retrieved May 14, 2013 from, http://www.cdc.gov/flu/avian/professional/infect-control.htm

Centers for Disease Control and Prevention. (2005a). Compendium of measures to prevent disease Associated with animals in public settings, 2005. *Morbidity and Mortality Weekly Report, 54*(RR04), 1–12.

Centers for Disease Control and Prevention. (2005b). Guidelines for the investigation of contacts of persons with infectious tuberculosis. *Morbidity and Mortality Weekly Report, 54*(RR15), 1–37.

Centers for Disease Control and Prevention. (2005c). Guidelines for using the QuantiFERON-TB gold test for detecting *Mycobacterium tuberculosis* infection, United States. *Morbidity and Mortality Weekly Report, 54*(RR15), 49–55.

Centers for Disease Control and Prevention. (2005d). Guidelines for preventing the transmission of *Mycobacterium tuberculosis* in health-care settings, 2005. *Morbidity and Mortality Weekly Report*, *54*(RR17), 1–141.

Centers for Disease Control and Prevention. (2005e). Controlling tuberculosis in the United States. Recommendations from the American Thoracic Society, CDC, and the Infectious Diseases Society of America. *Morbidity and Mortality Weekly Report*, *54*(RR12), 1–81.

Centers for Disease Control and Prevention. (2012). *Reported tuberculosis in the United States, 2011*. Atlanta, GA: U.S. Department of Health and Human Services.

Centers for Disease Control and Prevention. (2014). First confirmed case of Middle East respiratory syndrome coronavirus (MERS-CoV) infection in the United States, updated information. *Morbidity and Mortality Weekly Report*, *63*(19), 431–436.

Centers for Disease Control and Prevention. (2014, June 17). *Press release: MERS-CoV*. Retrieved June 26, 2014, from, http://www.cdc.gov/media/releases/2014/p0617 Mers.html

Centres for Health Protection (Hong Kong). (2014, May 25–June 7). *Summary of the second wave of human infections with avian influenza A (H7N9) virus* (Vol. 11, No. 12). Retrieved June 26, 2014, from http://www.chp.gov.hk/files/pdf.cdw_v11_12

Centers for Disease Control and Prevention. *2007 Guideline for isolation precautions: Preventing transmission of infectious agents in healthcare settings*. Retrieved June 4, 2013, from, http://www.cdc.gov/coronavirus/mers/downloads/Isolation2007.pdf

Centers for Disease Control and Prevention. *2009 H1N1: Overview of a pandemic*. Retrieved May 28, 2013, from http://www.cdc.gov/h1n1flu/yearinreview/

Centers for Disease Control and Prevention. *Airline guidance*. Retrieved from http://www.cdc.gov/quarantine//air/index.html

Centers for Disease Control and Prevention. *Babesiosis*. Retrieved June 27, 2014, from http://www.cdc.gov/parasites/babesiosis/health_professionals/index.html

Centers for Disease Control and Prevention. *Cases of Ebola diagnosed in the United States*. Retrieved from http://www.cdc.gov/vhf/ebola/united-states-imported-case.html

Centers for Disease Control and Prevention. *E. coli*. Retrieved June 8, 2013, from, http://www.cdc.gov/ecoli/general/index.html

Centers for Disease Control and prevention. *Ebola in Democratic Republic of the Congo*. Retrieved from http://www.cdc.gov/travel/notice/democratic-republic-of-the-congo.html

Centers for Disease Control and Prevention. *Epidemiologic risk factors for exposure to Ebola*. Retrieved from http://www.cdc.gov.vhf/ebola/exposure/risk-factors-when-evaluating-person-for-exposure.html

Centers for Disease Control and Prevention. *EVD diagnosis*. Retrieved from http://www.cdc.gov/vhf/ebola/diagnosis/index.html

Centers for Disease Control and Prevention. *EVD signs and symptoms*. Retrieved from http://www.cdc.gov/vhf/ebola/symptoms/index.html

Centers for Disease Control and Prevention. *How the flu virus changes*. Retrieved May 20, 2013, from, http://www.flu.gov/about_the_flu/virus_changes/index.html#

Centers for Disease Control and Prevention. *Infection prevention and control recommendations for hospitalized patients with known or suspected Ebola in U.S. hospitals*. Retrieved August 2, 2014, from, http://www.cdc.gov/vhf/ebola/hcp/infection-prevention-and-control-recommendations.htm

Centers for Disease Control and Prevention. *Infection prevention and control recommendations for hospitalized patients with known or suspected EVD in U.S. hospitals*. Retrieved August 1, 2014, from http://www.cdc.gov/vhf/ebola/hcp/infection-prevention-and-control-recommendations.html

Centers for Disease Control and Prevention. *Influenza: H7N9*. Retrieved June 27, 2014, from, http://www.cdc.gov/flu/h7n9-virus.htm

Centers for Disease Control and Prevention. *Lyme disease data*. Retrieved July 8, 2014, from, http://www.cdc.gov/lyme/stats/index.html

Centers for Disease Control and Prevention. *Lyme disease*. Retrieved July 8, 2014, from, http://www.cdc.gov/lyme/

Centers for Disease Control and Prevention. *Media release*. Retrieved from http://www.cdc.gov.media/releases/2014/p1022-post-arrival-monitoring.html

Centers for Disease Control and Prevention. *Middle East Respiratory Syndrome (MERS)*. Retrieved June 26, 2014, from http://www.cdc.gov/coronavirus/mers/hcp.html

Centers for Disease Control and Prevention. *Remembering SARS 10 years later.* Retrieved June 28, 2014, from, http://www.cdc.gov/about/history/sars/timeline.htm

Centers for Disease Control and Prevention. *TB Facts*. Retrieved May 23, 2013 from, http://www.cdc.gov/nchstp/tb/faqs/qa.htm

Centers for Disease Control and Prevention. *Travel health notices*. Retrieved from http://www.cdc.gov/travel/notices

Centers for Disease Control and Prevention. *Tuberculosis*. Retrieved June 8, 2013, from, http://www.cdc.gov/tb/

Centers for Disease Control and Prevention. *West Nile virus*. Retrieved May 16, 2013, from, http://www.cdc.gov/westnile/index.html

Department of Health and Human Services. (2000). *Healthy people 2010* (conference ed., Vol. 2). Washington, DC: Author.

Department of Health and Human Services. (2005a). *HHS pandemic influenza plan. Supplement 4: Infection control.* Washington, DC: Author.

Department of Health and Human Services. (2006). *State and local pandemic influenza planning checklist*. Washington, DC: Author.

Gao, R., Cao, B., Hu, Y., Feng, Z., Wang, D., & Hu, W., . . . Shu, Y. (2013). Human infection with a novel avian-origin influenza A (H7N9) virus. *New England Journal of Medicine*, *368*, 1888–1897.

Garrett, L. (1995). *The coming plague*. New York, NY: Penguin Group.

Gayer, M., Legros, D., Formenty, P., & Connolly, M. A. (2007, November). *Conflict and emerging infectious diseases* (Vol. 13, No. 11). Geneva, Switzerland: World Health Organization.

He, B., Zhang, Y., Xu, L., Yang, W., Yang, F., Feng, Y., . . . Tu, C. (2014). Identification of diverse alphacoronaviruses and genomic characterization of a novel severe acute respiratory syndrome-like coronavirus from bats in China. *Journal of Virology*, *88*(12), 7070–7082.

Hersh, M., Ostfeld, R. S., McHenry, D. J., Tibbetts, M., Brunner, J. L., Killilea, M. E., . . . Keesing, F. (2014). Co-infection of blacklegged ticks with *Babesia microti* and *Borrella burgdorferi* is higher than expected and acquired from small mammal hosts. *PLOS ONE*, *9*(6), e99348. Retrieved June 27, 2014, from, http://www.plosone.org

Hu, Y., Lu, S., Song, Z., Wang, W., Hao, P., Li, J., . . . Yuan, Z. (2013, May 28). Association between adverse clinical outcome in human disease caused by novel influenza A H7N9 virus and sustained viral shedding and emergence of antiviral resistance [Online]. *The Lancet*. Retrieved May 28, 2013, from, http://download.thelancet.com/flatcontentassets/pdfs/S0140673613611253.pdf

Institute of Medicine. (1992). *Emerging infections: Microbial threats to health in the United States*. Washington, DC: Author.

Institute of Medicine. (2010). *Infectious disease movement in a borderless world: Workshop summary*. Washington, DC: The National Academies Press. Retrieved May 15, 2013, from, http://www.nap.edu/catalog.php?record_id=12758

International Society for Infectious Diseases. (2013, June 13). Climate change, disease impact: Arctic spread. *ProMed Mail.* Retrieved June 15, 2013, from, http://www.promedmail.org/

Kilbourne, E. D. (2006). Influenza pandemics of the 20th century. *Emerging Infectious Diseases*, *12*(1), 9–14.

Krause, P. J., Narasimhan, S., Wormser, G. P., Barbour, A. G., Platonov, A. E., Brancato, J., . . . the Tick Borne Diseases Group. (2014). *Borelia miyamotoi senso lato* seroreactivity and seroprevalence in the northeastern United States. *Emerging Infectious Diseases*, *20*(7), 1183–1190.

references (continued)

Li, Q., Zhou, L., Zhou, M., Chen, Z., Li, F., Wu, H., . . . Feng, Z. (2014). Epidemiology of human infections with avian influenza A (H7N9) virus in China. *New England Journal of Medicine, 307*(6), 520–532.

Mutreja, A., Kim, D. W., Thomson, N. R., Conner, T. R., Lee, J. H., Kariuki, S., . . . Dougan, G. (2011). Evidence for several waves of global transmission in the seventh cholera pandemic. *Nature, 477*, 462–465.

National Fire Protection Association. (2013). *NFPA 1582 Standard on Comprehensive Occupational Medical Programs for Fire Departments*. Retrieved May 15, 2013, from, http://www.nfpa.org/aboutthecodes/aboutthecodes.asp?docnum=1582#

National Institute of Allergy and Infectious Diseases, National Institutes of Health. *Antigenic shift*. Retrieved May 25, 2013, from, http://www.niaid.nih.gov/topics/flu/research/basic/pages/antigenicshiftillustration.aspx

National Library of Medicine, National Institutes of Health. *Cholera on line*. Retrieved May 28, 2013, from http://www.nlm.nih.gov/exhibition/cholera/introduction.html

Nyamathi A., Nahid P., Berg, J., Burrage, J., Christiani, A., Agtash, S., . . . Leake, B. (2008). Efficacy of nurse case-managed intervention for latent tuberculosis among homeless subsamples. *Nursing Research, 57*(1), 33–39.

Russell, C. A., Fonville, J. M., Brown, A. E., Burke, D. F., Smith, D. L., James, S. L., . . . Smith, D. J. (2012). The potential for respiratory droplet–transmissible A/H5N1 influenza virus to evolve in a mammalian host. *Science, 336* (6088), 1541–1547.

Smolinski, M. S., Hamburg, M. A., & Lederberg, J. (2003). *Microbial threats to health: Emergence, detection, and response*. Washington, DC: The National Academies Press.

Steere, A. C., Coburn, J., & Glickstein, L. (2004). The emergence of Lyme disease. *Journal of Clinical Investigation, 113*, 1093–1101.

Tang, J. T. (2009, March). Fantastic voyage: Influenza [Another dimension]. *Emerging Infectious Disease* [Serial on the Internet]. Retrieved May 16, 2013, from http://www.cdc.gov/EID/content/15/3/512.htm

University of Minnesota Center for Infectious Disease Research and Policy. (2014, May 28). *H7N9 update*. Retrieved June 26, 2014, from http://www.cidrap.umn.edu/infectious-disease-topics/h7n9-avian-influenza.htm

Wang W., Song, Z., Guan W., Liu, Y, Zhang, X., Xu, L., . . . Hu, Y. (2014). PCR for detection of oseltamivir resistance mutation in influenza A (H7N9) virus. *Emerging Infectious Diseases, 20*(5), 847–849.

World Health Organization. (2007). *Infection prevention and control of epidemic- and pandemic-prone acute respiratory diseases in health care*. Geneva, Switzerland: Author. Retrieved June 8, 2013, from http://apps.who.int/iris/bitstream/10665/69707/1/WHO_CDS_EPR_2007.6_eng.pdf

World Health Organization. (2011). *Avian influenza fact sheet*. Geneva, Switzerland: Author. Retrieved June 8, 2013, from http://www.who.int/mediacentre/factsheets/avian_influenza/en/#history

World Health Organization. (2012). *Global tuberculosis report 2012*. Retrieved June 8, 2013, from http://apps.who.int/iris/bitstream/10665/75938/1/9789241564502_eng.pdf

World Health Organization. (2013, June 7). *WHO risk assessment: Human infections with avian influenza A (H7N9) virus*. Retrieved June 8, 2013, from http://www.who.int/influenza/human_animal_interface/influenza_h7n9/RiskAssessment_H7N9_07Jun13.pdf

World Health Organization. (2013, March 18). *Interim surveillance recommendations for human infection with novel coronavirus*. Retrieved June 4, 2013, from http://www.who.int/csr/disease/coronavirus_infections/InterimRevisedSurveillanceRecommendations_nCoVinfection_18Mar13.pdf

World Health Organization. (2013, May 6). *Infection prevention and control during health care for probable or confirmed cases of novel coronavirus (nCoV) infection interim guidance*. Retrieved June 4, 2013, from http://www.who.int/csr/disease/coronavirus_infections/IPCnCoVguidance_06May13.pdf

World Health Organization. (2013a). *Influenza at the human-animal interface*. Retrieved May 29, 2013, from http://www.who.int/influenza/human_animal_interface/Influenza_Summary_IRA_HA_interface_26Apr13.pdf

World Health Organization. (2013b). *Multidrug-resistant tuberculosis (MDR-TB), 2013 update*. Retrieved June 8, 2013, from http://www.who.int/tb/challenges/mdr/MDR_TB_FactSheet.pdf

World Health Organization. *Avian influenza*. Retrieved June 27, 2014, from http://www.who.int/influenza/human_animal_interface/Influenza_Summary_IRA_HA_interface_5_May14.pdf

World Health Organization. *Coronavirus infections*. Retrieved June 8, 2013, from http://www.who.int/csr/disease/coronavirus_infections/en/index.html

World Health Organization. *Ebola roadmap Apps*. Retrieved from http://apps.who.int/iris/bitstream/10665/137424/1/roadmapsitrep_31Oct2014_eng.pdf

World Health Organization. *Ebola virus disease update*. Retrieved July 11, 2014, from http://who.int/entity/csr/don/2014_07_10_ebola/en

World Health Organization. *Ebola virus disease*. Retrieved July 11, 2014, from http://who.int/mediacentre/factsheets/fs103/en

World Health Organization. *Global epidemics and impact of cholera*. Retrieved May 29, 2013, from http://www.who.int/topics/cholera/impact/en/

World Health Organization. *Human infection with avian influenza A (H7N9) virus update*. Retrieved June 27, 2014, from http://www.who/int/csr/don/2014_05_22_h7n9/en/

World Health Organization. *MERS-CoV Summary 9 May 2014*. Retrieved June 26, 2014, from http://www.who.int/csr/disease/coronavirus_infections/en/index

World Health Organization. *Middle East respiratory syndrome coronavirus (MERS CoV)—Update*. Retrieved June 27, 2014, from http://www.who.int/csr/don/2014_05_22_mers/en

World Health Organization. *Nigeria ends Ebola*. Retrieved from http://www.who.int/mediacenter/statements/2014/nigeria-ends-ebola/en/

World Health Organization. *Poliomyelitis*. Retrieved June 4, 2013, from http://www.who.int/mediacentre/factsheets/fs114/en/index.html

World Health Organization. *Poliovirus detected from environmental samples in Israel*. Retrieved June 4, 2013, from http://www.who.int/csr/don/2013_06_03/en/index.html

World Health Organization. *Revised interim case definition for reporting to WHO—Novel coronavirus*. Retrieved June 4, 2013, from, http://www.who.int/csr/disease/coronavirus_infections/case_definition/en/index.html

World Health Organization. *The five elements of DOT*. Retrieved June 8, 2013, from http://www.who.int/tb/dots/whatisdots/en/index2.html

web resources

Please visit thePoint® for up-to-date Web resources on this topic.

CHAPTER 16

Violence and Abuse

Annie Lewis-O'Connor and Karen Conley

If you and I are having a single thought of violence or hatred against anyone in the world at this moment, we are contributing to the wounding of the world.

Deepak Chopra

A tree never hits an automobile except in self-defense.

American proverb

You cannot shake hands with a clenched fist.

Golda Meir

From pacifist to terrorist, each person condemns violence—and then adds one cherished case in which it may be justified.

Gloria Steinem

Violence is immoral because it thrives on hatred rather than love. It destroys community and makes brotherhood impossible. It leaves society in monologue rather than dialogue.

Violence ends by defeating itself. It creates bitterness in the survivors and brutality in the destroyers.

Martin Luther King

chapter highlights

- Overview of violence in U.S. communities
- School violence
- Mandatory reporting of elder abuse, child maltreatment, and abuse of people with disabilities
- Intimate partner violence (IPV)
- Health consequences of exposure to IPV in children
- Model of care for victims of intentional crimes
- IPV as a major women's health problem, including impact on pregnancy
- Screening and intervention in IPV
- Risk and lethality assessment in IPV
- Role of healthcare providers: assessing for and intervening in violence and abuse

objectives

- Identify the incidence and prevalence of intimate partner violence (IPV).
- Understand the health consequences that violence has on the health of patients and families.
- Explain the effects of IPV on adults and children.
- Summarize the models of care that have evolved in caring for victims of intentional violence.
- Describe interventional strategies (screening) and the limitations of measuring the effects of these interventions.
- Summarize the tenets of mandatory reporting laws.
- Apply nursing process in caring for and screening for IPV.

key terms

Femicide: A term used to refer to a homicide of a female person that occurs in the context of intimate partner violence (IPV).

Gender-based violence: A term used to distinguish violence which targets people, or groups of people, on the basis of their gender from other forms of violence (United Nations Convention on the Elimination of All Forms of Discrimination against Women). It includes any act that results in, or is likely to result in, physical, sexual, or psychological harm such as rape, torture, mutilation, sexual slavery, forced impregnation, and murder.

Human rights: Basic rights and freedoms to which all humans are entitled.

Incidence: The number of cases of disease with an onset during a prescribed period of time; often expressed as a rate (e.g., the incidence of measles per 1,000 children 5 to 15 years of age during a specified year).

Intimate partner violence (IPV): A pattern of assaultive and coercive behaviors which may include inflicted physical injury, psychological abuse, sexual assault, progressive social isolation, deprivation, intimidation, and threats. These behaviors are perpetrated by someone who is, was, or wishes to be involved in an intimate or dating relationship with an adult or adolescent, and they are aimed at establishing control by one partner over the other (Family Violence Prevention Fund, 1999).

Lethality assessment: An assessment that identifies high-risk factors for IPV.

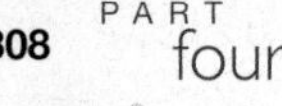

Case Study

References to the case study are found throughout this chapter (look for the case study icon). Readers should keep the case study in mind as they read the chapter.

Kathy is a 28-year-old married woman with three children who are all younger than 6 years. The middle child has autism. Last year, Kathy had a miscarriage at 20 weeks following a fall down the stairs. She has not worked outside the home since the birth of her first child and is financially dependent on her husband. Her relationship with her husband has always been emotionally abusive, and although signs of physical abuse have been present during visits to Laura, a nurse practitioner and healthcare provider, Kathy has denied serious physical abuse except for an occasional push or shove. Sometimes, she has presented with bruises, which she has always said were accidental. After the birth of each child, Kathy has become quieter and seems sadder, and she has been noticeably depressed since her miscarriage. Recently, Kathy has admitted to Laura that she trusts her and needs her help because her husband's behavior is becoming worse and she is not sure what to do. Kathy does not wish to go to the police at this point. She denies direct harm to her children, yet she says "they must hear us arguing and fighting."

- What should Laura do to help Kathy?
- What about the safety of her children?
- What should Laura do if she becomes ambivalent about her disclosure?

Kathy has voiced her concerns related to finances, housing, and fear of retaliation by her partner—very personal information. There are several questions to consider: Does the state Kathy lives in have a mandatory reporting law for abuse against women (only six states do)? If Kathy is not ready to report the intimate partner violence to the police, what safety precautions can Laura address? If Kathy does report the violence to the police and her husband is arrested, there will be no income—how should Laura help Kathy address her economic concerns? (Also, the state budget has recently cut many services that were once available for victims of abuse.) Kathy may become homeless and unemployed, with no income for three small children and a partner who may retaliate. In addition to safety issues, there are many ethical and legal responsibilities which Laura needs to consider in developing a plan of care with the patient. It is essential that she also respects Kathy's autonomy.

key terms (continued)

Perpetrate: To be responsible for; commit, as in a crime.

Prevalence: Number of cases of a disease, infected persons, or people with some other attribute present during a particular interval of time; often expressed as a rate (e.g., the prevalence of diabetes per 1,000 persons during a year).

Violence: Framed in the context of "intentional" violence, or stated another way, that which is carried out by a person or persons against another person or persons when there is a conscious choice to act in a violent manner.

OVERVIEW OF VIOLENCE

Violence in the United States is pervasive. In this chapter, **violence** is considered to be "intentional"; that is, violence is an act committed by a person or persons against another person or persons in which there is a conscious choice to act violently. When caring for the client's immediate needs, nurses should consider the cumulative exposures to violence over time and the far-reaching effects of violence on the family and the community at large. More than three decades of evidence is available to inform health practice and policy. The healthcare community is in a pivotal position to have a significant impact on the lives of clients affected by violence.

Violence has an adverse impact on society. It is estimated to cost billions of dollars per year (Dolezal, McCollum, & Callahan, 2009; Waters et al., 2004). These costs include direct medical care and rehabilitation and losses to the workforce (Corso, Mercy, Simon, Finkelstein, & Miller, 2007). The impact on families and the larger community is notable. *Healthy People 2020* has targeted injury and violence prevention as a priority. The injury prevention objectives of *Healthy People 2020* include (1) prevention and reduction of firearm-related deaths; (2) identification of improper firearm storage in homes; (3) surveillance of external causes of injury in emergency departments; (4) decreased incidents of homicide, child maltreatment, and physical assaults; (5) prevention and reduction of sexual assaults; and (6) elimination of weapon possession by adolescents on school property (Healthy People 2020). Such efforts require a multifaceted approach to public health that targets many settings and recognizes that social determinants of health such as exposures to violence result in poor health. Viewing violence from the many vantage points from which nurses deliver care (hospitals, home, clinics, schools, etc.) provides unique and complimentary healthcare to people experiencing violence and abuse.

Violence—look, we live in a violent world, man. This country was founded on violence. Who's kidding who?

Bruce Willis

All forms of violent behavior can be attributed to the need for power and control. A number of factors have contributed to the prevalence of violence in the United States.

Primary among those factors are the acceptability of violence in U.S. culture; racism, classism, and sexism; availability and accessibility of firearms; and lack of accountability.

Nothing is more despicable than respect based on fear.

Albert Camus

Guns

In May 2013, the Violence Policy Center released the most recent available data (2010) on gun-related deaths. In 2010, gun deaths (including gun suicides, homicides, and fatal unintentional shootings) outpaced motor vehicle deaths in Alaska, Arizona, Colorado, District of Columbia, Illinois, Louisiana, Maryland, Michigan, Nevada, Oregon, Utah, Virginia, and Washington. These data revealed that gun deaths outpaced automobile deaths in 12 states and in Washington, DC. There were 31,672 firearm deaths in 2010 and 35,498 motor vehicle deaths, and while motor vehicles deaths in aggregate are higher than firearms deaths, firearm-related deaths outpaced motor vehicle deaths (Box 16.1).

The data on firearms is daunting. Data from 2010 revealed that 17.5% of all injury deaths in that year were caused by a firearm (Murphy, Xu, & Kochanek, 2013). The two major component causes of all firearm injury deaths in 2010 were suicide (61.2%) and homicide (35.0%) (National Institute of Justice, 2010).

Dr. David Hemenway, director of the Harvard Injury Control Research Center, notes in his 2004 book *Private Guns, Public Health* "The time Americans spend using their cars is orders of magnitude greater than the time spent using their guns. It is probable that per hour of exposure, guns are far more dangerous. Moreover, we have lots of safety regulations concerning the manufacture of motor vehicles; there are virtually no safety regulations for domestic firearms manufacturers." Nurses should be vigilant in assessing whether there is a gun present in the home and whether it is safely stored away from children (Fig. 16.1). Nurses are in key positions—in schools, clinics, offices, and hospitals—to inquire about guns in the home and provide anticipatory guidance on safety when a gun is stored in the home.

Other factors that contribute to homicides related to guns are low income, discrimination, lack of education, and lack of employment opportunities. Most often, males are the victims as well as the perpetrators of homicides. African-

box 16.1 Gun-Related Deaths versus Motor Vehicle Deaths, by State, 2010

Alaska: 144 gun deaths, 71 motor vehicle deaths
Arizona: 931 gun deaths, 795 motor vehicle deaths
Colorado: 555 gun deaths, 487 motor vehicle deaths
District of Columbia: 99 gun deaths, 38 motor vehicle deaths
Illinois: 1,064 gun deaths, 1,042 motor vehicle deaths
Louisiana: 864 gun deaths, 722 motor vehicle deaths
Maryland: 538 gun deaths, 514 motor vehicle deaths
Michigan: 1,076 gun deaths, 1,063 motor vehicle deaths
Nevada: 395 gun deaths, 289 motor vehicle deaths
Oregon: 458 gun deaths, 324 motor vehicle deaths
Utah: 314 gun deaths, 274 motor vehicle deaths
Virginia: 875 gun deaths, 728 motor vehicle deaths
Washington: 609 gun deaths, 554 motor vehicle deaths

Source: Data from http://www.vpc.org/press/1305gunsvscars.htm

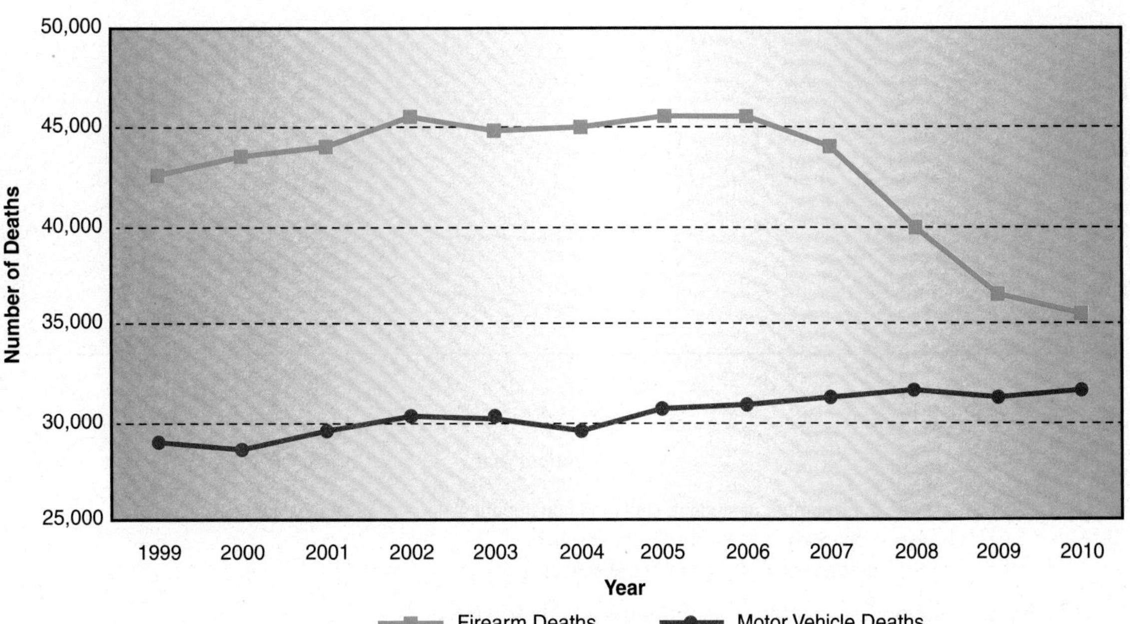

figure 16.1 Firearm and motor vehicle deaths, 1999 to 2010.
(From Centers for Disease Control and Prevention, National Center for Injury Prevention and Control, Division of Violence Prevention, 2008.)

American males are affected most frequently; in fact, African-Americans are six times more likely than White males to be murder victims (FBI, 2010). Although there has been a decline in the homicide of intimate partners, including spouses, partners, boyfriends, and girlfriends, over the past decade, this problem remains significant and warrants conscious attention.

Abuse a man unjustly, and you will make friends for him.

Douglas Horton

School Violence

Over the past decade, the unthinkable has happened; children have been killed while at school. In December of 2012, our Nation watched in horror as the news broke that Adam Lanza, 20, fatally shot 20 young elementary school children and six adult staff members in a mass murder at Sandy Hook Elementary School in Newtown, Connecticut. Before driving to the school, Lanza had shot and killed his mother Nancy at their Newtown home. As first responders arrived, he committed suicide by shooting himself in the head. This event stimulated new debates about gun control and safety and mental health.

Prior to this event, the literature states that from July 1, 2007, through June 30, 2008, 43 school-associated violent deaths occurred in the United States. Thirty-six of these violent deaths were homicides, 6 were suicides, and 1 was a legal intervention (National Center for Education Statistics, 2009). According to the data obtained from the well-known National Youth Behavioral Risk Survey in 2002 (Grunbaum et al., 2004), 7.9% of students reported being threatened or injured with a weapon such as a gun, knife, or club on school property in the preceding 12 months. Seven to eight percent of students in this same age group reported being bullied. Finally, 20% of all public schools experienced one or more serious violent crimes such as rape, sexual assault, robbery, and aggravated assault, and 71% of public schools reported violent incidents. Since 1992, the Centers for Disease Control and Prevention (CDC) in partnership with the Departments of Education and Justice has been conducting surveillance on school-related deaths (Fig. 16.2). Data from a number of the current national surveys are in process from collection to analysis to publication (Anderson et al., 2001; CDC, 2001, 2003).

Because in the two months since Newtown, more than a thousand birthdays, graduations, and anniversaries have been stolen from our lives by a bullet from a gun.

President Barack Obama

School nurses play a pivotal role in recognizing both children who are being victimized and those who are perpetrating violence. School nurses working with teachers, school administrators, and school psychologists are in a unique position to create an environment that promotes primary prevention and intervention. By addressing and discussing with students the root causes of violence through their educational curriculum, school nurses and educators might be able to shift the paradigm to a less violent one. Schools are fertile climates for education about prevention of violence. Violence prevention should start at home and continue in school (see Chapter 22).

Education is a vaccine for violence.

Edward James Olmos, Mexican American actor

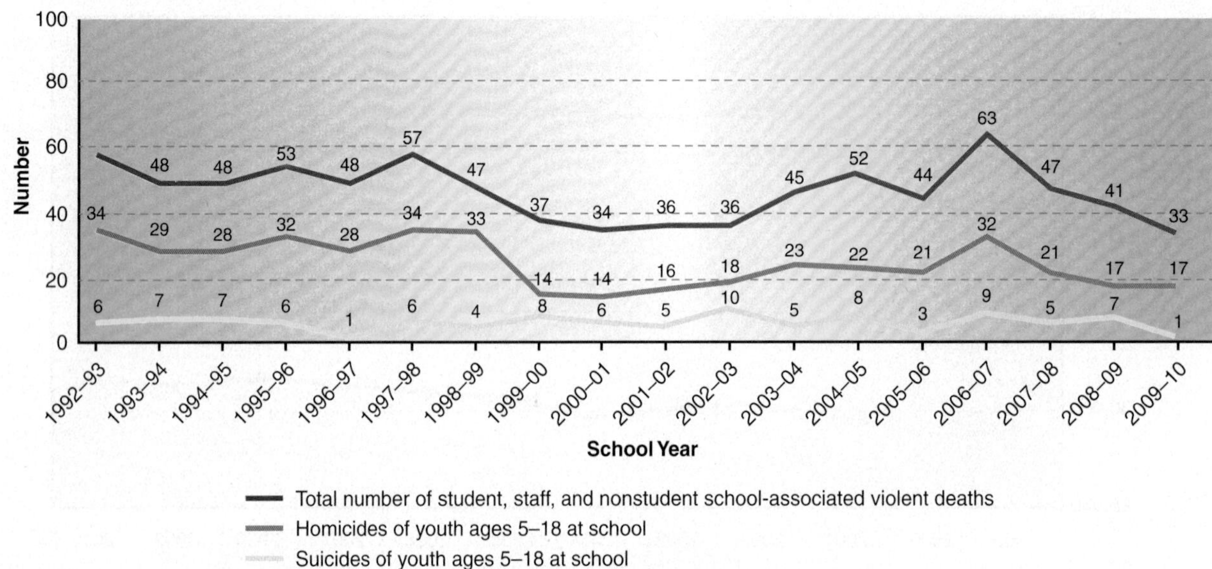

figure 16.2 Trends in school-associated violent deaths—1992 to 2010.
(Data from Centers for Disease Control and Prevention, National Center for Injury Prevention and Control (NCIPC), http://www.cdc.gov/violenceprevention/youthviolence/schoolviolence/savd.html)

PRACTICE POINT

Thinking about the root causes of violence helps nurses develop primary prevention strategies (raising awareness about violence), along with secondary (identifying those at risk for being abused or perpetrating abuse) and tertiary prevention interventions (identified victim or perpetrator).

INTIMATE PARTNER VIOLENCE

Intimate Partner Violence: A Major Women's Health Problem

The phenomenon of **intimate partner violence (IPV)** differs depending on culture, discipline, theoretical framework, and philosophical perspectives. Gradually, violence against women has been recognized globally as a **human rights** violation with significant consequences for the individual, family, and community. IPV does target an individual person, but the effects on bystanders are far reaching, affecting local, state, public, and private sectors through loss of productivity, and contributing to medical and mental health costs. Although data support the belief that men are generally the perpetrators of IPV, most healthcare providers and researchers recognize that women may also, though rarely, perpetrate violence against their intimate partner. In the early 1990s, the international community adopted the term **gender-based violence** when referring to violence against women and girls (United Nations, 1993). This terminology appears to reflect the evolution of researchers who have sought to understand the nature of abuse that is perpetrated against females. Although there have been variations in the definition of IPV among researchers, over the past decade these definitions have become increasingly similar. Healthcare providers see victims of IPV daily in their practice, and identification can lead to interventions that may help to decrease morbidity and mortality.

One of the speakers asked how many women had been harassed or abused sexually in their life? There were thousands of women in the audience, and almost every one of them raised her hand.

Cheryl James (Salt), American rapper

Investigators conducting population-based studies in the United States over the past several years have consistently reported a lifetime **prevalence** of IPV against women to be between 25% and 30%, with an annual prevalence between 2% and 12% (Black, Basile, & Breiding, 2011; Humphreys, Parker, & Campbell, 2001; Jones et al., 1999; Tjaden & Thoennes, 2000; Wilt & Olson, 1996). More recently, using a population-based national sample of women older than 18 years (n = 1,800) and calculating adult lifetime and prior-year prevalence of violent experiences, Moracco, Runyan, and Butts (2003) found that 60% of respondents experienced at least one form of violence since the age of 18, with 10% reporting violence in the previous year. Adult lifetime and prior-year prevalence varies by type of violence and respondents' socio demographic characteristics. Some of the inconsistencies reported in the literature are due to variations in defining the nature of the abuse (e.g., stalking, rape, emotional abuse, or verbal abuse) and limitations in sampling. Often, purposeful and convenient sampling was used in these studies.

Extent of Intimate Partner Violence

The literature on IPV is substantial and has evolved exponentially over the past two decades. The World Health Organization's World Report on Violence and Health (Krug, Dahlberg, Mercy, Zwi, & Lozano, 2002) found that in 48 population-based surveys from around the world, between 10% and 69% of women reported being physically assaulted by an intimate male partner at some point in their lives. This is important for nurses to recognize. Many women who have immigrated to the United States have long been exposed to violence in their country of origin, and awareness of this fact has significant implications for nursing plans of care. In addition, nurses need to know that although murder by an intimate partner is uncommon, approximately 1,181 women are victims of such murders annually in the United States, an average of about three women a day (Bureau of Justice Statistics, 2007).

Research in the area of homicides has helped to inform nursing practice, particularly in relation to the risk to children. In a ten-city study of risk factors for intimate partner **femicide** (murder of women) or attempted femicide, Lewandowski, McFarlane, Campbell, Gary, and Barenski (2004) found that 59% of domestic violence victims had children. About 33% of the children had witnessed the incident, and 43% were the first to find their mother's body. Nurses must be aware that some 35% to 60% of children who live in homes where there is IPV are themselves physically or sexually abused (Edelson, 1999), with fathers as the most common perpetrators (McCloskey, Figueredo, & Koss, 1995).

In the context of family-centered care, it is imperative that Laura considers the safety of the children. In the hopes of preventing further abuse in Kathy's situation, Laura should know about resources in the community. If Kathy has the phone numbers of local women's shelters, food banks, mental health agencies, unemployment offices, and the Women, Infants, and Children (WIC) program, she will be able to use these resources when she is ready to do so. By providing these resources, Laura hopes to give Kathy the confidence, with the support behind her, to make the right decisions for her family. Also, and equally important, Laura gains a better understanding of the factors that affect a victim's ability to make well-informed decisions.

Dr. Jacquelyn Campbell, a pioneer nurse researcher in the area of IPV, published the earliest data on the health consequences of IPV (Campbell, 2002) and has developed and implemented a multilanguage **lethality assessment** (Campbell, 1981, 1986, 1992, 1995a, b and c; Campbell et al., 2003a) tool for homicide. Dr. Campbell's research indicates that factors such as access to a firearm, the abuser's use of illicit drugs, unemployment, control of daily activities, stepchildren in the home, and threats to kill the victim pose serious risks for homicide for a woman (Table 16.1; Box 16.2). In particular, the presence of a firearm in the home is a risk factor for homicide in women (Campbell et al., 2003a; Kellerman & Heron, 1999; Sorenson & Wiebe, 2004; Wiebe, 2003). The majority of women killed with a gun were killed by their intimate partner (Hemingway, 2004; Bailey, Kellerman, & Somes, 1997; Moracco et al., 2003). These data underscore the necessity for nurses to screen clients for access to and/or presence of a gun in the home, and to provide education about safe storage.

box 16.2 Risk Factors That Indicate Significant Concern for the Safety of the Children

- Threats to kill the caretaker, children, and/or self; caretaker fears for the children's safety
- A child was physically injured in an incident where the caretaker was the target
- A child was coerced to participate in or witness the abuse of the caretaker
- A weapon was used or threats were made to use a weapon, and the caretaker believed that there was intention and ability to cause harm

table 16.1 Risk Factors for Intimate Partner Violence

Individual risk factors	• Low self-esteem • Low income • Low academic achievement • Young age • Aggressive behavior as a child • Heavy alcohol/drug use • Depression • Anger and hostility • Antisocial personality traits • Borderline personality traits • History of being physically abused • Few friends/isolation and abused • Unemployment • Emotional dependence and insecurity • Belief in strict gender roles • Desire for power and control • Perpetrating psychological aggression in relationships • Victim of physical or psychological abuse as a child • Experiencing poor parenting • Experiencing physical discipline as a child
Relationship factors	• Economic stress • Marital conflicts (e.g., fights) • Marital instability (e.g., divorce/separation) • Dominance/control of relationship by one partner over another • Unhealthy family relationships and interactions
Community factors/ societal factors	• Poverty and associated factors (e.g., overcrowding) • Low social capital—lack of institutions, relationships, and norms that shape a community's social interactions • Weak community sanctions against intimate partner violence (e.g., unwillingness of neighbors to intervene when violence is witnessed) • Traditional gender roles (e.g., women should stay at home, be submissive, not enter the workforce; men support the family and make the decisions)

While assessing how the abuse is affecting Kathy and her children, it is important to explore lethality risks (Box 16.3). Although the presence of lethality risk factors does not imply that Kathy is in imminent danger, the presence of these factors does warrant an in-depth assessment, such as a multilanguage danger assessment tool that is reliable and valid. Such in-depth assessments are dependent on the practice environment and the availability of social services. It is important to know what in-house and community referral resources are available.

In response to the evidence that IPV profoundly affects the health of victims and children, many professional organizations, such as the American Medical Association (1992), American Nurses Association (ANA) (1991), the American College of Obstetricians and Gynecologists (1993), and the Association of Women's Health, Obstetric, and Neonatal Nurses (AWHONN) established screening and routine assessment guidelines for IPV as the standard of practice. Valuable web sites include Futures Without Violence

box 16.3 Lethality Risks

- Is there a gun in the house?
- Is the woman's partner unemployed?
- What is the worst thing the partner has ever done to the victim?
- Does the victim feel that the partner is capable of hurting her? Of carrying out his threats?
- Has the woman's partner ever been arrested?
- Is the woman's partner using drugs? Drinking excessively?

(wwww.futureswithoutviolence.org), Academy on Violence (www.AVA.org), and National Health Collaborative on Violence and Abuse (www. Nhcva.org)—these three sites provide much information for healthcare providers.

STUDENT REFLECTION

I had never been involved in screening for routine assessment guidelines until I needed some minor surgery in my sophomore year in college. In the preoperative phase of the process, a nurse asked me whether I felt safe where I lived. (My boyfriend was waiting for me in a coffee shop at the medical center where I was having my surgery.) At first, I did not expect the question, but then I understood that the nurse was asking me about IPV, and whether I was at risk. It made me really happy to see that a nurse was asking such an important assessment question. Although this situation did not apply to me, I could see how this could be an opportunity for a client to obtain help or advice. However, I also realize that this could lead to breaking emotional or financial ties with another person or dealing with the children who resulted from a relationship that has become abusive.

High rates of IPV have long been detected in emergency departments (Abbott, Johnson, Koziol-McLain, & Lowenstein, 1995), prenatal clinics (Helton, McFarlane, & Anderson, 1987; Martin & Clements, 2002; McFarlane, Parker, Soeken, & Bullock, 1992), internal medicine practices, health maintenance organizations (Gin, Rucker, Frayne, & Cygan, 1992; Hamberger, Saunders, & Hovey, 1992; Jones et al., 1999), and hospitalizations when clients are admitted for behavioral health disorders, substance abuse, and suicidality (Kernic, Wolf, & Holt, 2000).

The literature has well documented the risks of IPV and pregnancy (Chang et al., 2005). Depression before, during, and after birth has been strongly correlated with IPV (Ogbonnaya, Macy, Kupper, Martin, & Bledsoe-Mansori, 2013). In a National Institutes of Health (NIH)-supported population analysis of 5 million records of California women over a 10-year period, researchers found that pregnant women who are assaulted by an intimate partner are at increased risk of giving birth to infants of reduced weight (NIH News, 2011). Although the results showed a pattern of low-weight births among women who experienced an assault, the study was not designed to establish cause and effect or explain the biologic factors for how violence against an expectant mother might cause her to deliver a lower-birth-weight infant. It is now standard of practice that all pregnant women are screened for IPV during each trimester of their pregnancy, following the birth of the infant, and in cases in which there are concerns (see ACOG, http://www.acog.org/Resources_And_Publications/Committee_Opinions/Committee_on_Health_Care_for_Underserved_Women/Intimate_Partner_Violence#11a).

Women victimized by abuse are more likely to be diagnosed with serious health problems, including depression and panic attacks, as well as migraine headaches, chronic pain, arthritis, high blood pressure, gastrointestinal problems, inconsistent use of birth control, and delayed entry into prenatal care (Weiss, Lawrence, & Miller, 2002; Campbell & Lewandowski, 1997). In fact, much has been learned about how reproductive coercion is a significant factor in relationships where IPV is of concern (Miller et al., 2010; Miller et al., 2010). It is essential to ask a woman about her ability to control her fertility issues and desires during reproductive healthcare visits.

In addition, women affected by IPV are more likely to engage in high-risk behaviors such as tobacco use, substance abuse, and sexual risk-taking (e.g., multiple sexual partners). (Silverman, Raj, & Clemens, 2004; Silverman, Raj, Mucci, & Hathaway, 2001). Nurses who recognize the significant impact of IPV, both acute and chronic, may be more influential in developing treatment plans with their patients that seek to intervene early, thus preventing some of the long-term mental and physical effects that are associated with IPV.

I had been, you know, held in the closet for two months and, you know, abused in all manner of ways. I was very good at doing what I was told.

Patty Hearst, kidnap victim

EVIDENCE FOR PRACTICE

Validation of many of the findings from research on the long-term effects of experiencing or witnessing IPV were validated by the Adverse Childhood Experiences (ACE) study, one of the largest studies of its kind. This study has been a decade-long collaboration between the Division of Adult and Community Health at the CDC and Kaiser Permanente's Department of Preventive Medicine in San Diego. The researchers designed the study to examine the health and social effects of adverse childhood experiences throughout the life span. It involved 17,337 middle-class members of the Kaiser Permanente Medical Care Program in San Diego who agreed to participate during the course of a comprehensive medical evaluation (Anda et al., 1999; Dube, Felitti, Dong, Giles, & Anda, 2003; Edwards et al., 2005; Felitti et al., 1998). It is important to note that this was a homogenous sample of middle-class Caucasians. However, the findings are significant and have important implications for practice (see www.acesconnections.com).

In this study, researchers assessed 10 categories of stressful or traumatic childhood experiences (Dong et al., 2004). They chose a broad range of ACEs that had been shown to have significant adverse health or social implications. Examples of ACEs are as follows:

- Childhood abuse (emotional, physical, and sexual)
- Neglect (emotional and physical)

- Growing up in a seriously dysfunctional household (battered mother, substance abuse, or mental illness in the home; parental separation or divorce; or a criminal household member)

In the case of participants who had a battered mother, 95% reported at least one additional ACE. The researchers also studied the relationship of childhood physical or sexual abuse, or growing up with a battered mother, to the risk of being a victim (among women) or perpetrator (among men) of IPV as an adult (Whitfield, Anda, Dube, & Felitti, 2003). Each of these three ACEs is associated with the risk of IPV; as the number of these violent childhood experiences increased, the risk of IPV also increased (CDC, 2005).

The history of Kathy's childhood or that of her husband is unknown. How an ACE score affects the ability to parent and to participate in healthy relationships is not known. The ACE score specifically considers the relationship between ACEs and health indicators, such as chronic obstructive pulmonary disease, hypertension, risky behaviors, weight, and mental health issues. It can be postulated from the ACE study that if Kathy's children remain in a home where violence is present, they would be at risk for health issues as adults.

Healthy People 2020 emphasizes a need to prevent violence and the sequelae known to result from exposure to violence, recognizing that violence leads to the following:

- Premature death
- Disability
- Poor mental health
- High medical costs
- Lost productivity

The objectives of Violence Prevention identified by *Healthy People 2020* are to reduce fatal and nonfatal injuries, reduce fatal and nonfatal traumatic brain injuries, reduce homicides, reduce firearm injuries, and reduce physical and sexual assaults. Preventing violence and recurrence of violence requires targeting efforts at all three levels of prevention: primary, secondary, and tertiary. There has been a great debate over the benefits of primary and secondary prevention because measuring the benefits of outcomes has intrinsic methodologic issues. However, when the United States Preventive Services Task Force (USPSTF) reviewed the literature on interventions in 2010 they found sufficient evidence to support inquiry and brief counseling for patients. The USPSTF (Moyer, 2013) recommends that clinicians screen women of childbearing age for IPV, and provide intervention services or refer women who screen positive to intervention services (http://www.uspreventiveservicestaskforce.org/uspstf12/ipvelder/ipvelderfinalrs.htm#summary).

It is well known that IPV occurs within all socioeconomic groups. Many victims and perpetrators of IPV differ in their opinions of what constitutes abuse. Opinions may be dependent on many factors: prior exposures, cultural identification, family and peer opinions, and education. Efforts to educate must be persistent, constant, multilingual, and culturally aware and must target both potential victims and potential perpetrators. Secondary prevention occurs through generalized screening and inquiry with high-risk populations.

Decades of research have indicated that some women have a higher risk of IPV (see Table 16.1). Risk factors include age less than 45, low income, lack of employment, recent separation or divorce, education at the high school level or less, and having young children (Campbell et al., 2003b). Currently under debate is how to implement policies and procedures for the identification of perpetration of violence. Issues such as safety, what to do when a person states he or she is hurting someone, and ethical considerations require in-depth discussions with collaborative community participation.

Kathy has risk factors for IPV: a long-term emotionally abusive relationship, isolation, stressors related to having a child with autism, and financial dependence on her husband. In the context of a healthcare setting, a woman may feel that she is able to trust her provider, and thus, with proper inquiry, interventions may be offered which would assist Kathy.

Tertiary prevention (caring for victims affected by, or currently experiencing, violence) has been a major focus in the health system, and has been driven by the Joint Commission. Prior to the Joint Commission's 1998 mandate to implement policies and procedures, victims of abuse received less than optimal care within the healthcare system (Joint Commission on Accreditation of Healthcare Organizations, 1995). Over several years, the Joint Commission required all clinical settings such as community health centers, primary care, emergency departments, and operating rooms to implement identification and interventions for victims of abuse. This was the catalyst for change within the healthcare system. Advocates working in healthcare found that this was the incentive they needed to move forward and to provide quality services for victims and their family members within the context of a healthcare environment. This movement continues to evolve today, with many hospitals and healthcare facilities employing advocates and organizing formal programs (Hathaway, Zimmer, Willis, & Silverman, 2008).

Victims of violence and abuse may often face barriers when seeking help, either immediately afterward or months or years later when the previous violence begins to affect their health. Successful programs in primary, secondary, and tertiary prevention are a critical element necessary for preventing abuse and helping victims recover while mitigating the health consequences.

Intimate Partner Violence: Health Consequences in Children Who Witness Abuse

It is alarming to consider how many children may be exposed to IPV. One of the first studies to look at the **incidence** and prevalence of children in the United States who were exposed to IPV estimated that 3.3 to 10 million children were witness to family violence each year (Edelson, 1999). The variation is due to dissimilarity in definitions of violence, sources of the data, and age of the children. Very young children are more likely to be disproportionately represented in studies because disclosure and identification are limited due to their development and age. These young children are not always able to get out of harm's way. Adolescents often try to intervene to protect the parent being abused. Younger children, from birth to 3 years of age, have received far less attention, and thus, their responses to the IPV directed toward their mothers are less well understood (Berman, Hardesty, & Humphreys, 2004). However, author and social worker Betsy McAlister Groves succinctly addressed the impact of violence on children 8 years of age and younger in her book *Children Who See Too Much* (2002). Groves found that young children exposed to IPV during this early period have experienced physical, intellectual, emotional, and behavioral problems.

The American Academy of Pediatrics' (1998) policy statement supports the recommendation that pediatric providers should screen mothers routinely for IPV in pediatric settings. However, safely carrying out screening in the pediatric setting requires exploration. Despite the implementation of policies and procedures to screen for IPV in pediatrics, few tools have been validated for use in pediatric settings. Pediatric providers face special issues in screening: the parent is not the client and documentation in the medical record may provide information to a potential abusive partner. Also, assessment of a caregiver with a child present, using tools validated in adult settings, may not be practical or safe. Creative strategies have been explored to address these issues and promising practices have been identified that include the following:

- Asking mothers indirectly (written questionnaire, computer survey)
- Asking mothers directly, without the child present
- Having providers inform parents about mandatory reporting laws prior to asking questions
- Being able to screen for safety and dangerousness of the situation
- Being aware of resources and referrals (Lewis-O'Connor, 2007)

The effects on adolescents are quite worrisome and have significant impact on nursing practice. Adolescent girls who reported experiencing sexual or physical assault were significantly more likely to report smoking, attempt suicide, use cocaine, become pregnant, and engage in unhealthy eating habits, compared with adolescents with no abuse history (Silverman et al., 2001). Researchers found that young women in their high school years to their mid-20s are nearly three times as vulnerable to an attack by a husband, boyfriend, or former partner when compared with women in other age groups.

PRACTICE POINT

Some strong evidence suggests that living in a violent home has detrimental effects later in life. Knowing this and integrating this into practice help the nurse recognize and prevent long-term healthcare issues.

Screening for Intimate Partner Violence

In 2012, the USPSTF revised recommendations from their controversial recommendation in 2004, in which they stated there was insufficient evidence to support screening for IPV (Neilson, Yuen, McKiernan, & Klein, 2004). The USPSTF now supports IPV screening and counseling. However, some researchers continue to have opposing views (MacMillan et al., 2009). For instance, there is no direct evidence that screening results in decreased disability or premature death.

The Affordable Care Act (ACA)—the health insurance reform legislation passed by Congress and signed into law by President Obama on March 23, 2010—helps make prevention affordable and accessible for all Americans. The ACA requires health plans to cover preventive services for women by eliminating cost sharing. Preventive services have proven evidence of improved health outcomes. Under the ACA, women's preventive healthcare screening and counseling for interpersonal and domestic violence are among eight preventive measures (http://www.hrsa.gov/womensguidelines/). The Institute of Medicine found that after reviewing the literature, there was sufficient evidence to support screening and brief counseling for IPV. When screening for IPV and assessing for risk, nurses need to make these questions a normal and routine part of healthcare assessment that fits in the context of the visit. Screening without being prepared for a positive disclosure could be more harmful than helpful. It is important to know what resources are available and how to respond to the needs of the client before asking questions. Box 16.4 presents a sampling of questions that can be asked. Ideal screening includes questions about emotional and physical abuse and forced sex. Nurses should use their own language in asking these questions, need to ensure that the questions are developmentally and culturally appropriate, and use language appropriate to the client's level of comprehension.

EVIDENCE FOR PRACTICE

Client-centered care "expands on the disease-oriented model by incorporating the patient's experience of illness, the psychosocial context, and shared decision making" (Stewart et al., 1995). This care requires that the healthcare provider is respectful and responsive to the individual client's preferences and needs. Working with victims of violence is best approached using the principles of care and intervention that are based on trauma care, are client-centered, and are conducted in a nonjudgmental manner that respects the client's autonomy while ensuring that safety issues are being addressed.

box 16.4 Inquiry and Assessment for Intimate Partner Violence

Assessment for intimate partner abuse

To begin the conversation about IPV, you may say "I now ask all my clients about past or current abuse in their lives because I recognize its impact on one's well-being. I ask so that I can help my clients identify help and support." Screening questions need to be culturally and developmentally framed. Such questions include the following:

- Are you currently or have you ever experienced physical or emotional harm/abuse in an intimate relationship? Has anyone ever forced you to engage in sexual activity that you did not want to participate in?
- Has your current partner ever pushed, shoved, slapped, or otherwise physically hurt you?
- Every couple has arguments and disagrees—what happens when you and your partner disagree?
- Does your partner ever make you feel afraid or scared? Tell me more.
- Are you currently being hurt by someone? Are you in a safe or unsafe situation? (When I see a client with a bruise such as this, I want to make sure he or she is safe.)

Follow-up questions when a woman states that she is being abused

- Can you tell me the worst thing that has ever happened? What happened? When did it happen? Where did it happen? Where were the children? Was a weapon used?
- Do you feel your partner is capable of hurting you or your children?
- What actions have you taken?
- What are your fears? What would you like me to help you with? Please help me understand what is happening, I would like to help.
- Are you in danger now? Can you tell me more about this?
- Have you ever needed emergency medical care as a result of how you were hurt? Can you tell me more about this?
- How has the abuse affected you? Do you ever think about hurting yourself, cutting, stopping eating, or purging food?
- Have you ever thought about or been granted a restraining order? What happened?
- Have you ever left? What happened? What obstacles did you face?
- What are your fears about your children? Are you worried about their safety?

People have all grown up with internalized myths, and it is imperative that healthcare providers be aware of clients' beliefs and work actively to dispel those myths so that healthcare interventions do not retraumatize clients. Victims and survivors of IPV are sensitive to nuances of words, tone of voice, and body language; so, providers must guard against making judgmental gestures, even if subtle and unintentional, because they may have an impact on the interaction between clients and providers. Healthcare professionals must take every precaution to avoid blaming victims of IPV. Victims have often lost trust in relationships, so nurses must work to build trust and not assume its existence.

Nurses can best implement the principles of trauma-sensitive care by actively listening, validating, and supporting clients as they tell their story (Box 16.5) (Elliott et al., 2005). It is imperative to keep safety issues for the victims (and children) in the forefront. Nurses should not try to "rescue" clients; rather, they should seek to empower clients to be able to make informed decisions. It is essential to always be honest about what nurses can and cannot do, especially regarding confidentiality and mandatory reporting. Nurses should never make promises about circumstances over which they have no control, as this may cause more harm than good.

PRACTICE POINT

The nurse's role needs to focus on sensitive communication, active listening, providing information and choices, risk assessment, medical and psychological treatment, safety planning, referral, and follow-up. Providers should be familiar with protocols that promote patient-centered assessment and interventions. When a client screens positive for IPV, it is imperative to assess for his or her safety and risk of harm. Communicating concern by validating the client's story builds trust between client and provider. Statements such as "Donna, I am so sorry that this is happening; help is available," "Thank you for sharing this with me; I would like to ask you some safety questions so that I can better understand your situation," "You are not alone and you deserve better," "This must be so difficult for you," "This is not your fault," and "I am here to help you unconditionally" are appropriate responses. We need to create systems with our patients rather than asking our patients to fit into our existing systems.

So many people suffer from abuse, and suffer alone.

Pamela Stephenson, Australian clinical psychologist

Safety Assessment and Planning in Intimate Partner Violence

How an in-depth safety assessment is conducted depends on the practice environment and staff model. Whoever is conducting the safety assessment needs to seek advanced training on risk assessment, and needs to be aware of community resources. The most validated and used instrument to assess

box 16.5 Trauma-Sensitive Care: Principles

- Demonstrate respect.
- Establish and maintain rapport.
- Share control.
- Share information.
- Respect boundaries.
- Foster a mutual learning process.
- Show compassion and avoid passing judgment.

for safety is the tool developed by Jacquelyn Campbell (1986), the Lethality Assessment tool. It is a 20-item tool available on the Internet in English, Spanish, Portuguese, and French Creole. Campbell developed this instrument to identify women at risk of being murdered by their intimate partner. It often heightens a women's awareness about her safety. Once the safety issues are identified, the healthcare provider can present intervention options to the client.

Safety planning involves nurse suggestions and client choices (e.g., does the client feel she is able to keep herself safe? Does she have friends or family members who could help? Does she have a supportive employer?). Components for safety planning include a crisis/disaster plan, a place to go, how to get there, and other considerations (e.g., if the abused victim stays and the abuser leaves, if victim and the abuser stay together, or if the victim decides to leave). Safety planning involves discussing measures that the client may not have considered. For example, if an argument occurs at home, the woman should stay away from (1) the kitchen because sharp instruments are there and (2) from the bathroom because the space is small and contains many hard surfaces. She should go to a room with a window or door, carry her cell phone with 911 set to speed dial, and tell family members and neighbors. Healthcare organizations should actively partner with local shelters and court advocates, as they can assist with safety plans.

MANDATORY REPORTING OF ABUSE

When any healthcare provider suspects that abuse of an elderly person, a child, or a person with a disability has occurred, he or she is mandated to report the abuse to the appropriate agency (Box 16.6). It must be kept in mind that the data reflects the number of reported cases and not actual number of abused people as some cases may have had multiple reports.

Elder Abuse

According to the U.S. Census bureau, 13.7% of the 313 million citizens are 65 years of age or older (http://quickfacts.census.gov/qfd/states/00000.html). Estimates of the frequency of elder abuse range from 2% to 10% on the basis of various sampling, survey methods, and case definitions (Lachs & Pillemer, 2004). Elder mistreatment (i.e., abuse and neglect) is defined as intentional actions that cause harm or create a serious risk of harm (whether or not harm is intended) to a vulnerable elder by a caregiver or other person who stands in a trust relationship to the elder. This includes failure by a caregiver to satisfy the elder's basic needs or to protect the elder from harm (Bonnie & Wallace, 2003). Valid incidence and prevalence rates for elder abuse and neglect are not available. From available data, it does appear that female elders (60 years and older) are abused at a higher rate than males and that the older one is, the more likely one is to be abused (Teaster, Dugar Mendiondo, Abner, Cecil, & Otto, 2004). The number of aging Americans will likely continue to increase. Therefore, concern for abuse and victimization of this population will require effective proactive programs to identify elder abuse, and provide the necessary resources to prevent and treat this vulnerable population.

box 16.6 Considerations When Making a Mandatory Report

- Talk with the adult victim about the possibility of filing a mandatory report.
- Consider the safety concerns of filing.
- Determine how the perpetrator may respond to a report being filed.
- Determine whether it will be safe to inform the children about the report.
- Identify resources available to victim (family, friends, clergy, coworkers).
- Consider filing in concert with the adult victim.
- Share concerns of safety with the Child Protective Agency.
- Address safety planning with the nonoffending victim.
- Ask about the perpetrator's behaviors: What is the worst thing he or she has done? Does he or she own a gun? Has he or she been arrested? Does he or she use drugs? Do you think he or she is capable of hurting you or your children?

As a nurse, it is essential to know both the mandatory reporting laws in the state in which the nurse practices, and the policies and procedures to be followed within the workplace. Although the nurse may view the decision to report as "damaging" to the nurse–client relationship, he or she has a duty to report the abuse as mandated by the state. It is necessary to regard mandatory reports in the context of acting for the safety of the abused person, rather than reporting against the alleged perpetrator.

Child Maltreatment

Although elder abuse has been acknowledged and addressed only more recently, child maltreatment has been prevalent for centuries. The federal Child Abuse Prevention and Treatment Act (CAPTA) (42 U.S.C.A. §5106g), as amended by the Keeping Children and Families Safe Act of 2003 (U.S. Department of Health and Human Services, 2003), defines child abuse and neglect as follows:

- Any recent act, or failure to act, on the part of a parent or caretaker which results in death, serious physical or emotional harm, sexual abuse or exploitation; or
- An act or failure to act which presents an imminent risk of serious harm

According to the U.S. Department of Health and Human Services Administration for Children and Families (2013) from 2008 to 2012, overall rates of victimization declined by 3.3%, from 9.5 to 9.2 per 1,000 children in the population. This results in an estimated 30,000 fewer victims in 2012 (686,000) compared with 2008 (716,000). Nationally, four-fifths (78.3%) of victims were neglected, 18.3% were physically abused, 9.3% were sexually abused, and 8.5% were psychologically maltreated. For 2012, a nationally estimated 1,640 children died of abuse and neglect, a rate of 2.20 children per 100,000 children in the national population (http://www.acf.hhs.gov/sites/default/files/cb/cm2012.pdf). School nurses, visiting nurses, public health nurses, and pediatric nurses must be familiar with signs and symptoms for children at risk. Early identification and intervention are key to mitigating the effects on child development and well-being.

Prevention strategies that address child maltreatment offer the best hope for reducing the incidence of child abuse or neglect. Early identification may help prevent significant morbidity and mortality. Over the past decade, much attention has been given to the effects of children witnessing violence in the home. Researchers indicate that witnessing violence in the home can have significant developmental and psychological sequelae and affect health subsequently, even into adulthood (Dube et al., 2003; Groves, 2002).

I was angry about the fact that my father would beat my mother on a daily basis, that my mother would take it in turn and beat on me. I was an abused child. I was mad about all those things, very bitter and very angry.

Rick James, American singer, songwriter, musician

Often, the strongest protective factor in the lives of children who are exposed to domestic violence is support for the nonoffending parent. Futures Without Violence produced a document entitled *The Facts on Children and Domestic Violence* (2008). This is an excellent resource for healthcare providers. A safe, stable, and nurturing relationship with a caring adult can help a child overcome the stress associated with IPV (Middlebrooks & Audage, 2008).

As the nurse caring for Kathy, Laura needs to assess the following, using observation skills and appropriate questioning:

- Her children's current functioning
- Changes in her children's behavior
- Changes in her children's functioning as a result of the perpetrator's actions

Laura uses Boxes 16.2 and 16.6 to assess whether there is significant concern about the safety of Kathy's children. After reviewing the data and consulting with team members, Laura may decide to file a report with the child protective agency.

Deciding whether a particular case may involve abuse that requires reporting is often difficult. Collaborating with others on the healthcare team ensures a well-informed decision. Nurses should remember that when they file a report for concern of child maltreatment, they are filing on behalf of the child, not against an individual person. If no report of child maltreatment is necessary, nurses should still encourage the affected mother to express her family's immediate needs, seek the support of a community domestic violence advocate, tell her about family services that meet their immediate needs, identify the family's support system, assist her in developing a safety plan, and consult with child protection experts and/or other domestic violence providers.

Abuse of Disabled People

Although overall trends in violence and abuse seem to be decreasing, Americans with disabilities seem to experience abuse disproportionately. In fact, research and the anecdotal experience of those who work with people with disabilities suggest that this population is experiencing a heightened risk of becoming victims of violence and abuse; however, research on this population is sparse.

Only limited and dated information that addresses the issues affecting this group can be found. One study found that more than 70% of women with developmental disabilities are sexually assaulted in their lifetime, which represents a 50% higher rate than the rest of the population (Sobsey & Doe, 1991; Sobsey, 1994). In another frequently cited study, Young, Nosek, Howland, Chanpong, and Rintala (1997) found that women with physical disabilities appear to be at risk of emotional, physical, and sexual abuse to the same extent as women without physical disabilities. It appears that people with cognitive disabilities, who have a desire to be accepted and "fit in," may acquiesce to behaviors they are not quite comfortable with because of fear of social isolation. Often, a person with a disability is dependent on another, and that dependency prevents him or her from recognizing abuse and seeking help. Even when a person with a disability reports a crime, the victim is often not believed, and is viewed as not creditable. It was only in 1998 that Congress passed the Crime Victims with Disabilities Awareness Act. This represented the first piece of national legislation in U.S. history to address the issue of abuse of persons with disabilities. Such legislature draws attention at many levels—policy, research, advocacy, and law enforcement.

Awareness of the risks to persons in the disabled population should guide nursing practice through the tasks of assessing clients at risk, discussing prevention strategies with clients and their caregivers, and reporting concern for abuse to the local designated social service agency. Knowing the risks to this vulnerable population may help detect early signs of abuse and provide services to intervene.

STUDENT REFLECTION

Long ago, I remember hearing in the news about a woman in a nursing home. Although she was in a coma, she became pregnant; a male attendant raped her. I was shocked, but thought how sensational and out of the norm this event really was. However, in thinking about vulnerability, it seems that abuse of people who are disabled, or of people who are unable to make their desires and needs known, is all too common. Becoming knowledgeable about how vulnerability can make certain groups of people more at risk for abuse helped me understand how assessment and follow-up is critical. It is as if nurses are the voice of the voiceless in many ways. Today, I asked an elderly person, who is wheelchair-bound in her private home, whether she felt safe; she thought I meant from burglars. I felt awkward in probing more about her physical, mental, and emotional safety, and I did not want to scare her. What I did do was help her develop a safety plan in the event she needed help, and helped her feel comfortable by giving her examples of how some community dwellers develop systems to protect their interests. Some useful examples might include sharing some routines with neighbors and having daily contact with a family member or friend via phone. I felt as though I had empowered her. It felt good.

INTERVENTION

Ideally, preventing exposures to violence and abuse offers the best outcomes for an individual's biopsychosocial well-being. Research on interventions has been predominately quasi-experimental and descriptive designs, as the research community is cautious about the use of randomized controlled trials (RCTs), since withholding services and/or interventions that could provide safety and well-being is contraindicated and possess ethical and moral discussions. Despite the limitations of RCT, there is notable evidence that supports interventions for women exposed to violence.

One rigorous longitudinal RCT is the Nurse Family Partnership program. The outcomes for mothers (first-time mothers) and babies have proven their effectiveness. Positive outcomes include improved prenatal health, fewer childhood injuries, fewer subsequent pregnancies, increased intervals between births, increased maternal employment, and improved school readiness.

A Research findings related to the effectiveness of home visiting programs with related improved health outcomes, safety, and well-being are worth replicating and implementing into practice (Eckenrode et al., 2000; Olds, Henderson, Chamberlin, & Tatelbaum, 1986; Olds et al., 2013). (See more at http://www.nursefamilypartnership.org/proven-results/published-research#sthash.k55hBbXe.dpuf.)

Dr. Phyllis Sharps and colleagues (2008) conducted research into targeted interventions for pregnant women experiencing abuse. The evidence from this synthesis review found that of the 80 potentially eligible studies, 17 met eligibility criteria. The majority of interventions recruited women from reproductive care sites. Interventions tended to be brief, delivered by nonphysicians, and focused on empowerment, empathetic listening, discussion of the cycle of violence and safety, and referral to community-based resources. Thirteen studies demonstrated at least one intervention-related benefit. Six of 11 articles measuring IPV persistence found reductions in future violence; two of five measuring safety-promoting behaviors found increases in safety; and six of 10 measuring IPV/community resource referrals found enhanced use. The majority of studies demonstrated patient-level benefit subsequent to primary care IPV interventions, with IPV/community referrals the most common positively affected outcome.

One major intervention that health providers can address with their patients is safety and risk for harm. Feder and associates (2011) conducted a cluster RCT aimed at IPV training for providers with a focus on identification and referral to improve safety (IRIS) for women experiencing domestic violence and seeking primary care. Researchers randomized 51 (61%) of 84 eligible general practices in Hackney (London) and Bristol (United Kingdom). Of these, 24 received a training and support program; 24 did not receive the program, and three dropped out before the trial began. Following the second training session, the 24 intervention practices recorded 223 referrals of patients to advocacy and the 24 control practices recorded 12 referrals (adjusted intervention rate ratio 22.1 [95% CI 11.5–42.4]). Intervention practices recorded 641 disclosures of domestic violence and control practices recorded 236 (adjusted intervention rate ratio 3.1 [95% CI 2.2–4.3). These findings strongly support training primary care clinicians on assessment of IPV, and referral to community resources that provide services to victims of IPV.

In an effort to build on earlier research of evidenced-based empowerment, researchers explored what facilitators and barriers exist to implementing home visiting interventions. Kilburn and colleagues (2008) developed and tested a "town and gown" partnership to assist pregnant women who were in a violent relationship based on the DOVE Program (Domestic Violence Enhanced Home Visitation) (Parker, McFarlane, Silva, Soeken, & Reel, 1999). This empowerment intervention utilized prenatal visitors (town partners) with a research-driven strategy (gown intervention). The DOVE intervention includes the following:

- A structured, tailored brochure with information regarding the cycle of violence, designed to meet each women's special needs
- Risk factors associated with increased risk of homicide
- Options available to women
- Safety planning
- IPV resources specific to their locale
- National hotline numbers

Barriers and facilitating factors to the working partnership were identified in focus groups conducted with home visitors. Barriers include the lack of knowledge and training received by healthcare professionals related to recognizing violence and warning signs, how to ask about violence, and legal options and social services. Also, issues related to the rural communities were identified, such as limited services, lack of anonymity, and the home visitor and the women knowing one another. The town/gown partnership provides home visitors with evidence-based knowledge and the hands-on experience needed to assist and empower the women they are working with.

Another promising practice is the use of in-clinic IPV advocates. Using a quasi-experimental design, investigators explored the efficacy of clinic-based advocacy for IPV to increase help-seeking, reduce violence, and improve women's well-being (Coker et al., 2012). Eligible and consenting women attending one of six selected clinics in the rural Southern United States were assessed for IPV. Consenting women disclosing IPV were offered either an in-clinic advocate intervention or usual care, depending on the clinic they attended and were followed for up to 24 months. Over follow-up time, both IPV scores and depressive symptoms trended toward greater decline among women in the advocate intervention clinics relative to the usual care. In some areas of the country, such as Boston, every teaching hospital employs in-house advocates.

MODEL OF CARE FOR VICTIMS OF INTENTIONAL CRIMES

In the past, approaches to acute care of sexual assault victims, domestic abuse victims, and victimized children were inconsistent and suboptimal. Victims of intentional violence often found provider services degrading and received victim-blaming treatment; these experiences would often exacerbate the victim's physical and mental distress (Campbell, Wasco, Ahrens, Sefl, & Barnes, 2001). However, in the past 25 years, significant reform in providing acute forensic medical examinations has occurred, and evidence-based practice has evolved exponentially. Caring for victims of sexual assaults has evolved with the development of nationally certified Sexual Assault Nurse Examiner (SANE) programs. There are now national standards in place for caring for pediatric victims (SANE-P) and adolescent and adult victims (SANE-A). In the United States today, there are more than 600 SANE programs (IAFN, 2009).

I can be changed by what happens to me but
I refuse to be reduced by it.

Maya Angelou

In response to child maltreatment, and in recognizing the special needs of these children, in June 2009 the American Academy of Pediatrics developed a clinical specialty leading to board certification in child maltreatment. Most pediatric academic hospitals in the United States have Child Protection or Children at Risk Teams made up of physicians, nurses, and social workers. Such teams evaluate cases for child maltreatment, work with state child social service agencies and law enforcement, provide education to a broad audience and conduct research. Over the next decade, this area of specialty practice is likely to expand significantly.

Assisting Kathy will require multiple practice disciplines coordinating and prioritizing her needs and those of her children. In Laura's institution, it is important that she be aware of policies and procedures related to IPV, child maltreatment, and abuse of the person with disabilities, as well as any resources for management of these problems. Knowing forensic nurse experts in the community will be useful for consultation.

FORENSIC NURSING

Nurses have been providing forensic-type services for centuries. From a formal educational perspective, it was not until recently that specific education in forensic nursing was offered through a traditional nursing college or university. Graduate programs in forensic nursing are growing (Burgess, Berger, & Boersma, 2004), and there will likely be a need for forensic nurses in the future. Some nurses in the SANE program have received broader instruction; trained as forensic nurse examiners, they care for victims of all types of intentional violence. Nurses working in these areas receive advanced training that includes a didactical component and clinical practicum which leads to eligibility for board certification.

Forensic nurses offer victims compassionate, evidence-based care. Advanced training focuses on taking a history of the assault, collecting evidence, and providing treatment and follow-up. The field of forensic nursing is growing rapidly, with forensic nursing programs developing in all regions of the country. Forensic nurses are employed in the following areas: emergency departments, police departments, medical examiners offices, homeland security offices, correctional institutions, and mental health facilities. As the evidence grows and the field of forensic nursing evolves, options for nurses to work within a collaborative community team offer interesting opportunities for nursing professionals. Forensic nursing focuses not only on providing client care, but its practitioners also collect evidence, counsel clients, and communicate with professionals in legal systems. Employers are asking for forensically prepared nurses who can screen and treat clients, as well as testify in court.

As with any relatively new science, it takes time to build a body of knowledge. The *Journal of Forensic Nursing*, a peer-reviewed journal, is now recognized as a scholarly scientific journal. The ANA and the International Association of Forensic Nurses (IAFN) released *Forensic Nursing: Scope and Standards of Practice (2009)*, a comprehensive reference guide that identifies and defines the expectations for the role and practice of the forensic nurse.

A panel of nurse experts convened by the ANA and the IAFN developed the standards for forensic nurses. The guide outlines six standards for forensic nursing practice and nine standards for professional performance. Forensic nurses are among the most diverse groups of clinicians in the nursing profession with respect to client populations served, practice settings, and forensic and healthcare services provided. Forensic nurses apply a unique combination of processes rooted in nursing science, forensic science, and public health to care for clients. In addition to recommended standards of professional performance, the IAFN book's summary discussion of the scope of forensic nursing practice—including characteristics, trends, education, practice environments, and its ethical and conceptual bases—lends an informative and broad context for the reader's understanding and use of these standards.

key concepts

- Violence against women is a form of gender-based violence that can result in physical, sexual, or psychological harm for both the direct victims and also their dependents (children).
- Intimate partner violence is fundamentally based on the desire for control on the part of the perpetrator.
- Empowering victims of intentional violence to care for themselves and get help is assumed to be a welcomed opportunity. For many, however, it is a difficult context that has brought them to violent, abusive relationships, and it is a difficult context which will release them from the situation.
- Although abuse and violence can be unintentional, it is the intentional violence which impels nurses to become members of a healthcare team involved in assessing and addressing policy as a way of decreasing the incidence of such acts in communities.

critical thinking questions

1. You live in a state that has no mandatory laws requiring professionals to report elder abuse. How would you develop support of the individual clients, families, and the community to work toward a system of mandatory reporting?
2. A mother in a pediatric setting becomes very upset when indirect questions are asked about her children's safety at home. How would you address her feelings?
3. Discuss the positives and negatives of domestic violence shelters for women and children.
4. Compare and contrast violence in the context of heterosexual and gay-lesbian-bisexual-transsexual relationships. Are preventive solutions the same in these groups?

community resources

Through networking and attending local conferences on domestic violence, one can begin to build a resource directory of community partners–knowing the following resources is imperative.

- Women's shelters
- Churches/synagogues/temples
- Food banks
- Women, Infants, and Children (WIC) program
- Mental health agencies
- Unemployment offices
- Law enforcement agencies
- Advocacy centers
- Justice centers
- Support groups
- Batterer's intervention groups
- Forensic nurses

references

Abbott, J. T., Johnson, R., Koziol-McLain, J., & Lowenstein, S. R. (1995). Domestic violence against women: Incidence and prevalence in an emergency department population. *JAMA, 273,* 1763–1767.

American Academy of Pediatrics, Committee on Child Abuse and Neglect. (1998). The role of the pediatrician in recognizing and intervening on behalf of abused women. *Pediatrics, 101,* 1091–1092.

American College of Obstetricians and Gynecologists. (1993). *The obstetrician-gynecologist and primary-preventive health care.* Washington, DC: American College of Obstetricians and Gynecologists.

American Medical Association Council on Scientific Affairs. (1992). Violence against women-relevance for medical practitioners. *JAMA, 267,* 3184–3189.

references (continued)

American Nurses Association. (1991). *Position statement on physical violence against women.* Kansas City, MO: American Nurses Association.

Anda, R., Croft, J., Felitti, V. J., Nordenberg, D., Giles, W. H., Williamson, D. F., & Giovino G. A. (1999). Adverse childhood experiences and smoking during adolescence and adulthood. *JAMA, 82,* 1652–1658.

Anderson, M., Kaufman, J., Simon, T. R., Barrios, L., Paulozzi, L., Ryan, G., … Potter, L.; School-Associated Violent Deaths Study Group. (2001). School-associated violent deaths in the United States 1994–1999. *JAMA, 286*(21), 2695–2702.

Bair-Merritt, M., Lewis-O'Connor, A., Goel, S., Amato, P., Ismailji, T., Jelley, M., … Cronholm, P. (2014). Primary care-based interventions for intimate partner violence: A systematic review. *American Journal of Preventive Medicine, 46*(2),188–194.

Berman, H., Hardesty, J., & Humphreys, J. (2004). Children of abused women. In J. Humphreys & J. Campbell (Eds.), *Family violence and nursing practice* (pp. 150–185). Philadelphia, PA: Lippincott Williams & Wilkins.

Black, M., Basile, K., & Breiding, M. (2011). The national intimate partner and sexual violence survey (NISVS): 2010 summary report. Atlanta, GA: Centers for Disease Control and Prevention.

Bonnie, R., & Wallace, R. (Eds.). (2003). *Elder mistreatment: Abuse, neglect and exploitation in an aging America.* Washington, DC: National Academies Press.

Bureau of Justice Statistics. (2007). *Intimate homicide victims by gender.* Retrieved April 30, 2010, from http://www.now.org/issues/violence/stats.html#endref1

Burgess, A. W., Berger, A., & Boersma, R. (2004). Forensic nursing: A graduate nursing specialty. *American Journal of Nursing, 104*(3), 58–64.

Campbell, J. C. (1981). Misogyny and homicide of women. *Advances in Nursing Science, 3,* 67–85.

Campbell, J. C. (1986). Nursing assessment for risk of homicide with battered women. *Advances in Nursing Science, 8,* 36–51.

Campbell, J. C. (1992). "If I can't have you, no one can": Power and control in homicide of female partners. In J. Radford & D. Russell (Eds.), *Femicide: The politics of woman killing.* New York, NY: Twayne.

Campbell, J. C. (1995a). *Assessing dangerousness.* Newbury Park, CA: Sage.

Campbell, J. C. (1995b). Prediction of homicide of and by battered women. In J. Campbell (Ed.), *Assessing the risk of dangerousness: Potential for further violence of sexual offenders, batterers, and child abusers.* Newbury Park, CA: Sage.

Campbell, J. C. (1995c). Homicide of and by battered women. In J. C. Campbell (Ed.), *Assessing dangerousness: Violence by sexual offenders, batterers, and child abusers* (pp. 96–113). Thousand Oaks, CA: Sage.

Campbell, J. C. (2002). Health consequences of intimate partner violence. *Lancet, 359,* 1331–1336.

Campbell, J. C., & Lewandowski, L. A. (1997). Mental and physical effects of intimate partner violence on women and children. *Psychiatric Clinics of North America, 20,* 353–374.

Campbell, J. C., Webster, D., Koziol-McLain, J., Block, C., Campbell, D., Curry, M. A., … Laughon, K. (2003a). Risk factors for femicide in abusive relationships: Results from a multicity case control study. *American Journal of Public Health, 93,* 1089–1097.

Campbell, J. C., Webster, D., Koziol-McLain, J., Block, C. R., Campbell, D., Curry, M. A., … Wilt, S. A. (2003b). Assessing risk factors for intimate partner homicide. *National Institute of Justice Journal, 250,* 14–19. Retrieved from http://ncjrs.org/pdffiles1/jr000250e.pdf

Campbell, R., Wasco, S., Ahrens, C., Sefl, T., & Barnes, H. (2001). Preventing the "second rape": Rape survivors' experiences with community service providers. *Journal of Interpersonal Violence, 16,* 1239–1259.

Centers for Disease Control and Prevention. *Adverse health conditions and health risk behaviors associated with intimate partner violence—United States, 2005.* Retrieved from http://www.cdc.gov/mmwr/preview/mmwrhtml/mm5705a1.htm

Centers for Disease Control and Prevention. (2001). Temporal variations in school-associated student homicide and suicide events—United States, 1992–1999. *Morbidity and Mortality Weekly Report, 50*(31), 657–660.

Centers for Disease Control and Prevention. (2003). Source of firearms used by students in school-associated violent deaths–United States, 1992–1999. *Morbidity and Mortality Weekly Report, 52*(09), 169–172.

Centers for Disease Control and Prevention. (2012). Youth risk behavior surveillance—United States, 2011. *Morbidity and Mortality Weekly Report* (Surveillance Summaries), 61(SS-4). Retrieved from www.cdc.gov/mmwr/pdf/ss/ss6104.pdf

Chang, J., Berg, C. J., Herndon, J., & Saltzman, L. (2005). Homicide: A leading cause of injury deaths among pregnant and postpartum women in the United States between 1991–1999. *American Journal of Public Health, 95,* 471–477.

Coker, A., Davis, K., Arias, H., Desai, S., Sanderson, M., Brandt, H. M., & Smith, P. H. (2002). Physical and mental health effects of intimate partner violence for men and women. *American Journal of Preventive Medicine, 23,* 260–268.

Coker, A., Smith, P., Whitaker, D., Le, B., Crawford, T., & Flerx, V. (2012). Effect of an in-clinic IPV advocate intervention to increase help seeking, reduce violence, and improve well-being. *Violence Against Women, 18*(1), 118–131.

Corso, P. S., Mercy, J. A., Simon, T. R., Finkelstein, E. A., & Miller, T. R. (2007). Medical costs and productivity losses due to interpersonal violence and self-directed violence. *American Journal of Preventive Medicine, 32*(6), 474–482.

Dolezal, T., McCollum, D., & Callahan, M. (2009). *Hidden cost in health care: The economic impact of violence and abuse.* Eden Prairie, MN: Academy on Violence and Abuse.

Dong, M., Anda, R., Felitti, V. J., Dube, S. R., Williamson, D. F., Thompson, T. J., … Giles, W. H. (2004). The interrelatedness of multiple forms of childhood abuse, neglect, and household dysfunction. *Child Abuse and Neglect, 28,* 771–784.

Dube, S., Felitti, V. J., Dong, M., Giles, W., & Anda, R. (2003). The impact of adverse childhood experiences on health problems: Evidence from four birth cohorts dating back to 1900. *Preventive Medicine, 37,* 268–277.

Eckenrode, J., Ganzel, B., Henderson, C., Smith, E., Olds, D., Powers;, J., … Sidora, K. (2000). Preventing child abuse and neglect with a program of nurse home visitation the limiting effects of domestic violence. *JAMA, 284*(11),1385–1391.

Edelson, J. (1999). Children's witnessing of adult domestic violence. *Journal of Interpersonal Violence, 14,* 839–870.

Edwards, V., Anda, R., Dube, S. R., Dong, M., Chapman, D., & Felitti, V. J. (2005). The wide-ranging health consequences of adverse childhood experiences. In K. Kendall-Tackett & S. Giacomoni (Eds.), *Child victimization: Maltreatment, bullying, and dating violence prevention and intervention.* Kingston, NJ: Civic Research Institute.

Elliott, D., Bjelajac, B., Fallot, R., Markoff, L., & Reed, R. (2005). Trauma-informed or trauma-denied: Principles and implementation of trauma-informed services for women. *Journal of Community Psychology, 33*(4), 461–477.

Family Violence Prevention Fund. (1999). *Preventing domestic violence: Clinical guidelines on routine screening.* San Francisco: Family Violence Prevention Fund. Retrieved November, 2, 2009, from http://endabuse.org/userfiles/file/HealthCare/dental.pdf

Federal Bureau of Investigation. (2010). *Supplementary Homicide Reports, 1976–2005.* Retrieved April 20, 2010, from http://bjs.ojp.

usdoj.gov/content/homicide/gender.cfm and http://bjs.ojp.usdoj.gov/content/homicide/race.cfm

Feder, G., Davies, R. A, Baird, K., Dunne, D., Eldridge, S., Griffiths, C., ... Sharp, D. (2011). Identification and referral to improve safety (IRIS) of women experiencing domestic violence with a primary care training and support programme: A cluster randomized controlled trial. *Lancet, 378,* 1788–1795.

Felitti, V., Anda, R., Nordenberg, D., Williamson, D. F., Spitz, A. M., Edwards, V., ... Marks, J. S. (1998). The relationship of childhood abuse and household dysfunction to many of the leading causes of death in adults. The Adverse Childhood Experiences (ACE) Study. *American Journal of Preventive Medicine, 14,* 245–258.

Gin, N. E., Rucker, L., Frayne, S., & Cygan, R. (1992). Prevalence of domestic violence among patients in three ambulatory care internal medicine clinics. *Journal of General Internal Medicine, 6,* 317–322.

Groves, B. M. (2002). *Children who see too much: Lessons from the child witness to violence project.* Boston: Beacon Press.

Grunbaum, J., Kann, L., Kinchen, S., Ross, J., Hawkins, J., Lowry, R., ... Collins J. (2004). Youth risk behavior surveillance—United States, 2003. *Morbidity and Mortality Weekly Report Surveillance Summary, 53*(2), 1–96.

Hamberger, L. K., Saunders, D. G., & Hovey, M. (1992). Prevalence of domestic violence in community practice and rate of physician inquiry. *Family Medicine, 24,* 283–287.

Hathaway, J., Zimmer, B., Willis, G., & Silverman, J. (2008). Perceived changes in health and safety following participation in a health care-based domestic violence program. *Journal Midwifery Womens Health, 53,* 547–555.

Healthy People 2020. *Understanding and Improving Health.* Retrieved from http://www.health.gov/healthypeople

Helton, A., McFarlane, J., & Anderson, E. (1987). Battered and pregnant: A prevalence study. *American Journal of Public Health, 77,* 1337–1339.

Hemingway, D. (2004). *Private guns, public health.* The University of Michigan Press.

Humphreys, J., Parker, B., & Campbell, J. C. (2001). Intimate partner violence against women. In D. Taylor & N. Fugate-Woods (Eds.), *Annual review of nursing research* (pp. 275–306). New York, NY: Springer Publishing Company.

International Association of Forensic Nurse. (2009). Retrieved from www.iafn.org

Joint Commission on Accreditation of Healthcare Organizations. (1995). *Accreditation manual for hospitals.* Oakbrook Terrace, IL: JCAHO.

Jones, A. S., Gielen, A. C., Campbell, J. C., Schollengerger, J., Dienemann, J. A., Kub, J., ... Wynne, E. C. (1999). Annual and lifetime prevalence of partner abuse in a sample of HMO enrollees. *Women's Health Issues, 9,* 295–305.

Kellerman, A., & Heron, S. (1999). Firearms and family violence. *Emergency Medicine Clinic North America, 17,* 699–716.

Kernic, M., Wolf, M. E., & Holt, V. (2000). Rates and relative risk of hospital admissions among women in violent intimate relationships. *American Journal of Public Health, 90,* 1416–1420.

Kilburn, E., Chang, C., Bullock, L., & Sharps, P. (2008). Facilitators and barriers for implementing home visit interventions to address intimate partner violence: Town and gown partnerships. *Nursing Clinics of North America, 43*(3), 419–435.

Krug, E., Dahlberg, L., Mercy, J., Zwi, A., & Lozano, R. (Eds.). (2002). *World report on violence and health.* Geneva, Switzerland: World Health Organization.

Lachs, M., & Pillemer, K. (2004). Elder abuse. *The Lancet, 364,* 1192–1263.

Lewandowski, L., McFarlane, J., Campbell, J. C., Gary, F., & Barenski, C. (2004). He killed my mommy: Children of murdered mothers. *Journal of Family Violence, 19,* 211–220.

Lewis-O'Connor, A. (2007). When push comes to shove: Screening mothers for intimate partner abuse during their child's pediatric visit (Doctoral Dissertation).

MacMillan, H. L., Wathen, C. N., Jamieson, E., Boyle, M. H., Shannon, H. S., Ford-Gilboe, M., . . . McMaster Violence Against Women Research Group. (2009). Screening for intimate partner violence in health care settings: A randomized trial. *JAMA, 302*(5), 493 -501.

Martin, S. E., & Clements, M. L. (2002). Young children's responding to interparental conflict: Associations with marital aggression and child adjustment. *Journal of Child and Family Studies, 11,* 231–244.

McCloskey, L. A., Figuerdo, A., & Koss, M. (1995). The effects of systemic family violence on children's mental health. *Child Development, 66,* 1239–1261.

McFarlane, J., Parker, B., Soeken, K., & Bullock, L. (1992). Assessing for abuse during pregnancy: Severity and frequency of injuries and associated entry into prenatal care. *JAMA, 26,* 3176–3178.

Middlebrooks, J. S., & Audage, N. C. (2008). *The effects of childhood stress on health across the lifespan.* CDC, NCIPC. Retrieved from http://www.cdc.gov/ncipc/pub-res/pdf/Childhood_Stress.pdf

Miller, E., Decker, M. R., Raj, A., Reed, E., Marable, D., Silverman, J. G. (2010). Intimate partner violence and health care-seeking patterns among female users of urban adolescent clinics. *Maternal Child Health Journal, 14*(6), 910–917.

Miller, E., Decker, M. R., McCauley, H., Tancredi, D. J., Levenson, R. R., Waldman, J., ... Silverman, J. G. (2010). Pregnancy coercion, intimate partner violence and unintended pregnancy. *Contraception, 81,* 316–322.

Miller, E., Decker, M. R., Raj, A., Reed, E., Marable, D., Silverman, J. G. (2010). Intimate partner violence and health care-seeking patterns among female users of urban adolescent clinics. *Maternal Child Health Journal, 14*(6), 910–917.

Moracco, K., Runyan, C., & Butts, J. (2003). Female intimate partner homicide: A population-based study. *Journal American Medical Women's Association, 58,* 20–25.

Moyer, V. A. (for U.S. Preventive Services Task Force). (2013). Screening for intimate partner violence and abuse of elderly and vulnerable adults: U.S. Preventive Services Task Force recommendation statement. *Annals of Internal Medicine, 158*(6), 478–486.

Murphy, S., Xu, J., & Kochanek, K. (2013). *Deaths: Final data for 2010.* National Vital Statistics Reports, 61(4). Retrieved from http://www.cdc.gov/nchs/data/nvsr/nvsr61/nvsr61_04.pdf

National Center for Education Statistics. (2009). *Indicators of school crime and safety: 2009.* Retrieved April 23, 2010, from http://nces.ed.gov/programs/crimeindicators/crimeindicators2009/ind_01.asp

National Institute of Justice. (2010). *Gun violence.* Retrieved May 1, 2010, from http://www.ojp.usdoj.gov/nij/topics/crime/gun-violence/welcome.htm

Neilson, H. D., Yuen, P., McKiernan, Y., & Klein, J.; U. S. Preventive Services Task Force. (2004). Screening women and elderly adults for family and intimate partner violence: A review of the evidence for the U.S. Preventive Services.

National Institute of Health News. (2011). *Violence during pregnancy linked to reduce birth weight.* Retrieved from http://www.nih.gov/news/health/sep2011/nichd-08.htm

Ogbonnaya, I. N., Macy, R., Kupper, L., Martin, S., & Bledsoe-Mansori, S. (2013). Intimate partner violence and depressive symptoms before pregnancy, during pregnancy and after infant delivery. *Journal of Interpersonal Violence, 28,* 2112–2133.

Olds, D., Henderson, C., Chamberlin, R., & Tatelbaum, R. (1986). Preventing child abuse and neglect: A randomized trial of nurse home visitation. *Pediatrics, 78,* 65–78.

Olds, D., Holmberg, J., Donelan-McCall, N., Luckey, D., Knudtson, M., & Robinson, J. (2013). Effects of home visits by paraprofessionals and by nurses on children: Follow-up of a randomized trial at ages 6 and 9 years. *JAMA Pediatrics,* E1–E8.

references (continued)

Parker, B., McFarlane, J., Silva, C., Soeken, K., & Reel, S. (1999). Testing an intervention to prevent further abuse to pregnant women. *Research in Nursing and Health, 22,* 59–66.

Robers, S., Zhang, J., Truman, J., & Synder, T. D. (2012). *Indicators of school crime and safety: 2011.* Washington, DC: National Center for Education Statistics, U.S. Department of Education, and Bureau of Justice Statistics, Office of Justice Programs, U.S. Department of Justice. Retrieved from http:// nces.ed.gov/pubs2012/2012002.pdf

Sharps, P., Campbell, J., Baty, M., Walker, K., & Bair-Merritt, M. (2008). Current evidence on perinatal home visiting and intimate partner violence. *Journal of Obstetric, Gynecologic and Neonatal Nursing, 37*(4), 480–491.

Silverman, J., Raj, A., Mucci, L., & Hathaway, J. (2001). Dating violence against adolescent girls, associated substance use, unhealthy weight control, sexual risk behavior, pregnancy, and suicidality. *JAMA, 286,* 572–579.

Silverman, J. G., Raj, A., & Clements, K. (2004). Dating violence and associated sexual risk and pregnancy among adolescent girls in the United States. *Pediatrics, 114,* e220–e225.

Sobsey, D. (1994). *Violence and abuse in the lives of people with disabilities.* Baltimore, MD: Paul H. Brookes Publishing Co.

Sobsey, D., & Doe, T. (1991). Patterns of sexual abuse and assault. *Journal of Sexuality and Disability, 9*(3), 243–259.

Sorenson, S. B., & Wiebe, D. J. (2004). Weapons in the lives of battered women. *American Journal of Public Health, 94,* 1412–1417.

Stewart, M., Weston, W., Brown, J. B., McWhinney, I. R., McWilliam C., & Freeman T. (1995). *Patient-centered medicine: Transforming the clinical method.* Thousand Oaks, CA: Sage.

Teaster, P. B., Dugar, T., Mendiondo, M., Abner, E. L, Cecil, K. A., & Otto, J. M. (2004). The 2004 survey of adult protective services: Abuse of adults 60 years of age and older. Washington DC: National Center on Elder Abuse.

Tjaden, P., & Thoennes, N. (2000). *Extent, nature and consequences of intimate partner violence: Findings from the National Violence against Women Survey* (Report publication No. NCJ-181867). Washington DC: U.S. Department of Justice, Office of Justice Programs.

United Nations. (1993). *Declaration on the elimination of violence against women, Geneva.* Universal Declaration of Human Rights. Retrieved November 2, 2009, from http://www.un.org/en/documents/udhr/

U.S. Department of Health and Human Services, Administration for Children and Families, Administration on Children, Youth and Families, Children's Bureau. (2013). *Child maltreatment 2012.* Available from http://www.acf.hhs.gov/programs/cb/research-data-technology/statistics-research/child-maltreatment.

U.S. Department of Health and Human Services, Administration for Children and Families, Children's Bureau. (2003). *Child abuse and neglect.* Retrieved from https://www.childwelfare.gov/can/

Waters, H., Hyder, A., Rajkotia, Y., Basu, S., Rehwinkel, J. A., & Butchart, A. *The economic dimensions of interpersonal violence.* Department of Injuries and Violence Prevention, World Health Organization, Geneva, 2004.

Weiss, H., Lawrence, B., & Miller, T. (2002). Pregnancy-associated assault hospitalizations. *Obstetrics & Gynecology, 100,* 773–780.

Whitfield, C., Anda, R., Dube, S., & Felitti, V. J. (2003). Violent childhood experiences and the risk of intimate partner violence in adults: Assessment in a large health maintenance organization. *Journal of Interpersonal Violence, 18,* 166–185.

Wiebe, D. (2003). Homicide and suicide risks associated with firearms in the home: A national case-control study. *Annals of Emergency Medicine, 41,* 771–778.

Wilt, S., & Olson, S. (1996). Prevalence of domestic violence in the United States. *Journal of the American Medical Women's Association, 51,* 77–82.

Young, M. E., Nosek, M. A., Howland, C., Chanpong, G., & Rintala, D. H. (1997). Prevalence of abuse of women with disabilities. *Archive of Physical and Medical Rehabilitation, 78,* S34–S38.

suggested readings

Bailey, J., Kellerman, A., & Somes, G. W. (1997). Risk factors for violence death of women in the home. *Annals of Internal Medicine, 157,* 777–782.

web resources

Please visit thePoint® for up-to-date Web resources on this topic.

CHAPTER 17

Substance Use

Judith Shindul-Rothschild

The basic thing nobody asks is why do people take drugs of any sort? Why do we have these accessories to normal living to live? I mean, is there something wrong with society that's making us so pressurized, that we cannot live without guarding ourselves against it?

John Lennon

Man is the only creature that refuses to be what he is.

Albert Camus

Drugs? Everyone has a choice and I choose not to do drugs.

Leonardo DiCaprio

Reality is just a crutch for people who can't cope with drugs.

Robin Williams

chapter highlights

- Factors affecting prevalence rates of substance use: age, gender, race, socioeconomic level, urban or rural settings
- Population-based interventions to decrease substance use
- Evidence-based treatment protocols for substance abuse that should be incorporated by community health nurses in all practice settings
- Self-help groups: a highly effective community-based treatment with proven efficacy in sustaining recovery

objectives

- Define substance use, substance abuse, and addiction.
- Describe the impact of substance abuse and addiction on individual people and their families, communities, and nations.
- Identify risk factors for substance misuse and abuse in individual people and populations.
- Apply evidence-based practice in the nursing care of populations most at risk for substance use disorders.
- Apply evidence-based interventions in providing nursing care in the community for clients with substance abuse.

key terms

The World Health Organization (WHO) has compiled a list of terms and definitions commonly used in population surveys and WHO research publications on substance use. The list is entitled "Lexicon of alcohol and drug terms published by the World Health Organization" and is available online. Other terms are defined by the *Diagnostic and Statistical Manual of Mental Disorders* (*DSM-5*) compiled by the American Psychiatric Association (APA, 2013)

Abstinence: No use of illicit substances or alcohol in the preceding 12 months; a person is considered "abstinent."

Addiction: A term, along with habituation, which the WHO recommends be substituted with substance dependence. However, clients and practitioners commonly use addiction.

Craving: A very strong urge or desire to seek the euphoric feeling achieved by using substances (*DSM-5*).

Intoxication: A reversible syndrome that appears after ingestion of a specific substance that results in clinically significant problematic behavioral or psychological changes (e.g., belligerence, mood lability, impaired judgment, disturbances of perception, psychomotor behavior, and interpersonal behavior [*DSM-5*]).

Remission: Early remission is defined in *DSM-5* as occurring when a person has previously met criteria for a substance use disorder but has not met the criteria for 3 to 12 months. Sustained remission occurs when a person no longer meets the criteria for substance use disorder for 12 months or more.

Substance use (in this chapter): The use of alcohol, illicit drugs, and nonmedical use of prescription medications. Illicit drugs include cannabis, cocaine, heroin, hallucinogens, inhalants, and methamphetamine. Prescription medications used nonmedically include pain relievers, tranquilizers, stimulants, and sedatives.

Substance use disorders (SUD): In *DSM-5*, SUD includes separate criteria for alcohol, anxiolytics, caffeine, cannabis, gambling, hallucinogens, hypnotics, opioids, phencyclidine, sedatives, stimulants, and tobacco.

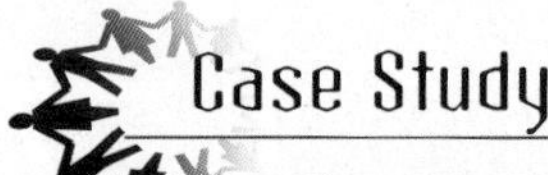

Case Study

References to the case study are found throughout this chapter (look for the case study icon). Readers should keep the case study in mind as they read the chapter.

James Campbell, a 63-year-old African-American man, is retired from the Boston Fire Department. His wife died 6 months ago from breast cancer, and he now lives alone next to his adult daughter. Since his wife died, Mr. Campbell has been increasingly relying on his daughter's assistance to manage his home. His daughter, who works full-time and has four children of her own, has not been able to spend as much time with her father as she would like, but she checks with him daily. Recently, she has noticed that her father's appetite seems to have decreased; he has lost so much weight that his pants are very loose around his waist. At his daughter's insistence, Mr. Campbell agrees to see a nurse practitioner at a Boston clinic for a thorough evaluation.

In the meeting with the nurse, the daughter says that she is worried about her father becoming depressed. Mr. Campbell does admit to having difficulty sleeping and says that he takes a "shot" of whiskey to help him relax. He injured his back before he retired, and sometimes, his back pain is so severe that he takes a "pain pill" that his wife was given to manage her cancer pain. Mr. Campbell's daughter believes that her mother took oxycodone (OxyContin). Mr. Campbell vehemently denies changes in mood but does admit that he gets the "jitters" during the day for no apparent reason and takes one alprazolam (Xanax), which his wife's physician prescribed for him when she was first diagnosed with cancer. His daughter says that it seems she has been filling the Xanax prescription more frequently lately.

key terms (continued)

Tolerance: Diminished physical and/or psychological response to effects of alcohol or illicit substances. A person develops tolerance when he or she needs to use higher doses of alcohol or illicit substances to achieve the desired euphoric effect (*DSM-5*).

Withdrawal: A reduction in prolonged substance use that results in problematic behavioral, physiologic, and cognitive changes. Withdrawal causes significant impairment in social, occupational, and interpersonal functioning and is usually associated with an urge to readminister the substance to reduce the symptoms (*DSM-5*).

INTERNATIONAL ASPECTS OF SUBSTANCE ABUSE

Substance use affects societies in many ways, and countries have used different models to address the impact on populations. Approaches range from strict prohibition and criminalization to the harm reduction model, which is based on public health principles. When substances that can alter mental states are believed to lead to **addiction** and social harms or dysfunction, some governments respond by enacting laws that support strict drug prohibition. The harm reduction approach focuses on the reduction of the harmful effects of drug use and addiction without necessarily achieving **abstinence**. Most countries actually apply a model combining both harm reduction strategies and criminalization (WHO, 2014a).

Scope of Substance Use

Worldwide, mental and substance use disorders are the leading cause of all nonfatal disease burdens, and most deaths (81%) are attributable to substance use disorders (Whiteford et al., 2013). These trends suggest that global disease burden is shifting from infectious to noninfectious disease and from premature death to years lived with disability (Whiteford et al., 2013). It is important for community health nurses to appreciate the cultural norms and differences in the use of illicit and licit substances. For example, in some cultures, such as the United States, alcohol use is viewed as normative, while in other cultures, the use of alcohol is strictly forbidden and viewed as a behavior that is one of the most stigmatized of all health conditions (WHO, 2014a). Globally, public health models that address drug and alcohol abuse focus on interventions at three points: the agent (the distributor of the substance), the host (the addicted person), and the environment (local, national, or international).

The real problems are cultural. The problems of the people who take drugs are a cultural trap—I think there's a real problem there, the crack stuff, the hopelessness of the junkie. The urban angst.

Jerry Garcia

Public Health Policies to Minimize Harms from Substance Use

Alcohol misuse is a global public health threat that poses significant social and economic costs to healthcare systems, criminal justice authorities, and social welfare systems (WHO, 2014a) (Fig. 17.1). Successful global and multinational policies aimed at reducing social harms associated with alcohol consumption focus on availability, marketing, pricing, drinking and driving, prevention, and treatment in healthcare systems (WHO, 2014a). These aspects of a public health model are reflected in the WHO's "Guiding public

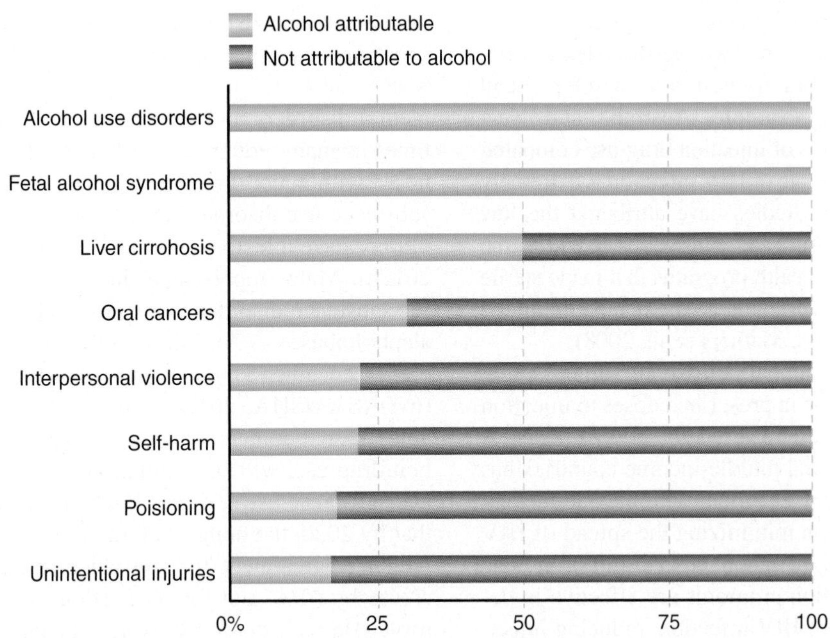

figure 17.1 Global alcohol attributable causes of death, disease, and injury, 2012. (From WHO. [2014]. *Global Status Report on Alcohol and Health* [p. 47]. Luxembourg: World Health Organization.)

health principles to reduce the harmful use of alcohol" (Box 17.1). The most common public health policies are national awareness campaigns that educate populations about the social harms associated with alcohol misuse, especially drinking and driving (WHO, 2014a).

Evidence-based policy options related to health services delivery include population screening and brief intervention with referral to treatment (SBIRT), especially for high-risk populations including children, adolescents, pregnant women, and older adults (WHO, 2014a). Population-based policies designed to limit the availability of alcohol include laws regulating the minimum drinking age, licensing restrictions, marketing restrictions, and increased pricing through taxation.

box 17.1 WHO Public Health Principles Guiding Development and Implementation of Alcohol Policies

a. Public policies and interventions to prevent and reduce alcohol-related harm should be guided and formulated by public health interests and based on clear public health goals and best available evidence.
b. Alcohol policies should be equitable and sensitive to national, religious, and cultural contexts.
c. Protection of populations at high risk for alcohol-related harm and those exposed to the harmful effects of drinking by others should be an integral part of public health policies.
d. Populations affected by the harmful use of alcohol should have access to affordable and effective prevention and care services.

Source: WHO. (2014). *Global Status Report on Alcohol and Health.* Luxembourg: World Health Organization.

Other examples of policies enacted by nations or states to minimize the harm to populations from alcohol use include blood alcohol limits on driving and warning labels on alcohol beverages about the adverse effects on health (WHO, 2014a).

At the community level, strategies to reduce the harmful use of alcohol include developing policies designed for specific community events such as sporting events or festivals where subpopulations, especially youth, maybe at risk for harm from excessive substance use. Community-based policies may include restrictions on public consumption of alcohol, restrictions on the hours establishments can serve alcohol, and mandatory training for hospitality providers.

Some of the key population factors associated with illicit drug use are the availability of illicit drugs and the perception of risk (UNODC, 2012). Unlike the use of alcohol, which is relatively stable across age cohorts, illicit drug use peaks among youth and then as a person matures, the illegal consequences of illicit drug use appear to have a mitigating effect on use in adulthood. The United Nations Office on Drugs and Crime (UNODC) sponsors two international projects to promote prevention of drug use targeting youth. The UNODC's Global Youth Network provides information and materials to prevent drug abuse at the individual, family, school, and community level. The UNODC/WHO's Global Initiative on Primary Prevention of Substance Abuse provides information on evidence-based practices to assess substance abuse, plan prevention programs, and evaluate effectiveness of programs on preventing substance abuse. More information is available at the UNODC's websites.

From a public health perspective, self-administered injection of illicit substances poses the greatest risk for population health and social harms (UNODC, 2012). Two public health programs, opioid substitution treatment and syringe-exchange programs, have been effective in lowering the rates of HIV infection among injection drug users in both developed and developing countries. For example, Australia and New Zealand have moderate levels of injection drug use compared with other countries, but the rate of HIV infection is extremely low (approximately 2.6%). Studies have attributed the low levels of HIV infection in Australia and New Zealand to the rapid introduction of public health programs that made sterile needles and syringes widely available to the population in the 1980s (Lawrinson et al., 2008; Mathers et al., 2008).

Opioid substitution treatment consists of administering methadone or buprenorphine in prescribed doses to injection drug users in programs administered by governments. A WHO study of eight low- and middle-income countries has demonstrated that outpatient treatment with methadone and buprenorphine is effective in minimizing the spread of HIV in developed countries (Lawrinson et al., 2008). It also found that opioid substitution programs are effective in decreasing the transmission of HIV infection, reducing injecting drug use, and improving the health of people addicted to opioids. There is widespread agreement among public health experts in both developed and developing countries that opioid substitution treatment programs are an effective public health strategy to reduce the social harms associated with illicit opioid use, such as prostitution, shoplifting, theft, and property crime.

National Scope of Substance Use

The United States leads the world in the portion of its citizens who abuse or are dependent on alcohol or illicit substances and is the country with the largest illicit drug market. Slightly more than half (52.1%) of all Americans older than 12 years drink alcohol and 9.2% use illicit drugs (Substance Abuse and Mental Health Services Administration [SAMHSA], 2013). The United States also leads the world in the percentage of drug users self-administering illicit substance by injection (UNODC, 2012). In the United States, substance use is highly correlated with a range of mental disorders and serious psychological distress. Three times as many youth 12 to 17 years of age who were diagnosed with major depression in the past year met criteria for substance use disorder (18.2%) as compared to youth who did not have a history of mental illness (5.8%) (SAMSHA, 2012b). Males represented three-fourths of all admissions for substance disorder treatment, with most admissions for alcohol abuse (41%), followed by opiates (23%), marijuana (18%), cocaine (8%), and methamphetamine/amphetamines (6%) (SAMSHA, 2012c) (Fig. 17.2). It is anticipated that aging baby boomers, the cohort with the highest rates of illicit drug use, will substantially increase demand for health and substance use services. Public health analysts anticipate that by 2020, the number of adults aged 50 to 59 years who will need treatment for substance abuse disorder will increase by 61%, and for older adults aged 60 to 69, it will triple (Han, Gfroerer, Colliver, & Penne, 2009) (Fig. 17.3).

In general, rates of substance use are higher among native-born populations than immigrants. Public health researchers theorize that the "immigrant paradox" for **substance use disorders** is related to protective factors, such as community safety and family cohesion, which contribute to lower rates of substance use among immigrants upon arrival to the United States (Qureshi et al., 2014; Salas-Wright & Vaughn, 2014; Savage & Mezuk, 2014). As immigrants' length of residence in the United States increases, the rate of substance misuse also increases, suggesting that sociocultural exposures, including acculturation and discrimination, play a direct role in increasing risk among immigrants (Savage & Mezuk, 2014). Immigrant youth in particular are more susceptible to peer influence and acculturation stress and are more likely to adopt unhealthy substance use behaviors than immigrant adults (Li & Wen, 2013).

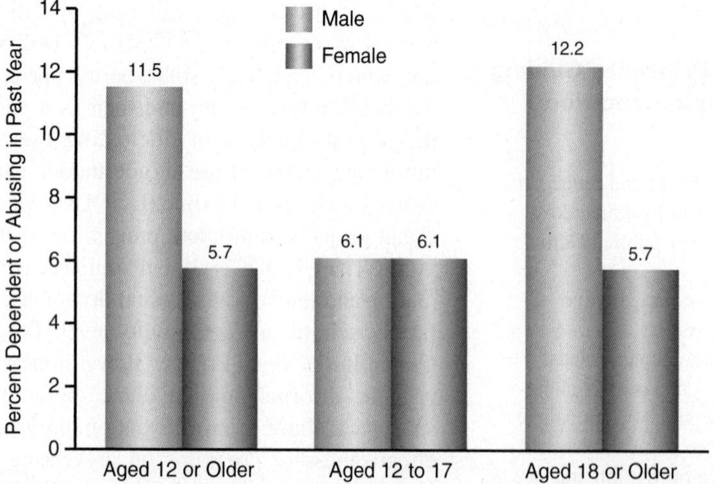

figure 17.2 Substance dependence or abuse by gender, 2012. (From Substance Abuse and Mental Health Services Administration. [2013]. *Results from the 2012 National Survey on Drug Use and Health: Summary of National Findings* [p. 81], NSDUH Series H-46, HHS Publication No. [SMA] 13-4795. Rockville, MD: Substance Abuse and Mental Health Services Administration, 2013.)

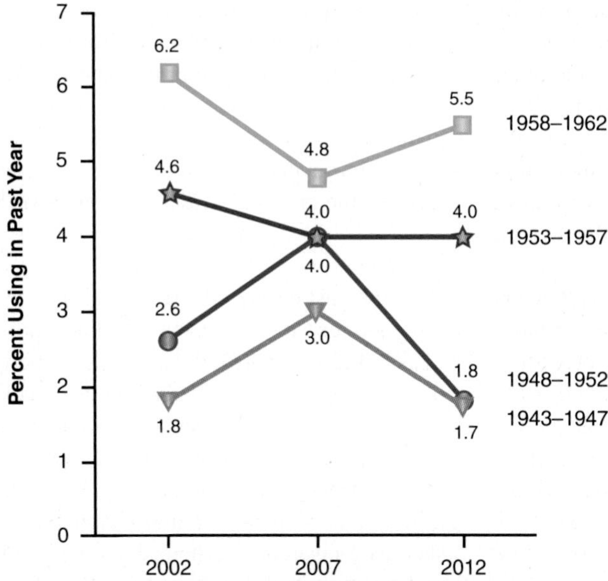

figure 17.3 Nonmedical use of prescription drugs by birth cohort, 2002, 2007, 2012. (From Substance Abuse and Mental Health Services Administration [2013]. *Results from the 2012 National Survey on Drug Use and Health: Summary of National Findings* [p. 102], NSDUH Series H-46, HHS Publication No. [SMA] 13-4795. Rockville, MD: Substance Abuse and Mental Health Services Administration, 2013.)

PRACTICE POINT

A challenge for community health nurses caring for immigrant populations, especially youth, is to preserve protective factors to minimize the risk of substance misuse associated with longer residency in the United States.

I bought a gun and chose drugs instead.

Kurt Cobain

EVIDENCE FOR PRACTICE

Lexicon for Behavioral Health and Primary Care Integration (Peek & The National Integration Academy Council, 2013).

WHAT: Integrated primary and behavioral healthcare that addresses mental health and substance use, health behaviors, and life stressors for a defined population. Medical, behavioral health, and substance use treatment are core components of primary care services and are integral to improving health outcomes.

GOAL: To integrate primary and behavioral healthcare to a population so there is "no wrong door" for seeking treatment

Role of Community Health Nurses in Collaborative Care Models:

1. Screening and implementation of prevention measures
2. Promotion of health behavior change
3. Psychological support and crisis intervention
4. Chronic or complex illness case management
5. Outcome measurement of clinical, functional, and quality of life
6. Outreach to patients or families who do not follow-up and to high-risk populations

Alcohol

Alcoholism is the only disease that you can get yelled at for having.

Mitch Hedberg

The age at which Americans first use alcohol is a significant risk factor for future dependence or addiction to alcohol. Children who initially use alcohol at 14 years of age or younger are seven times more likely to become dependent on alcohol or abuse it than those who initially use alcohol when they are 21 years of age or older. Rates of alcohol use are now equivalent in adolescent males and females (13.3% and 13.3%, respectively), and the rates of alcohol dependence and abuse are now equivalent in adolescents (SAMHSA, 2012a). Underage drinking is highest among those reporting two or more races as their ethnic heritage (17.5%), among Native Americans (15.2%), and among White youth (14.6) (SAMHSA, 2012a). Lower socioeconomic status and educational opportunities are two of the social factors associated with increased risk among Native Americans, but a comprehensive understanding of the root social causes is lacking (Stanley, Harkness, Swaim, Beauviask, 2014).

Drinking and driving is a serious public health concern. A positive trend is that the percentage of all Americans who reported drinking and driving continues to decline from 2002. Strict law enforcement and population-based strategies such as school-based education programs and community-based programs are credited with contributing to a decrease in the portion of Americans reporting they engaged in drinking and driving. Laws include mandatory alcohol testing for automobile drivers, sobriety checkpoints, social host laws to reduce teenage alcohol consumption by imposing liability on adults who provide alcohol to underaged drinkers, lower blood alcohol levels for driving under the influence (DUI), immediate license suspension for DUI, and age-21 minimum legal drinking age restrictions. A subpopulation that continues to be at high risk for drinking and driving is young adults (18 to 25 years of age) who have almost double the rate of driving impaired than the general population (18.6%) (SAMHSA, 2012a).

Binge drinking is defined by the National Institute on Alcohol Abuse and Alcoholism (NIAAA) as five or more drinks on the same occasion for 1 day during the preceding month for men and four or more drinks on the same occasion for women. Over the past decade, there has been a steady decline in binge drinking among youth who participated in substance prevention programs (SAMHSA, 2012a). Yet, almost one-fourth of all Americans over the age of 12 who drink alcohol (22.6%) still meet criteria for binge drinking (SAMHSA, 2012a).

Binge drinking peaks during young adulthood (ages of 18 and 25 years), with 39.8% of users reporting binge drinking behavior (SAMHSA, 2012a). Rates of binge alcohol use vary by race and ethnicity and are highest among American Indians or Alaska Natives (24.3%) (SAMHSA, 2012a). A major risk factor for problem drinking in young adults is enrollment in college. The significant difference ($p < 0.05$) in binge and heavy drinking between college students (39.1%) and their peers (35.4%) not enrolled in college has remained unchanged over the past decade and suggests campus cultural norms are a strong factor contributing to significantly higher health risks (SAMHSA, 2012a).

The nurse practitioner, Katherine, can see that Mr. Campbell has many of the risk factors for abuse of or dependence on illicit drugs but does not want to stereotype him or falsely assume that he has a drug problem. He may be depressed or in need of proper pain management. She determines that it would be appropriate to begin an evaluation of Mr. Campbell by assessing his mood, especially if he has had any suicidal ideation. In addition, he needs an evaluation for his back pain and sleep disorder.

Cannabis

Cannabis is the most frequently used illicit substance in the United States. In 2011, approximately 7.0% of the total U.S. population older than 12 years reported cannabis use in the preceding month (SAMHSA, 2012a). Past-month cannabis use was 10 times higher in youth who perceived there was moderate, slight, or no risk, compared to their peers who perceived great risk (SAMHSA, 2012a). Use of cannabis is six times higher in youth who perceive no parental disapproval compared to youth who perceive strong parental disapproval. In addition, the significant rise in cannabis use among youth since 2008 also corresponds with the legalization of medical marijuana in some states. In 2010, 87% of adolescent treatment admissions involved marijuana as a primary or secondary substance, and 41% of these marijuana-involved admissions were referred to treatment through the criminal justice system (SAMSHA, 2012c).

Tobacco

Over the past decade, the use of tobacco in the United States has continued to significantly decline from 30.4% in 2002 to 26.5% in 2011 (SAMHSA, 2012a). Importantly, the number of Americans reporting daily cigarette smoking, and cigarette smoking among adolescents, has continued to decline. Over 90% of adolescents strongly disapproved of cigarette smoking by their peers (SAMHSA, 2012a). However, a disturbing trend is the increasing use of nonconventional tobacco products, such as e-cigarettes or hookahs among youth. Public health experts attribute the increased use of nonconventional tobacco products to a lower perceived risk of harm and confusing public health messages (Mermelstein, 2014). In educating populations, especially youth, about the risks of tobacco use, community health nurses must expand their public health interventions to include nonconventional tobacco products.

Illicit Drugs

In 2012, 9.2% of Americans were current users of illicit substances, including cocaine, opioids (i.e., heroin), hallucinogens (i.e., lysergic acid diethylamide [LSD], phencyclidine [PCP], peyote, mescaline, psilocybin mushrooms, "ecstasy" [also known as MDMA]), inhalants (i.e., nitrous oxide, amyl nitrite, cleaning fluids, gasoline, spray paint, other aerosol sprays, and glue), pain relievers (i.e., oxycodone and propoxyphene), benzodiazepines (i.e., alprazolam and lorazepam), stimulants (i.e., methamphetamine), and sedatives (i.e., phenobarbital, seconal) (SAMHSA, 2013). The rate of illicit drug use peaks in adolescence and young adulthood and then declines with age (SAMHSA, 2013). Use of any illicit substance is highest among mixed-race Americans (23.3%), followed by native Hawaiians or Pacific Islanders (21.2%), Whites (15.1%), and Asian-Americans (6.8%) (Wu et al., 2013) (Fig. 17.4).

Although the rates of injection drug use in the United States are similar across ethnic groups, blacks comprised 50% of newly diagnosed injection drug users with HIV (Cooper, Friedman, Tempalski, Friedman, & Keem, 2005). People living in large metropolitan areas were twice as likely to use illicit drugs as those living in rural parts of America, and almost one-fourth of people in the criminal justice system were current illicit drug users. Over half of nonmedical users of stimulants, tranquilizers, sedatives, and pain relievers received the drug from a friend or relative for free, and four out of five stated that the drug was prescribed by one physician (SAMHSA, 2012a). Among adolescents, admissions for opiate use other than heroin rose 67% over the past decade (SAMHSA, 2012c).

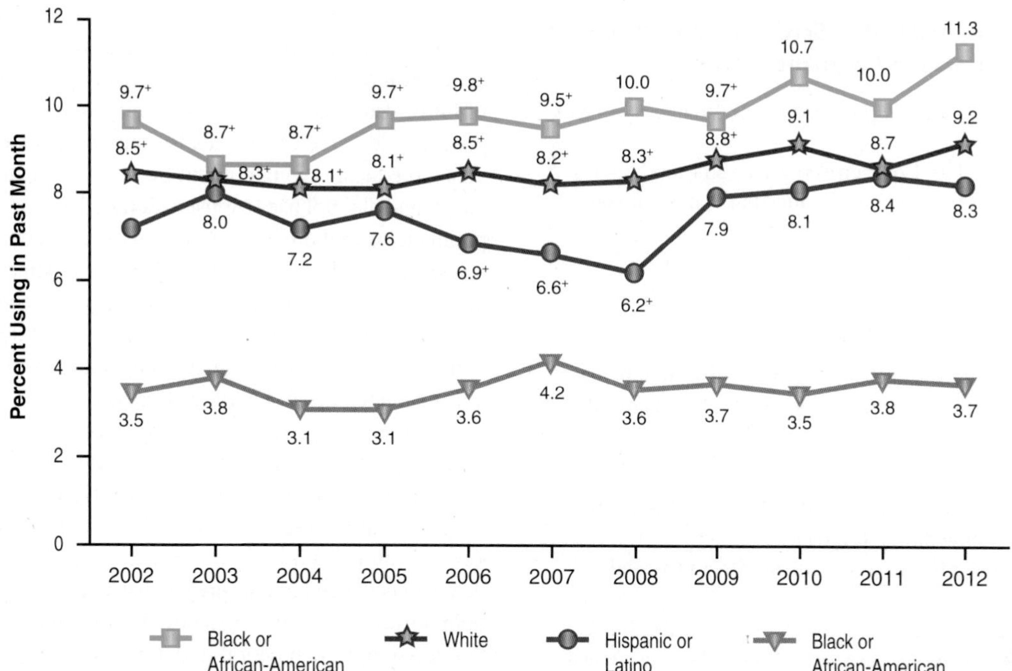

figure 17.4 Past-month use of illicit drugs by persons 12 years of age or older by race/ethnicity, 2002–2012. (From Substance Abuse and Mental Health Services Administration. [2013]. *Results from the 2012 National Survey on Drug Use and Health: Summary of National Findings* [p.25], NSDUH Series H-46, HHS Publication No. [SMA] 13-4795. Rockville, MD: Substance Abuse and Mental Health Services Administration, 2013.)

The most recent epidemiologic surveys on substance use in the United States help community health nurses identify populations at greatest risk for abuse and addiction. Some trends have remained stable over many years. But the latest surveys also warn of emerging trends that will pose new challenges for community health nurses. The rate of alcohol use by adolescents is now equivalent between males and females. Community health nurses, especially those in school settings, can anticipate that growing numbers of young women, who metabolize alcohol differently than men and who suffer the adverse health effects more acutely, will be in need of services for chronic alcohol abuse at even younger ages. One of the greatest challenges will be faced by nurses in the community who provide nursing care to at-risk populations. How community health nurses can identify people at risk across the life span and intervene with evidence-based programs aimed at prevention is the focus of the next section of this chapter.

HEALTH PROFILES AND INTERVENTIONS FOR HIGH-RISK POPULATIONS

Pregnant Women

Alcohol use during pregnancy is a serious public health concern because of the multiple deleterious, lifelong effects of alcohol on the fetus. These lifelong effects include low IQ, hyperactivity, short attention span, distinctive facial anomalies, and structural brain defects. Given the disability associated with fetal alcohol syndrome (FAS), the WHO (2014b) issued guidelines recommending that all healthcare providers ask all pregnant women about their use of alcohol and other substances as early as possible in the pregnancy and at every antenatal visit (Box 17.2). In the United States, the CDC Scientific Work Group on FAS also recommends that all women of childbearing age be screened for alcohol use in primary care settings. If pregnant women are using alcohol or drugs, the WHO (2014b) recommends brief intervention and immediate referral to detoxification services and psychosocial care.

Approximately 2 to 7 infants in 1,000 in the United States suffer from FAS (May et al., 2009). There is no clinically acceptable level of alcohol ingestion during pregnancy, and the U.S. Surgeon General advises all pregnant women to abstain from all alcohol use. Yet despite repeated public health warnings, the rate of alcohol use and binge drinking in pregnant women from 1991 to 2005 has remained unchanged at 14.1% (Denny, Tsai, Floyd, & Green, 2009). When screening women for alcohol use, nurses should ask women to respond to questions in the T-ACE questionnaire as they would before they learned that they were pregnant. Nurses should try to determine the stage of pregnancy at which the patient reduced or eliminated their alcohol consumption (Chang, 2005).

In 1981, the U.S. Surgeon General issued the first public health advisory warning about the association between

box 17.2 T-ACE Alcohol Screening Questionnaire for Use in Pregnant Women

1. Tolerance: How many drinks does it take to make you feel high?
   0 = None   1 = 1 or 2 drinks   2 = 3 or more drinks
2. Have people annoyed you by criticizing you about your drinking?
   0 = No   1 = Yes
3. Have you ever felt you ought to cutdown on your drinking?
   0 = No   1 = Yes
4. Eye-opener: Have you ever had a drink first thing in the morning to steady your nerves or get rid of a hangover?
   0 = No   1 = Yes

Scoring: With a score of 2 or more, nurses should use a brief intervention to discuss the risks to the fetus associated with alcohol consumption during pregnancy.

Referrals should be made if needed for treatment and counseling.

Source: Chang, G. (2005). Screening and brief intervention in prenatal settings. *Alcohol Research and Health, 28*(2), 83.

FAS and alcohol use during pregnancy. An act of Congress followed, ordering warning labels to be added to all products containing alcohol (Bertrand, Floyd, & Weber, 2005). Federal agencies have supported several public health measures to warn women about the serious adverse health effects of maternal drinking on unborn children. Given the marked risk for teratogenesis and obstetric complications, the American Society on Addiction Medicine recommends that pregnant women in need of substance use treatment be given the highest priority for admission and treatment (Haug, Duffy, & McCaul, 2014). Six new objectives have been added to *Healthy People 2020*, including abstinence from drinking or smoking in preconception.

EVIDENCE FOR PRACTICE

A study by Harrison and Sidebottom (2009) of pregnant women (n = 1,492) from 2005 to 2007 found that most women (87%) abstained from alcohol during their pregnancy. Continued alcohol use during pregnancy was strongly associated with women who were 30 years of age or older ($p < 0.001$), smoked two or more cigarettes the previous month ($p < 0.001$), had high rates of depression and intimate partner abuse ($p < 0.001$), and drank five or more alcoholic beverages on a weekly basis ($p < 0.001$) (Harrison & Sidebottom, 2009). Researchers found moderate associations between continued alcohol use during pregnancy and lack of social support ($p < 0.01$), low levels of child protection services involvement ($p < 0.01$), and physical or sexual abuse ($p < 0.01$).

Binge drinking behavior poses a significant risk to the neurodevelopment of the fetus because of the high concentration of alcohol crossing the placenta. The rising rates of binge drinking behavior, especially among college women, pose considerable challenges for nurses in student health services to educate women about the risks associated with pregnancy and alcohol use (Monsen, 2009). The fact that half of all pregnancies in the United States are unintended, coupled with an increase in the estimated number of women of childbearing age who binge drink, illustrates the urgent need for renewed public health efforts to identify women at risk and educate all women of childbearing age about the dangers of drinking during pregnancy (Tsai, Floyd, & Bertrand, 2006).

Two decades after giving birth, women who used alcohol during pregnancy had mortality rates 2.7 times higher ($p < 0.01$) than women who abstained (Berg, Lynch, & Coles, 2008). Clearly, continued alcohol use during pregnancy is a key indicator that a woman is at risk for multiple health disorders and is in need of comprehensive health and social services both during and after pregnancy. There is increasing evidence that integrating behavioral and substance use care within primary care settings expands access to comprehensive health services for pregnant women and improves retention along the continuum of treatment (Haug, Duffy, & McCaul, 2014).

Infants born with FAS have facial dysmorphia, growth problems, and central nervous system abnormalities, including neurologic problems and cognitive and functional deficits, which are lifelong impairments (Bertrand et al., 2005). Box 17.3 provides guidelines for assessing FAS. In 2001, the CDC-funded five community-based intervention projects across the United States for children with FAS to address their unique neurodevelopmental needs. Each of the CDC-funded initiatives provided children with a multidisciplinary assessment, referrals for specialized care (i.e., speech therapy), and education for families and caregiver support (Bertrand, 2009). Children with FAS typically have multiple neurocognitive impairments, and their ability to learn through observation and abstraction is compromised (Bertrand, 2009). In light of these neurocognitive deficits, a key element in all five programs that proved to be highly effective was parent education about FAS, and parent training on techniques of explicit instruction to the child. Importantly, each of these five community-based intervention projects demonstrated that it was possible to provide children and their families a variety of health and education services such as special education, mental health assistance, and educational counseling, using existing community resources.

EVIDENCE FOR PRACTICE

Unlike women who use alcohol prenatally, Harrison and Sidebottom (2009) found, only slightly more than half of drug-using women (55.6%) ceased to use cannabis or any drug not prescribed by a physician during their pregnancy. Continued drug use during pregnancy was strongly associated with women who were 20 to 24 years of age (p <0.001), Native American women (p <0.001), women who reporting weekly or daily drug use (p <0.001), and women who smoked two or more cigarettes the previous month (p <0.001) (Harrison & Sidebottom, 2009).

Substance use by mothers has been associated with an increased risk of substance use and mental health problems with their children (Toumbourou et al., 2007). Use of illicit drugs, including injected drugs, also poses hazards to an unborn child. Newborns exposed to cocaine in utero have varied symptoms at birth, depending on the extent of the mother's cocaine use as well as her nutritional and general health status. The most common signs seen at birth include low birth weight, smaller head circumference, autonomic instability, tremor, high-pitched cry, and irritability (Goldstein, DesLauriers, & Burda, 2009). Because mothers who use cocaine may also be polysubstance abusers, infants are at increased risk for contracting hepatitis, syphilis, and HIV (Goldstein et al., 2009). Although studies of the impact of these sequelae on neurocognitive development are mixed, prenatal exposure to cocaine has been associated with lower IQ and delayed language acquisition in children (Goldstein et al., 2009).

More than two decades ago, a study by Chasnoff, Burns, Schnoll, and Burns (1985) led to a public outcry about the perceived fate of what the media characterized as "crack babies." In the wake of the public's indignation, 30 states began prosecuting women who were alleged to be using cocaine while pregnant on a variety of criminal charges, including child abuse, neglect, and child endangerment (Tillett & Osborne, 2001). In the vast majority of states, higher courts reversed decisions in the lower courts and overturned the convictions of pregnant women who tested positive for cocaine. In the case of *Ferguson v. the City of Charleston (South Carolina) (99–936)*, the Fourth Circuit Court of Appeals upheld the conviction of a pregnant woman who tested positive for cocaine and was reported to law enforcement authorities on the basis of a hospital policy adopted at the University of South Carolina Medical Center. The case was ultimately heard by the United States Supreme Court.

Professional healthcare organizations such as the American Nurses Association (ANA), the American Public Health Association, and the American College of Obstetricians and Gynecologists submitted written testimony, termed an *amicus curiae* brief, in support of the defendant. Subsequent to the ruling of the U.S. Supreme Court, the ANA joined over 140 organizations and researchers in a public letter to the U.S. Surgeon General stating, "The ANA recognizes alcohol and other drug problems as treatable illnesses. The threat of criminal prosecution is counterproductive in that it prevents many women from seeking prenatal care and treatment for their alcohol and other drug problems" (Tillet & Osborne, 2001, p. 6). In 2001, the United States Supreme Court decided in a 6-to-3 ruling that the defendant's Fourth Amendment rights had been violated, and overturned the conviction. In an analysis of the Supreme Court ruling of *Ferguson v. the City of Charleston*, the noted medical ethicist George Annas (2001) observed that the more the lines between the professional duties of physicians and nurses are blurred with those of law enforcement, the more that trust between clients and healthcare providers is eroded, and the greater the likelihood that clients who are in need of prenatal care will not seek care at all.

The use of scientific findings to bolster criminalization of health behaviors raises serious ethical questions for scientists as well as for community health nurses who provide healthcare to people who may become targets of criminal investigations. Nurses must consider such important ethical questions as "What are the scientific findings regarding drug use in pregnancy that should influence public policy?" and "Should scientific evidence have any bearing at all on public policy?" Public health scientists must decide how to avoid unwittingly "crossing the line" and advancing a policy agenda that obscures the focus from unbiased scientific inquiry to value-laden maternal drug abuse public policies (Thompson, Levitt, & Stanwood, 2009). For community health nurses who rely on scientific evidence to identify populations at risk and provide evidence-based interventions to minimize harm to an unborn child, bridging the chasm between research and practice is a critical role that must not be relinquished to policy-makers. For example, researchers

box 17.3 Assessment Guideline for Identifying Fetal Alcohol Syndrome Disorder

Facial dysmorphia
- Smooth philtrum
- Thin vermillion border
- Small palpebral fissures

Growth problems
- Postnatal height, weight, or both <10th percentile

Central nervous system abnormalities

Structural
- Head circumference <10th percentile
- Reduced size or change in shape of corpus callosum, cerebellum, and basal ganglia seen on MRI

Neurologic
- Motor problems
- Seizures

Functional
- Cognitive or intellectual deficits <3rd percentile
- Functional deficits <16th percentile in three of the following:
  1. Cognitive development
  2. Executive functioning
  3. Motor functioning delays
  4. Problems with attention or hyperactivity
  5. Problems with social skills
  6. Sensory, language, or memory problems

Source: Bertrand, J., Floyd, R. L., & Weber, M. K. (2005). Guidelines for identifying and referring persons with fetal alcohol syndrome. *Morbidity and Mortality Weekly Report, 54*(RR11), 1–17.

have noted that scientific evidence indicates that alcohol, a legal substance, produces far more widespread and deleterious impairments in brain development in the fetus than cocaine (Thompson et al., 2009).

One of the most widely used and scientifically proven programs to improve health outcomes for at-risk first-time mothers is the Nurse-Family Partnership (NFP) program (Dawley, Loch, & Bindrich, 2007; Donelan-McCall, Eckenrode, & Olds, 2009). The NFP pairs at-risk new mothers with community health nurses who provide hour-long visits every 2 weeks in the home for the first 2 years of an infant's life. Health education and interventions provided by the community health nurses include avoiding alcohol and drug use, nutritional counseling, smoking cessation, parenting skills, case management regarding pediatric care for their infant and primary care for the mothers, and vocational counseling to promote economic self-sufficiency (Dawley et al., 2007).

Donelan-McCall et al. (2009) note that the NFP has the strongest support to date of any nurse home-visiting program; scientific evidence shows that it can improve the health outcomes of children born to at-risk mothers and is cost-effective. The savings realized by the NFP programs in decreased adverse health events, emergency department visits, and the like (approximately $18,000) are twice as much as the cost per family for 2 years of nurse home visits (approximately $9,000) (Donelan-McCall et al., 2009; Lee, Aos, & Miller, 2008). Begun in 1977 by Dr. David Olds with community health nurses in Elmira, New York, today NFP is in 350 counties nationally and is supported by funding from federal or state healthcare and social service grants as well as private foundations. NFP is a compelling example of how investing in preventive healthcare provided by community health nurses improves health outcomes in a cost-effective manner. SAMHSA has developed a National Registry of Evidence-based Programs and Practices, including NFP, to identify scientifically proven programs to prevent or treat mental and/or substance abuse disorders and facilitate their implementation in communities across the United States (Box 17.4). An example of a culturally tailored model using health educators indigenous to the population is Family Spirit, an organization in which trained health educators provide home-visiting intervention for American Indian teenage mothers (Box 17.5).

Substance Use at an Early Age

Individual, family, and community influences all contribute to the use of substances by underage children and adolescents. How much of the increased risk is due to nature (genetic vulnerabilities) or nurture (environmental influences) can partially be illuminated by studies of twins, adopted children, and genetic research. Monozygotic twin studies estimate the risk of inheritability of alcoholism at approximately 50% in both men and women (Prescott, Madden, & Stallings, 2006). Thus, at least half the risk of developing alcoholism may be due to factors in communities, schools, or families.

box 17.4 The Nurse-Family Partnership

Nurse–Family Partnership (NFP) is a prenatal and infancy nurse home visitation program that aims to improve the health, well-being, and self-sufficiency of low-income, first-time parents and their children. Nurses follow a detailed, visit-by-visit guide that provides information on (tracking) dietary intake; reducing cigarette, alcohol, and illegal drug use; identifying symptoms of pregnancy complications and signs of children's illnesses; communicating with healthcare professionals; promoting parent-child interactions; creating safe households; and considering educational and career options. Program objectives include decreased substance use, improved maternal economic self-sufficiency, fewer subsequent unintended pregnancies, reduced child abuse and neglect, and improved school readiness of the children. Individual programs serve a minimum of 100 to 200 families and are supported by four to eight trained registered nurse home visitors (each carrying a caseload of 25 families), a nurse supervisor, and administrative support. Nurse home visits begin early in pregnancy and continue until the child's second birthday. The frequency of home visits changes with the stages of pregnancy and infancy and is adapted to the mother's needs, with a maximum of 13 visits occurring during pregnancy and 47 occurring after the child's birth.

The NFP targets women in urban, suburban, rural, and frontier areas. Races and ethnicities who have received the NFP interventions include Asian, Black or African-American, Hispanic or Latino, and White.

Readiness for dissemination ratings by
criteria = 3.7 (0.0–4.0 scale)
Implementation materials = 3.5
Training and support = 4.0
Quality assurance = 3.5

Source: Substance Abuse and Mental Health Services Administration, National Registry of Evidence-Based Programs and Practices. (July 2008). Retrieved July 24, 2014, from http://www.nrepp.samhsa.gov/ViewIntervention.aspx?id=88

Developmental or peer influences also play a role. It is known that most adults with addiction or substance abuse disorders began using alcohol or illicit substances while in middle school. Alcohol use among 12- to 13-year-olds (2.2%) increases dramatically to 11.1% of 14- to 15-year-olds during this narrow window of vulnerability (SAMHSA, 2013). It is critical that community health nurses recognize that during middle school, risk is greatly increased if a child has any friends who have used alcohol in the past year (Strobbe, 2013). How individual vulnerabilities, social experiences, or community influences coalesce to the point where 12- to 14-year-olds are initiating alcohol use is the focus of both public health and basic science research.

The NIAAA has provided research funding since 1989 through the Collaborative Studies on Genetics of Alcoholism (COGA) to investigate how genetic factors interact with the environment to cause alcohol dependence (National Institute on Alcohol Abuse and Alcoholism [NIAAA], 2009). As of 2009, COGA genetic researchers have collected genetic analysis data on more than 300 families extensively affected

box 17.5 Family Spirit

Family Spirit is a culturally tailored home-visiting intervention for American Indian teenage mothers—who generally experience high rates of substance use, school dropout, and residential instability—from pregnancy through 36 months postpartum. The intervention is designed to increase parenting competence (e.g., parenting knowledge and self-efficacy), reduce maternal psychosocial and behavioral risks that could interfere with effective parenting (e.g., drug and alcohol use, depression, externalizing problems), and promote healthy infant and toddler emotional and social adjustment (i.e., internalizing and externalizing behaviors). It also aims to prepare toddlers for early school success, promote parents' coping and life skills, and link families to appropriate community services.

Family Spirit is based on Patterson's social interaction learning model, which suggests that a parent's stressful life circumstances (e.g., unstable housing, poverty, weak family support, mental health and substance abuse issues) trigger a high level of coercive parenting associated with early childhood behavior problems that predict poor outcomes in middle and later childhood. The intervention consists of 63 structured lessons delivered one-on-one by Health Educators in participants' homes, starting at about 28 weeks of gestation and continuing to 36 months postpartum. The lessons, designed to correspond to the changing developmental needs of the mother and child during this period, address topics such as prenatal care, infant care, child development, family planning, and healthy living. Each home visit lasts about an hour and includes a warm-up conversation, lesson content, question-and-answer period, and review of summary handouts. Health Educators, trained American Indian paraprofessionals, deliver the lessons using illustrated tabletop flipcharts. The bond formed between the Health Educator and mother is intended to facilitate the mother's progress toward goals. The 63 lessons can be delivered in 52 home visits, which occur weekly through 3 months postpartum and gradually become less frequent thereafter.

Family Spirit targets American Indian or Alaska native women in rural and frontier areas.

Readiness for dissemination ratings by criteria = 4.0 (0.0–4.0 scale)
Implementation materials = 4.0
Training and support = 4.0
Quality assurance = 4.0

Source: Substance Abuse and Mental Health Services Administration, National Registry of Evidence-based Programs and Practices. (November 2013). Retrieved July 24, 2014, from http://www.nrepp.samhsa.gov/ViewIntervention.aspx?id=361

by alcoholism. Even though the gene associated with alcoholism has not yet been identified, its inheritability accounts for about half of the risk for alcohol abuse disorders. To minimize the morbidity and mortality associated with substance misuse, it is critical for community health nurses to implement evidence-based programs for youth in community-based settings.

A thorough family history for substance use and screening youth for risk factors associated with early substance is a critical first step. The United States Preventive Services Task Force (USPSTF) (2014) recommends primary care and community-based health professionals screen youths to identify patients at risk for substance misuse. The American Academy of Pediatrics recommends the CRAFFT screening tool specifically designed for use in adolescent populations (Box 17.6). Integrative primary care and schools are ideal locations for nurses to introduce prevention and early intervention programs (Curtis, McLellan, & Gabellini, 2014).

Personality attributes such as poor impulse control, attention deficits, conduct disorders, and general psychological dysregulation are individual factors that have been associated with early-onset substance use (Clark, Thatcher, & Tapert, 2008). Often, these behaviors overlap with the early onset of anxiety disorders, post-traumatic stress disorder, and major depression, which have been associated with illicit substance use by age 15 years and dependence later in adulthood (Degenhardt et al., 2009).

Psychological dysregulation in children and adolescents has been theorized to be a function of neurobiologic influences in the prefrontal cortex—the "brakes" of the brain—where action based on primitive impulses from the midbrain is stopped. Development of white matter peaks in young adults and corresponds to the development of executive functioning, the ability to reason, and to anticipate the long-term implications of one's behavior more fully. It explains why, as the brain continues to develop throughout the 20s, the impulsivity that often characterizes adolescent behavior begins to subside.

In adolescents with alcohol use disorders, researchers have found that there are delays in neural substrates necessary for the frontal cortex to develop fully (Clark et al., 2008). Neuroimaging studies have shown that adolescents with alcohol use disorders, as well as those who are regular

box 17.6 CRAFFT Drug Screening Questionnaire for Use in Adolescents

1. Have you ever ridden in a **C**ar driven by someone (including yourself) who was "high" or had been using alcohol or drugs?
2. Do you ever use alcohol or drugs to **R**elax, feel better about yourself or fit in?
3. Do you ever use alcohol or drugs while you are by yourself, **A**lone?
4. Do you ever **F**orget things you did while using alcohol or drugs?
5. Do your family or **F**riends ever tell you that you should cut down on your drinking or drug use?
6. Have you gotten into **T**rouble while you were using alcohol or drugs?

Scoring: A "Yes" answer to two or more questions indicates the need for active intervention

Source: Substance Abuse and Mental Health Services Administration. *TIP 31: Screening and assessing adolescents for substance use disorders*. Retrieved July 30, 2009, from http://www.ncbi.nlm.nih.gov/books/bv.fcgi?rid=hstat5.chapter.54841

users of cannabis, have less prefrontal white matter than adolescents who do not abuse these substances (Clark et al., 2008). These neurobiologic findings have significant implications for community health nurses, who implement educational programs designed to teach youth about the dangers of substance and alcohol abuse on brain development. A key aspect of education for youth should include factual information about the neurobiologic impact of substance misuse on the developing brain.

Studies examining how social experiences influence adolescent drinking behavior have found associations between parental approval or initiation, peer influences, lack of interest in school, poverty, and community availability of alcohol to underage drinking behavior (Cleveland, Feinburg, Bontempo, & Greenberg, 2008). Although these factors affect adolescents at all developmental stages, it is critical for community health nurses to screen for family or social experiences that are associated with the use of alcohol in children and adolescents younger than 14 years. Nurses can ask whether there is excessive alcohol consumption by family members and by peers, if the adolescents have unrestricted access to alcohol, and if the adolescents have peers and family members who willingly provide them with access to alcohol. It is the early initiation of alcohol use that is most strongly predictive of alcohol addiction in adulthood.

I mean, I inherited the disease of alcoholism, and I learned early to get help when I needed it.

Liza Minnelli

EVIDENCE FOR PRACTICE

A survey of 3,592 adults between the ages of 18 and 39 years found that as the number of adverse childhood experiences increased, the age at which people began drinking decreased and the more likely they were to report they drank to cope (Rothman, Edwards, Heeren, & Hingson, 2008). After adjusting for age, gender, race, educational attainment, family attitudes about alcohol, and peer relationships, the adverse childhood events most strongly associated with drinking before age 15 years were sexual abuse, emotional neglect, physical abuse, substance abuse in the home, and a mentally ill family member (Rothman et al., 2008, p. 300). Violence in the home, a pattern also seen with women who continued alcohol use during pregnancy, puts youth under the age of 15 years at significant risk for drinking alcohol. A study of youth with inhalant use disorder found that they were significantly more likely to report high levels of trauma, self-harm behavior, psychiatric distress, antisocial disorders, and substance-related problems (Perron & Howard, 2009).

The difference in substance use among Native American youth and the general adolescent population is especially pronounced among the youngest adolescents. Substance misuse is a major public health concern for Native American youth on reservations where over half of eighth graders report alcohol and cannabis use, a pronounced increase from overall national prevalence rates for eighth graders of all ethnicities (Stanley et al., 2014). While there is no causal model to explain the higher rates of substance use among youth on reservations, social factors including greater availability from local cannabis farms, proximity to Mexico and drug gangs, lower socioeconomic status, and lower academic attainment are some of the social conditions that researchers have associated with this pronounced health disparity (Stanley et al., 2014).

There is debate in the literature about the "gateway effect" theory of substance abuse, which proposes that substance abuse is progressive and begins with tobacco, then moves sequentially to alcohol or cannabis, and ultimately to other illicit substances (Degenhardt et al., 2009). Studies of disadvantaged adolescents in impoverished areas or homeless youth have not found that these youth follow such a stepwise progression of substance use. The stepwise progression of use also does not hold true for the use of inhalants, with more eighth graders reporting use than high school students (Williams, Storck, & the Committee on Substance Abuse and the Committee on Native American Child Health, 2007).

The use of inhalants by middle school-aged children is strongly associated with living in rural areas in the United States, especially in white youth in Appalachia and in Mexican American youth in the rural west, where the rate of inhalant use is almost double that of youth residing in urban or metropolitan areas. For young adolescents, rates of inhalant use are highest for White females residing in the rural southeast (22.4%) and Mexican American females (22.7%) living in rural parts of western United States (Edwards et al., 2007).

Inhalants used by adolescents are common household items that contain volatile solvents such as glues or paint thinners; aerosols such as hair spray or air fresheners; and butane, propane, or gasoline. Fumes may be inhaled through the mouth, referred to by adolescents as "huffing," or the nose (sniffing), to achieve a state of **intoxication** similar to alcohol. Inhalants act as central nervous system depressants, and mortality of 22% has been reported during initial experimentation (Williams et al., 2007). Gasoline (45%), air fresheners (26%), and propane/butane (11%) are the inhalants associated with the majority of deaths (Williams et al., 2007).

EVIDENCE FOR PRACTICE

The LifeSkills Training program, an evidence-based program for prevention of drug and alcohol abuse, has been implemented in 33 rural public schools located in communities prone to methamphetamine abuse. Outcome studies of LifeSkills Training have reported statistically significant and sustained decreases in all forms of substance use, especially for higher-risk subpopulations of adolescents, including those in rural and frontier regions of the

United States (Spoth, Randall, Trudeau, Shin, & Redmond, 2008, p. 66). These scientifically validated prevention efforts appear to be having an effect. In 2011, the number of Americans 12 years of age or older who used methamphetamine for the first time (133,000) was less than half the number of the new users reported in 2012 (299,000) (SAMHSA, 2012a). These statistics suggest that comprehensive public health and law enforcement efforts are making a significant difference in decreasing the methamphetamine use in the United States. SAMHSA's National Registry of Evidence-Based Programs and Practices has given LifeSkills Training its highest rating for efficacy and readiness of dissemination (Box 17.7).

Population-based interventions to decrease substance use among adolescents can be conceptualized in four categories: regulatory, developmental prevention, early screening, and harm reduction (Toumbourou et al., 2007). Minimum age laws for drinking alcohol, strict enforcement of laws prohibiting drinking and driving, and enforcement of youth possession laws have proved to be effective deterrents to underage substance use (Toumbourou et al., 2007). Developmental prevention programs can be effective in deterring substance use in adolescents as well, if such prevention programs are sensitive to the significant variations in substance use in adolescence by age, ethnicity, geographic location, and gender.

Research shows that parents are the single biggest influence on children—if you are worried about your teen and drugs, talk to them.

John Walters

In contrast to screening and education of entire populations of adolescents, a public health approach demonstrating improved efficacy with adolescents is screening with the CRAFFT tool to identify youth at risk followed by tailored brief interventions and referral to specialty treatment based upon the severity score. This approach, termed SBIRT (screening, brief intervention, referral to treatment) has been implemented in primary care, emergency rooms, school-based settings, and in shelters with homeless youth (Mitchell, Gryczynski, O'Grady, & Schartz, 2013). In the SBIRT model, interventions are specifically targeted based on the severity of symptoms and it includes brief interventions for even mild symptoms in populations considered at-risk. The brief interventions in SBIRT consist of the chief components of motivational interviewing.

Motivational interviewing is particularly effective with adolescents because it respects the adolescents' developmental need for autonomy (Michell et al., 2013). The nurse partners with the adolescent to identify the harms associated with substance misuse in a nonjudgmental manner, and the nurse objectively points out inconsistencies with the adolescent's personal goals and aspirations. The nurse thoughtfully negotiates with the adolescent about the possibility of changing harmful behaviors and assists the adolescent in setting realistic goals achievable in a brief period of time. For example, a goal may be slightly decreasing the amount of alcoholic beverages consumed in a week or the weekend by a goal self-selected by the adolescent. In follow-up sessions, the nurse reinforces health promoting behaviors and the achievement of goals. Key to the successful implementation of brief interventions is that the goals be self-selected by the adolescent, that they be achievable, and that the nurse provides immediate reinforcement and encouragement for achieving the goal.

box 17.7 LifeSkills Training

LifeSkills Training (LST) is a school-based program that aims to prevent alcohol use, tobacco use, illicit substance use, and violence by targeting the major social and psychological factors that promote the initiation of substance use and other risky behaviors. LST addresses multiple risk and protective factors and teaches personal and social skills which build resilience and help youth navigate developmental tasks, including the skills necessary to understand and resist prodrug influences. LST is designed to provide information relevant to the important life transitions that adolescents and young teens face, using culturally sensitive and developmentally and age-appropriate language and content. Facilitated discussion, structured small group activities, and role-playing scenarios are used to stimulate participation and promote the acquisition of skills. Separate LST programs are offered for elementary school (grades 3–6), middle school (grades 6–9), and high school (grades 9–12).

LST targets adolescents in urban, suburban, rural, and frontier areas. Races and ethnicities who have received LST include American Indian or Alaska native, Asian, Black or African-American, Hispanic or Latino, and White.

Readiness for dissemination ratings by criteria = 4.0 (0.0–4.0 scale)
Implementation materials = 4.0
Training and support = 4.0
Quality assurance = 4.0

Source: Substance Abuse and Mental Health Services Administration, National Registry of Evidence-based Programs and Practices. (September 2008). Retrieved July 24, 2014, from http://www.nrepp.samhsa.gov/ViewIntervention.aspx?id=109

EVIDENCE FOR PRACTICE

SBIRT was implemented in two urban New York public schools during nonacademic classes (Curtis et al., 2014). All 6th- to 12th-grade students were screened with an interactive computer tool that included the CRAFFT scale. Adolescents with a CRAFFT score of zero (no use) would be given factual information and support for continuing health promoting behaviors. Those scoring 1 or 2 on the CRAFFT screen (low-risk use) would be given a motivational interview lasting between 15 and 30 minutes. Adolescents with a CRAFFT score of 3 or greater with significant levels of substance use were provided a brief intervention emphasizing the severity of substance use, telephone notification of parents, and options for referral to treatment.

In summary, community health nurses should follow the guidelines of the American Academy of Pediatrics that recommend all adolescents be screened for alcohol and drug use and that at-risk adolescents be given brief interventions and in the cases of severe misuse, referred for treatment by specialists (USPSTF, 2014). In formulating culturally appropriate evidence-based interventions, studies suggest that Hispanic youth have better outcomes when paired with Hispanic healthcare providers, and gang youths or youth with severe substance use and complex behavioral issues benefit from family-based therapies that broadly examine social issues within the family, school, peer relationships, and the juvenile justice system (Hogue, Henderson, Ozechowski, & Robbins, 2014).

College Students and Binge Drinking

In developed countries, 26.7% of all deaths in young adult men and women are alcohol-related (Toumbourou et al., 2007). The National Institute on Alcohol and Alcohol Abuse estimates that annually, almost 2,000 U.S. college students die from alcohol-related injuries. In 1 year alone, an additional 696,000 college students were victims of alcohol-related violence by another college student; some 599,000 were unintentionally injured while intoxicated; and 97,000 were victims of alcohol-related sexual assault or date rape (Hingston, Zha, & Weitzman, 2009). Because of the sheer magnitude of the harms associated with binge drinking on college campuses, it is considered one of the top public health problems in the United States.

Unlike their younger peers, who may use alcoholic beverages to cope with family dysfunction, violence, or painful emotions, college students are more likely to engage in heavy or binge drinking to enhance their mood or affective state. Rates of binge drinking vary by race, gender, and peer group affiliation, suggesting that cultural and environmental influences play a strong role in the patterns of drinking behavior by college students. High-risk drinking, defined as a consumption of alcohol that brings the blood alcohol level to 0.08% or above, is reported by 44% of college students. Such drinking is a leading cause of morbidity and mortality in this age group (Schaus et al., 2009).

That's all drugs and alcohol do, they cut off your emotions in the end.

Ringo Starr

In 2002, the NIAAA Task Force on College Drinking received a mandate to review and disseminate evidence-based strategies to decrease alcohol use on college campuses. The NIAAA Task Force compiled their findings in a report entitled *A Call to Action: Changing the Culture of Drinking at U.S. Colleges*, which was distributed to college administrators across the United States (DeJong, Larimer, Wood, & Hartman, 2009). The NIAAA Task Force continues to systematically review the scientific evidence for programs or initiatives with demonstrated efficacy and provides periodic updates of new evidence-based programs on its website (Table 17.1).

EVIDENCE FOR PRACTICE

Research compiled by the NIAAA (2007) has found that patterns of hazardous drinking varied by a number of demographic and environmental factors, including year in school, week in the semester, and whether the student was in residential housing on or off campus. For example, women drink more intensely in their freshman year, whereas men drink more intensely in their senior year (Kelly-Weeder, 2008). In both heavy and moderate college drinkers, drinking patterns are cyclical, with peaks 3 weeks into the semester, over holidays, and spring break (Greenbaum, DelBoca, Drakes, Wang, & Goldman, 2005). Despite the substantial patterns of alcohol abuse, studies have found that nurses and physicians screen for alcohol use in less than one-third of university health services and that only 12% use standardized instruments (Foote, Wilkens, & Vavkiakis, 2004).

PRACTICE POINT

One consequence of the failure to identify high-risk students is that although 67% of binge drinking college students acknowledge a need for mental health services, only 38% received such services. This indicates that many members of this high-risk population did not receive the support they needed to terminate their drinking behavior (Cranford, Eisenberg, & Serras, 2009).

The NIAAA (2007) has identified evidence-based interventions effective for the general population of college students (see Table 17.1). One of the recommended initiatives relevant to community health nursing practice is that alcohol screening be included as a standard practice in all university student health services (Schaus et al., 2009). To detect high-risk drinking in college students, nurses and physicians should specifically assess for the quantity and frequency of heavy episodic drinking, which is defined as five drinks in 2 hours for men or four drinks in 2 hours for women during the preceding month (this is termed "the 5/4 definition") (Schaus et al., 2009). Another suggestion is the addition of computerized screening surveys in routine health screening to more comprehensively identify students who may be at risk (NIAAA, 2007). One of the limitations of alcohol screening in a college health service is that it occurs at one point in time, and multiple studies have demonstrated wide variation among college students in their patterns of binge drinking behavior.

Nurses in university health services are ideally positioned to identify at-risk students and use motivational interviewing to ascertain the students' readiness to change their behavior (Kelly-Weeder, 2008). Motivational interviewing begins by establishing trust, being an empathic listener, and instilling hope and positive regard—communication skills familiar to nurses, which are the

table 17.1 **National Institute on Alcohol Abuse and Alcoholism (NIAAA) Evidence-based Programs to Decrease Binge Drinking on College Campuses**

Three-in-One Framework				
		Level of Operation		
Tier	Strategy	Individuals, Including At-risk and Dependent Drinkers	Student Population as Whole	Community
1. Effective among college students	Combining cognitive–behavioral skills with norms clarification and motivational enhancement intervention	Yes	No	No
	Offering brief motivational enhancement interventions in student health centers and emergency rooms	Yes	No	No
	Challenging alcohol expectancies	Yes	No	No
2. Effective with general populations	Increased enforcement of minimum drinking age laws	No	Yes	Yes
	Implementation, increased publicity, and enforcement of other laws to reduce alcohol-impaired driving	No	Yes	Yes
	Restrictions on alcohol retail density	No	No	Yes
	Increased price and excise taxes on alcoholic beverages	No	No	Yes
	Responsible beverage service policies in social and commercial settings	No	Yes	Yes
	The formation of a campus/community coalition	No	Yes	Yes
3. Promising	Adopting campus-based policies to reduce high-risk use (e.g., reinstating Friday classes, eliminating keg parties, establishing alcohol-free activities, and dorms)	No	Yes	No
	Increasing enforcement at campus-based events that promote excessive drinking	No	Yes	No
	Increasing publicity about enforcement of underage drinking laws/eliminating "mixed" messages	No	Yes	Yes
	Consistently enforcing campus disciplinary actions associated with policy violations	No	Yes	No
	Conducting marketing campaigns to correct student misperceptions about alcohol use on campus	No	Yes	No
	Provision of "safe rides" programs	No	Yes	Yes
	Regulation of happy hours and sales	No	Yes	Yes
	Enhancing awareness of personal liability	Yes	Yes	Yes
	Informing new students and parents about alcohol policies and penalties	Yes	Yes	No
4. Ineffective	Informational, knowledge-based, or values clarification interventions when used alone	N/A	N/A	N/A

Source: NIAAA. *College drinking: Changing the culture*. (July 11, 2007). Retrieved July 24, 2009, from http://www.collegedrinkingprevention.gov/StatsSummaries/4tier.aspx.

foundation of the nurse-client relationship. Once the nurse establishes rapport, brief motivational interviewing consists of specific cognitive strategies such as eliciting feelings about how the drinking behavior is affecting the student's life, noting discrepancies between attitudes toward alcohol and alcohol-associated harms, emphasizing strengths, supporting life goals, and empathically supporting the student on ways to implement change, or remaining neutral when met with ambivalence (Schaus, Sole, McCoy, Mullett, & O'Brien, 2009). Outcomes studies have demonstrated that at-risk students who received brief motivational interviewing at a university health service drink less alcohol and report fewer alcohol-related harmful incidents (Ehrlich, Hague, Swisher-McClure, & Helmkamp, 2006; Schaus et al., 2009).

Decreasing underage drinking requires sustained partnerships between government agencies, schools and colleges, parents, and local communities. The role of nurses in decreasing alcohol-related events involving students of all ages may begin in school-based health services. It also includes a coordinated effort among nurses in counseling services, health clinics, primary care offices, public health agencies, and hospital emergency departments to identify students' at-risk behaviors, implement evidence-based treatments, and educate students and others. Evidence-based programs most effective in decreasing alcohol-related harms to underage populations include (1) developmental prevention programs, (2) early screening and brief intervention, (3) government laws and school policies to reduce harmful incidents, and (4) tertiary treatments for those who meet criteria for substance use disorder or other associated mental disorders (to be reviewed later in this chapter) (Toumbourou et al., 2007). These are formidable challenges, as evidenced by the fact that despite concerted public health efforts, the final review of *Healthy People 2010* reported that there has been no change in the average annual consumption of alcohol by adults over 18 years of age and binge drinking among college students continues to rise (National Center for Health Statistics, 2012).

Older Adults

Katherine takes some time to ask Mr. Campbell how he thinks he is doing. She wants to begin with an open-ended question to assess how he feels about his health status. But he only responds by saying "I've got nothing to complain about" and smiles weakly. To Katherine, he appears sad and depressed. She asks him whether he has noticed that he has lost some weight, and he agrees that he has not been eating as he should. When she asks him why he thinks his appetite has changed, he says, "I really miss cooking for all the guys in the firehouse, and now that my wife is gone, I just don't have the motivation to cook for myself."

It is clear that Mr. Campbell is undergoing some major life transitions, which indicates to Katherine that she needs to screen for substance use using the Short Michigan Alcohol Screen Test–Geriatric Version (SMAST-G). She also asks Mr. Campbell's daughter to put all the prescription medications and over-the-counter medications that her father takes at home in a brown bag and bring them to his next appointment.

EVIDENCE FOR PRACTICE

The National Guideline Clearinghouse has 68 evidence-based treatment protocols for substance abuse, including screening and treatment of older adults. The protocols recommend screening for alcohol and prescription drug use yearly for all older adults and more frequent screening if there are any major life changes or transitions, or if physical symptoms suggestive of substance abuse appear. Recommended screening instruments for older adults include the Michigan Alcohol Screening Test—Geriatric Version (MAST-G), the CAGE questionnaire, and the Alcohol Use Disorders Identification Test (AUDIT) (Naegle, 2008). (Geriatric Nursing Resources for Care of Older Adults has more information available online.) Evidence-based practice protocols may be effective for evaluation of older adults for substance misuse or alcohol abuse (the National Guideline Clearinghouse's website has additional information). To assess prescription and nonprescription medication use among older adults, the protocols recommend the "brown bag approach"—asking the older adults to bring in all the medications they take to the practitioner in a brown bag.

The "baby boom" generation, the cohort with the greatest lifetime use and dependence on both alcohol and illicit substances, is now entering older adulthood. Not only will the "baby boomers" strain healthcare services because of their sheer numbers, but unlike previous generations, many will abuse or misuse substances, sometimes into old age (Oslin, 2005). Older adults who are most at risk of being diagnosed with substance abuse disorders are those who began drinking alcohol or using illicit drugs when they were 16 years of age or younger (Han et al., 2009). The number of older adults with substance abuse disorders is expected to more than double from approximately 2.8 million in 2002 to 5.7 million in 2020 (Han et al., 2009). An important aspect of this trend is the marked increase in the proportion older adults seeking treatment for illicit drug use (Lofwall, Schuster, & Strain, 2008).

EVIDENCE FOR PRACTICE

Trends over the past decade show that the only age cohort that had a significant increase in prescription drug use disorder ($p < 0.01$) were those 45 years of age or older. They had a significant increase ($p < 0.01$) in use of prescription tranquilizers (i.e., benzodiazepines such as alprazolam [Xanax], lorazepam [Ativan], and diazepam [Valium]) (McCabe, Cranford, & West, 2008). Almost 60% of clients prescribed benzodiazepines have comorbid alcohol use disorder (McCabe et al., 2008, p. 1301).

PRACTICE POINT

Benzodiazepines interact with alcohol (both of these substances are central nervous system depressants), with potentially fatal consequences. The combination of benzodiazepines and alcohol is particularly hazardous in an older adult, whose ability to metabolize and excrete substances may be compromised. Neurologic conditions, cardiac disorders, respiratory disorders, and kidney and liver function can all be adversely affected by drug and alcohol abuse, especially in an older adult. Drug and alcohol use also puts the older adult at greater risk for falls or other accidents that can cause skeletal injuries and hip fractures (Dowling, Weiss, & Condon, 2008).

For men, the NIAAA defines at-risk drinking as 14 or more standard drinks per week (no more than four drinks a day) and for women seven or more standard drinks per week (no more than three drinks a day) (NIAAA *Rethinking Drinking*, available online). The SAMHSA National Clearinghouse for Treatment Improvement Protocols advises that men older than 65 years drink no more than one drink a day, or two drinks in any one occasion, and that women older than 65 years drink even less (SAMHSA *Treatment Improvement Protocol for Substance Abuse Among Older Adults*, available online). However, comorbid medical conditions may substantially reduce levels of acceptable drinking in the older adult, and even much lower rates of alcohol consumption may put the older adult at risk.

Nurses should regularly screen for alcohol use using the MAST-G, which has been demonstrated to be a reliable and valid measure in older adult populations (Naegle, 2008). As of January 2008, the USPSTF concluded that there was insufficient evidence to recommend routine screening for illicit drug use across all age cohorts (USPSTF, Screening for Illicit Drug Use, available online). Nurses can assess for illicit and prescription drug use by conducting a thorough health history, examining urine and blood toxicology values, as well as systematically assessing older adults for symptoms suggestive of either intoxication or **withdrawal** symptoms from illicit substances and multiple classes of prescription medications, including benzodiazepines, opioids, and sedative hypnotics. In addition, nurses should inquire whether older adults are using over-the-counter preparations with caffeine (such as diet aids), cold remedies that have anticholinergic side effects or include alcohol, and herbal remedies that can have interactive effects with either prescription or nonprescription substances.

According to SAMHSA's *Treatment Protocols for Substance Abuse Among Older Adults*, benzodiazepines should not be prescribed for longer than 4 weeks, sedative hypnotics should not be prescribed for longer than 7 to 10 days, and antihistamines should be avoided completely because of changes in mental status that can result from anticholinergic effects. Misuse or excessive use of prescription as well as nonprescription medication may be a function of diminished cognitive capacity, poor vision, language barriers, lack of understanding about drug interactions, or the propensity for schedule II medications to cause dependence and **tolerance**.

SAMHSA has characterized substance abuse among older adults as an "invisible epidemic" (Lofwall et al., 2008, p. 898). *Treatment Improvement Protocol for Substance Abuse Among Older Adults* recognizes that there are many barriers to care for the older adult which are similar to those of other age groups such as language barriers, poor access to transportation, lack of health insurance, living in rural regions, and insensitivity of healthcare practitioners to the needs of racial and ethnically diverse populations (SAMSHA, 2012d). Other barriers noted by SAMHSA (2012d) as specific to older adults are a lack of substance disorder programs targeting the unique needs of older adults, as well as a lack of public awareness about the extent of substance abuse in older populations, including among healthcare providers.

EVIDENCE FOR PRACTICE

The USPSTF has found sufficient scientific evidence to recommend that positive screens for alcohol abuse be followed up with brief alcohol counseling in the primary care setting (USPSTF, 2013). It has described behavioral counseling of alcohol abuse in terms of the five As: (1) **as**sess using standardized screening instruments; (2) **a**dvise the older adult to reduce alcohol consumption to moderate levels; (3) **a**gree on goals for reducing alcohol use or for increasing abstinence; (4) **a**ssist clients with acquiring the motivations, self-help skills, or supports needed for behavior change; and (5) **a**rrange follow-up counseling and treatment (USPSTF, 2013).

PRACTICE POINT

Behavioral counseling interventions consist of the same principles as motivational interviewing (reviewed earlier in this chapter as an evidence-based treatment intervention for binge drinking in college students). Community health nurses and other primary care providers are encouraged to use this framework as an initial intervention for older adults who screen positive for alcohol abuse.

Nurses and other health providers may mistakenly attribute the presenting signs and symptoms of substance use disorder in older adults to depression, dementia, or other medical conditions. The nursing assessment of older adults may also be complicated by the inclination of many older adults to mask their symptoms and deny that they need treatment (Han et al., 2009). Nurses in all settings must be cognizant that the symptoms of delirium in the older adult may be related to polysubstance intoxication or withdrawal. The changing profile in substance use among older adults, from alcohol to polysubstance abuse, in combination with a precipitous increase in the sheer numbers of older adults needing substance use treatment, has profound clinical and public health implications (Lofwall et al., 2008, p. 902). As health educators, community health nurses have an important role in communicating to older adult populations that the national recommendations about acceptable levels of alcohol consumption decrease as they age. For example, nurses may use the confusion assessment method as a screening instrument to quickly and reliably assess for delirium (Waszynski, 2007).

Self-help programs are widely used community-based treatments that have proven efficacy in sustaining recovery for people with substance abuse disorders (Humphreys et al., 2004). Alcoholics Anonymous (AA) and Narcotics Anonymous (NA) are the two largest self-help groups for substance dependence or abuse, and both have local peer-support groups throughout the United States. Older adults may have higher dropout rates in AA or NA if there are few participants of the same age, if there are transportation difficulties, or if mobility is a problem (Oslin et al., 2005). To encourage participation by older adults, AA has developed an education pamphlet that includes testimonials by older adult members entitled *AA for the Older Alcoholic—Never Too Late* (available online).

Injection Drug Users

In 2007, the CDC reported that the total number of AIDS cases contracted from injection drug use was 255,859, which constitutes approximately one-fourth of all AIDS cases in the United States (Centers for Disease Control & Prevention [CDC], 2009). Of the new HIV infections reported in 2006, 12% were due to injection drug use and an additional 4% were due to a combination of injection drug use and male-to-male sexual contact (CDC, 2009). Hepatitis and other bloodborne pathogens are also primarily transmitted through injection drug use (National Center for Health Statistics, 2012).

Population surveys of injection drug use have consistently reported a racial and ethnic disparity, with Blacks and Latinos much more likely to suffer adverse health consequences than Whites (Cooper et al., 2005). The disproportionate burden of disease may be partially explained by the finding that blacks are significantly ($p < 0.001$) more likely to inject illicit drugs than whites (Cooper et al., 2005). In 2007, Blacks (37%), Latino (37%), and Native Americans (33%) were twice as likely as Whites (18%) to contract HIV from injection drug use (CDC, 2009).

EVIDENCE FOR PRACTICE

A study of injection drug use in 94 metropolitan statistical areas found considerable variation by area, suggesting that neighborhood characteristics may play a key role in the initiation of injection drug use behavior (Cooper et al., 2005). Neighborhoods where residents appear to be more at risk for injection drug use are those that are highly segregated and characterized by poverty, limited employment opportunities, substandard schools, poor access to health services, and questionable efficacy of police in containing the distribution of illicit drugs (Cooper et al., 2005).

In the 1980s, proponents of syringe-exchange programs argued that by providing sterile needles to injection drug users, pathogens transmitted by sharing needles would be lessened, slowing the spread of HIV, hepatitis, and other bloodborne diseases. In the ensuing years, as scientific evidence accumulated demonstrating the efficacy of syringe-exchange programs in decreasing the spread of HIV, the CDC, medical associations, public health agencies, and the ANA all formally endorsed syringe-exchange programs as a sound public health initiative (Bluthenthal, Heinzerling, Anderson, Flynn, & Kral, 2008; Villarreal & Fogg, 2006). Yet, as of July 2009, a federal ban on funding for syringe-exchange programs instituted in 1988 remains in place, hampering local efforts to expand the availability of sterile needles to injection drug users (Villarreal & Fogg, 2006). The schism between the scientific evidence that syringe-exchange programs are effective at reducing the spread of infectious disease, and those who view such programs as sanctioning the use of illicit drugs, illustrates the complexities in implementing public health programs with competing stakeholder interests.

The CDC estimated that, as of 2002, despite the lack of federal aid, there were approximately 184 syringe-exchange programs operating in 36 states, including the District of Columbia, Puerto Rico, and Native American-owned lands (CDC, 2005b). A study of syringe-exchange programs in California found that 11 new syringe-exchanges programs opened over the past 5 years but none were in high-need counties, suggesting that the effectiveness of syringe-exchange programs may be mitigated by difficulties in accessing those most at risk (Bluthenthal et al., 2008). Syringe-exchange programs typically work with illicit drug users who have complex healthcare needs and are not, or have not been, in treatment (Kidorf & King, 2008). Syringe-exchange programs can be the bridge for injection drug users to receive comprehensive substance abuse treatment and rehabilitation—one of the primary goals of *Healthy People 2010.*

Numerous studies have demonstrated that the safest and most effective treatment for injection drug users is opioid substitution treatment with long-acting opioids such as methadone or buprenorphine (Gerra et al., 2009; Mattick, Kimber, Breen, & Davoli, 2008). Unfortunately, access to opioid substitution treatment in the United States has been limited by a lack of methadone maintenance programs or waiting lists for those that do exist (*Healthy People 2010* Midcourse Review, 2006). Office-based treatment with buprenorphine can potentially expand the availability of opioid substitution treatment, but the number of physician providers is constrained by Food and Drug Administration (FDA) requirements for training and accreditation (*Healthy People 2010* Midcourse Review, 2006). *Healthy People 2010* (2006) reported an increase in admissions for injection drug use treatment and that 85% of the target of 256,680 admissions had been achieved—a strong indication that public health initiatives are having an impact on improving access to care for this highly at-risk population.

Methamphetamine Users

Methamphetamine is an addictive stimulant. Demographically, most methamphetamine users are white (71%), male (55%), and in their 30s (McGuinness, 2006). Admissions for methamphetamine treatment are in much higher concentrations in western regions and rural communities than in other parts of the United States. This contrasts with admissions for substance abuse treatment in other geographic regions of the United States, which are fairly uniform, with slightly higher rates reported in the Northeast (SAMHSA, February 7, 2008).

Methamphetamine is produced in home "laboratories" by cooking readily available ingredients (e.g., drain cleaner, fertilizer, starter fluid, and pseudoephedrine) at high heat (CDC, 2005a; Denehy, 2006; McGuinness, 2006). The process is extremely hazardous. Many of these so-called laboratories are located in remote rural areas, where noxious odors from the toxic chemicals released in the manufacturing process can disperse (Denehy, 2006).

In contrast to other incidents involving the release of hazardous fumes or materials in communities, adverse events associated with methamphetamine "laboratories" have a much greater percentage of injured victims (31%) with most being police officers (56%) and the general public (33%) (CDC, 2005a). First responders (60%) and the general public (34%) were also the most likely to require decontamination from hazardous toxins emanating from methamphetamine "laboratories" (CDC, 2005a).

It is important to note that children have been found in 20% of the homes containing methamphetamine "laboratories" (CDC, 2005a). Children who are chronically exposed to acetone or ammonia fumes are at grave risk for neurologic, psychological, and physical harm (Denehy, 2006; McGuinness, 2006). In addition to the signs of abuse and neglect, a distinguishing characteristic of children exposed to ammonia fumes released in methamphetamine production is a smell like the odor of cat urine (Denehy, 2006). Chemicals used in the manufacture of methamphetamine are highly explosive, and anyone in proximity to the methamphetamine "laboratory" is in danger of sustaining severe burns (Mitka, 2005). Toxic and hazardous chemicals used to manufacture methamphetamine may contaminate local neighborhoods and have necessitated the evacuation of surrounding residences (CDC, 2005a).

The danger methamphetamine poses to individual people, families, and communities requires a multifaceted prevention strategy that incorporates public health and law enforcement agencies. To disrupt the availability of ingredients needed to manufacture methamphetamine, in 2000, the Methamphetamine Anti-Proliferation Act put restrictions on the amounts of pseudoephedrine that could be purchased over the counter and regulated the distribution of other key ingredients used in the manufacture of methamphetamine (Birckmayer, Fisher, Holder, & Yacoubian, 2008). Departments of Health in states with high rates of methamphetamine manufacture and addiction, launched public health education efforts using media campaigns which depict the ravaged faces of young methamphetamine addicts to graphically illustrate the morbidity associated with methamphetamine use. A pamphlet available through the National Clearinghouse for Alcohol and Drug Information entitled *Tips for Teens: The Truth About Methamphetamine*, states bluntly in bold letters, "Methamphetamine can kill you. An overdose of meth can result in heart failure. Long-term physical effects such as liver, kidney, and lung damage may also kill you."

PRACTICE POINT

Denehy (2006) urges all school nurses to be part of the solution to the methamphetamine epidemic through education of children, families, and the community about the effects of methamphetamine use, and through advocacy for prevention and treatment programs.

IMPACT ON THE COMMUNITY

The economic cost to the United States from substance abuse is a staggering $510.8 billion annually (SAMHSA, 2008b). Communities hit hardest by substance use are often ill-equipped to combat the adverse effects on the quality of life in their neighborhoods, homes, and schools. The latest financing projections for substance abuse treatment indicate that it is expected that communities will need to shoulder more of the costs associated with substance abuse treatment (Levit et al., 2008). Public spending on substance abuse treatment is projected to swell to 83% by 2014 as public programs, as opposed to private insurers, are burdened with a larger share of the costs (Levit et al., 2008). The shifting of costs to state and local governments is the result of the stringent limits for substance abuse treatment that private insurance companies have written in their policies—limits that do not exist for other healthcare conditions. The states spend $81.3 billion on substance abuse-related services, including prevention programs, family assistance, mental health, public safety, criminal justice, and healthcare (SAMHSA, 2008b). Without added federal monies or private insurance reforms, the added burden on states and local government to assume the bulk of costs for substance abuse treatment may result in less access to services.

EVIDENCE FOR PRACTICE

SAMHSA (2008b) estimates that evidence-based prevention programs will save states and local governments $1.3 million on reduced costs to education, Medicaid, and criminal justice. The average return on investment in 10 evidence-based prevention programs implemented in schools, including the LifeSkills Training program referred to in this chapter, is $18 to $1 (SAMSHA, 2008, p.1).

PUBLIC HEALTH MODELS FOR POPULATIONS AT RISK

Community health nurses play a critical role in screening populations at risk for preventable disease. Population research suggests that there is a window of vulnerability for later development of addiction if initial substance use precedes age 15 (Crome & McLellan, 2014). The USPSTF is a multidisciplinary panel of experts within the Agency for Healthcare Research and Quality, whose mandate is to systematically evaluate scientific evidence regarding the efficacy of prevention interventions, and to make national recommendations to practitioners in primary care. Since its inception more than two decades ago, nationally recognized experts in community health nursing have served on the USPSTF (Trinite, Loveland-Cherry, & Marion, 2009).

A challenge in identifying people at risk for substance abuse is that many healthcare practitioners in primary care do not directly, or routinely, ask about alcohol or drug use across all age groups when collecting information about a person's health history. Reliable and valid screening instruments that are easy to administer are important tools to aid community health nurses in evaluating populations and individual people at risk for substance abuse. The USPSTF (2004) analyzed screening instruments for alcohol use on the ease of application in primary care settings, reliability, validity, and sensitivity to identifying diverse populations at risk for alcohol use. In 2004, the USPSTF issued a national recommendation that all adults in primary care should be routinely screened for alcohol use with the AUDIT-C or CAGE questionnaires (Box 17.8). The AUDIT-C, CAGE, and SMAST-G screening instruments are now available in a pocket-sized brochure to facilitate use in all primary care settings. (The Substance Abuse and Mental Health Services Administration website provide further information.)

Screening for substance use is the first step in assessing whether a person has substance use disorder. The efficacy of screening instruments is highly dependent on the candor of client responses. Putting the client at ease with a nonconfrontational request to ask a series of questions about health behaviors and beginning the conversation with less threatening questions about diet, sleep, and exercise are helpful transitions to questions pertaining to alcohol use.

The second step in assessing for substance use disorders is to determine whether there are maladaptive behaviors that have resulted in dysfunction in health and interpersonal, social, and legal domains. In conducting a complete biopsychosocial history, two of the key indicators for risk of substance dependence are age at first use and a family history of substance use disorder. Patterns of substance abuse often occur in the context of other high-risk behaviors such as driving while intoxicated or unsafe sex practices. Legal, employment, or academic difficulties that have resulted from misuse are an important gauge of how substance use is impairing the client's ability to fulfill normal role functions.

Specific questions about misuse or abuse of substances should include a list of all substances that can result in a change in behavior or mental status. Patterns of use for caffeine, nicotine, over-the-counter medications, and herbal treatments should also be assessed. To evaluate the degree of dependence on substances, it is critical to ascertain the last time the substance was used and how much was used. In situations in which the person has experienced withdrawal symptoms in the past, nurses should ask about the typical first signs of withdrawal and what medications or treatments he or she has found helpful.

Nurses should not only gather information about the patterns of substance use, but the social contexts in which the abuse occurs. Recognition of gender, ethnic, or cultural preferences and influences are at the core of fully understanding the individualized meaning of maladaptive behaviors. It is the environmental context of the substance use behavior that can guide the nurse in evaluating what prevention strategies or interventions will be the most effective in minimizing harm. In particular, nurses should carefully note whether the client has been a victim of trauma or whether there is any physical evidence of trauma. Children or the elderly in homes where there are adults with substance use disorders are at high risk for abuse and neglect. The ability of individual people to fulfill social role responsibilities at home, work, or school has implications not only for people with substance use disorders but for their dependents as well.

There is high comorbidity of substance use disorders with major mental illness. The mental status examination is a valuable tool in identifying signs and symptoms of major mental illness that co-occur with substance use. The mental status examination can alert the nurse to cognitive changes that are

box 17.8 AUDIT-C and CAGE Screening Instruments for Alcohol Abuse

1. How often do you have a drink containing alcohol?
   0 = Never
   1 = Monthly or less
   2 = 2–4 times per month
   3 = 2–3 times per week
   4 = 4 or more per week
2. How many drinks containing alcohol do you have on a typical day?
   0 = None
   1 = 1 or 2
   2 = 3 or 4
   3 = 5 or 6
   4 = 7 or more
3. How often do you have…
   [MEN]—five or more drinks on one occasion
   [WOMEN]—four or more drinks on one occasion
   0 = Never
   1 = <Monthly
   2 = Monthly
   3 = Weekly
   4 = Daily or almost daily
4. Have you ever felt you should cut down on your drinking?
   Yes/No
5. Have people annoyed you by criticizing your drinking?
   Yes/No
6. Have you ever felt bad or guilty about your drinking?
   Yes/No
7. Have you ever had a drink first thing in the morning to steady your nerves or to get rid of a hangover?
   Yes/No

Scoring: Refer client for further evaluation if

- Three or more points on questions 1 to 3
- Six or more drinks on one occasion
- "Yes" to questions 4 to 7 and drinking in 1 to 3

Source: Substance Abuse and Mental Health Services Administration. (2001). Alcohol use among older adults: Pocket screening instruments for health care and social service providers.

the result of chronic substance use and can help differentiate symptoms from other medical conditions, such as dementia or delirium. As a general rule, the more rapid the onset of symptoms is, the more likely it is that the symptoms are a product of substance use rather than a medical or psychiatric condition.

Urine and blood toxicology screens and physical assessments also aid in determining whether changes in behavior or mental status are a function of substance use or other health-care conditions. Vital signs are crucial in assessing impending withdrawal syndromes for central nervous system depressants, or intoxication on stimulants, both of which can be fatal. The Clinical Institute Withdrawal Assessment for Alcohol tool is commonly used to assess the degree of withdrawal, and to guide nurses in the appropriate administration of benzodiazepines used for the treatment of withdrawal symptoms of central nervous system depressants (Fig. 17.5). People who are grossly intoxicated or actively withdrawing from substances have pronounced positive signs and symptoms, such as gross motor skill impairment, slurred speech, marked disorientation, confusion, or even hallucinations (Table 17.2).

Clinical Institute Withdrawal Assessment - Alcohol (CIWA-A)

Patient: ______________ **Date:** (yy/mm/dd) ______________ **Time:** (24 hr) ______________

Pulse or heart rate: ______________ **Blood Pressure:** ______________

Nausea and Vomiting
Ask: *"Do you feel sick to your stomach? Have you vomited?"*
Observation:
- O 0—None
- O 1—Mild nausea with no vomiting
- O 2
- O 3
- O 4—Intermittent nausea with dry heaves
- O 5
- O 6
- O 7—Constant nausea, frequent dry heaves and vomiting

Paroxysmal Sweats
Observation:
- O 0—No sweat visible
- O 1—Barely perceptible sweating, palms moist
- O 2
- O 3
- O 4—Beads of sweat obvious on forehead
- O 5
- O 6
- O 7—Drenching sweats

Anxiety
Ask: *"Do you feel nervous?*
Observation:
- O 0—No anxiety, at ease
- O 1—Mildly anxious
- O 2
- O 3
- O 4—Moderately anxious, or guarded, so anxiety is inferred
- O 5
- O 6
- O 7—Equivalent to acute panic states as seen in severe delirium or acute schizophrenic reactions

Agitation
Observation:
- O 0—Normal activity
- O 1—Somewhat more than normal activity
- O 2
- O 3
- O 4—Moderately fidgety and restless
- O 5
- O 6
- O 7—Paces back and forth during most of the interview, or constantly thrashes about

Tremor
Arms extended and fingers spread apart
Observation:
- O 0—None
- O 1—Not visible, but can be felt fingertip to fingertip
- O 2
- O 3
- O 4—Moderate, with patient's arms extended
- O 5
- O 6
- O 7—Severe, even with arms not extended

Headache/Fullness in Head
Ask: *"Does your head feel different? Does it feel like there is a band around your head?"*
Do not rate diziness or lightheadedness. Otherwise rate severity.
Observation:
- O 0—Not present
- O 1—Very mild
- O 2—Mild
- O 3—Moderate
- O 4—Moderately severe
- O 5—Severe
- O 6—Very severe
- O 7—Extremely severe

Auditory Disturbances
Ask: *"Are you more aware of sounds around you? Are they harsh? Do they frighten you? Are you hearing anything that is disturbing to you? Are you hearing things that you know aren't there?"*
Observation:
- O 0—None
- O 1—Very mild harshness or ability to frighten
- O 2—Mild harshness or ability to frighten
- O 3—Moderate harshness or ability to frighten
- O 4—Moderately severe hallucinations
- O 5—Severe hallucinations
- O 6—Extremely severe hallucinations
- O 7—Continuous hallucinations

Tactile Disturbances
Ask: *"Do you have any itching, pins and needles sensations, any burning, numbness, or do you feel bugs crawling on or under your skin?"*
Observation:
- O 0—None
- O 1—Very mild itching, pins and needles, burning or numbness
- O 2—Mild itching, pins and needles,burning or numbness
- O 3—Moderate itching, pins and needles, burning or numbness
- O 4—Moderately severe hallucinations
- O 5—Severe hallucinations
- O 6—Extremely severe hallucinations
- O 7—Continuous hallucinations

Visual Disturbances
Ask: *"Does the light appear too bright? Is its color different? Does it hurt your eyes? Are you seeing things that you know aren't there?"*
Observation:
- O 0—None
- O 1—Very mild
- O 2—Mild
- O 3—Moderate
- O 4—Moderately severe
- O 5—Severe
- O 6—Very severe
- O 7—Extremely severe

Orientation and Clouding of Sensorium
Ask: *"What day is this? Where are you? Who am I?"*
Observation:
- O 0—Oriented and can form serial additions
- O 1—Cannot do serial additions or is uncertain about date
- O 2—Disoriented for date by no more than two calendar days
- O 3—Disoriented for date by more than two calendar days
- O 4—Disoriented for place and/or person

Rater's Initials: ______________

Total CIWA-A Score: ______________

Maximum Possible Score: 67

figure 17.5 Clinical institute withdrawal assessment of alcohol scale, revised (CIWA-Ar). (From http://www.ireta.org/ireta_main/webinarOnDemand-files/CIWA-Ar.pdf. This scale is not copyrighted and may be used freely.)

table 17.2 **Nursing Assessment and Implications for Alcohol and Illicit Drug Use**

Substance[a]	Dependence	Fatal in Overdose	Fatal in Withdrawal	Symptoms of Intoxication/ Overdose	Symptoms of Withdrawal	Nursing Implications in Community
Alcohol Beer Wine Spirits	Yes	Yes	Yes	Ataxia, slurred speech, disinhibition, drowsiness, hypotension, CNS depression, coma convulsions, death	Nausea, vomiting, hypertension, tachycardia, diaphoresis, tremors, delirium tremens, coma, death. Peaks 24–35 hours.	*In overdose if awake*, induce vomiting, give activated charcoal, vital signs q 15 min. *In overdose if unarousable*, maintain airway, seizure precaution, emergency transport to hospital. *In withdrawal early stage*, administer benzodiazepines. *In withdrawal late stage*, maintain airway, seizure precautions, emergency transport to hospital.
Illicit drugs Heroin	Yes	Yes	No	Constricted pupils, euphoria, slurred speech, CNS depression, coma, convulsions, death	Yawning, rhinorrhea, cramps, bone pain, chills, fever, diaphoresis, diarrhea, irritability, panic	*In overdose if unarousable*, administer IV Naloxone stat. *In withdrawal* administer buprenorphine, methadone. *In abrupt withdrawal* administer clonidine.
Nonmedical Pain relievers Oxycodone Fentanyl Morphine Codeine	Yes	Yes	No	Opioid analgesics have signs and symptoms similar to heroin, including death.	Opioid analgesics have signs similar to heroin. Peak symptoms depend on half-life.	Nursing implications are the same as for heroin.
Nonmedical Tranquilizers Diazepam Alprazolam Klonopin	Yes	Rare	Yes	Benzodiazepines are CNS depressants, and effects are similar to alcohol, including death.	Benzodiazepines are CNS depressants, and effects are similar to alcohol, including death.	Nursing implications are the same as for alcohol.
Nonmedical Sedatives Meprobamate Chloral hydrate	Yes	Yes	Yes	Sedative hypnotics are CNS depressants, and effects are similar to alcohol, including death.	Sedative hypnotics are CNS depressants, and effects are similar to alcohol, including death.	Nursing implications are the same as for alcohol.
Nonmedical Stimulants Amphetamine Adderall Concerta	Yes	Yes	No	Dilated pupils, insomnia, tachycardia, paranoia, hallucinations, assaultive, hyperpyrexia, coma, elevated BP, coma, stroke, death	Craving, agitation, hypersomnia, anxiety, depression	*In intoxication if awake,* antipsychotics, ambient cooling, seizure precautions. *In intoxication if severe,* emergency transport to hospital. *In withdrawal* administer antidepressants, dopamine agonist
Cocaine	Yes	Yes	No	Cocaine is a CNS stimulant, and the effects are similar to amphetamines.	Cocaine is a CNS stimulant, and the effects are similar amphetamines.	*Nursing implications* are the same as for amphetamines.

table 17.2 **Nursing Assessment and Implications for Alcohol and Illicit Drug Use (continued)**

Substance[a]	Dependence	Fatal in Overdose	Fatal in Withdrawal	Symptoms of Intoxication/ Overdose	Symptoms of Withdrawal	Nursing Implications in Community
Inhalants	Yes	Yes	Yes (chronic use)	Similar to alcohol and visual hallucinations, cardiac arrhythmias, sudden death	In chronic use, similar to alcohol and convulsions, delirium	*In intoxication,* rest, decrease stimulation, monitor for cardiac arrhythmias. *In overdose and withdrawal* emergency transport to hospital.
Hallucinogens LSD MDMA Mescaline Peyote	No	Yes	No	Dilated pupils, tremor, elevated vital signs, psychosis, death	None	*In intoxication if alert*, decrease sensory stimulation, administer benzodiazepines, or chloral hydrate.
PCP	No	Yes	No	Dilated pupils, nystagmus, hypertensive crisis, hyperthermia, death	None	*In intoxication if alert*, can be very violent, institute safety precautions, acidify urine, administer Haldol or diazepam, decrease stimuli.
Cannabis	No	No	No	Red eyes, dry mouth, increased pulse, panic, toxic psychosis	None	*In intoxication if psychotic*, administer antipsychotics.

CNS, central nervous system; IV, intravenous; PCP, phencyclidine; LSD, lysergic acid diethylamide; MDMA, 3,4-methylenedioxy-N-methylamphetamine; BP, blood pressure.
[a]Nine substance use categories are defined in 2007 National Survey on Drug Use and Health (NSDUH).
Source: From National Survey on Drug Use and Health (NSDUH).

In the community, nurses may encounter clients who are not seeking treatment and may deny a substance use problem, yet aspects of the history or behaviors suggest that their health status is at risk because of an underlying substance use disorder. This is particularly true for older adults whose misuse of substances can greatly exacerbate other chronic health conditions (Crome & McLellan, 2014). Fine motor tremors, shakiness, tremulous speech, sweaty palms, or restlessness may be misinterpreted as evidence of anxiety, when in fact the person is exhibiting subtle signs of withdrawal from central nervous system depressants. The condition of the person's skin is particularly illuminating about the extent and degree of substance use. Skin conditions seen with chronic substance use include dark shadows under the eyes, bruising, jaundice, burns between the fingers or inside the lips, scabs, bloody gums and nasal mucosa, decayed teeth, ascites, or needle track marks. A person's pupil size can reveal much about his or her current state of intoxication and the substances involved. Dilated pupils are seen with people intoxicated on stimulants, cocaine, or hallucinogens, whereas people intoxicated on opioids have constricted pupils.

A challenge for nurses in conducting a risk assessment for clients with substance use disorder is that the clients may mask symptoms or deny high-risk behaviors. More than half of clients with substance use disorders believed that primary care providers were not able to detect their dependence or abuse (Fleming, 2005). Sometimes, clients do not allow nurses to inquire with collateral informants (such as other healthcare providers, family, friends, or school personnel) about changes in behavior or evidence of high-risk behavior that suggest the person may have a substance use disorder. It is extremely useful in conducting a health assessment of a client who may have a substance use disorder if the client gives informed consent to elicit additional information from other people who know the client well.

Nurses must always ask directly if the client has any thoughts of harming himself or herself or others. All threats of self-harm or harm to others must be taken seriously. Nurses should ask clients who appear intoxicated or express suicidal ideation whether they have access to weapons. If a client responds affirmatively, the nurse must seek a responsible adult to secure any weapons. Clients who have substance use disorders may become less inhibited when they are intoxicated, or extremely despondent and agitated while withdrawing from substances. Any indication that the person is a danger to himself or herself or others warrants immediate referral to an emergency department for more thorough evaluation.

A person's readiness for substance use treatment varies greatly. Throughout the assessment, nurses should convey that they are a partner in helping the client access substance use services and achieve recovery. If clients disavow problems with substance use or the need for treatment, nurses can use the encounter as an opportunity to educate the clients and share concerns for their well-being. Throughout the encounter, nurses should follow the person's lead and work to problem-solve issues which they have identified are of immediate concern. An essential attribute of nurses who work with this population is the nurses' capacity to sustain unconditional positive regard as they partner with clients through an often-winding course of ambivalence, relapse, and recovery.

TREATMENT INTERVENTIONS FOR SUBSTANCE ABUSE

PRACTICE POINT

The main reason Americans who self-identify as needing treatment for alcohol or drug use and did not receive treatment stated that they had no health insurance and could not afford the cost (SAMHSA, 2013). Mandated coverage for essential services in the Patient Protection and Affordable Care Act includes substance use prevention, early intervention, treatment, and case management (Crome & McLellan, 2014). Federally qualified healthcare centers will take the lead in spearheading the integration of mental health and substance use treatment in primary care (Urada, Teruya, Gelberg, & Rawson, 2014). In response, the ANA has acknowledged that nurses must be clinically prepared to implement evidence-based screening, brief interventions and referrals for complex substance use treatment when indicated (Savage & Finnell, 2013).

In community settings, evidence-based treatments for substance use fall into two broad modalities, pharmacologic and psychosocial. Nurses should always ask women about their pregnancy status during the assessment because some medications used in treatment may be contraindicated in pregnancy. Co-occurring substance use disorder and major mental illness affect approximately half of all people with drug abuse, and about a third of people with alcohol abuse. Ideally, the treatments for co-occurring disorders, also termed *dual diagnosis*, are fully integrated in the multidisciplinary treatment plan. The substance use treatments reviewed in this chapter will be augmented with additional psychiatric treatments in cases where a person has a dual diagnosis.

Pharmacologic Treatments for Substance Use Disorders

Pharmacologic Treatments for Alcohol-Dependent Disorders

Based on empirical evidence, APA Practice Guidelines for Substance Use Disorders (2006) recommend treatment with naltrexone, acamprosate, or disulfiram. Naltrexone and acamprosate have pharmacologic properties that diminish **craving** for alcohol, whereas disulfiram induces aversive effects if alcohol is consumed. APA Guidelines (2006) note that pharmacologic studies sponsored by the NIAAA are under way to investigate if combinations of these three medications may improve outcomes for people who are dependent on alcohol.

NALTREXONE

Naltrexone (Vivitrol) mediates opiate receptors and diminishes the alcohol-induced release of dopamine thought to be involved in alcohol craving. The dosing is 50 mg a day orally or 380 mg intramuscularly (IM) every 4 weeks into alternating buttocks. Side effects associated with oral preparations of naltrexone include nausea, vomiting, and hepatotoxicity. The FDA approved a long-acting IM naltrexone in 2006 and issued a warning about adverse injection site reactions on August 12, 2008. (More information is available on the FDA's website.)

The warning reads, "Naltrexone IM should only be administered with the prepackaged 1.5-inch needle that is specifically designed for administration. Naltrexone IM should never be administered intravenously, subcutaneously, or inadvertently into fatty tissue. Nurses should not administer naltrexone IM to any client whose body habitus precludes a gluteal IM injection with the prepackaged 1.5-inch needle. Women are physiologically at higher risk for injection site reactions because of typically higher gluteal fat thickness. Nurses should advise clients to immediately report any signs of redness, pain, or swelling in the injection site."

ACAMPROSATE

Acamprosate is believed to normalize glutamate function that may contribute to craving or protracted withdrawal symptoms. Dosing is a maximum of 1,998 mg a day given in 333-mg tablets three times a day. Acamprosate is excreted through the kidneys. Creatine levels, blood urea nitrogen levels, and kidney function should be carefully monitored. Diarrhea is a common side effect.

DISULFIRAM

Disulfiram inhibits aldehyde dehydrogenase. When disulfiram is taken, and then alcohol is consumed, levels of aldehyde accumulate, which triggers flushing, nausea, and vomiting. Dosing is a maximum of 500 mg daily initially for 1 to 2 weeks followed by 250 mg daily. Clients must be carefully educated about the adverse symptoms that occur if they ingest alcohol. Nurses should alert clients that alcohol may be used in preparation of gravies, desserts, soups, ciders, mouthwash, cough syrups, and other common household items. Clients should avoid inhaling fumes from substances containing alcohol.

Pharmacologic Treatments for Opioid Use Disorders

The APA Treatment Guidelines (2006) recommend treatment with the opioid agonists methadone and buprenorphine for both withdrawal syndromes and maintenance. Methadone or buprenorphine should be given as maintenance medications only when the client has a history of opioid dependence exceeding 1 year. Methadone and buprenorphine are dispensed only in specially licensed facilities. As of 2009, there are approximately 1,200 opioid treatment programs operating nationwide which dispense methadone (Government Accountability Office [GAO], 2009). Buprenorphine is available in physicians' offices which have been licensed and approved by various states. Only physicians who meet qualifying requirements are authorized by the U.S. Drug Enforcement Agency to prescribe buprenorphine. Advanced practice nurses with prescriptive authority are not authorized to prescribe buprenorphine, and physicians do not have the authority to delegate authority to prescribe buprenorphine to these nurses. The SAMHSA Buprenorphine Information Center is available to answer any questions from nurses about buprenorphine. Nurses can assist clients in locating a provider of buprenorphine through the SAMHSA Center for Substance Abuse Treatment. SAMHSA's websites contain additional information.

METHADONE

Methadone binds to opioid receptors and blocks the euphoric and sedating effects of opiates, thus relieving the craving. The standard of once-a-day dosing of 60 to 120 mg by tablet, elixir, or diskette is followed in opioid treatment programs, which are located throughout the United States. Side effects include constipation, diaphoresis, and sexual dysfunction. Methadone prescriptions increased to 4.1 million in 2006. Levo-α-acetylmethadol (LAAM) is a form of methadone that has a longer half-life. Dosing of LAAM is 20 to 40 mg at induction, with gradual increases up to 10 days. Maintenance dose of LAAM is three times a week; each of the 3 days, the doses range from 60 to 180 mg.

Deaths associated with methadone overdose increased 262% from 2001 to 2007 to 10,361. At the request of Congress, in March 2009, the U.S. Government Accountability Office (GAO) completed a report analyzing factors associated with the steep rise in methadone deaths (GAO, 2009). It concluded that one factor associated with methadone fatalities was the increased use of methadone to treat chronic pain (GAO, 2009). To improve safety, the FDA has initiated a Risk Evaluation and Mitigation Strategy that restricts prescription authority of certain opioids to practitioners knowledgeable about the use of potent opioid medication.

Unlike when naltrexone is used in alcohol addiction, when naltrexone is used in the treatment of opioid addiction, the client should be opioid-free for at least 5 days after using heroin or 7 days after using methadone; otherwise, the naltrexone will trigger withdrawal symptoms. Dosing is oral 3 times a week, with 100 mg on Monday and Wednesday followed by 150 mg on Friday. There is poor compliance in opioid-dependent clients for the oral route of administration. The intramuscular route of administration has the advantage of being long-acting and promoting adherence (APA, 2006).

BUPRENORPHINE

Buprenorphine (Subutex) is considered a partial opioid agonist that enables opioid-dependent people to discontinue opioids without experiencing withdrawal symptoms. Initiation of maintenance treatment should be 12 to 24 hours after last use of opioids. On the first day of treatment, clients are given a dose of 2 to 4 mg and assessed for symptoms of withdrawal over a 2-hour period. If withdrawal symptoms occur, additional doses can be given in 2-hour intervals for a maximum daily dose of 8 mg. The average daily maintenance dose is 16 mg. For use in opioid withdrawal, buprenorphine can be withdrawn over a short (3 days), moderate (10 to 14 days), or long (180 days) period. Doses may be reduced by 50% per day. Buprenorphine can be abused, and in such cases, clients can be given a combination preparation of naloxone and buprenorphine (Suboxone). Side effects include hepatic failure and central nervous system depression when taken with benzodiazepines or alcohol. Nurses should caution clients that they should avoid driving during initial induction or with any dosing changes. This information is summarized from *Buprenorphine: A Guide for Nurses* (SAMHSA, 2009).

NALOXONE

Naloxone is an opioid antagonist that blocks the opioid receptors and temporarily reverses respiratory depression associated with opioid overdose. Over 10,000 potential opioid overdoses were reversed by community administered naloxone (CDC, 2012). Naloxone hydrochloride injection is available as a prescription treatment that can be used by family members or caregivers for the emergency treatment of an opioid overdose in a community setting. Once turned on, the handheld auto-injector provides verbal instruction to the user describing how to deliver the single dose of naloxone hydrochloride by injection to immediately reverse respiratory depression. Naloxone rescue kits include two mucosal atomization devises and two prefilled syringes with 2 mg/2 mL naloxone hydrochloride. Naloxone administered via the atomizer is given intranasally with 1 mL to each nostril (Doe-Simkins et al., 2014). Patients administered naloxone in community settings must seek emergency treatment in a medical center as the opioid antagonist effects dissipate and additional doses may be needed within 20 minutes. Currently 17 states and the District of Columbia have enacted laws permitting the distribution of naloxone rescue kits by injection or inhalation to first responders, family members, and opioid users (American Journal of Nursing [AJN], 2014).

Evidence-Based Psychosocial Treatments in Substance Use Disorders

In addition to brief motivational interviewing and social skills training (Box 17.9), additional evidence-based modalities for people with substance use disorders include cognitive behavioral strategies that focus on relapse prevention, behavioral therapy that uses community reinforcement and contingency contracting, and psychodynamic and

box 17.9 Project ASSERT

Project ASSERT (Alcohol and Substance Abuse Services, Education, and Referral to Treatment) is a screening, brief intervention, and referral to treatment (SBIRT) model designed for use in health clinics or emergency departments (EDs). Project ASSERT aims to reduce or eliminate unhealthy substance use through collaboration with trained nurses, peer educators, and other health professionals.

Patients with a positive screening result are engaged by interventionists with the Brief Negotiated Interview (BNI), a semiscripted, motivational interviewing counseling session that focuses on the negative consequences associated with drug use and unhealthy drinking. Using the BNI, the nurse builds rapport with the patient; asks the patient for permission to discuss drug and alcohol use; explores the pros and cons of the behavior associated with drug and alcohol use; discusses the gap between the client's real and desired quality of life; assesses the client's readiness for change in the targeted behavior; and develops an action plan, which includes direct referrals and access to substance abuse treatment.

On average, Project ASSERT is delivered in 15 minutes, although more time may be needed, depending on the severity of the patient's substance use problem and associated treatment referral needs. The face-to-face component of the intervention is completed during the course of primary care visit. After the nurse delivers the intervention, he or she follows up with each patient by telephone 10 days after the health clinic visit. This call serves as a 5- to 10-minute booster session to discuss what has transpired since the BNI and to find out whether new service referrals are needed.

Project ASSERT targets adults and adolescents in urban, suburban, rural, frontier, and tribal areas. Races and ethnicities who have received Project ASSERT interventions include Asian, Black or African-American, Hispanic or Latino, and White.

Readness for dissemination ratings by
criteria = 4.0 (0.0–4.0 scale)
Implementation materials = 4.0
Training and support = 4.0
Quality assurance = 4.0

Source: Substance Abuse and Mental Health Services Administration, National Registry of Evidence-based Programs and Practices. (May 2011). Retrieved July 24, 2014, from http://www.nrepp.samhsa.gov/ViewIntervention.aspx?id=222

box 17.10 Prize Incentives Contingency Management for Substance Abuse

Prize Incentives Contingency Management for Substance Abuse is a variation of contingency management and awards prizes for abstinence and treatment compliance, such as group attendance and healthy behaviors. Over a period of 3 months, urine and breath samples are collected two or three times a week for at least the first 6 weeks and once or twice weekly thereafter. For each sample that tests negative for the target drug, clients can draw slips of paper or plastic chips from a bowl for the chance of winning a prize valued from $1 to $100. Clients may also receive draws from the prize bowl for attending counseling/group therapy sessions and completing weekly activities designed to meet goals related to health (e.g., scheduling or attending a medical or nutritionist appointment, obtaining medications, recording daily medication or food consumption, exercising at a gym), sobriety (e.g., attending 12-step meetings), employment (e.g., creating a resume), and other areas. A drug-positive sample or an unexcused absence resets the number of draws to one.

Prize Incentives targets adults with substance use disorders and has also been applied to HIV-related risk behaviors. Races and ethnicities who have received Motivational Interviewing interventions include Asian, Black or African-American, Hispanic or Latino, and White. The program augments existing, usual care services in community-based treatment settings for adults who primarily abuse stimulants (especially cocaine) or opioids (especially heroin) or who have multiple substance use problems.

Readiness for dissemination ratings by
criteria = 4.0 (0.0–4.0 scale)
Implementation materials = 4.0
Training and support = 4.0
Quality assurance = 4.0

Source: Substance Abuse and Mental Health Services Administration, National Registry of Evidence-based Programs and Practices. (February 2013). Retrieved July 24, 2014, from http://www.nrepp.samhsa.gov/ViewIntervention.aspx?id=344

interpersonal therapies for people with dual diagnoses (APA, 2006). An example of contingency contracting is the "Prize Incentives Contingency Management for Substance Abuse" that is based upon operant conditioning principles, and use rewards to modify and change the occurrence of substance use behavior (Box 17.10).

Self-help group modalities and 12-step programs such as AA or NA are the primary source of support for people with substance use disorders. Research indicates that mutual-aid groups such as AA are also strongly associated with sustained recovery and improved health outcomes (Tusa & Burghoizer, 2013). The success of mutual self-help groups in helping these people sustain recovery is apparent by the sheer numbers of individuals with substance use disorders who use 12-step programs as their primary mode of treatment. Yet, AA does not consider itself a treatment but rather a fellowship of people who mutually support each other to sustain sobriety one day at a time. Addressing the spiritual needs of individual people and families is an essential component of comprehensive nursing care. A philosophy of spirituality and mutual support are the guiding principles of AA and NA and make it an important resource in recovery for two million people worldwide (Galanter, 2008) (Fig. 17.5).

The Mental Health Parity and Addiction Equity Act compelled health insurers to provide the same level of services for mental health and substance use treatment as physical disorders. In response, treatment for substance use has been transitioning from an episodic, disease model to a chronic care model (McLellan et al., 2014). Nurses have a key role in a chronic disease model to identify populations at risk, intervene early to prevent relapse, and use case management skills to sustain recovery.

One component of the chronic care model is teaching patients self-management skills to prevent relapse and self-harm. Self-management skills to sustain recovery include health promoting behaviors to improve nutrition and physical well-being, avoiding triggers and adopting healthy coping strategies to manage stress such as exercise or spiritual support (Bradbury-Golas, 2013; Walton-Moss, Ray, & Woodruff, 2013). Nurses apply a harm reduction approach to teach patients about sustaining sexual health to prevent HIV or other sexually transmitted diseases (Bartlett, Brown, Shattell, Wright, & Lewallen, 2013).

EVIDENCE FOR PRACTICE

A systematic review of 11 trials of nurse-conducted brief intervention for alcohol use was compared to usual treatment or physician-delivered brief intervention. In community settings, five studies found statistically significant reductions in alcohol consumption in nurse-delivered brief intervention and two trials found nurses were equally effective as physicians. Policy recommendations included adoption of nurse-delivered brief interventions for substance use as an essential standard of care by the International Council of Nurses (Joseph, Basu, Dandapani, & Krishnan, 2014).

In summary, nurses in the community can implement a wide range of evidence-based programs to decrease the morbidity and mortality associated with substance use. As healthcare educators and practitioners, nurses are leaders in ensuring that evidence-based prevention programs are available in schools and other community settings. Prevention programs are the first step in decreasing the use of substances in high-risk people, and some, such as NFP and LifeSkills Training, include motivational interviewing to address patterns of misuse or abuse. Motivational interviewing by nurses is an effective treatment intervention that can be delivered in a range of community settings such as primary care clinics or student health services (Kelly-Weeder, 2008) (Box 17.11). The National Registry of Evidence-based Programs and Practices lists programs that have demonstrated efficacy in treating individual people, couples, and families who are diagnosed with substance use disorder.

GOALS OF *HEALTHY PEOPLE 2010*

An estimated 23 million Americans are struggling with some form of substance use disorder in the United States—the highest proportion of any nation in the world. Community health nurses are at the forefront of strategic efforts to improve the health of Americans who abuse alcohol or illicit drugs in all segments of the population. Overall, almost two-thirds of the targets in *Healthy People 2010* for substance use were met or exceeded. An encouraging trend is that progress was made in achieving targets for decreasing substance use among youth. The *Healthy People 2010* Final Review (National Center for Health Statistics, 2012) found that the proportion of high school seniors who never used alcohol increased to 28%, just slightly below the target of 29%, and those who reported never using drugs increased to 53%, also just below the target of 56%. In addition, the proportion of high school students who reported riding in a car with a driver who had been drinking decreased and exceeded the *Healthy People 2010* target. While some progress has been made, there is notable work to be done especially among high-risk groups.

A goal of *Healthy People 2010* was to reduce the percentage of college students engaging in binge drinking by roughly half from 39% in 1998 to 20% in 2010. The proportion of adults who engaged in binge drinking in the past month actually changed very little, increasing 2.5% over the same tracking period, from 24.3% to 24.9%, and moving away from the 2010 target. Between 1998 and 2009,

box 17.11 Motivational Interviewing Interventions in Community Settings

Motivational Interviewing (MI) is a goal-directed, client-centered counseling style for eliciting behavioral change by helping clients to explore and resolve ambivalence. The operational assumption in MI is that ambivalent attitudes or lack of resolve are the primary obstacles to behavioral change, so that the examination and resolution of ambivalence becomes its key goal. MI has been applied to a wide range of problem behaviors related to alcohol and substance abuse, as well as health promotion, medical treatment adherence, and mental health issues. Although many variations in technique exist, the MI counseling style generally includes the following elements:

- Establishing rapport with the client and listening reflectively
- Asking open-ended questions to explore the client's own motivations for change
- Affirming the client's change-related statements and efforts
- Eliciting recognition of the gap between current behavior and desired life goals
- Asking permission before providing information or advice
- Responding to resistance without direct confrontation
- Encouraging the client's self-efficacy for change
- Developing an action plan to which the client is willing to commit

Motivational Interviewing targets adults and adolescents in urban and suburban areas. Races and ethnicities who have received MI interventions include Asian, Black or African-American, Hispanic or Latino, and White.

Readiness for dissemination ratings by criteria = 4.0 (0.0–4.0 scale)
Implementation materials = 4.0
Training and support = 4.0
Quality assurance = 4.0

Source: Substance Abuse and Mental Health Services Administration, National Registry of Evidence-Based Programs and Practices. (September 2013). Retrieved July 24, 2014, from http://www.nrepp.samhsa.gov/ViewIntervention.aspx?id=346

steroid use among high school seniors also moved away from the *Healthy People 2010* target and increased 29.4%. The increased perception of high risk was associated with exposure to public service announcements warning of the dangers of steroid use, lending support to the ability of professional athletes to influence healthy behavior among adolescents, especially among minority youth who had the highest perception of risk (Denham, 2009).

The *Healthy People 2010* Final Review (2012) found that the proportion of adults using illicit drugs in the past month did not change over the decade, and the disparity between non-Hispanic Whites, who had the highest rate of illicit drug use, and Asian or Pacific Islanders, who had the lowest rate of illicit drug use, increased by 269.3% points. Drug-induced deaths were also highest among non-Hispanic Whites, and increased 85.3% from 1999 to 2007. Consistent with these trends, drug-related emergency department visits moved away from the target and increased 27.4% between 2004 and 2009. The increase in mortality and emergency department visits may in part reflect the sharp increase in prescriptions for opioid medications and the precipitous rise in methadone-related deaths described in the GAO (2009) report discussed earlier. The fact that increasing numbers of Americans are currently having difficulty accessing specialty treatment for substance abuse is especially troubling, given predictions that there will be an even greater reliance on state and local revenues to support substance abuse treatment in the future.

> *Everybody needs a way out of that pain. Many people choose drugs and alcohol. Some people obsessively exercise or develop strange dietary habits, which is what I did. At least it got me toward a path of healthier living.*
>
> **Mariel Hemingway**

key concepts

- The United States leads the world in rates of substance use. Patterns of substance dependence vary by age, gender, race, ethnicity, and geographic location.
- Across the life span, the age cohorts at high risk for morbidity associated with substance use disorder include pregnant women, children younger than 14 years, college students, and older adults in the baby boom generation.
- Environmental factors, such as poverty, lack of access to health services, and the capacity of law enforcement to constrain supply, contribute to a disproportionate burden of harms associated with substance use among Native Americans, Alaskan Natives, and African-Americans.
- Biopsychosocial risk factors in substance use disorder include genetic history, family history, history of trauma, early initiation, and environmental factors such as poverty or group affiliation, sexual or other abuse.
- Substance use disorders have high comorbidity with major mental illness and increase the risk for chronic health conditions such as HIV.
- Evidence-based substance use prevention programs implemented in community settings are empirically proven to be effective in decreasing substance use in targeted populations.
- Substance use treatment need not be voluntary to help people achieve recovery. The most effective treatment involves a multimodal approach with interventions such as motivational interviewing, opioid substitution programs, family therapy or couples therapy, and 12-step self-help groups.

critical thinking questions

1. How do you think the values of different stakeholders such as the alcohol industry, local communities, law enforcement, public health organizations, nurse researchers, nurse clinicians in alcohol treatment facilities, and college students would affect the identification of "social harms" associated with alcohol abuse or misuse?
2. In what ways are the social harms associated with substance use different across the life span?
3. Why are some communities disproportionately impacted by the social harms associated with illicit drug use and what are the implications for nursing practice?
4. Do you think the general public's perception of the social harms associated with alcohol, tobacco, and cannabis has changed? Why?
5. What are the essential elements needed in prevention programs to change people's perceptions of the social harms associated with substance use?
6. Contingency management incentives give prizes, cash, or vouchers for substance abstinence. What are your views about providing pregnant women who are actively abusing teratogenic substances monetary incentives to abstain? In framing your response, consider the ANA Code of Ethics.

7. The United States prides itself on having the premier healthcare system in the world. Yet the "immigrant" paradox suggests the longer immigrants reside in the United States, the more likely they are to adopt substance use behaviors that result in the highest morbidity and mortality in world. How would you propose community health nurses intervene to mitigate acculturation influences on substance use?

8. How do you anticipate the legalization of cannabis in some states will impact that prevalence of cannabis use among children and adolescents? Discuss what, if any, effect there may be on development, academic attainment, and behavioral health.

community resources

- Local methadone treatment center
- NFP to help first-time mothers succeed
- LifeSkills training: evidence-based prevention program for schools, families, and communities
- Gatekeeper program: a proactive community training program to identify at-risk, home-dwelling older adults
- Alcoholics Anonymous
- Narcotics Anonymous

references

American Journal of Nursing. (2014). Heroin: Life, death and politics: A heroin epidemic spurs new laws as nurses work to prevent deaths. *American Journal of Nursing*, *114*(5), 22–23.

American Psychiatric Association. (2013). *Diagnostic and statistical manual of mental disorders (DSM-V)* (5th ed.). Arlington, VA: APA Press.

American Psychiatric Association. (2006). *Practice guidelines for the treatment of psychiatric disorders*. Arlington, VA: APA Press.

Annas, G. J. (2001). Testing poor pregnant women for cocaine—Physicians as police investigators. *New England Journal of Medicine*, *344*(22), 1729–1732.

Bartlett, R., Brown, L., Shattell, M., Wright, T., & Lewallen, L. (2013). Harm reduction: Compassionate care of persons with addictions. *MedSurg Nursing*, *22*(6), 349–358.

Berg, J. P., Lynch, M. E., & Coles, C. D. (2008). Increased mortality among women who drank alcohol during pregnancy. *Alcohol*, *42*, 603–610.

Bertrand, J. (2009). Interventions for children with fetal alcohol spectrum disorders (FASDs): Overview for findings for five innovative research projects. *Research in Developmental Disabilities*, *30*, 986–1006.

Bertrand, J., Floyd, R. L., & Weber, M. K. (2005). Guidelines for identifying and referring persons with fetal alcohol syndrome. *Morbidity and Mortality Weekly Report*, *54*(RR11), 1–17.

Birckmayer, J., Fisher, D. A., Holder, H. D., & Yacoubian, G. S. (2008). Prevention of methamphetamine abuse: Can existing evidence inform community prevention. *Journal of Drug Education*, *38*(2), 147–165.

Bluthenthal, R. N., Heinzerling, K. G., Anderson, R., Flynn, N. M., & Kral, A. H. (2008). Approval of syringe exchange programs in California: Results from a local approach to HIV prevention. *American Journal of Public Health*, *98*(2), 278–283.

Bradbury-Golas, K. (2013). Health promotion and prevention stratagies. *Nursing Clinics of North America*, *48*, 469–483.

Centers for Disease Control and Prevention. (2012). Community based opioid overdose prevention programs providing naloxone–United States, 2010. *Morbidity and Mortality Weekly Report*, *61*, 186–193.

Centers for Disease Control and Prevention. (2009). *HIV/AIDS surveillance report, 2007* (Vol. 19). Atlanta: U.S. Department of Health and Human Services, Centers for Disease Control and Prevention.

Centers for Disease Control and Prevention. (2005a). Acute public health consequences of methamphetamine laboratories—16 states, January 2000–June 2004. *Morbidity and Mortality Weekly Report*, *54*(14), 356–359.

Centers for Disease Control and Prevention. (2005b). Update: Syringe exchange programs—United States, 2002. *Morbidity and Mortality Weekly Report*, *54*(27), 673–676.

Chang, G. (2005). Screening and brief intervention in prenatal care settings. *Alcohol Research and Health*, *28*(2), 80–84.

Chasnoff, I. J., Burns, W. J., Schnoll, S. H., & Burns, K. S. (1985). Cocaine use in pregnancy. *New England Journal of Medicine*, *313*, 666–669.

Clark, D. B., Thatcher, D. L., & Tapert, S. F. (2008). Alcohol, psychological dysregulation, and adolescent brain development. *Alcoholism: Clinical and experimental research*, *32*(3), 375–385.

Cleveland, M. J., Feinberg, M. E., Bontempo, D. E., & Greenberg, M. T. (2008). The role of risk and protective factors in substance use across adolescence. *Journal of Adolescent Health*, *43*, 157–164.

Cooper, H., Friedman, S. R., Tempalski, B., Friedman, R., & Keem, M. (2005). Racial-ethnic disparities in injection drug use in large US metropolitan areas. *Annuals of Epidemiology*, *15*, 326–334.

Cranford, J. A., Eisenberg, D., & Serras, A. L. M. (2009). Substance use behaviors, mental health problems and use of mental health services in a probability sample of college students. *Addictive Behaviors*, *34*, 134–145.

Crome, L., & McLellan, A.T. (2014). Editorial: A new public understanding about addiction. *Public Health Reviews*, *14*(2). Online publication. Retrieved July 24, 2014, from http://www.publichealthreviews.eu/show/i/14

Curtis, B. L., McLellan, A. T., & Gabellini, B.N. (2014). Translating SBIRT to public school settings: An initial test of feasibility. *Journal of Substance Abuse Treatment*, *46*, 15–21.

Dawley, K., Loch, J., & Bindrich, I. (2007). The nurse-family partnership. *American Journal of Nursing*, *107*(11), 60–67.

Degenhardt, L., Chiu, W. T., Conway, K., Dierker, L., Glantz, M., Kalaydjian, A., ... Kessler, R. C. (2009). Does the 'gateway' matter? Associations between the order of drug use initiation and the development of drug dependence in the National Comorbidity Study Replication. *Psychological Medicine*, *39*, 157–167.

DeJong, W., Larimer, M. E., Wood, M. D., & Hartman, R. (2009). NIAAA's rapid response to college drinking problems initiative:

references (continued)

Reinforcing the use of evidenced-based approaches in college alcohol prevention. *Journal of Studies in Alcohol and Drugs*, (Suppl. 16), 5–11.

Denehy, J. (2006). The meth epidemic: Its effect on children and communities. *Journal of School Nursing, 22*(2), 63–65.

Denham, B. E. (2009). Determinants of anabolic-androgenic steroid risk perceptions in youth populations: A multivariate analysis. *Journal of Health and Social Behavior, 50*(3), 277–292.

Denny, C. H., Tsai, J., Floyd, R. L., & Green, P. P. (2009). Alcohol use among pregnant and nonpregnant women of childbearing age—United States 1991–2005. *Morbidity and Mortality Weekly Report, 58*(19), 529–536.

Doe-Simkins, M., Quinn, E., Xuan, Z., Sorensen-Alawad, A., Hackman, H., Al Ozonoff., & Walley, A. Y. (2014). Overdose rescues by trained and untrained participants and change in opioid use among substance-using participants in overdose education and naloxone distribution programs: A retrospective cohort study. *BMC Public Health, 14*, 297. Advance online publication. doi:10.1186/1471-2458-14-297.

Donelan-McCall, N., Eckenrode, J., & Olds, D. L. (2009). Home visiting for the prevention of child maltreatment: Lessons learned during the past 20 years. *Pediatric Clinics of North America, 56*, 389–403.

Dowling, G. J., Weiss, S. R. B., & Condon, T. P. (2008). Drugs of abuse and the aging brain. *Neuropsychopharmacology, 33*, 209–218.

Edwards, R. W., Stanley, L., Plested, B. A., Marquart, B. S., Chen, J., & Thurman, P. J. (2007). Disparities in young adolescent inhalant use by rurality, gender and ethnicity. *Substance Use and Misuse, 42*, 643–670.

Ehrlich, P. F., Hague, A., Swisher-McClure, S., & Helmkamp, J. (2006). Screening and brief intervention for alcohol problems in a university student health clinic. *Journal of American College Health, 54*, 279–287.

Fleming, M. F. (2005). Screening and brief intervention in primary care settings. *Alcohol Research and Health, 28*(2), 57–62.

Foote, J., Wilkens, C., & Vavgiakis, P. (2004). A national survey of alcohol screening and referral in college health centers. *Journal of American College Health, 52*, 149–157.

Galanter, M. (2008). Spirituality, evidence-based medicine and alcoholics anonymous. *American Journal of Psychiatry, 165*(12), 1514–1517.

Gerra, G., Maremmani, I., Capovani, B., Somaini, L., Berterame, S., Tomas-Rossello, J., … Kleber, H. (2009). Long-acting opioid-agonists in the treatment of heroin addiction. *Substance Use & Misuse, 44*(5), 663–671.

Goldstein, R. A., DesLauriers, C., & Burda, A. M. (2009). Cocaine: History, social implication and toxicity—a review. *Disease-a-Month, 55*(1), 6–38.

Government Accountability Office. (2009). *Methadone associated overdose deaths: Factors contributing to increased deaths and efforts to prevent them* (March. GAO-09–341). Washington, DC: U. S. Government Accountability Office.

Greenbaum, P. E., DelBoca, F. K., Darkes, J., Wang, C. P., & Goldman, M. S. (2005). Variation in the drinking trajectories of freshman college students. *Journal of Consulting and Clinical Psychology, 73*, 229–238.

Han, B., Gfroerer, J. C., Colliver, J. D., & Penne, M. A. (2009). Substance use disorder among older adults in the United States in 2020. *Addiction, 104*, 88–96.

Harrison, P. A., & Sidebottom, A. C. (2009). Alcohol and drug use before and during pregnancy: An examination of use patterns and predictors of cessation. *Maternal Child Health Journal, 13*, 386–394.

Haug, N. A., Duffy, M. & McCaul, M. E. (2014). Substance abuse treatment services for pregnant women: Psychosocial and behavioral approaches. *Obstetric and Gynecology Clinics of North America, 41*, 267–296.

Hingston, R., Zha, W., & Weitzman, E. R. (2009). Magnitude of and trends in alcohol-related mortality and morbidity among U. S. college students ages 18–24, 1998–2005. *Journal of Studies on Alcohol and Drugs*, (Suppl. 16), 12–20.

Hogue, A., Henderson, C. E., Ozechowski, T. J., & Robbins, M. S. (2014). Evidence base on outpatient behavioral treatments for adolescent substance use: Updates and recommendations 2007–2013. *Journal of Clinical Child & Adolescent Psychology*, Advance online publication. doi:10.1080/15374416.2014.915550.

Humphreys, K., Wing, S., McCarty, D., Chappel, J., Gallant, L., & Haberle, B. (2004). Self-help organizations for alcohol and drug problems: Toward evidence-based practice and policy. *Journal of Substance Abuse Treatment, 26*, 151–158.

Joseph, J., Basu, D., Dandapani, M., & Krishnan, N. (2014). Are nurse-conducted brief interventions (NCBIs) efficacious for hazardous or harmful alcohol use? A systematic review. *International Nursing Review, 61*, 203–210.

Kelly-Weeder, S. (2008). Binge drinking in college-aged women: Framing a gender-specific prevention strategy. *Journal of the American Academy of Nurse Practitioners, 20*(12), 577–584.

Kidorf, M., & King, V. L. (2008). Expanding the public health benefits of syringe exchange programs. *The Canadian Journal of Psychiatry, 53*(8), 487–495.

Lawrinson, P., Ali, R., Buavirat, A., Chiamwongpaet, S., Dvoryak, S., Habrat, B., … Zhao, C. (2008). Key findings from the WHO collaborative study on substitution therapy for opioid dependence and HIV/AIDS. *Addiction, 103*, 1484–1492.

Lee, S., Aos, S., & Miller, M. (2008). *Evidence-based programs to prevent children from entering and remaining in the child welfare system: Benefits and costs for Washington* (Document No. 08-07-3901). Olympia, WA: Washington State Institute for Public Policy.

Levit, D. R., Kassed, C. A., Coffey, R. M., Mark, T. L., Stranges, E. M., Buck, J. A., & Vandivort-Warren, R. (2008). Future funding for mental health and substance abuse: Increasing burdens for the public sector. *Health Affairs, 27*(6), 513–522.

Li, K., & Wen, M. (2013). Substance use, age at migration and length of residence among adult immigrants in the United States. *Journal of Immigrant Minority Health*. Advance online publication. doi:10.1007/s10903-013-9887-4.

Lofwall, M. R., Schuster, A., & Strain, E. C. (2008). Changing profile of abused substances by older persons entering treatment. *The Journal of Nervous and Mental Disease, 196*, 898–905.

Mathers, B. M., Degenhardt, L., Phillips, B., Wiessing, L., Hickman, M., Strathdee, S. A., … Mattick, R. P.; 2007 Reference Group to the UN on HIV and Injecting Drug Use. (2008). Global epidemiology of injecting drug use and HIV among people who inject drugs: A systematic review. *The Lancet, 372*, 1733–1745.

Mattick, R. P., Kimber, J., Breen, C., & Davoli, M. (2008). Buprenorphine maintenance versus placebo or methadone maintenance for opioid dependence. *Cochrane Database of Systematic Reviews, 16*(2), CD002207.

May, P. A., Gossage, J. P., Kalberg, W. O., Robinson, L. K., Buckley, D., Manning, M., & Hoyme, H. E. (2009). Prevalence and epidemiologic characteristics of FASD from various research methods with an emphasis on recent in-school studies. *Developmental Disabilities Research Review, 15*(3), 176–92.

McCabe, S. E., Cranford, J. A., & West, B. T. (2008). Trends in prescription drug abuse and dependence, co-occurrence with other substance use disorders, and treatment utilization: Results from two national surveys. *Addictive Behaviors, 33*, 1297–1305.

McGuinness, T. (2006). Methamphetamine abuse. *American Journal of Nursing, 106*(12), 54–58.

McLellan, A. T., Starrels, J. L., Tai, B., Gordon, A. J., Brown, R., Ghitza, U., … McNeely, J. (2014). Can substance use disorders be managed using the chronic care model? Review and recommendations from a NIDA consensus group. *Public Health*

Reviews, *35*(2). Advance online publication. Retrieved July 24, 2014, from http://www.publichealthreviews.eu/show/i/14

Mermelstein, R. J. (2014). Adapting to a changing tobacco landscape: Research implications for understanding and reducing youth tobacco use. *American Journal of Preventive Medicine*, *47*(2S1), S87–S89.

Mitka, M. (2005). Meth lab fires put heat on burn centers. *JAMA*, *294*(16), 2009–1010.

Mitchell, S. G., Gryczynski, J., O'Grady, K. E., & Schwartz, R. P. (2013). SBIRT for adolescent drug and alcohol use: Current status and future directions. *Journal of Substance Abuse Treatment*, *44*, 463–472.

Monsen, R. B. (2009). Prevention is best for fetal alcohol syndrome. *Journal of Pediatric Nursing*, *24*(1), 60–61.

Naegle, M. (2008). Screening for alcohol use and misuse in older adults. *American Journal of Nursing*, *108*(11), 50–58.

National Center for Health Statistics. (2012). *Final Report Healthy People 2010* (DHHS publication No. (PHS)2012–1038. 0276–4733). Hyattsville, MD.: U.S Government Printing Office. Retrieved May 28, 2013, from http://www.cdc.gov/nchs/data/hpdata2010/hp2010_final_review.pdf

National Institute on Alcohol Abuse and Alcoholism. (2009). *Collaborative studies on genetics of alcoholism (COGA)*. U.S. Department of Health and Human Services.

National Institute on Alcohol Abuse and Alcoholism. (2007). *What college need to know now: An update on college drinking research*. U.S. Department of Health and Human Services. National Institutes of Health Publication No. 07–5010.

Oslin, D. W. (2005). Evidence-based treatment of geriatric substance abuse. *Psychiatric Clinics of North America*, *28*, 897–911.

Oslin, D. W., Slaymaker, V. J., Blow, F. C., Owen, P. L., & Colleran, C. (2005). Treatment outcomes for alcohol dependence among middle aged and older adults. *Addictive Behavior*, *30*, 1431–1436.

Peek, C. J., & The National Integration Academy Council. (2013). *Lexicon for behavioral health and primary care integration: Concepts and definitions developed by expert consensus* (AHRQ Pub. No. 13-IP001-EF). Rockville, MD: AHRQ. Retrieved July 22, 2014, from http://integrationacademy.ahrq.gov/sites/default/files/Lexicon.pdf

Perron, B. E., & Howard, M. O. (2009). Adolescent inhalant use, abuse and dependence. *Addiction*, *104*, 1185–1192.

Prescott, C. A., Madden, P. A. F., & Stallings, M. C. (2006). Challenges in genetic studies of the etiology of substance use and substance use disorders: Introduction to the special issue. *Behavioral Genetics*, *36*, 473–482.

Qureshi, A., Campayo, G. J., Eiroa-Orosa, F. J., Sobradiel, N., Collazos, F., Febrel Bordejé, M., … Casas, M. (2014). Epidemiology of substance abuse among migrants compared to native born population in primary care. *American Journal on Addiction*, *23*, 337–342.

Rothman, E. F., Edwards, E. M., Heeren, T., & Hingston, R. W. (2008). Adverse childhood experiences predict earlier age of drinking onset: Results from a representative U.S. sample of current or former drinkers. *Pediatrics*, *122*, e298–e304.

Salas-Wright, C. P. & Vaughn, M. G. (2014). A "refugee paradox" for substance use disorders? *Drug and Alochol Dependence*. Advance online publication. doi:j.drugalcdep.2014.06.008

Savage, J. E., & Mezuk, B. (2014). Psychosocial and contextual determinants of alcohol and drug use disorders in the National Latino and Asian American study. *Drug and Alcohol Dependence*, *139*, 71–78.

Savage, C., & Finnell, D. (2013). Screening, brief intervention and referral to treatment (SBIRT). *Journal of Addictions Nursing*, *24*(3), 195–198.

Schaus, J. F., Sole, M. L., McCoy, T. P., Mullett, N., Bolden, J., Sivasithamparam, J., & O'Brien, M. C. (2009). Screening for high-risk drinking in a college student health center: Characterizing students based on quantity, frequency and harms. *Journal of Studies on Alcohol and Drugs*, (Suppl. 16), 34–44.

Schaus, J. F., Sole, M. L., McCoy, T. P., Mullett, N., & O'Brien, M. C. (2009). Alcohol screening and brief intervention in a college student health center: A randomized controlled trial, *Journal of Studies on Alcohol and Drugs*, (Suppl. 16), 131–141.

Spoth, R. L., Randall, G. K., Trudeau, L., Shin, C., & Redmond, C. (2008). Substance use outcomes 5 ½ years past baseline for partnership-based family-school preventive interventions. *Drug and Alcohol Dependence*, *96*, 57–68.

Stanley, L. R., Harness, S. D., Swaim, R. C., & Beauvais, F. (2014). Rates of substance use of American Indian students in 8th, 10th and 12th grades living on or near reservations: Update, 2009–2012. *Public Health Reports*, *129*, 156–163.

Strobbe, S. (2013). Addressing substance use in primary care. *The Nurse Practitioner*, *38*(10), 45–53.

Substance Abuse and Mental Health Services Administration. (2013). *Results from the 2012 National Survey on Drug Use and Health: Summary of national findings* (NSDUH Series H-46, HHS Publication No. (SMA) 13-4795). Rockville, MD: Substance Abuse and Mental Health Services Administration. Retrieved July 24, 2014, from http://www.samhsa.gov/data/NSDUH/2012SummNatFindDetTables/NationalFindings/NSDUHresults2012.pdf

Substance Abuse and Mental Health Services Administration. (2012a). *Results from the 2011 National Survey on Drug Use and Health: Summary of national findings* (NSDUH Series H-44, HHS Publication No. (SMA) 12-4713). Rockville, MD: Substance Abuse and Mental Health Services Administration.

Substance Abuse and Mental Health Services Administration. (2012b). *Results from the 2011 National Survey on Drug Use and Health: Mental health findings* (NSDUH Series H-45, HHS Publication No. (SMA) 12-4725). Rockville, MD: Substance Abuse and Mental Health Services Administration.

Substance Abuse and Mental Health Services Administration, Center for Behavioral Health Statistics and Quality. (2012c). *Treatment Episode Data Set (TEDS): 2000-2010. National admissions to substance abuse treatment services* (DASIS Series S-61, HHS Publication No. (SMA) 12-4701). Rockville, MD: Substance Abuse and Mental Health Services Administration.

Substance Abuse and Mental Health Services Administration, Center for Substance Abuse Treatment. (2012d). *Substance abuse among older adults*. Treatment Improvement Protocol (TIP) Series, No. 26, (HHS Publication No. (SMA) 12-3918). Rockville, MD: Substance Abuse and Mental Health Services Administration.

Substance Abuse and Mental Health Services Administration, Center for Substance Abuse Treatment. (2009). *Buprenorphine: A guide for nurses*. Technical Assistance Publication (TAP) Series 30, (DHHS Publication No. SMA 09-4376).

Substance Abuse and Mental Health Services Administration, Center for Abuse Prevention. (2008). *Substance abuse prevention dollars and cents: A cost-benefit analysis*. U.S. Department of Health and Human Services. (DHHS Pub. No. (SMA) 07–4298).

Substance Abuse and Mental Health Services Administration (SAMHSA), Office of Applied Studies (February 7, 2008). *The DASIS Report: Primary methamphetamine/amphetamine admissions to substance abuse treatment: 2005*. Rockville, MD.

Thompson, B. L., Levitt, P., & Stanwood, G. D. (2009). Prenatal exposure to drugs: Effects on brain development and implications for policy and education. *Nature Reviews in Neuroscience*, *10*, 303–312.

Tillett, J., & Osborne, K. (2001). Substance abuse by pregnant women: Legal and ethical concerns. *The Journal of Perinatal Neonatal Nursing*, *14*(4), 1–11.

Toumbourou, J. W., Stockwell, T., Neighbors, C., Marlatt, G. A., Sturge, J., & Rehm, J. (2007). Interventions to reduce harm associated with adolescent substance use. *The Lancet*, *369*, 1391–1401.

references (continued)

Trinite, T., Loveland-Cherry, C., & Marion, L. (2009). The U. S. Preventive Services Task Force: An evidenced-based prevention resource for nurse practitioners. *Journal of the American Academy of Nurse Practitioners, 21*, 301–306.

Tsai, J., Floyd, R. L., & Bertrand, J. (2006). Tracking binge drinking among U. S. childbearing-age women. *Preventive Medicine, 44*(4), 298–302.

Tusa, A. L. & Burghoizer, J. A. (2013). Came to believe: Spirituality as a mechanism of change in alcoholics anonymous. A review of the literature from 1992 to 2012. *Journal of Addictions Nursing, 24*(4), 237–246.

Urada, D., Teruya, C., Gelberg, L., & Rawson, R. (2014). Integration of substance use disorder services with primary care: Health center surveys and qualitative interviews. *Substance Abuse Treatment, Prevention and Policy, 9*(15). Advance online publication. doi:10.1186/1747-597X-9-15.

U.S. Preventive Services Task Force. (2014). Primary care behavioral interventions to reduce illicit drug and nonmedical pharmaceutical use in children and adolescents: Clinical summary of U.S. Preventive Services Task Force Recommendation. *Annals of Internal Medicine, 160*(9), 635–640.

U.S. Preventive Services Task Force. (2013). *Screening and behavioral counseling interventions in primary care to reduce alcohol misuse: Recommendation statement.* AHRQ Publication No. 12-05171-EF-3. Retrieved July 8, 2014, from: http://www.uspreventiveservicestaskforce.org/uspstf12/alcmisuse/alcmisusefinalrs.htm

United Nations Office on Drug and Crime. (2012). *World Drug Report*. Vienna: United Nations.

Villarreal, H., & Fogg, C. (2006). Syringe-exchange programs and HIV prevention. *American Journal of Nursing, 106*(5), 58–63.

Walton-Moss, B., Ray, E. M., & Woodruff, K. (2013). Relationship of spirituality or religion to recovery from substance abuse. *Journal of Addictions Nursing, 24*(4), 217–226.

Waszynski, C. M. (2007). The Confusion Assessment Method (CAM). *Best practices in nursing care to older adults, 13.* Retrieved from www.ConsultFeriRN.org

Whiteford, H. A., Degenhardt, L., Rehm, J., Baxter, A. J., Ferrari, A. J., Erskine, H., … Vos, T. (2013). Global burden of disease attributable to mental and substance use disorders: Findings from the Global Burden of Diseases Study 2010. *Lancet, 382*, 1575–1586.

World Health Organization. (2014a). *Global status report on alcohol and health*. Luxembourg: World Health Organization.

World Health Organization. (2014b). *Guidelines for the identification and management of substance use and substance use disorders in pregnancy*. Geneva: World Health Organization.

Williams, J. F., Storck, M., & Committee on Substance Abuse and the Committee on Native American Child Health. (2007). Inhalant abuse. *Pediatrics, 119*, 1009–1017.

Wu, L. T., Blazer, D. G., Swartz, M. S., Burchett, B., Brady, K. T.; NIDA AAPI Workgroup. (2013). Illicit and nonmedical drug use among Asian Americans, Native Hawaiians/Pacific Islanders and mixed race individuals. *Drug and Alcohol Dependence, 133*, 360–367.

suggested readings

Affordable Care Act Mandated Prevention Services. *Alcohol Misuse screening and counseling. Depression screening for adult. Tobacco Use screening for all adults and cessation interventions for tobacco users.* Retrieved on July 8, 2014 from: https://www.healthcare.gov/what-are-my-preventive-carebenefits/#part=1

SAMHSA – Substance Abuse and Mental Health Services Administration. *SBIRT–Screening, brief intervention, and referral to treatment.* Retrieved July 8, 2014, from Beta.samhsa.gov/sbirt

web resources

Please visit thePoint® for up-to-date web resources on this topic.

CHAPTER 18

Underserved Populations

Rosanna F. DeMarco

Being unwanted, unloved, uncared for, forgotten by everybody, I think that is a much greater hunger, a much greater poverty than the person who has nothing to eat.

Mother Teresa

No matter what people tell you, words and ideas can change the world.

Robin Williams

There is a lot that happens around the world we cannot control. We cannot stop earthquakes, we cannot prevent droughts, and we cannot prevent all conflict, but when we know where the hungry, the homeless and the sick exist, then we can help.

Jan Schakowsky, American Congresswoman

By trying we can easily endure adversity. Another man's, I mean.

Mark Twain

chapter highlights

- Vulnerable versus underserved populations
- Genomics and underserved populations
- Health priorities in rural areas, particularly elders
- Health priorities in gay, lesbian, bisexual, and transgender people; in people in correctional institutions; and in people who are homeless
- Access to quality care
- Chronic disease management
- Health personnel issues
- Risk, prevention, and health promotion in hard-to-reach populations

objectives

- Identify situations that make populations underserved.
- Apply recommendations from *Healthy People 2020* initiatives to meet individual, family, and population health needs.
- Discuss creative solutions such as increased use of Internet technologies to build participation and capacity in underserved populations.
- Compare and contrast population-based healthcare needs with unique needs of other population groups (urban, heterosexual, homeless dwellers).

key terms

Genomics: The study of DNA sequencing to analyze the function and structure of complete sets of DNA in a cell of an organism.

Health professional shortage area (HPSA): Geographic area, population group, or medical facility with shortages of healthcare professionals that may not allow a full complement of healthcare services.

Inmate: A person who is held in a jail or prison to protect the public.

Medically underserved area (MUA): Area that is determined through calculation of a ratio of primary medical care physicians per 1,000 population, infant mortality rate, percentage of the population with incomes below the poverty level, and percentage of the population aged 65 or older.

Medically underserved population (MUP): A U.S. federal designation for those populations that face economic barriers (low-income or Medicaid-eligible populations) or cultural and/or linguistic access barriers to primary medical care services.

Trimorbidity: Three common chronic illnesses of homeless people (i.e., mental illness, chronic physical illness, and substance addiction).

Underserved population: A subgroup of the population that has a higher risk of developing health problems due to a greater exposure to health risk because of marginalization in sociocultural status, access to economic resources, age, or gender.

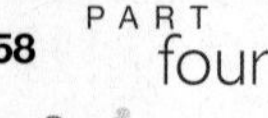

Case Studies

References to the case studies are found throughout this chapter (look for the case study icon). Readers should keep the case studies in mind as they read the chapter.

CASE 1

Lydie, an 80-year-old woman, was born in France. She came to the United States in her early 20s to be a cook for a wealthy family in a metropolitan area. She became a U.S. citizen, and when she retired in her mid-50s, she settled alone in a rural community in the United States along the Canadian border—unmarried, independent, and financially secure. She bought a small farm, raised goats, made goat cheese, and swore off any primary healthcare. She basically believed that she was in charge of her health; in reality, she found primary healthcare highly inconvenient. Although she did drive, seeing a physician or a nurse practitioner required a car ride of 90 minutes, and she had too much to do on the farm to be bothered with that commute.

Lydie fell one day while milking her goats. The mail carrier, who noticed that her mail was untouched for 3 days, found her and notified the local volunteer fire department. The moment she fractured her hip in the fall was a sentinel event that spiraled into many losses, including her farm, goats, and a life of solitude, because she had no immediate family, extended family, or friends who could help her, and little access to local healthcare that would have allowed her to stay home and enter a rehabilitation phase after surgery. Lydie died in a nursing home in a metropolitan area 150 miles away from her beloved farm 4 months after her fall. She was diagnosed with hypertension, diabetes, and congestive heart failure during her time in rehabilitation and died of complications from these comorbidities.

CASE 2

Saliha, a 15-year-old girl, has been in a youth detention facility, awaiting placement to foster care. She was arrested and brought to the center for selling marijuana in the neighborhood, as well as trading sex for money. Her home situation is less than ideal. Her mother is an active intravenous drug user and the single head of the household. Saliha is the only child living at home, and her mother, who is not a positive role model, often forgets to remind her daughter to attend school. Saliha has been living at friends' homes in the neighborhood for about 18 months, saving money she earns through selling marijuana and exchanging sex for money. She gets free healthcare at the local hospital, which has a clinic for people just like her, but she rarely follows through on any of the advice she receives from the nurses and doctors.

Saliha takes a positive step toward taking care of herself that often lasts for a month and then reverts to what she is most familiar with (i.e., a disruptive life on the streets). She frequents a place where she feels the safest, where she can get food, shower, and condoms. It is a harm reduction drop-in center. She is beginning to like and trust a nurse who volunteers there on Friday afternoons.

CASE 3

Reluctantly, Jan decides to make an appointment with her gynecologist to start having an annual Pap test. Her best friend has been diagnosed with cervical cancer, and she doesn't want this to happen to her. She has stopped seeing any sort of primary care physician, more from a sense of disillusionment than anything else. Although Jan, a bisexual woman, was once married to a man, she is now in a committed relationship with a woman. The female physician assistant (PA) who sees Jan begins to ask all the routine assessment questions, including whether Jan is sexually active and uses safe sex practices. Jan says "yes." Jan senses that the PA assumes that Jan is heterosexual, because she, the PA, refers to condoms when she discusses prevention of human immunodeficiency virus/acquired immunodeficiency syndrome (HIV/AIDS). Jan wonders why the PA doesn't ask her if she is having sex with men, women, or both, as at least a way to tailor her remarks. Jan is left feeling confused by assumptions and misdirected information.

THE CONTEXT OF HEALTH RISKS

We have a responsibility as a state to protect our most vulnerable citizens: our children, seniors, people with disabilities. That is our moral obligation. But there is an economic justification too—we all pay when the basic needs of our citizens are unmet.

John Lynch, American football player

Vulnerability

Discussions regarding the health risks of certain groups of people who have a greater disproportionate risk of poor health often identify the individual people who make up these groups as members of "vulnerable" populations. One definition of a vulnerable population comes from the seminal writing of Flaskerud and Winslow (1998)—that is, "social groups who have an increased relative risk or susceptibility to adverse health outcomes" (p. 69). Unfortunately, this definition is accurate in terms of negative outcomes complicated by struggles for the basic needs associated with a quality of life. However, vulnerability implies being a victim, with little recourse but to depend on others for help with healthcare goals and outcomes. Vulnerability seems to mean lacking sufficient ability to advance health and wellness, along with a greater need to look to others for solutions.

In reality, many people in certain groups are not served equitably by public and private healthcare infrastructures because of lack of access, racism, sexism, homophobia, and fear of what they do not understand. They constitute **underserved populations**. Here are some questions to consider about these populations.

- Why do some people have health insurance and others do not?
- Why do some have access to primary care and others end up in emergency departments for healthcare, with complex follow-up (Coddington & Sands, 2008)?
- How does shame contribute to decision-making involved in obtaining healthcare when one is ill (Rajabiun et al., 2007)?

Other people who are underserved from the perspective of healthcare include many who are not discussed in this chapter. The concept of vulnerability can apply to people with specific health conditions such as depression, schizophrenia, substance abuse, or HIV/AIDS. Even the benefits of living in a successful industrialized nation such as the United States may not include access to adequate healthcare. Unfortunately, some people continue to suffer from lack of basic assessment of their healthcare needs; from lack of assurance that the healthcare system is available and has trained professionals willing to help; and from lack of healthcare policies that specifically address the uniqueness of their needs. These people may include undocumented men, women, and children who migrate from their country to find work in rural areas; children and youth; populations with high rates of violence; frail elders who experience multiple organ failure and frequent rehospitalization; and children in foster care. In this chapter, discussion will focus on four groups of underserved people who are susceptible to adverse outcomes and, in some cases, health disparities: rural populations; prison inmates; lesbian, gay, bisexual, transgender (LGBT) people; and the homeless.

There is a hugely underserved population out there...those who are the least capable of paying pay the highest.

James Cameron, Canadian film director

Social Determinants of Health and Health Disparities

Levy and Sidel (2006) have defined social injustice as the denial of economic, sociocultural, political, civil, or human rights of certain populations or groups based on the belief of those with power that others are inferior. These authors have enhanced this definition of injustice by describing it as specific actions that fail to address what public health should be—what people do as a society to ensure existence of conditions conducive to health, or how people decide to keep everybody healthy. There are many groups that suffer social injustice related to a variety of basic needs—some may say "rights" (perhaps "inalienable rights," if one thinks about the Declaration of Independence). These groups include those classified by racial/ethnic status, age, socioeconomic status, sexual orientation, or other common characteristics. If people cannot obtain what they need from the healthcare infrastructure, or cannot enlist help when they try to build an infrastructure that addresses their needs, the results may be overwhelming. Examples of frustrations experienced by clients include long waiting periods to gain access to Medicaid coverage; negative, condescending attitudes by healthcare personnel; and complicated solutions to healthcare problems that are the antithesis of one-stop healthcare provision of services.

What is more alarming is when social injustice systematically denies equal healthcare to individual people, families, and communities while contributing to an attitude of "us and them"—those who deserve care and those who do not. The concept of health disparities is a form of systematic injustice and inequality in healthcare. According to *Healthy People 2020*, the term *disparities* often is interpreted to mean racial or ethnic disparities. However, many dimensions of disparity exist in the United States, particularly in health. "If a health outcome is seen in a greater or lesser extent between populations, there is disparity" (Healthy People 2020, 2010). Race or ethnicity, sex, sexual identity, age, disability, socioeconomic status, and geographic location all contribute to an individual's ability to achieve good health. The *Healthy People 2020* goals include a specific goal directed at eliminating heath disparities and healthcare inequities. A key operational definition, which was derived from consensus building during the construction of the *Healthy People 2020* goals, defines health disparities as systematic, plausibly avoidable health differences adversely affecting socially disadvantaged groups; they may reflect social disadvantage, but causality need not be established. This definition, grounded in ethical and human rights principles, focuses on the subset of health differences reflecting social injustice, distinguishing health disparities from other health differences also warranting concerted attention, and from health differences in general (Braveman et al., 2011). In the *Healthy People 2020* federal initiatives in the United States, the following groups are identified as needing special attention and creative solutions to live a healthy life in the face of the sobering health disparities and social injustices: (1) high-risk mothers, (2) chronically ill and disabled people, (3) people living with HIV/AIDS, (4) mentally ill people, (5) substance abusers, (6) homeless people, and (7) immigrants and refugees.

Until the great mass of the people shall be filled with the sense of responsibility for each other's welfare, social justice can never be attained.

Helen Keller

Genomics and Underserved Populations

Genomics is the study of DNA sequencing to analyze the function and structure of complete sets of DNA in a cell of an organism (Pevsner, 2009). Understanding the genetic predictors of disease through genomics is a determinant of how certain individuals, families, and communities may be disproportionately affected by illness, and why public health must be part of a practical strategy that addresses discoveries in this developing science. In many communities discussed in this chapter, screening, genetic differences, access to ethical treatment, patterns of disease prevalence, and care at secondary and tertiary levels of prevention are addressed. The application of epigenetics in these communities will affect other public health interventions.

Screening will need to be reconsidered related to specific populations who may have polygenic inheritance that is linked with what we thought were common diseases (Khoury, Janssens, & Ransohoff, 2013). For example, compared to age-based criterion for breast, colorectal, and prostate cancer screening, using polygenic risk and family history may be a more efficient way to screen, with an earlier start on screening for segments of the population at higher absolute risk (Khoury et al., 2013). According to Burton and colleagues (2013), a multidisciplinary program, which used results from the Collaborative Oncological Gene-Environment Study (COGS), identified genetic variants associated with breast, ovarian, and prostate cancers to model risk-stratified prevention for breast and prostate cancers. Implementing such strategies would require attention to the use and storage of genetic information, the development of risk assessment tools, new protocols for consent, and programs of professional education and public engagement as key in public health strategic plans of the future. Developing risk stratification will need to be changed to establish screening that is sensible and accessible, especially to those struggling with access from isolation or other barriers (Burton et al., 2013). We also know that different groups of people, based on gender or other key demographic characteristics, respond to preventive treatment differently because of their genetic makeup. For example, some genotypes may metabolize medications so differently that individuals, families, and communities might struggle with drug-seeking behaviors because accepted pain killers, such as codeine, may not work on common pain relief problems (Crews et al., 2012). Some populations may have specific vulnerability and may be subject to key environmental influences related to their health. Gomes and Pelosi (2013) discuss how the potential vulnerability to environmental changes can control gene expression in diseases of great interest in public health such as cancer, autoimmune diseases, and perhaps even the aging process. It is expected that in the future, epigenetics, the study of gene expression in the context of environment, will help guide lifestyle changes more precisely and modulate the development of disease, and thus will have a large role in prevention. Within this context of developing genomics, a variety of underserved populations are described in an attempt to understand the effects of a variety of factors that often yield outcomes fraught with challenges to public health. In the end, although genetics does not seem to fit with the notion of underserved populations, specialization in this area is evolving at the intersection of genomics with the specific diseases prevalent in populations currently underserved in the healthcare system. For example, there is a developing focus on highly prevalent chronic conditions (e.g., nicotine dependence, cancer, and obesity) which can help with the advances in treatment and prevention in communities of those who are underserved.

RURAL POPULATIONS

People who live in rural areas must fight social inequities and health disparities. The word "rural" can be a subjective interpretation of a geographic area, or it can be an area used to measure and compare predetermined characteristics established by the public and private sector. Definitions of rural areas can be based on administrative, land-use, or economic concepts, including variation of these three themes (Amber Waves, 2013; USDA, 20013b). Federal, state, and local public officials are interested in distinguishing rural from nonrural areas because they make decisions on resource distribution and other geopolitical needs. Therefore, creating a system that identifies the characteristics of an area with some level of fairness is imperative. For example, government agencies that use statistical criteria to identify areas as "rural" are the Office of Management and Budget (OMB), the U.S. Department of Commerce's Census Bureau, and the U.S. Department of Agriculture (USDA)'s Economic Research Service (ERS). In many cases, these offices categorize geopolitical sectors of the country to determine areas that need support whether from the perspective of financial backing, tax credits, or personnel.

According to the USDA, metropolitan or urban areas can be defined using several criteria (USDA, 2013b). Once this is done, nonmetropolitan (micropolitan statistical areas) or rural areas are defined by exclusion. Determining the criteria used has a great impact on the resulting classification of areas. According to the OMB (2013), each metropolitan statistical area must have at least one urbanized area of 50,000 or more inhabitants. Each micropolitan statistical area must have at least one urban cluster of at least 10,000 but less than 50,000 inhabitants. If specified criteria are met, a metropolitan statistical area containing a single core with a population of 2.5 million or more may be subdivided to form smaller groupings of counties referred to as "metropolitan divisions." As of June 6, 2003, there were 362 metropolitan statistical areas and 560 micropolitan statistical areas in the United States.

According to the United States Census Bureau (2013a), 61.7 million (25%) of the total population is rural, and according to the OMB, 55.9 million (23%) of the total population is nonmetropolitan. According to the Census Bureau (2013b), 97.5% of the total land area is rural, and according to the OMB definition, only 84% of the total land area is

table 18.1 **Urban, Urbanized Area, Urban Cluster, and Rural Population, 2010 and 2000, United States**

Area	Number of 2010 Urban Areas	Population 2010	Population 2000	Percentage of Total Population (%) 2010	Percentage of Total Population (%) 2000
United States	3,573	308,745,538	281,421,906		
Urban		249,253,271	222,360,539	80.7	79.0
Urbanized Areas	486	219,922,123	192,323,824	71.2	68.3
Urban Clusters	3,087	29,331,148	30,036,715	9.5	10.7
Rural		59,492,267	59,061,367	19.3	21.0

Source: United States Bureau of Census. (2014). Retrieved from http://www.census.gov/geo/reference/ua/urban-rural-2010.html

nonmetropolitan. The ERS estimates that, in 1990, 43% of the rural population in the United States lived in metropolitan counties. This classification of metropolitan does not truly consider the range of population density and land types between both of these extremes in populations and land area. It can be seen that determination of whether a geopolitical area is rural may vary depending on the viewpoint. See Table 18.1 for comparative data of rural and urban density between 2010 and 2000 and Box 18.1 for three primary definitions.

Rural towns aren't always idyllic. It's easy to feel trapped and be aware of social hypocrisy.

Bill Pullman, Actor

box 18.1 **Three Primary Definitions of Urban/Rural Areas**

1. The U.S. Census Bureau (http://www.census.gov/population/censusdata/urdef.txt) defines an urbanized area (UA) by population density. According to this definition, each UA includes a central city and the surrounding densely settled territory that together have a population of 50,000 or more and a population density generally exceeding 1,000 people per square mile. A "county" is a political distinction and is not incorporated in the U.S. Census Bureau classification scheme, so one UA may cover parts of several counties. Using this definition, all persons living in UAs and in places (e.g., cities, towns, and villages) with a population of 2,500 or more outside of UAs are considered the urban population. All others are considered rural.

Classification of Urban and Rural Areas (U.S. Census Bureau)

Question: How is my area classified, and where are the data?

Answer: If you want to find out the number of people within a designated area (e.g., place, county, and state) or whether it is urban or rural, do the following:

Go to https://ask.census.gov/. Select American FactFinder.

Select "Data Sets" from the listing on the left-hand side of the page.

Select "SF1" (default) on the left-hand side of the page and "Detailed Tables" on the right-hand side of the page.

Select your geographic preference (e.g., county, place, and metropolitan area) and place the exact geographic names in the box below.

Select "P2 Urban and Rural" from the table selection box and add it to the box below.

View the result.

The American FactFinder also lets users see the urban/rural components of the data shown in each of the tables found in the Summary Files. Once a user accesses a table in any of the four Summary Files, it is possible to view "Geo Components" in the "Options" menu. This lets the user see the urban/rural components, in many cases with other more narrow graduations (e.g., "Urban–in central place").

2. The Office of Management and Budget (OMB) (http://www.census.gov/population/www/estimates/metrodef.html) designates areas as metropolitan on the basis of standards released in January 1980. According to this definition, each metropolitan statistical area (MSA) must include at least one city with 50,000 or more inhabitants or an UA (defined by the Bureau of the Census) with at least 50,000 inhabitants and a total MSA population of at least 100,000 (75,000 in New England). These standards provide that each MSA must include the county in which the central city is located (the central county) and additional contiguous counties (fringe counties), if they are economically and socially integrated with the central county. Any county not included in an MSA is considered nonmetropolitan. The OMB periodically reclassifies counties on the basis of census data and population estimates.
3. The Economic Resource Service (ERS) (U.S. Department of Agriculture [USDA]) (http://www.ers.usda.gov/briefing/rurality/RuralUrbCon/) uses rural–urban continuum codes to distinguish metropolitan counties by size and nonmetropolitan counties by their degree of urbanization or proximity to metro areas. USDA defines codes 0 to 3 as metropolitan and 4 to 9 as nonmetropolitan (e.g., 4 = urban population of 20,000 or more, adjacent to a metropolitan area; and 9 = completely rural or urban population of fewer than 2,500, not adjacent to a metropolitan area).

PRACTICE POINT

It is important to remember that definitions of categories, such as urban or metropolitan and nonurban or rural, change with the new perspectives and calculations based on the census. The census data collected in 2010 will no doubt shift these classifications. This is important information for community and public health nurses to know because as leaders in health promotion, initiators of disease prevention projects, or as client advocates, nurses need to know where to access data that support the rationale of needed healthcare services or personnel. The U.S. Census Bureau has a useful area on its website that helps health professionals know how many persons live in a certain area.

Health Personnel Issues

Whether a geographic area consists of densely or less-densely populated segments, the notion of the public health core function of assurance (all people have access to healthcare) is of crucial importance in the role of the community and public health interprofessional team. A national survey supports the position that access to quality health services is the top-ranking priority among rural healthcare stakeholders and leaders, but with continued obstacles such as lack of healthcare providers and limited insurance access as a key struggle (Nelson & Gingerich, 2010). Unfortunately, healthcare providers enter rural settings in small numbers, primarily because many of them enter residency or postacademic training programs in the areas where they were educated or trained, which is often not in a rural setting (Garrison-Jakel, 2011). Programs like the Rural Health Workforce Development Program, which focuses on network development of recruiting and retaining health professionals in rural communities, may be a partial answer to the dilemma of lack of personnel (Wilkinson, 2010). Three key motivators to keep healthcare personnel engaged in coming to, and staying in, rural areas of practice must include a desire to live in a rural setting, good relationships with supervisors, and increased access with technology (Henry, Hooker, & Yates, 2012). Some feel the best way to begin to attract nurses and physicians to rural areas is to help balance urban exposure to patient care and education with rural exposure, and the best time to do this may be during student or residency years (Henry et al., 2011).

The Health Resources and Services Administration (HRSA) has developed a system for designating areas with a shortage of healthcare professionals based on certain criteria (HRSA, 2013). The HRSA then decides how to develop initiatives to train and secure health professionals to serve in these areas and to create networks of care that meet the unique needs of the populations. The use of the terms **health professional shortage areas (HPSAs)**, **medically underserved areas (MUAs)**, and **medically underserved populations (MUPs)** is part of the system that establishes a designation that becomes the focus of federal assistance. For example, if an area is designated as an HPSA or an MUA, then the HRSA can support programs to educate personnel who are needed in these areas and provide services to these areas with the help of tax dollars. It does this by soliciting grant proposals for healthcare models to meet population needs and by fiscally supporting training of healthcare personnel to meet these needs. See Box 18.2 for more information. Special attention is directed to MUPs. Underserved people may be living in the middle of a busy designated metropolitan area but are underserved for economic, cultural, or literacy reasons.

EVIDENCE FOR PRACTICE

1. The Interprofessional Rural Program of British Columbia (IRPBC) is an example of a pilot program created to recruit interprofessional health professionals for rural communities in British Columbia, Canada (Charles, Bainbridge, Copeman-Stewart, Kassam, & Tiffin, 2008). The program has given professional health training to students and has offered them the opportunity to evaluate whether this experience increases the likelihood of their working in nonurban settings after their education is complete. Researchers used interview and survey data to determine the impact of IRPBC on students and communities. The students who participated in it benefited not only from the chance to engage in rural practice but also from the opportunity to interact within an interprofessional context. The communities participating in the program profited from enhanced healthcare and the possibility of attracting new practitioners from these students.
2. Many of the interventions recommended to improve client safety have largely been based on research conducted in urban hospitals. Thornlow (2008) has demonstrated the extent and type of nursing research being conducted to advance rural-specific client safety research. The studies were conducted in various settings, with topics ranging from error reporting in hospitals to safety screening in the community. Guidance is offered for a future nursing research agenda to include the need for interprofessional research; cross-national and international collaboration; and, at a minimum, the necessity for nurse researchers to sample rural hospitals in larger studies of client safety.

Lydie lived in a nonmetropolitan, rural area that was technically classified as an MUA. As such, she inherited many prospective problems despite the numerous benefits. By moving to a less-populated area, she had more privacy, cleaner air, and less automobile traffic in a natural, country setting. However, when she became ill, shortages related to the availability of qualified, local healthcare personnel contributed significantly to primary, secondary, and tertiary prevention and her growing list of comorbid conditions and her eventual death.

- Can you determine what areas of this country are designated as a MUPs, MUAs, and HPSAs?
- Does the HRSA offer scholarships for healthcare personnel to obtain their respective degrees for entry to practice?
- If the HRSA does offer support, are there contingencies? What are they?
- How would a community and public health nurse begin to address the notion of assurance for a population of interest?

EVIDENCE FOR PRACTICE

Ligeikis-Clayton (2007) described an evening/weekend nursing program that was developed to respond to a nursing shortage and to give people an opportunity to attend school while working full-time. Advantages included small classroom settings with more interaction between students and faculty, as well as the program's serving as a vehicle for licensed practical nurses to go back to school. From a resource perspective, it was difficult to convince full-time faculty to rotate through the generic nursing program as well as this specific program. On weekends, staffing was problematic. Despite these resource issues, this program demonstrates a nontraditional way to improve access to educational opportunities and help fill a gap in health service to the community.

Morbidity and Mortality Issues

From an epidemiologic perspective, population trends indicate a primarily aging population over the past 18 years related to outward migration of youth (Faircloth, 2009). In rural areas, there is less racial diversity (residents are mostly Caucasian), although there are pockets of population diversity (Hispanics in Texas, Native Americans in Arizona and New Mexico). Other characteristics of people who live in rural areas are less college education, higher high school dropout rate, and decreased income (and thus lower socioeconomic status) (Goetzel, Liss-Levinson, Goodman, & Kennedy, 2009). On the other hand, the cost of living is lower. However, families struggle with homelessness and poverty. Females head many families. Employment opportunities are few. Because of the various constraints mentioned, women and children often are the most vulnerable and suffer the most in terms of lack of adequate healthcare. For example, women begin care in the last month of pregnancy, have babies categorized as low birth weight, and there is a larger incidence of infant mortality (Bailey & Byrom, 2007). See Box 18.3 for more detailed information.

Gamm (2007) has described rural health disparities and lack of access to care as significant but suggests that there is a need for a "meeting in the middle" of community health professionals concerning three areas: disease prevention, health promotion, and disease management. He has discussed a survey that was undertaken to gather information about key concerns that specifically relate to health in rural areas. The survey is part of the *Rural Healthy People 2020* and resembles the *Healthy People 2020* project established at the federal level, especially in terms of its priorities. The survey was undertaken by interviewing rural leaders regarding the health needs of rural communities and consequently

box 18.2 Health Professional Shortage Areas and Underserved Populations

Health professional shortage areas (HPSAs) may be designated as having a shortage of primary medical care, dental, or mental health providers. They may be urban or rural areas, population groups, or medical or other public facilities. As of March 31, 2009, there were

- **6,080 primary care HPSAs** with 65 million residents. It would take 16,585 practitioners to meet their need for primary care providers (a population-to-practitioner ratio of 2,000:1).
- **4,091 dental HPSAs** with 49 million residents. It would take 9,579 practitioners to meet their need for dental providers (a population-to-practitioner ratio of 3,000:1).
- **3,132 mental health HPSAs** with 80 million residents. It would take 5,352 practitioners to meet their need for mental health providers (a population-to-practitioner ratio of 10,000:1).

Medically Underserved Areas/ Populations:

- **Medically underserved areas (MUAs)** may be an entire county or a group of contiguous counties, a group of county or civil divisions, or a group of urban census tracts in which residents have a shortage of personal health services.
- **Medically underserved populations (MUPs)** may include groups of people who face economic, cultural, or linguistic barriers to healthcare.

Source: Health Resources and Services Administration. (2009). *Shortage designation: HPSAs, MUAs & MUPs.* Retrieved from http://bhpr.hrsa.gov/shortage

box 18.3 Health Factors and Effects of Living in Rural Geopolitical Areas

- Only about 10% of physicians practice in rural America despite the fact that nearly one-fourth of the population lives in these areas.
- Rural residents are less likely to have employer-provided healthcare coverage or prescription drug coverage, and the rural poor are less likely to be covered by Medicaid benefits than their urban counterparts.
- Although only one-third of all motor vehicle accidents occur in rural areas, two-thirds of the deaths attributed to these accidents occur on rural roads.
- Rural residents are nearly twice more likely to die from unintentional injuries, other than motor vehicle accidents, than are urban residents. Rural residents are also at a significantly higher risk of death by gunshot injuries than urban residents.
- Rural residents tend to be poorer. On the average, per capita income is $7,417 lower than in urban areas, and rural Americans are more likely to live below the poverty level. The disparity in incomes is even greater for minorities living in rural areas. Nearly 24% of rural children live in poverty.
- People who live in rural America rely more heavily on the federal Food Stamp Program, according to the Carsey Institute at the University of New Hampshire. The institute's analysis found that although 22% of Americans lived in rural areas in 2001, a full 31% of the nation's Food Stamp beneficiaries lived there. In all, 4.6 million rural residents received Food Stamp benefits in 2001, the analysis found.
- There are 2,157 health professional shortage areas (HPSAs) in rural and frontier areas of all states and U.S. territories compared with 910 in urban areas.
- Abuse of alcohol and use of smokeless tobacco is a significant problem among rural youth. The rate of driving under the influence (of alcohol) arrests is significantly greater in nonurban counties. Forty percent of rural 12th graders reported using alcohol while driving compared with 25% of their urban counterparts. Rural eighth graders are twice as likely to smoke cigarettes (26.1% vs. 12.7% in large metro areas.)
- Anywhere from 57% to 90% of first responders in rural areas are volunteers.
- There are 60 dentists per 100,000 population in urban areas versus 40 per 100,000 in rural areas.
- Cerebrovascular disease was reportedly 1.45 times higher in nonmetropolitan statistical areas (non-MSAs) than in MSAs.
- Hypertension was also higher in rural than in urban areas (101.3 per 1,000 people in MSAs and 128.8 per 1,000 people in non-MSAs.)
- Twenty percent of nonmetropolitan counties lack mental health services versus 5% of metropolitan counties. In 1999, 87% of the 1,669 mental health professional shortage areas in the United States were in nonmetropolitan counties and home to over 30 million people.
- The suicide rate among rural males is significantly higher than in urban areas, particularly among adult men and children. The suicide rate among rural women is escalating rapidly and is approaching that of men.
- Medicare payments to rural hospitals and physicians are dramatically less than those to their urban counterparts for equivalent services. This correlates closely with the fact that more than 470 rural hospitals have closed in the past 25 years.
- Medicare clients with acute myocardial infarction (AMI) who were treated in rural hospitals were less likely than those treated in urban hospitals to receive recommended treatments and had significantly higher adjusted 30-day post-AMI death rates from all causes than those in urban hospitals.
- Rural residents have greater transportation difficulties reaching healthcare providers, often traveling great distances to reach a doctor or a hospital.
- Accidents resulting in death and serious injury account for 60% of total rural accidents versus only 48% of urban. One reason for this increased rate of morbidity and mortality is that in rural areas, prolonged delays can occur between a crash, the call for emergency medical services (EMS), and the arrival of an EMS provider. Many of these delays are related to increased travel distances in rural areas and personnel distribution across the response area. National average response time from motor vehicle accident to EMS arrival in rural areas was 18 minutes, or 8 minutes greater than in urban areas.

Source: National Rural Health Association. (n.d.). *What's different about rural health care?* Retrieved from http://www.ruralhealthweb.org/go/left/about-rural-health/

establishing a ranking of rural health priorities based on many of the statistical trends previously shared (Box 18.4).

Identifying challenges is a critical aspect of rural health assessment. Creative solutions to key challenges related to access to care with the input and participation of the populations affected are critical. For example, veterans who are aging and live in rural areas are being served through a geriatric scholar program (GSP), a Department of Veterans Affairs' workforce development program directed to all disciplines working with veterans who are aging. The intent of the program is to infuse geriatric competencies in primary care using a multimodal educational program to target primary care providers and ancillary staff who work in Veteran Administration–sponsored rural clinics. GSP uses didactic presentations, webinars, audio conferences, clinical practica, and mentoring in these programs (Tumosa et al., 2012). Interprofessional teams that contain nurses are starting to make a difference in addressing the needs of people and their families in rural areas.

EVIDENCE FOR PRACTICE

1. Researchers tested a computer-based electronic screening tool (eScreening) for depression and alcohol use as a way to evaluate primary care needs of rural residents (Farrell et al., 2009). eScreening uses a portable

computer-based format. The study involved (1) a focus group with providers, (2) usability testing with selected rural clients using a computerized touch screen, and (3) implementation of the touch screen platform with a small sample in primary care to determine feasibility. Consumer response was extremely positive.

2. One study explored the incidence of depression in a sample of 48 people visiting a primary care clinic in rural southeastern North Carolina (Kemppainen, Taylor, Jackson, Kim-Godwin, & Kirby, 2009). Forty percent of the participants met the criteria of clinical depression according to the Center for Epidemiologic Studies Depression Scale (CES-D). Depression was highest in single, African-American men who were employed, with adequate health insurance. Researchers attributed this primarily to work-related stressors in dealing with overwhelming social problems of other rural residents and their own economic problems. Critical incident interviews identified self-management strategies for depression and sources of social support.
3. A program intended to encourage relationship building, called the Rural Health Roundtable Project, has prompted change in rural communities (Pennel, Carpender, & Quiram, 2008). This project involves identifying culturally relevant, sensitive topics. In an informal, social environment where participants feel comfortable sharing, targeted questions engage participants and empower local residents. Follow-up is part of the Rural Health Roundtable Project, which has demonstrated its value as an effective tool in working with rural communities. These communities, which have fewer human and financial resources at their disposal, can use the project strategies to identify and make the most of their unique strengths when responding to public health emergencies and natural disasters. Initiated in 1999, the methodology has been refined and enhanced over the past 8 years to more effectively reach participants, promote sharing and discussions, build stakeholder networks, and encourage continued communication and collaboration. The Rural Health Roundtable Project has significant potential for replication and application to all areas of rural public health.

Elderly People

Elders, who are diverse in culture and ethnicity, face many challenges as they age in rural settings. According to Krout and Kinner (2007), most elders do not live on farms. They may be isolated in a variety of housing situations, including family homes in which they brought up their families; the children may have left the area and the parents may live as widows or widowers. They have incomes that can be up to 20% lower than that of their urban counterparts because of lower social security payments, smaller levels of assets in the bank or in property, less pension coverage, and less

box 18.4 Ranking of Rural Health Priorities (*Healthy People 2010* and *Healthy People 2020* Goals)

1. Access to quality healthcare
2. Heart disease
3. Diabetes
4. Mental health and mental disorders
5. Oral health
6. Tobacco use
7. Substance abuse
8. Education and community-based programming
9. Maternal, infant, and child health
10. Nutrition and overweight
11. Cancer
12. Public health infrastructure
13. Immunization and infectious disease
14. Injury and violence prevention

Source: Office of Disease Prevention and Health Promotion, U.S. Department of Health and Human Services. (n.d.). *Healthy People 2010.* Retrieved from http://www.healthypeople.gov/

opportunity to make up the difference because of lack of part-time employment possibilities (Krout & Kinner, 2007). In many cases, fewer options for leisure and recreation are available to these older people.

What complicates these issues are the healthcare service components that are lacking, or are created on the basis of the primary mechanism of payment (i.e., Medicaid). Generally, there are fewer healthcare professionals—physicians, nurses, occupational therapists, and physical therapists—in rural areas, especially with expertise in gerontology, palliation, and end-of-life care. Lack of public transportation puts a burden on the elderly to find private transportation. If they are disabled or cannot drive, dependence for transportation rests on the network of friendships or connection to relatives that may or may not be in place.

It was once said that the moral test of government is how that government treats those who are in the dawn of life, the children; those who are in the twilight of life, the elderly; and those who are in the shadows of life, the sick, the needy, and the handicapped.

Hubert H. Humphrey

In Lydie's case, she had no relatives or friend networks available to help, primarily because she chose to live a solitary life that she thought was health-promoting for her. In the end, her approach isolated her so much that she had little recourse but to deal with her healthcare issues from a preventive perspective; she prided herself on "not needing those doctors and nurses" and not seeking any primary care treatment. In her mind, toughness in not doing this was a sign of personal and spiritual strength.

box 18.5 The Seven A's of Challenges to Elders in Rural Areas

1. Availability: Insufficient number and diversity of formal services and providers; lack of acceptable services and human service infrastructure
2. Accessibility: Shortages of adequate, appropriate, and affordable transportation; cultural and geographic isolation
3. Affordability: Poverty and inability to pay for services
4. Awareness: Low levels of information dissemination; literacy issues
5. Adequacy: Lack of service standards and evaluation; evidence-based practice compromised
6. Acceptability: Reluctance to ask for help
7. Assessment: Lack of basic information on what is needed using research rigor and analyses

Source: Krout, J. A., & Kinner, M. (2007). Sustaining geriatric rural populations. In L. L. Morgan & P. S. Fahs (Eds.), *Conversations in the disciplines: Sustaining rural populations* (pp. 63–74). Binghamton, NY: Global Academic Publishing.

When it comes to elder care in rural communities, seven factors compound disease prevention and health promotion efforts to identify and reduce modifiable risk: (1) availability, (2) accessibility, (3) affordability, (4) awareness, (5) adequacy, (6) acceptability, and (7) assessment. These are defined in Box 18.5. Community and public health nurses should discover how to deal with these issues. They should realize that they can use meeting places that seem to draw the greatest group of citizens to good effect. The nurses can work toward developing an education infrastructure to help rural citizens at least understand what modifiable risks they may be facing and how they may receive help if a coalition of requested services can be initiated. For example, in MUPs in inner cities, healthcare professionals often reach elders through churches. In rural areas, solutions may begin through education in a church, post office, or grocery store. In addition, public health nurses, in collaboration with interested citizens and other professional disciplines, can work together developing networks of volunteers to help with transportation needs or other needs that may be identified from a thorough assessment.

STUDENT REFLECTION

I will never forget my experience in the rural part of a county where I volunteered one summer to help the elderly. Although I was going into my senior year in nursing school and had explained that I wanted to help the elderly with healthcare teaching, I was initially dismayed to know that I would have to go door-to-door with a team of young adults like myself and ask whether there was any need for minor home repairs. My teammates were a physical therapy student and an occupational therapy student. The idea was to help in a practical way with minor issues in the elders' homes, and while doing this work, to take the opportunity to assess health needs and provide health education. It was the best time I had as a nursing student. I really felt as though we students were preventing problems from the beginning and dealing with problems that we found from a health and safety perspective, without shaming elders into thinking they were weak or unable to care for their needs.

Occupational and Environmental Health Problems

Occupational health is of particular concern in rural communities, where farmers live. Although the number of people who choose farming as a lifestyle choice has been decreasing steadily over the years, people who do select it as an occupation are exposed to many dangerous conditions in an environment that puts them at risk for injury or death (USDA, 2013a). Farming is a hazardous profession. The total number of agricultural fatalities has been decreasing in recent years, but according to the Bureau of Labor Statistics, 285 farmers and ranchers were killed on the job in 2007. The USDA's Cooperative State Research, Education and Extension Service (CSREES) addresses the issue of farm safety by supporting Cooperative Extension Service programs that train workers in appropriate field practices and equipment use and maintenance. In addition, CSREES supports the AgrAbility program, which reached 2,287 newly disabled farmers and ranchers through education, assistance, and networking from 2004 to 2008 (USDA, 2013a). This program used on-farm assessments and assistive technology implementation on work sites.

From a family perspective, it is often the case that parents and children help with the work on the farm so there is variability in experience and developmental knowledge. This lifestyle may contribute to injuries and a larger effect on families in general.

Finally, community and public health nurses evaluating safety must consider that farmers and their families work outdoors throughout the year in all sorts of weather and are exposed to a variety of conditions (extremes of heat and cold, snow, sleet, rain, tornados, and drought). Possible contact with chemical treatments applied to the land (e.g., pesticides, fertilizers) also adds variability to the direction of health promotion and injury prevention.

EVIDENCE FOR PRACTICE

One study has explored injuries to children that occur on farms (Morrongiello, Marlenga, Berg, Linneman, & Pickett, 2007). Researchers evaluated data to determine the interaction between risk factors for injury and actual injuries. Information about farm injuries to children in three age groups (<6 years, 6–12 years, 13+ years) was integrated with respect to factors such as the children's behavior, predictability of injury risk based on what the child had been doing, the unexpectedness of the injury, environmental events, and the level of environmental risk. Results revealed that in high-risk environments, unexpected child behavior correlated more frequently with injury risk when children younger than 6 years were injured than for older children, whereas in low-risk environments, unexpected child behavior had less effect on injury risk and showed no such age variation. With increasing age, the predictability of injury increased in a high-risk context, suggesting that children engage in increasingly hazardous activities as they develop. Consistent with this interpretation, unexpected environmental events increasingly contributed to injury in a high-risk context in the oldest age groups. The observed variations in risk factors suggest that interactions between behavioral and environmental factors are important to consider in studies of the etiology of pediatric farm injuries.

Although this chapter does not explicitly address migrant or seasonal workers' conditions on farms, these circumstances have come under scrutiny in terms of sanitation, emergency healthcare, and primary care during the time of high harvest intensity. Although workers and families who are involved in farming may vary by age and education, it is consistently the case that language barriers, health literacy, and generally lower educational status compound efforts to promote health and advance prevention by those involved with rural health initiatives.

EVIDENCE FOR PRACTICE

1. In many international settings, a relevant and sensitive approach to helping population groups obtain healthcare assistance and guidance, involves the use of health promoters. These key people can relate to specific groups with particular healthcare needs (Clark, Surry, & Contino, 2009). One study has discussed the use of this approach in rural areas. It is estimated that 9.3 million undocumented people are currently living in the United States. Not all people living within the U.S. borders benefit from the healthcare system in the United States; more than 47 million Americans have no health insurance coverage. For this reason, many use emergency departments for all of their health needs. Only one in five farm workers are able to obtain health insurance through either his or her employer or the state or federal government. The lack of health insurance makes it increasingly difficult for the uninsured and undocumented populations to obtain healthcare, and more than two-thirds of this population is living in poverty.
2. Another article has described a model of risk for HIV and problem drinking in Latino labor migrants in the United States (Organista, 2007). Specific risks that need to be addressed for this group include stressful living and working conditions, not just drinking behaviors that may compromise safe sex practices. The broader environmental risk in this unique population of Latinos needs to be addressed with a new model for interventions.

In most rural areas, the issue of access has been addressed with managed care organizations (MCOs) (Willging, Waitzkin, & Nicdao, 2008). MCOs build provider networks and encourage community health plans so that local providers of healthcare can control cost. Mobile clinics, school-based health programs, and telehealth systems (programs that use wireless and nonwireless electronic devices to communicate health information for educational or diagnostic purposes) are other ways by which distance between healthcare providers and family members can be addressed. At the local level, transportation volunteers and parish or church visitors can help decrease isolation and help families share health resources with adjacent rural areas. There needs to be a concentrated focus on prevention with particular emphasis on decreasing or eliminating smoking behaviors; decreasing sun exposure; reducing fat intake; and educating families about the signs and symptoms of depression, heart disease, diabetes, and cancer.

From a professional perspective, working in rural areas can have positive and negative aspects. In areas where people and communities have problems maintaining connections, it is important to create a way to interact, or network, with other professionals for professional support and diagnostic assistance. Working in a rural area offers opportunities to be creative and to "think outside the box" and not merely consider the usual care methodologies. Community and public health nurses have to use limited resources effectively.

The work of healthcare professionals in rural areas may not be as intensive as would be the case in a large medical center in an urban setting, or even in a community-based service in an urban setting. In areas where healthcare is intensive, there are also many opportunities to learn a specific discipline. What is intriguing and perhaps attractive in rural settings is the slower pace, with the opportunity to engage in relationships with communities that could be long-lasting and ultimately might prove more rewarding. Roles and disciplines are more blurred in rural areas because of lack of resources. So it may be the case that collaboration, interprofessional work, and self-care within the context of caregiving all become matters of pragmatic healthcare and intervention.

CORRECTIONAL HEALTH: UNDERSERVED POPULATIONS IN JAILS AND PRISONS

In the United States, detention centers, jails, and prisons are places that provide safety to the public by incarcerating people who have committed crimes and who are deemed a threat to society. There are a variety and levels of jails and prisons, ranging from detention centers, where **inmates** await arraignment or care decisions and where there is high turnover, to minimum- or maximum-security prisons, where there are longer lengths of stay for inmates in some cases. Generally, minimum- and maximum-security prisons are administered by the states, and penitentiaries are federally administered prisons in which inmates are incarcerated for crimes against the government. In correctional institutions, there is a disproportionate number of persons of color, regardless of youth, gender, and age (Zust, 2009). Incarceration may be socially determined, but in the final analysis, the health of the people in this system is compromised. Many reports contain evidence that illness and injury arrive at institutions with the inmates or detainees, occur in these areas, and recycle back into neighborhoods when inmates and detainees leave.

Maybe I won't stay out of prison. Who knows?

Jack Kevorkian

All levels of prevention need to be addressed for all people in correctional facilities. For example, the Children's Defense Fund (CDF) has taken a leadership role in addressing the issues of children being in a "pipeline" spiraling into lives of violence and crime because of a variety of negative contributing variables leading to arrest, conviction, incarceration, and death (CDF, 2009). The CDF supports initiatives at the individual, family, community, organizational, and government levels (Box 18.6). The Cradle to Prison Pipeline is a CDF campaign designed to bring public attention to this issue.

Where do you see community public health nurses contributing care and healing that relates to Saliha (see Box 18.5)? Give specific examples.

box 18.6 Solution Pyramid for Youth (Children's Defense Fund)

Individual People

- Mentor a child.
- Volunteer at an after-school program for youth.
- Vote in every election and advocate for children.
- Educate elected officials about the Cradle to Prison Pipeline.
- Host a house party to educate others about the Cradle to Prison Pipeline and what they can do to dismantle it.
- Volunteer with children who are homeless or in foster care.
- Organize a forum on incarcerated youth and the funding disparities between prisons and education in our nation.
- Volunteer your talents or professional services to help a single-parent, kinship care, or foster care family by babysitting, inviting them to events with their children, or providing transportation.
- Invite youth to events at the next educational level (i.e., taking a high school student to a college basketball game).

Families

- Spend quality time with your family (i.e., family game night, eating meals together).
- Join the Parents Teachers Association (PTA), a parent support group, or other school group.
- Attend school activities and/or volunteer in the classroom.
- Consistently praise your child's achievements in school and extracurricular activities.
- Establish and maintain a supportive home learning environment.
- Create daily homework routines and limit television viewing.
- Offer tutoring and homework help to your children or younger siblings.
- Offer to run errands or help around the house.
- Communicate with and listen to your child.
- Talk and actively listen to children within your extended family.
- Show affection, love, and respect to your child every day.
- Do something fun with your child or sibling.
- Adopt a foster child or become a foster parent.

Communities

- Institute a "cradle roll" within your faith-based institution or community, linking every child to a permanent, caring family member or adult mentor who can keep them on track and get them back on track if and when they stray.
- Promote learning by starting an after-school program for children.
- Ensure that at least one caring community member attends every public school student suspension meeting or court hearing.
- Encourage families to spend quality time together by hosting a movie or game night at your church.
- Start a support group for single-parent or kinship care families.
- Provide job opportunities and guidance for families and youth in need.
- Create college scholarships for children from disadvantaged, foster care, and kinship care families.
- Work with school officials to develop and adopt more child-appropriate discipline policies and procedures.
- Reach out to youth who are homeless or in foster care.
- Prepare care packages of new clothes, personal toiletries, and/or a welcome gift for children placed into foster care homes.
- Hold events to celebrate the strengths of our children and provide college scholarships and leadership opportunities to youth.
- Start a halfway house and counseling program for youth who have run away.
- Create a summer job opportunity for a youth.
- Create and distribute a community resource manual so that parents know where to turn for help for their families.

Organizations

- Invest in prevention and early intervention.
- Host a health fair to ensure that all children who are eligible for Medicaid or your state children's health insurance program are enrolled.
- Provide free tax filing assistance to low-income working families.

- Educate families about how they can apply for food stamps, Head Start, federal nutrition programs, and other similar benefits.
- Create and distribute a calendar of free family-friendly community events.
- Start a parent education program to familiarize parents about conflict resolution in the home and how to advocate for their children.
- Encourage alternatives to incarceration such as restitution, community service, electronic monitoring, drug rehabilitation treatment, or placement in a "staff secure" (but not locked) community corrections facility.
- Work to ensure that counseling, social services, education, and health and mental health services are provided to at-risk youth.
- Fund reinvestment in urban communities, such as parks, schools, and roads.
- Write annual child and gun violence reports to track the killing of children and call for effective gun control measures and nonviolent conflict resolution training.
- Host a Cradle to Prison Pipeline summit to connect and educate others about this "pipeline" and ways to dismantle it.

Government Agencies

- Bring other elected officials and leaders together to gain firsthand awareness of the status of your local children; demonstrate what is working and what is not.
- Ensure children in foster care and detention receive quality treatment to address their mental, behavioral, and emotional needs.
- Promote high-quality children's television programming and access to other quality electronic media.
- Provide high-quality early childhood development programs for all.
- Ensure all children and pregnant women access to affordable, seamless, comprehensive health coverage and services.
- Establish policies that emphasize prevention and rehabilitation to keep children out of or rescue them from the Pipeline.
- Expand "second chance" programs for high school dropouts, ex-offenders, and at-risk youth to secure General Equivalency Degrees (GEDs), job training, and employment.
- Reduce repeat offender rates by focusing on treatment- and family-oriented approaches.
- Make sure that every child can read at grade level by fourth grade and graduate from high school able to succeed in post-secondary education and/or work.
- Organize state and local leadership councils or committees to create strategic plans to address the learning and developmental needs of children.
- Invest money in community-based rehabilitation centers and treatment programs to serve as an alternative to juvenile detention and prison.
- Stop the criminalization of children at increasingly younger ages.
- Create partnerships with local businesses, schools, and/or churches to create quality exit programs for those leaving the juvenile justice system as a way to start them on the "Pipeline to Success."

Source: Children's Defense Fund. *Cradle to Prison Pipeline campaign—Key immediate action steps.* Retrieved from http://www.childrensdefense.org/helping-americas-children/cradle-to-prison-pipeline-campaign/action-steps.html

Most inmates are males who are African-American or Latino. The average age of inmates is 37. Prisoners who are incarcerated for violent crimes have been involved in rape, murder, sodomy, kidnapping, armed robbery, and sexual offenses, and 34% are in high- or maximum-security facilities, and 40% are serving sentences of more than 10 years. However, 75% of all prisoners are nonviolent and have been incarcerated for drug possession and trafficking, bribery, and extortion. Of those who are African-American, 14.5% are women and 52% are incarcerated primarily on drug possession or prostitution charges (U.S. Department of Justice, Bureau of Justice Statistics, 2011).

Many have conjectured that poverty, violence and abuse as children, lack of education, and poor self-esteem have made incarceration an area where those who are oppressed are further oppressed and exposed again to violence, mental health problems, and physical morbidities. Issues that face inmates, their families, and healthcare providers who work in prisons include security issues; despairing attitudes; overcrowding; and the increased risk of communicable diseases such as tuberculosis, HIV infection, sexually transmitted infections (STIs), and hepatitis C; and fragmentation of families. Community and public health nurses may find conflicts with the will of the warden or person in charge of the area of incarceration and the standards of nursing practice. For example, state nurse practice acts are in direct conflict with participation in the highly politicized issue of capital punishment. Despite the autonomous nature of nursing practice and medicine, the decision-maker in jails and prisons is often the warden or director. Thus, conflicts of interest and philosophy can and do occur (Nolan & Walsh, 2012).

After release from incarceration, inmates often face social injustices and economic problems. The ability to find appropriate shelter at a reasonable cost is becoming very difficult, as is finding social support that prevents recidivism. Trying to help families reconnect with adequate financial and rehabilitation support is extremely difficult. Literacy and job training are important family-centered approaches to maintaining a productive and financially stable life. Many men and women describe how repeating crimes that put them back in jail or prison is a way to bring them to a place where they feel protected and escape the painful realities they face on release (Zust, 2009).

What is critical to understand about those in prison returning to their home communities is how important it is to understand the integral connection and responsibility that is mutually shared. Those in charge of prison health and those in charge of health in communities need to help each other in creating the best opportunities for all types of success for citizens. Those citizens who have health problems "upstream" will bring them "downstream" and vice versa.

Probably the only place where a man can feel really secure is in a maximum security prison, except for the imminent threat of release.

Germaine Greer, Australian author

PRACTICE POINT

In the context of healthcare prevention education, one of the most important functions nurses can address when caring for people who have left correctional institutions is to discern whether the client has a health literacy challenge. Direction and encouragement of where to obtain support to advance education through a variety of extension programs and special projects can be important to preventive work at the individual, family, and community level.

Sixty percent of people entering prison today are illiterate.

Jeffrey Archer

EVIDENCE FOR PRACTICE

Out of concern that standards for pregnancy-related healthcare in jails and prisons need to be established, followed, and accredited regularly, a study specifically examined the healthcare practices of pregnant women in state prisons using a survey with 62 multiple choice questions and four open-ended questions. Wardens of 50 women's state correctional facilities were contacted to involve them in the process. Of the 50 contacted, 19 completed the survey, a 38% response rate. The findings of this study gave evidence that substandard care does exist for pregnant incarcerated women in correctional facilities. More specifically, nutritional recommendations for a healthy pregnancy are not met, adequate rest is compromised, and lower bunks are not required. Psychosocial support and education are minimal and the use of restraints, which can compromise the health and safety of the woman and her baby, continue, including during labor and delivery. A key finding found that best practices found was that best practices are not used generally and there is a serious need to address the unmet healthcare needs of this marginalized population, and support legislation to limit the use of restraints with pregnant incarcerated women (Ferszt & Clarke, 2012).

Criticism abounds in terms of the quality of care offered at correctional institutions. People who end up in prison systems almost always struggle with chronic, difficult-to-change healthcare problems such as chronic mental health issues, substance addiction, proclivity to violent acts, and risky behaviors, leaving them vulnerable to STIs in general and HIV/AIDS in particular. Although part of the reason for lack of quality care relates to maintaining qualified and inspired healthcare personnel, the more formidable issue is public financing of the growing numbers of inmates' healthcare needs. See Box 18.7 for commentary of a medical director in Michigan concerning prison inmates.

box 18.7 Summary of Study Criticizing Prison Healthcare

- The medical director for a Grand Rapids clinic serving low-income patients was the technical adviser to Michigan's prisons.
- Findings released indicate 32 changes needed to improve healthcare in the prisons.
- Infectious diseases, such as hepatitis C, need treatment.
- Inadequate care during incarceration must be addressed to face current burden in hospitals and other healthcare providers in the community on release.
- Report recommends reviving the Legislative Corrections Ombudsman, a position the legislature eliminated in 2003, and creating a permanent legislative committee to oversee prison medical care and mental healthcare.

Source: Adapted from Shellenbarger, P. (2008, February 6). Study criticizes prison health care. *The Grand Rapids [Michigan] Press.* Retrieved from http://blog.mlive.com/grpress/2008/02/study_criticizes_prison_health.html

According to van den Bergh, Gatherer, Fraser, and Moller (2011), from a local and global perspective there are also serious concerns related to the need for gender sensitivity directed to the care of women and their experience in prisons. Women prisoners, although a minority within all prison systems, have special health needs that are frequently neglected. The evidence in the literature includes a lack of gender sensitivity in policies and practices in prisons, violations of women's human rights and failure to accept that imprisoned women have more and different healthcare needs compared with male prisoners. Many of these violations are related to reproductive health issues, mental health problems, drug dependencies, and histories of violence and abuse. Additional needs stem from their frequent status as a mother and usually as the primary caregiver for her children.

In Michigan, a for-profit MCO called Correctional Medical Services has been hired to address the healthcare needs of inmates in the state's correctional system. Use of this kind of organization often occurs because many healthcare professionals find it difficult to work in the conditions of correctional institutions. From a community and public health perspective, students and licensed nurses should consider the contribution they could make in these settings with regard to primary, secondary, and tertiary prevention. Whatever improvements nurses engender concerning mental health, communicable disease, and physical wellness will eventually be a positive contribution to a family, a neighborhood, and a community.

STUDENT REFLECTION

It was really exciting to work with my nursing professor, who is not only a clinician but also a researcher in a project about the nursing care of incarcerated women, in a detention facility for women. We worked together over a 10-week period using yoga exercise as an intervention to effect perceptions of well-being. In the first week, we measured vital signs and completed a health history, measured depression on a self-report inventory, and also asked questions about perceptions of wellness. Then we met weekly and helped the women participate in yoga. Following these meetings, we took the measurements again. Some important changes took place in perceptions of wellness, especially mental health. But what really struck me was how happy the women were to be able to do something and accomplish something while they were in prison. As I got to know them, I felt very sad that many were in jail for crimes they committed to keep themselves from becoming even poorer (sex work, selling drugs). They were poor women trying to survive, not mass murderers. Many of them talked about their children, who were in foster care or with family members. All I could think was that these women not only had to heal themselves when they left jail but also their families, or the cycle will continue.

GAY, LESBIAN, BISEXUAL, AND TRANSGENDER PEOPLE

Not all people are attracted to people of the opposite sex all the time. Some belong to the LGBT group. People in this community have experienced many instances of discrimination within the healthcare system (Masiongale, 2009). Part of the discrimination is not intentional but comes from a lack of thoughtful sensitivity on the part of healthcare providers in not examining the assumptions made about lifestyles based on stereotypes. Some of the problem stems from assessing and offering interventions related to health issues using the standards of heterosexuals. Healthcare providers with LGBT clients need to understand that not all of these people are openly "out of the closet" and that confidentiality is extremely important in light of active discrimination. Such discrimination may involve work, housing, health insurance, and financial support if the client is in a domestic partnership with another person.

Gay people are the sweetest, kindest, most artistic, warmest, and most thoughtful people in the world. And since the beginning of time all they've ever been is kicked.

Little Richard

Jan is a good example of someone who is trying to approach her health in good faith, with a preventive orientation, but who may easily be persuaded to not to return to a primary care physician because of lack of consideration of her specific needs.

- How would you address the needs of healthcare professionals who wish to understand the specific needs of unique populations?
- Are there best practices that can help inform healthcare professionals related to how to assess what the specific needs may be?

STUDENT REFLECTION

Several months ago, I was involved as a leader in an education discussion about prevention of STIs with a group of women in a drop-in center in the inner city. Boy, was I embarrassed! I assumed that everybody in the group was heterosexual. In reality, four of the women there were lesbians and had brought their significant others with them. All of the information I shared was regarding risk related to intercourse or oral sex between a man and a woman alone. After the session was over, I was really horrified when the two couples told me about the sexual orientation of people in the group. I felt as though I perpetuated assumptions about sex and did not provide helpful statistics about risk.

My instructor and I came up with a solution. We were able, with these couples' permission, to recontact some members of the group who had attended originally and asked if they would like to bring some of their friends who may be in the same type of relationship with them so we could specifically address their needs in a tailored session of prevention messages. So about a month later, we had a lesbian/bisexual safe sex session that was uniquely constructed just for these people. It was so successful that many members of the group, who vary in age from 24 to 60 years, continue to meet in a supportive capacity. It has been a bonus to see the intergenerational sharing and support.

In the course of assessment, diagnosis, and treatment of LGBT people, community and public health nurses should be aware that partners need to be included in care decisions; be familiar with key health concerns of this population such as STIs, alcohol and substance abuse, depression, and suicide; and become comfortable with asking healthcare assessment questions that include LGBT lifestyles, so that key prevention opportunities are not missed. For example, during a physical assessment, it is essential to ask a client whether he or she has sex with men, women, or both; this information is critical in identifying further clarifying questions about high-risk behaviors and sex. No healthcare provider should assume that a client is homosexual or heterosexual based on appearance or other factors.

EVIDENCE FOR PRACTICE

1. One research article has examined the literature to provide clinicians with evidence-based recommendations for care of lesbian clients (Roberts, 2006). Data organization related to specific health problems was noted frequently in the research articles. Findings and conclusions include that lesbians have previously been invisible in health services and research. Lesbians are "coming out" more and more with healthcare providers, which means that data about them can be collected. Data now show that lesbians are at risk for cancer, heart disease, depression, and alcohol abuse. Adolescent lesbians are especially at risk for smoking, as well as depression and suicide. However, screening for these conditions continues to be low in lesbians.
2. In a world where healthcare needs of the LGBT population is increasingly important, healthcare professionals require appropriate academic and clinical training in preparation for the increased demand for culturally competent care. Nurses are of particular interest, as they are the core direct caregivers in many healthcare settings. This research study explored the national climate around LGBT individuals. The conclusion is that educators need to be committed to ensure the development of knowledgeable practitioners who will be able to implement best practices in LGBT patient care. Attention should be paid to providing students with diverse clinical placements, access to LGBT interest groups, and clear expectations for LGBT-sensitive nursing care plans and course outcomes selection that promote cultural competence (Lim, Brown, & Jones, 2013).
3. One qualitative study has used ethnography to identify, describe, and classify the effect of sociostructural factors on men who have sex with men and HIV transmission risk (Natale, 2009). Included are the perceptions of HIV risk in four subgroups: HIV-positive, Latino, Black, and young (18–24 years) men who have sex with men. Results classify participant-perceived transmission factors into sociostructural factors (e.g., social, health, economic, political, and mental health). This article also addresses significant areas of social stigma and discrimination—critical areas that need to be addressed to promote the general health of these men as well as their sexual health. It is also important to prevent and treat substance use in this population.
4. Families are of critical importance in Latino communities in the United States. Research has shown that familism—or the cultural ideal that involves reliance on nuclear and extended family members for emotional support, connectedness, honor, loyalty, and solidarity—reduces sexual health risks among heterosexual youth, yet this relationship has not been examined among Latino bisexual teenagers. A complex construct, familism has a strong potential for providing insights into sexual health practices of bisexual Latino adolescents. One study examined how familism shapes sexual decision-making regarding behavior and expressions of bisexuality in Latino adolescents living in New York City (Muñoz-Laboy et al., 2009). Twenty-five in-depth interviews and ethnographic observations in bisexual males and females (15–19 years of age) for 9 months were the basis for the study. Findings suggested that these bisexual Latinos value closeness to their families by maintaining family ties and seeking emotional and material support from their families. For those who wanted to keep their bisexuality private, the constant surveillance of the family network is a negative.

Bradford and Mayer (2008) have identified 10 summary points of great concern related to demographic information and the needs of LGBT people. These points include the following:

- The four different subgroups—gay, lesbian, bisexual, and transgender people—have unique needs. There is little demographic data tailored to each of these separate groups.
- Few population-based studies have been conducted in LGBT groups, with the exception of HIV-related research, particularly in men who have sex with men.
- Specific questions on surveys related to sexual orientation are lacking.
- Recognition of same-sex heads of households has not always been included in survey data.
- There is confusion regarding variability of expression of one's identity, behavior, and attraction.
- Cultural contexts vary across age and developmental staging about "coming out of the closet"; some people (e.g., older gays or lesbians) may not feel comfortable with the word "queer."
- Fluidity of gender and sexual identity changes over time.
- LGBT groups tend to experience more serious physical and mental health conditions, including interpersonal violence and substance addiction.
- Particular health concerns from a prevention perspective include obesity, injury, violence, and access to healthcare facilities.
- Health professionals are poised as confidants and trusted people to make significant preventive inroads at all levels if they approach LGBT groups informed, with data.

One of the key goals in community and public health nursing is to begin to understand the needs of LGBT people through specific training that addresses the needs of each particular group. The assumption that this information is included in healthcare training programs for all healthcare disciplines is often false. Many times, students need to attend extracurricular programs that are supported by local initiatives or institutions that care for these populations because of the unique nature of the information that needs to

box 18.8 Community Standards of Practice for the Provision of Quality Healthcare Services to Lesbian, Gay, Bisexual, and Transgender Clients

The Gay, Lesbian, Bisexual, and Transgender Health Access Project is a collaborative, community-based program funded by the Massachusetts Department of Public Health. The project's mission is to foster the development and implementation of comprehensive, culturally appropriate, quality health promotion policies and healthcare services for lesbian, gay, bisexual, and transgendered (LGBT) people and their families. Research has indicated that fear of discrimination and stigma cause many LGBT people to postpone or decline seeking medical care. Others, once in care, sometimes withhold from their providers personal information that may be critical to their well-being.

- Working closely with consumers and clinicians across the state, the Gay, Lesbian, Bisexual, and Transgender Health Access Project works to confront the insensitivity and ignorance that many LGBT people have experienced in accessing healthcare and related services.
- In addition, the project seeks to support LGBT people in understanding and acquiring the quality care they need.
- The need for community standards emerged from several sources, including a statewide provider survey and a 1997 Gay, Lesbian, Bisexual, and Transgender Health Access Project report, health concerns of the LGBT community. Among other things, these reports detailed a serious lack of LGBT awareness and understanding among healthcare providers in Massachusetts. Some believed that they had no LGBT clients or staff in their facilities; many were unsure about what their role should be in identifying and addressing LGBT issues; and a few had policies in place to guide personnel or consumers.
- To address these concerns, the Gay, Lesbian, Bisexual, and Transgender Health Access Project convened a community working group of more than 60 consumers, providers, public, and private agency administrators and staff. The group worked to develop a framework to improve LGBT access to quality care and to assist clinicians and their facilities in creating responsive environments. This group's efforts were guided by four principles: (1) the elimination of discrimination on the basis of sexual orientation and gender identity, (2) the promotion and provision of full and equal access to services, (3) the elimination of stigmatization of LGBT people and their families, and (4) the creation of health service environments where it is safe for people to be "out" to their providers.
- The community standards of practice and quality indicators outlined in this document will guide and assist providers in achieving these goals. The standards address both agency administrative practices and service delivery components, including the following areas:
  1. Personnel
  2. Client's rights
  3. Intake and assessment
  4. Service planning and delivery
  5. Confidentiality
  6. Community outreach and health promotion
- LGBT people live in and seek healthcare and prevention services in every community in Massachusetts. Eliminating barriers to care requires both an educated and empowered consumer base and a skilled, culturally competent, sensitive, and welcoming provider community that is openly supportive of LGBT people and their families. These standards are one tool for achieving greater healthcare for all.

Source: Massachusetts Department of Health. (2013). *Gay, lesbian, bisexual and transgender health access project.* Retrieved from http://www.lgbthealth.org

be shared. For example, Transgender Awareness Training and Advocacy is an initiative started by Sam Lurie. He is a transgendered man, or transman, who has used his own experience as a way to help inform others of the needs of the transgender community (Transgender Awareness Training and Advocacy, 2009).

Training is meaningful only if community standards are developed so that evidenced-based practice can progress to assist people in these groups. See Box 18.8 for a LGBT health access project developed and supported by the Massachusetts Department of Public Health (Massachusetts Department of Public Health, 2013).

PRACTICE POINT

When taking a sexual history, always ask whether a client is having sex with men, women, or both. This clarification is critical in offering prevention, health promotion, and risk advice. It is crucial that healthcare providers also be respectful by using the term "sexual orientation" versus "sexual preference." Although many LGBT people are not ashamed of their lives, many would also admit that their identity, behaviors, and attractions have caused a significant amount of personal pain related to stigma and isolation (i.e., sexual orientation may not have been their choice).

It is critical for community and public health nurses to ask questions in order to be sensitive to the LGBT community. This method is a healing approach that may decrease stigma and isolation.

HOMELESS POPULATIONS

Was I always going to be here? No I was not. I was going to be homeless at one time, a taxi driver, truck driver, or any kind of job that would get me a crust of bread. You never know what's going to happen.

Morgan Freeman

Homeless people include single men, families with children led by single heads of households (women), single women (bag ladies), and children (<18 years) who lack adult supervision. In developed countries, the majority of homeless people are male and more likely to be black, veterans, unemployed, struggle with mental health challenges and/or addictions, and are victims of domestic violence (National Coalition for the Homeless, 2013). Many of these people take refuge in homeless shelters, and others live in abandoned buildings, jails, hospitals, parks, airports, and bus/train stations, as well as under bridges or in the entries to buildings.

Homelessness has many causes. Reasons for homelessness include the deinstitutionalization efforts of the 1960s to mainstream the mentally ill into society, unemployment and underemployment, domestic violence, abandonment, natural disasters and fires, disability, substance abuse and addiction, immigration, and political unrest and wars (Shelton, Taylor, Bonner, & van den Bree, 2009). Historically, many circumstances have led to homelessness, including freedom from slavery, westward expansion, lumber and railroad work, the Great Depression, and the aftereffects of war. In recent years, the shortage of affordable housing has been a key reason (Kirkpatrick & Byrne, 2009).

I lived rough, by my wits, was homeless, lived on the streets, lived on friends' floors, was happy, was miserable.

Ben Okri, Nigerian poet and novelist

Reaching homeless people is difficult. It is not easy to provide care with trained and experienced interprofessional teams because of the inability to locate clients in the community by address or phone. Many homeless people have complications from decreased hygiene, hypothermia, and hyperthermia; suffer from lice and scabies; and have diseases or conditions such as tuberculosis, HIV infection, substance abuse and addiction, and dental problems. Even **trimorbidity** (i.e., substance addiction, mental illness, and another chronic health problem such as hypertension) is common in the homeless.

It takes much time and energy to build trust with the homeless before the many comorbidities with which they are burdened can be addressed. Some approaches to administering healthcare to the homeless have included not just offering shelter, but also offering harm reduction as a way to keep clients alive without further complicating their serious situations. For example, offering needle cleaning kits to users of intravenous drugs may decrease the use of dirty needles at the individual and population level, or providing mobile homeless units may make healthcare more accessible. Even with these efforts, homeless people may refuse assistance. To promote accessibility to healthcare for these people, community and public health nurses should approach homeless people in the following ways:

- Show respect and use a positive approach, which builds trust.
- Support primary (advocacy), secondary (tuberculosis screening), and tertiary ("detox" treatment) prevention to make it easier to cope with difficult, challenging lives.

EVIDENCE FOR PRACTICE

1. Needle exchange programs, although controversial, offer a harm reduction approach to intravenous drug users by offering clean needles for use. Operational and systematic limitations exist, including acceptable hours of operation, the location of the programs, and transportation needs. Researchers have described a novel backpack needle exchange outreach model implemented in Providence, Rhode Island (Hebert et al., 2008). Backpack exchange appears to be a feasible method for providing needle exchange services and referrals to hard-to-reach injectors.
2. One qualitative study has explored how people who are homeless perceive outreach practices and available services (Kryda & Compton, 2009). Researchers conducted interviews with 24 people who had been homeless for 1 year or more and who consistently resided on the streets of New York City. Reasons why these people refuse services include a pervasive mistrust of outreach workers and the agencies that employ them, as well as a prominent lack of confidence in available services. The findings suggest a need for an approach to outreach that incorporates giving individualized attention from outreach workers, using an empathetic listening approach, minimizing stereotyping, providing greater choices, and employing formerly homeless people as outreach workers.
3. Using data from the National Survey of Homeless Assistance Providers and Clients (NSHAPC), researchers have identified predictors of current alcohol and drug-misuse problems among homeless, previously homeless, and marginally housed older adults. Childhood sexual assault, victimization, and neglect, being male, being younger, being homeless or previously homeless, being a minority, and having income below $499 per month increased the odds of reporting a drug problem. Being male, being younger, being homeless, and having mental illness increased the odds of reporting an alcohol problem. Reporting any type of substance use problem increased the odds of reporting the other problem (Dietz, 2009).

box 18.9 Common Themes of Underserved Populations

- Blaming the victim, healthcare professionals, and others assuming abuse/neglect/incompetence
- Making poor choices and having the wrong priorities on the part of individuals, families, and populations
- Powerlessness and vulnerability
- Nobody cares about injury, infection, screening, preventive care.

key concepts

- In discerning community/public health practices as a nurse, one of the fundamental issues that needs to be faced are the biases and prejudices that can be barriers to understanding the needs of populations.
- Community and family assessments need to be grounded in trusting approaches that are mutually defined between health professionals and those living in situations that are less than ideal.
- Being a caregiver in a community where rural access, prison isolation, sexual discrimination, and continuity of care are all struggles of great magnitude allows nurses to do what they do best: heal, and not necessarily fix, healthcare situations.
- A key suggestion in carrying out the core values of public health may be to check the common themes or biases that each of these groups experience "at the door" (Box 18.9).

critical thinking questions

1. What are the ethical and moral issues that present themselves when communities/cities/states choose to address or not address the health needs of the populations covered in this chapter?
2. Are there legal obligations that you can identify in relation to rural, correctional, LGBT, or homeless health? Give specific examples and what your recourse would be to address these issues.
3. Community violence is reported as an issue in all four of the populations described in this chapter. Identify a coalition-building approach that could unify these communities regarding this issue (refer to Chapter 16 to assist you with this answer).
4. Why is it the case that single men are prominently represented in the homeless? Is there a primary prevention program that could be a part of a public health initiative that would address this cohort specifically?

community resources

- Rural health
  - Emergency medical services
  - Faith-based initiatives
- Correctional/prison health
  - Local jails, correctional facilities
  - Police departments
  - Detention centers for youth
  - Outreach programs directed to correctional facilities
  - Foster care agencies
- Gay, lesbian, transgender, and bisexual populations
  - Community health and neighborhood centers
  - Local HIV/AIDS services
- Homeless populations and health
  - City and state housing authorities
  - Hunger and food assistance programs
  - Health programs and clinics targeted at this group

references

Amber Waves. (2013). *Rural America*. Retrieved May 23, 2013, from http://www.ers.usda.gov/AmberWaves/June08/Features/RuralAmerica.htm

Bailey, B. A., & Byrom, A. R. (2007). Factors predicting birth weight in a low-risk sample: The role of modifiable pregnancy health behaviors. *Maternal & Child Health Journal, 11*(2), 173–179.

Bradford, J. B., & Mayer, K. H. (2008). Demography and the LGBT population: What we know, don't know, and how the information helps to inform clinical practice. In H. J. Makadon, K. H. Mayer, J. Potter, & H. Goldhammer (Eds.), *Fenway guide to lesbian, gay, bisexual, and transgender health* (pp. 25–44). Philadelphia, PA: American College of Physicians.

Braveman, P. A., Kumanyika, S., Fielding, J., LaVeist, T., Borrell, L. N., Manderscheid, R., & Troutman, A. (2011). Health disparities and health equity: The issue is justice. *American Journal of Public Health, 101*(Suppl. 1), S149–S155.

Burton, H., Chowdhury, S., Dent, T., Hall, A., Pashayan, N., & Pharoah, P. (2013). Public health implications from COGS and potential for risk stratification and screening. *Nature and Genetics, 45*, 349–351. doi:10.1038/ng.2582

Charles, G., Bainbridge, L., Copeman-Stewart, K., Kassam, R., & Tiffin, S. (2008). Impact of an interprofessional rural health care practice education experience on students and communities. *Journal of Allied Health, 37*(3), 127–131.

Children's Defense Fund. (2009). Retrieved June 6, 2009, from http://www.childrensdefense.org

Clark, P. A., Surry, L., & Contino, K. (2009). Health care access for migrant farmworkers: A paradigm for better health. *Internet Journal of Health, 8*(2), 7.

Coddington, J. A., & Sands, L. P. (2008). Cost of health care and quality outcomes of patients at nurse-managed clinics. *Nursing Economics, 26*(2), 75–83.

references (continued)

Crews, K. R., Gaedigk, A., Dunnenberger, H. M., Klein, T. E., Shen, D. D., Callaghan, J. T., … Skaar, T. C. (2012). Clinical pharmacogenetics implementation consortium (CPIC) guidelines for codeine therapy in the context of cytochrome P450 2 D6 (CYP2D6) genotype. *Clinical Pharmacology Therapies*, *91*(2), 321–326. doi:10.1038/clpt.2011.287

Dietz, T. L. (2009). Drug and alcohol use among homeless older adults: Predictors of reported current and lifetime substance misuse problems in a national sample. *Journal of Applied Gerontology*, *28*(2), 235–255.

Faircloth, S. C. (2009). Revisioning the future education for native youth in rural schools and communities. *Journal of Research in Rural Education*, *24*(9), 1–4.

Farrell, S. P., Zerull, L. M., Mahone, I. H., Guerlain, S., Akan, D., Hauenstein, E., & Schorling, J. (2009). Electronic screening for mental health in rural health care: Feasibility and user testing. *Computers, Informatics, Nursing*, *27*(2), 93–98.

Ferszt, G. G., & Clarke, J. G. (2012). Health care of pregnant women in U.S. state prisons. *Journal of Health Care for the Poor & Underserved*, *23*(2), 557–569.

Flaskerud, J., & Winslow, B. (1998). Conceptualizing vulnerable populations in health-related research. *Nursing Research*, *47*(2), 69–78.

Gamm, L. (2007). Keynote address: Rural Healthy People 2010 and sustaining rural populations. In L. L. Morgan & P. S. Fahs (Eds.), *Conversations in the disciplines: Sustaining rural populations* (pp. 1–12). Binghamton, NY: Global Academic Publishing.

Garrison-Jakel, J. (2011). Patching the rural workforce pipeline—Why don't we do more? *Journal of Rural Health*, *27*(2), 239–240.

Goetzel, R. Z., Liss-Levinson, R. C., Goodman, N., & Kennedy, J. X. (2009). Development of a community-wide cardiovascular risk reduction assessment tool for small rural employers in upstate New York. *Preventing Chronic Disease*, *6*(2), A65.

Gomes, M. V., & Pelosi, G. G. (2013). Epigenetic vulnerability and the environmental influence on health. *Exploratory Biological Medicine (Maywood)*, *238*(8), 859–865.

Health Resources and Services Administration. (2013). *Find shortage areas*. Retrieved May 23, 2013, from http://hpsafind.hrsa.gov/

Healthy People 2020 (2014). Disparities retrieved from http://www.healthypeople.gov/2020/about/foundation-health-measures/Disparities

Hebert, M. R., Caviness, C. M., Bowman, S. E., Chowdhury, S. P., Loberti, P. G., & Stein, M. D. (2008). Backpack needle exchange: Background, design, and pilot testing of a program in Rhode Island. *Journal of Addictive Diseases*, *27*(3), 7–12.

Henry, L.R., Hooker, R.S., & Yates, K.L. (2011). The role of physician assistants in rural health care: a systematic review of the literature. *J Rural Health, 27*(2), 220-9.

Kemppainen, J. K., Taylor, J., Jackson, L. A., Kim-Godwin, Y. S., & Kirby, E. (2009). Incidence, sources, and self-management of depression in persons attending a rural health clinic in southeastern North Carolina. *Journal of Community Health Nursing*, *26*(1), 1–13.

Khoury, M. J., Janssens, A. C., & Ransohoff, D. F. (2013). How can polygenic inheritance be used in population screening for common diseases. *Genetics and Medicine*, *15*, 437–443. doi:10.1038/gim.2012.182

Kirkpatrick, H., & Byrne, C. (2009). A narrative inquiry: Moving on from homelessness for individuals with a major mental illness. *Journal of Psychiatric & Mental Health Nursing*, *16*(1), 68–75.

Krout, J. A., & Kinner, M. (2007). Sustaining geriatric rural populations. In L. L. Morgan & P. S. Fahs (Eds.), *Conversations in the disciplines: Sustaining rural populations* (pp. 63–74). Binghamton, NY: Global Academic Publishing.

Kryda, A. D., & Compton, M. T. (2009). Mistrust of outreach workers and lack of confidence in available services among individuals who are chronically street homeless. *Community Mental Health Journal*, *45*(2), 144–150.

Levy, B. S., & Sidel, V. W. (2006). *Social injustice and public health*. New York, NY: Oxford University and American Public Health Association.

Ligeikis-Clayton, C. (2007). Meeting the rural nursing shortage needs: An evening/weekend nursing program. In L. L. Morgan & P. S. Fahs (Eds.), *Conversations in the disciplines: Sustaining rural populations* (pp. 75–84). Binghamton, NY: Global Academic Publishing.

Lim, F. A., Brown, D. V., Jr., & Jones, B. H. (2013). Lesbian, gay, bisexual, and transgender health: Fundamentals for nursing education. *Journal of Nursing Education*, *52*(4), 198–203.

Masiongale, T. (2009). Ethical service delivery to culturally and linguistically diverse populations: A specific focus on gay, lesbian, bisexual, and transgender populations. *Perspectives on Communication Disorders & Sciences in Culturally & Linguistically Diverse (CLD) Populations*, *16*(1), 20–30.

Massachusetts Department of Health. (2013). *LGBT health access project*. Retrieved May 23, 2013, from http://www.glbthealth.org

Morrongiello, B. A., Marlenga, B., Berg, R., Linneman, J., & Pickett, W. (2007). A new approach to understanding pediatric farm injuries. *Social Science & Medicine*, *6*(7), 1364–1371.

Muñoz-Laboy, M., Leau, C. J., Sriram, V., Weinstein, H. J., del Aquila, E. V., & Parker, R. (2009). Bisexual desire and familism: Latino/a bisexual young men and women in New York City. *Culture, Health & Sexuality*, *1*(3), 331–344.

Natale, A. P. (2009). Denver MSM sociostructural factors: Preliminary findings of perceived HIV risk. *Journal of HIV/AIDS & Social Services*, *8*(1), 35–56.

National Coalition of the Homeless. (2013). Retrieved May 24, 2013, from http://www.nationalhomeless.org/factsheets/who.html

Nelson, J. A., & Gingerich, B. S. (2010). Rural health: Access to care and services. *Home Health Care Management & Practice*, *22*(5), 339–343.

Nolan, G., & Walsh, E. (2012). Caring in prison: The intersubjective web of professional relationships. *Journal of Forensic Nursing*, *8*(4), 163–169.

Office of Management and Budget (U.S.). (2013). *Statistical programs and standards*. Retrieved May 23, 2013, from http://www.whitehouse.gov/omb/inforeg_statpolicy/

Organista, K. C. (2007). Towards a structural-environmental model of risk for HIV and problem drinking in Latino labor migrants: The case of day laborers. *Journal of Ethnic & Cultural Diversity in Social Work*, *16*(1/2), 95–125.

Pennel, C. L., Carpender, S. K., & Quiram, B. J. (2008). Rural health roundtables: A strategy for collaborative engagement in and between rural communities. *Rural & Remote Health*, *8*(4), 1054.

Pevsner, J. (2009). *Bioinformatics and functional genomics* (2nd ed.). Hoboken, NJ: Wiley-Blackwell.

Rajabiun, S., Mallinson, R. K., McCoy, K., Coleman, S., Drainoni, M. L., Rebholz, C., & Holbert, T. (2007). Getting me back on track: The role of outreach interventions in engaging and retaining people living with HIV/AIDS in medical care. *AIDS Patient Care & STDs*, *21*(Suppl. 1), S20–S29.

Roberts, S. J. (2006). Health care recommendations for lesbian women. *Journal of Obstetric, Gynecologic, and Neonatal Nursing*, *35*(5), 583–591.

Shelton, K. H., Taylor, P. J., Bonner, A., & van den Bree, M. (2009). Risk factors for homelessness: Evidence from a population-based study. *Psychiatric Services*, *60*(4), 465–472.

Tumosa, N., Horvath, K. J., Huh, T., Livote, E. E., Howe, J. L., Jones, L. I., & Kramer, B. J. (2012). Health care workforce development in rural America: When geriatrics expertise is 100 miles away. *Gerontology & Geriatrics Education, 33*(2), 133–151.

Thornlow, D. K. (2008). Nursing patient safety research in rural health care settings. *Annual Review of Nursing Research, 26*, 195–218.

Transgender Awareness Training and Advocacy. (2009). Retrieved from http://www.tgtrain.org/

United States Bureau of Census. (2013a). *Health insurance data.* Retrieved May 23, 2013, from http://www.census.gov/hhes/www/hlthins/hlthins.html

United States Bureau of Census. (2013b). *We the people of more than one race: Census 2000 special report*. Retrieved May 23, 2013, from http://www.census.gov/prod/2005pubs/censr-22.pdf

United States Department of Agriculture. (2013a). *Farm safety*. Retrieved May 24, 2013, from http://www.csrees.usda.gov/farmsafety.cfm

United States Department of Agriculture. (2013b). *What is rural*? Retrieved June 6, 2009, from http://www.nal.usda.gov/ric/ricpubs/what_is_rural.shtml#define

United States Department of Justice, Bureau of Justice Statistics. (2011). Retrieved May 24, 2013, from http://www.bjs.gov/index.cfm?ty=pbse&sid=40

van den Bergh, B. J., Gatherer, A., Fraser, A., & Moller, L., (2011). Imprisonment and women's health: Concerns about gender sensitivity, human rights and public health. *Bulletin of the World Health Organization, 89*(9), 689–294.

Wilkinson, K. (2010, September 15). *HHS funding looks to meet challenges of providing health care in rural areas* [Transcript and Audio File]. Retrieved October 18, 2010, from http://origin.eastbaymedia.com/~advisoryboard/podcast_media/iHBSpecialReportTranscript091510.pdf

Willging, C. E., Waitzkin, H., & Nicdao, E. (2008). Medicaid managed care for mental health services: The survival of safety net institutions in rural settings. *Qualitative Health Research, 18*(9), 1231–1246.

Zust, B. L. (2009). Partner violence, depression, and recidivism: The case of incarcerated women and why we need programs designed for them. *Issues in Mental Health Nursing, 30*(4), 246–251.

web resources

Please visit thePoint® for up-to-date web resources on this topic.

CHAPTER 19

Environmental Health

Tarah S. Somers*

TEARS OF NATURE
(A villanelle)

I think I just heard Mother Nature cry,
Or was it one more broken, falling tree?
You'd think we'd learn as time goes speeding by.

They tell us there's a big hole in the sky,
We won't believe in something we can't see,
I think I just heard Mother Nature cry.

Coal-fired chimneys reaching up so high,
Even though the solar power's free,
You'd think we'd learn as time goes speeding by.

We develop rocket ships that fly,
But still can't stop pollution of the sea,
I think I just heard Mother Nature cry.

Headlines: One more species set to die,
Keep it quiet...use diplomacy,
You'd think we'd learn as time goes speeding by.

Worry on the future? Pass it by!
How can preservation start with me?
I think I just heard Mother Nature cry.
You'd think we'd learn as time goes speeding by.

Graeme King

chapter highlights

- Human health and the environment
- Assessing contaminants in the environment
- Exposure pathways
- Assessing the environment of a community
- Planning interventions to make communities healthier
- Evaluating interventions
- Environmental epidemiology
- Working toward healthy communities
- Environmental justice
- Global environmental health issues

*The findings and conclusions in this report are those of the author and do not necessarily represent the views of the Agency for Toxic Substances and Disease Registry.

objectives

- Comprehend the links between human health and the environment.
- Understand how the nursing process of using assessment, intervention, and evaluation can be used to examine the impact of the environment on human health.
- Describe the concept of an exposure pathway.
- Describe several environmental conditions to consider when assessing the environment of a community.
- Understand the concept of environmental justice.
- Identify major global environmental health issues.

key terms

Bioavailability: The amount of a substance that is absorbed or becomes available at the site of physiological activity.
Biomonitoring: Process of using medical tests such as blood or urine collection to determine whether a person has been exposed to a contaminant and how much exposure he or she has received.
Environmental epidemiology: Field of public health science that focuses on the incidence and prevalence of disease or illness in a population from exposures in their environments.
Environmental health: A field of public health science that focuses on how the environment influences human health.
Environmental justice: The belief that no group of people should bear a disproportionate share of negative environmental health consequences (regardless of race, culture, or income).
Exposure: The total amount of a contaminant that comes in direct contact with the body.
Exposure estimate: Factors that determine a person's level of exposure to a contaminant.
Exposure pathway: Method by which people are exposed to an environmental contaminant that originates from a specific source.
Exposure history: Process to help determine whether an individual has been exposed to environmental contaminants.
Precautionary principle: If something has the potential to cause harm to humans or the environment, then precautionary measures should be taken even if there is a lack of scientific evidence for cause and effect.

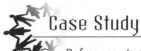

Case Study

References to the case study are found throughout this chapter (look for the case study icon). Readers should keep the case study in mind as they read the chapter.

Chris is a public health nurse in a coastal town with a long, proud history of commercial and recreational fishing. Throughout the 20th century, many industries lined the edges of the harbor, creating additional economic opportunities for the town. From 1940 to the 1970s, polychlorinated biphenyls (PCBs) were used at the transformer facility that manufactured electrical capacitors and transformers. As a result, soil and groundwater at the site, as well as at the building, are heavily contaminated with PCBs. This facility is considered the major source of historic PCB contamination of the harbor.

The facility is now fenced, and there is no public access to the contaminated soil and buildings. The community is supplied by public drinking water sources which are not connected to the site's groundwater. Commercial fishing in the harbor is banned, and all commercial fishing takes place out at sea. However, some members of the community frequently fish in the harbor, and they eat the fish they catch to supplement their diets.

The community around the harbor enjoys seasonal recreational activities along the water and sometimes boats on the water, but swimming in the harbor is difficult, since the shores are steep and rocky and there is no beach area. Access to the water can really only happen from community-owned piers.

key terms (continued)

Healthy communities: Communities that optimize the physical, social, and economic environments of the community.

Risk assessment: Process to determine the likelihood or probability that adverse effects such as illness or disease will occur in a group of people because of an exposure to an environmental contaminant.

Toxicology: The study of the adverse effects of chemical, physical, or biological agents on people, animals, and the environment.

The environment can be considered as anything outside of ourselves whether human-made or natural. **Environmental health** is the branch of public health science that focuses on how the environment influences human health.

HUMAN HEALTH AND THE ENVIRONMENT

The environment can affect human health in many ways. Some of these effects are immediate and obvious, such as when drinking water supplies are contaminated by sewage and flood water after a hurricane. Other effects, such as contamination of a private well by arsenic, may be more difficult to discover. Where people live, work, and spend time can have direct consequences on their health. For example, living and working in highly urban environments may expose people to higher concentrations of some air pollutants, but living and working in an agricultural setting may expose them to more pesticides. **Exposure** occurs when there is contact between people and an environmental contaminant.

Peoples' environment can have positive or negative effects on their health. Conditions in the environment may exacerbate existing health conditions. For example, people with asthma may experience more asthmatic episodes on days when air quality is poor. The poor air quality may not cause asthma, but it may induce more frequent and severe asthma attacks in people who already have asthma.

The environment can also help improve people's health. If residents of a certain town believe that they can safely walk in their community, they may choose to walk instead of drive to the store or to schools. This can help increase their activity levels and decrease obesity or other chronic diseases. It could also lead to less pollution from cars, which, in turn, improves air quality. In some ways, the built environment can be intentionally designed to help make people healthier.

What is the use of a house if you haven't got a tolerable planet to put it on?

Henry David Thoreau

History of Environmental Health

Historically, people often did not clearly understand the links between environment and health and did not recognize how humans influenced their environment. As nations became industrialized, the effects on the quality of air and water became more apparent. People also began to take note of the impact on ecosystems as plants, animals, or other wildlife began to disappear. Many industries were loosely, if at all, regulated, and disposal practices of hazardous materials and industrial by-products were shortsighted. Disposal of waste materials often simply involved burying or dumping the waste into lakes, rivers, or oceans in the belief that the "solution to pollution is dilution." The intent of this improper disposal of contaminants was not always malicious—people did not understand the impact that the contaminants could have on human health and ecosystems. Materials such as PCBs and asbestos were commercially available, essential to certain manufacturing processes, and were not believed to be harmful. Over time, with the development of more research and understanding, we now realize that many contaminants and hazardous materials have adverse impacts on human health.

The quality of the environment became a popular topic in the mid- to late 20th century. Books such as *Silent Spring* by Rachel Carson (1962) brought to public attention how human actions and pollution were affecting the quality of air, water, and land. In 1969, because of debris and oil in the river, the Cuyahoga River in Ohio caught on fire. The river had caught fire many times in the past, but the 1969 event caught the public's attention and helped increase awareness of how polluted some places had become. In July 1970, the White House and Congress established the Environmental Protection Agency (EPA) in response to the growing public demand for cleaner water, air, and land. The EPA had the daunting task of repairing the damage already done to the natural environment and to establish new criteria to making a cleaner environment a reality. For more information on the creation and current role of EPA, visit the EPA website. Several important pieces of legislation that helped highlight the importance of environmental health and protection are still used to help enforce environmental health and protection (Box 19.1).

box 19.1 Influential Environmental Laws

Clean Air Act

The Clean Air Act (CAA), passed in 1970, created a national program to control the damaging effects of air pollution. The Clean Air Act Amendments of 1990 went further to ensure that the air Americans breathe is safe. The CAA protects and enhances the quality of the nation's air by regulating stationary and mobile sources of air emissions. More information is available at http://www.epa.gov/compliance/civil/caa/index.html.

Clean Water Act

The Clean Water Act, passed in 1972, focuses on improving the quality of the nation's waters. It provides a comprehensive framework of standards, technical tools, and financial assistance to address the many causes of pollution and poor water quality, including municipal and industrial wastewater discharges, polluted runoff from urban and rural areas, and habitat destruction. More information is available at http://www.epa.gov/compliance/civil/cwa/index.html.

Superfund

Superfund is the name given to the environmental program established to address abandoned hazardous waste sites. It is also the name of the fund established by the **Comprehensive Environmental Response, Compensation and Liability Act** of 1980. It allows the Environmental Protection Agency to clean up such sites and compel responsible parties to perform cleanups or reimburse the government for EPA-led cleanups. More information is available at http://www.epa.gov/superfund/about.htm.

> *Love Canal started it all. I visited the canal area at that time. Corroding waste disposal drums could be seen breaking up through the grounds of backyards. Trees and gardens were turning black and dying. One entire swimming pool had been popped up from its foundation, afloat now on a small sea of chemicals.... Everywhere the air had a faint, choking smell. Children returned from play with burns on their hands and faces.*
>
> **Eckardt C. Beck, EPA Regional Administrator**

Today, the public has better understanding of the impact of human actions on the environment and how the environment can in turn affect human health. However, there are still many environmental health challenges that people must face, including cleaning up past, as well as ongoing contamination, deciding what to do about newly recognized issues such as climate change and energy production, and dealing with emerging scientific advances such as nanotechnology. Even though new research and developments are occurring at a historically rapid pace, there are still large gaps in peoples' knowledge about certain subjects:

- How do certain contaminants affect human health?
- How do we assess exposures to contaminants?
- How does the environment influence health?
- How do we live as a population while maintaining a healthy environment?

> *Loads of chemicals and hazardous wastes have been introduced into the atmosphere that didn't even exist in 1948. The environmental condition of the planet is far worse than it was 42 years ago.*
>
> **Gaylord Nelson, politician and principal founder of Earth Day, 1990**

The Community Environment

The environment and its effect on human health is often considered in two ways. The first focuses on how contaminants in the environment, such as asbestos, lead, or radon, influence human health. The second focuses on how the entire environment surrounding the community, such as neighborhood safety, climate, access to grocery stores, and community design, affects health. These two ways of considering the effect of the environment on human health frequently relate to each other.

For example, lead was used in paint until the 1970s and is often found in houses built earlier. As the old paint breaks down, lead can be found in dust and old paint chips in homes (CDC, 2009a). In communities with older, deteriorating housing, children can be exposed to lead. In many cases, such housing is found in poorer communities. Many low-income communities also have fewer full-service grocery stores, and all residents do not have access to necessary healthy, iron-rich foods. Sufficient blood iron can protect against some of the effects of lead exposure (EPA, 2001). Some research suggests that the combination of iron deficiency and elevated blood lead levels may work synergistically to create greater neurological impacts in children than just iron deficiency or elevated blood lead levels. The impact of the contaminant, the lead, on children's health may be greater because of characteristics of the children's community environment (CDC, 2002).

In the case of lead-based paint in the environment, it is fairly easy to determine the link between the environment and health. Sometimes, it can be challenging to determine which environmental factors have the greatest impact on health. Information about the way many contaminants affect humans is very limited. People are exposed to thousands of different things in their environment every day. One person may come into contact with a number of personal care products (e.g., shampoo, toothpaste, lotions, clothing detergent), food products (artificial colors, pesticide residue on foods, preservatives), other commercial products (e.g., inks, gasoline, dry cleaned clothing, flame retardants), and environmental contaminants (e.g., diesel particles) every day. In the modern world, it is nearly impossible to isolate people from all of the exposures they have every day.

The American Chemical Society, which provides the Chemical Abstracts Service (CAS) database for chemicals, had as of March 2013 over "71 million unique organic and inorganic chemical substances, such as alloys, coordination compounds, minerals, mixtures, polymers and salts" (American Chemical Society, 2013). Even if only a fraction of these chemicals eventually find their way into the environment and humans, the burden of chemical exposure to everyone in the United States is enormous.

Only a small number of these chemicals have ever been tested to see how they affect human health. Many groups have called for the use of the **precautionary principle** when it comes to the use of contaminants that find their way into the environment and humans. The precautionary principle maintains that if something has the potential to cause harm to the environment or humans, then precautionary measures should be taken if there is a lack of scientific evidence concerning cause and effect (Kriebel et al., 2001). Applying the precautionary principle to new technology and chemicals may help protect the environment and human health. For example, there is a concern that use of cell phones may create health effects, including changes in brain activity. The scientific evidence is not yet certain, but by applying the precautionary principle, nurses can encourage people to use their cell phones on speakerphone mode or with earpieces to decrease the exposure caused by holding the phone against their heads.

It can also be challenging to prove the existence of direct links between the environment and health status of community residents. It seems logical that if sidewalks are built, people will use them, thus improving their cardiovascular health. But is it possible to measure sidewalk use? If a community could measure sidewalk use, how could it show that using the sidewalks significantly improves cardiovascular health? Often, there is a lack of scientific data to determine how exactly the community environment impacts human health. It is also difficult to determine how genetic and behavioral factors shape the health of an individual or a population.

PRACTICE POINT

Proving causal links between exposure to environmental contaminants and health outcomes, or links between the community environment and health outcomes, is often very difficult.

Genetic and Behavioral Factors

Understanding the interaction between the environment and genetics as it relates to expression of disease is still an evolving science. The challenge for environmental health nurses is to use the best science available to assess how the environment affects human health, to formulate evidence-based or best practice interventions, and to evaluate the effectiveness of these interventions.

Hereditary factors may play an important role. Many scientists believe that there are people who are more genetically susceptible to a specific disease but that environmental triggers play a role in determining who actually develops the disease. The interaction between genetics and the environment may help explain why some people who are exposed to specific contaminants develop certain health effects but others do not. Genetic alterations to glutathione-S-transferase, which codes for a protein that enables chemicals to be excreted in urine, affect the body's ability to rid itself of toxins. People with this genetic alteration may have increased cancer risks when exposed to certain chemicals in the environment (Goodman, 2009).

Individual human behaviors may also interact with environmental exposures to influence human health. For example, radon, a naturally occurring radioactive compound, can be found in the basements of many homes. Exposure to this substance has been linked to lung cancer. Research has shown that people who live in a home with radon and who smoke have a greater risk of developing lung cancer than do nonsmokers who live in homes with radon. The exposure to cigarette smoke and radon seem to interact to increase the risk of lung cancer. More information about radon and health can be found on the EPA website.

Nursing and Environmental Health

Scientific understanding of how the environment affects human health has evolved since the days of Florence Nightingale, but nurses have long recognized that people's surroundings can influence their health. Even in the 19th century, nurses realized that clients who had clean food and water and fresh air had better outcomes than did those who were left in squalid conditions. Nurses can help lead the way in healthcare by understanding that clients are part of the environment and that the health of the environment has a direct impact on their health. Nurses are in a strong position to advocate for healthier environments in both the workplace and community.

Across the country, there are great examples of nurses working with communities, conducting research, and leading programs to help promote healthy people in healthy

box 19.2 Principles of Environmental Health for Nursing Practice

1. Knowledge of environmental health concepts is essential for nursing practice.
2. The Precautionary Principle guides nurses in their practice to use products and practices that do not harm human health or the environment and to take preventive action in the face of uncertainty.
3. Nurses have a right to work in an environment that is safe and healthy.
4. Healthy environments are sustained through multidisciplinary collaboration.
5. Choices of materials, products, technology, and practices in the environment that affect nursing practice are based on the best evidence available.
6. Approaches to promoting a healthy environment respect the diverse values, beliefs, cultures, and circumstances of clients and their families.
7. Nurses participate in assessing the quality of the environment in which they practice and live.
8. Nurses, other healthcare workers, clients, and communities have the right to know relevant and timely information about the potentially harmful products, chemicals, pollutants, and hazards to which they are exposed.
9. Nurses participate in research of best practices that promote a safe and healthy environment.
10. Nurses must be supported in advocating for and implementing environmental health principles in nursing practice.

Source: From American Nurses Association. (2007). *Principles of environmental health for nursing practice with implementation strategies.* Silver Spring, MD: American Nurses Association.

environments. Nurses are also involved in helping to ensure that the environmental impact of healthcare practices in the clinical setting and community setting are considered. For example, the group Health Care Without Harm has worldwide membership from health providers to raise awareness on issues such as safer chemicals (disinfectants, solvents in laboratories) in healthcare, green purchasing (less toxic, minimal packaging), and medical waste management. More information about their work can be found at the Health Care Without Harm website (Health Care Without Harm, 2014).

The American Nurses Association (ANA) has created the *ANA's Principles of Environmental Health for Nursing Practice with Implementation Strategies.* These principles can help nurses incorporate principles of environmental health into nursing practice (Box 19.2). Nurses can use their core skills of assessment, intervention, and evaluation when considering the environment and its impact on individual patients or communities.

ASSESSMENT

Assessing Contaminants in the Environment

Frequently, public health professionals are asked to help assess whether a specific contaminant or contaminants in the environment are making a person or community sick.

The state public health agency asks Chris to assist with an environmental health assessment when media attention on PCBs starts drawing public concern. People start calling their local and state health departments and asking if the PCBs are making their families sick.

Chris starts by doing research on PCBs. These substances are not naturally occurring, tend to be heavy, and quickly settle out of the air to the ground or water. Being hydrophobic, once in the water, they also settle out of water into sediment. They are slow to break down, and unless they are removed, they remain in soil or sediment for a very long time. The PCBs can build up in small animals and fish. As larger fish and animals eat the smaller ones, the PCBs become increasingly concentrated in the food chain. In general, what would be good sources of information to find out more about PCBs?

If ever we had proof that our nation's pollution laws aren't working, it's reading the list of industrial chemicals in the bodies of babies who have not yet lived outside the womb.

Louise Slaughter, U.S. Congresswoman

People in communities often want to know their risk of getting sick from known or suspected exposure to a contaminant. In other words, they want a **risk assessment**—a process to determine the likelihood or probability that adverse effects such as illness or disease will occur in a group of people because of exposure to an environmental contaminant. The amount of risk can be a difficult thing to determine. There are different methods for conducting risk assessment for environmental contaminants. A simple way to understand risk is that the amount of risk equals the hazard plus exposure (risk = hazard + exposure).

The presence of a hazard alone does not determine the amount of risk the hazard poses. If a substance is hazardous, but there is no exposure to the substance, then a person is not at risk. For example, think of the sun. It is well known that exposure to too much sun can cause sunburns and put people at risk for skin cancer. However, if a person eliminates exposure by staying indoors or in the shade, he or she eliminates the risk. If a person puts on sunscreen or a hat or stays out of the sun in the middle of the day, he or she modifies the amount of risk by taking measures to reduce the exposure.

To assess exposure, one method is to think about exposure pathways. An **exposure pathway** is a process by which someone is exposed to a contaminant that originates from a specific source (Agency for Toxic Substances and Disease Registry, 2005). Understanding exposure pathways is important because *if the pathway is not complete or if it can be disrupted, the contaminant of concern should not affect human health.* Frequently, people incorrectly assume that if a contaminant is near their home, work, or school, they will automatically experience adverse health effects from the substance. An exposure pathway helps illustrate that proximity to a contaminant is not the deciding factor in determining its effect on humans. An exposure pathway consists

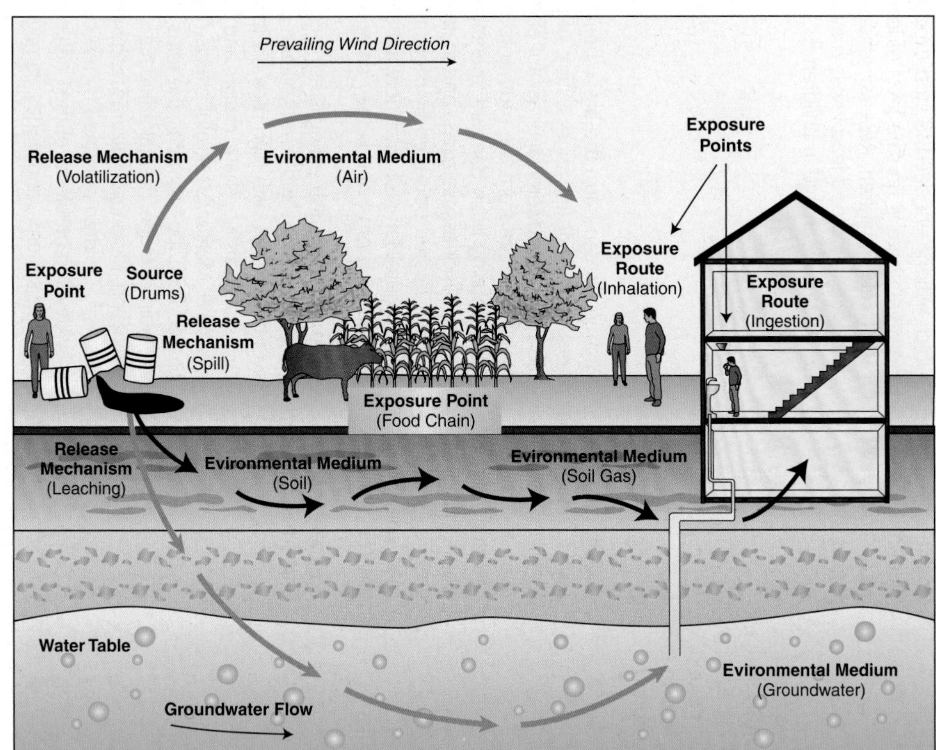

figure 19.1 Exposure pathway. (Data from Agency for Toxic Substances and Disease Registry. [2005]. *Public health assessment guidance manual*. Available at http://www.atsdr.cdc.gov/HAC/phamanual/ch6.html)

of five parts: (1) source of contamination, (2) environmental media and transport, (3) point of exposure, (4) route of exposure, and (5) receptor population. Figure 19.1 shows how each of these components is related, and the following discussion describes them in more detail.

Source of Contamination

The source of contamination is used to describe what the contaminants are and from where they originate. Sometimes, a source of contamination is easy to identify (e.g., mercury coming from a former thermometer factory site). Other sources can be more difficult to identify, such as vapor intrusion into a home from contaminated groundwater. Sources of contamination can come from point or nonpoint sources. Nonpoint sources consist of many diffuse sources while a point source tends to be one specific identified source. For example, a nonpoint source of contamination could be if gasoline drips on parking lots and roads from thousands of cars and then is washed into a neighboring lake when it rains. A tanker truck carrying gasoline that crashed and spilled its contents into a pond is an example of a point source of contamination.

Knowing the type of contaminant is important to understanding its possible effect on human health. Some contaminants quickly break down in the environment, whereas others are very persistent. Contaminants that stay longer in the environment may influence health over a greater period of time. Generally, contaminants can be thought of in three categories: chemical (lead, mercury, volatile organic compounds), biologic (mold, anthrax, ricin), and radiologic (radium, radon). Table 19.1 lists some common environmental contaminants.

Environmental Media and Transport Mechanisms

Environmental media include groundwater, surface water (lakes, ponds, rivers), air, surface soil, subsurface soil, sediment, and biota (plants and animals). The environmental medium that the contaminant is in helps determine who is exposed and how they are exposed (Agency for Toxic Substances and Disease Registry, 2005).

Transport mechanisms describe how the contaminant moves from the source to the point of exposure to people. For example, if an old drum full of a contaminant is buried and leaking, knowing how that contaminant moves through the environment helps determine if only the surrounding soil is contaminated or if the contaminant is volatile and will disperse into the air or if the contaminant is likely to get into ground water (Agency for Toxic Substances and Disease Registry, 2005).

Point of Exposure

The point of exposure is the place where people come in contact with the contaminated medium, which may include food or another item (Agency for Toxic Substances and Disease Registry, 2005). An exposure point can be a home, a playground, a lake, a business, a cloud of diesel fumes, an abandoned lot, a fish to be eaten, or a park.

Route of Exposure

The route of exposure is how the contaminant enters the body. Environmental contaminants enter the body primarily by ingestion, inhalation, or skin contact. Contaminants can come from groundwater, surface water, soil, and food (Agency for Toxic Substances and Disease Registry, 2005). Most adults do

table 19.1 **Common Exposure Pathways for Selected Environmental Contaminants**

Contaminant	Most Common Sources	Media and Transport	Most Common Point of Exposure	Route of Exposure	Populations of Most Concern	Health Effect
Lead	Paint before 1978. Homes built before 1978 may have lead paint on walls, windows, or other painted surfaces inside and outside the home.	As paint deteriorates, it can chip and create dust that contains lead. The chips and dust can accumulate in the house or be deposited into soil around the house.	Inside the house as chips or dust Soil outside the house	Ingestion	Children frequently have greater exposures because they put their hands and other objects in their mouths, they may eat paint chips, and they play outside in the soil more and may ingest the soil.	Children's brains and nervous systems are sensitive to the damage done by lead. Elevated levels of lead can damage the nervous system and brain development, slow growth, create learning problems such as hyperactivity, and cause hearing problems and headaches. A blood lead level of 5 μg/dL or greater is a level at which action is needed to stop exposure. However, there is no safe level of lead in the blood of children. Research shows that even low blood lead levels may cause neurological damage in children.
	Dust can get into air. Lead vapor if lead is heated (as if with a heat gun used to remove paint).	Inside the house	Inhalation	Children have faster respiratory rates and their breathing zone is closer to the ground, which may lead to a greater exposure.		
Mercury	Thermometers used in industry, batteries. Burning coal releases it into the air.	Intentional or accidental spills of elemental mercury	In area near a mercury spill, indoor levels can become unsafe with even small mercury spills.	Inhalation	People near the spill. Children have faster respiratory rates and their breathing zone is closer to the ground, which may lead to a greater exposure.	High levels can harm the brain, heart, kidneys, lungs, and immune system of people of all ages. Mercury's harmful effects may be passed from the mother to the fetus, causing brain damage, mental retardation, blindness, seizures, and inability to speak. Children poisoned by mercury may develop problems of their nervous and digestive systems, and kidney damage.
		Can enter the environment, settle into water, and bioaccumulate in fish	Fish	Ingestion	Pregnant women and small children	For most adults, fish eating is not a concern. Pregnant women and small children should avoid eating fish with high mercury levels such as swordfish, shark, tilefish, and king mackerel. Mercury's harmful effects may be passed from the mother to the fetus, causing brain damage, mental retardation, incoordination, blindness, seizures, and inability to speak. Children poisoned by mercury may develop problems of their nervous and digestive systems, and kidney damage.

Radon	Naturally occurring radioactive gas. Product of decaying uranium and found in soils	Moves into houses through cracks and holes in foundations	Indoor air	Inhalation	People living in homes with radon present. People who smoke	Can damage lungs. Exposure has been linked to lung cancer. Smoking combined with radon exposure is a serious health risk.
Polychlorinated biphenyls (PCBs)	Family of human-made organic chemicals, PCBs were domestically manufactured from 1929 until their manufacture was banned in 1979. They were used in hundreds of industrial and commercial applications, including electrical, heat transfer, and hydraulic equipment; as plasticizers in paints, plastics, and rubber products; in pigments, dyes, and carbonless copy paper; and many other industrial applications.	PCBs do not readily break down and therefore may remain for long periods of time cycling between air, water, and soil. They can be carried long distances and have been found in snow and sea water in areas far away from where they were released into the environment. As a consequence, PCBs are found all over the world. In general, the lighter the form of PCB, the further it can be transported from the source of contamination. PCBs can bioaccumulate in fish.	Fish Water Air near hazardous sites or if burning	Ingestion Inhalation	Women of childbearing age and children People living near a contaminated site or near where PCBs may be burning	PCBs have been shown to cause a number of serious noncancer health effects in animals, including effects on the immune system, reproductive system, nervous system, endocrine system, and other health effects. PCBs have been shown to cause cancer in animals. Women who were exposed to relatively high levels of PCBs in the workplace or ate large amounts of fish contaminated with PCBs had babies who weighed slightly less than babies from women who did not have these exposures. Babies born to women who ate PCB-contaminated fish also showed abnormal responses in tests of infant behavior. Some of these behaviors, such as problems with motor skills and a decrease in short-term memory, lasted for several years. The most likely way infants will be exposed to PCBs is from breast milk.
Tetrachloroethylene (perchloroethylene [PERC])	Another name from tetrachloroethylene is PCE. Tetrachloroethylene has been found in at least 771 of the 1,430 National Priorities List sites identified by the Environmental Protection Agency (EPA). PERC is a manufactured chemical used for dry cleaning and metal degreasing.	Much of the PERC that gets into water or soil evaporates into the air, but it can contaminate groundwater and drinking water supplies.	Clothes from the dry cleaners, vapor intrusion—when vapors can come from contaminated groundwater or soil into a building or home.	Inhalation	People who live or work in a building with vapor intrusion	High concentrations of the PERC (particularly in closed, poorly ventilated areas) can cause dizziness, headache, sleepiness, confusion, nausea, difficulty in speaking and walking, unconsciousness, and death. In industry, most workers are exposed to levels lower than those causing obvious nervous system effects. The health effects of breathing in air or drinking water with low levels of PERC are not known. Tetrachloroethylene has been shown to cause liver tumors in mice and kidney tumors in male rats.
			Drinking water containing tetrachloroethylene	Ingestion	People who drink water contaminated by PERC	

(continued on page 386)

table 19.1 **Common Exposure Pathways for Selected Environmental Contaminants** (continued)

Contaminant	Most Common Sources	Media and Transport	Most Common Point of Exposure	Route of Exposure	Populations of Most Concern	Health Effect
Mold	Thousands of different types of molds can grow indoors and outdoors. They thrive in moist conditions.	Mold spores can travel in the air. When the spores land in favorable conditions, they will grow and produce mold.	Indoor and outdoor air	Inhalation	People who are sensitive to mold can become sick with respiratory symptoms. At high-enough levels, even people with no previous reactions to mold may experience symptoms.	Respiratory symptoms can be severe in people who are sensitive to molds. Symptoms generally will be better once exposure to mold stops. Since everyone's sensitivity to mold is different, there is no standard "safe" level of mold. When mold is seen growing in an indoor environment, it should be properly cleaned.
Anthrax spores	Anthrax is an acute infectious disease caused by the spore-forming bacterium *Bacillus anthracis*. The *B. anthracis* spores can live in the soil for many years, and humans can become infected with anthrax by handling products from infected animals or by inhaling anthrax spores from contaminated animal products. Anthrax spores can be used as a bioterrorist weapon, as was the case in 2001, when *B. anthracis* spores had been intentionally distributed through the postal system, causing 22 cases of anthrax, including 5 deaths.	Naturally occurring spores can be spread from people handling animal products infected with spores. Weaponized anthrax spores can be distributed in a variety of ways. Once the spores are in the environment, they can remain viable for long periods of time. Weaponized anthrax spores are designed to cause more illness and death because the spores have been altered to make them travel through the environment differently than naturally occurring spores.	Handling contaminated animal products Exposure to anthrax used as a weapon; may look like a white powder	Dermal Inhalation Dermal Inhalation	People working with animals or animal hides—such as drum makers, ranch workers People targeted by terrorists or people living or working in an area where weaponized anthrax is released	Cutaneous: Most (about 95%) anthrax infections occur when the bacterium enters a cut or abrasion on the skin, such as when handling contaminated wool, hides, leather, or hair products (especially goat hair) of infected animals. Skin infection begins as a raised itchy bump that resembles an insect bite. Inhalation: initial symptoms may resemble a common cold—sore throat, mild fever, muscle aches, and malaise. After several days, the symptoms may progress to severe breathing problems and shock. Inhalation of anthrax is usually fatal.

Benzene	Benzene is a colorless liquid with a sweet odor. It evaporates into the air very quickly and dissolves slightly in water. It is highly flammable and is formed from both natural processes and human activities. Benzene is widely used in the United States; it ranks in the top 20 chemicals for production volume. Some industries use benzene to make other chemicals that are used to make plastics, resins, and nylon and other synthetic fibers. Benzene is also used to make some types of rubbers, lubricants, dyes, detergents, drugs, and pesticides.	Benzene can pass into the air from water and soil. It reacts with other chemicals in the air and breaks down within a few days. Benzene in the air can attach to rain or snow and be carried back down to the ground. It breaks down more slowly in water and soil and can pass through the soil into underground water.	Outdoor air contains low levels of benzene from tobacco smoke, automobile service stations, exhaust from motor vehicles, and industrial emissions. Air around hazardous waste sites or gas stations contains higher levels of benzene.	Inhalation	People who smoke. People who live near sites with benzene contamination	The major effect of benzene from long-term exposure is on the blood. Benzene causes harmful effects on the bone marrow and can cause a decrease in red blood cells, leading to anemia. It can also cause excessive bleeding and can affect the immune system, increasing the chance for infection. Long-term exposure to high levels of benzene in the air can cause leukemia, particularly acute myelogenous leukemia, often referred to as AML. This is a cancer of the blood-forming organs. It is not known whether children are more susceptible to benzene poisoning than are adults. Benzene can pass from the mother's blood to a fetus. Animal studies have shown low birth weights, delayed bone formation, and bone marrow damage when pregnant animals breathed benzene.
Asbestos	Asbestos is the name given to a group of six different fibrous minerals (amosite, chrysotile, crocidolite, and the fibrous varieties of tremolite, actinolite, and anthophyllite) that occur naturally in the environment. Asbestos has been used for a wide range of manufactured goods, mostly in building materials (roofing shingles, ceiling and floor tiles, paper products, and asbestos cement products), friction products (automobile clutch, brake, and transmission parts), heat-resistant fabrics, packaging, gaskets, and coatings. Some vermiculite or talc products may contain asbestos.	Asbestos fibers can enter the air from the breakdown of natural deposits or manufactured asbestos products. Renovation of older homes or facilities containing asbestos can release it into the air.	Indoor or outdoor air	Inhalation	Workers who have worked with asbestos. Family member of people who work with asbestos. People who live or work in areas where asbestos fibers are being released into the indoor or outdoor environment.	Asbestos mainly affects the lungs and the membrane that surrounds the lungs. Breathing high levels of asbestos fibers for a long time may result in scar-like tissue in the lungs and in the pleural membrane (lining) that surrounds the lung. This disease is called asbestosis and is usually found in workers exposed to asbestos, but not in the general public. Breathing lower levels of asbestos may result in changes called plaques in the pleural membranes. Pleural plaques can occur in workers and sometimes in people living in areas with high environmental levels of asbestos. It is known that breathing asbestos can increase the risk of cancer in people. There are two types of cancer caused by exposure to asbestos: lung cancer and mesothelioma. Cigarette smoke and asbestos together significantly increase your chances of getting lung cancer.

(continued on page 388)

table 9.1 **Common Exposure Pathways for Selected Environmental Contaminants (continued)**

Contaminant	Most Common Sources	Media and Transport	Most Common Point of Exposure	Route of Exposure	Populations of Most Concern	Health Effect
Pesticides	These chemicals are used to kill pests. There are thousands of registered pesticides in the United States. Pesticides are applied commercially and privately to protect plants and crops from pests.	Once pesticides are used on crops or to control pest infestations, they can move through the environment in a variety of ways. They may end up in water. Pesticides must be carefully used to protect human health and the environment.	Indoor or outdoor air	Inhalation Dermal contact	People who work or live close to where pesticides are applied either in an indoor or outdoor environment. People can have health effects from an exposure that occurs long after the pesticides are applied because pesticides are designed to "stick around" and rid an area of pests.	The Environmental Protection Agency regulates pesticides that are commercially available in the United States; however, there are thousands of products each with unique formulation. Without knowing the specific chemicals used in the formulation, it is impossible to predict health effects for pesticides as a group. Some pesticides have been linked to a variety of health problems. Some pesticides, such as the organophosphates and carbamates, affect the nervous system. Others may irritate the skin or eyes. Some pesticides may be carcinogens. Others may affect the hormone or endocrine system in the body.
			Drinking water Eating foods with pesticides applied or accidentally ingesting pesticides	Ingestion	People drinking water contaminated with pesticides. People who ingest pesticides when they eat foods that have had pesticides applied. Adults and more likely children who accidentally ingest pesticides	

Arsenic	Arsenic is a naturally occurring element widely distributed in the earth's crust. In the environment, arsenic is combined with oxygen, chlorine, and sulfur to form inorganic arsenic compounds. Inorganic arsenic compounds are mainly used to preserve wood. Copper chromate arsenate (CCA) is used to make "pressure-treated" lumber. CCA is no longer used in the United States for residential uses; it is still used in industrial applications. Organic arsenic compounds are used as pesticides, primarily on cotton fields and orchards. Arsenic was used in many industries and many former industrial sites may have arsenic contamination. Arsenic has been found in at least 1,149 of the 1,684 National Priority List sites identified by the EPA.	Arsenic occurs naturally in soil and minerals and may enter the air, water, and land from wind-blown dust and may get into water from runoff and leaching. Many common arsenic compounds can dissolve in water. Most of the arsenic in water ultimately ends up in soil or sediment.	Indoor or outdoor air Drinking water	Inhalation Ingestion	Burning of treated wood that contained CCA People whose drinking water contains high amounts of arsenic	Ingesting very high levels of arsenic can result in death. Exposure to lower levels can cause nausea and vomiting, decreased production of red and white blood cells, abnormal heart rhythm, damage to blood vessels, and a sensation of "pins and needles" in hands and feet. Ingesting or breathing low levels of inorganic arsenic for a long time can cause a darkening of the skin and the appearance of small "corns" or "warts" on the palms, soles, and torso. Skin contact with inorganic arsenic may cause redness and swelling. Almost nothing is known regarding the health effects of organic arsenic compounds in humans. Several studies have shown that ingestion of inorganic arsenic can increase the risk of skin cancer and cancer in the liver, bladder, and lungs. Inhalation of inorganic arsenic can cause increased risk of lung cancer.

For a list of up-to-date online resources on these substances, please visit thePoint (http://thepoint.lww.com/Harkness).

not ingest large amounts of soil. However, children may ingest soil while playing, from mouthing objects, from not washing their hands, or from pica behaviors. Contaminants can be inhaled from soil (dust), air, and aerosolized water (e.g., during showering). Dermal contact from contaminants can come from soil, water, sediment, air, or food.

Receptor Population

The receptor population is the population of people who are likely to be exposed (Agency for Toxic Substances and Disease Registry, 2005). It is necessary to carefully consider and accurately identify the exposed population. For example, if a contaminant is in the groundwater, then only people with drinking wells supplied by that groundwater are exposed to the contaminant. People whose wells were fed by another source or people who use public water systems are not exposed.

When thinking about populations, it is also important to think about whether people are currently being exposed, whether people were exposed in the past, and whether people will continue to be exposed in the future. Thinking about when a population was or is exposed can help determine what interventions may be useful. The exposure pathway is illustrated in Figure 19.1.

Determining the Health Impact of a Completed Exposure Pathway

A completed exposure pathway does not guarantee that people will become sick. The exposure may not be great enough to cause a health effect. It is also possible we might not know enough about the toxicology of certain contaminants to understand their health effects. Given what experts know about medicine and science, it is difficult to imagine that we cannot determine with certainty whether exposure to a contaminant will lead to illness. There is often "an understandable misconception among the public that modern-day health scientists and medical professionals can precisely determine at what environmental level a particular contaminant presents a clear and predictable risk to human health future" (De Rosa, Holler, & Mehlman, 2002, p. 149). For most contaminants, toxicologic data are too limited to say for sure whether an exposure will have an effect. **Toxicology** is the study of the adverse effects of chemical, physical, or biological agents on people, animals, and the environment (Society of Toxicology, 2009). Many of the guiding principles of toxicology will seem familiar to nurses who are familiar with pharmacology. Toxicology and pharmacology are very similar, since both require knowledge of the "dose" needed to effect a change (either positive or negative) on a human system.

To determine any possible health effects from a contaminant, an **exposure estimate** is created. An exposure estimate determines a person's level of exposure to a contaminant. Several factors are taken into account when calculating the exposure estimate, including the duration of the exposure, the frequency of exposure, and the bioavailability of the contaminant. **Bioavailability** is the amount of a substance that is absorbed or becomes available at the site of physiological activity. In pharmacology, the bioavailability of a drug helps clinicians determine the necessary dose to ensure that the drug is effective. In toxicology, bioavailability helps toxicologists determine the "dose" of a certain contaminant that will cause a health effect.

Once toxicologists give an exposure estimate, health professionals compare it with standard health guidelines. If an exposure estimate is greater than the health guideline, there is a greater chance that the exposure can cause adverse health effects. Health guidelines are set to protect the whole population, including those who are most sensitive to potentially hazardous substances, such as children or the elderly. Health guidelines include safety factors designed to protect even the most sensitive members of a population; therefore, an exposure estimate above a particular health guideline does not guarantee that an exposure will cause harm. State health agencies, as well as federal health and environmental agencies such as the Agency for Toxic Substances and Disease Registry (ATSDR) and the EPA, develop the health guidelines.

The field of toxicology is always evolving. Nurses can consult with professionals trained in the field of toxicology to help determine whether a specific exposure can lead to a health effect. State or local health departments usually have an office that deals with environmental health issues. They are a useful resource for nurses who believe they have identified an environmental health concern or who need more information about the toxicology of a specific contaminant.

Frequently, when individuals learn they have been exposed to a contaminant, they will ask their medical provider to "test" them. For some contaminants, clinical tests can determine whether someone has been exposed. For example, a blood test or urine test can determine the level of

Chris considers if there is an exposure pathway that can link the contaminant to people who live in her town. She creates a table to help her determine if there are completed exposure pathways of PCBs into people. What would the exposure pathway table below look like for this site?

Source	Media and Transport	Point of Exposure	Route of Exposure	Receptor Population	Duration of Exposure

mercury in blood or urine. These levels provide information about how much mercury a person has in his or her body. These types of tests, referred to as **biomonitoring**, can be helpful for determining exposures to individual people and communities. Technology allows medical professionals to test for many chemicals in the body; however, our understanding of toxicology has not evolved as quickly as our ability to test for chemicals in a person. As health professionals we may be able to test for and find a chemical in a person, but we do not have the ability to tell the person how that level of chemical in them will affect their health. If biomonitoring for a chemical exposure is being considered, medical professionals first need to be sure that the testing will provide useful clinical information for treatment of the patient.

If biomonitoring is possible, the results need to be carefully interpreted. For example, many states require at least one blood lead level be checked in young children (ages 1–5 years old) as part of their wellness visits for children to attend school. A single child's elevated blood lead level can alert a nurse to the lead exposure and can allow the nurse to determine whether the blood lead level is dangerously high. However, the test cannot tell exactly when or where exposure occurred or what form of lead was involved (e.g., paint chips, lead in soil, lead in drinking water, lead paint on a toy). If many children in a community have elevated blood lead levels, it alerts health professionals to a problem in that community, but again, the test alone cannot determine where exactly the children were exposed. Much information about how lead affects children is available, and medical professionals know the significance of an individual blood lead level in terms of the child's health. However, for many contaminants, even if a medical test can detect a certain level of a contaminant, data to determine whether detected levels cause an adverse health effect may be insufficient.

EVIDENCE FOR PRACTICE

Young children in Maine are routinely screened for elevated blood lead levels. As a report by the Centers for Disease Control and Prevention (CDC, 2009c) shows, between 2003 and 2007, the Maine Childhood Lead Poisoning Prevention Program (MCLPPP) identified 55 children with elevated blood lead levels. For 90% of the children, lead exposure was linked to lead hazards in the children's homes. However, for six children, there was no evidence of lead exposure inside the home. As the investigation expanded to outside of the home, researchers discovered that the six children were exposed to lead dust in their family vehicles and in child safety seats. Investigators believed that the lead dust entered the vehicles by cross contamination from family members who had high-risk lead exposure occupations (e.g., construction, painting and paint removal, metal recycling). The lead dust on the seats likely came from contamination from either clothing or articles that family members had placed in the vehicles. This was the first documented report of child lead poisoning caused by a child's exposure to lead while in a child safety seat.

Public health nurses can apply this type of information when dealing with families of children who have elevated blood lead levels. Although lead sources in the house (e.g., old chipping paint, old lead plumbing fixtures) may be the cause of the majority of lead exposure in children, nurses may need to consider other unique sources when trying to determine how children have been exposed. Asking parents about their occupations or hobbies might help a nurse discover an unexpected exposure pathway.

The CDC's National Exposure Report describes exposures among the U.S. population to many environmental contaminants. This continuously updated biomonitoring report is a valuable resource for environmental health professionals. It establishes a reference range for typical U.S. population exposures which can be compared to individual and population measurements made in other contexts. The report also provides information about trends in U.S. exposures over time and helps environmental health professionals learn more about the various chemicals to which Americans are exposed. In addition, it establishes a reference range that these health professionals can use for comparative purposes (i.e., is an exposure low, medium, or high), determines whether exposures are higher in certain groups in the United States, and provides information about trends in the levels of contaminants in humans over time (CDC, 2009e). The complete report, titled *Fourth National Report on Human Exposure to Environmental Chemicals*, can be found on the CDC website. Caution needs to be taken if a nurse wants to compare an individual's test results to data found in the CDC report to ensure laboratory analysis and collection of the samples for the individual were done with the same methodology as the CDC data.

For many contaminants, there are no medical tests to determine whether an exposure has occurred or what the health effect of the exposure might be. There are resources and professionals who work in the field of environmental and occupational health who can help a nurse decide whether medical testing is necessary or useful for an individual client or for a community. For example, the Association of Occupational and Environmental Health Clinics (AOEC) and the Pediatric Environmental Health Specialty Units (PEHSU) are staffed with medical providers who specialize in occupational and environmental health. These providers can provide expert advice when there is a question about a possible environmental exposure and its effects (Box 19.3.).

After determining that there is at least one complete exposure pathway, the next step for Chris is to determine whether people are being exposed to high-enough levels of PCBs to make them sick. Chris meets with a member of the state environmental agency and a toxicologist from the state health department. The state has received data from fish collected in the harbor. Chris helps the toxicologist try to determine how many fish from the harbor are being eaten. With her knowledge of the local population, Chris believes that people who supplement their diets with fish from the harbor probably eat two to four fish meals a week during the warmer weather. Based on the PCB levels in the fish, Chris and the toxicologist determine that if people eat fish from the harbor two to four meals a week for 5 months a year, their exposure to PCBs is high enough to cause concern.

Some people may want to be tested to determine if they have been exposed to PCBs from the harbor. What could you do as a public health nurse to answer their questions about being tested?

EVIDENCE FOR PRACTICE

Firefighters use flame-retardant clothing for personal protection while fighting fires. Antimony oxides are often used in the production of these textiles. In 2008, the CDC received a report from a fire department chief that there was an outbreak of antimony toxicity among 30 firefighters who had elevated antimony levels detected in hair samples (CDC, 2009d). The fire department believed that exposure to the antimony in the firefighters' protective clothing caused the outbreak. The CDC administered questionnaires and collected urine antimony samples from two different groups of firefighters—one group whose clothing contained antimony and one group whose clothing did not contain antimony. The CDC found that both the groups had urine antimony levels that were not clinically significant and that wearing clothing made with antimony did not increase urine antimony levels. It should be noted that hair testing is *not* reliable or valid for measuring exposure to metals and levels of metals in the body.

Public health nurses can apply this information to practice by understanding that only valid methods of testing for metals or other chemicals in the body should be used to determine whether people are being exposed to dangerous levels of a substance. Invalid tests may make people fearful that they are ill now or will be in the future. They may also lead people to seek inappropriate treatment or delay proper care. Nurses can distribute timely and accurate risk communication and health communication materials that provide useful, specific information about environmental exposure and its effects on health.

Assessing the Environment of a Community

Knowing what contaminants are in the environment and whether there are completed exposure pathways are key steps in determining how people's health is affected by the environment. However, many other environmental conditions, aside from environmental contaminants, can influence disease and injury rates. Some environmental conditions that may be important when reflecting on the potential impact of the environment on a community's health are presented in Table 19.2. This table was designed to consider many different types of communities—urban and rural, developed and developing—regardless of socioeconomic status.

box 19.3 Association of Occupational and Environmental Clinics, Pediatric Environmental Health Specialty Units, and American College of Medical Toxicologists

Established in 1987, the Association of Occupational and Environmental Clinics (AOEC), a nonprofit organization, has grown to a network of more than 60 clinics and more than 250 individuals committed to improving the practice of occupational and environmental medicine through information sharing and collaborative research. All AOEC member clinics are multidisciplinary in staff and meet specific criteria that promote providing high-quality healthcare and patient rights. More information is available at http://www.aoec.org.

The Pediatric Environmental Health Specialty Units (PEHSU) form a respected network of experts in children's environmental health. The PEHSU were created to ensure that children and communities have access to, usually at no cost, special medical knowledge and resources for children faced with a health risk due to a natural or human-made environmental hazard. More information is available at http://aoec.org/PEHSU/index.html.

The American College of Medical Toxicologists (ACMT) is a professional nonprofit association that is dedicated to advancing medical toxicology. ACMT has physicians with expertise in medical toxicology and aims to advance the quality of care for patients poisoned with chemicals or other toxins. ACMT professionals can help medical providers by providing expert and timely advice on how to care for patients with poisoning or chemical exposures. More information is available at www.acmt.net.

If a man walks in the woods for love of them half of each day, he is in danger of being regarded as a loafer. But if he spends his days as a speculator, shearing off those woods and making the earth bald before her time, he is deemed an industrious and enterprising citizen.

Henry David Thoreau

Assessing the many ways that the environment of a community can impact health is helpful to consider before interventions are developed and implemented. For example, even if community members know that exercise such as walking can help improve their health, if the town streets lack sidewalks, this discourages walking. Creating a community program to increase awareness of the benefits of exercise will not do much to increase activity levels until the issue of the sidewalks or alternative safe exercise spaces, such as parks, is addressed.

table 19.2 **Community Environment and the Potential Effects on Health**

Environmental Condition	Effects on Health and Examples
Access to healthy housing	Age and condition of housing can expose people to contaminants (lead, asbestos, radon, or mold), pests (cockroaches, rodents, or mosquitoes), and injuries (falls, electrocution, fire, or carbon monoxide). One major concern with housing is the quality of indoor air, which can have a direct effect on diseases such as asthma (see "Indoor air" below). Location of housing can also encourage or discourage how community members get around in their communities. For example, houses built on streets that do not connect or streets without sidewalks may encourage people to drive rather than walk even short distances—this can decrease a person's physical exercise, which increases people's risk for obesity and other health issues.
Access to potable water	Most drinking water in the United States comes from public water or private water supplies such as wells. Public drinking water supplies are tested frequently and must meet federal standards. Private water supplies are not tested regularly unless done so by the person who owns or uses the water. Both public and private water supplies can be contaminated with bacteria or chemicals; however, because public water supplies are tested regularly, contamination is likely to be identified quickly. Contaminated water can make people sick quickly or more slowly, depending on the type of contamination. In some rural communities in the United States and around the world, access to potable water is still a significant health issue. An association has also been made between lack of modern water sources and lower respiratory tract infections in young children. Droughts and floods can also impact water supplies. Floods may bring contamination into public or private water supplies and drought can limit the availability of water to communities.
Sanitation and waste removal	In most parts of the United States, sanitation services and waste removal services are taken for granted. However, there are some areas where these services are lacking. For example, in some communities that lack public sewer services, there is also a lack of septic systems because of cost or difficulty in installing a septic system. Improper disposal of human waste can create health problems from direct contact with the waste or can contaminate drinking water supplies. In some poorer countries, there are virtually no sanitation or waste removal systems. People live in and around sewage and trash. Improper disposal of trash can also encourage pests, which can carry diseases and may expose people to contaminants that leach out of the trash.
Access to green spaces	Green spaces such as parks and playgrounds can help encourage people to exercise and play. Exercise can have a positive impact on health by helping to control obesity and providing other health benefits. Exercise can also promote social development in children and provide a place for the community to gather. Green space may also help people feel better about the community they live in and have positive effects on mental health.
Ambient air	Tiny airborne particles and ground-level ozone can trigger respiratory problems, especially for people with asthma. Air pollution can aggravate health problems for the elderly and others with heart or respiratory diseases. Things to consider for ambient air include potential pollution from a variety of sources, including industry, power plants, waste sites, and vehicle traffic. Other issues to consider for ambient air include local sources of particulate matter from things such as wood burning or dust from unpaved roads or construction. Air quality is an important issue worldwide. Many poorer countries lack laws, resources, and programs to help eliminate air pollution sources, whereas more affluent countries may produce more air pollution from manufacturing, making electricity, and driving automobiles. Both situations can create air quality issues that need to be addressed on a global scale.
Indoor air	Indoor air quality can often be worse than ambient air quality. Indoor air can contain high levels of particulate matter from combustion of heating and cooking fuels, cigarette smoke, and can also contain chemical contaminants from products used in the home for cleaning and painting or even from items such as carpet or furniture. Other contaminants such as mold spores and other asthma triggers such as dust and dust mites are often also found in indoor air. Poor indoor air quality can affect both poorer and more affluent homes.
Abandoned buildings, vacant lots, or facilities	Abandoned properties can create physical hazards such as structurally unsound buildings and trenches where children could be hurt. These places can also increase criminal activities and may be fire risks. Abandoned cars, tires, or piles of trash create similar risks. Abandoned properties or trash can also impact resident's pride in their community and their sense of well-being. How community pride or a sense of well-being affects health can be difficult to quantify, but it does affect quality of life.

(continued on page 394)

table 19.2 **Community Environment and the Potential Effects on Health (continued)**

Environmental Condition	Effects on Health and Examples
Access to healthy and safe foods	Full-service grocery stores are more likely than small convenience stores or fast food restaurants to stock healthy foods and fresh fruits and vegetables. If grocery stores are within easy access, then people may be able to include more healthy foods and fewer fast foods or processed foods into their diets. Farmers' markets and community-supported gardens may be a good source of healthy foods in a community. Food that is hunted, fished, or gathered may also be a source of healthy foods. However, all food that is purchased, grown, or gathered can be contaminated with bacteria or chemicals that can make people sick. Food safety is a challenge in all communities, and in the United States, there are programs in place to help keep consumer food products safe. Chemicals used in food production such as pesticides and herbicides can impact workers and community members where the chemicals are applied and may end up being consumed by those who eventually eat the produce. Modern food production using Concentrated Animal Feeding Operations (CAFOs) can increase the need for farmers to use chemicals and to treat and prevent animal pests and diseases that tend to spread when many animals are concentrated into small areas. Waste production from CAFOs can also pollute the environment. Worldwide, food quality and safety are critical health issues.
Access to physical activity such as biking, or other public spaces that encourage physical activity	A community that has safe sidewalks, bike paths, and/or jogging trails encourages people to exercise more, which can have positive health benefits. An absence of safe ways to walk or bike encourages dependence on automobiles, which can affect air quality and the amount of exercise that people get during the day. Also, if people are forced to walk or bike along unsafe streets or highways, there is a greater risk of pedestrian injuries.
Location of schools, public facilities, public transportation, and entertainment	Schools and other facilities such as libraries, theaters, or stores can help encourage people to walk or use public transportation rather than driving. Decreasing car dependency can improve air quality and increase the amount of exercise people engage in during the day.
Safety and crime	If people feel it is unsafe in their community, they may not walk as much or allow their children to play outside. The impact of stress from living in a community that is unsafe may also affect people's physical and mental health.
Animals—strays or pests	Stray animals can discourage people from exercising in and around their communities. Other animal pests such as rodents may help spread disease.
Vectors	Vectors such as mosquitoes or ticks can transmit diseases such as those caused by the West Nile virus or Lyme disease. Changes in the environment can help decrease the number of vectors. For example, getting rid of standing or stagnant water can help decrease the number of mosquitoes.
Access to healthcare (primary care providers and services such as pharmacies)	If a community can easily access primary healthcare services, they may be better able to manage chronic and acute health issues. For example, if people need to drive long distances or if public transportation is difficult to use or does not exist, they may postpone receiving healthcare.
Climate	The climate may influence health in many ways. For example, very hot or very cold weather conditions may affect how often people leave their homes to exercise. Hot weather may also lead to problems with ambient air quality, which can affect people with respiratory problems. Cold climates may also affect indoor air quality if heating sources are not clean and safe. Severe storms, droughts, and flooding can also create hazards that impact people's health.
Noise	Unwanted sound can have impacts on sleep, concentration, or even conversation. Some problems related to noise include sleep disruption, high blood pressure, and loss of productivity.
Ultraviolet (UV) radiation	UV radiation comes from the sun. Exposure to UV radiation is directly linked to skin cancers. Some areas of the world have a greater UV index. Some communities also spend a greater amount of time outside, which exposes them to greater amounts of UV radiation.
Subsistence or supplemental food gathering and hunting	Some communities may subsist on or supplement their diets with locally gathered animals or plants. These food sources can help create a healthy diet if the foods are safe but may also be a source of exposure to contaminants if the foods are not safe. For example, fish is a good source of healthy protein and fats but fish caught in contaminated waters may have a negative impact on health.
Cultural practices and traditions	Some cultural practices such as using herbs or cosmetics can expose people to contaminants in those products. In some countries, manufacturing processes may not be carefully regulated to monitor for contaminants being added either intentionally or unintentionally to the products. Cultural traditions may also expose some communities to contaminants. For example, a tradition in a community might be to gather local plants or materials to create products for sale or personal use. The collection of these items may cause people to be exposed to contaminants if the plant used to make a product naturally grows in a wetland area and the wetland water is contaminated.

table 19.2 **Community Environment and the Potential Effects on Health (continued)**

Environmental Condition	Effects on Health and Examples
Natural and human-made hazards	Some communities are more vulnerable to natural hazards such as hurricanes, tornadoes, earthquakes, or other storms. These natural events can present physical hazards or chemical hazards and create community stress. Often, when power is lost, people use generators to try to heat, cool, or light their homes. Carbon monoxide poisoning after disasters, although easy to prevent with proper use of generators, and other CO generating equipment, continues to be a challenge in the United States.
Community concerns	Listening to the concerns of the community about their environment and health can provide important insight into how the environment impacts the health of the community. Listening to and addressing the concerns is vital when helping determine intervention strategies to create healthier community environments.
Recreational waters	Recreational waters can be an excellent resource for communities to engage in recreational activities for exercise, pleasure or even as a food source such as fishing. Unfortunately, sometimes recreational water sources can be a place where people are exposed to chemical (fuel oils, metals, etc.) or biological contaminants (such as red tide or bacteria from sewage) that can cause harm. In pools, sometimes misuse/overuse of chemical pool cleaners can cause chemical exposures.

For a list of up-to-date online resources on these topics, please visit thePoint (http://thepoint.lww.com/Harkness).

The state health department asks Chris to help it discover the steps necessary to develop interventions to disrupt the exposure pathway and keep people from being exposed to the PCBs in fish from the harbor. She determines that assessing the environment of the community may be helpful in planning successful interventions. Chris thinks about the community who eats fish caught in the harbor. For many people who fish in the harbor, fish is a major protein source in their traditional diet and a way to supplement their diets. In the harbor area, there are several small, locally owned grocery stores that carry other traditional foods, and there is also a larger national grocery store. English is a second language spoken by many of the people who patronize these stores.

Why is it important to understand more about the entire environment of the community and not just about the contaminated site?

Assessment of Individuals: Taking an Exposure History

Often when clients visit a clinic or health provider, the healthcare professional does not ask them about exposures to hazardous substances or contaminants. Many people also do not associate exposures at work or home with how they are feeling, and they may not think to tell a provider about an exposure. For example, a man may come to the clinic complaining about an increase in the number of times per week that he must use his rescue inhaler for asthma. Unless he is asked by the clinician about changes at home, work, or with hobbies, he may simply not think to mention that his hobby of building model planes is occupying more of his time. Without this knowledge, the practitioner may not know about the increasing exposure to glues and paints, which could irritate the client's airways, leading to more asthma symptoms.

Taking an **exposure history** can help nurses identify current or past exposures, eliminate exposures, and try to mitigate or reduce a client's adverse health effects from exposures. The basic elements of an exposure history are found in Table 19.3.

If an exposure history reveals an exposure of concern, or if a client's illness is still possibly linked to an environmental exposure, it is important to refer that client to the appropriate resources. For example, the AOEC and the PEHSU have many useful documents and guidelines on their websites (see Box 19.3).

Local and state health departments may also have staff who can assist in finding resources for community members who have an exposure that warrants additional follow-up. In addition, a poison control center may also be able to assist with a client who has medical problems related to a suspected acute exposure, such as exposure to a pesticide.

PRACTICE POINT

Poison control centers are staffed by trained professionals who can help you evaluate a client and also help a medical professional decide on treatment options for specific exposures. The national phone number is 1-800-222-1222.

INTERVENTIONS

Planning an intervention to address environmental health issues is similar to planning any other nursing intervention. After assessing the situation, the nurse decides which intervention will best help protect and improve health. When thinking about contaminants in the environment and completed exposure pathways, the intervention is most often something designed to interrupt or break the exposure

table 19.3 **Taking an Exposure History**

Subject	Types of Questions
Present work	Where do you work? At your present work, are you exposed to any types of dusts, fumes, solvents, radiation, loud noises, pesticides, or other chemicals? Do you wear personal protection equipment? Do you wear the clothing you wear at work to home? Are there any coworkers with similar symptoms?
Past work	Where are all the places you have worked in the past? What was the longest job you held? In your past jobs, were you ever exposed to any dusts, fumes, solvents, radiation, loud noises, pesticides, or other chemicals?
Home/residence	When was your home/residence built? What type of heating do you have? Have you recently done any remodeling? Where does your drinking water come from? What types of chemicals do you use at home or in the yard? Do you have mold, mildew, or water damage issues in your home?
Activities/hobbies	In what activities or hobbies do you or your family participate? Do you hunt or fish? Do you grow any of your own foods? Do you burn or melt anything? Are there any cultural practices or traditional foods?
Concerns	Do you have any concerns about current or past exposures? Do you feel like your health is being affected by past or current exposures? Have you ever felt sick after coming into contact with chemicals or other substances? Do any of your symptoms get better when you are away from home or work?

pathway. For example, if children are playing in an area with contaminated dirt or soil, placing a fence around the site to keep them away from the site is a reasonable and likely successful intervention.

From working at the local health department, Chris knows many of the clients who come to prenatal clinic and the local Women, Infants, and Children (WIC) program are members of the harbor community. Chris works with the WIC staff to determine whether women who use WIC services know about the state fishing ban in the harbor. Chris thinks about possible interventions to prevent people from eating contaminated fish from the harbor. Engineering controls such as building a fence or blocking all fishing in the harbor would be impossible to construct or enforce. The state has already banned fishing within the harbor, so new fishing bans are not likely to prevent fishing by members of the local community. State and federal environmental agencies are working to dredge the PCB-contaminated sediment and remove the PCBs from the harbor, but the process may take decades to complete.

What types of interventions could be used to help stop people from being exposed from this site?

When thinking about interventions to improve the environment of the entire community, it can be difficult to craft interventions to address some problems. For example, it would be nearly impossible to replace all the older deteriorating housing in a community, for reasons such as cost, even if housing quality seems to have a negative impact on health. It would also be very difficult to rebuild all roads to include sidewalks and bike lanes. Interventions to make a community's environment healthier need to include the community input, be as evidence based as possible, and be feasible given the political and economic limitations.

Some interventions produce measurable results quickly, whereas other interventions might take years to produce changes. For complex or large environmental health problems, the assistance of many different community agencies and organizations, as well as local, state, tribal, or federal government support may be necessary. It is important to remember that it may take years for the community to identify a problem, develop a program to solve it (e.g., plan an intervention), and find the necessary resources, such as state or federal grants, for this program.

For example, consider a community concerned about air quality near schools. One identified source of air pollution impacting the schools is diesel exhaust from school buses. To address the problem, the community may not have the money to purchase a fleet of new less-polluting buses.

Working with the local health department, the school board, and the company that is contracted to run the school buses, the community decides that it can quickly decrease diesel emissions by implementing a "no idling" policy for school buses. Now buses parked and waiting to pick up children will no longer idle. For a longer-term solution, the community decides that it would like to engage in a program such as one suggested by EPA's website for Clean School Bus USA. In this example, the community was able to create a quick, cost-effective intervention to mitigate some exposure while also working on a more permanent solution.

With Chris's help, the health department decides that an education program aimed at letting people know why harbor fish are not safe to eat while also providing alternatives to eating harbor fish could help interrupt the exposure pathway. The education program will target women of childbearing age and children because they may be most susceptible to the effects of the PCBs and because work with the WIC staff revealed that many of the clients who come to WIC were not aware of the hazards of eating fish caught in the harbor.

What information should the educational materials for this education program include? What other consideration needs to be given to how the materials should be produced? Who should receive the materials and how will they receive them? How can Chris have community members participate in the development of the materials?

EVALUATION

Trying to evaluate the effectiveness of an intervention that stops exposures or makes an environment healthier can be challenging. As previously stated, some interventions may result in immediate, measurable changes, whereas others may not lead to changes for years. Here are two examples of measurable interventions:

- Suppose a city adopts a program to screen houses for lead and make the homes as lead-free as practically possible. By the end of a year, the city will be able to determine how many homes were screened and made safer.
- Suppose a town identifies contaminated private wells and decided to bring public water to supply the homes. At the end of the year, the town could count the number of people who have a safe water supply.

However, even if it is possible to measure some positive changes, it may be very difficult to measure how the intervention positively impacted people's health. Think of the lead in housing example above and consider how a program might be viewed if, after the program was in place for a year, there was an increase in the total number of children living in the city who had elevated blood lead levels. Would the increase in numbers indicate the program was a failure? Or could the increase be caused by an increased awareness of lead as a hazard and a willingness by parents to have their children's blood lead levels tested. As more children were tested, more elevated blood lead levels were discovered. Using only the total number of children with elevated blood lead levels within the city might not be the best indicator to prove the intervention is successful.

An evaluation performed for any intervention should help decide whether the intervention has achieved its goals and whether improvements or changes need to be made. When interventions are being funded either from private or public funding sources, the entity funding the intervention often requires that some type of evaluation be performed. Sometimes, no matter how successful a program or project is, if the people running the program cannot evaluate it and communicate the results of their evaluation, the program or project may not receive the funding needed to continue.

Some types of questions to consider when evaluating an intervention include the following:

- Has the exposure pathway been interrupted?
- What does the community think about the intervention—are people satisfied?
- How has health improved?
- How many people did the intervention affect?
- Can the intervention demonstrate any cost savings?
- Is the intervention sustainable?

It is helpful to consider how an intervention will be evaluated in the process of developing the intervention. This way, it is possible to think about how to collect the necessary data either quantitatively or qualitatively to determine whether the intervention resulted in the intended outcome.

Chris tests the effectiveness of educational materials with the help of the local clinic and WIC staff. They ask clients for feedback about the materials and ask them whether they have been able to avoid eating fish from the harbor. A community member suggests that if information was available in the grocery store, more people might be able to make safer fish choices while shopping. As a result, there is outreach to owners of local grocery stores, who are asked if the educational materials can be located in the stores. The grocery store owners are receptive to posting information because fish sold in their stores is obtained from commercial fishing sources (not caught in the harbor).

Chris also works with the WIC staff to keep data on the number of clients who receive information about safe fish consumption. Why is it important to test materials before using them? Why would you want to keep data about the materials used? What other ways could be used to determine if the intervention is effective?

ENVIRONMENTAL EPIDEMIOLOGY

Epidemiology is a field of public health science that focuses on the incidence and prevalence of disease or illness in a population. This field of study is most well known for helping to identify outbreaks of infectious diseases. Many basic principles of epidemiologic studies can be applied to the field of environmental health. **Environmental epidemiology** can help determine whether the environment is affecting people's health. One challenge in environmental epidemiology is that it is nearly impossible to create an experimental study that is generally considered the most conclusive form of epidemiologic study. In an experimental study, one group is exposed to something while another group is not exposed. It is unethical to expose a person or population to an environmental hazard or contaminant intentionally for the purposes of conducting an experimental study. For example, if we suspect that a chemical used in water treatment is harmful to health but do not know how much of an exposure would cause a health effect, it would be unethical to put various amounts of the chemical in the water supply of different communities to watch and see when people become ill. Since experimental designs cannot be used for most environmental studies, cohort studies, case-control studies, or cluster investigations are generally used for environmental epidemiology.

Case-control studies and cluster investigations are retrospective studies that first identify people who have an adverse health condition and then try to determine what exposure or exposures caused the health effect. Cohort studies are prospective studies that go forward in time and document the characteristics or the health effects that occur (see Chapter 7). The information gained from environmental epidemiologic studies can be very helpful in trying to identify whether particular exposures have made people ill.

Major challenges to most environmental epidemiology studies include the following:

- Limited availability of data on many contaminants and their effect on health
- Limited understanding about how exposures to multiple contaminants may sicken people
- Latency between exposure and illness can be very long (e.g., even decades).

In addition, studies in environmental epidemiology may be

- Time-consuming to perform
- Resource-intensive in terms of personnel and money
- Inconclusive in determining whether X contaminant caused Y illness

Disease clusters occur when there seem to be an elevated number of diseases in a family, in a community, among coworkers, or among classmates. Epidemiologists who have knowledge of disease, biostatistics, and public and environmental health investigate these suspected clusters. Frequently, state or local health departments conduct these investigations. A healthcare professional should report any suspected disease cluster to the local or state health department. A variety of factors can create the appearance of a cluster where there is no increased rate of disease.

Cancer is a frequent concern for community members. For example, the local health department might receive a report that a specific neighborhood has "a lot of cancer." When the health department investigates, it finds that in the neighborhood there are many cases of cancer but that all the cancers are different types, including breast cancer, bladder cancer, prostate cancer, leukemia, and colon cancer. Unfortunately, these cancers are common, and to community members, there is a perception that their community has more cancer than other areas, but the etiology of each of these cancers is different and not linked to a common cause.

Most states have cancer registries that track all cancers diagnosed within the state. These registries can be helpful for epidemiologists to determine if a specific area has a higher-than-expected rate of cancer. However, the information from the registry needs to be considered carefully. For example, when someone is diagnosed with cancer, where they lived at time of diagnosis is put into the registry. The registry does not track whether someone just moved to that location or whether they lived their entire life at one location. Since many environmental exposures which cause cancer can take years or decades to develop, cancer registries cannot reliably show a link between cancer and exposure where people live. Other registries are also sometimes available for birth defects and diseases such as multiple sclerosis (MS) or amyotrophic lateral sclerosis (ALS). These registries, such as cancer registries, can be used by public health nurses to gather useful data. Circumstances that point to a potential true cluster include the occurrence of (1) large number of cases of one type of cancer rather than several different types, (2) rare types of cancer rather than common types, and/or (3) increased numbers of cases of a certain type of cancer in an age group usually not affected by that type of cancer (National Cancer Institute, 2011). For many suspected cancer clusters, ultimately no evidence is found to indicate that the cases of cancer represent a true cluster. A 2012 study reviewed 487 investigations for cancer clusters reported from 1990 to 2010. Only three of the investigations could link an increase in the number of cancers to a hypothesized exposure and only one investigation found a clear cause (Goodman, Naiman, Goodman, & LaKind, 2012). Because cancer is not one but many diseases, trying to find a true cancer cluster and link it to a specific environmental exposure is very challenging.

PRACTICE POINT

When thinking about environmental epidemiologic studies, it is important to remember how they differ from assessing an exposure pathway. An epidemiologic study often starts with people who are ill or who had a known exposure. The studies try to determine whether the illness was caused by an environmental exposure or whether people with a known exposure became sick. Assessing an exposure pathway starts with looking at specific contaminants in the environment and determining if there is a completed exposure pathway to humans.

WORKING TOWARD HEALTHY ENVIRONMENTS

Healthy Communities

Healthy communities can help mitigate exposure to harmful contaminants and also encourage good health by incorporating design principles that optimize the physical, social, and economic environment of the community. In the 20th century, builders of communities did little planning and did not consider the impact on human health and ecology from this type of development. As areas around urban centers expanded, the term "urban sprawl" or just "sprawl" described how communities edged away from urban centers. The concept of sprawl included nonexistent land use planning, dependence on automobiles, and widespread commercial development along major roads and residential areas with low population densities. Communities developed as part of sprawl often lacked sidewalks or bike routes, and there were no routes between residential developments to allow for walking between neighborhoods.

Healthy communities help combat sprawl, and their design is gaining attention and acceptance. Terms such as *smart growth*, *healthy communities*, *green development*, *built environment*, and *healthy community design* all try to promote the concept that when health considerations are incorporated into the planning or redevelopment, the community design itself can work to make people healthier. Researchers have discovered that well-planned community growth can help lessen the environmental impacts of development.

The combination of buildings and transportation make up to 71% of the country's greenhouse gas emissions (EPA, 2009b). By working to build communities where people can decrease their transportation needs and by creating more energy-efficient buildings, communities can create healthier environments for local community members and positively impact the health of the larger national or global community. Planned, smart-growth communities can improve water quality by designing green infrastructure for storm water runoff. When rain and storm water hit impermeable structures such as paved roads, parking lots, and other surfaces, water runs off into sewer systems or directly into lakes, streams, rivers, and oceans, often taking contamination with it. Encouraging landscape design and minimizing impervious surfaces can help to keep water cleaner. Green roofs, shaded sidewalks and streets, and building with solar reflective materials can also help mitigate the "heat island" effect that makes cities and urban areas hotter than surrounding green areas.

As new communities are built or older communities are being redeveloped, nurses and public health professionals can work with planners, political leaders, developers, bankers, local boards of public health, and community groups to help ensure that the health impacts (both positive or negative) of the development are considered. Often, simple design changes can have significant health effects. For example, if a new school site is being considered, choosing a site that encourages children to safely walk to school will help increase children's activity levels and create less vehicular traffic in the community. Selection of building materials and considering the entire life cycle of materials (from where and how they are created to how they will eventually be disposed of) can also help to make communities healthier. More information on healthy communities and smart growth can be found at the CDC and EPA websites.

Healthy Homes

Like the concept of healthy communities, the central premise of the healthy homes concept is that the home has a direct influence on health. The CDC has started a Healthy Homes Initiative, which is a coordinated, comprehensive, and holistic approach to preventing diseases and injuries that result from housing-related hazards and deficiencies. The focus of the initiative is to identify health, safety, and quality-of-life issues in the home environment and to act systematically to eliminate or mitigate problems (CDC, 2009b). The initiative seeks to provide resources, such as healthy home inspection guidelines, to educate public health professionals and to promote cross-disciplinary activities at the local, state, tribal, and federal levels to eliminate housing deficiencies and hazards.

In the past, issues such as lead (paint) and radon dominated discussions about environmental issues and housing. These topics are still very important and deserve attention, but the more holistic healthy homes concept has continued to expand. Now, considerations about the environment and individual homes or community housing involve topics such as indoor air quality, mold and mildew mitigation and control, green building and green cleaning techniques, and integrated pest management. In addition, information is available about how older citizens can safely continue to live in their homes and communities, with new technologies and assistance that reduce hazards (such as falls and remote medical monitoring) in the home. The CDC has created a Healthy Housing Reference Manual that is available at the CDC website.

CHILDREN'S HEALTH AND THE ENVIRONMENT

Vulnerability to the Environment

Children may be more vulnerable to environmental exposures than are adults. Several factors increase children's vulnerability, including the following:

- Children's body systems are still rapidly developing.
- Children eat, drink, and breathe more in proportion to their body size than do adults.
- Children's breathing zone is closer to the ground compared with adults.
- Children's bodies may be less able to break down and excrete contaminants.

- Children's behaviors can expose them to more contaminants. For example, young children, especially, spend time crawling and placing their hands or other objects in their mouths (EPA, 2013).
- Children spend time in places (school, day care, play spaces, gyms) outside of their homes where environmental hazards may exist. For example, children often spend more time playing outside in the dirt compared with adults (EPA, 2013).

Nurses should consider children's unique vulnerabilities to contaminants when assessing an exposure pathway. For example, lead poisoning is a problem that largely affects young children. Children living near a site with lead in the soil would likely be at greater risk from lead poisoning than the adults in the community because, as previously stated, they tend to put their hands or other objects, which may be contaminated with lead dust, into their mouths. Children who live in a community with older housing and close to a site with lead-contaminated soil may be exposed to the metal from multiple exposure pathways. Data show that children living at or below the poverty line who live in older housing are at greatest risk. There are approximately 500,000 children in the United States aged 1 to 5 with blood lead levels above 5 micrograms per deciliter (μg/dL), the reference level at which CDC recommends public health actions be initiated (CDC, 2013). The CDC has online resources relating to lead poisoning and its prevention.

Older children and adolescents may also be at risk for exposure to environmental hazards in a way which adults are not. For example, mercury is a metal that comes from a variety of sources, including old thermometers and blood pressure cuffs. Metallic mercury is fun to play with because of the way it rolls around and forms beads. Children who find mercury frequently like to play with mercury and inadvertently track it from place to place as they share it with their friends. Most adults realize that mercury can be harmful, but most children may not realize how dangerous an object of play can be. Unfortunately, mercury has well-known health effects, and even at low levels, metallic mercury can cause health problems.

Metallic mercury exposure can cause harm before symptoms arise (Agency for Toxic Substances and Disease Registry [n.d.], National Alert). The vapor from the mercury when inhaled can cause serious health problems. Even a small amount of liquid mercury can create enough mercury in the air to close a school, take buses out of circulation, or force evacuations of homes. There have been incidents where schools have been forced to stay closed for days while a mercury cleanup, which is difficult and expensive, took place. The *Don't Mess with Mercury* project, a collaboration between ATSDR and EPA, has short videos aimed at teens to help them realize the danger of mercury. The videos and other materials on mercury can be found at the website www.dontmesswithmercury.org.

When an entire community is being assessed, it is important to consider how the environment affects children specifically. For example, a lack of safe places to play may affect children more directly than adults. Children may be at risk for more injuries if they are playing in streets or other areas that were not designed for safe play. Teens may be more likely to trespass on contaminated abandoned sites to hang out with friends or engage in activities like riding bikes. In low-income areas, the playgrounds may have more trash, rusty play equipment, and damaged surfaces, which could all contribute to an increased injury rate (CDC, 2011).

In 2013, EPA released *America's Children and the Environment*, third edition, which has valuable information on environmental stressors' effect on children. This document and many others on children's health can be found at the EPA website. The World Health Organization (WHO) also has information on children's environmental health from a global perspective that is available online.

STUDENT REFLECTION

In many respects, I don't think many of my classmates understand the impact of contaminants in the home environment. My community health practicum was in an elementary regional school in a rural setting. One little 7-year-old girl, Rebecca, who did well in school last year, was reported to have recent attention problems, and difficulty breathing, especially after recess. After talking to the family, my preceptor and I decided to make an environmental home assessment to gather more information. We found that the small two-bedroom, old farmhouse was extremely littered and crowded. All three adults in the family smoked. The only heat came from a wood stove and a small, old electric heater. There were four younger children in the house who looked frightened. While we were there, Rebecca had a coughing spell and looked very pale. Several interventions were necessary. Ultimately, Rebecca saw a physician who diagnosed asthma, and smoke was a significant trigger for her attacks. A referral to the county asthma prevention program led to a thorough assessment there. Health professionals presented an educational program about asthma, its triggers, use of inhalers, and warning signs for complications to both Rebecca and her parents. By the time my practicum was finished, Rebecca was having much less trouble breathing on exertion and was doing better in the classroom.

Healthy Schools

More than 50 million children attended school in more than 99,000 public school buildings in the United States in 2009 (National Center for Education Statistics, 2009). Many of these buildings, which are old and in poor condition, may contain environmental conditions that inhibit learning and pose increased risks to the health of children and staff. Many programs and materials are available to help schools create healthy environments. These programs and materials deal with issues such as lead to green cleaning techniques, chemical management, indoor and outdoor air quality, and school site selection. The EPA has a website devoted to healthy school environments and in 2011 released the EPA Voluntary School Siting Guidelines to help communities determine the best location for schools. The U.S. Department of Education also suggests online how to provide safe school environments. In addition, the CDC has many resources available online for schools.

ENVIRONMENTAL JUSTICE

Environmental justice is the belief that no group of people should bear a disproportionate share of negative environmental health consequences regardless of race, culture, or income. In 1994, a White House executive order required that each federal agency make environmental justice part of its mission. The Interagency Workgroup on Environmental Justice, established by the executive order, is charged with reducing disparities in community exposure to lead, toxic wastes, air pollution, and pesticides. It defines environmental justice as

> . . . the fair treatment and meaningful involvement of all people regardless of race, color, national origin, or income with respect to the development, implementation, and enforcement of environmental laws, regulations, and policies. Fair treatment means that no group of people, including a racial, ethnic, or a socioeconomic group, should bear a disproportionate share of the negative environmental consequences resulting from industrial, municipal, and commercial operations or the execution of federal, state, local, and tribal programs and policies. (CDC, 2008)

More information about the Interagency Workgroup on Environmental Justice is available online.

Many poorer or minority communities that lack political and economic power bear a disproportionate burden of environmental hazards. For example, in 2005, Hurricane Katrina hit the city of New Orleans. The storm caused massive flooding of several parishes when some of the city's levees broke. The parishes most affected by the flooding were among the poorest in the city. Some experts have argued that years of city growth and development and neglect of the levees, without adequate consideration of environmental justice, created a situation where the most economically disadvantaged communities were in areas most vulnerable to devastation from a major storm.

Another example that illustrates environmental justice concerns farm workers. Approximately 90% of the 2 million farm workers in the United States are people of color. Through direct exposure to pesticides, farm workers and their families may face serious health risks. It has been estimated that as many as 313,000 farm workers in the United States may suffer from pesticide-related illnesses each year (Environmental Protection Agency, 2009a). These illnesses may make the workers and their families even more vulnerable to extreme poverty if their illness prevents them from working. Many farm workers and their families tend to live close to their work because they have few resources to travel to and from work. Living close to the field they work in often means they are exposed to pesticides while working in fields and while at home. Children may also be exposed because they live close to where the pesticides are applied. The workers may lack opportunities that would enable them to seek jobs in other industries. In addition, they may lack resources to make moving possible and if they complain, they may lose their jobs.

When we talk about environmental justice, we mean calling a halt to the poisoning and pollution of our poorest communities, from our rural areas to our inner cities. When our children's lives are no longer cut short by toxic dumps, when their minds are no longer damaged by lead paint poisoning, we will stop wasting energy and intelligence that could build a stronger, more prosperous America.

Former President Bill Clinton

Environmental justice is also an important consideration when working with tribal communities. Tribal communities often bear a disproportionate burden of impact from pollution on their tribal lands. Many tribal communities still continue to practice traditional tribal life ways, including eating traditional foods for either a majority or a portion of their diets. These traditional practices are often negatively affected by contaminated land and water. For example, if a tribal community's traditional fishing grounds are polluted, a state may issue a "no fishing" advisory, and the community may lose a large part of its traditional diet. The "no fishing" advisory may affect the tribal community more than it does the nontribal community whose diet is not as dependent on fish.

GLOBAL ENVIRONMENTAL HEALTH CHALLENGES

Climate change is happening, humans are causing it, and I think this is perhaps the most serious environmental issue facing us.

Bill Nye, American science educator and television personality

In the 21st century, there is a greater focus on world health. Modern travel and communication systems make it possible for people to go to all parts of the world. As people begin to feel more connected to their world, they may also feel more vulnerable, because environmental health issues in one country can affect others. Contamination created in one country does not abide by map boundaries and may affect neighboring countries. Consumption patterns may also create a situation where one country contaminates its air, water, or land while manufacturing goods for other countries. If we want to all live in a healthy environment as society moves forward, people will be forced to confront difficult issues with global consequences.

Clean Water and Sanitation

In the United States, most citizens have access to clean water and sanitation services and often take these services for granted. Worldwide, however, clean water and sanitation are not standard. According to the WHO, in 2010, 783 million people lacked access to improved water sources. Improved water sources are water sources that are considered likely to be safe. About 2.5 billion people globally also lacked access to adequate sanitation and 1.1 billion people still practice open defecation. The regions with the lowest access were sub-Saharan Africa (31%), southern Asia (36%), and Oceania (53%). (*Oceania* is the term used for the geographical region consisting of numerous countries and territories, mostly islands, in the Pacific Ocean.) Studies show that improved sanitation reduces death from diarrhea by one-third (WHO, 2011a). A major killer, diarrhea is largely preventable; it is responsible for 1.5 million deaths every year, mostly among children living in developing countries (WHO, 2011a). Hygiene education and the promotion of simple interventions such as hand washing can help decrease diarrheal diseases. As the world's population continues to expand, access to clean water and sanitation services is likely to remain a challenge.

Air Quality

Outdoor and indoor air quality affects people in all countries. However, people in developing countries bear more than half of the burden from air pollution on human health. Exposure to particulate matter and ozone carries serious risks to health. By reducing air toxins, it is possible to reduce the morbidity and mortality of illnesses such as lung cancer, asthma, respiratory tract infections, and heart disease (WHO, 2009a). As the relationship between air quality and health has become clearer, the WHO has established guidelines for countries to help decrease air pollution–related illnesses.

Indoor air quality is a problem, especially in homes where biomass fuel and coal are burned for heat or cooking. In some areas, people are forced to burn fuels such as animal dung for heat or cooking. Many fuel sources, including animal waste, wood, and coal, do not combust well and create high levels of particulate matter. The indoor air concentrations of particulate matter can be 10 to 15 times higher in indoor air than in outdoor air. Chronic exposure to particulate matter can increase the risk of cardiovascular and respiratory diseases. In developing countries, exposure to particulate matter from indoor heating and cooking sources can also increase the risk of acute lower respiratory tract infections and associated deaths in young children (WHO, 2009a).

Weather forecast for tonight: dark.

George Carlin

Chemical and Contaminant Exposure

Worldwide, people may be exposed to chemicals and other contaminants in ways that are very different than in the United States. Many countries lack environmental and occupational protections that we have come to appreciate. For example, mining practices in Nigeria led to an outbreak of lead poisoning in at least six villages. In this part of Nigeria, people use rudimentary tools to break apart ore to find pieces of gold. The process creates lots of lead-contaminated dust, since the ore has a high lead concentration. Much of the work is done near or in family compounds. In 2010, a multidisciplinary team surveyed two of the affected villages and collected blood from children younger than 5 years. The team found in just two villages, in the 12 months before the team arrived, 118 out of 463 (26%) children younger than 5 years had died. Parents reported that 82% of the children who died had convulsions before death, a sign of severe lead poisoning. Blood samples collected from 205 living children found that 97% had blood lead levels greater than 45 µg/dL. In the United States, children with a blood lead level of 45 µg/dL would immediately have chelation therapy started to reduce their blood lead levels. The blood lead concentrations in the children ranged from 33.3 to 445 µg/dL (CDC, 2010). The total number of deaths across all villages is not known, but according to the WHO, an estimated 2,000 children need chelation therapy. The WHO has stated of the crisis, "[S]ome children will require chelation for many months…In addition, capacities within Nigeria for the diagnosis and management of lead poisoning need further strengthening and support. A further challenge is the purchase of sufficient chelating agents: these are expensive drugs that are not available as generics" (WHO, 2011b).

This story from Nigeria illustrates the potential deadly consequences when there exists a combination of limited environmental protections, lack of knowledge concerning environmental dangers by local community members, and the community members' need to earn an income. As we become a more globalized community with natural resources and materials being produced, shipped, and moved around the world faster than ever before, we need to consider the impact on the communities that produce those resources and materials and strive to protect their health as we protect ours in the United States. Just as we consider environmental justice within the United States, we must consider it on the global scale.

Climate Change

Although the extent and severity of climate change are still topics under debate, most scientists and governments agree that human activities are influencing global climate. Climate variability and change affect human health in a variety of ways. Climate change will likely cause a shift in the number and severity of natural disasters, such as heat waves, floods, and droughts. These natural disasters will have an immediate, direct impact on human health, but they will also have wider-ranging impacts on water and food supplies. Food security, already a problem for many poorer areas, will continue to be a challenge as climate change affects crop patterns.

Changes to water supplies and increased flooding may make some areas more vulnerable to diarrheal diseases. In addition, many diseases are highly sensitive to changes in climate. Experts predict that common vector-borne diseases such as malaria and dengue fever will affect larger geographic areas, as the vectors that carry the diseases find agreeable climates in expanding areas. Climate change will also affect air quality. The WHO estimates that 300,000 million people have asthma and will face increased disease burden from climate change.

It is necessary to realize that the effects of climate on human health will not be evenly distributed around the world. Populations in developing countries, particularly in the Small Island Developing States, arid and high mountain zones, and densely populated coastal areas, are considered to be particularly vulnerable (WHO, 2009b). However, it is not only developing countries that will be affected. For example, a heat wave in Western Europe in 2003 caused approximately 70,000 more deaths that year than had been caused in previous years. Countries in Europe and the United States will feel the impact of changes to storm patterns and may also face water and food supply issues if patterns of drought or excessive rain affect agricultural areas (WHO, 2012).

Climate change has helped illustrate that humans live in a world where the health of all environments is connected. It is nearly impossible to view global environmental issues as something that happens "over there." The industrialization of countries such as China and India will have a direct impact on the environmental health of the entire planet. To tackle these issues, global cooperation and planning are essential. Information about climate change and what one person can do is available at the EPA's Climate Change website.

key concepts

- The environment has a direct impact on human health.
- The nursing process of using assessment, intervention, and evaluation can be used when thinking about how the environment affects human health.
- Proximity to a contaminant or hazard is not the only factor in determining whether there is a risk to human health. For a contaminant to pose a risk, there must be a completed exposure pathway.
- When assessing a community's environment, it is helpful to think about the whole environment to determine what components are influencing human health.
- Environmental justice is important to consider when looking at the impact of the environment on a community.
- A community environment can be built to help positively influence the health of those living in the community.
- Globally, there are still many environmental health challenges that must be faced.

critical thinking questions

1. You are a public health nurse and receive a call from a resident who stated "many people on Spruce Street near the old junk yard have cancer." The resident is concerned. What types of questions would you think about to begin to determine whether there could be a connection between the cancer and the site?
2. As a local public health nurse, a family is referred to you because their 3-year-old child has a blood lead level of 26 μg of lead per deciliter. Is this a high lead level? What are the likely sources of lead exposure for the child? What type of education would you likely do for the family? Consider looking at the Center for Disease Control and Prevention's website on lead.
3. The town you live in is considering using a multiacre abandoned site to build a mixed-use development (it will have retail facilities, residential buildings, and public space). As a public health nurse, what would you suggest the designers consider to optimize the environmental health of the development? Consider looking at the Environmental Protection Agency's website on smart growth and green building.
4. Think of the community surrounding your school of nursing. Pick two environmental conditions and assess these conditions. Where do you think you could locate data to support your observations?
5. Why do you think it is important for the government to monitor human exposures across the United States?
6. Consider an environmental health challenge facing a developing country. What are some economically feasible interventions that could help protect community members? (Websites such as the CDC Safe Water System or the WHO Environmental Health websites might help provide some ideas.)

references

Agency for Toxic Substances and Disease Registry. (2005). *Public health assessment guidance manual*. Retrieved June 21, 2010, from http://www.atsdr.cdc.gov/HAC/phamanual/ch6.html

Agency for Toxic Substances and Disease Registry. (n.d.). *A warning about continuing patterns of metallic mercury exposure*. Retrieved December 15, 2009, from http://www.atsdr.cdc.gov/alerts/970626.html

American Chemical Society. (2013). *CAS registry—The gold standard for chemical substance information*. Retrieved March 28, 2013, from http://www.cas.org/content/chemical-substances

Carson, R. (1962). *Silent spring*. New York, NY: Houghton Mifflin Harcourt

Centers for Disease Control and Prevention. (2002). *Managing elevated blood lead levels among young children: Recommendations from the Advisory Committee on Childhood Lead Poisoning Prevention*. Retrieved December 15, 2009, from http://www.cdc.gov/nceh/lead/CaseManagement/caseManage_main.htm

Centers for Disease Control and Prevention. (2008). *Environmental justice*. Retrieved December 15, 2009, from http://www.cdc.gov/omhd/AMH/EJ.htm

Centers for Disease Control and Prevention. (2009a). *National surveillance data for lead 1997–2006*. Retrieved December 15, 2009, from http://www.cdc.gov/nceh/lead/data/national.htm

Centers for Disease Control and Prevention. (2009b). *CDC's health homes initiative*. Retrieved December 15, 2009, from http://www.cdc.gov/nceh/lead/healthyhomes.htm

Centers for Disease Control and Prevention. (2009c). Childhood lead poisoning associated with lead dust contamination from family vehicles and child safety seats—Maine, 2008. *Morbidity and Mortality Weekly Report, 58*(32), 890–893.

Centers for Disease Control and Prevention. (2009d). Pseudo-outbreak of antimony toxicity in firefighters—Florida, 2009. *Morbidity and Mortality Weekly Report, 58*(46), 1300–1302.

Centers for Disease Control and Prevention. (2009e). *Fourth national report on human exposure to environmental chemicals*. Atlanta, GA: Department of Health and Human Services, Centers for Disease Control and Prevention. Retrieved March 4, 2013, from www.cdc.gov/exposurereport/pdf/fourthreport.pdf

Centers for Disease Control and Prevention. (2010). Notes from the field: Outbreak of acute lead poisoning among children aged <5 Years—Zamfara, Nigeria, 2010. *Morbidity and Mortality Weekly Report, 59*(27), 846.

Centers for Disease Control and Prevention. (2011). School health guidelines to promote healthy eating and physical activity. *Morbidity and Mortality Weekly Report, 60*(RR05), 1–17.

Centers for Disease Control and Prevention. (2013). *Lead*. Retrieved July 11, 2014, from, http://www.cdc.gov/nceh/lead/

De Rosa, C. T., Holler, J. S., & Mehlman, M. A. (2002). *Impact of hazardous chemicals on public health, policy and service*. Princeton, NJ: International Toxicology Books.

Environmental Protection Agency. (2001). *Fight lead poisoning with a healthy diet*. Retrieved December 15, 2009, from http://www.epa.gov/lead/pubs/nutrition.pdf

Environmental Protection Agency. (2007). *Plain English guide to the Clean Air Act* (Publication No. EPA-456/K-07-001). Research Triangle Park, NC: Office of Air Quality Planning and Standards. Retrieved from http://www.epa.gov/oar/caa/peg/peg.pdf

Environmental Protection Agency. (2009a). *Environmental justice frequently asked questions*. Retrieved December 15, 2009, from http://www.epa.gov/compliance/resources/faqs/ej/index.html#faq20

Environmental Protection Agency. (2009b). *Smart growth guidelines for sustainable design and redevelopment*. Retrieved from http://www.epa.gov/smartgrowth/sg_guidelines.htm

Environmental Protection Agency. (2013). *Fast facts on children's environmental health*. Retrieved March 8, 2013, from http://yosemite.epa.gov/ochp/ochpweb.nsf/content/fastfacts.htm

Goodman, J. E. (2009). Overview: Gene–environment interactions. *Gradient Trends Risk Science and Application, 46*, 1–4.

Goodman, M., Naiman, J. S., Goodman, D., & LaKind, J. S. (2012). Cancer clusters in the USA: What do the last twenty years of state and federal investigations tell us? *Critical Reviews in Toxicology, 42*(6), 474–490.

Health Care Without Harm. (2014). *What we do*. Retrieved February 13, 2014, from http://www.noharm.org/all_regions/about/

Kriebel, D., Tickner, J., Epstein, P., Lemons, J., Levins, R., Loechler, E. L., . . . Stoto, M. (2001). The precautionary principle in environmental science. *Environmental Health Perspectives, 109*(9), 871–876. Retrieved June 21, 2010, from http://ehp.niehs.nih.gov/members/2001/109p871-876kriebel/kriebel-full.html#def

National Cancer Institute. (2013). *Facts on cancer clusters*. Retrieved March 7, 2013, from http://www.cancer.gov/cancertopics/factsheet/Risk/clusters#p2

National Center for Education Statistics. (2009). *Fast facts*. Retrieved December 15, 2009, from http://nces.ed.gov/fastfacts/

Society of Toxicology. (2009). Retrieved July 7, 2010, from http://www.toxicology.org

World Health Organization. (2009a). *Air quality and health. Factsheet No 313*. Retrieved December 15, 2009, from http://www.who.int/mediacentre/factsheets/fs313/en/index.html

World Health Organization. (2009b). *Climate change and human health*. Retrieved July 7, 2010, from http://www.who.int/globalchange/en/

World Health Organization. (2011a). *10 facts on sanitation*. Retrieved March 4, 2013, from http://www.who.int/features/factfiles/sanitation/en/index.html

World Health Organization. (2011b). *Nigeria: Mass lead poisoning from mining activities, Zamfara State—Update 1*. Retrieved March 7, 2013, from http://www.who.int/csr/don/2011_11_11/en/index.html

World Health Organization. (2012). *10 facts on climate change*. Retrieved March 4, 2013, from http://www.who.int/features/factfiles/climate_change

web resources

Please visit thePoint® for up-to-date web resources on this topic.

CHAPTER 20

Community Preparedness: Disaster and Terrorism

Joy Spellman and Gail A. Harkness

DOWN*

down
it came
down
from
the
autumn
sky
down
it came
down
& every
one
rose
& wept
in the
city
(my
city)
& some
were flying
& some
were falling
& some
were running
& some
were burning
where
were
you
listening
watching
then?
in the
shattered
earth?
in the
broken air?
in the
oily fire?
in the
tainted
sea?
where
were
you
listening
watching
then
when
everyone
rose
& lookt
at the
sky
lookt
at the
sky
where
they
stood
in my
city
& wept?

Jesse Glass

chapter highlights

- Public health nurses and disaster response
- Types of disasters
- Disaster management
- Public health response
- Role and responsibility of nurses in disasters
- Classification of agents
- Field response
- Skill building for field activity

objectives

- Identify disaster types.
- Explain the disaster planning process and nursing participation.
- Understand nursing participation in a disaster.
- Promote increased competency levels through the use of simulation technology and field drills, and exercises.
- Differentiate between biologic, chemical, and radiologic agents and response to exposure.
- Describe the public health response.

key terms

After-action report: Retrospective analysis used to evaluate emergency response drills.
Decontamination: Process of cleaning to remove biologic, chemical, or radiologic agents.
Evacuation: Moving people from a dangerous place to safety.
Incident command system (ICS): Common organizational structure implemented to improve emergency response.
Invacuation: Moving people from one area to another within the same facility.
National Response Framework (NRF): Framework that guides how the nation conducts all-hazards incident response.
National Incident Management System (NIMS): Structured, flexible framework that guides the response to disasters at all levels of government, the private sector, and nongovernmental organizations.
Personal protective equipment (PPE): Clothing and/or equipment used to protect the body from injury and illness.
Point of distribution (POD): Centralized location where the public picks up emergency supplies following a disaster.
Real time: The actual time in which something occurs.

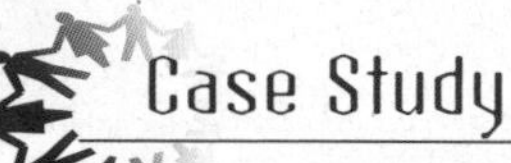

Case Study

References to the case study are found throughout this chapter (look for the case study icon). Readers should keep the case study in mind as they read the chapter.

After September 11, 2001, emergency management departments in the United States began to develop disaster response plans that called for a multidisciplinary, team-training approach. Focusing on biologic, chemical, and radiologic agents not normally seen in practice, local health department personnel, including public health nursing departments, became active participants. Although well versed in infection control, disease prevention, and health promotion activities, nurses expressed concerns about clinical skills needed to conduct field triage when dealing with agents outside the scope of their day-to-day practice.

Geoff, a nurse educator at New Jersey's Public Health Nurses Association, has played an active role in providing education and hands-on experiences involving disaster-based scenarios among community-based nurses throughout the state. Nurses require more specific knowledge about harmful agents and situations not usually seen in their practice. With state support, the Public Health Nurses Association, with Geoff's leadership, decides that a certificate on biologic, chemical, and radiologic terrorism will be offered with expanded content that will build new skill sets needed in a field response. Lessons learned from the response to the aftermath of Hurricane Sandy along the coast of New Jersey in November 2012 will be incorporated into the certificate curriculum.

The goal of the 40-hour course is to provide community and public health nurses with an introduction to a new practice dimension. Geoff decides to continue to incorporate human simulation technology in a field exercise setting that will stimulate critical thinking capacity, sharpen decision-making skills, and apply knowledge in a safe, nonthreatening, **real-time** field setting. The human patient simulators (HPS) are programmed with realistic agent-specific crisis scenarios that represent a variety of disasters of increasing complexity, threat, and pressure. Participants will develop emergency policies, plans, and procedures to ensure an effective response. Based on evacuation activities during Sandy, Geoff will include a module on preparedness operations while working with diverse communities. The program will be delivered in the spring, followed by an emergency exercise designed to test the capability of a large city's response to a deliberate chemical attack. The community and public health nurses enrolled in the course will be key players in the planning, execution, and evaluation phases of the drill.

key terms (continued)

Scenario: The sequence of possible events or circumstances.
Shelter in place: The protective action of taking cover in a building.
Simulation: The imitation of the features of an object or anticipated response.
Surveillance: A process to document and track changing information to prevent injury and illness.
Terrorism: The use of threats and/or violence to intimidate or coerce society for political purposes.

The only difference between reality and fiction is that fiction has to make sense.

Tom Clancy

Public health nurses have been responding to disasters for more than a century. Historically, nursing evolved from the actions taken by Florence Nightingale in the Crimean War. Long before the nursing process was theorized, researched, and established as part of the nursing profession, Nightingale used her skills of observation and critical thinking to improve health outcomes. McDonald (2001) has suggested that Nightingale implemented principles of evidence-based nursing at that time. As she strolled through hospital wards, Nightingale was actually documenting environmental conditions and their impact on clients she was charged to keep well. Nightingale's analysis of health-related statistics, used to track outcomes, introduced epidemiology to the healthcare setting (see Chapter 6). Since that time, the public health nurse has continued to expand competencies by utilizing interventions that are enlightened by an evidence-based approach to improve population health. With a public health nursing workforce that understands and implements evidence-based public health practice, local health department officials and policy-makers will see the benefits of decision-making during a disaster. The *Healthy People 2020* initiative issues a call to action "to strengthen policies and improve practices that are driven by the best available evidence and knowledge" (Healthy People, 2020). Additionally, the Patient Protection and Affordable Care Act of 2010 mentions "evidence based" throughout the document and will provide $900 million in funding to communities to implement the practice in an effort to improve population health (Patient Protection and Affordable Care Act, 2010).

Community and public health nursing has a broad scope of practice. For example, population-based practice has a narrow focus (e.g., six students with diabetes in a middle school) or a broad one (e.g., a potential H7N9 pandemic). Managing a client load of six certainly seems reasonable.

Doing the same within a county of 400,000 people is quite different. The role of nurses within the community is to assess the needs of the populace and ensure that service breaches are addressed. Nurses accomplish this by calling on existing agencies and institutions to find ways to serve the needs of the citizens. Collaborative effort is a significant part of response. For example, local health department nursing personnel, school nurse organizations, and volunteers from the Medical Reserve Corps (MRC) have worked in concert to provide in-school H1N1 immunization as well as engaging in **surveillance** activities. From that experience, public health nurses in New Jersey are working at putting the knowledge and skills gained from the 2009 pandemic into evidence-based policies that may be implemented during the next event. Jacobs, Jones, Gabella, Spring, and Brownson (2012) point out that when evidence-based tools are applied, evaluated rigorously, and shared, improvements in population health will yield measurable outcomes. A well-prepared cadre of community and public health nurses is essential to minimize the effects of both immediate and long-range disasters.

The aftermath of the destruction of the World Trade Center in 2001 identified a lack of trained leaders and workers in all areas of public health service. The event also stimulated a growing appreciation of those who respond to large-scale events. Increased competency in disaster response became a new dimension to nursing practice. The Centers for Disease Control and Prevention (CDC) has called for the mobilization of the public health workforce to ensure the training and education of communities across the nation regarding biologic, chemical, radiologic, and explosive device attacks. It is necessary to learn how to prepare for events that are difficult to imagine, and it is even more challenging to mount a response. Recent disasters in New Jersey and Boston illustrate the importance of having a coordinated, multidisciplinary response to a culturally diverse population.

There cannot be a crisis next week. My schedule is already full.

Henry A. Kissinger

EVIDENCE FOR PRACTICE

A "Ready and Willing" (Alexander & Wynia, 2003) survey asked physicians and nurses whether they would be willing to respond to a biologic, chemical, or radiologic disaster. The study revealed that although 80% of professionals polled were willing to act in response to such an event, only 20% believed that they had the knowledge and appropriate skills to respond with competency. This served as a stimulus for the development of educational programs for health professionals. In an effort to update the evidence of the willingness of health professionals to participate in a disaster response, Chaffee (2009) conducted a systematic review of literature addressing this issue. The review outlined the clinical and nonclinical factors (e.g., family situation) that influenced the physicians' and nurses' decision to participate, their perception of responder safety, and the nature of the incident itself. A follow-up to Ready and Willing (Crane, McCluskey, Johnson, & Harbison, 2010) shows that classroom study and field exercise participation among community-based nurses, physicians, and pharmacists resulted in a significant increase in their ability and willingness to respond effectively in a disaster.

What kind of data does Geoff gather in his disaster training needs assessment?

How can these new findings affect the emergency planning process for healthcare facilities and the community at large? How will the needs of a diverse community be addressed in the new plan?

EMERGENCIES, DISASTERS, AND TERRORISM

Response to emergencies and disasters has been a part of the human experience since humans first walked on the earth. A nation's capacity to respond to these threats depends in part on the ability of healthcare professionals and public health officials to rapidly and effectively detect, manage, and communicate during an event resulting in mass casualties. Emergencies are considered events that require a swift, intense response on the part of existing community resources. Disasters are often unforeseen, serious, and unique events that disrupt essential community services and cause human morbidity and mortality that cannot be alleviated unless assistance is received from others outside the community. Disasters vary by (1) the type of onset (they often occur without warning), (2) the duration of the immediate crisis, (3) the magnitude or scope of the incident, and (4) the extent to which the event affects the community.

There are three types of disasters: natural, accidental, and terrorist attacks. Nature can wreak havoc when a tornado touches down or a hurricane obliterates a once-wide sandy beachfront. Natural disasters are widespread throughout the world. The 2010 catastrophic earthquake in Haiti, killing more than 230,000 people and injuring even more, remains in the news. Ongoing cholera outbreaks remain an issue on the island as a slow rebuilding and recovery process continues. Hurricane Sandy destroyed over 375,000 homes and displaced millions of people over a 6-month period beginning in November 2012, while an avalanche in northeastern Afghanistan destroyed a village of 200 in March 2012. The "Chelyabinsk Meteor," as it has become known, resulted in 1,500 injuries caused by broken glass, burns, and the effects of shock waves as the asteroid fell to earth in northern Siberia in February 2013. To prove the point that natural disasters can occur by many natural forces, a cyclone striking Madagascar created optimal conditions for locusts to overbreed, resulting in 50% of the country's farmlands being infested by swarms (Foley, 2012). Accidents include human-made disasters such as the Chernobyl meltdown in the former Soviet Union, which remains a constant reminder of the devastating effects of such a radiologic event. The near meltdown that occurred in post-tsunami Japan in 2011 has been deigned to be a human-made disaster based on evidence that revealed faulty design elements in the placement of reactor cooling tanks. Terrorist attacks continue to occur throughout the world on a daily basis, and in the United States, the April 2013 Boston Marathon bombings reminds us to be prepared for the unexpected.

Natural Disasters

Natural disasters are the result of naturally occurring events that have an impact on the environment, the economy, and the people who live in the area. Examples include earthquakes, extreme heat, floods, hurricanes, landslides, tornadoes, tsunamis, volcanic eruptions, wildfires, and winter weather. All of these conditions are threats to health.

Although many natural disasters are not predictable, it is possible to assess the circumstances that increase vulnerability to a natural disaster ahead of time and take steps to prevent complications. For example, as reports of a strengthening tropical storm in October 2012 came in to New Jersey's state incident command center, experts tracking the storm agreed that "Sandy" would soon assume full hurricane status. With 127 miles of ocean front coast and 10 counties exposed to coastal waters, a storm evacuation plan has been in place and exercised over the years. Previously identified sites to be used as shelters were activated 2 days before the hurricane made land fall. County and state health departments, the Red Cross, local and state law enforcement, and public health nurses worked closely to accept the storm victims and assess their needs. On-site triaging resulted in the transfer of many storm victims for hypothermia and complications from existing chronic illnesses. In this instance, rapid assessment of an impending natural disaster, resource identification, and activation of an often exercised scenario resulted in saving scores of lives. As public health practitioners gather evidence for practice, it is becoming clear that in many disaster scenarios, the displacement of people before, during, and after the event must be considered as plans are developed. In 2010, 45 million people were forced to flee their homes due to sudden-onset natural disasters (Halff, 2011).

PRACTICE POINT

Many natural disasters are anticipated, such as hurricanes, rising flood waters, and temperature extremes. Include these events when planning for emergencies—a response can begin before the onset of disaster. Become familiar with locally designated shelter sites.

Accidental Disasters

Accidental incidents, broadly defined, are those that happen as a result of circumstantial factors (e.g., road conditions, human error, and physical plant deterioration) and are usually not deliberate. For example, a truck containing a toxic chemical being transported on a major highway system overturns when the driver fails to negotiate a clearly marked warning of the steep incline of the exit ramp. Evacuation of the area takes place. "Accident" implies that the incident is uncontrollable and/or unpreventable, usually with a negative outcome. But, do accidents just happen? Or can they be prevented? Over time, epidemiologists have identified ways to prevent the negative outcomes of unanticipated events by improving preparedness and awareness training and education. For instance, research findings may suggest that road signage located well before the steep incline, or consistent driver evaluation, could prevent vehicle accidents, or at least minimize their severity.

Like natural disasters, accidents may also have an impact on the environment, cost millions, and affect the lives of those involved. The 2010 collapse of the oil rig in the Gulf of Mexico and the consequent destruction of a vast, sensitive ocean environment is a good example. Preparing for accidental disaster is difficult, largely because of the possibility of human error and the setting in which it occurs. Certainly, the accidental release of nuclear materials affecting 1,000,000 people may not be seen in the same light as a medication error on the part of a nurse. In both cases, assessment of vulnerabilities with subsequent correction, followed by implementation of a preventive action, might have prevented the accident. Forgetting to complete a task can also contribute to a disastrous situation. For example, during review of an evacuation of a long-term care facility as part of a mandatory yearly exercise, administrators find that contracts with medical transport companies were not renewed, making effective evacuation impossible. **Simulation** training, discussed later in this chapter, may be an effective tool to identify human error potential. Regular review of emergency plans and twice yearly tabletop or functional drills will also point out needed areas of improvement and gaps in competency.

EVIDENCE FOR PRACTICE

Carrier, Yee, Cross, and Samuel (2012) points out that given the fragmentation of the healthcare system, diversity of community stakeholders, and limited resources, it is becoming more challenging to maintain coalitions that are committed to preparedness planning and execution of those plans. The authors suggest that policy-makers might consider providing incentives that encourage more community-based practitioners and organizations to participate in the planning process. Although the development of planning documents is essential to preparedness activities, planning leaders might consider defining outcomes expected within the collaboration in the event of a disaster. Clear identification of roles and responsibilities as the process develops lends itself to effective response. By broadening the scope of participants in the planning process, details previously overlooked have a better chance to be included in the disaster response, preventing accidental injury to community members. Coordination within a wider community coalition assures a workable, relatable mass casualty **scenario**.

In New Jersey, the use of simulation supports an evidence-based approach to disaster planning by identifying methods to use empirical data in the decision-making process. This process will help emergency response planners to identify hazards and vulnerabilities through a wide variety of scenarios, learn responses to each, and develop principles or best practices that apply to a broad spectrum of disaster scenarios. Ultimately, the promotion of injury and disease prevention programs and practices will be enhanced.

Terrorism

Terrorism, such as that experienced in New York City and Boston, is relatively new to America but not to the rest of the world. Although there are difficulties in defining global definition of **terrorism**, the United Nations described it as "any action intended to cause death or serious bodily harm to civilians or noncombatants with the purpose of intimidating a population or compelling a government or an international organization to do or abstain from doing any act" (United Nations, 2013). As the risk of catastrophic disasters increase, so too, the need to mitigate suffering and physical damage from these events also increases (Koenig & Schultz, 2010). As of early 2013, there still is no single agreed-upon definition of terrorism that is accepted globally. Nevertheless, it can be stated that terrorism is the deliberate use of violence or the threat of violence to coerce others for political purposes. The main goals of terrorism are creating fear, causing casualties, and rendering sites unusable. Fear and intimidation are potent concepts for the human psyche to process. The threat potential for continued acts witnessed worldwide underlies the need to develop and maintain society's response capabilities (Berkshire Publishing Group, 2011).

Part of this new world of completely improvisational terrorism is that there were codes of war that disintegrated in the face of terrorism.

Diane Sawyer

DISASTER PREPAREDNESS IN A CULTURALLY DIVERSE SOCIETY

It is important to integrate a community's ethnicity, race, culture, and language into emergency preparedness response and recovery plans (Andrulis, Siddiqui, & Purtie 2011). Outreach to diverse members of every community is critical to assure effective, inclusive strategies to protect all citizens. Public health nurses are well versed in identifying vulnerable populations within the districts in which they serve. Efforts to assure that health professionals and emergency responders become more culturally competent have gained momentum in the past few years. An increasing awareness of inequities visited upon ethnically diverse communities has emerged since Hurricane Katrina hit the Gulf Coast early in the morning of August 29, 2005. The Office of Minority Health, U.S. Department of Human Services, has developed a Cultural Competency Curriculum for Disaster Preparedness and Crisis Response that offers continuing education for those looking to enhance their skills toward the provision of competent care in disaster situations (U.S. Department of Health and Human Services, 2009). The courses will be offered through 2015.

Culture is the learned knowledge of values and beliefs of a particular group that are passed down through generations. These belief systems influence a person's view of the world, decisions made, and behaviors tied into those beliefs. The latest data collected in New Jersey has identified over 4 million non-white citizens, of a total population of 9 million, calling the state home. These numbers clearly illustrate the importance of addressing multicultural influences during a disaster. A person's culture is a comforting and reassuring system at the best of times. The degree of community cohesion can be seen as a determinant in survivor support. For instance, a disrupted community will not be able to provide the same level of support as one that is viewed as cohesive (Rutgers University, 2012). Given the benefit of advanced warning as Hurricane Sandy fast approached the New Jersey coastline, public health leaders and emergency response teams identified designated shelters for specific coastal county residents in an attempt to try to maintain a neighbor-to-neighbor environment. Separated family members were given the opportunity to move to a shelter where they could reunite with family and friends.

Social and economic inequality plays a large part in all areas of life; however, special attention to minority and disadvantaged neighborhoods must be given during the planning process. By most accounts, the poor and disenfranchised live in the less-desirable sections of the city, and the dwellings they occupy are not as resistant to time and natural weather extremes. Public health nurses recognize that many immigrant populations are not only unfamiliar with existing community resources but are reluctant to disclose their immigration status for fear of deportation.

In developing an inclusive community preparedness plan, it is important to become familiar with those community institutions that can meet the mental health needs of a diverse population. Language, and the potential barriers it may present during a disaster response, must be considered as a first step when mounting a field intervention during an event. As part of state and local planning in New Jersey, colleges and universities have identified volunteers who will act as interpreters for specific ethnic communities. As planning progresses, identify who the cultural brokers are within a community. By establishing solid working relationships with trusted organizations, and various cultural group leaders, public health nurses can begin to educate the citizenry about plans, intended response, and community resources well before the beginning of a disastrous event. Invite leaders to participate in all phases of disaster preparedness, response, and recovery operations.

A committee of nursing researchers has formed to establish standards of practice for cultural competency to guide nurses in their practice across the world to provide "culturally congruent nursing care" (Douglas et al., 2009). These standards are applicable to all nursing disciplines but are especially useful to public health nurses whose focus is community and populations at large. Standard 12, "Evidence-Based Practice," stresses the importance of implementing interventions that have proved successful among diverse populations. In terms of disaster response, although evidence is building within the scope of public health practice, nurse researchers have a fresh opportunity to test interventions used during the events surrounding Hurricane Sandy with a focus on the reduction of disparities in health outcomes among the poorest citizens.

Geoff decides to integrate evidence-based knowledge from his Hurricane Sandy experiences in 2012 into the preparedness certificate curriculum. Based on the multicultural makeup of the displaced population he cared for, he is asking each nurse participant to select two distinct cultural and ethnic groups from within the community he or she serves. What vulnerabilities, hazards, and special needs will you have identified during the community planning process? If an evacuation order is given, how will this message be conveyed to these sectors in the community? Cite specific and special needs these community members may need once transported to a shelter.

PRACTICE POINT

During any disaster scenario, identify yourself as a nurse immediately upon making contact with a victim. Nurses are recognized globally for their caring attitude and competency in difficult times.

DISASTER MANAGEMENT

Disasters have a timeline, often referred to as a life cycle or phases. These include the preimpact phase (before), the impact phase (during), and the postimpact phase (after). Actions taken during these phases will affect the illness, injury, and death that occur following the incident. Although disasters vary significantly, the response to each is similar. All disaster response begins at the local level—all communities must be prepared for emergencies. The disaster management continuum illustrates the essential steps in the process (Fig. 20.1).

Just as there are distinct phases of a disaster, so too are there phases of an emergency management response. These are preparedness, mitigation, response, recovery, and evaluation. It is important to remember that during the management of any disaster, the activities carried out will frequently overlap phases. During a disaster, duties and their associated activities often cross boundaries in order to complete a task at hand.

Preparedness

Disaster preparedness plans are action plans developed in anticipation of disaster scenarios, providing a framework for response to emergency situations. They are proactive planning efforts that provide structure to a disaster response before it happens. In an all-hazards event plan, the response must be a coordinated community effort. This means engaging members of the community in ongoing preparedness activities. Working relationships can be strengthened by formalizing mutual aid agreements with regional health, police, and fire departments; volunteer organizations such as the Red Cross and other local planning groups; healthcare organizations; schools; and state response coordinators.

To ensure a successful response, steps must be taken before any incident, however minor, occurs. In this process, the risk for a given disaster is assessed, and the potential impact is evaluated. Planning for disasters involves data collection in three areas: (1) identification of hazards, (2) analysis of vulnerability, and (3) assessment of risk. The effectiveness of the disaster plan is only as good as the data that underlie the planning efforts and the assumptions (Veenema, 2012).

The identification of all existing and potentially dangerous situations before disasters occur is the first step in planning for an effective response. The types and combination of hazards are unique to a community. They may involve propensity for natural disasters, chemical or radioactive spills, transportation accidents, congregation of large groups of people, and numerous other situations. Different circumstances result in different types of injuries or illness, damage, and disruption of communication and transportation. Gathering historical data about previous disasters is helpful, and proven successful nursing interventions can be noted in the growing practice of evidence-based public health. Aerial photography, satellite imagery, wireless remote sensing devices, and geographic positioning systems are tools commonly used in hazard identification. Computer-generated pluming software is a proven means of indicating the direction in which a wind-driven chemical release is heading. Once the hazards are identified, the extent of damages, interruption of services, and threats to health can be estimated. This information can be used in designing a community emergency plan.

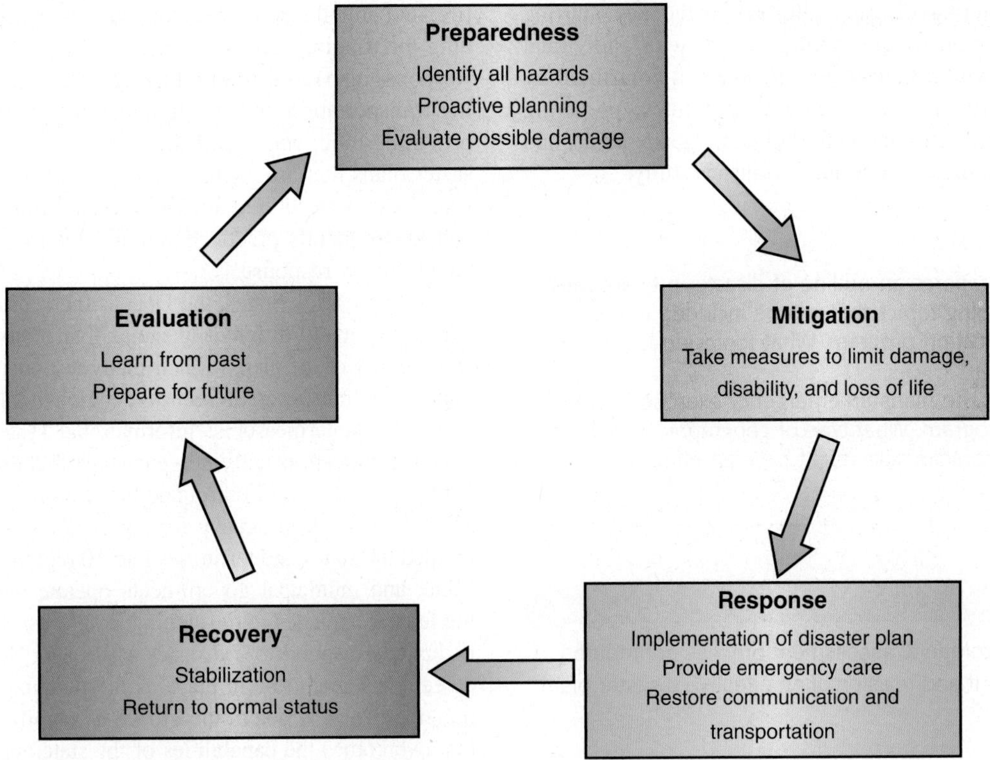

figure 20.1 The disaster management continuum. (Adapted from Veenema, T. G. [2009]. *Ready RN handbook for disaster nursing and emergency preparedness* [pp. 3–25]. St. Louis: Mosby Elsevier.)

Analysis of Vulnerability

The community disaster planning team should also identify those groups of people who are most likely to be affected in a variety of disaster events. Vulnerability varies according to the type of hazard involved, and people who are most likely to suffer injury, death, or loss of property should be identified for each hazard. In addition, the ability or capacity of the community to respond to the effects of specific disasters should be assessed. Vulnerability analysis predicts who will be affected the most and identifies community resources that are available for a response. To keep emergency plans up-to-date, population and environment changes need to be documented with changes made to the plan accordingly.

Assessment of Risk

Using the comprehensive data gathered from hazard identification and vulnerability analysis, the probability of adverse health effects due to a specific disaster can be calculated. This is often represented as a low, medium, or high risk. In this process, the resources of the community that would reduce the impact of a given hazard should be identified and plans made to strengthen those resources if necessary. Disaster prevention measures may be instituted that involve the removal of identified hazards, relocation of at-risk people away from the hazard area, provision of educational materials, institution of sensors, and development of community early warning systems.

National Response Framework

When the scope of a disaster extends beyond the capability of local and state governments to respond, the federal government is asked to provide assistance. The **National Response Framework** (NRF), established by the U.S. Department of Homeland Security (DHS), guides the overall conduct and coordination of all-hazards incident responses. These include all disasters, whether natural, human-made, or a result of terrorism, including threats to resources such as information technology and energy sources. The NRF presents a unified response that depends on the mutually supporting capabilities of federal, state, and local resources—all levels of government—working together. Federal leadership responsibilities are outlined in the NRF; however, the states have the primary responsibility for coordinating resources and capabilities and obtaining support from other states and the federal government.

The role of state government is to supplement and facilitate local efforts before, during, and after incidents. Although the state has a crucial coordination role, local officials have the primary responsibility for community preparedness and response. Local officials are responsible for ensuring public safety and the welfare of people of that jurisdiction. The local emergency manager has the day-to-day authority and responsibility for overseeing emergency management programs and activities. Local hospitals also need to develop an emergency operations plan (EOP) that will guide the activation of resources in the event of either an internal or external disaster. Ultimately, the key starting points for emergency preparedness rest with individual people, often within households. People can contribute by reducing hazards in and around their homes, preparing emergency supply kits and household emergency plans, and monitoring emergency communications carefully.

Geoff prepares an outline of disaster preparedness planning topics that will be included in the certification program. What topics does he choose?

In addition, he plans an emergency exercise for the end of the program. What type of geographic and demographic characteristics might have an effect on program content?

PRACTICE POINT

An ongoing community assessment process contributes to the development and revision of an effective disaster plan.

Mitigation

Mitigation is a prevention process with two components. First, mitigation is an effort to prevent identified risks from causing a disaster. By focusing on implementation of preventive measures for reducing and eliminating identified risks before the event occurs, mitigation becomes a cost-effective primary prevention. Structural mitigation involves creation or removal of structures or alteration of the environment to remove or modify risks. An example is the installation of a generator to be used during a power failure. Nonstructural mitigation includes disaster training for healthcare personnel, the establishment of emergency evacuation regulations, land use planning, legislation, and insurance.

Second, mitigation involves efforts to lessen the impact of a disaster by initiating measures to limit damage, disease, disability, and loss of life among the members of a community (tertiary prevention). In this case, mitigation refers to a broad range of activities that are only accomplished satisfactorily by planning prior to the event.

PRACTICE POINT

Disasters occur locally, but their impact can extend globally.

Response

All response begins at the local level, where the disaster management plan is implemented and responders are deployed. This mobilization is multidisciplinary, and the first people on the scene will more than likely be law enforcement, fire, and ambulance crews. Reaching the victims and beginning the triaging process is essential to prevent loss of life. Response also refers to minimizing, improvising, and restoring transportation and communication systems, as well as providing food, water, and shelter to those affected. The disaster plans that are most effective are clear, easy to understand, use a structured **incident command system** (ICS), and are frequently practiced and updated to ensure a coordinated, timely response.

In the United States, the DHS is the central organization overseeing many different agencies that focus on the safety and security of the nation. Their many responsibilities include border and transportation security; chemical, biologic, and radiologic countermeasures; informational systems and infrastructure protection; and emergency preparedness and response (Centers for Disease Control and Prevention, 2002/2013). The FEMA, as the lead agency for emergency management, has divided the states and territories into 10 regions. State, county, tribal, and municipal governments operate independently of the federal agencies in developing programs. Surrounding jurisdictions respond to a disaster as needed; thus, mutual aid agreements should be in place as the planning progresses. If the emergency is determined to be of significant magnitude that overcomes the capabilities of the state and local governments, the Secretary of Homeland Security will initiate the NRF to release federal resources to local jurisdictions. Health departments and emergency management offices use the **National Incident Management System** (NIMS) to develop a coordinated response to the disaster.

National Incident Management System

The NIMS is a structured, flexible framework that guides the response to disasters of governments at all levels, private companies, and nongovernmental organizations. Its goal is to reduce the loss of life, property, and harm to the environment by helping departments and agencies work seamlessly to prepare for, prevent, mitigate, respond to, and recover from the effects of incidents—regardless of cause, size, location, or complexity. This process involves coordination and cooperation between public and private organizations in various emergency management and incident response activities. The NIMS is not an operational incident management or resource allocation plan. It represents a core set of doctrines, concepts, principles, terminology, and organizational processes that enable effective, efficient, and collaborative incident management. The ICS, coordinated by the NIMS, is the on-scene organization and management structure that may be followed in planned community events as well as disaster incidents. Governments of all levels—federal, state, tribal, and local—as well as many nongovernmental organizations and private companies use ICS.

Incident Command System

When a disaster occurs, there is an immediate need for organization and management at the scene of the incident. The ICS is an on-site, flexible, all-hazards system that provides a set of personnel, policies, procedures, facilities, and equipment integrated into a common organizational structure that is designed to improve emergency response operations of all types, sizes, and complexities.

The ICS designates common titles and roles to be used in all organizations and agencies that respond to disasters. It organizes emergency response in five major functional areas: command, planning, operations, logistics, and finance and administration (Fig. 20.2). These temporary management hierarchies control funds, personnel, facilities, equipment, and communications until the requirement for management and operations no longer exists. Operations can be expanded or contracted as required. Participants are trained and approved by legitimate authorities before incidents occur so that personnel from a wide variety of agencies, jurisdictions, and backgrounds can meld rapidly into a common management structure using common terminology. The result is a unified, centrally authorized, legitimate, cost-effective emergency organization that facilitates communication and coordination of response efforts. Nurses and other healthcare professionals are encouraged to become a part of their local ICS. Basic level courses (ICS 100–200) are available online at the FEMA website.

Most countries have national agencies that oversee response in that country. Western Europe, India, Russia, the United Kingdom, Australia, and Canada refer to disaster phases as outlined above. New Zealand uses different terminology; disaster phases are known as the four Rs (reduction [mitigation], readiness [preparedness], response, and recovery).

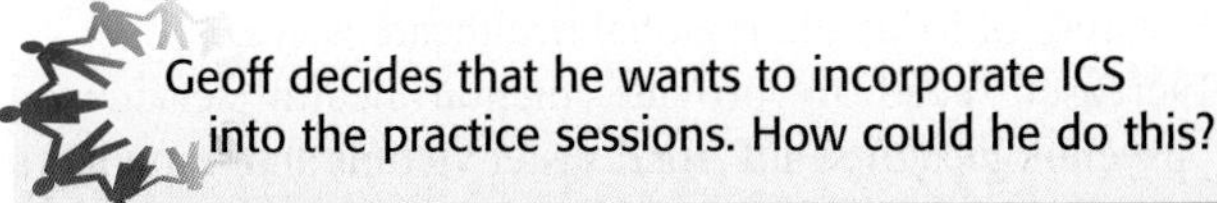

Geoff decides that he wants to incorporate ICS into the practice sessions. How could he do this?

PRACTICE POINT

Participate in your local multidisciplinary ICS network as a part of your disaster response activities.

Recovery

Recovery is the stabilization of the community and the return of the disaster area to its previous status. The response phase deals with immediate needs, whereas the recovery phase focuses on those activities that will protect the health of the public and restore buildings and services. The threats to life have passed. An epidemiologic analysis of adverse health effects after any kind of disaster identifies factors that

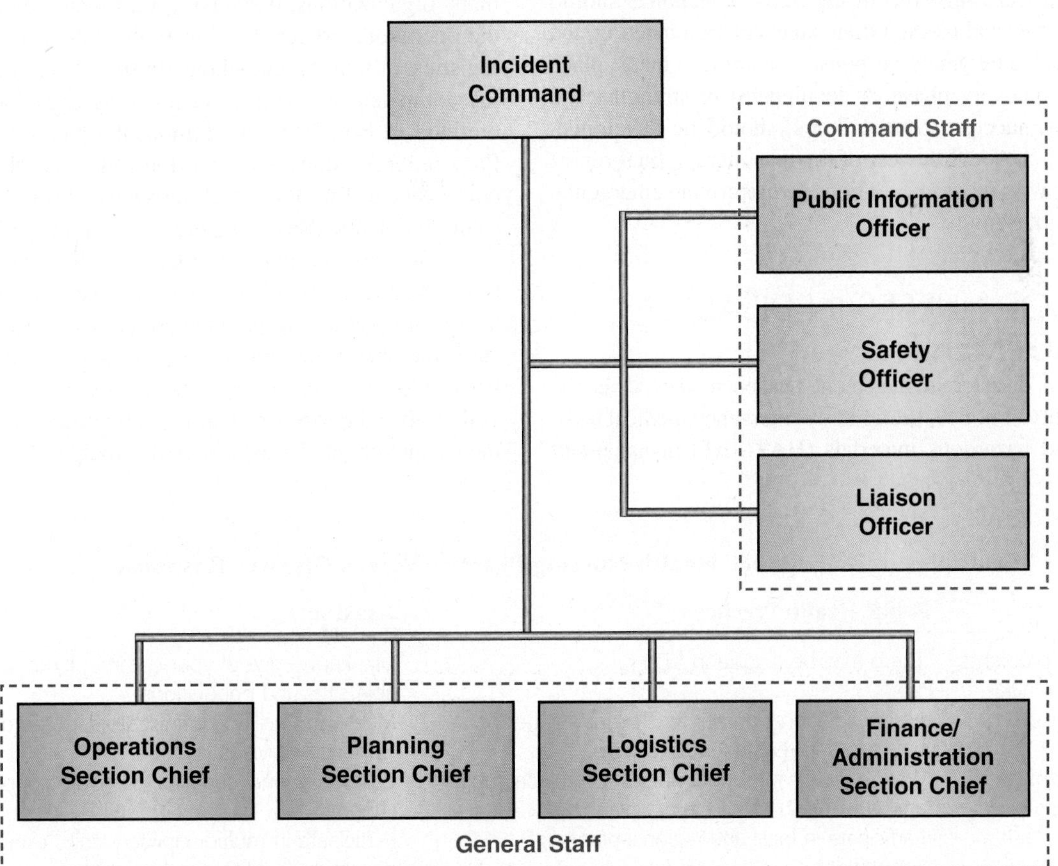

figure 20.2 Incident command structure. (Adapted from Federal Emergency Management Agency. [2008]. *National incident management system*. Retrieved February 21, 2010, from http://www.fema.gov/pdf/emergency/nims/NIMS_core.pdf.)

influence the health status of the community on a long-term basis. Some of these factors are as follows:

- Continuing death, chronic illness, and/or disability
- Population shift if recovery is prolonged
- Contamination of food and water supplies, with an increased risk of infectious diseases
- Collapse of local and regional healthcare access
- Increased need to provide mental health services—"psychological first aid" for disaster victims and responders

The timeline for recovery varies widely, depending upon the type and extent of the disaster. The institution of stress debriefing and mental health services is essential in most cases. However, recovery may also involve rebuilding damaged buildings, transportation systems, and communication systems, as well as the relocation of those affected by the disaster. Communities that perform a hazard risk assessment to predict the effects of disasters on a community, and have a targeted disaster plan in place, are better prepared to address recovery issues.

Evaluation

Evaluation is the foundation for evidence-based disaster response. By analyzing specific aspects of the plan and assessing the effectiveness of the plan in action, future planning efforts are enhanced. All agencies, organizations, and personnel who were involved in the disaster response should take part in the evaluation. Often, an evaluation meeting, led by the local emergency response committee, takes place during the recovery phase. A detailed list of strengths and weaknesses, successes and failures, should be developed. Following a thorough review of the responses, a final report is prepared with recommendations for improving emergency response in the future.

ROLES OF NURSES IN DISASTER MANAGEMENT

Historically, disaster management has been viewed as the responsibility of police, firefighters, emergency medical technicians, and hazardous materials (HAZMAT) management teams. Traditionally the first to arrive on the scene, they act to save lives, protect property, and meet basic human needs. However, nurses, particularly public health nurses, can play a crucial role in all phases of disaster management. Nurses have a diverse knowledge base, well-developed risk assessment and clinical skills, and a strong commitment to public welfare that brings depth to the disaster management process.

The ability of nurses to be calm, creative, and responsive to emergency situations is an asset, and it is imperative that roles be clearly articulated. Public health nurses are experts in providing health education for the various populations in a community setting. They can be proactive in providing information and developing educational materials for dissemination to an anxious public, especially for disasters that can be anticipated, such as hurricanes or tornadoes. Table 20.1 presents the "prepare, respond, and recover" steps that occur in daily practice versus disaster situations.

For most nurses, disaster preparedness planning is usually associated with the workplace. One of the first questions a nurse may ask is, "What is my role if an emergency occurs?" Nurses should be familiar with the EOP in their workplace and understand how their practice may change during an emergency or disaster. For example, a long-term care facility may become a shelter, or nurses in home healthcare agencies may be expected to be first responders. In many organizations, the nursing staff would be deployed by the operations officer. They may also take part in planning, logistics, or finance and administration. A summary of nursing competencies for disaster planning and management is outlined in Box 20.1. In addition, the Nursing Emergency Preparedness Education Coalition (NEPEC) has developed competencies for entry-level nurses in response to mass casualty incidents; these competencies can be found online.

Also, some normal workplace activities will likely continue. Knowing in advance exactly what is expected of the healthcare facility during an emergency or disaster gives all staff members the opportunity to acquire the pertinent knowledge and to practice necessary skills beforehand. Today, the majority of healthcare facilities, health departments, and private industry include emergency preparedness

table 20.1 **Examples of Daily Public Health Nursing Practice Versus Disaster Response**

	Public Health Practice	Disaster
Anticipate problems and emergencies	There may be a spike in STIs.	Use knowledge of your community to target vulnerable sites and populations.
Develop plans	Assign additional nurses to STI clinics. Offer nurse hours to answer student questions.	Meet with facility administrators to coordinate response activities.
Build system-wide partnerships	Work closely with school nurses to provide support and guidance. Refer to family planning.	Call on regional contacts to ensure cooperation and support.
Practice!	Participate in local and regional planning committees.	Participate in multidisciplinary drills, exercises, becoming familiar with key players.

STIs = Sexually transmitted infections.

box 20.1 Disaster Preparedness and Management Competencies

- Participate in all aspects of the planning process.
- Contribute to the hazard assessment in the community.
- Conduct vulnerability and risk assessments, especially with special populations.
- Identify and locate the agency's emergency response plan.
- Understand the agency's role in responding to emergencies.
- Understand your role in an emergency.
- Ensure that the plan is reviewed and updated frequently.
- Describe the communication process in emergency response both within the agency, with the general public, and with personal contacts.
- Recognize deviations from the norm that might indicate an emergency and describe appropriate action.
- Participate in the development of a data, gathering system that addresses morbidity, mortality, mental health, and infectious disease.
- Apply creative problem-solving skills and flexible thinking to emergency situations, within the confines of your role.
- Identify the limits of your own knowledge, skills, and authority, and referring matters that exceed these limits.
- Evaluate the effectiveness of every drill and after-action response.

Source: Adapted from Gebbie, K.M., & Qureshi, K. (2002). Emergency and disaster preparedness: Core competencies for nurses. *American Journal of Nursing, 102*(1), 46–51.

information as part of the orientation process for new employees. They should know the communication structure inherent in the ICS that has been established for the organization.

Disaster response can involve fear of the unknown and the daunting prospect of serving entire communities during a very difficult time. However, by their nature, all types of disasters do not occur regularly. This is an opportunity for nurses to embrace the opportunity to test skills, practice disaster plans, and assert themselves as key members of state, regional, county, and local response organizations.

Public Health Nurses as First Responders

Public health nursing practice focuses on the provision of comprehensive public health services to ensure that community members have access to preventive care, immunizations, safe food and water, and assistance with services that may go beyond medical needs. An extensive knowledge of the community is the foundation for these services. Therefore, the public health nurse's expertise is valuable in all phases of the disaster management continuum, whether anticipating potential emergencies, developing appropriate plans, building system-wide partnerships, practicing implementation of disaster management plans and skills on a regular basis, or evaluating outcomes. By increasing clinical knowledge and skill sets associated with specific biologic, chemical, radiologic and explosive agents, public health nurses are better prepared to apply their upgraded proficiencies in the field. The responsibilities of public health nurses in disaster management are outlined in Box 20.2. Even though there will be clutter, clamor, and confusion during a disaster, public health nurses are not expected to function as critical care nurses in a disaster setting.

EVIDENCE FOR PRACTICE

Although public health nurses assume the lead in conducting disease surveillance activities in daily practice, their roles during a disaster response have become clearer. Working closely with members of multidisciplinary response and planning teams has secured the public health nurse's position on the disaster team. Clinical skills aside, general management skills possessed by public health nurses are a value to the team.

Public–private collaboration is essential in effecting a solid emergency plan. Archer and Cameron (2013) point out that collaborative leadership is necessary when working within a multidisciplinary framework. Skill at building relationships, handling conflict that may arise from these relationships, and the ability to share control of the collaborative task are essential qualities. These characteristics are part of the daily practice of public health nursing.

PRACTICE POINT

Know your limitations and understand your role in the field.

Just-in-Time Training

The foremost concern voiced by public health nurses is the fear that they do not possess the necessary skills to function in a disaster. Just-in-time training (JITT) is given immediately before it is used so that the least amount of resources is expended in producing the final result. There is a shortened period of time between learning and application. For

box 20.2 Responsibilities of Public Health Nurses in Disaster Management

- Assess the needs of the community as the events unfold.
- Conduct surveillance for communicable disease and unmet needs.
- Prevent and control the spread of disease.
- Maintain communication channels to ensure accurate dissemination of information to colleagues and the public.
- Organize and manage points of distribution centers and mass immunization sites as required.
- Provide on-site triage as needed.
- Manage behavioral responses to stress.
- Ensure the health and safety of self, colleagues, and the public.
- Document events and interventions.

example, in 2009, JITT for nasal H1N1 immunization administration was conducted for volunteers just before the clinics began. In most cases, three options were made available to nurses, physicians, and MRC volunteers: formal, 1-hour scheduled classroom sessions; an online video demonstration; or an on-site, show one–do one presentation.

However, emergencies and disasters are unpredictable. The challenge is to identify new, creative ways to educate and engage all nurses to increase their competencies in responding to disasters. There are many options both online and in residence educational settings for unique, flexible courses that address disaster management. The DHS is committed to helping first responders nationwide by ensuring that emergency response professionals are prepared, equipped, and trained for any situation. Through FEMA's Emergency Management Institute, more than 125 courses are offered to help build critical skills that first responders need to function effectively. The CDC offers many online JITT training sessions, and many states and localities have developed their own training programs. By establishing an internal train-the-trainer program, JITT access is ensured as the need presents itself.

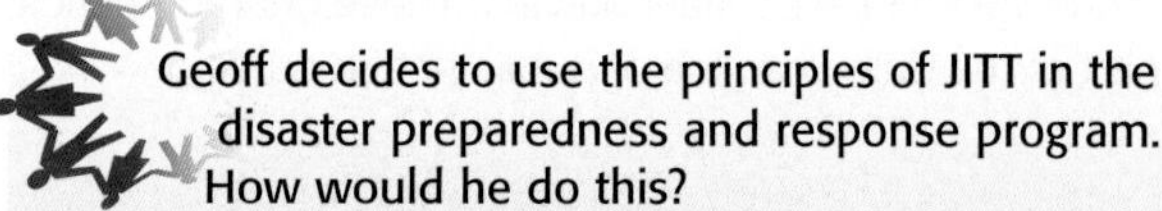

Geoff decides to use the principles of JITT in the disaster preparedness and response program. How would he do this?

STUDENT REFLECTION

During my community health practicum, Hurricane Sandy struck the New Jersey shore. Along with some classmates, I had the opportunity to work with the county health department's nursing staff and local MRC nurses who volunteered to provide care to the displaced shore residents. It was a great experience. I learned a lot about rapid assessment of needs from the public health nurses and how to quickly set up a sick bay and make it operational.

The shelter I worked in housed 200 people from one shore community. Many of the residents knew each other from the neighborhood. The shelter residents ranged in age from 4 months to 87 years of age and came from many ethnic groups. Most people brought a small trash bag of belongings with them. Residents brought their medications with them and gave them to the nurses to store and administer as needed. Sick bay operations were activated immediately and my classmates assisted the nurses in taking brief histories and filling out basic paperwork. Everyone was so grateful for our help, and they really liked the fact that we were student nurses! Residents who couldn't speak English were identified, and the local college sent teachers and students to the shelter who were fluent in the native language. Education majors set up a play area for the children.

The lead nurse from the health department and the county emergency management coordinator provided JITT to the students and MRC volunteers on the principles and practices of ICS under which the shelter operated. Maybe the best part of the experience was visiting residents throughout the shift to ask how they were doing and listening to them as they spoke of their sadness or frustration or fear about the future.

I was given the responsibility to direct a clinic that was set up at a high school. With my preceptor, I assigned a number of different jobs to the staff nurses from the Visiting Nurse Association and the volunteer nurses: drawing up the vaccine, checking clients' paperwork, distributing supplies, and administering the nasal spray or injections, or both. Although I thought I was organized, there were lots of questions that I had not answered in my orientation.

The shelter stayed open and busy for 6 days and then the residents were moved to a shelter closer to their home county. While there I was able to really see what it means to work as a member of a multidisciplinary team. Law enforcement, elected officials, Red Cross representatives, and nurses conferred at a daily team meeting to update each other on concerns and successes shared. While there I signed up to be an MRC volunteer and have my first meeting as a member next month.

My class was invited to the preliminary after-action review meeting. Because there was a 2-day warning before the storm hit, the county was prepared to operationalize its coastal evacuation plan and shelter activation plan. The major weakness was maintaining up-to-date communication between the many agencies involved. A date to meet with FEMA representatives has been initiated, and the shelter has once again resumed being a community sports center.

Field Triage

When a mass casualty incident occurs, rapid assessment and treatment of the victims is the utmost priority. On a disaster site, the process of field triage identifies and assesses those people who need medical care and prioritizes their needs. Triaging soldiers on the battlefield has been in practice for quite some time. In fact, field disaster response is based on evidence gained by measuring successful outcomes during combat. Triage is used in mass casualty situations and in any disaster event. The victims are assessed by their presenting condition and are then color-coded as to the severity of the case. A triage tag, colored tape, or ribbon is placed on each injured person after being prioritized to indicate status (Table 20.2, Fig. 20.3).

Basic triage and rapid treatment (START) is a simple, prehospital triage system that was developed in California to assist emergency responders for use in earthquakes. Evidence-based and field-proven, the system separates injured people

table 20.2 **Color Coding for Prehospital Triage**

Red	Critical	Unstable, requiring immediate intervention
Yellow	Urgent	Stable, but may deteriorate
Green	Delayed	Injured or ill but stable and not likely to deteriorate (walking wounded)
Black	Expectant	Dead or nonsalvageable given available resources

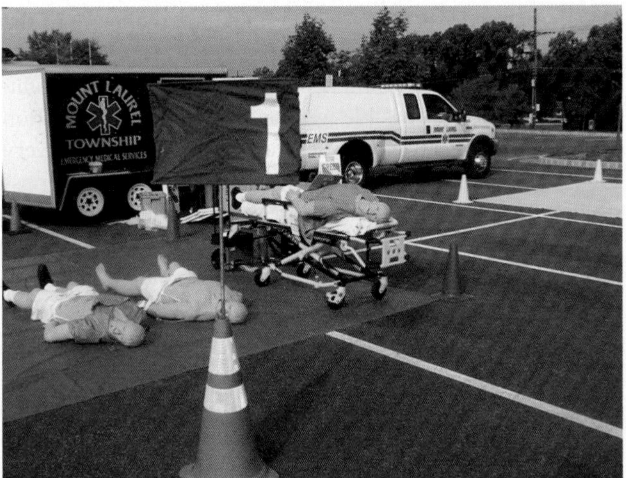

figure 20.3 **Triage.**

into four groups according to the severity of their injuries or illnesses (Box 20.3). Other triaging systems have been developed to address the needs of vulnerable or special populations, such as The JumpSTART system for triaging children and the Start/Save system for triaging victims over a long period. The latter would be used when disasters are of such a nature that evacuation of the person to a field hospital is impossible (Glarum, Birow, & Cetauk, 2010).

From a global perspective, prevention and treatment of injuries in a mass casualty disaster is a leading public health priority. Emergency responders throughout the world use a variation of the START model. The primary difference in use of the model is the interpretation of the triage scale and the qualifications of the people who classify the victims. In Western Europe, as in the United States, paramedics, field physicians, ambulance crews (emergency medical services), and nurses implement the system on-site.

During a mass casualty incident, wherever it may occur, many different local, national, and international agencies work together in the initial rescue phase. These agencies must be able to communicate information, especially critical information about the condition of victims, effectively. With the increase of international disasters, naturally occurring and otherwise, preparedness professionals have called for a global standardized triage system with well-defined categories and instructions. This universal triage classification

box 20.3 **Simple Triage and Rapid Triage: The START Model**

1. Those who have died
2. Injured, requiring immediate transfer
3. Injured, who can wait to be transferred
4. Injured, with minor less urgent needs

system includes a standardized approach to chemical, biologic, and radiologic agents as well as injuries sustained from an explosion that provides prompt information to medical providers, increasing their ability to care for victims promptly and efficiently. The CDC has published guidelines for field triage for the injured, but worldwide adoption has not taken place. A study conducted in California shows a large variation between regions in both the frequency of use and type of field triage criteria used (Barnett et al., 2013). The conclusions drawn from this suggest that aggressive dissemination of revised criteria guidelines will be an effective step in establishing some level of uniform adoption.

Field triage is an essential topic for the nurses in the disaster management training program. What are the essential components of field triage? How does Geoff use this information in planning specific hands-on experiences?

PRACTICE POINT

Identify yourself as a nurse during an event. This helps establish your credibility as a competent responder and establishes you as part of the multidisciplinary emergency response team.

Point-of-Distribution Plans

A **point of distribution** (POD) is a centralized location where the public picks up emergency supplies, including food, water, and medications (if necessary), following a disaster. The plan details the staffing required and procedures to be followed in the setup and deactivation of a POD.

Local departments of public health determine the need, the staffing, and the location of the POD, as well as the commodities that are to be distributed. FEMA has developed training programs to assist in planning for the execution and subsequent deactivation of PODs as a part of disaster relief efforts. This training helps states and communities coordinate with federal and nongovernmental groups as they provide much needed supplies to the public in a timely and consistent manner during and after a disaster event.

PRACTICE POINT

Become familiar with the POD plan for your facility and for your community. Make sure POD location agreements are current.

Personal Protective Equipment

Personal protective equipment (PPE) has been used in healthcare for a century. PPE primarily refers to the use of respiratory equipment as well as gloves, gown, and/or goggles. The purpose of PPE is to prevent the transfer of the hazardous agent from the victim or the environment to healthcare practitioners. The type of agent present determines the kind of PPE required. Generally biologic, chemical, and radiologic exposures occur by breathing contaminated air, dermal contact, and/or by eating or drinking adulterated products. Nurses who have been prepared as active response team members are often issued "Go Kits" that contain various useful items, such as gloves, surgical masks, N95 masks, goggles, pencils and paper, and large trash bags. A fit-tested respirator also may be included.

The Occupational Safety and Health Administration (OSHA) has outlined four levels of personal protection and the types of equipment that should be worn in various emergency situations (Table 20.3). The agent involved and the risk of exposure are the primary determinants of the level of PPE required. If PPE is to be used, a PPE program should be implemented that addresses the hazards present; the selection, maintenance, and use of PPE; the training of employees; and monitoring of the program to ensure its ongoing effectiveness. JITT videos are available for PPE training purposes.

PRACTICE POINT

To ensure your safety during an emergency event, learn where PPE is located in your facility and how to use and dispose of it properly. Include your local or county HAZMAT unit at a yearly inservice on proper use of equipment.

Documentation in a Disaster

During an emergency event, it is not possible or expected that normal documentation standards and protocols will be maintained. When responding to an emergency, the time, place, general assessment of the field, and the name of the Incident Commander should be noted. Events move quickly, and documentation of observations is important. However, it is not possible to document all the information that is normally required, such as victims' names. Every event is organized differently. For example, during a possible anthrax "white powder" site investigation, there were enough nurses so that one could be assigned to be the site scribe. This nurse circulated among responders and took notations as reported to her. She became the primary contact for the medical care director, an absolute necessity to obtain an accurate clinical report (see Incident Command System). Due to the number of victims in a mass casualty event, taking names and identifying information is not an effective action. When necessary, record the location and a very general description of the victim, then continue your assessment activities. After the event, coordinate notes and appoint a nurse to participate and report findings and recommendations at the "hotwash" or postevent gathering. Although circumstances of the incident may make it impossible to assign a central scribe, the notes and observations from the field are invaluable when preparing the **after-action report** and conducting an evaluation.

table 20.3 **Levels of Personal Protection in Disasters: A–D**

Level of Protection	Equipment
Level A Highest protection for respiratory tract, skin, eyes, and mucous membrane	SCBA, fully encapsulated water- and vapor-proof suit with a cooling system, boots, gloves, hard hat, and a two-way communication device
Level B Highest protection for respiratory tract; skin, and eye splash–resistant protection	SCBA, liquid splash–resistant clothing, hood, gloves, hard hat, boots, two-way communication device
Level C Same level of protection for skin and eyes as level B, air-purifying system for respiratory tract	Full face, air-purifying respirator rather than SCBA, liquid splash–resistant clothing, hood, gloves, hard hat, boots, two-way communication device
Level D Standard work protection from splashes, minimal skin protection, no respiratory protection	Cover suits, safety glasses, gloves, boots, and face shield

SCBA = self-contained breathing apparatus.
Source: Occupational Safety and Health Administration Standards—29-CFR Standard number 1910—132 Personal Protective Equipment. Retrieved May 20, 2010, from http://www.osha.gov.

Geoff requires a plan for documentation of events during the hands-on practice sessions. What does he include and how does he plan to implement documentation in the practice sessions?

PRACTICE POINT

Time is a factor in a disaster. Note unusual incidents and appropriate essential observations and report immediately.

Skill Building for Disaster Response

Planning and practicing for a crisis is the foundation for successful communication and response. A well-trained front-line response team reduces the impact of an event. HPS models, such as those Geoff used in the training program, are increasingly used in medical and nursing education. With this technology, trainees are assisted in applying the techniques learned in the classroom laboratory to actual situations. A HPS incorporates sophisticated computer technology, including mathematical models of complex human anatomy, physiology, and pharmacology, into a realistic model of the human body (Fig. 20.4). The system demonstrates clinical signs such as heart, breath, and bowel sounds; palpable pulses; chest excursion and airway patency; pulmonary artery pressure; and cardiac output. Pupils automatically dilate and constrict in response to light, respiratory gas exchange is monitored, and automatic recognition and response to administered drugs occurs. A wide variety of preprogrammed clinical experiences are simulated, and real physiologic monitoring equipment is used. Simulator use can involve a simple task, such as transporting a disabled employee to an alternative care center, or be a complex scenario requiring a multidisciplinary response. A number of factors influence the use of simulation. These include the quality and safety of simulation use, the incorporation of new technology as it evolves, the integration of a variety of ways of learning within the existing educational systems, and the resolution of ethical issues as they arise.

During actual drills, a successful exercise using simulation is one in which weaknesses, mistakes, and ineffective plans are exposed. As a practice event, the opportunity to make corrections, improve certain skills, or revise disaster response plans should also be seen as a means to become a competent responder and leader. Nonclinical responders can benefit from inclusion in a simulation experience with nurses. Incident command, communication systems testing, and a clearer understanding of the importance of the role of the nurse in an emergency event make the multidisciplinary team approach an effective use of simulation as a competency and confidence builder. Frequent, specific-scenario-formulated training prepares the public health nurse responder to take the lead in emergency events.

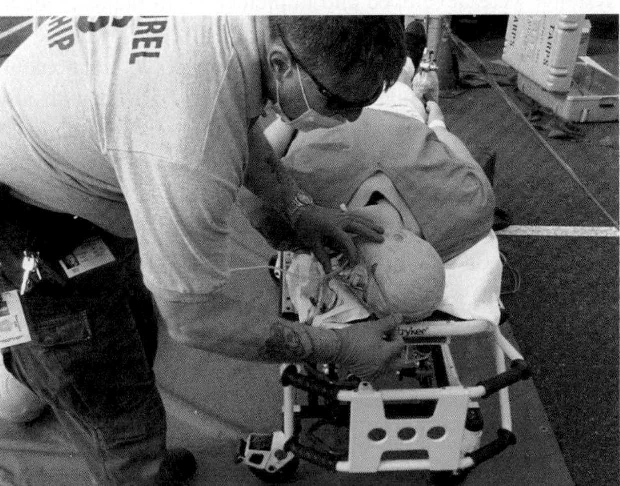

figure 20.4 First responder with a human patient simulator.

BIOTERRORISM

A bioterrorism event involves the intentional release of viruses, bacteria, fungi, or toxins from living organisms into the environment for the purposes of causing illness or death. Although agents may result in familiar diseases, someone intent on harming others can engineer agents to make them more deadly or to extend their life on a variety of surfaces. Biologic agents are air- or waterborne and are inhaled or ingested (Centers for Disease Control and Prevention, 2002/2012). The United States Committee on the Prevention of Weapons of Mass Destruction Proliferation and Terrorism released a report in 2009 indicating that terrorists are more likely to obtain and use biologic agents than nuclear weapons. For terrorists, there are some distinct advantages to using biologic versus chemical agents. The incubation periods of live agents afford the terrorist time to leave the scene of the crime before detection, whereas releases of chemicals are evident almost immediately, regardless of the circumstances. Box 20.4 presents the advantages of biologic agents as weapons.

box 20.4 Advantages of Biologics as Weapons

- Infectious via aerosol
- Organisms fairly stable in the environment
- Civilian populations are susceptible
- High morbidity and mortality rates
- Person-to-person transmission (smallpox, plague, viral hemorrhagic fever)
- Difficult to diagnose and/or treat
- Easy to obtain
- Inexpensive to produce
- Potential for dissemination over large geographic area
- Creates panic
- Can overwhelm medical services
- Perpetrators escape easily
- Previous development of organisms for biologic weapons

Terrorism has once again shown it is prepared deliberately to stop at nothing in creating human victims. An end must be put to this. As never before, it is vital to unite forces of the entire world community against terror.

Vladimir Putin

History of Bioterrorism

The world has become aware that bioterrorism is not a new tactic. History will reveal that as early as 1346, the Tartar army hurled corpses of plague victims over the walls of Caffa, a seaport on the Crimean coast, and 400 years later, Russians used the same tactic against Sweden. Using infected people as "weapons" may have contributed to the spread of plague across Europe in the 14th century. People who became victims ultimately became weapons themselves; a smallpox or plague victim approaching a village must have been a fearsome sight. Later, during the Pontiac Rebellion in 1763, the British army provided the Delaware Indians with blankets and handkerchiefs from a smallpox hospital (Handysides, 2009).

The word *terrorism* was first used in 1795 during the French Revolution, when the "reign of terror" was unfolding on the streets and hillsides of France. During World War I, Germany used biologic agents to infect livestock hindering troop movement. In the United States, the development of biologic warfare agents began in 1942, under President Franklin D. Roosevelt, and was not discontinued until the late 1960s. The former Soviet Union began a massive program to develop biologic weapons in the 1970s. In 1979, there was an accidental release of anthrax at a Soviet military facility, resulting in 68 deaths, and it is believed that this ultimately led to the end of the program.

Since the 1990s, worldwide bioterrorist attacks have been carried out by relatively small radical political factions (Box 20.5). However, a number of nations have acquired, or are seeking to acquire, biologic weapons. There are concerns that individual terrorists or terrorist groups may acquire the technologies and expertise to use these agents. Weaponized forms of some agents have been used against civilian populations in recent memory, as was the case when anthrax-contaminated mail was circulated in New Jersey, New York, and Washington, DC. Biologic agents may be used for an isolated assassination or to cause the injury or death of thousands of people. Environmental contamination could be a long-term threat.

An eye for an eye, and the whole world would be blind.

Khalil Gibran

Categories of Bioterrorism Agents

The CDC (2006c/2011) has divided biologic agents into three categories (Box 20.6): A, B, and C. The high-priority agents in category A include organisms that pose a risk to national security. These agents (1) can be easily disseminated or transmitted from person to person, (2) result in high mortality, (3) have the potential for major public health impact, (4) might cause public panic and social disruption, and (5) require special action for public health preparedness. "Category A" agents are discussed in the following section.

box 20.5 Bioterrorist Attacks by Small Radical Political Factions, 1984–2001

1984, United States: Rajneeshee bioterrorist attack using *Salmonella* bacteria to contaminate salad bars in 10 restaurants in Oregon. The objective of the group was to incapacitate the residents of the area during local elections with the hope of taking over political control. The attack sickened 751 people but caused no fatalities. This is the first known biologic attack in the United States in the 20th century, in Oregon, 1984.

1993, Japan: Aum Shinrikyo anthrax release in Tokyo without infecting anyone

1995, Japan: Sarin released in a Tokyo subway

2001, United States: Anthrax spores were mailed to several news media offices and two Democratic U.S. senators, killing five people and infecting 17 others. It has subsequently been shown that the total number of harmed people should be raised to 68.

Detection of a Bioterrorism Event

Early detection of a biologic event is often difficult. The first recognition of a bioterrorism event may result from routine surveillance activities. However, a single case or a few cases of bioterrorism-related disease may not be identified. Surveillance for infectious diseases is a continual process, conducted on an everyday basis by clinicians and laboratory staff. All personnel in any healthcare-related activity should be aware of the diseases that may be associated with bioterrorism. In actuality, all people should be involved in reporting unusual events or illnesses to the local public health department. Public health nurses are important resources in collecting and analyzing symptoms before a diagnosis is made. By identifying unusual spikes in disease, deliberate biologic attacks will be revealed in a timely manner. Public health nurses also use their system-wide relationships with their communities to track illness. Automatic biosurveillance systems were developed and implemented in major cities in the United States following the events of 2001, with the intent to improve the response time to a potential incident. Although the systems have not yet been utilized with any regularity in this country and across the world, situational awareness of the need for early detection has been established. Linking syndromic data to triage activities and clinical documentation would increase the value of biosurveillance as a tool to fight morbidity and mortality (Kaydos-Daniels, Rojas, & Farris, 2013). Box 20.7 presents clues indicating that a deliberate biologic attack has occurred.

PRACTICE POINT

Report higher-than-normal cases of infectious disease, unusual occurrences, and clusters of illnesses to the local department of public health.

box 20.6 Categories of Bioterrorism Agents

Category A Agents

- Pose the greatest risk to the public because they
  - Spread easily
  - Result in a high mortality rate
  - Cause public panic
  - May impact national security
  - Require special training and response and may be unfamiliar to the responding community
  - Easy to obtain and "weaponize"
  - Can overwhelm existing medical resources
- High-priority agents include organisms that pose a risk to national security because they
  - Can be easily disseminated or transmitted from person to person
  - Result in high mortality rates and have the potential for major public health impact
  - Might cause public panic and social disruption
  - Require special action for public health preparedness

Agents/diseases include the following:

- Anthrax (*Bacillus anthracis*)
- Botulism (*C. botulinum* toxin)
- Plague (*Y. pestis*)
- Smallpox (variola major)
- Tularemia (*F. tularensis*)
- Viral hemorrhagic fevers (filoviruses [e.g., Ebola, Marburg] and arenaviruses [e.g., Lassa, Machupo])

Category B Agents

Pose less of a threat to the public. However, they are a danger because

- They are easily available.
- Can be reproduced and disseminated easily
- Surveillance and tracking will still require an intense response.
- Mortality, though lower than that with classified "A" agents, still poses a serious public health threat.

Agents/diseases include the following:

- Brucellosis (*Brucella* species)
- Epsilon toxin of *Clostridium* perfringens
- Food safety threats (e.g., *Salmonella* species, *Escherichia coli* O157:H7, *Shigella*)
- Glanders (*Burkholderia mallei*)
- Melioidosis (*Burkholderia pseudomallei*)
- Psittacosis (*Chlamydia psittaci*)
- Q fever (*Coxiella burnetii*)
- Ricin toxin from *Ricinus communis* (castor beans)
- Staphylococcal enterotoxin B
- Typhus fever (Rickettsia prowazekii)
- Viral encephalitis (alphaviruses [e.g., Venezuelan equine encephalitis, eastern equine encephalitis, western equine encephalitis])
- Water safety threats (e.g., *Vibrio cholerae*, *Cryptosporidium parvum*)

Category C Agents

Include emerging pathogens and share these attributes:

- They are easily engineered for mass production and dissemination.
- Their potential for high morbidity and mortality rates is significant.
- Diseases include the following:

Emerging infectious diseases

- Nipah virus
- Hanta virus
- Multiple drug–resistant infectious diseases

Source: From National Center for Environmental Health. Retrieved from http://www.cdc.gov/nceh/; Agency for Toxic Substances and Disease Registry. Retrieved from http://www.atsdr.cdc.gov/; Coordinating Center for Environmental Health and Injury Prevention. Retrieved from http://www.cdc.gov/about/organization/ccehip.htm

Bioterrorism Agents

Anthrax

Anthrax results from infection with spore-forming bacillus bacteria (*Bacillus anthracis*) that occur naturally in the soil. The resulting noncontagious acute infectious disease occurs primarily in cattle and sheep. Contact with infected animals or contaminated animal products may lead to infection in humans. In the past, anthrax, considered a woolsorter's disease, was prevalent among tanners. Cutaneous anthrax occurs from inoculation of spores under the skin, gastrointestinal and oropharyngeal anthrax occurs from ingesting contaminated meat, and inhalation anthrax occurs from spores entering the respiratory tract while breathing (Table 20.4). Without swift diagnosis and treatment, inhalational anthrax is usually fatal in approximately 90% of the cases. In 2001, weaponized anthrax spores were sent through the U.S. postal system, resulting in 22 cases and 5 deaths.

box 20.7 Clues of a Biologic Attack

- Case clusters of similar clinical presentation and timelines
- Case cluster of unexplained illness
- Unusually severe disease or higher mortality for a given agent
- Uncommon transmission of an agent
- Multiple outbreaks of different diseases in a given population
- Disease unusual for a given age
- Disease unusual for a region or season
- Case clusters of same illness in various locations
- Case clusters of illness and deaths of animals in the timeframe shared by humans

Source: From United States Army Medical Reserve Institute of Infectious Diseases. (2005). *USAMRID's medical management of biological casualties handbook* (6th ed.). Frederick, MD: USAMRID.

Once infection has been diagnosed, antibiotic treatment usually runs a 60-day course. Researchers have developed a protective vaccine against anthrax. Military personnel and people at high risk, such as workers in research laboratories

table 20.4 **Bioterrorism Agents**

Anthrax	
Agent	*Bacillus anthracis* Aerobic, spore-forming bacterium
Forms of disease/systems affected	Cutaneous Inhalational Gastrointestinal Oropharyngeal
Transmission	Skin: direct contact with spores Respiratory: inhalation of aerosolized spores Gastrointestinal: ingestion of undercooked meat of infected animals No person-to-person spread
Reporting	Report suspected cases to local/state health departments
Incubation	1–7 days
Signs and symptoms	Fever, fatigue, body aches Inhalational: cough, chest pain, dyspnea Gastrointestinal: nausea, bloody diarrhea Cutaneous: necrotic ulcer, edema
Laboratory	Serology Ulcer exudate
Treatment	Ciprofloxacin or doxycycline Additional antimicrobials for 60 days
Postexposure prophylaxis	Ciprofloxacin or doxycycline
Mortality	High (80%–90%), inhalational form
Botulism	
Agent	Toxin produced by *Clostridium botulinum* Spore-forming bacterium found in soil and contaminated food
Forms of disease/systems affected	Neuroparalytic illness Food-borne ingestion of preformed toxin Infant ingestion of soil-producing toxin in gastrointestinal tract Wound infection by toxin
Transmission	Not spread from person to person
Reporting	Report suspected case to local/state health department
Incubation	12–72 hours
Signs and symptoms	Difficulty swallowing, speaking Double or blurred vision, dilated pupils Constipation (infant botulism) Descending flaccid paralysis
Laboratory	Stool, vomitus, suspect food samples
Treatment	Prompt diagnosis Antitoxin, ventilator support
Postexposure prophylaxis	None
Mortality	Low
Plague	
Agent	Bacterium *Yersinia pestis* Found in rodents and their fleas; found throughout the world
Forms of disease/systems affected	Pneumonic (lungs) Bubonic (lymph glands) Septicemic (blood)
Transmission	Pneumonic: inhalation of aerosolized spores; spread person to person Bubonic: bite by an infected flea; not spread person to person Septicemic: multiplication of bacteria in blood; not spread person to person
Reporting	Report suspected cases to local/state health department
Incubation	1–6 days
Signs and symptoms	Pneumonic: chest pain, dyspnea, hemoptysis, sepsis, respiratory shock Bubonic: tender, swollen lymph glands (buboes), bacteremia, fever Septicemic: fever, bacteremia, sepsis
Laboratory	Blood, sputum, bubo culture
Treatment	Streptomycin, gentamicin, tetracyclines
Postexposure prophylaxis	Ciprofloxacin or doxycycline
Mortality	High (pneumonic) if untreated within 24 hours

Smallpox	
Agent	Smallpox virus
Systems affected	General viral infectious disease
Transmission	Person to person, aerosolized spread Contact with infected body fluids
Reporting	Declared eliminated by World Health Organization in 1980; one confirmed case constitutes an outbreak. Report case to local/state health departments
Incubation	7–12 days (12-day average)
Signs and symptoms	Influenza-like, high fever, body aches Early rash, raised bumps (most contagious) Pustular rash, raised firm bumps (contagious) Pustules with scab formation (contagious) Resolving scabs (contagious) Scabs resolved (noncontagious)
Laboratory	Pharyngeal or nasal swab Scab examination Serology
Treatment	Supportive intravenous therapy Antibiotics for secondary infections
Postexposure prophylaxis	Smallpox vaccine within 4 days of exposure
Mortality	Moderate (20%–40%), unvaccinated
Tularemia	
Agent	*Francisella tularensis* Found in rodents, rabbits, hares (also known as rabbit fever)
Forms of disease/systems affected	Pulmonary Cutaneous Gastrointestinal
Transmission	Not spread person to person Cutaneous Gastrointestinal Inhalational
Reporting	Report cases to local/state health departments
Incubation	3–4 days average (up to 14)
Signs and symptoms	Fever, chills, body aches Dry cough Joint pain Ulcers on skin and mouth
Laboratory	Sputum, blood cultures
Treatment	Streptomycin, gentamicin
Postexposure prophylaxis	Ciprofloxacin or doxycycline
Mortality	Low, 5%–15%, untreated
Viral Hemorrhagic Fevers (VHFs)	
Agent	Highly contagious virus; Ebola, Marburg, Lassa fever, and arenaviruses
Systems affected	General viral infectious disease Gastrointestinal Cutaneous Cardiovascular
Transmission	Field rodents, arthropod ticks Vectors not known for Ebola, Marburg Person-to-person spread greatest as disease progresses
Reporting	Report suspected cases to local/state health departments
Incubation	2–21 days, agent dependent
Signs and symptoms	High fever, headache, body ache Bloody diarrhea, mucous membrane hemorrhage Shock, circulatory collapse
Laboratory	Serology
Treatment	Ribavirin for Lassa fever Supportive therapy for other VHFs
Postexposure prophylaxis	None
Mortality	High 80%–90% Ebola-Zaire 50%–60% Ebola-Sudan Variable for other VHFs

who handle anthrax bacteria routinely or those who work with imported animal hides or furs from areas where standards are insufficient to prevent exposure, are most likely to receive the vaccine.

Postexposure prophylaxis, which combines 60 days of antibiotics plus three doses of vaccine, is effective in preventing anthrax disease from occurring after an exposure. In an attack, public health nurses may set up PODs in their communities to administer prophylactic medications. Nurses also have the responsibility to educate the public about anthrax by managing "hotlines," answering questions, providing factual information, and offering reassurance.

Botulism

Botulism is a muscle-paralyzing disease caused by the bacterium *Clostridium botulinum,* which is found in the soil worldwide. The toxin produced by the bacterium is the most potent lethal substance known to humans. The disease is relatively uncommon; in the United States, there are approximately 100 reported cases per year. Botulism is probably familiar to most consumers: beware of canned food with "popped" tops. Table 20.4 summarizes the three forms of botulism. Botulism is not spread person to person in any of its forms.

Food-borne botulism occurs when the preformed toxin is ingested and can affect people of any age. As cases are identified and confirmed, health departments have environmental inspectors, guided by epidemiologic data patterns, who work diligently to ensure that contaminated foods are removed from stores to protect against further illness.

In botulism, muscle weakness begins and descends through the body. At the point where breathing muscles are involved, ventilator assistance becomes necessary. Antitoxin must be administered because a toxin produced by *C. botulinum* is the cause of the paralysis. A supply of this antitoxin is maintained by the CDC (CDC, 2012).

Plague

Plague, believed to have first emerged in Egypt about 540 AD, is an infectious disease caused by the bacterium *Yersinia pestis*, found globally in rodents and their fleas. The World Health Organization (WHO) reports the occurrence of 1,000 to 3,000 cases yearly throughout the world, with approximately 15 cases in the western United States (CDC, 2003, 2012). Most cases are of the bubonic form, which is the most common of the three forms of plague (see Table 20.4).

Pneumonic plague occurs when *Y. pestis* infects the lungs. Airborne transmission from person to person makes this form of plague a possible agent of choice as a bioweapon. The incubation period, 1 to 6 days, makes it possible for the bacteria to spread to others before symptoms present. Considering this incubation period and the mobile society of the developed world, pneumonic plague can spread easily from state to state, country to country. The gap between infection and diagnosis also makes early treatment more difficult. The bacterium occurs naturally and, therefore, could be engineered as a weapon by an organization technologically savvy enough to create an aerosol.

Without early treatment, pneumonic plague has a high mortality rate. Several types of antibiotics are effective in the treatment of all forms of plague. Should there be a confirmed bioterrorism attack, prophylactic distribution of antibiotics to the public will occur through POD sites.

Smallpox

Smallpox is an acute, contagious, and possibly fatal disease caused by the variola virus. Humans are the only known reservoirs. The virus is contagious and spreads from person to person by contact or through inhalation of aerosols. In America, smallpox last occurred in 1949, and in the world, it last occurred in Somalia in 1977. In 1980, the WHO declared the disease eradicated. For further scientific research on the smallpox virus, the CDC has maintained stockpiles of the virus at its laboratories. Before the dissolution of the former Soviet Union, stockpiles existed at sites throughout that country. After the tragic events of September 11, 2001, officials in the United States became concerned that smallpox could become a biologic weapon.

No treatment exists for smallpox, and the only prevention available is vaccination. The vaccine is made from a virus called vaccinia, which is a "pox"-type virus related to smallpox. Unlike many other vaccines, the smallpox vaccine contains live vaccinia virus. For that reason, it is necessary to care for the vaccination site carefully to prevent the virus from spreading. In 2003, several states initiated a smallpox immunization campaign to protect citizens. For example, in New Jersey, JITT training for smallpox immunization techniques began. Public health nurses operated PODs throughout the state to administer vaccination to first-line healthcare workers and clinically oriented first responders. Currently, the United States has stockpiled enough smallpox vaccine to vaccinate everyone in the United States in the event of a biologic event that involves smallpox. The disease itself has been eliminated for more than three decades; therefore, the report of just one confirmed case of smallpox would be declared an outbreak. Table 20.4 gives more information about smallpox.

Tularemia

Tularemia is a potentially serious illness caused by the bacterium *Francisella tularensis*, which occurs naturally in the Northern Hemisphere. Approximately 200 cases of tularemia are reported yearly in rural and semirural areas of the United States, mostly in the southern, central, and western states. Summer outbreaks also often occur on Martha's Vineyard in Massachusetts. The bacterium is not spread person to person, but a low infectious dose, 1 to 10 organisms, is spread by aerosol or the intradermal route. People who are infected can die if not treated quickly with the correct antibiotic. *F. tularensis* occurs naturally; thus, it could be harvested and reengineered as a bioweapon (see Table 20.4). If the organism can be aerosolized, severe respiratory illness would result.

PRACTICE POINT

Unusual, out-of-season spikes in infectious disease cases may indicate a bioterrorism attack.

Viral Hemorrhagic Fevers

Viral hemorrhagic fevers (VHFs) are a group of illnesses caused by several distinct RNA virus families. The survival of these viruses is dependent on host vectors, usually rodents, mosquitoes, and ticks. The viruses are found only in geographic areas where their host species live. However, the hosts of two VHFs, Marburg fever and Ebola fever, are unknown. Humans are infected when they accidentally come into contact with infected hosts. In some instances, humans can transmit the virus to one another.

The diseases appear to be global; however, VHFs do not occur naturally in the United States. Outbreaks are sporadic and cannot be easily predicted. In general, the term *viral hemorrhagic fever* is used to describe a severe multisystem syndrome that damages the vascular system throughout the body, and the body's ability to regulate itself is impaired. Hemorrhaging occurs, but the bleeding itself is rarely life-threatening. Although some types of hemorrhagic fever viruses can cause relatively mild illnesses, many cause severe, life-threatening conditions, and mortality is high. For example, Ebola hemorrhagic fever is a severe, often fatal viral disease in humans, and it is one of the most virulent viral diseases known to humankind (Fig. 20.5). No treatment or vaccine is available, and death occurs in 50% to 90% of all cases of clinical illness. Prevention involves rodent and insect control.

The CDC classifies VHF viruses as biosafety level four (BSL-4) pathogens (Box 20.8). Once illness is confirmed, isolation is enforced along with strict infection control techniques. The CDC, in partnership with the WHO, has produced hospital-based guidelines, *Infection Control for Viral Hemorrhagic Fevers in the African Healthcare Setting* (CDC, 2003, 2012). Researchers have identified containment, treatment, and vaccine development as goals to address the threat of VHFs (Croddy, E., & Ackerman, G., 2013).

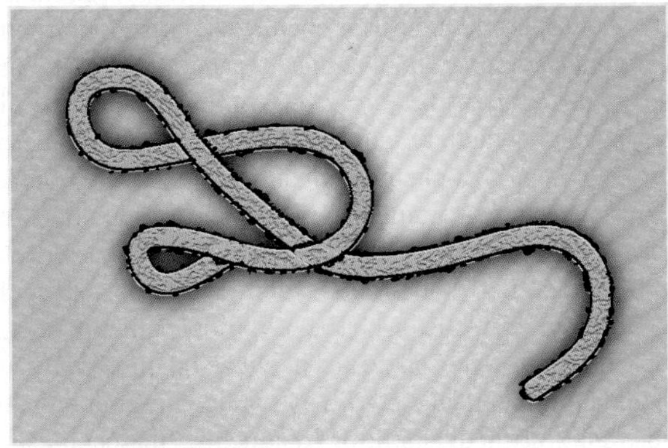

figure 20.5 Ebola virus.

box 20.8 Biosafety Levels for Infectious Agents

1. Not known to consistently cause disease in healthy adults
2. Associated with human disease
3. Hazard from percutaneous injury, ingestion, mucous membrane exposure
4. Indigenous or exotic agents with potential for aerosol transmission
5. Disease may have serious or lethal consequences
6. Dangerous/exotic agents that pose high risk of life-threatening disease, aerosol-transmitted laboratory infections; or related agents with unknown risk of transmission

Source: From the Centers for Disease Control and Prevention. Retrieved June 30, 2010, from Centers for Disease Control and Prevention, Office of Health and Safety (Biosafety information page), http://www.cdc.gov/od/ohs/biosfty/bmbl4/bmbl4s3t.htm

PRACTICE POINT

Maintain a library of biologic, chemical, and radiologic fact sheets from the CDC website to provide clear, accurate information to the public and fellow clinicians.

CHEMICAL DISASTERS

The intentional or accidental spill of chemical substances can have a devastating effect both on the environment and on human health. In 1984, the release of toxic gases at Union Carbide's pesticide plant in Bhopal, India, resulted in approximately 8,000 deaths and 150,000 injuries. Severe contamination with heavy metals and toxic cancer-producing chemicals occurred at the factory site, on the surrounding land, and in the groundwater. This disaster brought the horror of industrial development to people's attention worldwide and stimulated development of environmental policy and legislation throughout the world. In response, the U.S. Congress passed the Emergency Planning and Community Right-to-Know Act (EPCRA) to address concerns about storing and handling of toxic chemicals.

Multiple chemical environmental disasters have occurred, such as the spill of 11 million gallons of crude oil into Prince William Sound by *Exxon Valdez* and the collapse of the BP oil rig that spewed huge amounts of oil from the ocean floor, to contaminate the Gulf Coast of the United States. Oil from this disaster entered the Gulf Stream and spread to the Atlantic Coast and beyond. The toxic chemical waste landfill used by Hooker Chemical in Love Canal, Niagara Falls, NY, affected hundreds of people who lived there before cleanup plans were initiated. OSHA is now responsible for developing programs to prevent chemical incidents. The Environmental Protection Agency requires all companies that use flammable and toxic substance to develop a risk management program that includes hazard assessment, a prevention program, and an emergency response program. The CDC categorization of hazardous chemicals is outlined in Table 20.5, and the characteristics

table 20.5 **Centers for Disease Control and Prevention Categorization of Hazardous Chemicals**

Category	Action	Example
Biotoxins	Poisons that come from plants or animals	Ricin
Blister agents/vesicants	Chemicals that severely blister the eyes, respiratory tract, and skin on contact	Mustard gas
Blood agents	Poisons that affect the body by being absorbed into the blood	Cyanide
Caustics (acids)	Chemicals that burn or corrode people's skin, eyes, and mucus membranes (lining of the nose, mouth, throat, and lungs) on contact	Hydrogen fluoride
Choking/lung/pulmonary agents	Chemicals that cause severe irritation or swelling of the respiratory tract (lining of the nose and throat, lungs)	Chlorine
Incapacitating agents	Drugs that make people unable to think clearly or that cause an altered state of consciousness (possibly unconsciousness)	Fentanyl
Long-acting anticoagulants	Poisons that prevent blood from clotting properly, which can lead to uncontrolled bleeding	Super warfarin
Metals	Agents that consist of metallic poisons	Mercury
Nerve agents	Highly poisonous chemicals that work by preventing the nervous system from working properly	Sarin
Organic solvents	Agents that damage the tissues of living things by dissolving fats and oils	Benzene
Riot control agents/tear gas	Highly irritating agents normally used by law enforcement for crowd control or by individuals for protection	Mace
Toxic alcohols	Poisonous alcohols that can damage the heart, kidneys, and nervous system	Ethylene glycol
Vomiting agents	Chemicals that cause nausea and vomiting	Adamsite

Source: From National Center for Environmental Health (NCEH)/Agency for Toxic Substances and Disease Registry (ATSDR); Coordinating Center for Environmental Health and Injury Prevention (CCEHIP).

of individual chemical agents can be reviewed in depth at the CDC website.

A chemical's persistence, the length of time a chemical remains potent after its dissemination, is a factor that contributes to the classification of, and response to, a given agent. Nonpersistent chemicals lose their effectiveness in a few minutes to a few hours. For example, chlorine and other pungent gases are nonpersistent chemicals that might be used by terrorists whose goal is to take control of a site of interest. In contrast, persistent chemicals remain in the environment for weeks. For example, liquids such as blister agents and certain nerve agents are oily, and **decontamination** procedures are difficult.

Geoff works with the public health department, hospitals, and other community organizations in planning the disaster management exercise. It will be conducted in a New Jersey city of 100,000 residents where a deliberate release of anhydrous ammonia via a large explosive device has occurred.

Determine the characteristics of the chemical release and the type of cases that may appear for triage.

Chemicals have been used as tools of war for centuries. However, the destructive qualities of chemicals are not primarily the result of their explosive qualities. Modern chemical warfare began in World War I. At that time, available gases such as chlorine and phosgene were in use. Trench warfare was the main military formation, and soldiers were particularly vulnerable to this form of attack. In effect, attackers simply opened canisters of the gas and let prevailing winds disseminate the chemicals. During the 20th century, the development of chemical munitions, such as artillery shells, projectiles, and bombs, increased a chemical's capacity to kill and maim (Organization for Prohibition of Chemical Weapons, 2012).

Although living organisms can be biologic warfare agents, nonliving toxins produced by living organisms (e.g., botulinum and ricin) can be considered chemical agents according to the Chemical Weapons Convention. Similar to bioterrorism agents, these chemical agents can affect health through inhalation, ingestion, or skin absorption. Examples are nerve agents such as sarin and VX, gases such as the sulfur and nitrogen mustard agents, and choking agents such as phosgene (CDC, 2006a/2013). In an attempt to reduce the amount of chemical weapons, the Department of Defense began incinerating weapons at eight U.S. sites beginning in 2005. Additionally, industrial chemicals, poisonous chemicals found in nature, and chemicals made from compounds in everyday use can be released intentionally. Unlike biologic agents, which require an incubation period before symptoms appear, a chemical agent, when released, makes its presence known immediately through observation (explosion), self-admission (accidental), or the occurrence of rapidly emerging symptoms, such as burns, difficulty breathing, or convulsions (Fig. 20.6) (Spellman, 2013). People may be exposed to a chemical in three ways: by breathing the chemical directly; by swallowing contaminated food, water, or medication; or by touching the chemical or coming into contact with contaminated clothing or objects.

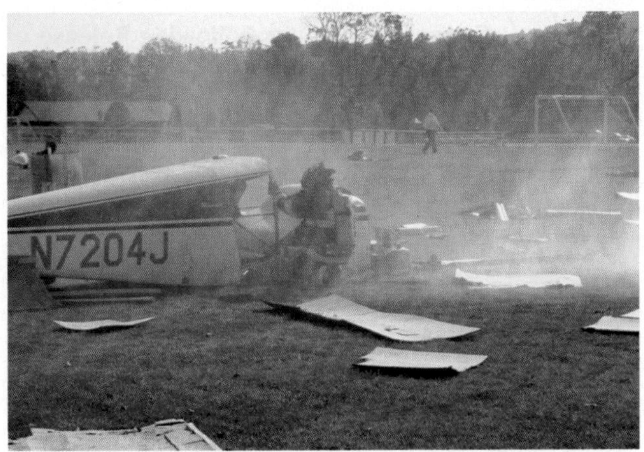

figure 20.6 Cleanup of the crash of a small airplane. This firefighter is trying to prevent the highly volatile aviation fuel from exploding and causing a fire.

General treatment guidelines are found in Table 20.6 (Croddy Ackerman, 2013).

PRACTICE POINT

You may be exposed to chemicals, even though you may not be able to see or smell anything unusual.

Fear is a defining element of chemical and biologic terrorism. In 1995, after the sarin attack in the Tokyo subway system, the "worried well" descended on the Japanese healthcare system in far greater numbers than those who were actually affected. In 2001 to 2002, the anthrax events in a New Jersey postal facility resulted in a similar response by the community. The New Jersey health department received approximately 100 calls daily, reporting "white powder" events in schools, banks, gas stations, and even doughnut shops. Recognizing that perception is reality to many people, authorities dispatched teams to investigate the reports. A nursing contingent provided telephone support for concerned citizens. No retrieved samples turned out to be anthrax, but for the 700 plus people who called in, the testing of the samples and the presence of a public health nursing team to answer questions and allay fears was an important step toward restoring public confidence in the face of a real, or thought-to-be-real, anthrax attack. The reaction by the public, fueled by fear, would seem to be a catalyst to encourage "copycat" events. However, every report called in required a response that involved sampling, testing, and community education. To do less would not meet the standards of public health practice and disease investigation. This serves as another example of how the process itself is time-consuming and costly but essential.

table 20.6 **Established Treatment Guidelines for Chemical Exposures**

Chemical Agent	Treatment
Nerve agents	Atropine, diazepam
Incapacitating agents	Fresh air and basic decontamination
Pulmonary agents	Oxygen, restricted activity
Vesicants	Fresh air, removal of clothing, skin decontamination, oxygen, eye irrigation
Blood agents	Amyl nitrate, sodium nitrate

Source: From Centers for Disease Control and Prevention, Agency for Toxic Substances. Retrieved from http://www.atsdr.cdc.gov/

The only thing we have to fear is fear itself.

Franklin D. Roosevelt

Role of Nurses in a Chemical Disaster

In the field, the public health nurse's response to a chemical incident is summed up in two words: "act quickly." HAZMAT experts report to the hot zone on notification of the release of the chemical. The nurse may be asked to report to a temporary evacuation site where people exposed to the chemical are awaiting triage (Fig. 20.7). Donning PPE must be the first priority. Then assessment of the victim's ability to breathe is necessary. Maintaining adequate respiratory function tops the list for effective client management in a chemical event. Keeping the victims in a sitting position with constrictive clothing loosened or removed is necessary. If the client cannot sit, the torso should be elevated.

In the citywide disaster management drill at the end of the program on emergency preparedness that Geoff has designed, PPE is necessary. What PPE is required for exposure to anhydrous ammonia?

PRACTICE POINT

After donning PPE, the first action in a chemical incident is to maintain adequate ventilation for the victims.

Field decontamination of the victim requires removal of as many outer layers of clothing as possible and placing the victims at a good distance from unaffected population. Washing with soap—or at least water—should follow. Rinsing of the eyes is necessary; bottled water works. For more thorough decontamination, field tents may be erected nearby. Victims who have been severely compromised by the chemical release will be transported to the hospital; there, they will undergo decontamination on the facility grounds before being admitted into the emergency department. The nurse leader is responsible for maintaining communication, especially updating the receiving institutions on client transfer and clinical status. Before leaving the field, nurses should decontaminate themselves before entering their vehicles and returning to the workplace.

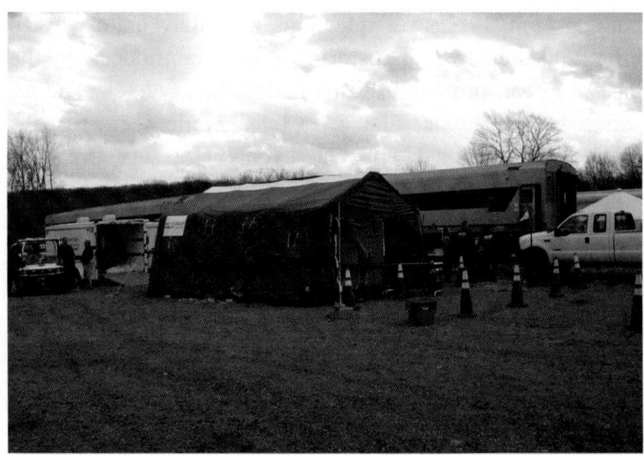

figure 20.7 Decontamination tent. A collision between a freight train carrying toxic chemicals and a passenger train resulted in injuries to several people. Before they were transported to a local hospital, emergency medical personnel carried out on-site decontamination in this temporary facility.

During the day of the disaster management scenario, 75 "victims" plus six high-fidelity HPS replicas are on site. Various levels of chemical injuries are represented, with the HPS models representing the most seriously injured. Arrangements are made for field triage and victim transfer to four medical centers in the area. The nurse responders, the majority of whom were participants in the certificate program, don PPE and assist in the prioritizing of clients in the streets. As the triage activities begin, the nurses facilitate effective client transfer to emergency departments. There are more than 1,000 response participants, including county and local public health department personnel.

Stay or Go?

The decision to stay or go should be made quickly; as time passes, options are reduced. The decision should be made by evaluating factors specific to the event:

- The HAZMAT involved
- The population threatened
- The time span involved
- The current and predicted weather conditions
- The ability to communicate emergency information

The toxicity of the released factor influences the decision to move. Radio stations and the websites of local health departments will report information about the event. Generally speaking, once toxicity has been determined, actions are taken according to the level of toxicity and the duration of the event (Table 20.7).

Shelter in Place

Shelter in place is used for short-duration incidents, when moving would result in a greater hazard, or it is impractical to evacuate. People should stay inside their home, place of business, or nearest building available. It is a protective action that provides a suitable place to stay until the threat from a hazardous agent has passed. Guidelines for sheltering in place are presented in Box 20.9.

table 20.7 **Suggested Actions Following Release of a Hazardous Chemical**

Nature of Exposure	Action
High toxicity and short duration	Shelter in place
Low toxicity and long duration	Evacuate
High toxicity and long duration	Calculate indoor concentrations (done by HAZMAT) Evacuate, if necessary

HAZMAT = hazardous materials.

PRACTICE POINT

Ensure that your place of employment has an effective shelter in place and evacuation plan and that it is included in orientation for new employees.

Evacuation

Evacuation occurs when there is potential for massive explosions and fire as well as for long-duration events. People must leave their homes and go to a safer area. In localized, internal events, **invacuation**, where people in a hospital or residential facility may be moved to another floor or area within the facility, may occur. Natural disasters and industrial accidents require people to evacuate, sometimes on a large scale. Based on the characteristics of the emergency, a combination of evacuation and in-place protection measures may be appropriate. People in areas downwind and in proximity to a chemical release, where concentrations are likely to be higher and less time is available for response, might be advised to shelter in place. At the same time, areas that are

box 20.9 **Guidelines for Sheltering in Place**

- Remain inside your home or office.
- Shut down heating, ventilation fan, and air conditioning systems.
- Close and lock all windows and exterior doors.
- Stuff a towel tightly under each door and tape (aluminum foil or waxed paper) around the sides and top of the door.
- Cover each window and vent in the room with a single piece of plastic sheeting, seal edge with duct tape, and fill any cracks or holes with clay or similar material, such as those around pipes entering a bathroom.
- Close the fireplace damper.
- Go to an interior room without windows that is above ground level. Some chemicals are heavier than air and may seep into basements.
- Get your disaster supplies kit.
- Listen to your radio or television until you are told all is safe or you are told to evacuate.

box 20.10 Guidelines for Evacuation

- Wear long-sleeved shirts, long pants, and sturdy shoes.
- Take your pets with you.
- Lock your home.
- Take your disaster supplies kit.
- Use travel routes specified by local authorities: do not use shortcuts because certain areas may be impassable or dangerous.
- Stay away from downed power lines.

upwind or farther from the release might be evacuated. Evacuating upwind areas makes sense as a precautionary measure because a wind shift could rapidly place these areas in jeopardy. In fact, evacuation is most effective when it is used as a precautionary measure; thus, it is necessary to practice evacuation plans. Guidelines for evacuation are presented in Box 20.10.

EVIDENCE FOR PRACTICE

Evacuation is considered an important strategy to limit victim exposure to hazardous chemical release (HCR). However, because of the wide range of possible disaster scenarios, there is little evidence-based research to guide evacuation or sheltering decisions. A baseline study, conducted by Preston et al. (2008), evaluated the impact of evacuation on the number of victims resulting from different types of HCR. Researchers used the Hazardous Substances Emergency Events Surveillance database to test the hypothesis that evacuation is associated with a reduced victim risk. They developed a series of logistic regression models in which the presence or absence of a victim was the primary outcome, with the specific chemical agent as the predictor.

Of the recorded HCR events, 7.77% resulted in evacuation. Compared with no evacuation order, evacuation was associated with a significantly lower number of victims, per HCR, when the chemical involved was acid, ammonia, or chlorine. Findings indicated that evacuation remains the mainstay for prehospital care to limit the number of victims of an HCR. A more recent broadly focused study by Sengul, Santell, and Steinberg (2010) on accidental chemical releases suggests that several factors, including evacuation as well as improved employee training and advanced safety standards, contribute to a decrease in injury during such an event.

PRACTICE POINT

Maintaining close contact with local HAZMAT teams guides the decision-making process for evacuation/shelter-in-place activities.

RADIOLOGIC DISASTERS

Radiation is energy that moves in the form of particles or waves, such as heat, light, radio waves, and microwaves. Ionizing radiation is a high-energy form of electromagnetic radiation. People benefit from it daily through the warmth of the sun and the use of X-ray technology. In fact, small amounts of radioactive materials are in the air, drinking water, food, and human body. It is known that excessive radiation affects the body in many ways, and often those results do not become evident for several years. The health outcome depends on (1) the amount or dose of radiation absorbed, (2) the type of radiation, (3) the route of exposure, and (4) the length of time exposed to the dose.

When large doses are released accidentally (e.g., from a nuclear power plant) or intentionally (e.g., in a terrorist act), there is an increased risk that health effects will occur. The combined disasters of an earthquake, a tsunami, and a radiologic release in the Iwate Prefecture in Japan in 2011 is an example of a multidimensional disaster that serves as an example of a local disaster with global implications. Within days, the CDC activated their emergency operations center to respond to the health issues related to the three different disasters recorded (CDC, 2010; CDC, 2011; CDC, 2011a; Noto et al., 2013; Centers for Disease Control and Prevention, 2002b/2011). Very often, the terms *exposure* and *contamination* are used incorrectly or interchangeably. Internal exposure occurs when the radioactive materials enter the body by eating or drinking, whereas external exposure occurs when the radioactive source is outside the body. Contamination occurs when particles of radioactive material are deposited where they are normally not found. The Environmental Protection Agency provides additional information on radiologic risks on its website (Centers for Disease Control and Prevention, 2011b).

"Dirty" Bombs

Deliberate release of a radioactive agent, the use of "dirty" bombs, has become a concern. This is a radiologic dispersion device that uses explosives as well as radioactive materials. The act of explosion disseminates the radioactive agent. Unlike a nuclear explosion, fission does not occur. The range of a "dirty" bomb is relatively small. Security at nuclear plants is high, and it is thought that the materials used in making a "dirty" bomb come from low-level sources found in hospitals, at construction sites, and at food irradiation plants (Medalia, 2011).

PRACTICE POINT

In a radiologic emergency, it is necessary to decrease time spent near the source, increase distance from the source, and increase shielding from the source.

With low-level radiation, the greatest risk to the population is the blast itself. The radiation levels released are not likely to cause severe illness. For this reason, "dirty" bombs often are not considered weapons of mass destruction. Dealing with the fear that such an event would instill in the public could very well be the greatest challenge facing first responders. In addition, the economic impact of a "dirty" bomb, involving cleanup efforts and decontamination of the site, is significant.

Iraq is a long way from the U.S., but what happens there matters a great deal here. For the risks that the leaders of a rogue state will use nuclear, chemical, or biological weapons against us or our allies is the greatest security threat we face.

Madeleine Albright

Role of Nurses in a Radiologic Disaster

In a radiologic event, people should leave the area quickly (distance, time); enter the nearest building (shielding); cover their noses and mouths; remove their clothes and seal them in double-thickness trash bags; shower as soon as possible (decontamination); clean and cover any open wounds; and listen to the radio, watch the television, or access the state's website. Community-based nurses are not called to the actual location. However, nurses working in a receiving station may observe dust on arrivals. It must be assumed that dust on victims is radioactive. PPE should be worn, and HAZMAT should be notified. People should remove their clothing and be referred for decontamination. Physical injuries are more acute than radioactive contamination. Stable victims should be moved out of the area quickly, and the people in surrounding facilities should be notified. Information should be documented; it will be used to monitor long-term health consequences. Accurate information regarding appropriate protective actions should be made available to the public.

EVIDENCE FOR PRACTICE

Although there has been increased government and public awareness of the threat of a radiologic emergency from either a terrorist attack or an industrial accident, there has been little emphasis on preparation of healthcare personnel for such an event. Balicer et al. (2011) conducted a survey of hospital workers at Johns Hopkins University, including nurses and physicians, to measure their willingness to respond to a dirty bomb radiologic terrorist event. Forty percent of respondents were unwilling to respond to duty during the event. Perceived willingness of peers to respond, personal safety, and their perceived ability to care for victims appropriately were found to be important factors associated with their willingness to respond. The level of perceived threat had minor impact. It appears that the evidence needed to guide preparedness planning points to the importance of training and an increase of knowledge in dealing with radiologic incidents. A study conducted in Japan (Kitamiya, 2011) 2 years before the near nuclear meltdown surveyed public health nurses assigned to health centers in districts with nuclear power plants. They voiced anxiety with regard to their lack of knowledge in radiologic response and concern for personal safety given their location and perceived risk for an accident given their location.

PRACTICE POINT

Being exposed to or contaminated by radioactive materials is *not* treatable in the emergency department immediately after an incident.

BLAST INJURIES

In the blink of an eye, an explosion and its subsequent blast can create chaos and lay waste to an area previously untouched. Explosions can occur as a result of an industrial accident, such as the fertilizer plant explosion and fire that happened in Texas, or when used as a weapon of choice by a terrorist, as witnessed during the Boston Marathon bombings in April 2013. Construction directions for makeshift devices are readily available on the Internet. Such a mechanism can be inexpensive to build while producing many casualties with injuries not normally seen after naturally occurring disasters. Injuries sustained in an explosion are multisystem threatening and "war-like" in their presentation: mutilation, shrapnel wounds to bone, soft tissue, and vascular structures, and dismemberment. In the Boston attack, it has been reported that all victims who were evacuated to a hospital survived. Aside from the courage of fellow marathon runners, volunteers and the rapid response of medical first responders, on view for the word to see was a community effort to practice and exercise response to a mass casualty event (Centers for Disease Control and Prevention, 2011b).

During a field response in an explosion-based event, there are some considerations to weigh (CDC, 2012):

- Explosions in confined spaces are associated with higher morbidity and mortality.
- Communication with victims may be difficult due to sudden temporary deafness.
- Many injuries are not life-threatening due to blunt force trauma from flying debris.
- Open wounds have an increased chance to become infected.
- Triage and life-saving efforts should not be delayed because of the possibility of a dirty bomb detonation.
- Detailed assessments and on-site evaluations are counterproductive to decreasing mortality.

The improvisational use of tourniquets on bombing victims on-site has been documented to be an effective intervention to stop bleeding and ultimately save lives. Field stabilization of bombing victims can be incorporated into professional and volunteer responder training to sustain the survival rate of victims seen in Boston.

Geoff decides to include two HPSs who have sustained typical blast-related injuries from the plant explosion. What will the field response nurse have to do to minimize field mortality?

PRACTICE POINT

The most important aspect of field response to an explosion victim in the field is stabilization and rapid transfer to a hospital.

PUBLIC HEALTH DISASTER RESPONSE

Every state department of health has established reporting requirements to ensure accurate surveillance of infectious diseases. All disasters originate as local events, and historically, local health departments respond accordingly, through stepped up surveillance activities or communication with their respective state health department. It is part of a larger emergency response effort within the region. The Health Alert Network is a nationwide integrated information and communication system that links local and state health and safety departments. This network broadcasts and receives health alerts, offers distance learning opportunities, and provides electronic laboratory reporting and disease surveillance. In an emergency, the Health Alert Network provides essential information for an appropriate response from public health officials. People will be informed of the type of health hazard, area(s) affected, self-protection measures, evacuation routes, shelter locations, the type and location of medical facilities, and telephone numbers to call if extra help is needed.

Key factors in an effective disaster response are summarized in Box 20.11.

Scope and Magnitude of Response

The scope of the disaster should become evident within the first hours of the emergency, and the magnitude of a public health response can be assessed. An act of terrorism will involve large numbers of innocent people, with a sudden increased demand for health-related services. Triage, transport, medical care, and mental health services for victims, their families, responders, and the community may be necessary. Also, recovery, transportation, and storage of human remains may be required. It is necessary to know what other agencies are involved, if an incident command post has been established and commander identified, and if state, local, or tribal operations centers have been activated. A large-scale emergency response could involve dozens of agencies at various levels of government, working together in accordance with mutual aid agreements and written emergency plans.

The public health response should be implemented in accordance with existing EOPs and procedures. As part of this joint effort, all participants should function within the incident management system adopted by the community. Once the need for the participation of the health department and public health nurses has been established, key personnel should be notified. It will be necessary to coordinate with area healthcare partners and document efforts to contact participants, including unsuccessful attempts. A representative from the health department should be assigned to establish communications and act as liaison to others in the emergency operations center. The health department will take steps to ensure the safety of the response team. This will probably include the use of PPE and ongoing safety reports throughout the day. Throughout the event, documentation of activities should be maintained.

It is essential to constantly verify the status of the response effort. Asset and resource allocation plans will be made in response to the disaster. The mutual agreements among providers can be implemented, calling on partners to assist in the evacuation of residents, the provision of temporary shelter and food, or the transfer of injured to hospitals outside of the affected community.

A response is always a dynamic process; therefore, an ongoing assessment of the situation should be in place. Once the health department and the regional public health system have been activated, health surveillance systems should be initiated. The needs of special populations within the jurisdiction should be addressed. The state authorities are involved at this stage, and local health authorities must confirm that the state laboratories are available so that the process of specimen collection and analysis can begin. A contact person should be identified for updates. Additional consideration should be given to the jurisdiction's policy on using volunteers during a disaster response. Often, the MRC is activated. If the incorporation of volunteers is used, the MRC contact person should be included in the communication effort.

Depending on the scope of the disaster and its nature—natural or intentional—state and, perhaps, federal representatives may be at the operations site. Specially trained response teams may be brought into the region if required. The public health authorities have the responsibility to request additional staff, supplies, and other resources as soon as the need is identified. Monitoring of health resources is essential to maintain a sustained response.

box 20.11 Dos and Don'ts in Disaster Response

Dos

Plan now!
Respond quickly—the first 24 hours are critical.
Emphasize that the response process is in place and activated.
Respond in a straightforward manner, giving anticipatory guidance.
Reassure your clients by giving them accurate information.
Acknowledge people's fears, not panic.
Give people things to do.

Don'ts

Assume "it won't happen here."
Allow your issues and standards as a nurse to be defined by someone else.
Talk down to people of any age.
Overreassure.

As assessment and updates continue, the characteristics of the response may begin to change. The support of response personnel must be a priority. Backup shift personnel should be mobilized at the outset and deployment to the site arranged. After the acute phase of a disaster passes, specific activities related to the nature of the event should be addressed. These may include agent identification, laboratory collection and analysis, dissemination of educational materials, evacuation plans, health status assessment of responders as well as the general public affected by the event, infectious disease protocol implementation, and assessment of water supply, food safety, and vector control. The importance of veterinary services during an emergency event cannot be overlooked. Professionals in this field should be included in disaster plan development. During Hurricane Sandy, several pet shelters were opened by the ASPCA and other charities. As evacuation proceeded in shore towns in New Jersey, domestic pets were admitted to the designated shelter. The goal was to reunite families with their pets as soon as possible.

The difficult we do immediately. The impossible takes a little longer.

The United States Army–Air Force

Communication during a Disaster

Communication is one of the most important aspects of maintaining a detailed, dynamic, and broad-based response to a disaster. "Risk communication" is defined as a science-based discipline that provides an interactive exchange of information and opinions among individuals, groups, and institutions in a disaster setting. The risk communication plan is an important component of the disaster preparedness plan; it involves identifying key decision-makers, a risk communication team, representatives for talking to media contacts, a clinical spokesperson, and a venue for conducting media updates. High-concern situations can change the rules of communication. Similar to emergency preparedness planning, effective risk communication relies on three keys to success: anticipation, preparation, and practice (Covello & Milligan, 2010).

Risk communication often involves multiple messages between multiple groups concerning the nature of risk. The perception of the risk depends on the circumstances. For example, although a voluntary evacuation may produce anxiety, it is more acceptable than one imposed on citizens. Earning trust and credibility is essential for effective risk communication. It is especially important when dealing with the fear factor associated with a deliberate attack. During this process, public health officials, nurses, and other representatives must provide clear, accurate information while minimizing the fear that may be associated with the event.

With heightened emotion, there is potential for an already bad situation to get worse. Rumors and unreliable information can create an unstable environment. Reassurance in times of crisis is essential. It is essential to listen and not interrupt. Simple statements such as "The risk is low" or "Nurses are available to answer your questions at this toll-free number…" are very effective. Depending on the situation, nurses can suggest actions to decrease risk of illness or suggest that people call their primary care provider if they become ill. Trust and credibility will be compromised if these emotions are not addressed effectively. It is important to remember that feelings of fear, frustration, and anger in a crisis are to be expected, and the resulting behavior should not be taken personally. To do so will make it difficult to work with the public and address their concerns. Covello (2010) points out that in emergency situations, people want to know that someone cares about them before they care about what you know. Public health nurses are well placed to reassure frightened citizens.

For example, in the initial phases of the immunization effort for H1N1 in 2009 and 2010, the demand for vaccine far outweighed the supply. Nurses often had the task of dealing with frustrated and angry people who were being told to obtain their immunizations yet could not succeed in finding available vaccine. There should be backup plans in this type of situation. In this case, the 1,100 people turned away were given appointments over the next 2 weeks as vaccine supplies increased.

Sometimes, important information is not available or cannot be verified. In that case, the information should not be communicated to the public. "I don't know" is acceptable and may even increase a nurse's credibility. Under no circumstances should a nonclinical person convey or interpret clinical data. A field nurse should be identified, who will receive client reports from another clinician in the receiving facility or surge site. Medical terminology can be badly misinterpreted by someone who is unaccustomed to working in the medical professions. Erroneous messages, even if innocently transmitted, derail efforts to keep the public well informed. During a crisis, messages should be reiterated frequently. When interacting with the media, a clinician should be present to answer any questions or clarify information. Fact sheets regarding the crisis should be prepared for informing the public and shared with public information officers. The biologic, chemical, and radiologic fact sheets from the CDC should be distributed if needed.

During the disaster preparedness drill in New Jersey, nurses conduct triage activities and communicate with receiving hospitals to facilitate swift transfer of victims. What underlying principles are practiced when communicating with the receiving hospitals?

It takes me two weeks to prepare an impromtu speech.

Mark Twain

Recovery and After-Action Evaluation

The recovery phase begins as the disaster ends. Although normal operations may return, critical incident stress debriefing for staff members is important. Responders may have been exposed to traumatic situations or worked for lengths of time that left them exhausted. An after-action evaluation is conducted following the event that includes the responders and agencies involved. Each step of the disaster event is reviewed, and a report is compiled that describes the scenario, response activities, participants, what went well, and what problems occurred. The financial, manpower, and other resources are determined. A list of detailed recommendations is made for revisions to the emergency response plan. Arrangements are then made to follow the progress of making the recommended changes. The final report assists with closure of the event and demonstrates that emergency preparedness is valued (Veenema, 2013).

Geoff creates an evaluation tool to use following the disaster management exercise. What topics did Geoff include in the after-action analysis?

Results of Geoff's evaluation indicate that the use of agent-specific simulation training in the classroom enabled the nurses to increase their competency skills while raising their confidence in a nonthreatening setting. These practice sessions enable them to perform effectively in the field.

key concepts

- Nurses play an important role in all phases of disaster response.
- All practicing nurses should become familiar with disaster phases and their role during an event.
- Public health nurses practice principles of disaster response on a daily basis.
- Although disasters do not occur with frequency, planning with vulnerability assessment can reduce their impact on the community.
- Properly implemented triage models minimize the morbidity and mortality of people affected by the event.
- Disaster phases and the nursing process are closely aligned.
- Biologic agents have an incubation period, which delays the investigation of the use of such agents as weapons.
- Chemical agents cause illness and/or death shortly after release. Decontamination is required for most chemical exposures.
- Fear and intimidation are a terrorist's strongest tools in orchestrating an attack.
- During a biologic, chemical, or radiologic event, the "worried well," in addition to the injured, can overwhelm and immobilize the healthcare system.
- Policies and procedures for mass immunization clinics should be in place to adapt to an emergency POD operation.
- Unless wounded by the explosive force of a "dirty" bomb, radiologic exposure alone is not treatable in an emergency department immediately after the event.
- Public health nurses' clinical skills in agent identification, triage, and field activities may be greatly enhanced through the use of simulation technology in repeated training experiences.

critical thinking questions

1. Identify a disaster scenario, outline the disaster preparedness steps that should be used, and relate them to the nursing process.
2. Both your local and state health departments have confirmed reports of 16 cases of pneumonic plague among students at a large suburban college campus.
   a. Develop a just-in-time training (JITT) program on standard and droplet infection control practices for health department staff members and college residents and staff. Use the boxes, tables, and figures found in this chapter, and if necessary, consult other resources.
   b. Prepare a postexposure antibiotic prophylaxis distribution plan for your community.
3. Identify several roles that a public health nurse can function in, within the framework of a multidisciplinary planning committee. Consider how his or her assessment, implementation, and evaluation skills can be utilized in a nonclinical role.
4. Conduct a vulnerability assessment using a community of choice, or review a disaster event taken from recent history, and identify weaknesses that contributed to the emergency. Could the event have been minimized or even prevented with accurate assessment?
5. List the emergency plans that must be in place before, during, and after a hazardous chemical release to provide essential care for clients and the community at large following the disaster.

community resources

- Local, county, and state public health departments
- Local Visiting Nurse Associations
- Local town hall
- Local fire department
- Local police department
- Regional Red Cross
- Regional Medical Reserve Corps (Homeland Security)
- U.S. Homeland Security regional offices

references

Alexander, G. C., & Wynia, M. K. (2003). Ready and willing? Physicians' sense of preparedness for bioterrorism. *Health Affairs, 22*(5), 189–197.

Andrulis, D. P., Siddiqui, N. J., & Purtie, J. (2011). Integrating language, culture and community into planning for and providing effective emergency healthcare during disasters: Challenges and opportunities from the California experience. *Prehospital and Disaster Medicine, 24*(2), s133–s134.

Archer, D., & Cameron, A. (2013). *Collaborative leadership: Building relationships, handling conflict and sharing control.* Burlington, MA: Elsevier.

Balicer, R. D., Catlette, C. L., Barnett, D. J., Thompson, C., Hsu, E. B., Morton, M. J., . . . Links, J. M. (2011). Characterizing hospital workers willingness to respond to a radiologic event. *PLOS One, 6*(10), e25327.

Barnett, A. S., Wang, N. E., Sahni, R., Hsia, R. Y., Haukoos, J. S., Barton, E. D., . . . Newgard, C. D.;WESTRN Investigators. (2013). Variations in prehospital use and uptake on the national field triage decision making scheme. *Prehospital Emergency Care, 17*(2), 135–148.

Berkshire Publishing Group. (2011). *Patterns of global terrorism 2011–2012. US Department of State Report with supplementary documents and statistics.* Retrieved from www.state.gov/j/ct/ris/crt/2011

Carrier, E., Yee, T., Cross, D., & Samuel, D. (2012). Emergency preparedness and community coalitions: Opportunities and challenges. *Research Brief,* (24), 1–9.

Centers for Disease Control and Prevention. (2002/ 2012). *Bioterrorism.* Retrieved April 26, 2013, from www.emergency.cdc.gov/bioterrorism

Centers for Disease Control and Prevention. (2002/2013). *Chemical emergencies.* Retrieved April 26, 2013, from www.emergency.cdc.gov/chemical

Centers for Disease Control and Prevention. (2002b/2011). *Revised recommendations on radiation control.* Retrieved April 26, 2013, from www.emergency.cdc.gov/radiation

Centers for Disease Control and Prevention. (2006a/2013). *Biological agents of concern.* Retrieved April 26, 2013, from http://www.bt.cdc.gov/Agent/AgentlistBio.asp

Centers for Disease Control and Prevention. (2006c/2011). *Hospital-based infection control for viral hemorrhagic fevers in the African healthcare setting.* Retrieved April 27, 2013, from http://www.who.int/csr/resources/publications/ebola/WHO_EMC_ESR_98_2_EN/en/

Centers for Disease Control and Prevention. (2011a). Biological and chemical terrorism: A national strategic plan for public health preparedness and response. Recommendations of the CDC Strategic Planning Workgroup. *Morbidity and Mortality Weekly Report, 49,* No. RR-4. Retrieved from www.cdc.gov/phpr/publications

Centers for Disease Control and Prevention. (2011b). *Blast injuries.* Retrieved May 1, 2013, from www.emergency.cdc.gov/blastinjury

Centers for Disease Control and Prevention. (2012). *National Center for Injury Prevention and Control: Division of unintentional injury report, 2012,* 1–9.

Chaffee, M. (2009). Willingness of health care personnel to work in a disaster: An integrative review of the literature. *Disaster Medicine and Public Health Preparedness, 3*(1), 42–56.

Covello, V., & Milligan, P. (2010). *Protecting People and the Environment.* Presentation to the Unites States Nuclear Regulatory Commission.

Crane, J. S., McCluskey, J. D., Johnson, G. T., & Harbison, R. D. (2010). Assessment of community healthcare providers ability and willingness to respond to emergencies resulting from bioterrorist attacks. *Journal of Emergencies, Trauma and Shock, 3*(1), 13–20.

Douglas, M., Uhl Pierce, J., Rosenkoetter, M., Callister, L., Hattar-Pollara, M., Lauderdale, J., . . . Pacquiao, D. (2009). Standards of practice for culturally competent nursing care: A request for comments. *Journal of Transcultural Nursing, 20*(3), 257–269.

Foley, J. A. (2012). Biblical locust plagues threatens Madagascar. *Nature World News.* Retrieved May 1, 2013, from www.natureworldnews.com

Glarum, J., Birow, D., & Cetauk, E. (2010) . *Hospital emergency response teams: Triage for optimal disaster response.* Burlington, MA: Elsevier.

Halff, K. (2011). *Increased number of people displaced by disasters* (Press release). Retrieved May 1, 2013, from http://www.internaldisplacement.org

Handysides, S. (2009). The history of bioterrorism: Old ideas, new word, continuing tabool. In L. I. Lutwick, & S. M. Lutwick (Eds.). *Beyond Anthrax.* Clifton, NJ: Humana Press.

Healthy People 2020, Framework: the vision, mission and goals of Healthy people 2020. United States Department of Health and Human Services, Office of Disease Prevention and Health Promotion. Retrieved March 22, 2013, from http:// www.healthypeople.gov/2020/consortium/HP2020Framework

Horton, R. (2012). Global burden of disease 2010: Understanding disease, infection and risk. *The Lancet, 380*(9859), 2053–2054.

Iserson, K.V. (2012). *Providing care in extreme environments.* New York, NY: Mc Graw Hill.

Jacobs, J. A., Jones, E., Gabella, B. A., Spring, B., & Brownson, R. C. (2012). Tools for implementing an evidence based approach to public health practice. *Preventing Chronic Disease, 9,* 110324.

Kaydos-Daniels, S. C., Rojas, S. L., & Farris, T. R. (2013). Biosurveillance in outbreak investigations: Biosecurity and bioterrorism. *Biodefense Strategic Practice and Science, 2,* 20–28.

Kitamaya, C. (2011). Exploratory study on the preparation required for public health nurses responding to a radiation accident. *Radiation Emergency Medicine, 1*(1–2), 84–85.

Koenig, K. I., & Shulz, C. H. (2010). *Disaster medicine: Comprehensive principles and practice.* New York, NY: Cambridge University Press.

McDonald, L. (2001). Florence Nightingale and the early origins of evidence-based nursing. *Evidence-Based Nursing, 4,* 68–69.

Medalia, J. (2011). Dirty bombs: Technical background, attack prevention and response. *Issues for Congress, the Congressional Research Service.* Retrieved April 14, 2013, from www.crs.gov

Noto, Y., Kitamiya, C., Itaki, C., Urushizaka, M., Kidachi, R., & Yamabe, H. (2013). Role of nurses in a nuclear disaster: Experience in the Fukushima dar-ici nuclear power plant accident. *International Nursing Review, 60*(2), 196–200.

Nuclear Threat Initiative. (2012). *Organization for prohibition of chemical weapons*. Retrieved November 10, 2014, from http://www.nti.org/treaties-and-regimes/organization-for-the-prohibition-of-chemical-weapons/on

Patient Protection and Affordable Care Act (2010). 124, Statute 119, 111–148.

Preston, R. J., Marcozzi, D., Lima, R., Pietrobon, R., Braga, L., & Jacobs, D. (2008). Effect of evacuation on the number of victims in a hazardous chemical release. *Pre-Hospital Emergency Care, 12*(1), 18–23.

Rutgers University. (2012). *The cultural impact on disaster relief.* School of Social Work. Retrieved December 11, 2012, from www.nj.ptc.org

Sengul, H., Santella, N., & Steinberg, L. G. (2010). Accidental hazardous materials release with human impact in the United States. *Journal of occupational and Environmental Medicine, 52*(9), 920–925.

Spellman, J. (2013). The role and preparation of the public health nurse for disaster response. In T. Veenema (Ed.), *Disaster nursing and emergency preparedness for chemical, biological, and radiological terrorism and other hazards* (pp. 588–599). New York, NY: Springer.

United Nations. (2013). *Report of the ad hoc committee on internationally agreed upon definition of terrorism* (A/66/37), April 12, 2013.

United States Department of Defense. (2010). *Multi-service tactics, techniques and procedures for nuclear, biological, chemical (NBC) protection.* (ATTP3-11.361MCRP3-37B1NTTP3–11.34/AFTTP(1) 3–20.70. Retrieved April 15, 2013, from www.us.army.mil.

United States Department of Health and Human Services, Centers for Disease Control and Prevention. (2001). *The public health response to biological and chemical terrorism: Interim planning guidance for state public health officials*. Retrieved July 7, 2014, from http://www.bt.cdc.gov/Documents/Planning/PlanningGuidance.pdf

United States Department of Health and Human Services, Office of Minority Health. (2009). *Culturally competent curriculum for disaster response.* Retrieved December 26, 2012, from https://cccdpcr.thinkculturalhealth.org

Veenema, T. G. (2012). *Disaster nursing and emergency preparedness for chemical, biological, and radiological terrorism and other hazards*. New York, NY: Springer.

web resources

Please visit thePoint® for up-to-date Web resources on this topic.

Specialty Practice

PART

five

CHAPTER 21

Community Mental Health

Judith Shindul-Rothschild

ALONE

From childhood's hour I have not been
As others were; I have not seen
As others saw; I could not bring
My passions from a common spring.
From the same source I have not taken
My sorrow; I could not awaken
My heart to joy at the same tone;
And all I loved, I loved alone.
Then—in my childhood, in the dawn
Of a most stormy life—was drawn
From every depth of good and ill
The mystery which binds me still:
From the torrent, or the fountain,
From the red cliff of the mountain,
From the sun that round me rolled
In its autumn tint of gold,
From the lightning in the sky
As it passed me flying by,
From the thunder and the storm,
And the cloud that took the form
(When the rest of Heaven was blue)
Of a demon in my view.

Edgar Allan Poe

chapter highlights

- Epidemiology of mental illness from a public health perspective
- Early intervention in the treatment of schizophrenia
- Strategies to enhance treatment adherence
- Public health implications for children with behavioral disorders
- Evolution of community mental health
- Policy development and legislation for mental health services
- Role and responsibilities of the community mental health practitioner

objectives

- Interpret the meaning of mental illness in the context of societal and cultural norms about behavior.
- Describe the scope of mental illness and the effects on morbidity and mortality worldwide.
- Describe the side effects of antipsychotic medication and its implications for nursing assessment and long-term treatment.
- Analyze emerging models of treatment that offer promise in improving the quality of life for the chronic mentally ill in communities.
- Identify the social and biologic factors associated with the incidence of mood and anxiety disorders.
- Describe public health programs to decrease the incidence of suicide, especially among youth.
- Differentiate the key signs and symptoms of attention-deficit/hyperactivity disorder and bipolar disorder in children as members of families in communities.
- Identify the motor, language, and social characteristics of infants and toddlers that are early signs of autism spectrum disorders as members of families in communities.
- Describe the policy implications in the shift in locus of care to community mental health centers for the chronic mentally ill.
- Identify the key components of psychological first aid.

key terms

Autism spectrum disorders: Also known as pervasive developmental disorders; cause severe and pervasive impairment in thinking, feeling, language, and the ability to relate to others.

"Black box" warning: Warning by the Food and Drug Administration (FDA) to advise clients and caregivers of dangers related to the use of a drug or treatment alone or in combination.

Community mental health centers: Primary care centers and neighborhood-based centers in communities with the goal of serving populations and aggregates in need of follow-up care and counseling.

Culturally competent mental health services: Mental health services by professionals who demonstrate knowledge in group values, traditions, and the cultural expression of mental illness.

Deinstitutionalization: The phenomenon of allowing patients who leave care in large, complex healthcare systems to receive care in neighborhoods and communities on an outpatient basis.

***Diagnostic and Statistical Manual*, 5th edition (*DSM-5*):** The standard classification of mental disorders, published by the American Psychiatric Association and used by mental health professionals in the United States, it is intended to be applicable in a wide array of contexts and used by clinicians and researchers of many different orientations.

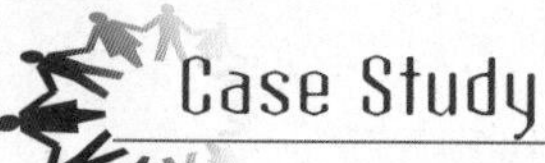

Case Study

References to the case study are found throughout this chapter (look for the case study icon). Readers should keep the case study in mind as they read the chapter.

Carmen, a 48-year-old immigrant from Peru, is brought to the emergency department by her daughter after taking 10 mg of lorazepam (Ativan) in less than 4 hours. Her daughter describes her mother as acting "crazy" and not making any sense. Carmen lives with her mother, her husband, her two sons, her daughter, and her daughter's child. Until 2 years ago, Carmen worked cleaning houses when she sustained a back injury. She has been taking 5 mg of hydrocodone/acetaminophen (Vicodin) prn every 6 hours, but her supply ran out, and she claims that her nurse practitioner would not send in another prescription to the pharmacy. Carmen speaks some English and explains to the psychiatric nurse that she was in such pain from her back that she just wanted the pain to end. The psychiatric clinical nurse specialist contacted a primary care provider in the community, who expressed concern that Carmen was suicidal and needed additional medical evaluation for her back injury. After consulting with the primary care providers, her family, and Carmen herself, the psychiatric mental health clinical specialist admitted Carmen to a locked psychiatric unit for evaluation.

In the psychiatric unit, Carmen begins to wail loudly, slap her head with her hands, and throw her head in a backward motion against a wall. She stands rigidly against a wall and appears unresponsive to a nurse's inquiries in English about what she is experiencing. Given her daughter's concern about her mother's mental status on admission, and her current behavior and unresponsiveness to the nurses' inquiries, an order is requested for an as-needed dose of olanzapine (Zyprexa) 5 mg. When a student nurse asks Carmen in Spanish what is wrong, she replies that her pain is unbearable and she needs Vicodin; otherwise, she just wants to be dead.

key terms (continued)

Early intervention programs: Specialized teams of professionals whose primary goal is to maintain the individual's current level of educational and vocational functioning through early treatment.

First-generation antipsychotics: Medications developed and used early in the science of psychiatric therapeutics.

Nonadherence: The choice to not follow directions for care; can include medications, follow-up healthcare appointments, or wellness checkups.

President's New Freedom Commission on Mental Health: Expert panel created to advise Congress and the President on how policy-makers could improve mental health services for both the chronic mentally ill and children with serious mental illnesses.

Prodromal stage: Earliest stage of beginning pathology.

Psychological first aid: An evidence-informed intervention in the immediate aftermath of a disaster.

Second-generation antipsychotics: Medications developed more recently in the science of psychiatric therapeutics.

Tardive dyskinesia: Twisting movements of tongue, limbs, and torso; irreversible; often a side effect of psychotropic medication.

CULTURAL CONTEXT OF MENTAL ILLNESS

Mental health and, conversely, mental illness are concepts bound by culture. Understanding of what connotes mental health is shaped by social norms that evolve from generation to generation. In Western cultures, medical science interprets any deviation from normative function of the five senses as indicative of a psychotic disorder. Hearing a voice, claiming to see an object, or having certain tactile sensations are viewed as pathologic states to be treated by psychiatric professionals. In some parts of the world, spiritual possession or healers with special powers and beliefs are culture-bound syndromes (Hwang et al., 2008). Whenever health professionals are tempted to label behavior as "abnormal," it is important to always be cognizant of the values of the health professional and how these values may be in conflict with community norms. Differences in incidence by race, gender, and ethnicity are evident in many mental illnesses. It is important to determine whether these differences are a product of better surveillance and access to treatment or whether psychiatric professionals are more apt to label a behavior deviant in a certain population. Because of the stigma associated with mental disorders, many people and their families are reticent to speak publicly of their experiences and need for services. It is crucial that advocates are cognizant of the epidemiologic findings that describe the needs, trends, risk factors, and effectiveness of community mental health services. Sound epidemiologic research, both nationally and internationally, is the foundation policy-makers need to formulate, plan, and implement effective community-based programs that address the needs of the mentally ill.

In Western cultures, emotional distress is most often expressed verbally, whereas in Asian or Latino cultures, somatization, specifically, physical complaints of pain, headache, or stomach aches can be a prominent symptom of depression and anxiety

(Hwang et al., 2008). For Carmen, both her emotional and physical pain warrants nursing intervention and careful assessment. By alleviating her physical pain, nurses can more comprehensively assess her mental status and what, if any, symptoms of mood or psychosis would benefit from psychotropic medication.

DEFINITIONS OF MENTAL ILLNESS

Although there is no universally accepted definition of mental health, for practical purposes, widely accepted parameters of the types of behaviors that connote psychopathology must be used to measure the incidence, morbidity, and mortality of mental illness in a population. The first challenge for epidemiologists who study the prevalence of mental illness is to develop valid operational definitions and standardized measurement instruments. Since 1952, the American Psychiatric Association (APA) has been refining the diagnostic criteria that describe mental illness. This nomenclature is compiled in a text titled the *Diagnostic and Statistical Manual of Mental Disorders* (*DSM-5*) (APA, 2013). The National Comorbidity Survey (NCS) is a nationally representative survey that assesses the prevalence of major mental illnesses according to the criteria in the *DSM-5* (Kessler & Wang, 2008). Internationally, the World Mental Health initiative replicated the NCS; this allowed researchers to examine cross-cultural prevalence of major mental illnesses (Kessler & Wang, 2008).

"Normal" is just a setting on the dryer.

Barbara Johnson, author

PRACTICE POINT

Epidemiologic studies describe the social costs of mental illness and are essential to target programs to populations in greatest need. *Healthy People 2010* identified the following key objectives in measuring progress toward improving mental health: suicide, adolescent suicide attempts, serious mental illness in homeless adults, employment of homeless adults, and the employment of people with serious mental illness and eating disorder relapses. The Centers for Disease Control and Prevention (CDC) tracks epidemiologic data to determine the extent to which target objectives for mental health and mental disorders have been reached (Fig. 21.1).

SCOPE OF MENTAL ILLNESS

There is no difference in lifetime prevalence rates of major mental illness between developed and developing countries. However, the projected lifetime risk of developing a major mental illness is highest in countries where the population is subject to sustained violence (Kessler et al., 2007). A disturbing trend is that the prevalence rate of major mental illness is increasing in younger populations (Kessler et al., 2007).

Psychiatric disorders are the leading cause of disability worldwide. Every year, approximately one-third of the world's population suffers from a major mental illness, yet almost two-thirds does not receive any mental health treatment (Thornicroft, 2007). Countries that spend a larger portion of their gross domestic product on healthcare are also those countries where individuals are most likely to receive treatment for mental illness (Wang et al., 2007). Despite the prevalence of disability associated with major mental illness, these disorders are much more likely to be untreated than physical illness at every income level (Ormel et al., 2008). Those suffering from alcoholism and addictive disorders are most likely to go untreated (78%), followed by anxiety disorders (57%), depression (56%), and bipolar disorder (50%) (Thornicroft, 2007). Young African-Americans and the elderly have the highest rates of unmet psychiatric care (Neighbors et al., 2007).

The mind is like an iceberg, it floats with one-seventh of its bulk above water.

Sigmund Freud

Stigma, inequities in mental health benefits, and fragmentation in the delivery system have prevented many people, especially the elderly, those in rural areas, and ethnic minorities, from receiving appropriate mental health treatment. The failure to identify and treat young people for mental illness can have profound social consequences, including truancy, incarceration, addiction, unplanned pregnancy, poverty, and suicide.

EVIDENCE FOR PRACTICE

Access to mental health services for children and adolescents is problematic even in developed countries. Studies have demonstrated that protective factors in the community can mitigate the risk factors that contribute to maladaptive behaviors by adolescents, such as truancy and substance abuse. Protective factors in the community include healthy role models, involvement with community groups and rewards for involvement, and connection with school and affirmation of achievements (Patel et al., 2007). Population-based programs targeting adolescents and children in school- or community-based settings are under way in several countries to educate youth about health risk behaviors and help them develop more adaptive ways of coping with stress. Examples include *HealthWise* in the Republic of South Africa, which engages community resources, especially schools, to teach youth strategies for productively using their free time and decrease high-risk behavior, and *The Federal National Youth Mental Health Initiative* in Australia, which partners with youth organizations in the community, such as sports teams, to provide for youth with access to drug and alcohol programs.

LEGEND — Moved away from target | Moved toward target | Met or exceeded target

Objective	Percent of target change achieved (%)	2010 Target (%)	Baseline (Year) (%)	Final (Year) (%)	Baseline vs. Final: Difference (%)	Baseline vs. Final: Statistically significant	Baseline vs. Final: Percent change (%)
18-1. Suicide, age-adjusted, per 100,000 population)	(moved away)	4.8	10.5 (1999)	11.3 (2007)	0.8	Yes	7.6
18-2. Suicide attempts by students who required medical attention (grades 9–12)	43.8	1.0	2.6 (1999)	1.9 (2009)	−0.7	Yes	−26.9
18-3. Homeless adults with mental health problems who receive mental health services (18+ years)	766.7	30	27 (2000)	50 (2009)	23	Not tested	85.2
18-5. Students engaging in disordered eating (grades 9–12)	166.7	16	19 (2001)	14 (2009)	−5	Yes	−26.3
18-6. Primary care facilities that provide mental health treatment	133.3	68	62 (2000)	70 (2009)	8	Not tested	12.9
18-7. Treatment for children with mental health problems (4–17 years)	128.6	67	60 (2001)	69 (2008)	9	Yes	15.0
18-8. Juvenile residential facilities that screen admissions for mental health problems	160.0	55	50 (2000)	58 (2006)	8	Not tested	16.0
18-11. Community-based jail diversion programs for adults with serious mental illness (SMI)	1028.6	7.6	6.9 (2004)	14.1 (2010)	7.2	Not tested	104.3
18-12. State tracking of consumer satisfaction with mental health services (no. states and DC)	94.1	51	34 (2002)	50 (2009)	16	Not tested	47.1
18-13. State mental health plans addressing cultural competence (no. states and DC)	33.3	32	29 (2004)	30 (2009)	1	Not tested	3.4
18-14. State mental health plans addressing care of elderly persons (no. states and DC)	12.1	51	18 (2001)	22 (2009)	4	Not tested	22.2

NOTE: See the Reader's Guide for more information on how to read this figure. See DATA2010 at http://wonder.cdc.gov/data2010 for all *Healthy People 2010* tracking data. Tracking data are not available for objectives 18-4, 18-9a through d, and 18-10.

figure 21.1 Final review *Health People 2010* mental health and mental disorders.

Source: National Center for Health Statistics [2012]. *Final Report Healthy People 2010* [DHHS publication No. (PHS)2012–1038. 0276–4733]. Hyattsville, MD: U.S Government Printing Office. Retrieved May 28, 2013, from http://www.cdc.gov/nchs/data/hpdata2010/hp2010_final_review.pdf

SOME MAJOR MENTAL ILLNESSES

Worldwide there has been a global shift in disease burden from communicable diseases to noncommunicable diseases, including mental and behavioral disorders (Murray et al., 2012). Data from the NCS and the Epidemiologic Catchment Area studies suggest that approximately 50% of all Americans will suffer from a mental disorder during their lifetime (Kessler & Wang, 2008) (Table 21.1). Major mental illness may be broadly grouped into three categories: thought disorders, mood disorders, and anxiety disorders. Often, the dysfunction that a person is experiencing in his or her thinking or mood is further complicated by substance abuse, dementia, or a medical condition. One of the top 10 causes of disability worldwide is schizophrenia, a thought disorder characterized by psychotic thinking and profound social apathy or withdrawal.

EVIDENCE FOR PRACTICE

In 2008, the Mental Health Gap Action Programme (mhGAP) in the World Health Organization (WHO) conducted a systematic review of evidence on the treatment of major mental illness in resource-poor countries. On the basis of this scientific review, the WHO released the "*mhGAP Intervention Guide for mental, neurological and substance use disorders in non-specialized health settings*" (WHO, 2010). The intent of the intervention guide is to provide nonspecialist healthcare providers evidence-based protocols to expand mental healthcare in resource-poor settings (WHO, 2010).

table 21.1 **Prevalence of Mental Disorders in the United States, 2011**

Mental Disorders	12-Month Prevalence Rates in the United States (%)
Anxiety disorders[a]	**22.2**
Specific phobia	12.1
Social phobia	7.4
Post-traumatic stress disorder (PTSD)	3.7
Generalized anxiety disorder (GAD)	2.0
Panic disorder	2.4
Agoraphobia	1.7
Obsessive–compulsive disorder (OCD)	1.2
Mood disorders[a]	**9.4**
Major depressive disorder	7.1
Bipolar I–II	1.8
Impulse control disorders[b]	**8.9**
Attention-deficit/hyperactivity disorder (ADHD)	4.1
Psychotic disorders[c]	**1.5**
Schizophrenia	1.3
Nonaffective psychosis	0.2
Other[c]	
Antisocial personality disorder	2.1
Anorexia nervosa	0.1
Severe cognitive impairment	1.2

[a] Kessler, R. C., Petukhova, M., Sampson, N. A., Zaslavsky, A. M., & Wittchen, H. U. (2012). Twelve-month and lifetime prevalence and lifetime morbid risk of anxiety and mood disorders in the United States. *International Journal of Methods in Psychiatric Research, 21*(3), 169–184.
[b] Kessler, R. C., & Wang, P. S. (2008). The descriptive epidemiology of commonly occurring mental disorders in the United States. *Annual Review of Public Health, 29,* 115–129.
[c] U. S. Department of Health and Human Services. (1999). *Mental health: A Report of the Surgeon General.* Rockville, MD: US Department of Health and Human Services, Substance Abuse and Mental Health Services Administration, Center for Mental Health Services, National Institutes of Health, National Institute of Mental Health. Retrieved June 3, 2013, from http://www.surgeongeneral.gov/library/mentalhealth/home.html

Schizophrenia

Epidemiology

About 1% of the world's population suffers from schizophrenia. Symptoms of schizophrenia typically first appear in late adolescence or young adulthood and persist throughout a person's life, causing significant impairment in all aspects of a person's psychosocial functioning. The exact etiology is unknown; however, genetic studies have found a high concordance of schizophrenia (40% to 50%) among monozygotic twins (Clarke, Kelleher, Clancy, & Cannon, 2012). Complications in pregnancy, delivery, viral infections, early childhood stress, head injuries, and cannabis abuse have all been implicated in increasing the risk of developing schizophrenia. Although the onset of symptoms of the disease is similar across a range of countries and cultures, there is debate among epidemiologists about cross-cultural comparisons, suggesting that the functional status of people with schizophrenia is higher in developing rather than developed countries.

It might be presumed that greater access to pharmacologic treatments and a range of mental health services in developed countries would result in a higher quality of life and better outcomes for people who have schizophrenia. However, three multinational WHO studies have reported that the outcomes for people with schizophrenia are better in developing rather than in developed countries (Craig et al., 1997). Specifically, the International Pilot Study of Schizophrenia found that over 5 years, only 6% of the patients with schizophrenia in the United States and England had no residual symptoms, compared with 42% of the patients in India and 34% in Nigeria (Messias, Chen, & Eaton, 2007). Although the WHO studies suggest that outcomes for schizophrenics are more favorable in developing countries, other epidemiologists in cross-cultural psychiatry have criticized these conclusions, noting that evidence of improved outcomes and quality of life between developed and developing countries is complicated by differences in social norms (Cohen, Patel, Thara, & Gureje, 2008).

EVIDENCE FOR PRACTICE

In the WHO studies, researchers found that employment, marital status, and residing with one's family were associated with improved social outcomes. However, Cohen et al. (2008) noted that evidence from research other than the WHO suggests that the data collected by the WHO may not be reliable indexes of occupational or social function. Specifically, these investigators reported that unemployment may be higher in developed countries because of the availability of unemployment and disability benefits, which do not exist in developing countries. Cohen et al. (2008) also argued that there is little empirical evidence to support the assumption that living with one's family is predictive of better outcomes when conflict within the family can exacerbate psychotic symptoms and have the opposite effect.

PRACTICE POINT

Cohen et al. (2008) appropriately critiqued the conclusions of the WHO outcomes studies on schizophrenia, by questioning how employment and marital status can be valid measures of prognosis for countries with vastly different expectations for work and the family. Nurses in Western cultures need to be mindful of the fact that there are societies and cultures whose beliefs about what connotes abnormal behavior are very different from those in the United States. All social indicators are culture-bound, so when epidemiologists conduct cross-cultural comparisons of mental illness and disability, they need to take these cultural differences into account.

Carmen receives a prn dose of hydrocodone/acetaminophen (Vicodin) for pain and olanzapine (Zyprexa) for agitation. Mary, a student nurse, stays with Carmen as she rested in her room, and within an hour, her restlessness, agitation, and emotional distress markedly diminished. Mary converses with Carmen in Spanish and asks her about how she manages her pain at home. Carmen explains that she believes her son, who lives with her and recently became unemployed, has been taking her Vicodin and selling it. She tearfully shares with Mary that she has been running out of Vicodin before she can refill the prescription, and her nurse practitioner has refused to prescribe additional pills. Carmen says that she has repeatedly pleaded with her son to stop, to look and see what he was doing to his mother, but he continues to take her pain medication. In desperation, Carmen admits to Mary that she took an overdose of lorazepam because she could no longer stand the pain and could see no other way out of the situation.

PRACTICE POINT

All states have laws mandating that licensed healthcare professionals report elder abuse and neglect. In Carmen's case, the treatment team reported Carmen's claims of drug diversion by her son to the Department of Elder Protection. Prior to Carmen's discharge, the Department of Elder Protection conducted an investigation and prohibited Carmen's son from living in the home with his mother.

Early Intervention Programs for First-Episode Psychosis

One of the most promising advances in the treatment of schizophrenia has been the use of **early intervention programs** for people at risk for psychosis. Developed countries, such as the United States, Australia, and the United Kingdom, have established early intervention teams (Tyrer et al., 2005). Detailed descriptions of the mission, goals, and services of the early intervention programs of Canada and Norway, in addition to Australia, are available on the Internet (Table 21.2). Developing countries, such as Cyprus and India, also have early intervention treatment (Tyrer et al., 2005). All these programs typically consist of specialized teams of nurses, occupational and rehabilitative therapists, and physicians, whose primary goal is to maintain the person's current level of educational and vocational functioning.

The early intervention programs are based on the theory that repeated episodes of psychosis are toxic to the brain, producing debilitating cognitive effects that may be minimized with early treatment. The hope is that if the initial treatment occurs during the first episode of psychosis, the less likely the person will be incapacitated by the disease during his or her life. Researchers are also examining whether intervening even prior to the onset of psychotic behavior will improve treatment responsiveness to antipsychotic medication. The first goal of early intervention programs is to identify at-risk people prior to the onset of hallucinations, delusions, and other symptoms of disordered thinking. Early identification is complicated by the fact that, on average, adolescents and their families delay seeking psychiatric treatment until 1 to 5 years after the onset of frank psychotic symptoms.

Ideally, early intervention programs identify young adolescents at risk during the **prodromal stage** and immediately begin treatment with a low dose of a second-generation antipsychotic. Psychotropic medication treatment is also supplemented by psychoeducation, cognitive-behavioral therapy, and family therapy. Studies suggest that both psychopharmacologic and psychotherapy interventions are essential to minimize the social disruptions that characterize schizophrenia, such as dropping out of school, withdrawal from friends and family, and loss of employment.

The specialized teams of mental health practitioners intervene across the entire spectrum of the illness, including outreach, early identification, treatment, and long-term follow-up. Occupational and rehabilitation counselors work with clients to maintain role functioning at work or school during the treatment phase. Psychotherapists provide family therapy, family self-help groups, and peer support to help

table 21.2 **Early Intervention Programs for First Psychotic Episode**

Country	Program	Internet Link
Australia	Australian Early Intervention Network for Mental Health in Young People (AusEinet)	http://auseinet.flinders.edu.au
	Melbourne—Early Psychosis Prevention and Intervention Centre (EPPIC)	www.eppic.org.au
Canada	British Columbia—Early Psychosis Initiative (EPI)	www.mheccu.ubc.ca/projects/EPI
	Calgary—Early Psychosis Program (EPP)	www.ucalgary.ca/cdss/epp
	Vancouver—Helping Overcome Psychosis Early (HOPE)	www.hope.vancouver.bc.ca
Finland	Detection of Early Psychosis (DEEP Project)	http://www.med.utu.fi/tutkimus/tutkimusprojektit/psykiatria3.html
France	Paris—PREPSY	http://prepsy.free.fr/
Germany	Cologne—Early Recognition and Intervention Center	http://www.kompetenznetz-schizophrenie.de/rdkns/index.htm
Ireland	Dublin—Detection, Education and Local Team Assessment (DELTA)	http://www.deltaproject.ie/
Netherlands	Amsterdam—People with Increased Vulnerability to Psychosis (PSILON)	http://www.ypsilon.org/hulp/advies/preventi/index.htm
New Zealand	Takapuna—Early Intervention National Training Program	http://www.werrycentre.org.nz/
Norway	Program to Reduce the Duration of Untreated Psychosis (TIPPS)	www.tips-info.com
Singapore	Early Psychosis Intervention Program (EPIP)	http://www.epip.org.sg/
Switzerland	Basil—FEPSY Project	http://www.fepsy.ch/
United Kingdom	NHS—Early Intervention in Psychosis	http://www.iris-initiative.org.uk/
United States	Albuquerque—Early Assessment and Resource Linkage for Youth (EARLY)	http://www.earlyprogram.org/
	Boston—First Episode and Early Psychosis Program (FEPP)	www.massgeneral.org/allpsych/Schizophrenia/
	Chicago—First Episode Psychosis Program	http://uillinoismedcenter.org/content.cfm/psychosis
	Los Angeles—Center for the Assessment and Prevention of Prodromal States (CAPPS)	http://www.capps.ucla.edu/
	Manhattan—Center of Prevention and Evaluation (COPE)	http://cumc.columbia.edu/dept/pi/research/clinics/pc.html
	New Haven—Prevention Through Risk Identification and Prevention (PRIME)	www.ynhh.org/ynhph/ynhph.html
	Pittsburgh—Services for the Treatment of Early Psychosis (STEP)	http://www.upmc.com/services/behavioral-health/pages/early-psychoses.aspx
	Portland, Maine—Prevent Mental Illness with Early Detection	http://www.preventmentalillness.org/pier_home.html
	Salem, Oregon—Prevent Mental Illness With Early Detection	http://www.preventmentalillness.org/pier_home.html

Source: Schizophrenia.com. Retrieved on June 3, 2013, from http://www.schizophrenia.com/earlypsychosis.htm#ill; National Alliance for the Mentally Ill. Retrieved on May 28, 2013, from http://www.nami.org/FirstEpisode/clinics_psychosis.jpg

manage the symptoms of the illness and enhance treatment adherence, especially with low-dose atypical antipsychotics. Community health nurses, too, have an integral role to play in each facet of the early intervention treatment model. In the predisease phase, primary care nurses who work in schools or pediatrician's offices are well positioned to identify youth who may be at risk. During the acute phase, nurses assess the therapeutic efficacy of antipsychotic treatment and educate clients and their families about how antipsychotic medication can help alleviate symptoms of the illness and the importance of treatment adherence. During the maintenance phase, nurses play a critical role in helping families and clients adhere to treatment recommendations and manage some of the residual symptoms of the disease.

The prodromal signs and symptoms suggesting that a young adolescent is at risk for developing psychosis are not unlike those behaviors exhibited during normal adolescent development. In light of these similarities, some practitioners have raised ethical questions about the appropriateness of medicating young people with low-dose atypical antipsychotics prior to the onset of overt psychotic symptoms. Although these reservations may have delayed the widespread adoption of early intervention programs, outcome studies suggest that the long-term disability associated with schizophrenia can be significantly lessened if people at risk are treated with medication and provided with services prior to the onset of delusions or hallucinations (Amminger et al., 2006).

Screening tools to identify adolescents at risk for developing schizophrenia have been developed by practitioners in Germany, Australia, the United Kingdom, and the United States. The Structured Interview for Prodromal Symptoms and the Scale of Prodromal Symptoms are two widely used scales in the United States developed by researchers at Yale University (Miller et al., 2002). Specific prodromal signs and symptoms manifested in adolescence include sleep disturbance, anxiety, irritability, deterioration in role function, depressed mood, social withdrawal, poor concentration, suspiciousness, loss of motivation, and perceptual disturbances (Yung et al., 2007). Early identification of psychosis and administration of low-dose antipsychotic medication may help mitigate the chronic, debilitating course of schizophrenia and significantly improve long-term outcomes.

EVIDENCE FOR PRACTICE

Outcome studies have uniformly concluded that assertive community treatment (ACT) teams are more effective than case management alone in reducing rehospitalizations, shortening the length of stay, improving social functioning, and increasing satisfaction for both patients and their families (Beebe, 2007). Nurses in "ACT teams" enhance adherence to the medication regime by providing around-the-clock support for families and clients in the community, which includes psychoeducation, transportation to appointments or pharmacies, cognitive-behavioral interventions (such as positive reinforcement) for achievement of treatment goals, referrals to self-help groups, respite for families, and opportunities for socialization for the client.

Primary Prevention Programs

One of the challenges for researchers is to better understand the relationship between substance abuse, the onset of psychotic symptoms, and relapse. Originally, it had been presumed that adolescents who are susceptible to mental illness abuse cannabis or other illicit substances as a means of self-medication. There is empirical evidence that cannabis use is a component cause of schizophrenia and increases the risk two- to fourfold (Clarke et al., 2012). The possibility that the amount, duration, and strength of cannabis may be a precursor to the development of schizophrenia has significant implications for both drug education programs and early intervention programs for the treatment of adolescents at risk for psychosis. Public health education campaigns should continue to educate adolescents about the potential adverse effects of cannabis use, especially on mental health.

Up until the legalization of marijuana for medical use, there had been a downward trend in the use of marijuana by youth that was attributed to the success of drug educational programs. Since the late 2000s, cannabis use precipitously increased by a significant 19% among high school students. The pronounced rise in cannabis use among youth coincided with states' legalization of medical marijuana and a perception among youth of diminished risk (National Institute on Drug Abuse, 2012). Cannabis remains the most widely used illicit substance with over one-third (36.4%) of high school seniors reporting using cannabis during the past year and 6.5% reporting daily use (National Institute on Drug Abuse, 2012). A future area for epidemiologic research will be to examine whether the rise in the use of cannabis and synthetic cannabinoid substances is correlated with an increase in the prevalence and morbidity of schizophrenia in the United States.

The lead investigator of the National Institute of Drug Abuse survey credits the media primary prevention campaign undertaken by the White House Office of Drug Control Policy as significantly influencing the perceptions of adolescents about the dangers of cannabis use (Johnston, Malley, Bachman, & Schulenberg, 2005). Research studies will need to examine whether a continued decline in the use of cannabis, combined with widespread adoption of early intervention programs, is correlated with a decrease in the prevalence and morbidity of schizophrenia in the United States.

Enhancing Treatment Adherence in Schizophrenia

Nonadherence with medication is the most common factor associated with relapse and recurrence of psychotic symptoms. One of the largest studies of treatment efficacy for patients diagnosed with schizophrenia, the Clinical Antipsychotic Trials of Intervention of Effectiveness (CATIE) study, found that 74% of the patients discontinued their medication before 18 months (Levine, Rabinowitz, Faries, Lawson, & Ascher-Svanum, 2012). The longer and more frequently patients diagnosed with schizophrenia experience psychotic symptoms, the greater the gray matter atrophy in the prefrontal cortex and the greater the impairment of executive cognitive function (Morton & Zubek, 2013). A common feature of all early intervention programs is to educate the client and the family about how nonadherence to the medication regime can lead to relapse. To be maximally effective, both the client and the family must be educated about the morbidity associated with untreated psychotic symptoms, especially in light of growing evidence that the more frequent the psychotic episodes, the greater and more lasting the negative effects on cognitive function (Pekkala & Merinder, 2005).

Nursing interventions to enhance medication adherence applicable to those with chronic mental illness may include oral and written reminders, self-monitoring tools, cues, and positive reinforcements by both the nurse and the family. Psychoeducation by community health nurses should teach clients and families about the signs of impending relapse, how medication can help remit the more debilitating negative symptoms of the disease, and the importance of lifestyle changes, especially avoiding use of illicit substances. Psychosocial interventions for clients with chronic mental illness also include employment or vocational training, social skills development, and coaching, with an emphasis on problem-solving and motivational interviewing. Family support groups, training in cognitive-behavioral approaches, and basic communication strategies are particularly helpful for families who are trying to manage medication administration in the home.

In addition to psychosocial interventions, which can be prohibitively expensive and difficult to implement in resource-poor countries, long-acting injectable antipsychotic (LAI) medications are another strategy to enhance treatment adherence. However, no long-acting injectable form of antipsychotic should be administered until it is clear how the client responds to oral forms of the medication. The first-generation antipsychotics haloperidol decanoate and fluphenazine decanoate, and the second-generation antipsychotic depot risperidone are presently the only antipsychotics available as long-acting preparations. They are given by injection every 2 to 4 weeks.

EVIDENCE FOR PRACTICE

Studies using electronic monitoring of oral medication adherence have found that approximately 78.2% of patients with schizophrenia do not take their antipsychotic medication as prescribed (Byerly, Nakonezny, & Lescouflair, 2007). There is sufficient empiric evidence supporting a correlation between LAIs and treatment adherence for first-episode psychosis or recent-onset schizophrenia (Kim, Lee, Yang, Park, & Chung, 2012). Registered nurses and prescribers can immediately follow up to reinforce the importance of adherence if the patient fails to appear for the injection. Yet there are wide cross-cultural variations in prescribing LAIs with over half of the mental health prescribers in the United Kingdom likely to prescribe LAIs in first-episode psychosis compared to less than half of the prescribers in the United States (Kim et al., 2012).

STUDENT REFLECTION

In the following conversation, two nursing students discuss the use of antipsychotic medication.

Student 1: Obviously, all patients have the right to refuse treatment, especially injections of antipsychotic medication, unless they pose an immediate danger to themselves or others. But it seems inhumane not to offer chronic mentally ill patients the option of taking their antipsychotic medication by injection, especially those who become so impaired they can't take care of themselves and put themselves at risk.

Student 2: I heard that some community outreach programs in England provide financial incentives for patients to receive their injections (Claassen, 2007).

Student 1: Don't you think that is unethical, to bribe a patient to take the medication by offering money or gifts?

Student 2: Well, what is the alternative, the community has rights, too, and what if a chronic mentally ill person is so psychotic that he or she is wandering the streets intimidating people? If I worked in a mental health center and I was directed to give a gift to entice a patient to take medication, I wouldn't have any problem with doing that—the patient can refuse both if he or she wants to.

Student 1: I think it would be better to go to court and seek a court order on the basis of the medical evidence and the patient's mental health history rather than to offer the patient a bribe, especially since most of the patients receiving the injectable medication are disproportionately incarcerated, uninsured, or poor people, who may belong to ethnic minorities (Glazer, 2007).

Medication adherence is also complicated in clients with schizophrenia because all antipsychotic medications have side effects that can interfere with normal daily functioning. Some side effects, especially with **first-generation antipsychotics** (e.g., haloperidol and fluphenazine), can be life-threatening and physically debilitating. Of particular concern with the first-generation antipsychotics is the risk of developing **tardive dyskinesia** (TD). This condition, which is irreversible, is characterized by twisting movements of tongue, limbs, and torso. The longer clients are on the first-generation antipsychotics, the greater the risk of acquiring TD. Because TD is permanently disfiguring, nurses in the community should routinely screen patients for subtle symptoms of TD using the Abnormal Involuntary Movement Scale (Guy, 1976). Some of the other debilitating side effects of the first-generation antipsychotics include akathisia (extreme restlessness in the limbs), dystonia (severe stiffness in muscles, most prominently the neck), blurred vision, urinary retention, and neuroleptic malignant syndrome.

The **second-generation antipsychotics** have fewer extrapyramidal symptoms and are much less likely to cause TD but have greater risks of metabolic syndrome. Metabolic syndrome is an adverse effect of treatment with second-generation antipsychotics (such as clozapine, olanzapine, quetiapine, risperidone, and ziprasidone) that develops as a result of pronounced weight gain, dyslipidemia, and hyperglycemia. Clients may experience weight gain on all of the antipsychotics; however, almost half of all patients on the second-generation antipsychotics experience a 20% increase in weight. Evidence is mounting that the second-generation antipsychotics, in particular clozapine and olanzapine, may increase the risk of developing new-onset type 2 diabetes.

At this time, regulations mandating regular monitoring of the client's weight and other symptoms associated with type 2 diabetes have not been promulgated by the Food and Drug Administration (FDA). In 2004, the APA and the American Diabetes Association (ADA) developed consensus guidelines to screen clients on second-generation antipsychotics for the development of cardiovascular diseases and type 2 diabetes (Table 21.3). The ADA and the APA emphasize that given the significant risk for developing hyperglycemia, the consensus guidelines should be considered a basic standard of care for all schizophrenic patients prescribed the second-generation antipsychotics.

Studies have shown that neither class of antipsychotics is superior in treating the positive and negative symptoms of schizophrenia and both have risks of adverse effects. One exception is clozapine, which has been shown to be superior in treating both the positive and negative symptoms of schizophrenia. It is important to note that clozapine has been associated with life-threatening agranulocytosis. The FDA has established a national clozapine registry and mandates white blood cell (WBC) counts within 24 hours of the initial dose, weekly for 6 months, and then every 2 weeks. Pharmacists may only dispense enough clozapine until the next WBC count test and must receive notification of the laboratory results prior to dispensing any additional medication. Like the other second-generation antipsychotics, clozapine causes weight gain, which is one of the most common side effects of the drug that contributes to nonadherence. The World Psychiatric Association has recommended that government funding agencies provide coverage for a broad array of medication treatment options to allow individualized treatment based on safety, tolerability, and efficacy of first- and second-generation antipsychotics (Tandon et al., 2008).

PRACTICE POINT

All antipsychotics have untoward effects that can compromise treatment adherence and physical health. Community health nurses must carefully monitor clients especially for TD, agranulocytosis, and metabolic syndrome, which can be a precursor to type 2 diabetes. Metabolic syndrome affects one in four patients treated for schizophrenia, and it is a major public health concern for this population (Rejas et al., 2008).

High-Risk Populations

The unemployed, the poor, and the homeless all report higher levels of depression, anxiety, schizophrenia, and substance abuse than the general population (WHO, 2008). Whether these social conditions trigger the symptoms of depression, anxiety, and psychosis or the debilitating effects of these illnesses lead to loss of employment, housing, and subsequent poverty is a source of debate within the field of epidemiology. The rising number of mentally ill clients who are homeless has steadily increased in the United States as state governments embarked on a systematic plan to "deinstitutionalize" the mentally ill. The goal of **deinstitutionalization** is to replace state hospitals with smaller group homes, half-way houses, or other supported living arrangements that integrate, rather than separate, the chronic mentally ill in the community. Tragically, the services available in the community seldom have kept pace with the demand for services. The gap in community-based services persists in all developed countries because of fiscal and political constraints.

In the United States, local officials resist proposals to site-supported living arrangements in their community. At the state level, mental health appropriations for community-based care are rarely fully funded. At the federal

table 21.3 **Recommendations for Monitoring Patients Taking Second-Generation Antipsychotics**

	Baseline	4 weeks	8 weeks	12 weeks	Quarterly	Annually	5 years
Personal and family history	X					X	
Body mass index (weight)	X	X	X	X	X	X	X
Waist circumference	X					X	
Blood pressure	X			X		X	
Fasting plasma glucose	X			X		X	X
Fasting lipid profile	X			X			

Source: American Diabetes Association, American Psychiatric Association Consensus Conference, American Association of Clinical Endocrinologists. (2004). North American Association for the study of obesity. Consensus development conference on antipsychotic drugs and obesity and diabetes. *Journal of Clinical Psychiatry, 65*, 267–272.

level, both Congress and the White House have continued to tighten eligibility criteria for social security disability—the primary financial resource for the chronic mentally ill who cannot work. Other federal programs in the Departments of Health and Human Services, Labor, Education, and Veterans Affairs that target homeless people have been "level funded." Therefore, funding has not kept pace with inflation. As government resources for the poor and disabled erode, shelters have been transformed from temporary to permanent housing. On the streets of any urban area, the failure to integrate the chronic mentally ill is glaringly apparent.

EVIDENCE FOR PRACTICE

Studies have demonstrated that the emotional well-being of the chronic mentally ill is enhanced when affected people live in socially and economically diverse neighborhoods that contain a mixture of commercial and residential real estate (Newman & Goldman, 2008). Outcomes for the mentally ill in the community also are improved when they reside in housing with an occupancy of less than 20 tenants and where a greater percentage of occupants also are mentally ill. Newman and Goldman (2008) note that housing combined with case management or ACT appears to be associated with decreased rehospitalization and homelessness; however, there is insufficient empiric evidence to identify which subgroups of patients can best benefit from specific housing configurations and support services to achieve successful treatment outcomes.

Role of Community Mental Health Teams in the Treatment of Schizophrenia

Prior to the community mental health movement and the deinstitutionalization of the mentally ill, people with chronic mental illness would be "warehoused," or confined to state hospitals for prolonged periods, many for life. Deinstitutionalization began as a humane initiative to end this "warehousing." But tragically, insufficient housing and the lack of other social supports in the community often results in homelessness for people with chronic mental illness. The burden of providing supportive care for the severe and persistently mentally ill has increasingly fallen to community agencies and families.

As a person with schizophrenia becomes less capable of managing social role responsibilities, families are faced with the burden of assuming the locus of care and support. Respite services, day-treatment facilities, and sheltered workshops are a few of the outpatient services that help alleviate the daily burden of care for families. Within families, caregiver burden is disproportionately shouldered by women, often the mother of the person with chronic mental illness. Women at greatest risk for burnout from the burden of care are Caucasian mothers caring for young adults with bipolar disorder in the home (Zauszniewski, Bekhet, & Suresky, 2008).

Families of people with chronic mental illness assume many of the economic costs associated with custodial care, but significant costs are also incurred by federal and local governments. People with schizophrenia are one of the largest beneficiaries of the federal and state welfare system. Federal, state, and local funds support care for people with chronic mental illness in homeless shelters, jails, long-term care facilities, and state mental hospitals. Too often, clients with chronic mental illness slip into no-care zones, adrift between the social welfare and healthcare sectors. The fragmentation of care among a myriad of institutions and professionals makes collaboration and continuity of care a major challenge for providers.

To address these shortcomings in the delivery of care, the WHO (2008) recommends the use of community mental health teams to coordinate both the psychosocial and psychopharmacologic needs of clients with schizophrenia. Unlike standard treatment approaches, community health teams provide mental health services in the client's home instead of in an office or clinic. Ideally, community mental health teams are composed of a variety of mental health professionals, including nurses, physicians, social workers, and occupational and rehabilitation therapists. Studies in the United States and Australia indicate that use of community health teams for people with chronic mental illness decreases rehospitalizations and significantly improves the overall quality of life (Mueser & McGurk, 2004).

Internationally, several studies are evaluating the effectiveness of community mental health teams and early intervention programs, including the EDIE study in the United Kingdom, the LifeSPAN study in Australia, the OPUS study in Denmark, the PRIME study in the United States, and the TIPS study in Norway (Marshall & Lockwood, 2005). ACT is an evidence-based treatment for the chronically mentally ill that includes interdisciplinary teams, with a focus on medication management, housing, and rehabilitation. Findings thus far indicate that the most effective aspects of ACT are those that target psychosocial functioning, including vocational skills and supported employment, activities of daily living, and social relationships (Mueser, Deavers, Penn, & Cassisi, 2013).

Clients with schizophrenia often have a myriad of comorbid chronic health conditions. Obesity, hypertension, and severe cardiac and metabolic complications all are prevalent to much higher degrees in people with schizophrenia due to higher rates of smoking, poor nutrition, and lack of exercise. The social apathy associated with the disease, limited access to healthcare services, and social stigma make it difficult for clients with schizophrenia to advocate for their healthcare needs. As client advocates, an important role of the community health nurse is to ensure that the primary healthcare needs of the chronic mentally ill are met in a variety of community-based agencies.

PRACTICE POINT

A promising research initiative from the National Institute of Mental Health (NIMH), the Recovery After an Initial Schizophrenia Episode (RAISE), is a network approach to integrate early intervention models with ACT (Narayan, Mohwinckel, Pisano, Yang, & Manji, 2013). The goal of RAISE is to integrate community-based biopsychosocial treatment in the early stages of schizophrenia to minimize relapse, morbidity, and disability associated with chronic mental illness.

Mood and Anxiety Disorders

Epidemiology

SOCIAL FACTORS

Unlike schizophrenia, for which the incidence is stable across cultures worldwide, there is substantial variation in the incidence of mood disorders and suicide. Noted sociologist Emile Durkheim wrote in 1925, "Man is the more vulnerable to self-destruction the more he is detached from any collectivity. The extent that familial society is more or less cohesive, tightly-knit and strong—man is more or less strongly attached to life" (Durkheim, 1972, p. 13). By the end of the century, epidemiologic studies empirically validated Durkheim's theories that social factors do play a prominent role in the incidence of mood and anxiety disorders.

Across all cultures, the two most consistent social factors associated with the incidence of depression and anxiety are education and employment status. Specifically, the lower the educational level and the greater the incidence of unemployment are, the higher the risk is of developing symptoms of depression and anxiety (Melzer, Fryers, & Jenkins, 2004). People who have two or more chronic physical illnesses, or who have experienced two or more stressful life events, have a six times greater risk than the general population of developing symptoms of depression and anxiety. The social factors with the lowest impact are lack of social support and being a single parent (Melzer et al., 2004). The effect of social class is inconsistent: some studies report an association with depression and anxiety, others do not.

BIOLOGIC THEORIES OF DEPRESSION AND ANXIETY

One of the first researchers to analyze the impact of stress on the biologic function of the brain was Hans Selye in the early 1900s. In the middle of the 20th century, researchers found that a person's behavior could be markedly altered by the administration of adrenocorticotropic hormone and cortisone. These discoveries prompted further research on the neurophysiologic effects of stress on combat veterans. Some of the greatest advances in the field of psychiatry and in the understanding of the relationship between the biology of the brain and behavior were discovered as clinical researchers attempted to treat soldiers exhibiting the symptoms of post-traumatic stress disorder (PTSD).

More recently, studies have uncovered important links between trauma, levels of cortisol in the brain, and feelings of anxiety, depression, and even psychosis. Although researchers have significantly increased the current understanding of the links between neurophysiology and behavior, many questions remain unanswered. Indeed, to highlight the importance of continuing this area of research, in 1990, President George Bush and Congress proclaimed the last 10 years of the 20th century to be the "Decade of the Brain."

Over the past two decades, there has been a dramatic increase in the number of somatic treatments for depression. Total Medicaid expenditures in 45 states for antidepressants rose from $500 million in 1995 to $985 million in 1998—an average increase of 25% per year, for an overall increase of 96%. Much of this increase can be attributed to increased expenditures for three antidepressants classified as selective serotonin reuptake inhibitors (SSRIs). SSRIs limit the reuptake of serotonin, an enzyme in the brain that has been found to be lower in people suffering from depression. While still under patent, the costs for paroxetine (Paxil) increased to $128 million over 4 years; costs for fluoxetine (Prozac) went up 73%, to $120 million; and for sertraline (Zoloft), costs went up 64%, to $84 million, for a total increase of 240% over 5 years (Lewin Group, 2000). The dramatic rise in the cost of pharmaceuticals triggered widespread shortfalls in states' Medicaid budgets. In response, many states have attempted to balance their Medicaid budgets by slowing rising pharmaceutical costs, especially those associated with psychiatric prescriptions. Some states have attempted to eliminate prescription drug coverage for certain classes of medications, and others have mandated generic prescribing or "first fail" policies that direct practitioners to order less-expensive SSRIs before prescribing more expensive alternatives. Specialty organizations such as the APA and the American Psychiatric Nurses Association have warned that policies restricting access to psychotropic medications could have the paradoxical effect of increasing Medicaid costs when clients who cannot afford the out-of-pocket expense for their psychotropic medications decompensate and are rehospitalized.

Populations at Risk for Suicide

Worldwide, suicide rates rise gradually with age, and in the United States, suicide now surpasses motor vehicle accidents as a leading cause of death (Centers for Disease Control and Prevention, 2013a). In addition to age, gender differences are significant, with rates of completed suicides more than twice as high for men than for women, and retired, divorced, white men at highest risk (Fig. 21.2). In the United States, American Indian youth and youth in lower socioeconomic groups have the highest rates of mortality from suicide (Fig. 21.3). While differences in suicide rates

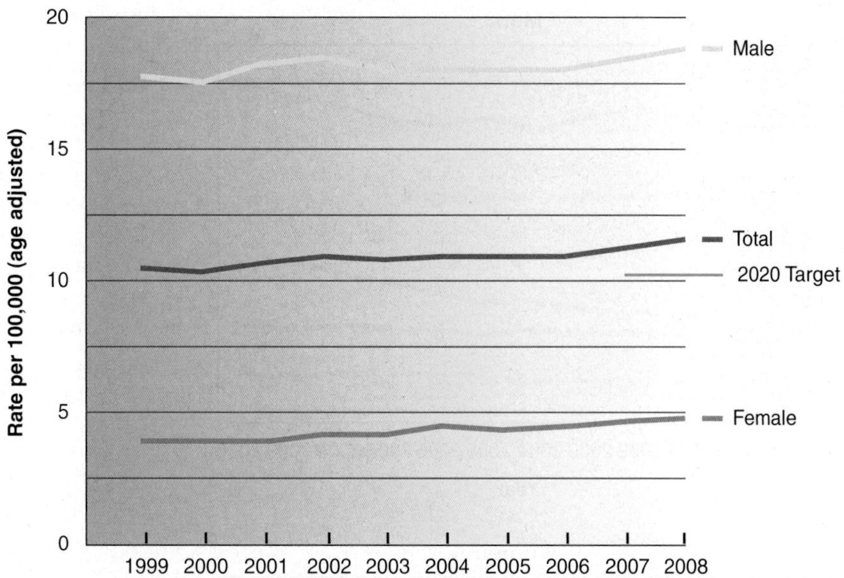

figure 21.2 *Healthy People 2020* target to decrease suicide by gender
Source: National Vital Statistics System–Mortality [NVSS-M], CDC/NCHS. Retrieved May 29, 2013, from http://www.healthypeople.gov/2020/topicsobjectives2020/nationalsnapshot.aspx?topicId=28

between youth of different races and ethnic backgrounds is narrowing, the gender gap between males and females persists, with far more females making nonlethal suicide attempts and males having higher rates of death from suicide (Joe, Canetto, & Romer, 2008) (Fig. 21.4).

One of the most pressing challenges for community mental health nurses is to address the precipitous increase in the rate of suicide, especially among young adults (Box 21.1). Worldwide, suicide among adolescents is the second leading cause of death (Centers for Disease Control and Prevention, 2013b; World Health Organization, 2012). The WHO recommends three evidenced-based population strategies to reduce suicide, including

1. Restrict access to means of self-harm/suicide
2. Develop policies to reduce harmful use of alcohol as a component of suicide prevention
3. Encourage the media to provide information about where to seek help and avoid sensationalizing suicide (World Health Organization, 2012)

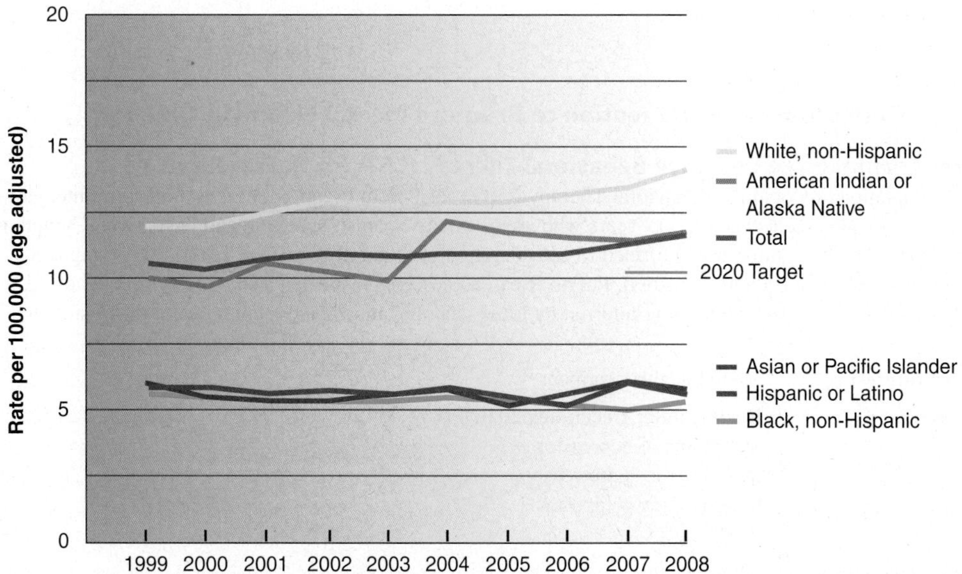

figure 21.3 *Healthy People 2020* target to decrease suicide by ethnicity.
Source: National Vital Statistics System–Mortality (NVSS-M), CDC/NCHS. Retrieved May 29, 2013, from http://www.healthypeople.gov/2020/topicsobjectives2020/nationalsnapshot.aspx?topicId=28

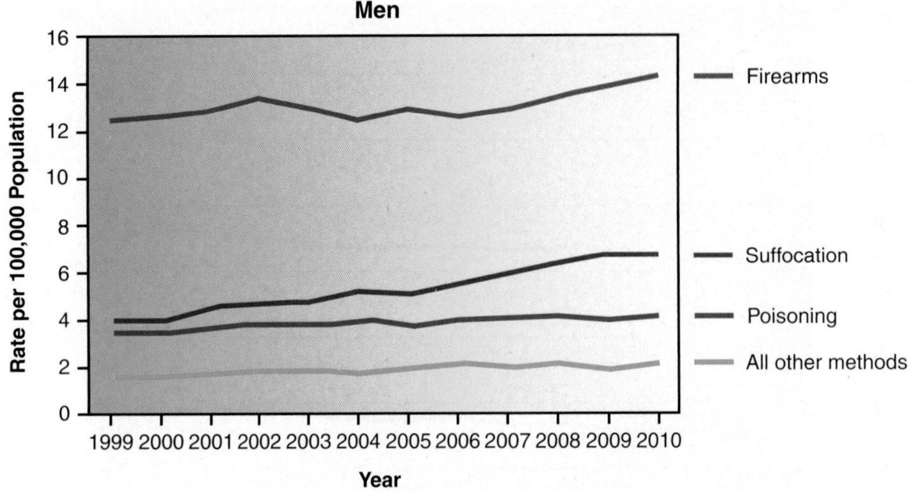

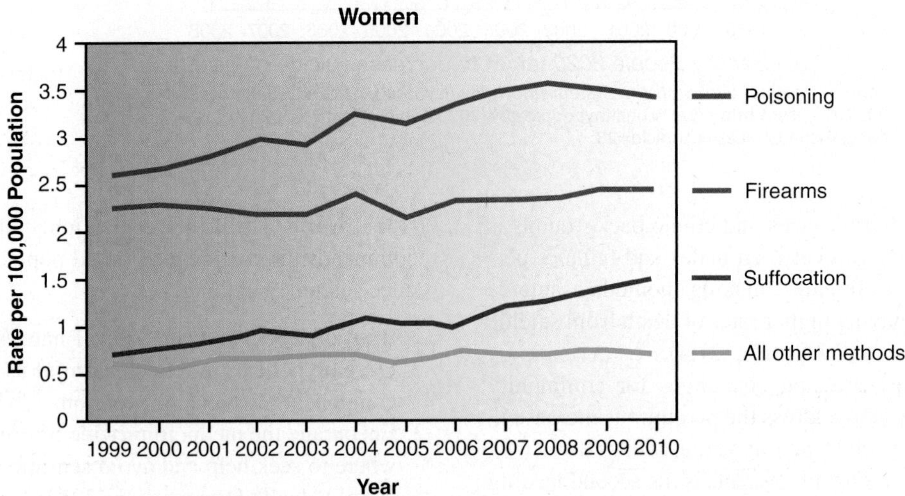

figure 21.4 Trends in suicide rates by gender and means 1999 to 2010.
Source: Centers for Disease Control and Prevention [2013]. Suicide among adults aged 35–64 Years—United States, 1999–2010. *Morbidity and Mortality Weekly Report, 62*(17), 325.

box 21.1 Evidence-Based Intervention to Promote Mental Health in Children

Cultural Adaptation of Cognitive Behavioral Therapy (CBT) for Puerto Rican Youth

Cultural Adaptation of Cognitive Behavioral Therapy (CBT) for Puerto Rican Youth is a short-term intervention for Puerto Rican adolescents aged 13–17 years who are primarily Spanish-speaking and have severe symptoms of depression. The intervention was informed in consideration of culturally sensitive criteria (i.e., language, developmental, and socioeconomic factors). Puerto Rican adolescents identified as having symptoms of depression received the intervention after being referred by local schools, clinics, and mental health professionals.

Areas of interest	Mental health treatment
Outcomes	**Review date: December 2010** Symptoms of depression Internalizing symptoms Externalizing symptoms Self-concept
Outcome categories	Mental health Social functioning

Ages	13–17 (Adolescent)
Genders	Male Female
Races/ethnicities	Hispanic or Latino
Settings	Outpatient Other community settings
Geographic locations	Urban
Implementation history	This intervention was first implemented in 1992 at the University of Puerto Rico, Río Piedras Campus. Since then, 198 Puerto Rican adolescents have received this intervention.
NIH funding/CER studies	Partially/fully funded by National Institutes of Health: Yes Evaluated in comparative effectiveness research studies: Yes

Source: *SAMHSA's National Registry of Evidence-based Programs and Practices*. Retrieved May 28, 2013, from http://www.nrepp.samhsa.gov/ViewIntervention.aspx?id=219

The National Strategy for Suicide Prevention (NSSP) is a public health initiative launched by the federal government to prevent suicide through public health education and community-wide interventions that restore cohesiveness among community members (National Strategy for Suicide Prevention, 2001). A key feature of the NSSP is to disseminate public health programs about suicide prevention widely, among a wide range of institutions in society, especially schools. Community health nurses, who may practice in nontraditional settings (i.e., parish nurses, senior or recreational centers, and people's workplaces), are ideally positioned to implement many of the proposed program initiatives.

A man who has not passed through the inferno of his passions has never overcome them.

Carl Jung

A recent study of the findings of the Third National Health and Nutrition Survey found that after adjustment for other risk factors, a history of major depressive disorder was the strongest risk factor associated with attempted suicide for both men and women (Zhang et al., 2005). Other risk factors include a history of substance abuse, suicide or self-mutilating behaviors, chronic pain, social isolation, stress, unemployment, and poverty. In the United States, Native American youths and youths from lower socioeconomic groups have the highest rates of mortality from suicide. Although differences in suicide rates among youths of different races and ethnic backgrounds is narrowing, the gender gap between males and females persists, with far more females making nonlethal suicide attempts and males having higher rates of death from suicide (Joe et al., 2008). The NSSP hopes that with early identification of individuals at risk, coupled with crisis intervention and ongoing treatment, the incidence of suicide in the United States can be lowered. Ideally, to meet this goal, all at-risk clients in community settings should be routinely screened by community health nurses for suicide.

Another objective of NSSP is to limit access to lethal means of attempting suicide. Firearm access is a risk factor for suicide in the United States (U.S. Department of Health and Human Services, 2012). Often, suicide is an impulsive act that may be prevented if the means of completing the suicide was removed. The rate of completed suicides has been significantly reduced in many countries by a public health strategy termed *means restriction* (U.S. Department of Health and Human Services, 2012). One of the goals of the 2012 NSSP is to promote efforts to reduce access to lethal means of suicide among individuals with identified suicide risk. A higher number of firearm laws in a state are associated with a lower rate of suicides from firearms fatalities (Fleegler, Lee, Monuteaux, Hemenway, & Mannix, 2013). Unfortunately, in American society, the power of the National Rifle Association, the availability of firearms, and the cultural value of personal freedom have thwarted enacting any meaningful restrictions on firearms.

Community health nurses can promote "means restriction," especially in families where there is a member at risk for suicide. Families who own firearms should be encouraged to secure firearms using trigger locks and locking bullets in a separate location from the firearm. If a client informs the nurse that he or she is having thoughts of taking an overdose, then prescription or over-the-counter medications that may be fatal in overdose should be removed or secured in a safe location. Although families might presume that removing the instrumental means of harm is an ineffective gesture, the community health nurse must reassure the family that their actions are sending a strong, unambiguous message to the potential victim that people care about them and will take any necessary steps to ensure their safety.

Suicide prevention strategies have traditionally focused on identifying individuals at risk through mental health assessments or screening tools. Screening tools are designed specifically to identify individuals who are depressed, socially isolated, or have a history of substance abuse. There are also variations in the rate of suicide due to population factors such as cultural values and beliefs, the rate of industrialization, poverty, war, and social upheaval. The NSSP represents an effort in the United States to meld public health strategies that target both individual people and entire populations for intervention. Because social or cultural attributes contribute as much as individual risk factors in the incidence of suicidal behavior, the WHO recommends that all suicide prevention programs incorporate population-based risk reduction approaches (Knox, Conwell, & Caine, 2004).

Worldwide, suicide rates rise gradually with age. In addition to age, gender differences are significant, with rates of completed suicides more than twice as high for men than for women, with retired, divorced, white men at highest risk. Other individuals at risk for suicide are those with a family history of suicide (Goodwin, Beautrais, & Fergusson, 2004) and those with comorbid substance abuse disorder (Grant et al., 2004).

I spent a year in a 12-step program, really committed, because I could not believe what had happened— that I might have killed myself.

Carrie Fisher

EVIDENCE FOR PRACTICE

Although epidemiologic studies have identified the risk factors for suicide based on a variety of demographic and social factors, the role of culture in the prevention or exacerbation of the phenomenon of suicide is not well understood. Joe et al. (2008, p. 358) suggest that future research on protective and risk factors for suicide consider discrimination, poverty, acculturation, differences in social supports among ethnic groups, spirituality, and sexuality. Gun control laws are one of the few proven suicide prevention policies (Miller & Hemenway, 2008). In conducting suicide assessment, nurses should always inquire about access to lethal means of attempting suicide.

PRACTICE POINT

Social and cultural factors are significantly associated with the incidence of suicide, yet the primary treatment, especially in Western cultures, is somatic, specifically antidepressant or antianxiety medication. Medication treatment may alleviate the symptoms of depression and anxiety of many individuals, but it is also important to attend to the social and cultural factors that play a significant role in the incidence of suicide throughout the developed and developing world. Goldston et al. (2008) summarize cultural differences in suicide among African-American, American Indian, Asian-American, Pacific Islander, and Latino adolescents that provide nurses with useful insights about protective factors, the role of religion, family cultural mistrust, and help-seeking behavior.

Nursing Interventions for Mood and Anxiety Disorders

Approximately 80% of people diagnosed with major depression have a remission of symptoms on antidepressant medications. In general, the SSRIs are the first line of treatment because they are well tolerated and easy to administer in once-a-day dosing. An older class of antidepressants, the tricyclic antidepressants (TCAs), is a second-line treatment because these antidepressants have strong anticholinergic side effects and dosing has to be gradually titrated before a client reaches a therapeutic level. Both the SSRIs and the TCAs can take 4 to 6 weeks before reaching therapeutic blood levels—a serious concern when working with acutely suicidal clients. For that reason, electroconvulsive therapy (ECT) may be used for clients who are acutely suicidal or exhibiting profound neurovegetative signs of depression.

In the acute care setting, ECT is administered every other day for 9 to 12 treatments. Maintenance ECT may be given weekly or monthly on an outpatient basis for clients who are resistant to treatment with antidepressants. Clients who receive ECT experience short-term memory loss for events that occurred immediately prior to the treatment, so nurses and family members should be prepared to reorient the client if necessary. Over-the-counter analgesics may be prescribed if a person complains of headache immediately after the treatment. As with any same-day surgery, clients scheduled for ECT should be NPO after midnight and not drive themselves home from the hospital or clinic. Rest is also advised for the first few hours after receiving ECT.

Adherence issues may arise for clients on antidepressants because of side effects such as nausea, headaches, and diarrhea. One of the most common side effects of SSRIs is sexual dysfunction, which causes erectile dysfunction or difficulty achieving orgasm in approximately 6% to 30% of clients. Weight gain, although not as prominent as is the case with the atypical antipsychotics, can also occur. In general, the most frequently expressed concern of clients on antidepressants is if, and when, they can discontinue their medication.

In a first-episode depression, it is reasonable to consider a gradual lowering of the dose of antidepressants a year to 18 months after symptoms have remitted, assuming the client's life is relatively stable. Approximately 50% of all clients diagnosed with major depression have a recurrence of symptoms. For clients who have a second episode of depression, 70% will experience a third episode, and of that group, 90% will continue to be incapacitated by periodic episodes of depression. In a case where a person has experienced a recurrence of major depressive illness, community health nurses should encourage the client to continue taking antidepressant medication. If a client is experiencing intolerable side effects and is insisting on stopping the medication, the community health nurse should inform the prescribing physician or nurse practitioner and suggest switching to a different antidepressant to promote long-term adherence.

SSRIs are also prescribed for the long-term treatment of generalized anxiety and obsessive-compulsive disorders. Anxiety disorders encompass a range of syndromes, including phobias (i.e., fear of heights), obsessive thoughts (i.e., "I will get a sexually transmitted disease from using a public restroom"), compulsive behaviors (i.e., repeated handwashing), and panic attacks. Calm, simple, and reality-centered communication is the most immediate therapeutic response to a person experiencing anxiety or panic attack. The nurse should direct the client to engage in deep breathing by inhaling through the nose and exhaling slowly through pursed lips to a count of 10. If a person is hyperventilating, a paper bag may be placed over the mouth. Longer-acting benzodiazepines (i.e., clonazepam [Klonopin]) may be administered to treat acute symptoms but should be discontinued after 2 to 3 weeks because of the potential for developing tolerance.

The symptoms of major depression or anxiety commonly seen in community settings are fatigue, headache, backache, gastrointestinal complaints, anhedonia, and sleep and appetite disturbance. Clients who are exhibiting these somatic signs as well as mood symptoms should be asked directly if they have had any thoughts of harming themselves. If a client responds in the affirmative, the nurse needs to ascertain if the client has a specific plan and the means to carry out the plan. Suicide is a significant public health problem. Community mental health nurses can play an important role in implementing new federal initiatives to prevent suicide, especially among youth. For community health nurses, it is important to note that African-Americans are much more likely than other ethnic minorities to seek care of mood and anxiety symptoms through faith-based organizations and ministers than psychiatric professionals (Neighbors et al., 2007).

PRACTICE POINT

In clients with somatic and mood symptoms, nurses must always directly inquire if the client has had any thought of harming himself or herself.

Attention-Deficit/Hyperactivity Disorders and Emotional Disorders in Children

Mental disorders are evident across the life span, beginning in childhood. Rates of major mental illness in adolescents range from 8% in the Netherlands to 57% in one county in California (Patel et al., 2007). Rates of pediatric bipolar disorder have dramatically increased in the past decade, doubling in the primary care setting (6%) and quadrupling in child psychiatric units in hospitals (Leibenluft & Rich, 2008). Children with behavioral disorders incur healthcare costs that on average are higher ($1,492) than chronic medical conditions ($1,245) and, as is the case with adults who have chronic major mental illness, most of the costs are accounted for by a small group of children (Guevara et al., 2003). Because of the significant morbidity associated with untreated mental disorders in childhood, both the President's Commission on Mental Health (2003) and the WHO (2008) emphasize the essential role of schools in early identification of children at risk for mental disorders.

School nurses have always screened students for common medical conditions and administered medications for chronic health conditions such as asthma, diabetes, and epilepsy. Increasingly, school nurses are administering psychotropic medications to younger students and to a greater number of students than ever before. Studies examining medication administration practices of school nurses have estimated the prevalence of administering attention-deficit/hyperactivity disorder (ADHD) medication from 1.91% of students in a Kansas school system to 9.9% of students in two schools in Virginia—rates that are roughly equivalent to the administration rates for asthma medication by school nurses (Weller et al., 2004).

School nurses and other education professionals may be responsible for caring for students with multiple overlapping mental disorders. The overlap in symptoms among ADHD, bipolar disorder, and conduct disorder makes it more difficult for the school nurse to identify correctly students at risk and make referrals for appropriate treatment. Hyperactivity and impulsivity, hallmarks of ADHD, may also be displayed by children with bipolar disorder. A review of clinical records at a mood disorder clinic in New York found that prior to being diagnosed with bipolar disorder, most children are incorrectly diagnosed with ADHD (60%), and an additional 21% are diagnosed incorrectly with conduct or oppositional-defiant disorder (Faedda, Baldessarini, Glovinsky, & Austin, 2004). Because the pharmacologic treatment for both conditions is vastly different—in ADHD, children are prescribed stimulants and in bipolar disorder, children are prescribed second-generation antipsychotics and mood stabilizers—it is important that clinicians recognize the subtle features that distinguish the two disorders.

The main characteristics that help healthcare practitioners, including school nurses, differentiate ADHD from bipolar disorder are the pervasiveness of the symptoms and the predominant symptoms. In children with ADHD, hyperactivity and impulsivity are evident in all spheres of the child's life. There is a constancy and pervasiveness of the hyperactivity in school, at home, and in activities. Distractibility and unrelenting motor behavior (e.g., always being in motion, begin unable to sit still and attend to a task) are the symptoms that cause the most distress for parents and teachers. Unlike bipolar disorder, mood and anxiety symptoms are not predominant in ADHD; generally, teachers and parents do not characterize the child with ADHD as angry, irritable, and moody.

In contrast, almost 75% of the children diagnosed with bipolar disorder have a predominance of mood symptoms such as irritability, sleep disturbances, and anxiety (Faedda et al., 2004). In most cases, the prodromal symptoms of bipolar disorder are evident when the child is younger than 3 years of age. For a child with bipolar disorder, the slightest frustration can set off a flood of crying, screaming, or anxiety symptoms. Unlike toddlers who have temper tantrums that are time-limited, children with bipolar disorder can have rage episodes that can last from 2 to 3 hours. Generally, children who are angry and frustrated can be comforted by adults. However, children with bipolar disorder appear inconsolable. Angry or aggressive outbursts are unpredictable and episodic, varying from day to day and moment to moment.

Family history may also alert the clinician to the possibility a child has bipolar disorder rather than ADHD. Almost all (90%) children with bipolar disorder had a family history of mood disorder or substance use (Faedda et al., 2004) compared with 4.4% of mothers who have children with ADHD (Lesesne, Visser, & White, 2003). If parents or siblings report that they have experienced performance difficulties in school or work, it is important for the diagnostician to determine whether the poor performance was due to mood symptoms (such as depression) or motor behavior (such as impulsivity). If the social role functioning of a family member was disrupted primarily by mood symptoms, this may suggest that the child is more at risk for bipolar disorder than for ADHD.

Finally, clinicians, as well as school nurses, should carefully observe for improvement in target symptoms with medication treatment. With ADHD, there should be some improvement in symptoms after an adequate trial of psychostimulants. Similarly, with bipolar disorder, there should be an improvement in symptoms after treatment with second-generation antipsychotics. The danger in failing to make a proper diagnosis is that if children with bipolar disorder are prescribed antidepressant or stimulant drugs, there can be an exacerbation of suicidality, hostility, and agitation (Faedda et al., 2004). Current estimates are that 20% to 40% of children initially diagnosed with depression will develop bipolar disorder. It is crucial for school nurses to carefully monitor any child on antidepressants for a worsening of symptoms, especially any indications of disinhibition.

In October of 2004, the U.S. FDA mandated the following warning to be added to the drug information insert included in all antidepressant packaging:

- Antidepressants increase the risk of suicidal thinking and behavior (suicidality) in children and adolescents with major depressive disorder and other psychiatric disorders.
- Anyone considering the use of an antidepressant in a child or adolescent for any clinical use must balance the risk of increased suicidality with the clinical need.
- Patients who are started on therapy should be observed closely for clinical worsening, suicidality, or unusual changes in behavior.
- Families and caregivers should be advised to closely observe the patient and to communicate with the prescriber.

Up until the issuance of what is termed by the FDA as a **"Black box" warning**, there had been a steady rise in the use of SSRIs by pediatric practitioners. One study in California found that the use of SSRIs in children and adolescents doubled from 1994 to 2003 (Hunkeler et al., 2005). In the wake of the FDA warning, there are recent indications that the number of adolescents being prescribed antidepressants is beginning to decline. Now the concern expressed by pediatric practitioners is how to best weigh the risks and benefits of treatment with antidepressants so that the gains achieved over the past decade in lowering the rates of suicide among youth are not reversed. In response, the APA is in the process of developing guidelines for primary care providers on the clinical management of the depressed adolescent.

Multidisciplinary collaboration among teachers, therapists, and primary care providers is a central feature of comprehensive treatment for the child with any behavioral disorder. Psychotherapies, specifically cognitive-behavioral therapy and family therapy, have been demonstrated to be effective in the management of depression but not as effective as antidepressants alone. Self-help groups for families are of enormous benefit in helping families cope with the child's disruptive behaviors that can quickly lead to caregiver burnout.

The role of the school nurse is integral to helping the child or adolescent understand the nature of the disorder; the purpose and side effects of medication; and the importance of maintaining a healthy lifestyle, including good sleep hygiene, avoidance of caffeine, relaxation techniques, and abstinence from illicit drugs. It may sound like a tall order for the school nurse, but there is compelling evidence that young adults and children respond positively to primary interventions, education, and support from caring adults. Often, a depressed child will come to the health office with somatic complaints such as headache, gastrointestinal upset, or fatigue. The school nurse's office can be an oasis of calm and comfort in the midst of the daily demands of school life. Empathy, active listening, and unconditional positive regard are the cornerstones to developing a therapeutic alliance—an alliance that can make a significant positive impact on the quality of a child's experience in school.

PRACTICE POINT

Careful assessment of mood and motor symptoms by school nurses is essential in ensuring early and accurate diagnosis of ADHD, bipolar disorder, and major depression in school-age children.

The Precipitous Rise in Autism—A Public Health Crisis

Throughout the world, there has been an increase in the prevalence rate of autism that is not explained by improved screening or changes in diagnostic criteria. Epidemiologic surveys of autism in America, western Pacific, and Europe do not statistically differ with a global mean prevalence of 1 child out of 160 having a pervasive developmental disorder

(Elsabbagh et al., 2012). Based on parent self-report, in 2013 the CDC estimates that 1 in 50 children in the United States has autism, which represents a 2% increase in all age groups in 5 years (Blumberg et al., 2013). Given the public health implications of the growing numbers of children worldwide diagnosed with autism, the foundation, "Autism Speaks" has partnered with the WHO and the CDC to enhance collaboration among researchers investigating the causes of pervasive developmental disorders and improve healthcare services, especially in developing countries (Elsabbagh et al., 2012).

Etiologic factors under investigation include genetic, biologic, developmental, and environmental agents. The heritability of autism is high, with an increased recurrence risk of 12% to 20% in siblings of a child diagnosed with autism (Chase & Leboyer, 2012). A genetic test for autism in a population of central European decent has been developed with a level of diagnostic accuracy and offers promising insights in genetic testing research for other ethnic populations (Skafidas, Testa, Zantomio, Chana, Everall, & Pantelis, 2012). While specific alleles contribute to risk, there is growing research evidence that environmental factors and the interaction between the environment and genes also play an important role in the etiology of autism. For example, epidemiologic studies of unaffected siblings find fewer prenatal and perinatal exposures and complications than with the affected sibling (Chase & Leboyer, 2012).

Given the upsurge in autism cases, epidemiologists are investigating potential exposures that effect entire populations. The list of causative environmental agents includes exposures in utero, to the mother, and in infancy. Exposures during pregnancy associated with increased risk of developing autism include medications such as antibiotics, valproic acid, SSRIs, and misoprostol as well as substances such as ethanol, thalidomide, and the insecticide chlorpyrifos (Atladóttir, Henriksen, Schendel, & Parner, 2012; Chase, & Leboyer, 2012; Croen, Grether, Yoshida, Odouli, & Hendrick, 2011; Duchan & Patel, 2012).

While the genetic risks to offspring of older mothers has been known for some time, recent studies have identified the role of paternal age in the occurrence of genetic mutations that can lead to autism. The role of paternal age in a U.S. sample was first reported in the *American Journal of Epidemiology* by lead author Dr. Maureen Durkin who found that the risk of autism increased by 30% if the mother was over 35 years of age and 40% if the father was over 40 years of age (Durkin et al., 2009). The increased risk of a child developing autism with parents over 35 to 40 years of age has been replicated in Swedish, Danish, and Israeli populations (Dchan & Patel, 2012). The interaction between genetic mutations and the environment was confirmed by Kong et al. (2012), who found two or more mutations for every year in paternal age, or a doubling in the number of mutations every 16.5 years. The genetic mutations were theorized to be due to environmental influences or by errors in maintaining DNA integrity over time. Collectively, these epidemiologic studies suggest that the increase in couples delaying childbearing may be contributing to the increase in the incidence of autism.

Given the profound public health implications for the rising rate of autism among U.S. children, in 2006 Congress created a federal advisory committee, the Interagency Autism Coordinating Committee (IACC) to accelerate progress in autism research and services. In 2011, Congress reauthorized the IACC, which is assisted by the Office of Autism Research Coordination (OARC), to communicate directly to Congress, other government agencies, and the public the latest information about federally supported autism research. The 2012 IACC Strategic Plan documents the magnitude of groundbreaking research and advances in treatment with the explicit goal of improving the quality of life for autistic children and their families (Interagency Autism Coordinating Committee, 2012).

Most research investigating the genetic and environmental risk factors for autism has been conducted with populations in developed countries. Yet unlocking the clues about the role of parental age, complications in pregnancy or medications taken in pregnancy can best be elucidated with cross-cultural comparisons for these and other associated risk factors. Even in the United States, prevalence rates of autism are higher in more affluent communities (Durkin et al., 2010). The Global Autism Public Health Initiative has partnerships in 42 nations to expand epidemiologic research globally in an effort to identify how genes and the environment may interact to increase the risk for autism. Epidemiology research on environmental factors associated with autism, both in the United States and abroad, is critical in providing public health nurses specific targets for education and prevention with at-risk populations.

PUBLIC HEALTH INITIATIVES IN AUTISM

Public health organizations have an important role in promoting screening programs and providing information about treatment resources. In the past, diagnosis of autism was often delayed until preschool because clinicians would look for evidence of language impairments before making a definitive diagnosis. More recently, the emphasis is on screening for prodromal symptoms in infancy with the hope that some of the more debilitating features of the disorder might be mitigated with early intervention and treatment. A goal of *Healthy People 2020* is to increase the proportion of young children with an **autism spectrum disorder** (ASD) and other developmental delays who are screened, evaluated, and enrolled in early intervention programs. The CDC's "Learn the Signs—Act Early" is a health education campaign targeting parents, educators, and healthcare providers promoting awareness of child development and information about early intervention programs. In the United States, Hispanic and African-American children have been diagnosed later and enter treatment for autism later than Caucasian children. The CDC's "Learn the Signs—Act Early" education effort includes parent-friendly materials that are customizable for populations with health disparities to improve case finding and referral. The foundation "Autism Speaks" has partnered with the Ad Council to create Spanish-language educational ads for the media, church groups, and other community organizations to also enhance outreach to Latino and black communities.

PRACTICE POINT

In 2013, the diagnostic criteria for autistic disorder in *DSM-5* eliminated the diagnosis of Asperger syndrome, and the category of pervasive developmental disorders was replaced with ASD (APA, 2013). Public health and school nurses should be aware of parents' heightened concerns that the more precise diagnostic criteria will be used to deny their child special education services (Halfon & Kuo, 2013). When educating parents of newborns about normal developmental milestones, it is important for community health nurses to encourage parents to report any concerns they may have about their child's social or language development.

EVOLUTION OF COMMUNITY MENTAL HEALTH

In the United States, community-based treatment of the mentally ill gained momentum as World War II veterans returned home exhibiting the symptoms of PTSD. There was a recognition that witnessing or experiencing a horrific traumatic event could have debilitating effects on the mind. The stigma associated with mental illness also began to subside in the wake of the tragic 1942 Cocoanut Grove fire in Boston, in which hundreds of trapped victims died and scores of survivors and their families sought mental health services. Through his pioneering work with people traumatized by the Cocoanut Grove fire, Dr. Erich Lindemann developed the concept of crisis intervention and promoted the notion that those suffering from mental illness can be best healed with their own communities among family and social institutions who cared and supported them.

By the early 1960s, a scathing report by the Joint Commission on Mental Health and Illness about conditions in state-supported psychiatric hospitals prompted the adoption of the Community Mental Health Center (CMHC) Act and federal initiatives to revamp mental healthcare delivery (Dixon & Goldman, 2004). Initially, the populations to be served by community mental health centers were those suffering from acute, not chronic, mental illnesses (Dixon & Goldman, 2004). In the coming decades, more than 700 community mental health centers funded by the federal government were created, and through outreach services, many younger and less-debilitated individuals received mental health services than ever before (Feldman, 2004). One of the distinctive features of these mental health centers was that treatment was to be population-based. Each **community mental health center** was responsible for providing a range of mental health services to people who lived in a specific geographic area that was not to exceed 200,000 people. The services mandated by the CMHC Act included inpatient, outpatient, day treatment, and emergency treatment, as well as consultation and education to the community (Feldman, 2004). It was a sweeping agenda, with profound implications for the continued viability of state-run psychiatric hospitals.

Aided by advances in the development of pharmacologic treatment of the mentally ill, the numbers of patients treated in state mental hospitals precipitously declined. Coupled with changes in involuntary commitment regulations that made the confinement of patients against their will unlawful except in extreme instances of a clear danger to themselves or others, more and more mentally ill found themselves homeless. Community mental health centers had paved the way for mental health services to be provided for those who were acutely ill. However, few resources were in place at these centers to provide the range of supportive care needed by the overwhelming numbers of mentally ill who were rapidly being discharged from state hospitals.

The deinstitutionalization trend began as a humane effort to reduce the stigma associated with mental illness and reintegrate those suffering from mental illness into community-based settings. Indeed, some of the patients with chronic mental illness who qualified for income support through Social Security Disability were transferred to long-term care facilities, half-way houses, and supportive housing. However, in all too many cases, vast numbers of those discharged from state hospitals fell into a no-care zone—homeless, living on the streets or in shelters.

In hindsight, as originally conceived, the community mental health centers were ill prepared, financially or organizationally, to meet the housing, income, employment, and rehabilitation needs of people with chronic mental illness. By the 1980s, the President's Commission for Mental Health offered a new agenda to the community mental health centers that shifted the funding to rehabilitation, affordable housing, and vocational training (Geller, 2000). The shift to a more pragmatic treatment model recognized that clients with severe mental illness would likely have a lifelong dependency on services aimed at sustaining their independence and social functioning.

Based on recommendations from the President's Commission on Mental Health, the NIMH allocated $3.5 million to develop Community Support Programs (CSPs) that would target employment, supportive housing, and social rehabilitation to those with persistent mental illness (Dixon & Goldman, 2004). But the ability of the CSPs to engage the chronically ill and help them achieve the goal of independence remains a challenge. Dixon and Goldman (2004) believe that the CSPs have not realized greater gains in helping the chronic mentally ill integrate successfully in the community primarily because of two factors. First, in addition to having a major mental illness, such as schizophrenia, many of the chronic mentally ill are also addicted to alcohol or other illicit substances. Second, in many CSPs, there is pressure to prematurely discharge clients to keep down the overall costs of the program (Dixon & Goldman, 2004).

In 2002, the **President's New Freedom Commission on Mental Health** was created to advise Congress and the President on how policy-makers could improve mental health services for both the chronic mentally ill and children with serious mental illnesses. The interim report of this commission confirmed what many practitioners and clients had long known, that fragmentation of services among 42 federal programs has made continuity of care a major obstacle (President's New Freedom Commission on Mental Health's website). Although the chronic mentally ill receive $21 billion in income support through Social Security Disability and $24 billion in Medicare and Medicaid benefits, approximately 25% of the homeless still do not have access to mental health services (Iglehart, 2004). On the state level, community health nurses responsible for case management must negotiate with separate agencies for mental health services, criminal justice, substance abuse, and housing services. Coupled with the split at the federal level between the Social Security Administration, Medicare, and Medicaid, it is easy to see how a family or provider would have difficulty accessing or coordinating care. One of the proposals from the President's New Freedom Commission on Mental Health (2003) is the development of a comprehensive state mental health plan that would create new partnerships among federal, state, and local officials. By reallocating federal expenditures to the state level, it is hoped that the states will be able to provide a comprehensive model of care that encompasses the entire spectrum of services for the chronic mentally ill within one entity.

Since deinstitutionalization began, there has been an outcry of frustration from nurses in the community about the lack of supportive services to meet the needs of people with chronic mental illness. Community mental health nurses have been forceful advocates at the state, national, and local level to ensure that policies and programs are in place to provide a safe haven for those no longer confined to state-run psychiatric hospitals. These state hospitals remain the provider of last resort for clients with intractable symptoms. Over a decade ago, Geller (2000) warned that by solely focusing on the locus of care or where the care is given, without regard to the humane character, appropriateness, or quality of care, there is a risk that the very conditions deinstitutionalization sought to ameliorate will be recreated. One of the future goals for community health nurses will be to find innovative ways to partner with families in designing and implementing mental health programs that reflect the values, traditions, and beliefs of their community.

Carmen's treatment team begins planning for the psychiatric care she will need in the community from the day she is admitted. The case manager contacts day programs near Carmen's home and negotiates with Medicare disability reviewers to approve outpatient treatment for 2 weeks. At discharge, Carmen's mood is much improved, and she is reassured that a referral to a pain specialist is pending. Although the day-treatment program is near her residence, she has to rely on family members for rides. She is hesitant to ask her family for them, and at home, unexpected financial expenses mean that she does not fill her prescriptions for both pain management and depression. Carmen is readmitted to the hospital less than a month after her original discharge. She returns in severe pain, saying that she is "too much of a burden" to her family and "what is the point of living." During the second hospitalization, the case manager is able to arrange for transportation to and from day treatment and enroll Carmen in a low-cost medication administration program offered by a pharmaceutical company to improve her adherence with the treatment plan.

LEGISLATION FOR PARITY IN MENTAL HEALTH INSURANCE BENEFITS

The United States maintains the unique distinction of having a private health insurance system that allocates benefits based on where a person is employed. Because health insurance is a substantial cost to employers, myriad strategies have been used to contain healthcare costs. One of these strategies is that traditionally, in private health insurance, there have been different benefits, co-pays, and insurance limits for mental health versus medical health conditions. Beginning in 1993, Congress debated the merits of legislating equal benefits for all healthcare conditions. Proponents of parity cite research evidence that many mental disorders are more responsive to treatment than common medical conditions and that with early treatment, the more chronic, residual effects of mental disorders maybe lessened. More than 365 organizations representing a wide array of public interest groups, local governments, and healthcare providers, including the American Psychiatric Nurses Association and the American Nurses Association, support mental health parity.

After 3 years of debate, the Mental Health Parity Act (MHPA) was enacted, requiring that lifetime and annual ceilings on expenditures for mental healthcare not be lower than those for physical illness. In an important concession, MHPA only applied to employer-based insurance that served 50 or more employees, exempting small businesses or people who were self-insured, and it excluded certain psychiatric conditions. As can be found with all public policies, ingenious strategies were devised to thwart the spirit of the 1996 parity law. For example, some private insurance plans set limits on inpatient days for psychiatric treatment or increased the co-pays and deductible charges for mental healthcare.

In the original legislation, it was stipulated that the provisions of the MHPA would expire, or "sunset", in 6 years. After a 12-year battle on Capitol Hill and in the White House, in October of 2008, the Paul Wellstone and Pete Domenici Mental Health Parity and Addiction Equity Act of 2008 was passed by Congress and signed by President Bush. The

MHPA of 2008 expands the MHPA of 1996 and mandates that by January 1, 2010, health insurance plans covering 50 or more employees provide equal benefits for medical, surgical, mental health, and substance use treatment. All health insurance coverage, including deductibles, co-payments, coinsurance, and out-of-pocket expenses, and all treatment limitations, including frequency of treatment, number of visits, days of coverage, or other similar limits, will be the same regardless of health need or diagnosis. Those opposed to the MHPA argued that health insurance costs to employers and individuals would increase significantly if benefits for mental and medical conditions were equal. To date, mental health parity has not led to increased health insurance costs (Mark, Vandivort-Warren, & Miller, 2012).

ROLES AND RESPONSIBILITIES OF THE COMMUNITY MENTAL HEALTH PRACTITIONER

Throughout this chapter, the roles of the community health nurse as teacher, clinician, and advocate have been described. Mental health is a leading health indicator in the U.S. *Healthy People 2010* program (see Fig. 21.1), and mental health promotion and disease prevention are an integral part of nursing practice. Box 21.2 outlines selected primary, secondary, and tertiary levels of prevention that help reduce risk, identify and limit disabilities, and reduce complications of mental health problems.

Providing population-based care that addresses the cultural diversity of a community remains one of the most pressing challenges facing all health providers. The WHO and the Affordable Care Act have cited the application of culturally sensitive care for people suffering from mental illness as one of the most pressing goals in the new millennium. There is not a single path to achieve this objective, although there is unanimity on the importance of providing mental health services that are sensitive to the cultural needs and expectations of clients and their families.

box 21.2 Levels of Prevention in Community Mental Health

Primary

- Educate families and community groups about mental health issues, symptoms of stress, and barriers to seeking help.
- Foster availability of support services for community groups, such as prenatal and parent education sessions, bereavement sessions, and caregiver support.

Secondary

- Screen for mental health disorders.
- Refer high-risk people for diagnostic services.
- Provide mental health services following stressful community events.

Tertiary

- Promote support groups for people with mental health disorders.
- Initiate health promotion activities as a part of rehabilitation services.

Developing a therapeutic alliance is the cornerstone to culturally sensitive nursing care. The Substance Abuse and Mental Health Services Administration (SAMHSA) has developed cultural competence standards for mental healthcare services (see link). For example, one of the implementation guidelines is that bilingual mental health staff be certified in language proficiency and cultural competence. The outcome benchmark recommended by SAMHSA is that 90% of racial/ethnic consumers of mental health services be satisfied with the communication styles of mental health specialists. In addition, culturally competent nursing care plans must identify and involve a range of community resources, including native societies, healers, spiritual leaders, and community organizations. Culturally competent community health nurses must demonstrate knowledge in group values, traditions, and the cultural expression of mental illness. In turn, therapeutic interventions described in the treatment plan should reflect the client's cultural values. Education and outreach programs must be designed to include specific information that addresses the unique cultural needs of a community.

In California, cultural competency plans and standards are part of statewide mental health programs and managed care plans (Dougherty, 2004). In Pennsylvania, treatment plans in the Community Connections for Families program incorporate recreational and social activities to keep the family and child integrated with members of their community (Dougherty, 2004). The President's New Freedom Commission on Mental Health (2003) cites a culturally competent school-based mental health program as a model for implementing **culturally competent mental health services**.

Almost a decade ago, the Surgeon General's Report on Mental Health (U.S. Department of Health and Human Services, 1999) urged researchers to investigate differences in access to care and treatment response by culture, race, or ethnicity. More recently, the Affordable Care Act also highlighted the importance of expanding access to culturally competent mental health services (Nardi, Waite, & Killian, 2012). It is important to acknowledge that health insurance reform alone will not be sufficient to erase racial and ethnic healthcare disparities. Disparities in access and response to mental health treatment exist by age, gender, race, ethnic background, socioeconomic status, and geographic location (Dougherty, 2004). Clinic hours, transportation, stigma, and the availability of culturally competent mental health providers are some of the roadblocks marginalized populations face when attempting to access mental health services (Alegria, Lin, Chen, Duan, Cook, & Meng, 2012). Community health nurses can play a critical role in advancing nursing knowledge and understanding of how models of nursing care can be developed that account for cultural differences in access to care, treatment responsiveness, and adherence. Mental health parity will never be fully realized until systems of culturally sensitive care meet the needs for treatment in every community (McCarty, 2013).

PRACTICE POINT

Community health nurses should seek certification in cultural competence and incorporate the standards of cultural competence developed by SAMHSA into treatment plans and programs that provide mental health services.

PSYCHOLOGICAL FIRST AID

Populations Traumatized by Disasters

Since 1970, the incidence of natural disasters throughout the world has been rising and irrespective of the socioeconomic status of the country, lifetime exposure to natural disasters is high, ranging from 4.4% to 7.5% (Kessler, McLaughlin, Koenen, Petukhova, Hill, & The WHO World Mental Health Consortium, 2012). Globally, there were 168 natural disasters and 150 human-made disasters, resulting in 20 million fatalities, 50 million casualties, and 2000 million homeless in 2012 (Sigma, 2013). Population's hardest hit were in Asia where over 1,900 people died or were missing from Typhoon Bopha and Africa where 3 million people were displaced from floods. The same year, more than 45,000 people, the majority of whom were civilians and children, were victims of terrorist attacks with 64% of all attacks occurring in Afghanistan, Iraq, and Pakistan (U.S. Department of State, 2012).

In the United States, the incidence of natural disasters has been increasing since 1998, peaking in 2011 with 242 disaster declarations by Federal Emergency Management Administration (FEMA, 2013). Of all the natural disasters occurring in the past 5 years, Hurricane Sandy triggered the greatest response with the American Red Cross providing more than 103,000 health and emotional support visits (American Red Cross, 2012). "Rampage shootings," characterized by a male engaging in a shooting spree within institutions familiar to him, but toward victims that may be unknown, have also been increasing in the United States since the 1990s (Harris & Harris, 2012, p. 1054). Four terrorist attacks, including the First World Trade Center bombing in 1993, the Oklahoma City bombing in 1995, the 9/11 attacks in 2001, and the Boston Marathon bombing in 2013, resulted in over 3,000 deaths and 2,000 injuries to U.S. civilians (National Consortium for the Study of Terrorism and Responses to Terrorism, 2012).

Populations at Risk for Psychological Trauma

Natural and human-made disasters inflict psychological impacts on populations that are 4 to 50 times greater than the number of physical injuries (McCabe, Barnett, Taylor, & Links, 2010).

Studies of the psychological effects of disasters find considerable variation in prevalence rates among populations, ranging from 14% to 76% for prolonged grief reactions, to 5% to 68% for PTSD, and to 10% to 45% for major depression (Kristensen, Weisaeth, & Heir, 2012). Population risk factors for developing disaster-associated PTSD include female gender; older adult age; Hispanic ethnicity; lower education level; personal injury; witnessing in injury or death, especially among family or friends; and prior history of psychiatric illness, especially PTSD, major depression, or panic disorder (North, Oliver, & Pandya, 2012). Psychological harms are also greater when a community is victimized by a terrorist attack or a rampage shooting rather than a natural disaster. The challenge for public health nurses is how best to intervene to minimize psychological harms when an entire community or a population has been traumatized.

In the 1950s, the federal government requested that the APA develop guidelines for providing psychological support to communities impacted by disasters. Building on the principles of crisis intervention originated by Eric Lindeman, a brief therapeutic intervention was developed termed *psychological first aid* (Forbes, 2011). Psychological first aid is designed to be delivered by disaster relief workers, including nurses who are often on the front lines of a disaster in a variety of community-based settings.

The core features of psychological first aid are to protect, connect, and direct (Fig. 21.5). Nurses can protect victims of a disaster by, first and foremost, providing food, clothing, and shelter. **Psychological first aid** is the fundamental principles of therapeutic communication such as active listening, allowing silence, allowing the expression of emotions, and paraphrasing these reactions to convey understanding and compassion. Similar to the nursing process, the first steps of psychological first aid include assessment of physical and psychological well-being, coping skills, and social supports. Victims should be assessed for severe psychological reactions especially suicidal or homicidal ideation and directed to mental health disaster specialists.

The second stage of psychological first aid mirrors the intervention phase of the nursing process. The most immediate concern for many survivors is their desire to be reunited with friends, family, and social and spiritual supports. Connection with family and loved ones can be challenging in the aftermath of a disaster. Relief workers have developed innovative strategies to reunite families and friends as quickly as possible. Disaster mental health nurses may meet with families to gather information for the identification process in the event of death. Nurses can minimize retraumatization by limiting the number of individuals, victims and survivors, interact with to "tell their story" and the number of individuals who witness the horror of aftermath.

In the third stage of psychological first aid, nurses act as advocates and direct survivors to relief agencies. Nurses actively partner with survivors in practical problem-solving to address specific, immediate concerns. It is critical that nurses not make promises or conjecture about the

Psychological First Aid for First Responders

Information Clearinghouses

National Mental Health Information Center (NMHIC)
P.O. Box 42557, Washington, DC 20015
(800) 789-2647 (English and Español)
(866) 889-2647 (TDD)
www.mentalhealth.samhsa.gov

National Clearinghouse for Alcohol and Drug Information (NCADI)
P.O. Box 2345, Rockville, MD 20847-2345
(800) 729-6686 (English and Español)
(800) 487-4889 (TDD)
www.ncadi.samhsa.gov

Treatment Locators

Mental Health Services Locator
(800) 789-2647 (English and Español)
(866) 889-2647 (TDD)
www.mentalhealth.samhsa.gov/databases

Substance Abuse Treatment Facility Locator
(800) 662-HELP (4357) (Toll-Free, 24-Hour English and Español Treatment Referral Service)
(800) 487-4889 (TDD)
www.findtreatment.samhsa.gov

Hotlines

National Suicide Prevention Lifeline
(800) 273-TALK (8255)
(800) 799-4889 (TDD)

SAMHSA National Helpline
(800) 662-HELP (4357) (English and Español)
(800) 487-4889 (TDD)

Workplace Helpline
(800) WORKPLACE (967-5752)
www.workplace.samhsa.gov/helpline/helpline.htm

When you work with people during and after a disaster, you are working with people who may be having reactions of confusion, fear, hopelessness, sleeplessness, anxiety, grief, shock, guilt, shame, and loss of confidence in themselves and others. Your early contacts with them can help alleviate their painful emotions and promote hope and healing.

Your goal in providing this psychological first aid is to promote an environment of safety, calm, connectedness, self-efficacy, empowerment, and hope.

DO:

Promote Safety:

- Help people meet basic needs for food and shelter, and obtain emergency medical attention.
- Provide repeated, simple, and accurate information on how to get these basic needs.

Promote Calm:

- Listen to people who wish to share their stories and emotions, and remember that there is no right or wrong way to feel.
- Be friendly and compassionate even if people are being difficult.
- Offer accurate information about the disaster or trauma, and the relief efforts underway to help victims understand the situation.

Promote Connectedness:

- Help people contact friends and loved ones.
- Keep families together. Keep children with parents or other close relatives whenever possible.

Promote Self-Efficacy:

- Give practical suggestions that steer people toward helping themselves.
- Engage people in meeting their own needs.

Promote Help:

- Find out the types and locations of government and nongovernment services and direct people to those services that are available.
- When they express fear or worry, remind people (if you know) that more help and services are on the way.

DO NOT:

- Force people to share their stories with you, especially very personal details.
- Give simple reassurances like "everything will be OK" or "at least you survived."
- Tell people what you think they should be feeling, thinking, or how they should have acted earlier.
- Tell people why you think they have suffered by alluding to personal behaviors or beliefs of victims.
- Make promises that may not be kept.
- Criticize existing services or relief activities in front of people in need of these services.[1]

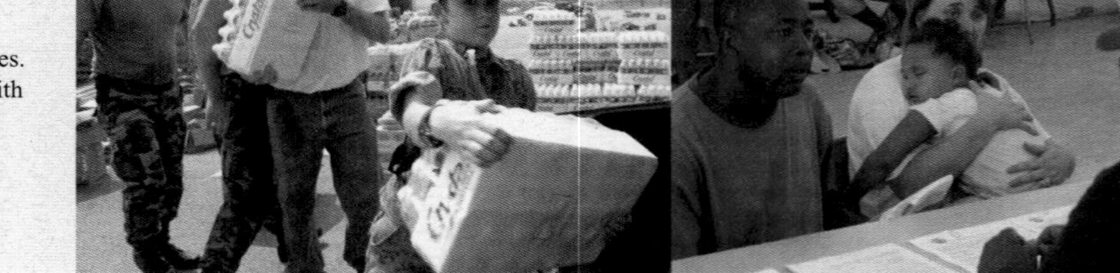

figure 21.5 SAMSHA psychological first aid for first responders.
Source: SAMHSA psychological first aid for first responders: Tips for emergency and disaster workers. U.S. Department of Health and Human Services. NMH05-0210. Washington, DC: U.S. Government Printing Office. Retrieved May 29, 2013, from http://store.samhsa.gov/shin/content/NMH05-0210/NMH05-0210.pdf

availability of resources. Information to survivors must be credible, culturally and linguistically appropriate, timely, and specific as to where and when resources may arrive, such as transportation, assistance for dependents, medical care, or housing. During this stage, nurses provide psychoeducation on bereavement for individuals, families, and communities who are coping with multiple losses.

Families, survivors, and first responders benefit from education about expected behavioral responses to avoid pathologizing normal grief reactions. Expected psychological reactions may include guilt or shame, anger, frequent crying or blunting of emotions, difficulty concentrating, uncharacteristic social isolation, and inability to forget sensory images of trauma. Expected physical reactions may include headaches, fatigue, gastrointestinal disturbance, pain, disrupted sleep, and disrupted eating (too much or too little). Deep breathing, yoga, prayer, and spiritual reflection can help diminish anxiety for those exhibiting expected psychological responses. As much as possible, encourage individuals to engage in group activities to facilitate social cohesion, hope, and resilience.

Survivors or first responders experiencing moderate to severe psychological reactions, including suicidal or homicidal ideation, should be directed to disaster mental health specialists. Moderate psychological reactions include nightmares, intrusive daytime images, bodily sensations related to traumatic experience, excessive physical startle reflex, extreme anxiety alternating with numbing, and difficulty modulating anger. Cognitive behavioral therapies are evidence-based interventions that can help individuals cope with the moderate symptoms of emotional distress (Everly, Barnett, & Links, 2012). Symptoms of major mental illness such as dissociation, panic attacks, agoraphobia, depression or substance abuse, in addition to the inability to perform basic self-care, or threats of violence against others or self would warrant immediate emergency treatment.

In disasters, ordinary people emerge as innovative problem-solvers who are responsive to the needs of others around them. This prosocial response has been documented by researchers over several decades in countless disasters and highlights the resilience of communities even in the face of horrific traumatic events (McCabe et al., 2012). Resilience is built on the self and community perception of having the ability to cope and respond flexibly to the unexpected. Faith-based organizations, social clubs, and local schools are a few of the indigenous community supports that provide extraordinary services in disasters and are vital to long-term psychological recovery (McCabe, Perry, Azur, Taylor, Bailey, & Links, 2011) (Table 21.4).

EVIDENCE FOR PRACTICE

In 2009, a scientific review by the Advisory Council to the American Red Cross determined that psychological first aid was an evidenced-informed intervention that can be used effectively by trained volunteers to address the basic needs of individuals in the immediate aftermath of a disaster (Fox, Burkle, Bass, Pia, Epstein, & Markenson, 2012). The same year, the WHO Mental Health Guidelines Development Group concluded that psychological first aid, and not psychological debriefing, should be provided to populations impacted by disaster (WHO, 2011) (Box 21.3). The U.S. Medical Reserve Corps training manual on psychological first aid (Brymer et al., 2006) and the WHO state there is insufficient evidence on the efficacy of debriefing and caution there is a risk that the systematic ventilation of feelings maybe triggering and hinder, rather than support, the recovery of survivors and first responders.

box 21.3 WHO Psychological First Aid in Different Cultures

Consider the Following Questions as You Prepare to Offer PFA in Different Cultures:

Dress	Do I need to dress a certain way to be respectful? Will impacted people be in need of certain clothing items to keep their dignity and customs?
Language	What is the customary way of greeting people in this culture? What language do they speak?
Gender, Age and Power	Should affected women only be approached by women helpers? Who may I approach? (In other words, the head of the family or community?)
Touching and Behaviour	What are the usual customs around touching people? Is it all right to hold someone's hand or touch their shoulder? Are there special things to consider in terms of behaviour around the elderly, children, women or others?
Beliefs and Religion	Who are the different ethnic and religious groups among the affected people? What beliefs of practices are important to the people affected? How might they understand of explain what has happened?

Source: World Health Organization. (2011). *Psychological first aid: Guide for field workers.* War Trauma Foundation and World Vision International, Geneva: WHO. Retrieved May 28, 2013, from: http://whqlibdoc.who.int/publications/2011/9789241548205_eng.pdf

table 21.4 **Evidence-Based Psychological Interventions for Mass Casualties**

Phase	Preincident	Impact (0–48 hours)	Rescue (0–1 week)	Recovery (1–4 weeks)	Return to life (2 weeks–2 years)
Goals	Preparation, improve coping	Survival, communication	Adjustment	Appraisal/planning	Reintegration
Behavior	Preparation vs. denial	Fight/flight, freeze, surrender, etc.	Resilience vs. exhaustion	Grief, reappraisal, intrusive memories, narrative formation	Adjustment vs. phobias, post-traumatic stress disorder, avoidance, depression, etc.
Role of all helpers	Prepare, train, gain knowledge	Rescue, protect	Orient, provide for needs	Respond with sensitivity	Continue assistance
Role of mental health professionals	**Prepare** TrainGain knowledgeCollaborateInform and influence policySet structures for rapid assistance	**Basic Needs** Establish safety/security/survival Ensure food and shelter Provide orientationFacilitate communication with family, friends, and community Assess the environment for ongoing threat/toxin **Psychological First Aid** Support and "presence" for those who are most distressed Keep families together and facilitate reunion with loved ones Provide information and education (i.e., services), foster communication Protect survivors from further harm Reduce physiological arousal **Monitoring the Impact on Environment** Observe and listen to those most affected Monitor the environment for stressors **Technical Assistance, Consultation, and Training** Improve capacity of organizations and caregivers to provide what is needed to reestablish community structure, foster family recovery/resilience, and safeguard the communityProvide to relevant organizationsother caregivers and responders leaders	**Needs Assessment** Assess current status, how well needs are being addressed Recovery environment What additional interventions are needed for Group Population IndividualTriage Clinical assessment Refer when indicatedIdentify vulnerable, high-risk individuals and groups Emergency hospitalization or outpatient treatment **Outreach and Information Dissemination** Make contact with and identify people who have not requested services (i.e., "therapy by walking around") **Outreach and Information Dissemination** Inform people about different services, coping, recovery process, etc. (e.g., by using established community structures, fliers, web sites) **Fostering Resilience and Recovery** Social interactions Coping skills training Education about stress response, traumatic reminders, coping, normal vs. abnormal functioning, risk factors, services Group and family support Foster natural social supportLook after the bereaved Repair organizational fabric Operational debriefings, when this is standing procedure in responder organizations Spiritual support	**Monitor the Recovery Environment** Observe and listen to those most affected Monitor the environment for toxins Monitor past and ongoing threats Monitor services that are being provided	**Treatment** Reduce or ameliorate symptoms or improve functioning via • Individual, family, and group psychotherapy • Pharmacotherapy • Short-term or long-term hospitalization

Source: National Institute of Mental Health. (2002). Mental health and mass violence: Evidence-based early psychological interventions for victims/survivors of mass violence. A workshop to reach consensus on best practices (NIH Publication No. 02-5138). Washington, DC: U.S. Government Printing Office.

key concepts

- Genetic, biologic, and environmental risk factors all influence the incidence of mental illness.
- Early intervention can minimize the morbidity associated with mental illness.
- Adherence to psychopharmacology and psychotherapy enhances recovery from mental illness.
- The continuum of care for the chronic mentally ill includes community services, such as supportive housing and employment.
- Public health initiatives to educate communities about mental health can be effective in lowering the incidence of high-risk behaviors such as suicide.
- Psychological first aid is recommended to help support survivors and first responders to natural and intentional disasters.

critical thinking questions

You are a school nurse in a middle school when Jamal comes to the nurse's office requesting medication for a headache. You notice that his eyes are red, and it appears as if he has been crying. You ask if he is hurt, but he denies it. The phone rings in the office, and a teacher tells you that a female student has approached her concerned about Jamal. The teacher tells you that Jamal sent her a text message saying that he flunked his biology examination and wished he was dead.

1. What is the most immediate nursing assessment that should be evaluated?
2. If Jamal is hesitant to share his thoughts with you, what could you say or do to develop a therapeutic alliance?
3. What other collateral sources of information would you contact to evaluate the risk of suicide associated with the text message? Would you leave Jamal alone to discuss the situation with other colleagues?
4. If Jamal shared with you a suicide plan that including harming himself with a weapon, what would be your first nursing intervention?
5. If you determined Jamal was at risk for self-harm, to whom would you refer Jamal?
6. How would you continue to assess Jamal's mental health while he was a student in the middle school?
7. How might health insurance, transportation, and family circumstances influence Jamal's ability to access mental health services?
8. What educational program would you develop for the middle school to educate students about ways to cope with stress and how to respond if a friend needs support?

community resources

- Local public health departments
- Town and county departments of human services
- Community homeless shelters
- Community mental health organizations
- Community public schools

references

Alegria, M., Lin, J., Chen, C. N., Duan, N., Cook, B., & Meng, X. L. (2012). The impact of insurance coverage in diminishing racial and ethnic disparities in behavioral health services. *Health Services Research*, *47*(3, Pt. 2),1322–1344. doi:10.1111/j.1475-6773.2012.01403.x

American Psychiatric Association. (2004). *Practice guidelines for the treatment of psychiatric disorders, compendium 2004*. Arlington, VA: American Psychiatric Association.

American Psychiatric Association. (2013). *Diagnostic and statistical manual of mental disorders*. (5th ed.). Arlington, VA: American Psychiatric Publishing.

American Red Cross. (2012, December 19). *Red Cross recovery efforts to help Sandy survivors*. Retrieved May 25, 2013, from http://www.redcross.org/news/article/Red-Cross-Recovery-Efforts-to-Help-Sandy-Survivors

Amminger, G. P., Leicester, S., Yung, A. R., Phillips, L. J., Berger, G. E., Francey, S. M., … McGorry, P. D. (2006). Early-onset of symptoms predicts conversion to non-affective psychosis in ultra-high risk individuals. *Schizophrenia Research*, *84*(1), 67–76.

Atladóttir, H. O., Henriksen, T. B., Schendel, D. E., & Parner, E. T. (2012). Autism after infection, febrile episodes, and antibiotic use during pregnancy: An exploratory study. *Pediatrics*, *130*(6), e1447–e1454.

Beebe, L. H. (2007). Beyond the prescription pad: Psychosocial treatments for individuals with schizophrenia. *Journal of Psychosocial Nursing and Mental Health Services*, *45*(3), 35–43.

Blumberg, S. J., Bramlett, M. D., Kogan, M. D., Schieve, L. A., Jones, J. R., & Lu, M. C. (2013). Changes in prevalence of parent-reported autism spectrum disorder in school-aged U.S. children:

references (continued)

2007 to 2011–2012. *National Health Statistics Reports, 65*. Hyattsville, MD: National Center for Health Statistics.

Brymer, M., Jacobs, A., Layne, C., Pynoos, R., Ruzek, J., Steinberg, A., Watson, P. (2006). *Psychological First Aid: Medical reserve corps field operations guide*. Washington, DC: National Child Traumatic Stress and Network National Center for PTSD. Retrieved November 18, 2014 from: http://www.naccho.org/topics/emergency/MRC/resources/upload/MRC-PFA-Field-Operations-Guide.pdf

Byerly, J. J., Nakonezny, P. A., & Lescouflair, E. (2007). Antipsychotic medication adherence in schizophrenia. *Psychiatric Clinics of North America, 30*(3), 437–452.

Centers for Disease Control and Prevention. (2013a). Suicide among adults aged 35–64 Years—United States, 1999–2010. *Morbidity and Mortality Weekly Report, 62*(17), 321–342.

Centers for Disease Control and Prevention. (2013b). Mental health surveillance among children—United States, 2005–2011. *Morbidity and Mortality Weekly Report, Supplement, 62*(2), 1–32.

Charles, J. M., Carpenter, L. A., Jenner, W., & Nicholas, J. S. (2008). Recent advances in autism spectrum disorders. *International Journal of Psychiatry in Medicine, 38*(2), 133–140.

Chase, P., & Leboyer, M. (2012). Autism risk factors: Genes, environment and gene-environment interactions. *Dialogues in Clinical Neuroscience, 14*(3), 281 -292.

Claassen, D. (2007). Financial incentives for antipsychotic depot medication: Ethical issues. *Journal of Medical Ethics, 33*(4), 189–193.

Clarke, M. C., Kelleher, I., Clancy, M., & Cannon, M. (2012). Predicting risk and the emergence of schizophrenia. *The Psychiatric Clinics of North America, 35*(3), 585–612. doi:10.1016/j.psc.2012.06.003

Cohen, A., Patel, V., Thara, R., & Gureje, O. (2008). Questioning an axiom: Better prognosis for schizophrenia in the developing world? *Schizophrenia Bulletin, 34*(2), 229–244.

Craig, T. J., Siegel, C., Hopper, K., Lin, S., & Sartorius, N. (1997). Outcome in schizophrenia and related disorders compared between developing and developed countries: A recursive partitioning re-analysis of the WHP SOSMD data. *British Journal of Psychiatry, 170*, 229–233.

Croen, L. A., Grether, J. K., Yoshida, C. K., Odouli, R., & Hendrick, V. (2011). Antidepressant use during pregnancy and childhood autism spectrum disorders. *Archives of General Psychiatry, 68*(11), 1104 -1112.

Dixon, L., & Goldman, H. (2004). Forty years of progress in community mental health: The role of evidence-based practices. *Administration and Policy in Mental Health and Mental Health Services Research, 31*(5), 381–392.

Doughtery, R. H. (2004). Reducing disparity in behavioral health services: A report from the American College of Mental Health Administration. *Administration and Policy in Mental Health, 31*(3), 253–270.

Duchan, E., & Patel, D. R. (2012). Epidemiology of autism spectrum disorders. *Pediatric Clinics North America, 59*(1), 27 -43.

Durkheim, E. (1972). *Selected writings* [Introduction by A. Giddens]. New York, NY: Cambridge University Press.

Durkin, M. (2009). Advancing parental age and the risk of autism spectrum disorder. *The American Journal of Epidemiology, 168*(11), 1268–1276.

Durkin, M. S., Maenner, M. J., Meaney, F. J., Levy, S. E., DiGuiseppi, C., Nicholas, J. S., … Schieve, L. A. (2010). Socioeconomic inequality in the prevalence of autism spectrum disorder: Evidence from a U.S. cross-sectional study. *PLOS ONE 5*(7), e11551. doi:10.1371/journal.pone.0011551

Elsabbagh, M., Divan, G., Koh, Y., Kim, Y. S., Kauchali, S., Marcin, C., … Fombonne, E. (2012). Global prevalence of autism and other pervasive developmental disorders. *Autism Research, 5*, 160–179.

Everly, G. A., Barnett, D. J., & Links, J. M. (2012). The Johns Hopkins model of psychological first aid (RAPID-PFA): Curriculum development and content validation. *International Journal of Emergency Mental Health, 14*(2), 95–103.

Faedda, G. L., Baldessarini, R. J., Glovinsky, I. P., & Austin, N. B. (2004). Pediatric bipolar disorder: Phenomenology and course of illness. *Bipolar Disorders, 6*(5), 305–313.

Feldman, S. (2004). Reflections on the 40th anniversary of the Community Mental Health Centers Act. *Administration and Policy in Mental Health and Mental Health Services Research, 31*(5), 369–380.

Federal Emergency ManagementAdministration. (2013). *Disaster declarations by year*. Retrieved May 25, 2013, from http://www.fema.gov/disasters/grid/year

Fleegler, E. W., Lee, L. K., Monuteaux, M. C., Hemenway, D., & Mannix, R. (2013). Firearm legislation and firearm-related fatalities in the United States. *Journal of the American Medical Association Internal Medecine, 173*(9), 732–740. doi:10.1001/jamainternmed.2013.1286

Forbes, D., Lewis, V., Varker, T., Phelps, A., O'Donnell, M., Wade, D. J. . . . Creamer, M. (2011). Psychological first aid following trauma: Implementation and evaluation framework for high-risk organizations. *Psychiatry, 74*(3), 224 -239.

Fox, J. H., Burkle, F. M., Bass, J., Pia, F. A., Epstein, J. L., & Markenson, D. (2012). The effectiveness of psychological first aid as a disaster intervention tool: Research analysis of peer reviewed literature from 1990–2010. *Disaster Med Public Health Preparedness, 6*, 247–252.

Geller, J. L. (2000). The last half-century of psychiatric services as reflected in Psychiatric Services. *Psychiatric Services, 51*(1), 41–67.

Glazer, W. M. (2007). The depot paradox. *Behavioral Healthcare, 27*(5), 44–46.

Goldston, D. B., Molock, S. D., Whitbeck, L. B., Murakami, J. L., Zayas, L. H., & Hall, G. C. (2008). Cultural considerations in adolescent suicide prevention and psychosocial treatment. *The American Psychologist, 63*(1), 14–31.

Goodwin, R. D., Beautrais, A. L., & Fergusson, D. M. (2004). Familial transmission of suicidal ideation and suicide attempts: Evidence from a general population sample. *Psychiatry Research, 126*(2), 159–165.

Grant, B. F., Stinson, F. S., Dawson, D. A., Chou, S. P., Dufour, M. C. Compton, W., … Kaplan, K. (2004). Prevalence and co-occurrence of substance use disorders and independent mood and anxiety disorders: Results from the National Epidemiologic Survey on Alcohol and Related Conditions. *Archives of General Psychiatry, 61*(8), 807–816.

Guevara, J. P., Mandell, D. S., Rostain, A. L., Zhao, H., & Hadley, T. R. (2003). National estimates of health services expenditures for children with behavioral disorders: An analysis of the Medical Expenditure Panel Survey. *Pediatrics, 112*(6), 440–446.

Guy, W. (1976). *ECDEU assessment manual for psychopharmacology: Revised* (DHEW publication number ADM 76-338). Rockville, MD: U.S. Department of Health, Education and Welfare, Public Health Service, Alcohol, Drug Abuse and Mental Health Administration, NIMH Psychopharmacology Research Branch, Division of Extramural Research Programs.

Halfon, N., & Kuo, A. A. (2013). What DSM-5 could mean to children with autism and their families. *Journal of the American Medical Association Pediatrics*. Advance online publication. doi:10.1001/jamapediatrics.2013.2188

Harris, J. M., & Harris, R. B. (2012). Rampage violence requires a new type of research. *American Journal of Public Health, 102*(6), 1054–1057.

Hunkeler, E. M., Fireman, B., Lee, J., Diamond, R., Hamilton, J., He, C. X., … Hargreaves W. A. (2005). Trends in use of antidepressants, lithium and anticonvulsants in Kaiser Permanente-insured youths, 1994–2003. *Journal of Child and Adolescent Psychopharmacology*, *15*(1), 26–37.

Hwang, W.-C., Myers, H. F., Abe-Kim, J., & Ting, J. Y. (2008). A conceptual paradigm for understanding culture's impact on mental health: The cultural influences on mental health (CIMH) model. *Clinical Psychology Review*, *28*(2), 211–227.

Iglehart, J. K. (2004). Mental health maze and the call for transformation. *New England Journal of Medicine*, *350*(5), 507–514.

Interagency Autism Coordinating Committee. (2012, December). *IACC strategic plan for autism spectrum disorder (ASD) research—2012 update*. Washington, DC: U.S. Department of Health and Human Services. Retrieved May 27, 2013, from http://iacc.hhs.gov/strategic-plan/2012/index.shtml

Joe, S., Canetto, S. S., & Romer, D. (2008). Advancing prevention research on the role of culture in suicide prevention. *Suicide and Life Threatening Behavior*, *38*(3), 354–362.

Johnston, L. D., O'Malley, P. M., Bachman, J. G., & Schulenberg, J. E. (2005). *Monitoring the future national results on adolescent drug use: Overview of key findings*, 1975 -2004. Bethesda MD: National Institute on Drug Abuse.

Kessler, R. C., & Wang, P. S. (2008). The descriptive epidemiology of commonly occurring mental disorders in the United States. *Annual Review of Public Health*, *29*, 115–129.

Kessler, R. C., Angermeyer, M., Anthony, J. C., De Graaf, R., Demyttenaere, K., Gasquet, I., … Üstün, T. B. (2007). Lifetime prevalence and age of onset distributions of mental disorders in the World Health Organization's World Mental Health Survey Initiative. *World Psychiatry*, *6*(3), 168–176.

Kessler, R. C., McLaughlin, K. A., Koenen, K. C., Petukhova, M., Hill, E. D., & The WHO World Mental Health Survey Consortium. (2012). The importance of secondary trauma exposure for post-disaster mental disorder. *Epidemiology and Psychiatric Sciences*, *21*(1), 35–45.

Kim, B., Lee, S. H., Yang, Y. K., Park, J. I., & Chung, Y. C. (2012). Long-acting injectable antipsychotics for first-episode schizophrenia: The pros and cons. *Schizophrenia Research and Treatment*. Advance online publication. doi:10.1155/2012/560836

Knox, K. L., Conwell, Y., & Caine, E. D. (2004). If suicide is a public health problem, what are we doing to prevent it? *American Journal of Public Health*, *94*(1), 37–45.

Kong, A., Frigge, M. L., Masson, G., Besenbacher, S., Sulem, P., & Magnusson, G., … Stefansson, K. (2012). Rate of de novo mutations and the importance of father's age to disease risk. *Nature*, *488*(7412), 471–475.

Kristensen, P., Weisaeth, L., & Heir, T. (2012). Bereavement and mental health after sudden and violent losses: A review. *Psychiatry*, *75*(1), 76–97.

Leibenluft, E., & Rich, B. A. (2008). Pediatric bipolar disorder. *Annual Review of Clinical Psychology*, *4*, 163–187.

Lesesne, C. A., Visser, S. N., & White, C. P. (2003). Attention-deficit/hyperactivity disorder in school-aged children: Association with maternal mental health and use of health care resources. *Pediatrics*, *111*(5), 1232–1237.

Levine, S. Z., Rabinowitz, J., Faries, D., Lawson, A. H., & Ascher-Svanum H. (2012). Treatment response trajectories and antipsychotic medications: Examination of up to 18 months of treatment in the CATIE chronic schizophrenia trial. *Schizophrenia Research*, *137*(1–3), 141–146. Retrieved from http://dx.doi.org.proxy.bc.edu/10.1016/j.schres.2012.01.014

Lewin Group. (2000). *Access and utilization of new antidepressant and antipsychotic medications* [Submitted to: The Office of the Assistant Secretary for Planning and Evaluation and The National Institute of Mental Health, U. S. Department of Health and Human Services]. Washington, DC: Government Printing Office.

Mark, T. L., Vandivort-Warren, R., & Miller, K. (2012). Mental health spending by private insurance: Implications for the mental health parity and addiction equity act. *Psychiatric Services*, *63*(4), 313–318. doi:10.1176/appi.ps.201100312

Marshall, M., & Lockwood, A. (2005). Early intervention for psychosis. In *The Cochrane Collaboration*. New York, NY: John Wiley.

McCabe, O. L., Barnett, D. J., Taylor, H. G., & Links, J. M. (2010). Ready, willing, and able: A framework for improving the Public Health Emergency Preparedness System. *Disaster Medicine and Public Health Preparedness*, *4*, 161–168.

McCabe, O. L., Marum, F., Mosley, A., Gwon, H. S., Langlieb, A., Everly, G. S., … Links, J. M. (2012). Community capacity building in disaster mental health resilience: A pilot study of an academic/faith partnership model. *International Journal of Emergency Mental Health*, *14*(2), 112–122.

McCabe, O. L., Perry, C., Azur, M., Taylor, H. G., Bailey, M., & Links, J. M. (2011). Psychological first-aid training for paraprofessionals: A systems-based model for enhancing capacity of rural emergency responses. *Prehospital and Disaster Medicine*, *26*(4): 251–258.

McCarty, D. (2013). Parity: An ongoing challenge and research opportunity. *American Journal of Psychiatry*, *170*(2),140–142. doi:10.1176/appi.ajp.2012.12101334

Melzer, D., Fryers, T., & Jenkins, R. (2004). *Social inequalities and the distribution of the common mental disorders*. New York, NY: Psychology Press.

Messias, E. L., Chen, C. Y., & Eaton, W. W. (2007). Epidemiology of schizophrenia: Review of findings and myths. *Psychiatric Clinics of North America*, *30*(3), 323–338.

Miller, M., & Hemenway, D. (2008). Guns and suicide in the United States. *New England Journal of Medicine*, *359*(10), 989–991.

Miller, M., Azrael, D., & Hemenway, D. (2004). The epidemiology of case fatality rates for suicide in the northeast. *Annals of Emergency Medicine*, *43*(6), 723–730.

Miller, T. J., McGlashan, T. H., Rosen, J. L., Somjee, L., Markovich, P. J., Stein, K., & Woods, S. W. (2002). Prospective diagnosis of the initial prodrome for schizophrenia based on the structured interview for prodromal syndromes: Preliminary evidence of interrater reliability and predictive validity. *American Journal of Psychiatry*, *159*, 863–865.

Morton, N. K., & Zubek, D. (2013). Adherence challenges and long-acting injectable antipsychotic treatment in patients with schizophrenia. *Journal of Psychosocial Nursing*, *51*(3), 13–18.

Mueser, K. T., Deavers, F., Penn, D. L., & Cassisi, J. E. (2013). Psychosocial treatments for schizophrenia. *Annual Review of Clinical Psychology*, *9*, 465–497.

Mueser, K.T., & McGurk, S. R. (2004). Schizophrenia. *The Lancet*, (363), 2063 -2072.

Murray, C. J. L., Vos, T., Lozano, R., Naghavi, M., Flaxman, A. D., Michaud, C., … Memish, Z. A. (2012). Disability-adjusted life years (DALYs) for 291 diseases and injuries in 21 regions, 1990–2010: A systematic analysis for the Global Burden of Disease Study 2010. *Lancet*, *380*, 2197–2223.

Narayan, V. A., Mohwinckel, M., Pisano, G., Yang, M., & Manji, H. K. (2013). Beyond magic bullets: True innovation in health care. *Nature Reviews. Drug Discovery*, *12*, 85–86. doi:10.1038/nrd394

Nardi, D., Waite, R., & Killian, P. (2012). Establishing standards for culturally competent mental health care. *Journal of Psychosocial Nursing and Mental Health Services*, *50*(7), 3–5. doi:10.3928/02793695-20120608-0

National Consortium for the Study of Terrorism and Responses to Terrorism. (2012). *Global terrorism database 1993–2012*. Retrieved May 25, 2013, from http://www.start.umd.edu/gtd

National Institute on Drug Abuse. (2014). *High school and youth trends*. Retrieved on November 18, 2014 from: http://www.drugabuse.gov/sites/default/files/drugfactsmtf.pdf

references (continued)

Neighbors, H. W., Caldwell, C., Williams, D. R., Nesse, R., Taylor, R. J., Bullard, K. M., … Jackson, J. S. (2007). Race, ethnicity and the use of services for mental disorders: Results from the National Survey of American Life. *Archives of General Psychiatry, 64*(4), 485–494.

Newman, S., & Goldman, H. (2008). Putting housing first, making housing last: Housing policy for persons with severe mental illness. *American Journal of Psychiatry, 165*(10), 1242–1248.

North, C. S., Oliver, J., & Pandya, A. (2012). Examining a comprehensive model of disaster-related posttraumatic stress disorder in systematically studied survivors of 10 disasters. *American Journal of Public Health, 102*(10), e40–e48. doi:10.2105/AJPH.2012.300689

Ormel, J., Petukhova, M., Chatterji, S., Aguilar-Gaxiola, S., Alonso, J., Angermeyer, M. C., … Kessler, R. C. (2008). Disability and treatment of specific mental and physical disorders across the world. *British Journal of Psychiatry, 192*, 368–375.

Patel, V., Flisher, A. J., Hetrick, S., McGorry, P. (2007). Mental health of young people: A global public-health challenge. *The Lancet, 369*(9569), 1302–1313.

Pekkala, E., & Merinder, L. (2005). Psychoeducation for schizophrenia [Review]. In *The Cochrane Collaboration*. New York, NY: John Wiley.

President's New Freedom Commission on Mental Health. (2003). *Achieving the promise: Transforming mental health care in America* (Final Report. No. SMA-03-3832). Rockville, MD: Department of Health and Human Services.

President's New Freedom Commission on Mental Health (2003). Retrieved on November 18, 2014 from: http://govinfo.library.unt.edu/mentalhealthcommission/reports/FinalReport/downloads/FinalReport.pdf

Rejas, J., Bobes, J., Arango, C., Aranda, P., Carmena, R., & Garcia-Garcia, M. (2008). Concordance of standard and modified NCEP ATPII criteria for identification of metabolic syndrome in outpatients with schizophrenia treated with antipsychotics: A corollary from the CLAMORS study. *Schizophrenia Research, 99*(1), 23–28.

Sigma. (2013, February). *Natural catastrophes and manmade disasters in 2012: A year of extreme weather events in the US* (No. 2). Zurich, Switzerland: Swiss Re Ltd. Retrieved from http://media.swissre.com/documents/sigma2_2013_EN.pdf

Skafidas, E., Testa, R., Zantomio, D., Chana, G., Everall, I. P., & Pantelis, C. (2012). Predicting the diagnosis of autism spectrum disorder using gene pathway analysis. *Molecular Psychiatry, 19*(4), 504–510. doi:10.1038/mp.2012.126

Tandon, R., Belmaker, R. H., Gattaz, W. F., Lopez-Ibor, J. J., Jr., Okasha, A., Singh, B., … Section of Pharmacopsychiatry, World Psychiatric Association. (2008). World Psychiatric Association Pharmacopsychiatry Section statement on comparative effectiveness of antipsychotics in the treatment of schizophrenia. *Schizophrenia Research, 100*(1–3), 20–38. doi:10.1016/j.schres.2007.11.033

Thornicroft, G. (2007). Most people with mental illness are not treated. *The Lancet, 370*(9590), 807–808.

Tyrer, P., Coid, J., Simmonds, S., Joseph, P., & Marriott, S. (2005). Community mental health teams (CMHTs) for people with severe mental illnesses and disordered personality [Review]. In *The Cochrane Collaboration*. New York, NY: John Wiley.

U.S. Department of Health and Human Services. (1999). *Mental health: A report of the Surgeon General*. U.S. Department of Health and Human Services, Substance Abuse and Mental Health Services Administration, Center for Mental Health Services, National Institutes of Health, National Institute of Mental Health.

U.S. Department of Health and Human Services. (2012, September). Office of the Surgeon General and National Action Alliance for Suicide Prevention. *National Strategy for Suicide Prevention: Goals and Objectives for Action*. Washington, DC: Author.

U.S. Department of State. (2012). National Counterterrorism Center: Annex of Statistical Information. Office of the Coordinator for Counterterrorism. *Country reports on terrorism, 2011*. Retrieved May 25, 2013, from http://www.state.gov/j/ct/rls/crt/2011/195555.htm

Wang, P. S., Aguilar-Gaxiola, S., Alonso, J., Angermeyer, M. C., Borges, G., Bromet, E. J., … Wells, J. E. (2007). Use of mental health services for anxiety, mood, and substance disorders in 17 countries in the WHO world mental health surveys. *Lancet, 370*(9590), 841–850.

Weller, L., Fredrickson, D. D., Burbach, C., Molgaard, C. A., & Ngong, L. (2004). Chronic diseases medication administration rates in a public school system. *Journal of School Health, 74*(5), 161–165.

World Health Organization. (2008). *Mental Health Gap Action Programme: Scaling up care for mental, neurological, and substance use disorders*. Geneva: Author.

World Health Organization. (2010). *mhGAP intervention guide for mental, neurological and substance use disorders in non-specialized health settings: Mental Health Gap Action Programme (mhGAP)*. Geneva: Author.

World Health Organization. (2011). *Psychological first aid: Guide for field workers*. Geneva: Author.

World Health Organization. (2012). *Public health action for the prevention of suicide*. Geneva: Author.

Yung, A. R., McGorry, P. D., Francey, S. M., Nelson, B., Baker, K., Phillips, L. J., … Amminger, G. P. (2007). PACE: A specialised service for young people at risk of psychotic disorders. *Medical Journal of Australia, 187*(Suppl. 7), S43–S46.

Zauszniewski, J. A., Bekhet, A. K., & Suresky, M. K. (2008). Factors associated with perceived burden, resourcefulness and quality of life in female family members of adults with serious mental illness. *Journal of the American Psychiatric Nurses Association, 14*(2), 125–135.

Zhang, J., McKeown, R. E., Hussey, J. R., Thompson, S. J., & Woods, J. R. (2005). Gender differences in risk factors for attempted suicide among young adults: Findings from the Third National Health and Nutrition Examination Survey. *Annals of Epidemiology, 15*(2): 167–174.

web resources

Please visit thePoint® for up-to-date web resources on this topic.

CHAPTER 22

School Health

Pamela DiNapoli

Computers are useless. They can only give you answers.

Pablo Picasso

Education is what remains after one has forgotten what one has learned in school.

Albert Einstein

Home computers are being called upon to perform many new functions, including the consumption of homework formerly eaten by the dog.

Doug Larson

chapter highlights

- Historical perspectives of school health
- Components and organization of school health programs
- School health scope of services
- Health assessment and screening of school-aged children
- Development, implementation, and evaluation of preventive health programs
- Common health concerns in schools

objectives

- Trace the history of school health practice.
- Explain the scope of the school nurse's role in the provision of healthcare.
- Identify useful sources for tracking epidemiology of common health concerns.
- Use best practice guidelines to address common preventable health concerns of the student population.

key term

Americans with Disabilities Act (ADA): Wide-ranging federal legislation enacted in 1990 that is intended to make American society more accessible to people with disabilities.

Coordinated School Health: A systematic approach to school health recommended by CDC as a strategy for improving students' health and learning in the nation's schools.

Community school model: Collaborative design that uses the resources of a community to provide structured preventive services such as after-school programs, parent outreach, and crisis intervention.

Council on School Health: Coalition of a wide range of community stakeholders, including family and student representatives, who contribute to the development of action plans designed to improve the health and safety of the students.

Cyberbullying: Any kind of repeated aggression perpetrated through information technology, such as the Internet, to intentionally harm or harass another individual.

Early Periodic Screening, Diagnosis, and Treatment (EPSDT): Program mandated by a federal law passed in 1969 that required that children and adolescents younger than 21 have access to periodic screenings.

FAAMA: Food Allergy and Anaphylaxis Management Act: Requires the U.S. Secretary of Health and Human Services to develop and make available to schools a voluntary policy to manage the risk of food allergy and anaphylaxis in schools and provide for school-based food allergy management incentive grants to support implementation of food allergy management guidelines in public schools.

Individual Education Plan (IEP): A plan developed by a multidisciplinary team to provide education and services to any student that has an identified disability to correspond with individual needs in the least restrictive environment.

Individuals with Disabilities Education Act (IDEA): Federal law enacted in 1990 and reauthorized in 1997, designed to protect the rights of students with disabilities by ensuring that everyone receives a free appropriate public education, regardless of ability. IDEA strives to grant equal access to students with disabilities and to provide additional special education services and procedural safeguards.

School Health Index: Is an online self-assessment and planning tool that schools can use to improve their health and safety policies and programs.

School health nursing: Specialized practice of nursing that integrates wellness, safety, growth, learning, and development in the lives of school-aged children and adolescents within the context of their school, and with the coordinated alliance of the family and the medical home.

Youth Risk Behavior Surveillance Survey (YRBSS): Biannual report of the common risk behaviors that influence the health of youth in the United States.

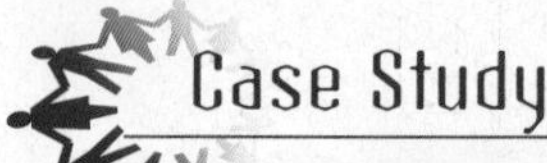

Case Study

References to the case study are found throughout this chapter (look for the case study icon). Readers should keep the case study in mind as they read the chapter.

Susan is the school nurse in a rural elementary school for children in kindergarten through grade 5. The school has approximately 300 students, who present Susan with many challenges. One, a child with special health needs, is in a wheelchair, is catheterized twice a day while at school, and receives a tube feeding at lunch. Two children who have type 1 diabetes—one requires blood sugar monitoring and insulin injections at a minimum of once daily, while the other has a continuous insulin pump. Several children have allergies ranging from severe peanut allergies to bee stings. In addition, Susan administers daily medications to 18 students at various times; these medications include methylphenidate (Ritalin), gabapentin (Neurontin), carbamazepine (Carbatrol), and Lactaid.

Susan uses a computerized database to track the visits of the children to her office, which average 30 per day. Reasons for visits include playground injuries and acute illnesses with symptoms such as vomiting, fever, or headache.

Many people outside of the school environment have little understanding of the varied roles and responsibilities of the school nurse. Currently, there are well over 75,000 licensed professionals providing healthcare in the school environment in the United States (HRSA, 2010). The role of the school nurse, first introduced in the early 1900s, has changed dramatically over the years. These changes closely parallel the increasing number of complex health issues being seen within the school system. Although the school nurse is often seen merely as someone who simply applies adhesive bandages or one who is a parent substitute for children having difficulty adjusting to the school setting, the role of the school nurse has evolved to where it is now recognized as a specialty area in nursing. The scope of the role in promoting wellness includes administrative, educational, clerical, and supportive responsibilities, along with encouragement of school wellness policies such as physical activity in daily practice (Avery, Johnson, Cousins, & Hamilton, 2013). This chapter describes **school health nursing** and illustrates how the school nurse has become a cornerstone in providing healthcare and health promotion to school-aged children and their families. Based on the needs of certain school regions and the availability of funding, a single school nurse may be responsible for providing care in more than one school.

The National Association of School Nurses (NASN) (Council on School Health, 2008) has defined school nursing as "an integration of wellness, safety, growth, learning, and development in the lives of school-aged children and adolescents within the context of their school, and with the coordinated alliance of the family and the medical home." School nurses

- Help encourage positive responses to normal development.
- Help promote health and safety.
- Help solve actual and potential problems.
- Provide case management services.
- Work with others to develop student and family capacity for adaptation and self-management.

HISTORICAL PERSPECTIVES

The history of school nursing can be traced back to 1902, when Lillian Wald, working in a New York City public school, saw that school nursing services were a way to decrease excessive absenteeism (see Chapter 6). At that time, the role of nurses in schools was limited to the treatment of minor contagious diseases, the conduct of health education programs, and the use of home visits to demonstrate recommended treatments to family. However, soon the first citywide school nursing program in the world was established. Lina Rogers (Struthers) became the first school nurse in New York City and is credited with providing evidence-based nursing care across the city.

During the following decades, there was a dramatic increase in the number of school nurses in the United States. With that increase, the role of the school nurse became more focused on screening and referral. This practice change came largely as a result of the **Early Periodic Screening, Diagnosis, and Treatment (EPSDT)** program provided for by Section 1905(a) in Title XIX of the Social Security Act, which was passed in 1965. This act recognized that schools can be a focal point from which to identify children with problems, to increase students' access to both preventive and curative health services, and to ensure appropriate use of healthcare resources for children and adolescents who received Medicaid and were younger than 21 (http://www.cms.gov/Regulations-and-Guidance).

The biggest change in school nursing practice came with the passage of the Education for All Handicapped Children Act of 1975 (Public Law 94-142). Children who had previously not been able to attend school because of chronic or complex medical issues were now entitled to a public education, and they began attending public schools. School nurses were now providing more complex care for conditions such as seizure disorders, asthma, cardiac conditions, cystic fibrosis, quadriplegia, and life-threatening allergies (Robert Wood Johnson Foundation, 2010). For example, peanut allergy, the most common cause of anaphylaxis, is a medical emergency that requires immediate treatment with an epinephrine (adrenaline) injector (EpiPen, Twinject) and a trip to the emergency department.

Today, it is not uncommon for school nurses to record up to 100 visits in a single day. With these complex diagnoses came the need for high-tech skills to perform procedures such as tube feedings, catheterizations, and suctioning. The impact of these requirements on school nursing has been considerable, given that historically, the scope of school health services was often the function of public health nurses contracted through municipal health departments. The inclusion of children with special needs led to a change in the EPSDT program. The School Health-Related Services Plan Section 1905(r)(5) of the Social Security Act (the Act) requires that any medically necessary healthcare service listed in Section 1905(a) of the Act be provided to an EPSDT recipient even if the service is not available under that state's Medicaid plan. An amendment required identification of children who have a learning problem due to a medical problem that requires special services. Once the child is identified, an **Individual Education Plan (IEP)** or 504 plan, which lists services needed, is completed by the school. The schools employ people with special training to assist children with special needs. The services reimbursable by Medicaid when performed by the school are listed in Box 22.1.

The **Individuals with Disabilities Education Act (IDEA),** originally the Education for all Handicapped Children Act, has undergone several legislative amendments in recent years. Lawmakers made these changes to accommodate the changing climate for disabled people in the United States and to promote the belief that "improving educational results for children with disabilities is an essential element of our national policy of ensuring equality of opportunity, full participation, independent living, and economic self-sufficiency for individuals with disabilities" (Individuals with Disabilities Education Improvement Act of 2004). The IDEA website gives more information about provisions of the act. The most recent change came in 2004 to align with the No Child Left Behind Act of 2003, which attempts to ensure success by focusing on the best teaching and learning strategies for the disabled. Reforms to these standards were enacted in 2009 and continue to the present time.

You have got to keep autistic children engaged with the world. You cannot let them tune out.

Temple Grandin

box 22.1 **Services Reimbursable by Medicaid**

Speech/language therapy and evaluations
Occupational therapy and evaluations
Physical therapy and evaluations
Psychological evaluations
Psychotherapy services

Danielle is a student with special health needs who attends the school where Susan works as a nurse. Susan must catheterize her twice daily while at school, and while Danielle's aide can assist with her tube feedings, Susan has primary responsibility for programming and attaching the pump to Danielle's "MIC-KEY button."

ROLE OF THE SCHOOL NURSE

The school nurse provides a critical link between the child, the family, and the education and healthcare systems. Each of the 50 states has state nurse practice acts that regulate the profession of nursing, including school nursing. *The Scope and Standards of Professional School Nursing Practice* (ANA/NASN, 2011) defines the practice of school health nurses. In addition, Centers for Disease Control and Prevention (CDC) recommendations define the components and organization of school health programs. However, it should be acknowledged that many school health programs suffer as a result of inconsistency and ambiguity in the practice of school nursing. The eight recommended components of a comprehensive school health program are summarized in Table 22.1.

Provision of health services by the school nurse is the anchor of the school health program. To address the diverse needs of students, the school nurse must adopt the central management position for all children and adolescents in the school. The role that emerges within the context of this management position requires that the nurse have skills in health assessment, with skills in the identification of common problems that impact a child's learning such as vision impairment, attention-deficit/hyperactivity disorder (ADHD), and scoliosis. Screening is also a valuable tool in identifying and treating problems that may result in a child being excluded from school, such as infestation with lice. Health promotion, health education, and child health advocacy are key components of the school nurse's role. Many nurses take on the expanded role of certified health educator and function increasingly as valuable classroom teachers. The nurse needs to collaborate with members of the school health services team and school district wellness team to ensure the existence of comprehensive wellness policies and practices (http://www.nasn.org/ToolsResources/SchoolWellnessPolicies). These teams often include a school health physician, in addition to the clerical staff, school counselors, school administration, and families.

Hugs can do great amounts of good—especially for children.

Diana, Princess of Wales

PRACTICE POINT

School nursing requires autonomous practice and independent decision-making.

table 22.1 **Comprehensive School Health Programs**

Recommended Components	Description
K-12 health education curriculum	Should discuss personal health, family health, community health, consumer health, environmental health, sexuality education, mental and emotional health, injury prevention and safety, nutrition, prevention and control of disease, substance use and abuse
K-12 physical education curriculum	Should promote optimum physical, mental, emotional, and social development, as well as activities and sports that all students enjoy and can pursue throughout their lives
Health services	Should provide primary healthcare services, foster appropriate use of primary healthcare services, prevent and control communicable disease and other health problems, provide emergency care for illness or injury, promote and provide optimum sanitary conditions for a safe school facility and school environment, and provide educational and counseling opportunities for promoting and maintaining individual, family, and community health
Nutrition services	Should ensure access to nutritious and appealing meals that accommodate the health and nutrition needs of all students
Health promotion for staff	Should encourage staff to pursue a healthy lifestyle that contributes to their improved health status, improved morale, and develop a greater personal commitment to the school's overall coordinated health program
Counseling and psychology services	Should include individual and group assessments, interventions, and referrals
Healthy and safe school environment	Should include the physical, emotional, and social conditions that affect the well-being of students and staff
Family/community involvement	Should include school health advisory councils, coalitions, and broadly based constituencies for school health

Source: Centers for Disease Control and Prevention. *Healthy youth! Coordinated school health program*. Retrieved May 23, 2013, from http://www.cdc.gov/healthyyouth/cshp/

Health Assessment

Typically, there are three types of school health service visits that require the nurse to use assessment skills. The first type of visit is for acute illness (e.g., vomiting, fever, or headache) and playground injury. The nurse can easily use physical assessment skills and knowledge of first aid to address these issues. The second type is for typical screenings, often begun when the child enters school (immunization status) and may be continued as the child grows and is at risk for problems that may impact learning, such as vision impairment. The third type of visit is for counseling. Students may seek out the school nurse for advice and support regarding daily stressors encountered in the social framework of the school, such as being picked on or bullied by others. These visits require that the nurse assess the child individually. In addition, there are visits that are part of population-based screening programs that may include periodic vision and hearing tests, height and weight measurements (e.g., to calculate body mass index), or immunization checks.

Individual Health Assessment

The individual assessment of the child is specific to the need for the visit and may not occur in the health office. In any case, health assessment should be the responsibility of a licensed healthcare professional in the school setting. Within the school, a variety of data sources are available to the nurse to use in completing a thorough assessment of the child's chief complaint. The nurse should begin by collecting subjective data gathered from the child, teacher, or parent, or any other witness to the complaint. Data should include location, frequency, duration and severity, quality, quantity, setting, associated symptoms, and factors that make the symptom better or worse. Objective data provide information that makes the nurse's job of understanding the complaint easier. These data should include any information or signs pertinent to the illness, such as fever.

PRACTICE POINT

The child's chief complaint may only be the tip of the iceberg. Use all data sources available to assess the problem.

Collectively, this information guides the actions taken by the nurse. These actions might include treatment, referral to a healthcare provider, and notification of a parent and/or sending the child home. Individual school policy dictates the extent to which the nurse is able to treat the presenting symptoms.

Danielle also receives occupational and physical therapy services while at school. Susan must incorporate data gathered from the treatment notes, as well as from the special medical services treatment providers who monitor Danielle's medical care within her home. It is important that Susan maintains frequent communication with this team to ensure close monitoring of Danielle's healthcare needs.

Population-based Assessment

There are no federal laws requiring that periodic screening be provided by the schools, although as a public health concern consistent with EPSDT, these screenings are often a major part of the school health program. The screenings may be essential to the early detection of, and intervention in, problems that may affect academic success.

In addition, people often ask a school nurse why he or she performs periodic screening and how schools use this information. Screening programs typically begin when the child enters school and may continue in different forms throughout the child's education. Before implementing a screening program, schools should address these questions. For example, it is helpful if the health education curriculum addresses the conditions being assessed in the screening process. That way everyone, including the school staff, students, and families, is fully informed. It is necessary to develop clear procedures that evaluate the results of screening tests and stipulate how the results will be reported. In addition, it is essential to establish what the desired screening outcomes are and to emphasize those that fall outside of the targeted benchmarks.

The school nurse should play a major role in planning these screenings and will need to spend the required time to develop a successful program. For example, in response to the obesity epidemic, many schools are implementing walking programs or similar programs to encourage the recommended 60 minutes a day of physical activity. Box 22.2 outlines the guidelines for organizing a screening program.

box 22.2 Guidelines for Implementing a Screening Program

- Determine the purpose of the screening program.
- Define the population to be screened.
- Decide which screening procedure or test to use.
- Ensure that adequate resources are available for equipment and supplies; staff training; and staff time to conduct tests and retests, record results, interpret them to students and families, and conduct follow-up.
- Determine referral criteria using evidence-based standards for screenings.
- Collaborate with members of the school health team, including community health providers, regarding the following: criteria used for referral for diagnosis and treatment, decisions regarding who will be treated, and what resources are available for follow-up, especially for those who are uninsured.
- Plan the mechanics of the actual screening program, including determination of time required for screening, designating screening personnel, and deciding who will do the following:
  - Order supplies
  - Ensure that the equipment is in good working order
  - Obtain parental consent
  - Train personnel
  - Recruit, orient, and train volunteers, if used
  - Arrange for space that is appropriate, quiet, and private
  - Record findings
- Rescreen students with borderline or questionable results.
- Plan and complete the follow-up procedures.

Source: Minnesota Department of Health. Retrieved November 2, 2010, from http://www.health.state.mn.us/divs/fh/mch/webcourse/devscrn/.

PRACTICE POINT

Screening should only be performed if there are options for intervention that will potentially improve the health of the child.

Health Promotion and Assessment of School Health Needs

Healthy People 2020 has acknowledged the need for targeted data collection and health promotion efforts regarding the common health concerns of children and adolescents (U. S. DHHS, *Healthy People 2020*). One tool, the **Youth Risk Behavior Surveillance Survey (YRBSS)**, is a biannual report of the common risk behaviors influencing the health of the nation's youth. These risk behaviors are identified because of their potential impact on the long-term health and well-being of youth. Box 22.3 illustrates the six behavior categories for which statistics are typically reported. The CDC's YRBSS website is a source of additional information about this data collection tool.

A second data collection tool is the **School Health Index**, which focuses on how schools can promote physical activity, healthy eating, adopting a tobacco-free lifestyle, and a wide range of safety-related behaviors in an attempt to counter common risk behaviors (CDC, 2012d). There are two versions of the index, one for elementary schools and the other for middle schools and high schools. These can be obtained in print form or can be used online. The importance of the School Health Index is its ability to help schools identify the strengths and weaknesses of a particular school's policies and programs for promoting health and safety. On the basis of this assessment, school personnel can develop an action plan, which is then incorporated into a school's overall improvement plan to improve the health and safety of the students. The CDC developed the School Health Index Self-Assessment and Planning Guide for the following purposes (CDC, 2014):

- Enabling schools to identify the strengths and weaknesses of health and safety policies and programs
- Enabling schools to develop an action plan for improving student health, which can be incorporated into the school improvement plan
- Engaging teachers, parents, students, and the community in promoting health-enhancing behaviors and better health

box 22.3 Youth Risk Behavior Surveillance Survey Risk Behavior Categories

Unintentional injury
Violence
Tobacco use
Alcohol use
Drug use
Sexual behaviors
Unhealthy dietary behaviors
Physical inactivity

EVIDENCE FOR PRACTICE

Along with the School Health Index, the CDC has several standardized adolescent and school health tools that assist in assessment, planning, implementing, and evaluating school health programs. The Summary of Adolescent and School Health Tools website provides more information. These tools include the following:

- *Food-Safe Schools Action Guide (FSSAG),* which helps schools work with Cooperative Extension, health departments, and families in efforts to make schools food-safe
- *Health Education Curriculum Analysis Tool (HECAT),* which helps schools, school districts, and other school personnel responsible for curricular redesign to analyze health education curricula on the basis of alignment with national health education standards and characteristics of effective health education curricula
- *Improving the Health of Adolescents and Young Adults: A Guide for States and Communities,* which helps guide people and organizations through public health processes that address the 21 Critical Health Objectives identified in *Healthy People 2010* for adolescents and young adults
- *Physical Education Curriculum Analysis Tool (PECAT),* which enables users to analyze written physical education curricula based on alignment with national standards, guidelines, and best practices for quality physical education programs
- *Making It Happen!,* which provides examples and success stories of 32 schools and school districts that have implemented innovative approaches to improve the nutritional quality of foods and beverages sold outside the school meals program

The CDC recommends that action plans can be best accomplished through the development of school health advisory councils. Membership on the **council on school health** should consist of a wide range of community stakeholders. Most important, the council should have family and student representation. Approximately one-third of the nation's schools have school health councils. The development of these councils has significantly improved the odds that schools have comprehensive policies and programs that address common health concerns.

The establishment of school-based health centers (SBHCs) and services, a model of primary healthcare in the schools specifically designed to fill gaps in health services, including those to prevent teen pregnancy, began to appear in the early 1980s. Today, more than 2,000 SBHCs exist in over 43 states, the Obama administration's new health law appropriated $200 million through 2013 for the centers, to build new facilities, purchase equipment, and expand services (Wall Street Journal, 2012). The definition of SBHC is a "partnership created by schools and community health organizations to provide on-site medical and mental health services that promote the health and educational success of school-aged children and adolescents" (National Assembly on School-Based Healthcare, Principles and Goals from SBHCs). The SBHCs do not take the place of existing nursing services, but they enhance health services by decreasing barriers to needed healthcare. The National Association of Pediatric Nurse Practitioners advocates SBHCs as a necessary component of comprehensive healthcare for children. The SBHCs are located where the children are and can effectively treat problems affecting children's health.

PRACTICE POINT

Establishing a school health council, whether it is called a school health council, school wellness team, or school health advisory team, is the most important step that schools can take to improve their school health program.

Susan is the chair of the School District Wellness Committee. The Wellness Committee was formed primarily to oversee the nutrition and physical activity needs of school community as part of an overall commitment to wellness. The committee has recently implemented a before-school walking program to encourage children to engage in at least 60 minutes of physical activity per day.

The School Nurse as Health Educator

Schools, where children and adolescents spend one-third of their day, present an ideal setting for providing health education. A health education curriculum is an important part of a comprehensive kindergarten to grade 12 school health program. Successful evidence-based programs vary in their approach but should be age-appropriate and should focus on strengthening what have been termed "the developmental assets of the population" (Wholechildeducation.org). Programs that serve to increase self-esteem, develop social skills, and increase understanding of issues such as peer influence and decision-making should be considered. Some professionals have recommended that the school nurse's role in health education should be that of a resource person or consultant and not necessarily that of a teacher. This opinion is contrary to that of the NASN, which considers health education an important intervention to be implemented as a primary responsibility of the school nurse.

Whether or not the school nurse is in the classroom, health education is a priority. The school nurse must seek to accomplish health teaching in encounters with students and families, in the classroom, in individual counseling sessions (e.g., teaching a child how and when to use his or her EpiPen), and in group meetings. It is recommended that the focus of health education be health promotion based on concerns addressed in the National Health Objectives of *Healthy People 2020.* These issues include use of drugs and alcohol, sexual behavior, tobacco use, nutrition, physical activity, and violence prevention.

Emergency Preparedness

An essential role of the school nurse is to be prepared for emergencies, yet as few as 75% have any specialized training in emergency care beyond basic life support. Emergency preparedness does not address a specific hazard but addresses the planning, response, and recovery needs within a local community such as a school. Currently, there are three organizations that provide training for school nurses in emergency management of school emergencies: The NASN and both the Illinois and the New Mexico Emergency Medical Services for children. It is imperative that school nurses continue to gain knowledge, skills, and attitudes to lead in times of emergency (Elgie, Sapien, Fullerton, & Moore, 2010).

COMMON HEALTH CONCERNS

It is easier to build strong children than to repair broken men.

Frederick Douglass

Substance Use: Drugs and Alcohol

Epidemiology

The Office of Applied Studies (OAS) in the Substance Abuse and Mental Health Services Administration (SAMHSA) is responsible for the National Survey on Drug Use and Health (NSDUH), formerly called the National Household Survey on Drug Abuse (NHSDA)(Office of Applied Studies, 2009). SAMHSA is the primary source of data on drug and alcohol use in the civilian population. From 2002 to 2008, the prevalence of current illicit drug use among youth 12 to 18 years of age dropped significantly, from 11.2% to 9.6%, and has remained stable. Of all persons admitted to publicly funded treatment centers, 7.5% were aged 12 to 17 years. The most commonly reported illicit drug used in this age group is marijuana. In the most recent 2008 survey, on an average day 3,695 Americans used marijuana for the first time. About two-thirds (69%) of these new users were younger than 18, and about half (53%) were female. In 2008, approximately half (51.1%) of youth aged 12 to 20 reported drinking alcohol in the month prior to the survey. Of these, 23.3% were binge drinkers. Binge drinking is defined as having five or more drinks on the same occasion on at least 1 day in the past 30 days, and 2.3 million (6.9%) were heavy drinkers, defined as five or more drinks on the same occasion on 5 or more days in the past 30 days.

Best Practices: Drug and Alcohol Prevention

There is an extensive body of research related to the effectiveness of school-based substance abuse programs. The SAMSHA has collated a series of evidence-based programs with the potential to produce sustained behavior change (National Registry of Evidence Based Programs and Practices). The NREPP website (www.nrepp.samhsa.gov) is a searchable database of interventions that have been evaluated in comparative effectiveness research. These interventions include the following:

1. Introducing interventions during the three periods when they are most likely to produce results: (1) the primary prevention or inoculation phase, which is designed to introduce knowledge; (2) the secondary prevention or early relevance phase, when information is likely to have meaning and applicability to students; and (3) the tertiary prevention or later relevance phase, when young people are actually being exposed to new situations involving experimentation. Programs and booster sessions should be implemented throughout these periods.
2. Providing school drug education programs that are meaningful and interesting to the participants. It is important to assess the needs and interests of the group carefully prior to the selection of any program.
3. Integrating the goals of the school with those of the prevention program. For example, is the goal of the program nonuse, delayed use, or harm minimization?
4. Using teaching and learning principles that are developmentally appropriate and using interactive techniques that give students an opportunity to practice new skills
5. Designing programs that are behavior-focused rather than knowledge-based

PRACTICE POINT

Classroom-based drug education should be made routinely available in schools as a cost-effective method for the prevention of drug abuse.

It is clear that the majority of adolescents will experiment with substances and that given the limited funding available in many schools for prevention programming evidence-based prevention strategies must be initiated as early as elementary school to prevent initiation (Singh, Jimerson & Renshaw, 2011).

Substance Use: Smoking

Epidemiology

Among students nationwide, the prevalence of current cigarette use increased during 1991 to 1997 (27.5–36.4%) and then decreased during 1997 to 2011 (36.4–18.1%). The prevalence of current cigarette use did not change significantly from 2009 (19.5%) to 2011 (18.1%). During the late 1990s, the overall downward trend in current cigarette smoking among high school students began to slow, as observed by the National Youth Tobacco Survey (NYTS) and other national surveys. Overall, white male students had the greatest prevalence of cigarette use among all racial/ethnic groups and grade levels. Among female students, current cigarette use declined significantly from 18.4% to 16.1%. This downward trend can be attributed to interventions that prevent and reduce tobacco use among youths, including media campaigns, limiting advertisements and other promotions, increasing the price of tobacco products, and reducing the availability of tobacco products for purchase by youths (CDC, 2012b). Cigarette smoking is a primary risk factor for the development of coronary artery disease and stroke, and it is estimated that the rise in adolescent smoking in the 1990s will result in more adult smokers. Using statistical models that factor in age of initiation and quitting, it is predicted that this could mean that about 250,000 to 500,000 additional people will live shorter lives due to smoking, at a cost of billions in value of life years.

The *Healthy People 2020* objectives also specifically target adolescent tobacco use. Specific objectives include reducing the reported use of tobacco products in the previous 12 months from 7.7% to 5.7%. Also included are objectives to decrease the initiation of smokeless tobacco and cigars among children and adolescents aged 12 to 17 years. *Healthy People 2020* suggests that effective prevention approaches for improving health behaviors in adolescents must include school-based prevention programs as well as community-wide strategies that address the overall social context of health risk behaviors.

Best Practices: Smoking Prevention

In 1996, the extent of youth tobacco use in Texas became particularly high, coinciding with increasing Medicaid costs due to smoking-related illnesses among the impoverished residents. The state of Texas then initiated a lawsuit that was joined by three other states—Florida, Mississippi, and Minnesota—against five tobacco companies, seeking reimbursement for its medical expenses. This lawsuit resulted in settlements representing an enormous sum of money. The tobacco industry made a legal agreement to put an end to all marketing efforts that primarily target minors. In 1998, the Attorneys General of the 46 remaining states signed the Multistate Settlement Agreement (MSA) with the four largest tobacco companies in the United States to settle state suits that were initiated to recover costs associated with treating smoking-related illnesses. Conditions of the agreement included restrictions on tobacco advertising and marketing. The MSA also required the tobacco industry to deposit $300 million a year for 5 years into a newly created foundation. These funds were to be used for public education in an attempt to decrease underage tobacco use. The agreement provides for a $200 billion distribution of these funds to the 46 states, and there was no specification about how this money was to be spent. (The actual per-state allocation is based on estimated Medicare expenditures for tobacco-related illness and estimated number of current smokers.) The full text of the MSA can be accessed at the Tobacco Free Kids website.

An article in the 1994 *Morbidity and Mortality Weekly Report (MMWR)*, published by the CDC, stated that youths spend up to 25% of their waking hours in school and are thus a captive audience for tobacco prevention programming. This same report recommended that programming should start with tobacco prevention education before students begin to smoke. The CDC Division of Adolescents and School Health established guidelines for school-based tobacco prevention and control programs, which still exist today, although with some modifications. These guidelines are available to all school districts nationwide and are available on the CDC website. The CDC's *Guidelines for Preventing Tobacco Use Among Young People* include recommendations for "a coordinated, multicomponent campaign involving policy changes, taxation, mass media, and behavioral education [which] can effectively reduce the onset of tobacco use among adolescents." These guidelines include seven recommendations for school-based tobacco prevention (Box 22.4).

PRACTICE POINT

Strategies to prevent tobacco use in schools should begin with specific training of both the school personnel, who interact with the adolescents on a daily basis, and the student peer leaders involved with the program.

Sexual Behavior and Teenage Pregnancy

The American Psychological Association has recommended annual screening for sexual activity and condom use in adolescents. Unfortunately, there are many barriers to this type of preventive healthcare. One study of adolescents who had received health supervision visits reported that only 42.8% females and 26.4% of males reported having discussions of sexual behavior that included content about teen pregnancy and sexually transmitted infections (STIs) (formerly known as sexually transmitted diseases [STDs]) (Burstein, Lowry, Klein, & Santelli, 2003). This clearly represents missed opportunities for important dialogues that may prevent detrimental outcomes of sexual behavior. Students attending school should have the opportunity to receive knowledgeable and accessible sexual behavior education and counseling.

box 22.4 Recommendations for School-Based Tobacco Prevention Programs

1. Develop and enforce a school policy on tobacco use.
2. Provide instruction about the short- and long-term negative physiologic and social consequences of tobacco use, social influences on tobacco use, peer norms regarding tobacco use, and refusal skills.
3. Provide tobacco-use prevention education in kindergarten through 12th grade; this instruction should be especially intensive in junior high or middle school and should be reinforced in high school.
4. Provide program-specific training for teachers.
5. Involve parents or families in support of school-based programs to prevent tobacco use.
6. Support cessation efforts among students and all school staff who use tobacco.
7. Assess the tobacco-use prevention program at regular intervals.

Source: From Centers for Disease Control and Prevention. *Guidelines for school health programs to prevent tobacco use and addiction.* Retrieved May 26, 2013, from http://www.cdc.gov/mmwr/PDF/RR/RR4302.pdf

Epidemiology

Childbearing among teenagers fell to historical lows in 2010. Birth rates in the United States fell 11% for women aged 15 to 17 years and 7% for women aged 18 to 19 years. The rate of teen pregnancy has dropped 45% since 1991. While reasons for the declines are not clear, teens seem to be less sexually active, and more of those who are sexually active seem to be using birth control than in previous years. Long-acting reversible birth control can be a good option for a teenaged woman. Implants and intrauterine devices (IUDs) are two types. These do not require her to do anything on a regular basis, such as take a pill each day. For the past 10 years, the prevalence of adolescent pregnancy has been declining, but the ramifications for those teenagers who do become mothers are long-lasting, keeping adolescent pregnancy on the list of major public health problems. In 2011, a total of 329,797 babies were born to women 15 to 17 years old. Many of these births are unintended and occur outside of marriage (MMWR, 2000). There is a strong association between teenage pregnancy and child well-being. Morbidity associated with children of teenage pregnancy includes preterm birth, low birth weight, child abuse, neglect, poverty, and premature death. Infant mortality is higher in children of teenage mothers than in other children (CDC, 2012a).

Best Practices: Pregnancy Prevention

A number of public programs have been initiated in the country to prevent teen pregnancy.

The Adolescent Family Life (AFL) program, created in 1981 (Title XX of the Public Health Service Act), was the first federal program to focus on adolescents. From 1998 to 2009, the program relied heavily on abstinence-only education. In 2010, a new Teen Pregnancy Prevention program was funded to provide "medically accurate and age-appropriate programs that reduce pregnancy." The Patient Protection and Affordable Care Act (ACA) enables states to operate a new Personal Responsibility Education Program (PREP), which is a comprehensive approach to teen pregnancy prevention that educates adolescents on both abstinence and contraception to prevent pregnancy and STDs. Finally, the Title V Abstinence Education Block Grant is available to states specifically for abstinence-only education. Successful strategies for preventing adolescent pregnancy vary from responsible sexual behavior education, which includes abstinence education, to improved contraceptive counseling and confidential reproductive services (Solomon-Fears, 2013). A complete list of 28 evidence-based, abstinence-based curricula can be accessed at the Resource Center for Adolescent Pregnancy Prevention's website. Comprehensive sex education teaching aims to reduce risky sexual behaviors by teenagers. These programs may include not only abstinence as a method to prevent pregnancy but also discussions of contraception for those who are already sexually active.

The American Academy of Pediatricians, the American Academy of Family Physicians, and the American Medical Association all endorse sex and contraceptive counseling performed by healthcare professionals as the model to be used to promote responsible sexual behavior and reduce teen pregnancy. The YRBSS reports that the prevalence of sexual intercourse among high school students nationwide is 47.4%. Nationwide, 6.2% of students report a sexual debut prior to 13 years of age. Of those students reporting they are currently sexually active (33.7%), 60.2% report using condoms regularly and 18% report using birth control pills regularly (CDC, 2012d). In previous surveys, the reasons that female students gave for not using contraceptives consistently included the belief that pregnancy will not affect them, the desire to become pregnant, "cultural" beliefs, and fear.

The ACA of 2010 provides significant funding for SBHCs, particularly those that serve Medicaid-eligible populations. SBHCs may be helpful; most available on-site services include abstinence counseling (84%), pregnancy testing (81%), and counseling for birth control (70%). About 60% are prohibited from dispensing contraception. Although there is no direct evidence that SBHCs have decreased teen pregnancy, intermediate measures suggest that these centers do play a role in improving academic success as a result of improved health status (Ethier et al., 2011).

PRACTICE POINT

A multidisciplinary team consisting of nurse practitioners, educators, school nurses, social service workers, and other professionals should collaborate to meet the needs of children and adolescents.

STUDENT REFLECTION

My community health clinical experience was in a city high school in Massachusetts. During my time there, I became acutely aware of the student issues regarding STIs, teen pregnancy, and the lack of sexual health information. The statistics of STI rates are frightening: one in four of American girls have had an STI, and in 1 year in Massachusetts, syphilis increased by 20%, gonorrhea by 12%, and chlamydia infections by 8.3%. An annual questionnaire given in high schools around the state found that in 2011, 64% of teens have had intercourse by the time they graduate from high school, and many more engage in a range of other sexual activities. Only 50% of the students said that their parents had talked to them about sex!

There also were a high number of teenage pregnancies in the high school. Along with my teacher, I became involved in presenting seminars for students who were currently pregnant or had recently had a child. The groups were small to create an intimate nonjudgmental or nonthreatening atmosphere. The teen mothers-to-be learned what to expect in pregnancy and the changes that their bodies would be going through. They learned how to stay healthy—about the right things to eat, things to avoid eating, when to see a doctor, how to know when to go to the hospital, and seeking father and family support. We also discussed the labor process and postpartum issues, in particular postpartum depression and shaken baby syndrome. Then the group learned about lifestyle changes when the baby arrives. This included feeding and sleeping patterns, along with crying issues. We demonstrated changing a diaper and washing the baby and practiced using dolls. At all times, the students had the opportunity to ask questions and clear up any misconceptions or concerns. We also supplied information about STIs, contraception, and safe sex. Pamphlets, magazines, posters, fact sheets, contact information, and other resources were available.

I believe that a nurse has a responsibility to be proactive by encouraging clients to make healthy decisions and live a healthy lifestyle without pressuring them. By providing students with information, we empowered students and gave them the opportunity to make their own informed decisions. In the evaluations completed by the students, they found the interventions "catchy, current, and something that they could relate to."

Sexually Transmitted Infections

Epidemiology

Sexually transmitted infections, once called venereal diseases or STDs, are among the most common infectious diseases nationwide. Teens and young adults have the highest rates of STIs of any age group: 27% of all new cases of gonorrhea were among teens 15 to 19 years of age. Ninety percent of all newly diagnosed STIs are genital wart-associated human papillomavirus (HPV) which can be prevented by vaccination. Of 15- to 19-year-olds, 8.3% are diagnosed with chlamydia, 2.5% with trichomoniasis, and 1.9% with herpes simplex virus type 2. Among the teenage girls who had an STI, 15% had more than one (CDC, 2012c). Together, the three STIs (HPV, trichomoniasis, and chlamydia) accounted for 88% of all new cases of STIs in adolescents and young adults 15 to 24 years of age, although accurate measures of STIs in this population are difficult to obtain because many affected people have few, if any, identifiable symptoms. Additional information can be found in Chapter 14.

PRACTICE POINT

Making HIV testing a routine part of healthcare for adolescents and adults 13 to 64 years of age is one of the most important strategies recommended by the CDC for reducing the spread of HIV (Centers for Disease Control and Prevention, 2013a).

School Relevance

The school nurse's role as a case finder is very important because the nurse is in a good position to provide the necessary counseling and referral for STI treatment. However, school health personnel should know that symptomatic adolescents who are suspected of having an STI cannot be excluded from school. In addition, health personnel should also be aware that federal law stipulates that adolescents can go directly to a health department-operated STI clinic for diagnosis and treatment of their disease without parental consent. In some cases where communication with parents does not occur, the student may choose not to seek treatment for what could ultimately result in long-term consequences of the infection. If this is the case, school health personnel should preserve the student's privacy while assisting the student with contacting the health department and arranging for necessary diagnosis and treatment. Finally, health professionals should assist in the identification of all sexual contacts involved so they can be warned and treated. In many cases, it may be easier to locate and speak with these students at school (Newton et al., 1997).

PRACTICE POINT

It is rare for a person to contract an STI without some form of sexual contact. Although as many as 50% of teens are sexually active by the end of high school, not all are engaging in heterosexual contact. Sexual contact may involve mouth-to-genital contact, either homosexual or heterosexual.

Nutrition

Epidemiology

Obesity in children and adolescents is a serious health concern. Trends indicate that an estimated 17% of children and adolescents aged 2 to 19 are obese, and that about 1 in 7 low-income, preschool-aged children are obese. This is largely a result of overeating and insufficient exercise, which lead to an energy imbalance. Obese children and adolescents are at risk for health problems as children and adults. They are more likely to have conditions such as high blood pressure, high cholesterol, and type 2 diabetes that are risk factors for cardiovascular disease (CDC, 2012b). In addition, children and adolescents who are obese are more likely to remain obese as adults. Although in recent years the obesity epidemic in children and adolescents appears to be stabilizing, it remains at an unacceptably high level.

Continued obesity in children may result in an epidemic of cardiovascular disease and type 2 diabetes in the adolescent population. Cardiovascular disease is already the fifth leading cause of preventable death among adolescents, and there has been a marked increase in insulin resistance and type 2 diabetes. The National Health Objectives of *Healthy People 2020* address cardiovascular disease prevention in adolescents by focusing on physical inactivity and obesity. The 2011 YRBSS report states that 49.5% of children in the United States engage in exercise that results in sweating or hard breathing for the recommended 60 minutes per day, 5 or more days per week (CDC, 2012d). Exercise can be linked to both physical and emotional well-being by decreasing cardiovascular risk factors, reducing feelings of depression and anxiety, and stimulating an overall improvement in psychological health and academic functioning.

This might be the first generation where kids are dying at a younger age than their parents and it's related primarily to the obesity problem.

Judy Davis, Australian actress

Adolescents, both in school and out, have wide access to foods with low nutritional value and high levels of fat and calories through vending machines, à la carte lunches, and snack bars. Although the USDA school-based nutrition programs have played a key role in contributing to improvement in overall health indicators in adolescents, there is no legislation banning foods sold outside of the cafeteria. The food environment in schools often serves to reinforce poor eating habits. Schools are the primary setting for engaging children in the establishment of lifelong positive behaviors. However, the matter of food choices should also be addressed using broad-based environmental and public health policy approaches.

Best Practices: Nutrition

In the Child Nutrition and WIC Reauthorization Act of 2004, the U.S. Congress established a requirement that all school districts with a federally funded school meals program develop and implement wellness policies that address nutrition and physical activity by the start of the 2006 to 2007 school year (Section 204). The CDC has established a self-assessment and planning tool (School Health Index) and guidelines that can be used in school health programs in an effort to improve the food environments of school-aged children and adolescents. These current CDC guidelines focus on changing the social norms and environments of adolescents. In addition to school-based prevention, the guidelines recommend policy and regulatory strategies, community participation, establishment of public and private partnerships, strategic use of media, development of local programs, coordination of statewide and local activities, linkage of school-based activities to community activities, and use of data collection and evaluation techniques, such as the School Health Index (described previously), to monitor program impact.

PRACTICE POINT

An extension of the CDC website gives access to the School Health Index at no cost to the school. Based on the results of the assessment, a school can strengthen existing school health programs. For example, a school may choose to implement *CDC Guidelines to Promote Lifelong Healthy Eating*, which identify strategies most likely to be effective in promoting lifelong healthy eating among young people. Alternatively, it may choose to implement *CDC Guidelines to Promote Lifelong Physical Activity*, which identify strategies most likely to be effective in helping young people adopt and maintain a physically active lifestyle.

Joe, who is 10 years old, is in the fifth grade in the school where Susan works. When he was 8, he was diagnosed with ADHD. Joe also has a severe peanut allergy and must avoid any contact with peanuts and peanut-containing products. Using yearly height and weight screenings, Susan has found that Joe's body mass index is in the 99th percentile, which indicates obesity.

Using the CDC Guidelines for School Health Programs to Promote Lifelong Healthy Eating (CDC, 1996) and the CDC Guidelines for School and Community Programs to Promote Lifelong Physical Activity Among Young People (CDC, 1997), identify Joe's needs and plan interventions to address each of these nutritional issues. (See the References for specific information.)

STUDENT REFLECTION

During my clinical rotation in community health, I encountered several high school students struggling with eating disorders, a common problem in this age group. One particular case that I found interesting involved a senior boy on the wrestling team who came to the health office because he was not feeling well. He complained of being tired and feeling worn out; he said that he just felt like he needed to go home and rest. After calling his mother, he transferred the call to the nurse. The nurse explained to his mother that her son was not feeling well and asked whether he could be dismissed. The mother stated "I know what is wrong with him…the wrestling coach told him to only drink water for the past two days because of the match tomorrow… that's why he is not feeling well." The mother said that she was very concerned about this practice. However, she did not want to make a big deal out of the situation because she did not want the coach to bully her son, who loves wrestling. She agreed to let her son come home. However, I couldn't help but think of this boy, who was putting wrestling ahead of eating; he was at risk for an eating disorder.

This is a disturbing situation. However, no matter how much education is provided to students, I do not think the situation will change unless the teachers and coaches are involved and see the necessity of promoting healthy eating.

Violence

I have a theory because I was being beaten up a lot by people outside of school, it was almost like if I could make myself sick enough they'd take sympathy on me.

Daniel Johns, Australian musician

Violence was declared a public health emergency in 1985, and since then, violence prevention has been a national health promotion objective. However, the incidence of youth violence remains higher in the United States than in most developed countries. The YRBSS (CDC, 2012d) measures a number of manifestations of violence, including carrying a weapon (e.g., gun, knife, or club) (16.6%), carrying a gun (5.1%), physical fighting (32.8%), dating violence (9.4% of students had been hit or slapped by a boyfriend or girlfriend), bullying (20.1% of students had been bullied on school property), and feeling unsafe (5.9% of students reported not going to school because they felt unsafe). These numbers did not change significantly from 2009 to 2011.

The tongue like a sharp knife…Kills without drawing blood.

Buddha

In response to an increased awareness to bullying—specifically defined as unwanted, aggressive behavior among school-aged children that involves a real or perceived power imbalance—numerous prevention and intervention programs have been implemented that have now made children and adolescents safer in school than anywhere else. In 2007, the Office of Juvenile Justice and Delinquency Prevention commissioned a study to examine the impact of bullying in schools. The report released in 2011 discusses connections between bullying in schools, school attendance and engagement, and academic achievement and presents recommendations for prevention strategies. Box 22.5 contains information from that report that identifies successful prevention strategies.

Traditional violence is not the only problem. Adolescents are fascinated with cell phones, computers, and tablets, and they quickly develop an expanded vocabulary, by using instant messaging (IMing), blogging, and texting. Although new technology has many social and educational benefits, it has been used to harass and intimidate others. **Cyberbullying** is a relatively new phenomenon, defined as any kind of deliberate and repeated aggression perpetrated through any type of information technology. It includes harassment, bullying, teasing, telling lies, making fun of someone, making rude or mean comments, spreading rumors, or making threatening or aggressive comments that occur through e-mail, a chat room, IMing, a website, blogs, or text messaging. The majority of young people report little or no involvement in electronic aggression, but 9% to 35% say that they have been a victim. Rude or nasty comments are most frequently experienced by victims, followed by rumor spreading and then threatening or aggressive comments (Hertz & David-Ferdon, 2008). Although the news media has recently devoted much attention to the potential dangers of technology, face-to-face verbal and physical aggression is still far more common than cyberbullying.

Caregivers and educators have expressed concern about the dangers young people can be exposed to through these technologies. To respond to this concern, some states and school districts have, for example, established policies about the use of cell phones on school grounds and developed policies to block access to certain websites on school computers. The CDC convened the first expert panel to address these issues in 2006. Suggestions for educators, policymakers, caregivers, and parents to address this problem are summarized in Boxes 22.6 and 22.7.

box 22.5 Bullying Prevention

Model caring behavior.
Increase student engagement.
Offer mentoring programs.
Provide opportunities for community service.
Start prevention programs early.
Address difficult transitions between elementary and middle school.

Source: http://www.ojjdp.gov/pubs/234205.pdf

box 22.6 Cyberbullying: Suggestions for Educators

1. **Explore current bullying prevention policies and work collaboratively to develop new policies.** States, school districts, and boards of education must work in conjunction with attorneys to develop policies that protect the rights of all students and also meet the needs of the state or district and those it serves. In addition, it is also helpful to involve representatives from the student body, students, families, and community members in the development of the policy. The policy should also be based upon evidence from research and on best practices.
2. **Explore current programs to prevent bullying and youth violence.** Many of the programs developed to prevent face-to-face aggression address topics such as school climate and peer influences that are likely to be important for prevention of electronic aggression.
3. **Offer training on electronic aggression for educators and administrators.** The training should include the definition of electronic aggression, characteristics of victims and perpetrators, related school or district policies, information about recent incidents of electronic violence in the district, and resources available to educators and caregivers if they have concerns.
4. **Talk to adolescents.** Providing young people opportunities to discuss their concerns through, for example, creative writing assignments is an excellent way to begin a classroom dialogue about using electronic media safely and about the impact and consequences of inappropriate use. Technology safety could easily be integrated into the standard health education curricula. Educators and researchers should explore with adolescents how electronic media can be used as tools to prevent electronic aggression and other adolescent health problems.
5. **Work with information technology (IT) personnel and support staff.** Administrators must create the infrastructure and support necessary for classroom teachers to work with IT staff to keep abreast of issues affecting young people and develop strategies to minimize risk.
6. **Create a positive school atmosphere.** Research indicates that students who feel connected to their school, who think their teachers care about them and are fair, and who think

the school rules are clear and fair are less likely to perpetrate any type of violence or aggression, including electronic aggression.

7. **Have an action plan in place to address incidents.** Be proactive in developing a thoughtful plan to address problems and concerns. Having a plan in place may make young people more likely to come forward with concerns and may support the appropriate handling of a situation when it arises. Create an atmosphere that encourages a dialogue between educators and young people and between families and young people about their electronic experiences.

Source: Hertz, M. F., & David-Ferdon, C. (2008). *Electronic media and youth violence: A CDC issue brief for educators and caregivers*. Atlanta, GA: Centers for Disease Control and Prevention.

box 22.7 Cyberbullying: Suggestions for Parents and Caregivers

1. **Talk to your child.** Just as you would ask children where they are going and whom they are going to be with whenever they leave the house, ask where they are going and whom they are with when they are on the Internet. Talk with teens to come up with a solution to prevent or address victimization that does not punish the teen.
2. **Develop rules.** Together with your child, develop rules about acceptable and safe behavior for all the electronic media they use and what they should do if they become a victim of electronic aggression or they witness or know about another teen being victimized.
3. **Explore the Internet.** Visit the websites your child frequents. Remember that young people can learn new information on the Internet, interact with and learn about people from diverse backgrounds, and express themselves to others who may have similar thoughts and experiences. Technology is not going away, so forbidding young people to access electronic media may not be a good long-term solution. Together, parents and youth can come up with ways to maximize the benefits of technology and decrease its risks.
4. **Talk with other parents and/or caregivers.** Discuss strategies that are effective as well as those that do not work.
5. **Encourage your school or school district to conduct a class for caregivers about electronic aggression.** Review school or district policies on the topic, recent incidents in the community, and resources available to caregivers who have concerns.
6. **Keep current.** Keep current on what new devices and features your child is using. You need to know "where they are going" and explore these websites yourself. Ask your teenager to educate you. This may help strengthen parent–child communication and bonding, which is important for other adolescent health issues as well.

Source: Hertz, M. F., & David-Ferdon, C. (2008). *Electronic media and youth violence: A CDC issue brief for educators and caregivers*. Atlanta, GA: Centers for Disease Control and Prevention.

EVIDENCE FOR PRACTICE

Using data (YRBSS), one study examined the associations among physical dating violence (PDV), sexual dating violence (SDV), and selected health risk behaviors in high school students in southeastern North Carolina (Kim-Godwin et al., 2009). Participants totaled 747 students, 375 in 2005 and 372 in 2007. The findings indicate that PDV increased slightly from 2005 (11.6%) to 2007 (12.5%), while SDV remained approximately the same (10.4% in 2005 and 10.3% in 2007). PDV was strongly associated with SDV in the students. Significant associations also exist among dating violence and sexual behavior, substance use, violence, psychological health, and unhealthy weight control. School nurses should be actively involved in promoting healthy lifestyles and healthy choices in high school students through interdisciplinary efforts with parents, teachers, school districts, and communities.

PRACTICE POINT

Ineffective programs are characterized by assumptions about the cause-and-effect relationships that result in violence in schools. For example, there is an assumption that exposure to media violence causes violence. In fact, the problem of youth violence extends beyond the exposure to media into the social context of youth. School health programs must work instead to construct a culture of nonviolence.

Susan has become aware that some of the children have been making fun of Joe because of his daily visits to the nurse's office. Joe confides in her that children sometimes pick on him because he takes medicine and cannot eat peanuts. Today, a student pushed a peanut butter sandwich into his face and laughed when he got upset. Identify specific interventions that should be taken to stop this bullying.

STUDENT REFLECTION

During my clinical rotation in community health, I assisted a school nurse at an elementary school. I worked with many emotionally distressed students in need of emotional support. Often, they were homesick, frustrated with an assignment, or just needed time away from the stress of the classroom. I listened to the children's worries, offered advice on how to cope with their sadness, and called their parents if necessary. However, everything I had been taught and all the experience I had could not have prepared me for a visit I received.

A teacher entered the nurse's office, looking rather disturbed, and asked to speak to myself and my teacher (the school nurse) in a separate room. The teacher said that a student, very upset, had told the teacher that her father hits her and that she is too scared to go home because he might hit her again. The teacher calmed the student down, telling her that she would be protected. The nurse called the social worker, and everyone met to decide the best action to take to protect this child.

First, the nurse called the Department of Children and Families (DCF) so it could file a report. The DCF said that because its staff believed that the current situation could be one where it was unsafe for the student to return home, a representative was going to come to the school. The DCF requested that the nurse call the student to the office and that the child was to be inspected for any signs of physical abuse.

It was very difficult for the teacher/nurse to have to ask the child, who trusts the nurse and had developed a relationship with the nurse, to take off her clothes so that we could observe for signs of abuse. During the examination, the student was tearful; however, it appeared that she trusted us and she provided more information about the potential abuse. She said "he hits me but I hate when I see the blood coming from there (her bottom)." This made me very concerned, since it was unclear whether she was talking about blood from where she got hit on the bottom, or if there was some kind of sexual abuse involved. We did not see any signs of physical abuse.

The DCF wanted information about both her and her brother, including their friends, their demeanor in the nurse's office, medical record information, and the nurses' interactions with the parents of the children. I was not able to be very helpful, since I had not had a lot of interactions with the children, but my teacher had a wealth of information. She was able to look back at her electronic log and see that the boy had visited the nurse's office on five occasions, tearfully seeking emotional support. The nurse also said that the father was "difficult to deal with," and on one occasion left a message threatening to call the nurse's boss because the nurse was requesting records that the children had received a physical examination.

During the next 10-day period, the DCF investigators visited the children's home, talked with both the children and parents, and decided not to open the case. I had a lot of different feelings and mixed emotions during this time, and this case helped shape my philosophy and value system regarding community and public health nursing. First, I was horrified. I wanted the father to be locked up immediately and the children to be protected. However, soon I realized there were DCF procedures and nursing procedures that had to be followed. Having to check the child for hit marks really upset me. I thought that it was unfair that the nurse had to break this child's trust, which might affect the student's willingness to come to the nurse's office in the future. However, we worked hard to make the examination as painless as possible.

THE SCHOOL NURSE AS A CHILD ADVOCATE

Advocacy plays a central role in school health personnel's responsibility for the overall physical and emotional well-being of the children and adolescents they serve. Advocacy involves both teaching children and empowering others who care for the children to ensure quality care. Key components of the advocacy role include collaboration and policy-making. School nurses often spend more time with specific students than any other adult during the school day (Alexandropoulou, 2013). The advocacy role emerges from this caregiving process.

As an advocate, the school nurse needs to find a balance between empowering parents and others external to the school to pursue healthcare for the child. The child with a chronic health condition presents a unique challenge for nurses as advocates. The nurse must often mediate between educators, parents, and physicians to ensure children with chronic health conditions can function to their maximum potential. As many as 10% to 15% of children in schools are affected with chronic conditions, such as asthma, diabetes, and seizure disorders, that require daily treatment (U.S. DHHS, National Heart Lung and Blood Institute, n.d.). The nurse as advocate has two important roles: spreading knowledge and networking. Spreading knowledge does not ensure health, but a person's sense of being able to control his or her own healthcare does promote healthy behaviors. This sense of control comes from the provision of adequate resources. Networking is also important. Working together, the school nurse, parents, teachers, and healthcare providers can ensure that the child with special healthcare needs has access to all educational resources and opportunities. Knowledge of federal laws, including the **Americans with Disabilities Act (ADA)**, IDEA, Section 504, Family Educational Rights and Privacy Act of 1974 (FERPA), and **FAAMA: Food Allergy and Anaphylaxis Management Act** is essential (see definitions at the beginning of the chapter). If the school nurse has identified a pupil in the school who has special healthcare needs, a meeting should be arranged to provide health accommodations—a 504 plan, IEP, or other school plan. Children may represent themselves in these meetings if appropriate but at a minimum should have representation by the family, school health staff, special education coordinator, and any person trained to assist the student or who has primary responsibility for the student. As an advocate, the school health staff should (U.S. DHHS, National Heart Lung and Blood Institute) do the following:

- Provide education and communication necessary to ensure that the student's health and educational needs are met.
- Implement strategies to reduce disruptions in the student's school activities.
- Communicate with families and healthcare providers as authorized.

- Ensure the student receives prescribed medications and treatments and that staff who interact with the student on a regular basis are knowledgeable about these needs.
- Provide a safe and healthy school environment to promote learning.

Today, in addition to her routine activities, Susan is participating in a transition-planning meeting about Joe. He will be going to the middle school next year, and his parents have asked for a transition-planning meeting. For his ADHD, he currently takes 20 mg of Ritalin in the morning before school and 10 mg at lunch time. His severe peanut allergy requires that an EpiPen be kept in the nurse's office. His 504 plan, which was developed when he was diagnosed, allows Joe to take his medication midday, provides for a peanut-free lunch environment, and suggests that Joe's desk be positioned in such a way that distractions are limited.

- Who should be included in the planning meeting?
- What topics should be discussed? Prepare an anaphylaxis algorithm for Joe.
- What are Susan's responsibilities regarding this transition meeting?

Joe's parents are hoping that he can stop taking his medication. Lately, Susan has had to send a messenger to remind him to take it. She knows that Joe's transition into middle school will be important in the development of his self-esteem. A strong sense of self-esteem will be a protective factor against engaging in health risk behaviors in middle school. What recommendations can Susan make that would help resolve this situation?

PRACTICE POINT

With the attention and scrutiny given to personal health information in all settings, and as a result of federal legislation, it is imperative for school nurses to revisit policies and procedures for protecting the privacy of student and family health information.

THE FUTURE OF SCHOOL HEALTH: THE COMMUNITY SCHOOL MODEL

For each of the common health problems discussed in this chapter, it should be made clear that a single focused approach to prevention based only on education, that is, one that is approached only by teaching, has a minimal effect. In some cases, researchers believe that this type of programming may, in fact, contribute to experimentation (Berk, 2013). For example, if students are given knowledge about tobacco use, they may be motivated to experiment with tobacco.

One solution for the provision of comprehensive school health services is called the **community school model** (http://www.communityschools.org/about/default.aspx). This model is a collaborative design that uses the resources of a community to provide structured preventive services such as after-school programs, parent outreach, and crisis intervention. These preventive services are designed to promote changes throughout the school environment. Consistent with a social change model, the philosophy of the community school model is to create culture change that promotes a healthy learning environment for children. This ultimately has both academic and nonacademic positive outcomes; it builds social capital (Looman & Lindeke, 2005). Nurses have long been aware of the importance of practicing within context to implement and sustain change. As a result of the groundbreaking findings at the time from the National Longitudinal Study of Adolescent Health, school connectedness has become a key focus point in the provision of primary healthcare (CDC, 2009b). Research has identified the importance of the link between schools and community within a prevention framework. Community-driven programs that encourage key stakeholders, including students, to set the agenda and create solutions are more likely to create a supportive environment for engaging in health promoting behaviors.

In the political sphere of the No Child Left Behind Act of 2003 and subsequent 2009 Reform as part of the American Accountability and Reform Act, schools have been challenged to rethink and redesign efforts to educate children. These reforms will undoubtedly present new challenges to the school nurse. The success of any reform must be linked to the social environment. School nurses have the expertise in assessment, education, and advocacy necessary to play a major role in meeting the needs of children and adolescents to ensure academic success.

key concepts

- Since the passage of PL 94-142 in 1975, school nurses provide more complex care for conditions such as seizure disorders, asthma, cardiac conditions, cystic fibrosis, quadriplegia, and life-threatening allergies.
- The role that emerges within the context of this management position requires the nurse to have skills in health assessment, health promotion, skills as a health educator, and the ability to work as a child health advocate.
- Data from the Youth Risk Behavior Surveillance Survey (YRBSS), a biannual report of the common risk behaviors influencing the health of our nation's youth,

can be used by the school nurse as a tool for monitoring trends both locally and nationally.

- There are online clearinghouses of school-based, evidence-based programs for the prevention of common health risk behaviors.
- School nurses play a key advocacy role that includes collaboration and policy-making, often participating in school district wellness committees.
- The future of school nursing is providing a prevention framework that links the community and the school.

critical thinking questions

The school nurse has a unique role in the provision of school health services for children with special health needs, including children with chronic illnesses and disabilities with various degrees of severity. This case describes the role of the school nurse caring for a child with type 1 diabetes.

Susan has two students with type 1 diabetes in her school, one requires blood glucose monitoring and daily insulin injections, while the other has a continuous insulin infusion pump. The incidence of type 1 diabetes presents a complex challenge to school healthcare providers. Type 1 diabetes ranks as the second most common chronic illness in childhood, second only to asthma. The American Diabetes Association (ADA, 2013) reports that about 125,000 children younger than 19 live with diabetes and 13,000 more are diagnosed annually. Children with diabetes are considered disabled and as such are protected under federal laws that prohibit discrimination against children with disabilities. Studies show that the majority of school personnel have an inadequate understanding of effective diabetes management. It is best for the student to monitor blood glucose and respond to the results as quickly as possible to avoid possible complications.

1. What are the essential elements of a diabetes medical management plan for each student with diabetes in the school?
2. When the school nurse is unavailable, who is legally responsible for providing care to a child with diabetes?
3. What expectations should the school nurse have of the students in diabetes care?

community resources

- Local and county public health departments
- State and local police departments
- Local community centers
- Town parks and recreation departments
- Primary care physicians
- Advanced nurse practitioners
- YMCA and YWCA programs
- Local amusement centers

references

Alexandropoulou, M. (2013). The health promoting school and the school nurse: A content analysis of school staff's views. *British Journal of School Nursing*, *8*(3), 134–141.

American Academy of Pediatrics Council on School Health, Magalnick, H., & Mazyck, D. (2008). Role of the school nurse in providing school health services. *Pediatrics*, *121*(5), 1052–1056.

American Diabetes Association. (2013). New evidence linking adiponectin and gestational diabetes mellitus. *Diabetes Care*, *36*(6), 1431–1432. doi:10.2337/dc13-ti06

American Nurses Association & National Association of School Nurses. (2011). *Scope and standards of practice—School nursing* (2nd ed.). Silver Spring, MD: Nursesbooks.org.

Avery, G., Johnson, T., Cousins, M., & Hamilton, B. (2013). The school wellness nurse: A model for bridging gaps in school wellness programs. *Pediatric Nursing*, *39*(1), 13–17.

Berk, B. (2013). *Effective substance use prevention*. Retrieved from http://www.ca-cpi.org/docs/Publications/Other/EffectiveSubstanceAbusePrevention_March2013.pdf

Burstein, G. R., Lowry, R., Klein, J. D., & Santelli, J. S. (2003). Missed opportunities for sexually transmitted diseases, human immunodeficiency virus, and pregnancy prevention services during adolescent health supervision visits. *Pediatrics*, *111*(5), 996.

Centers for Disease Control and Prevention. (1996). CDC guidelines for school health programs to promote lifelong healthy eating. *Morbidity & Mortality Weekly Report*, *45*(RR-9), 1–33. Retrieved from http://www.cdc.gov/HealthyYouth/nutrition/guidelines/index.htm

Centers for Disease Control and Prevention. (1997). CDC guidelines for school and community programs to promote lifelong physical activity among young people. *Morbidity & Mortality Weekly Report*, *46*(RR-6), 1–36. Retrieved from http://www.cdc.gov/HealthyYou.th/physicalactivity/guidelines/index.htm

Centers for Disease Control and Prevention. (2009a). *How much physical activity do children need*? Retrieved May 10, 2013, from http://www.cdc.gov/physicalactivity/everyone/guidelines/index.html

Centers for Disease Control and Prevention. (2009b). *School connectedness: Strategies for increasing protective factors among youth*. Atlanta, GA: U.S. Department of Health and Human Services.

Centers for Disease Control and Prevention. (2012a). Births: Final data for 2010. *National Vital Statistics Report*, *61*(1). Retrieved May 26, 2013, from http://www.cdc.gov/nchs/data/nvsr/nvsr61/nvsr61_01.pdf

Centers for Disease Control and Prevention. (2012b). *National youth tobacco survey*. Retrieved May 26, 2013, from http://www.cdc.gov/mmwr/preview/mmwrhtml/mm6131a1.htm?s_cid=%20mm6131a1.htm_w

Centers for Disease Control and Prevention. (2012c). *Sexually transmitted disease surveillance 2011*. Atlanta, GA: U.S. Department of Health and Human Services.

Centers for Disease Control and Prevention. (2012d). *Youth risk behavior surveillance survey*. Retrieved May 26, 2013, from hhttp://www.cdc.gov/mmwr/pdf/ss/ss6104.pdf

Centers for Disease Control and Prevention. (2013a). *Bringing high quality HIV and STD prevention to youth schools*. Retrieved from http://www.cdc.gov/healthyyouth/about/pdf/hivstd_prevention.pdf

Centers for Disease Control and Prevention. (2013b). *Childhood overweight and obesity*. Retrieved April 29, 2013, from http://www.cdc.gov/obesity/childhood/

Centers for Disease Control and Prevention. (n.d.). *The school health index (SHI): Self-assessment & planning guide 2014. Retrieved November 11, 2014, from http://www.cdc.gov/healthyyouth/shi/*

Elgie, R., Sapien, R., Fullerton, L., & Moore, B. (2010). School nurse online emergency preparedness training: An analysis of knowledge, skills, and confidence. *Journal of School Nursing*, *26*(5), 368–376. doi:10.1177/1059840510372090

Ethier, K. A., Dittus, P. J., DeRoas, C. J., Chung, E. Q., Martinez, E., & Kerndt, P. R. (2011). School-based health center access, reproductive health care, and contraceptive use among sexually experienced high school students. *Journal of Adolescent Health*, *48*, 562–565.

Health Resources and Services Administration. (2010). *The registered nurse population*. Retrieved from http://bhpr.hrsa.gov/healthworkforce/rnsurveys/rnsurveyinitial2008.pdf

Hertz, M. F., & David-Ferdon, C. (2008). *Electronic media and youth violence: A CDC issue brief for educators and caregivers*. Atlanta, GA: Centers for Disease Control and Prevention. Retrieved from http://www.cdc.gov/ViolencePrevention/youthviolence/electronicaggression/index.html

Kim-Godwin, Y. S., Clements, C., McCuiston, A. M., & Fox, J. A. (2009). Dating violence among high school students in Southeastern North Carolina. *Journal of School Nursing*, *25*(2), 141–151.

Looman, W. S., & Lindeke, L. L. (2005). Health and social context: Social capital's utility as a construct for nursing and health promotion. *Journal of Pediatric Health Care, 19*(2), 90–94.

Newton, J., Adams, R., & Marcontel, M. (2010). *The new school health handbook* (3rd ed). Hoboken, NJ: John J. Wiley Co.

Office of Applied Studies. (2009). *Results from the 2008 National Survey on Drug Use and Health: National findings* (HHS Publication No. SMA 09-4434, NSDUH Series H-36). Rockville, MD: Substance Abuse and Mental Health Services Administration. Retrieved from http://oas.samhsa.gov/nsduh/2k8nsduh/2k8Results.cfm

Robert Wood Johnson Foundation. (2010). *Unlocking the potential of school nursing: Keeping children healthy, in school, and ready to learn*. Retrieved from http://www.rwjf.org/files/research/cnf14.pdf

Singh, R., Jimerson, S., & Renshaw, T. (2011). A summary and synthesis of contemporary empirical evidence regarding the effects of the Drug Abuse Resistance Education Program (D.A.R.E.). *Contemporary School Psychology*, *15*, 93–102.

Solomon-fears, C. (2013). Teenage pregnancy prevention: Statistics and strategies. congressional research service, 7-5700. Retrieved May 26, 2013, from http://www.fas.org/sgp/crs/misc/RS20301.pdf

U.S. Department of Health and Human Services, National Heart Lung and Blood Institute. (n.d.). *Health information for the public*. Retrieved May 24, 2013, from http://www.nhlbi.nih.gov/health

U.S. Department of Health and Human Services. *Healthy People 2020*. Retrieved from http://healthypeople.gov/2020/topicsobjectives2020/objectiveslist.aspx?topicId=11

Wall Street Journal. (2012, September 24). *School Nurses' New Role in Children's Health*. Retrieved from http://online.wsj.com/article/SB10000872396390444358804578016221407143166.html

suggested readings

National Assembly on School-Based *Health Care. Health care for special populations: Children with special health care needs.* Retrieved May 26, 2013, from http://www.nasbhc.org/site/c.ckLQKbOVLkK6E/b.7505827/k.7C4D/About_NASBHC.htm

U.S. Department of Health and Human Services. Healthy people national health objectives. Retrieved November 11, 2014, from http://www. hhs.gov

web resources

Please visit thePoint® for up-to-date Web resources on this topic.

CHAPTER 23

Faith-Oriented Communities and Health Ministries in Faith Communities

Susan K. Chase

Faith is taking the first step even when you don't see the whole staircase.

Martin Luther King Jr.

Fear knocked at the door. Faith answered. No one was there.

Author unknown

CIRCLES

We are circles, in circles
Brushing and touching
Reaching and breaching
Our narrow confines
Giving and needing
Following, leading
Calling and heeding
Reciting our lines

Anonymous

chapter highlights

- Faith communities as centers for community health
- Cultural and developmental features of faith community work
- Integration of body, mind, and spirit in whole person health
- Health promotion in faith communities

objectives

- Differentiate faith community nursing from community health nursing.
- Describe various models of faith community nursing practice.
- Explain scope and standards of faith community nursing practice.
- Give examples of community assessments and interventions used by faith community nurses.

key terms

Congregation: An organized group of people who share religious beliefs, customs, or practices. The congregation has an internal governance structure and may be independent or affiliated to local or national denominations. It is a community within the larger community.

Congregation-based model: A faith community nurse serving a particular faith community by virtue of a contract or job description; supports the concept of a faith community nurse who can be paid or serve as a volunteer.

Faith community nursing: Equivalent to parish nursing; term used in settings in which the word "parish" may have no meaning or association. This broader term is the preferred term, but many original documents used "parish nursing" as the title for the role.

Institution-based model: The faith community nurse serves a health system with assignment to particular congregational settings. In this model, the parish or faith community nurse serves as liaison and helps plan and coordinate care, particularly at times of transition.

Parish nursing: A specialty practice of nursing having registered nurses contribute to the health and wholeness of people in the context of a faith community. The parish nurse is part of the ministry staff of the congregation and serves the illness needs of individual people, families, and the entire faith community. The original term describing the practice.

Spiritual care: Care of the human spirit that may include dealing with the meaning of health, illness or loss, relationships with God and others, and which has the goal of peace.

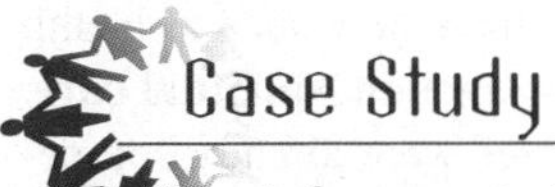

Case Study

References to the case study are found throughout this chapter (look for the case study icon). Readers should keep the case study in mind as they read the chapter.

Mary is the faith community nurse in a medium-sized suburban congregation. She conducted a monthly blood pressure screening session between the two services on Sunday morning. Matilda Swenson, a 76-year-old Swedish immigrant, who is active in the church despite the fact that she does not drive, has Mary check her blood pressure every month. The readings and notes for the past several months are shown below:

Medications: Advil for arthritis; no known drug allergies
Primary MD: Dexter Smith
June: 154/92 mm Hg; instructed pt to call her physician and notify him of the reading; gave pt a copy of her readings
July: 148/88 mm Hg; asked whether pt had called her physician and she had not. Repeated importance of contacting MD. Pt reported that she only went to rheumatologist for arthritis and they never checked her BP. Instructed pt to reconnect with primary care MD and report BP readings
September 2 (Labor Day weekend): 184/98 mm Hg; asked whether Mary could contact MD with pt present. Pt agreed. Drove pt home and called on-call service for advice. Learned that primary care physician had left the service but that the covering MD was available. Discussed with MD whether to go to the ER, but MD tells Mary to have pt call first thing Tuesday AM for an appointment. Called a friend of pt who was a member of the congregation who agreed to drive pt to MD Tuesday AM. Reported plan to clergy to support follow-up
September 4: Called to follow up on appointment. Learned that MD had switched pt from Advil to Tylenol for her arthritis pain and started her on atenolol for BP management. Planned to call in 3 days to check on pain level and medication compliance
October: 134/78 mm Hg. Reviewed mild exercise and low-salt diet; reinforced following medication plan. Pain control acceptable

Mrs. Swenson had been most bothered by her arthritis pain and had not found a new primary care physician when her previous physician left the practice. Her hypertension was causing her no symptoms, and arranging appointments was difficult. By assisting her in activating appropriate care, Mary helped Mrs. Swenson control her hypertension. Medications (nonsteroidal anti-inflammatory drugs), smoking, or alcohol consumption sometimes exacerbates elevated blood pressure. At least in part, because of Mary's efforts, Mrs. Swenson has felt better cared for by her new healthcare team, and her new treatment plan helps to increase her comfort and function and to reduce her health risks.

Mary records the number of home and hospital visits that she makes and keeps track of services used for referrals. She also keeps track of how many seniors in the congregation are able to maintain independent living with her support. She compiles an annual report showing who had access to health ministry in the year, including the numbers of people who belong, and who do not belong, to the congregation. Some health-related programs are open to the community, which is seen as an outreach for the congregation. Documenting participation by both members and nonmembers of the congregation is important in sustaining support for faith community nursing programs.

NURSING IN FAITH COMMUNITIES

Faith community nursing is a specialty practice of nursing that sees the faith community as a source of health, healing, and wholeness, and that sees the entire community as the recipient of care. Faith community or parish nurses have specialized education in spiritual care and health promotion in working in the faith community setting. They see the faith community as the focus and context of care, and their work has a goal of providing health promotion, health screening, and health teaching as well as caring for individuals and groups associated with the congregation. The faith community nurse does not replace activities that a community health or visiting nurse service would provide. There are no direct care activities such as dressing changes or injections regularly performed. The faith community nurse considers the needs of congregation members and makes referrals and advocates for quality care from a variety of sources for congregation members. Additionally, the faith community provides a context that allows the values, beliefs, and cultural practices of a community to support and enhance the experience of health. In addition to providing health promotion activities, the faith community nurse provides guidance to members of the faith community as they act out their faith and provide care to other members of the community. In this way, the faith community nurse supports the ministry of the faith community itself. Nursing in faith communities combines the worlds of ministry and community nursing. The faith community nurse meets the needs of a particular community—the faith community. This chapter will focus on the activities of faith community nurses as providers and supporters of health in the particular community organized around a faith stance.

Faith consists in believing when it is beyond the power of reason to believe.

Voltaire

For community nurses, health is not the mere absence of disease. The faith community nurse "focuses on the intentional care of the spirit, as well as on the promotion of holistic health, and prevention or minimization of illness within the context of a faith community" (American Nurses Association [ANA], 2012, p. 5). Faith community nurses also establish programs that support health promotion for individual people and groups in the congregation.

PRACTICE POINT

When a faith community member is diagnosed with a new chronic illness such as diabetes, consider the mental and spiritual issues that might be raised as the entire family deals with the new diagnosis. Assess the family for signs of stress and help them work through what the diagnosis means to them spiritually.

HISTORY OF FAITH COMMUNITY NURSING

Faith community nursing is a fairly recent concept; however, in ancient times, families and religious communities served as a primary source of health and illness care. Religious groups and monasteries established the first hospitals that were designed to provide "hospitality." Religious orders of both men and women delivered healthcare to the poor as they acted out their faith. For the individual person, the faith tradition provides the basis for many health beliefs and practices. Understanding a person's religious and spiritual background is important in establishing healthcare priorities.

Diseases of the soul are more dangerous and more numerous than those of the body.

Cicero

Granger Westberg, a Lutheran minister and hospital chaplain, began "parish nursing" in the 1980s. He had been involved in grant-funded holistic health programming, hospital chaplaincy, and community outreach by the healthcare system. He made the observation that all churches had a number of nurses as members and that these nurses formed an informal network of advice and support because congregation members looked to them as sources of advice and information.

The Lutheran General Hospital established an interfaith outreach program where nurses from several Chicago area congregations were paid in part by their congregations and in part by a grant to provide services in their congregations and to come together for regular training and support. This holistic care model was linked to the hospital through the chaplaincy program. The hospital saw the **parish nursing** program as a kind of outreach to the community. The role was new, so no organized curriculum existed. As part of a grant-funded program, the nurses met regularly and asked for help on issues that arose during their care, such as health counseling, grief and loss, health promotion, **spiritual care**, and leading prayer. The parish nurses were already competent nurses, but they needed additional training in community health concepts and principles. In addition, they needed more knowledge and skill in spiritual care because this was part of their role. Over the years, the congregations assumed more responsibility for the financial support of the nurses, who eventually received full support from the congregation.

MODELS OF FAITH COMMUNITY PRACTICE

Currently, faith community nurses work either on a volunteer basis or in paid positions. Some work in an individual congregation, and others are based in a healthcare system which has links to several congregations. In any case, the principles of parish or faith community nursing apply. Table 23.1 shows the variety of faith community nurse models (Solari-Twadell & McDermott, 1999).

In a paid, congregation-based model, the nurse is hired by the faith community to provide faith community nursing services. There is a job description, a clear list of resources or advisors, and a plan for evaluation. The advantage of this model is that the congregation clearly commits to supporting the program, and the nurse is a named member of the congregational staff. Potential problems can exist if the congregation staff members do not understand the role of the nurse. The role of the faith community nurse is different from that of (1) a chaplain who conducts hospital and home visits, in that the faith community nurse can help interpret and advocate for healthcare services, or (2) a visiting nurse service, in that the faith community nurse knows the members of the congregation over time and sees them in states of illness and health and in that the faith community nurse is not employed to do specific technical skills that congregation members might need. Overall, the strength of this model is that the faith community nurse is committed for a set number of hours to develop the faith-based nursing program for the entire faith community.

The parish pays Mary to work 20 hours a week for the parish, and she has an office on the church property. She can conduct individual assessments and teaching in this space or use larger meeting rooms for educational programs.

In an unpaid, **congregation-based model**, a faith community nurse volunteers his or her services in a congregational setting. Even though unpaid, this faith community nurse provides the same standard of care in the services as those provided by a paid nurse. Just as with the paid model, the congregation should have an advisory committee, with a

table 23.1 **Models of Faith Community Nursing Practice**

	Paid	Unpaid
Based in congregation	Paid and based in congregation	Volunteer and based in congregation
Based in health system	Paid and affiliated with health system	Volunteer and affiliated with health system

job description and evaluation method, so that the program can develop. The faith community nurse might need to ask for these things or develop them for the congregation. Even unpaid faith community nurses require a budget for supplies, resources, and continuing education. One disadvantage to having an unpaid faith community nurse is that this person may not be recognized as a member of the ministry team, and will probably have fewer hours to offer in service. One advantage is that the faith community nurse can limit how much time he or she offers, and can maintain other employment. This allows nurses who work in clinical or educational settings to offer their services to the congregation as both a professional volunteer activity and as a lay ministry. It also allows a congregation that cannot financially support a faith community nursing program to receive some of its benefits.

Often, new programs are started using an unpaid, congregation-based model. After the benefit of the program is demonstrated, a paid model can be supported. Both paid and unpaid congregation-based models share a disadvantage. The nurse usually operates independently, with little assistance from other nurses, and there is little support for developing new approaches to care. Faith community nurses often form informal networks to offer such encouragement to independent faith community nurses.

PRACTICE POINT

In an unpaid congregation-based model, the faith community nurse must be creative in securing resources to support the program. Obtaining small-grant funding can help, and making a case for an item in the parish budget can help obtain blood pressure equipment, including large-sized cuffs, health reference books, and teaching handouts for specific conditions.

In a paid institution-based model, a faith community nurse is employed by a health system, hospital, or community agency. The benefit to the agency is that the faith community nurse can serve as an ambassador and referral agent for the institution. For example, a religiously-affiliated hospital can support the services of faith community nurses in key feeder congregations, so that clients discharged from the hospital have coordinated transition to the home congregation setting. Discharge coordination can result in smoother transitions for patients and can reduce costs for the hospital system. The faith community nurse does not provide direct nursing care services, but supports the patient and family members in assuming self-care and in engaging the healthcare system appropriately. The faith community nurse serves as a health advisor, and he or she can recommend services which the hospital or health system provides. One advantage of this model is that the faith community nurse is connected to other healthcare providers for clinical and personal support. Reports and accountability for practice lie with the healthcare system. The faith community nurse who works within this model may not be considered by members of the congregation to be "one of their own" as much as with the congregation-based community model.

In an unpaid **institution-based model**, which is the least often used, some hospitals or care systems may support their nursing staff by paying for their time as these nurses volunteer their time in congregation settings. This can be an advantage for the nurse who wants to have time to offer services to his or her own congregation, but also wants to maintain primary identification with a healthcare institution. This can be an advantage for the institution, since community nursing activities are consistent with its mission, it receives referrals, and patients discharged from the institution benefit from coordinated transitional care.

Whatever the practice setting or the organizational structure of the faith community nurse, having a theoretic model for driving practice can help to organize both activities and reports. A model is useful when explaining a new practice to audiences such as congregation councils and members themselves. One model was developed by conducting a grounded theory analysis of case reports of faith community nurse network in a southern U.S. state. The analysis revealed a multistep model of practice: "(1) entering the private world, (2) connecting to faith, (3) mutually transforming experience, and (4) sustaining health" (Dyess & Chase, 2012, p. 224). Nurses reported that, at times, a task such as the relationship between patient and nurse was taking a blood pressure, and doing this task opened the door to deeper conversations. The encounter almost always had a faith component which included reflection or prayer. The experience transformed both patient and nurse in sharing their human experience in a faith context, and finally, health was supported through comfort as well as active intervention.

THE UNIQUENESS OF FAITH COMMUNITIES

Regardless of the model chosen, the prospective faith community nurse must consider certain factors when setting up a faith community nursing program. A **congregation** is a group of people with its own structure, and the faith community nurse must work within this structure. Where the program will fit into the congregation in organizational terms is one of the first things to consider. The faith community nurse must discover whether there is already a committee or commission which focuses on health concerns. Perhaps there is a social ministry group or an outreach group in the congregation. Understanding the structure of the congregation as a whole is important to support coordination with ongoing ministry activities in the congregation. Otherwise, long-time volunteers or leaders might be offended. This is part of the assessment process that will be discussed in more detail later in this chapter.

The pastor, rabbi, or other congregational leader can be a great source of information about structure. If no suitable group exists, the faith community nurse needs to assemble an advisory board (Garity & Ryan, 2002). The advisory board offers leadership, establishes policy, and helps develop guidelines. Having the support of an advisory board is essential for solving problems and avoiding pitfalls. Membership of the board can vary but might include the pastor, a spiritual director, designated health professionals, and interested lay people. The advisory board can help develop support for a budget for the program. When new members join the advisory board, they will need orientation about the faith community nursing program. By providing new members of the board with articles about faith community nursing, past annual reports of the congregation, and written job descriptions and evaluation forms, the faith community nurse assists the new member in becoming an active participant in the program. Meetings can take place as often as once a month. Meeting less than six times a year means that members will not have as much participation as they might like, and support for the faith community nurse might be diminished.

Relationship with the Clergy

Supportive relationships with the spiritual head of the congregation are important for the success of a faith community nursing program. Unless the pastor has worked with a faith community nurse before, repeated explanations will most likely be necessary. One common misconception is that the faith community nurse is a private visiting nurse for the congregation. The faith community nurse provides confidential professional nursing and refers to the ANA's *Faith Community Nursing: Scope and Standards of Practice* (2012) for guidance. If a member of the congregation is in need of visiting nurse services, the faith community nurse provides an appropriate referral.

EVIDENCE FOR PRACTICE

One interview study explored the experiences of chronically ill seniors who were members of an established faith community nurse's practice in a large suburban congregation. Despite the fact that individuals had from two to nine different diseases and were taking two to nineteen different medications, the seniors reported that their lives were connected to others, and that they felt they were living well. They were connected to the goodness of God in their lives, and most were caregivers for others, which gave their life meaning (Dyess & Chase, 2010).

In another study, researchers developed a survey that explored clergy members' commitment to health-related programming, and their experience with "congregational health ministers," a term used to include faith community nurses and other health professionals such as social workers, therapists, or pharmacists who were working in the congregational setting. Nearly 350 pastors from 80 different denominations returned the survey. The pastors fell into five main categories: mainline Protestant, conservative Protestant, African-American Protestant, Roman Catholic, and other (Catanzaro, Meador, Koenig, Kuchibhatla, & Clipp, 2006). The groups with the most experience with congregational health ministers were mainline Protestant and Catholic, and congregations that were large, suburban, and financially well off. Pastors with congregational health ministries in place in their settings reported more frequent health promotion programming in their setting. The most common reported reason for starting a health program in the church was that a nurse who was a member proposed it (Catanzaro et al., 2006). This study shows that individual nurses can influence health programming in their own faith communities.

A church is a place in which gentlemen who have never been to heaven brag about it to persons who will never get there.

H. L. Mencken, author

In the case study presented at the beginning of the chapter, the morning that Mary detects the highest blood pressure reading, she communicates her concern about Mrs. Swenson's health issue to the pastor, Mr. Dryden. She wants him to be fully informed about his parishioner. Being new in her position, Mary wants him to develop trust in how the program is operating. This way, if Mrs. Swenson needed to be admitted to hospital, he would not be surprised. He would also be able to set up a clergy visit.

Faith Community as Community

Faith community nursing is focused on the entire community of faith, not just on individual people who happen to be members of the community. This is consistent with most models of community healthcare. To assess the health of the faith community, principles of epidemiology, which were discussed earlier in this book, can be applied. The faith community group may be smaller than some other aggregate groups, but the same principles are appropriate. Although epidemiology began with tracing the patterns of infectious disease in the community at large, within the faith community, goals such as reducing disease risk factors, reducing the burden of chronic illness, and promoting health become more prominent than infectious disease. Nevertheless, principles of epidemiology can be used as a method to determine patterns of illness for the faith community, and risk factor assessment helps the nurse decide what programs to provide.

One of the major tools of epidemiology is statistics. Florence Nightingale was an early user of statistics to gather support for the changes she wanted to make in the British healthcare system. Similarly, faith community nurses can use statistics in two ways. First, the nurse should gather general demographic data about the faith community, including age, family structure, and proximity of residence to a healthcare facility and other health resources. These data can be summarized with descriptive statistics that can be used to generate reports and to assist planning. Second, the nurse should use data about various diseases from comparison groups, such as public health prevalence data. Is swine flu (H1N1) or methicillin-resistant *Staphylococcus aureus* infection becoming more prevalent in the area? County health departments publish data on certain reportable diseases which can be useful in planning screening or educational programs. It helps to compare the rate of cardiac events or strokes in a faith community which has wellness programs with rates for the same conditions in the region or nation. Using these data, the faith community nurse can demonstrate both the need for programming and the effectiveness of the programs conducted.

EVIDENCE FOR PRACTICE

A research review of faith community health promotion for African-Americans pointed out that using practice sites away from traditional healthcare systems can increase access to effective diabetes health education programs. Fourteen studies were reviewed. Overall, these studies showed the effectiveness of using culturally appropriate messages with the faith community as the recruitment source and the place for delivering the material. The studies used a collaborative approach in designing and carrying out their activities. Patient outcomes included increased vegetable usage, weight loss, and lowered HbA1c levels (Newlin, Dyess, Allard, Chase, & Melkus, 2011).

PRACTICE POINT

Developing a needs-and-skills inventory is a good way to determine what kinds of programs a congregation might value. Do people want information regarding specific high-impact conditions such as diabetes or heart disease risk, or do they care more about learning how to support the function of their aging parents? Sometimes, people are reluctant to admit to having weaknesses, but they want to help the health ministry. For example, a homebound person could have the "job" of writing cards to people who are in the hospital or who are having birthdays.

Another way to consider a congregation's social patterns is to explore the various ways members relate to one another, both individually and in groups. Faith communities often develop around ethnic groups. Roman Catholic parishes might be predominantly Irish, Italian, Polish, or Hispanic. Lutheran congregations might be German, Swedish, Finnish, or Norwegian. Jewish congregations share ethnic as well as religious commonalities. Are gatherings planned around major life events such as weddings, funerals, baptisms, or other entry rituals? (Are regular feast or holy days important to the group?) Understanding ethnic roots can help the parish nurse understand preferences and traditions that might affect health issues (Bigby, 2003). In all cases, the faith community nurse needs to be careful to avoid stereotyping, and to assess each individual person's perspective. However, celebrating ethnic background is a wonderful way to build community and make all people feel welcome.

The secret of health for both mind and body is not to mourn for the past, nor to worry about the future, but to live the present moment wisely and earnestly.

Buddha

Faith community nurses engage in primary, secondary, and tertiary prevention activities in their congregations. Primary prevention activities include programs on exercising to maintain health, smoking cessation programs, and heart-healthy eating programs. Secondary prevention includes screening for hypertension and setting up screenings such as mammogram vans or other tests to diagnose problems early. Tertiary prevention is another important focus where faith community nurses work to minimize the effect of health problems and maximize function for people with such conditions such as diabetes, stroke, or injury.

Faith communities are also part of a larger geographic or public community. Federal support for faith initiatives has increased in recent years. The congregation can be a site for health-related programming for entire communities. For some people in these communities, this may be the only health resource. One such program in central Texas organized a coalition that included state health departments, healthcare organizations, faith communities, county and city health departments, and local colleges and universities (Patillo, Chesley, Castles, & Sutter, 2002). Working together over 3 years, the coalition offered workshops to more than 1,000 nurses and prepared 54 nurses with the full parish nurse educational programs. The work of this coalition allowed the number of active congregational programs to increase from 5 to 53, established Web links to state health department resources, and offered services to Hispanic migrant families without health insurance. Students from local colleges and universities gained experience in conducting events such as health fairs.

ROLES OF THE FAITH COMMUNITY NURSE

Faith community nurses perform several roles which are similar to nurses' roles in many settings, but which often have a different emphasis. For example, as many community health nurses do, faith community nurses maintain lists of community and healthcare referrals. On the other hand, the faith community nurse's role as patient advocate may be unique because the faith community nurse has an ongoing relationship with the congregation member, may know family members, and can directly follow up on recommendations and additional referrals. Faith community nurses do health teaching in a variety of settings. These may include group settings for topical areas such as general health promotion, end-of-life planning or healthy lifestyle activities. Faith community nurses may also do individual teaching for congregation members with specific health conditions. The ministry to the congregation as a whole often leads the faith community nurse to organize and support volunteer groups, such as home visitors, drivers to appointments, or volunteers to provide meals to families who have members just home from the hospital. Faith community nurses can also lead or convene groups with specialty leaders such as bereavement or family caregiver groups. Perhaps more importantly, faith community nurses provide spiritual care based in the belief structures of the congregation. This may include assisting the congregation member to discern God's presence in a difficult time or to use spiritual resources as a support. The roles and activities of faith community nurses are varied. One of the functions of the health cabinet or other congregational group is to assist the faith community nurse in planning and evaluating activities.

Mary has several roles as a faith community nurse. Her primary responsibility is to empower Mrs. Swenson to make healthcare choices that promote better long-term health. Describe four roles that Mary assumes as a faith community nurse.

EVIDENCE FOR PRACTICE

1. One study reported on the activities and roles of parish nurses. A statewide survey was completed by 72 parish nurses, most of whom were volunteers who worked less than 10 hours a week. The largest denominations represented were Catholic (25) and Methodist (23) (King & Tessaro, 2009). Activities reported by the parish nurses were blood pressure screening (70%), physical health counseling (45%), health education relating to exercise (31%), and nutrition (29%). The nurses also provided counseling on spiritual health (28%) and bereavement (21%), and they offered support to clients engaged in weight control (25%) and stress reduction (25%). The range of services and support provided by parish nurses in this study reflects a balance of body, mind, and spiritual concerns. In the parish setting, nurses can truly provide holistic care.
2. An additional survey of nurses in a large Catholic healthcare system (McGinnis & Zoske, 2008, p.179) revealed that parish nurses, in addition to health promotion, "provide chronic disease management that is often lacking in our current healthcare systems." These activities included case management, advocacy, collaborating with other health professionals, and assisting clients in adapting to functional limitations.

HEALTHY PEOPLE 2020 PRIORITIES

Where do faith community nurses obtain guidance for planning, programming, and prioritizing their activities? Some of the best sources are national guidelines to support health such as *Healthy People 2020* (U.S. Department of Health and Human Services, n.d.). *Healthy People 2020* is the program sponsored by the federal government to help set health goals for the United States as a whole. Leading health indicators are listed in Box 23.1.

Most of these health indicators are issues that can be addressed in congregation-wide health promotion programs. Church groups can address local environmental quality issues as they arise. Physical activity for all age groups in the congregation can be supported through hiking clubs, senior exercise programs, or by sponsoring an aerobics group in one of the church rooms. Denominationally related weight management programs are available which a church could sponsor. Smoking cessation materials can be prominently displayed. Alcohol and substance abuse problems can be addressed individually, or by having the church be the site of a 12-step program. Parental groups can develop and support the teaching of healthy sexuality. In any congregation, the parish nurse must be alert to signs of domestic violence which can include child abuse or neglect, elder abuse or neglect, or partner violence. Individual referrals

box 23.1 *Healthy People 2020* Leading Health Indicators

- Physical activity
- Overweight and obesity
- Tobacco use
- Substance abuse
- Responsible sexual behavior
- Mental health
- Injury and violence
- Environmental quality
- Immunization
- Access to healthcare

Source: Office of Disease Prevention and Health Promotion, United States Department of Health and Human Services. Retrieved from http://www.healthypeople.gov/

and support can be important. Mental health is often a hidden health problem. Knowledge of risk, and insight into high-risk situations, can assist the faith community nurse in appropriate assessment and response. To ensure that each member of the congregation obtains appropriate care, the nurse can counsel members individually about access to care, or offer resources in a reading area or library at the faith community.

PRACTICE POINT

Periodically review the *Healthy People 2020* or other such initiatives and reflect on what health programming suggested by these groups would benefit the congregation. Would adding a senior exercise group help maintain both socialization and improve function? Would a youth group focused on safety reduce the risk of traumatic injury or death for the younger members of the congregation?

STUDENT REFLECTION

In community health, we try to think of ways of reaching people with health programs before they get sick and need acute care. When I was placed with a faith community for my experience, I realized that this is real community care. This is where people come together regularly, and there is always a chance for a health program, either with new mothers or with senior citizens. At my site, we sponsored a new mothers' group, and used the church nursery for child care for the toddlers, so that the mothers could focus on the classes on nutrition. They shared a lot of wisdom with each other, too.

SCOPE AND STANDARDS OF PRACTICE

Faith community nurses function by virtue of their license to practice nursing. The vast majority of nurses in the United States are employees of hospitals, long-term care facilities, or home care agencies. In contrast, the faith community nurse functions more independently. The resources of the nursing profession as a whole, including the ANA's *Faith Community Nursing: Scope and Standards of Practice* (2012) are important guides to the faith community nurse. In terms of well-developed policies or procedures, the faith community nurse may not have the same level of structure as the nurse who works in a complex healthcare system. The ANA Standards of Care for Faith Community Nursing Practice are organized around the steps of the nursing process (Table 23.2).

How do faith community nurses actually spend their time? Using focus groups, researchers have conducted studies of parish nurses themselves. This method brings together people who have shared an experience to discuss and share their impressions of that experience with a researcher. The researcher then analyzes the discussion and presents the

table 23.2 **Standards of Care for Parish Nursing Practice**

Standard	Sample Criteria
Assessment	Collects comprehensive, appropriate data Collaborates with others in selecting and collecting data Data may include the following: Demographics, including living arrangements Health and illness incidence Functional status Spiritual issues Psychological issues Social issues in the community Community services and resources Assessment is an ongoing process Assessment data are used to form diagnoses
Diagnosis	Identifies actual and high-risk diagnoses and potential areas for growth, with attention to strengths Makes holistic diagnoses that include body–mind–spirit issues Uses accepted standardized nomenclature in documentation Diagnoses are recorded and communicated to support health and healing
Outcome identification	Expected outcomes are determined for each diagnosis, preferably with the client's participation Outcomes are measurable Outcomes are adapted to the particularities of the client, including cultural aspects and are achievable
Planning	Plans for health promotion are developed at every opportunity Plans specify activities and who should perform them Plans include evidence-based approaches Particular strengths and weaknesses of each client/family/group are considered Plans include a consideration of the client's values/beliefs/customs Plans include follow-up activities
Implementation	Interventions are mutually developed with the people involved Interventions are within the legal, professional, and contractual scope of practice Activities include the use of appropriate technology Interventions are recorded in standardized language to provide for continuity of care
Evaluation	Evaluation includes care of individuals, families, and groups using outcome criteria Evaluation of the major programs of the parish nurse is ongoing Revisions of plans and programs are based on evaluation data

Source: Adapted from American Nurses Association. (2012). *Faith community nursing: Scope and standards of practice* (2nd ed.). Silver Spring, MD: American Nurses Association.

findings. One study involved 17 faith community nurses from a hospital-sponsored program of volunteer nurses. These nurses discussed the attributes of the care that they delivered in their parish settings. Investigators used a focus group and telephone interviews (Chase-Ziolek & Iris, 2002). The faith community nurses reported that their most important contributions to their congregation were health promotion and prevention of disease, advocacy, health education, health counseling, psychosocial support, and spiritual care. They stated that the congregational setting provided a personal relationship which extended over time, and which integrated faith and health in a way that was rewarding to them and their patients. The nurses also reported that having the time to meet such a wide range of needs, and contend with differences in beliefs, even in the congregational setting, presented a challenge.

To determine the perceptions of members of the congregation about parish nursing, researchers conducted an ethnographic study of faith community nursing in two congregations, one predominantly African-American and one predominantly White (Tuck & Wallace, 2000; Wallace, Tuck, Boland, & Witucki, 2002). Ethnographic studies consider the language and culture of a particular group of people. This study showed that congregants were grateful for the easy access to health information that the faith community nurse provided. They also reported that the parish nurse was able to combine health and spirituality issues, and helped people more actively promote their own health. Specifically, many congregants described a successful, faith community approach to weight loss.

THE NURSING PROCESS IN FAITH COMMUNITY NURSING

In all interactions, the faith community nurse should keep in mind that the nursing process is the basis of the caring relationship (ANA, 2012). Individual assessments may include blood pressure, gait stability, home assessment for safety, assessing for distress related to grieving for the recently widowed, and assessment of knowledge regarding self-management of medical diagnoses and chronic illness. Family assessments might include stress assessment for the family with a new baby, support of the wife who is transporting her husband for chemotherapy, or strategizing with parents of teenagers whose behavior has been troubling. Community assessments can include assessing whether healthcare is accessible to members of the congregation, and determining whether a recent industry closing will create personal or financial stress for members of the congregation.

Assessment and Diagnosis

Epidemiologic principles are useful in planning faith community nurse programming. When assessing the health of a faith community, the community as a whole is the target of concern. Several key questions need to be addressed:

- What are the common health problems experienced by members of this community? The faith community nurse visits members in the hospital, and in counseling individual members, he or she begins to see patterns that affect the congregation as a whole.
- What are the chief demographic groups in the congregation? A large number of elderly people means that health programs need to be planned with an understanding of major health problems of the elderly, and should include support for maximizing functional status. A large number of young families means that programs need to include parenting support. Young mother's groups can provide socialization and encouragement to an important segment of the congregation. An active youth group means that health programs can be woven into activities in which the youth group participates.
- What are the health assets of the faith community? Churches and synagogues have a rich group of volunteers who can assist their communities by providing meals after hospitalization, transportation to physician's visits or treatments, hospital visits by specially trained visitors, and support groups for a variety of conditions. Assessing for strength is the key focus of community health assessment.
- What environmental health concerns exist in the congregation? The congregation is rooted in a local community. Members include people who have lived in the community for generations, as well as newcomers. By being active in the particular community, members become active in environmental health concerns. For example, the first meeting to address an observation of a cluster of cases of childhood leukemia was in a church in the community. A successful book and movie, *A Civil Action* (Harr, 1995), tells how a toxic waste dump endangered the health of a Massachusetts community. The book shows how members of the community came together in a faith community setting to begin to address their concerns about the safety of their local environment.

The purpose of an assessment is to provide baseline data and support reporting and planning. A health assessment can be thought of as a needs assessment for developing congregational programming. Faith community nursing is often misunderstood because concepts of community health are frequently not understood by the general public, who see healthcare as physician-dominated and disease-focused. Fortunately, the importance of self-care and active participation in maintaining a person's own health has become widely accepted today. Faith community assessment can lead to important health programming in a rich community setting. North American Nursing Diagnosis Association-International (NANDA-I) regularly updates the list and organization of nursing diagnoses (NANDA-I, 2012). Many of these are applicable to the community as a whole. Domains of nursing diagnoses include Health Promotion, Nutrition, Activity/Rest, Role-Relationships, Coping/Stress Tolerance, and Life Principles. Diagnoses under the domain of Life Principles include Decisional Conflict, Readiness for Enhanced Spiritual Well-Being, and Spiritual Distress. These domains are clearly aligned with the practice of faith community nurses.

Mary maintains records of blood pressure trends and current medications for all church members who come for blood pressure screening. This assists her in detecting patterns of concern. What other assessment data would Mary gather that would be helpful, particularly for the senior citizens in the congregation? A monthly senior luncheon held at the church hall allows for socializing among the senior members of the congregation as well as those in the surrounding community. A program is associated with the luncheon, and every year Mary presents a talk about a health-related topic related to her activities. Suggest three possible topics for Mary to consider for her presentation.

● PRACTICE POINT

Ask a faith community nurse to share his or her best practices. Find out what documentation system the local health department uses. Does this nurse use a similar type? Perhaps if all nurses used a common format, they could combine reports and better evaluate the health of the community.

Diagnoses for faith community nurses should include nursing diagnoses as identified by organizations such as the NANDA (NANDA-I, 2012), the Omaha system (Martin, 2005), or some other recognizable nomenclature system. Diagnoses can be made for individual people, families, or the entire faith community. Table 23.3 lists diagnoses that would be appropriate for each of these three levels.

Mary identifies that Mrs. Swenson has several diagnoses that need intervention. Based on what you know about Mrs. Swenson from this case study, name three of these nursing diagnoses.

Interventions and Outcomes

Outcomes may seem to be the end point in the nursing process, but before choosing interventions, it is necessary to determine which outcomes are desirable and achievable (Bulechek, Butcher, & Dochterman, 2008). This choice must include preferences of the client, family, and community and must include consideration of people's values and beliefs and resources as well as best available evidence for what actions are likely to have positive benefits for the patient. Nurses should individualize outcomes for diagnoses based on these factors. For example, for the diagnosis of Ineffective Therapeutic Regimen Management, the outcome for one person might involve independent management of diabetic testing and medication management. The outcome for another person might involve following the advice of a visiting nurse and taking medications as prescribed. Outcomes for the community as a whole might include acceptance of health status, caregiver emotional health, pain level control, decision-making, or self-care (Moorhead, Johnson, Maas, & Swanson, 2008). When nurses have determined outcomes, they can select interventions that support attainment of those specific outcomes.

Planning in the context of the faith community includes care of individual people, as well as care of the entire faith community. For example, the faith community nurse might assess the health risk factors of members of the community as high risk for cardiovascular illness and plan programs for heart health, including (1) nutrition programs using the church kitchen to plan and prepare healthy, tasty food; (2) hypertension screening; and (3) an exercise program in the church basement.

Faith and prayer are the vitamins of the soul; man cannot live in health without them.

Mahalia Jackson

table 23.3 **Nursing Diagnoses Appropriate to the Faith Community Setting**

Individual	Family	Community
Ineffective health maintenance	Impaired home maintenance	Lack of health-seeking behaviors
Impaired swallowing	Risk for imbalanced nutrition: more than body requirements	Imbalanced nutrition: more than body requirements
Impaired physical mobility	Risk for activity intolerance	Deficient diversional activity
Impaired memory	Deficient knowledge: asthma management	Deficient knowledge: resources for Alzheimer's caregivers
Chronic low self-esteem	Caregiver role strain	Powerlessness
Death anxiety	Chronic sorrow	Diminished readiness for enhanced community coping
Risk-prone health behavior	Compromised family coping	Ineffective protection
Risk for loneliness	Decisional conflict	Risk of other-directed violence

Source: Adapted from North American Nursing Diagnosis Association-International. (2012). *Nursing diagnoses: Definitions and classification 2012–2014* (H.Herdman, ed.). Philadelphia, PA: Author

EVIDENCE FOR PRACTICE

1. Ann Solari-Twadell, one of the key leaders in parish nursing, has conducted research on the interventions that active faith community nurses most often use. This study used a detailed survey based on the current version of the Nursing Intervention Classification (NIC) (Solari-Twadell, 2002; Solari-Twadell & Hackbarth, 2010), including interventions from the behavioral domain such as coping assistance, patient education, communication enhancement, and cognitive therapy. Physiologic interventions reported by nurses included activity management and nutrition education. One intervention not included in the NIC which faith community nurses reported as essential was "prayer." Prayer was listed as an activity in the NIC under the intervention labeled *spiritual growth facilitation*. One intervention listed under community was program development. This groundbreaking research is the most extensive report to date of the specific interventions that faith community nurses actually use, and it can be the basis for documentation systems, as well as for faith community nurse educational program development.
2. Weis, Schank, Coenen, and Matheus (2002) conducted a research study to examine the most frequent diagnoses and interventions reported by faith community nurses when working with groups of parishioners. They collected data from 22 faith communities over a 5-month period. The groups represented a variety of ages and included both men and women. In addition to quantitative data recorded by the faith community nurses, 10 participated in a focus group interview about what it is like working with groups of congregation members and whether documentation labels fit. The majority of group activities (56%) were for disease prevention, such as smoking cessation. Eighteen percent of group sessions were for illness management concerns, such as asthma or arthritis.

Although this study did not use as extensive a data collection instrument as the Solari-Twadell study, it showed that the nursing diagnoses selected for the group activities include health-seeking behavior, potential for spiritual well-being, knowledge deficit, anxiety, social isolation, and altered family processes. The interventions selected included active listening, health screening, support system enhancement, and presence. Other interventions for the groups included spiritual and emotional support. The nurses in the focus groups validated that these labels were a good description of their activities with congregation groups (Weis et al., 2002).

Community-Level Interventions

Of particular concern in community health is the disparity that some groups experience in gaining access to appropriate care. Faith community settings can be a unique and powerful approach to filling gaps in care. Recent immigrants and people without English language skill are particularly vulnerable to health risks. One parish nursing intervention project focused on 100 Mexican American women with gestational diabetes (Mendelson, McNeese-Smith, Koniak-Griffin, Nyamathi, & Lu, 2008). Participants in the study completed the Health Promoting Lifestyle Profile (HPLP-II), which was used to measure the effect of a randomized trial of a parish nurse intervention program. This program consisted of a 9-hour educational program regarding nutrition, with a spiritual message related to health and wholeness consistent with the belief system of the participant. Participants not selected for the intervention received the usual care. Outcomes were scores of the HPLP-II 3 weeks after the session, maternal glucose (hemoglobin A1C [Hgb A1C]) on admission for delivery, and birth weight of the infant to detect macrosomia, a common result of gestational diabetes. The study showed that scores on the HPLP-II for the parish nurse intervention group were significantly higher in stress management, health responsibility, physical activity, and spirituality. The study did not show differences in Hgb A1C or macrosomia. The sample size may have been too low to show an effect, and the intervention may need to be designed for more of a nurse "dose," that is, more engagement to show lasting effect.

Implementation requires carrying out interventions in ways that are well supported by nursing textbooks, clinical evidence, or national guidelines. Interventions classified by the NIC (Bulechek et al., 2008) or the Omaha system (Martin, 2005) can target individual people, families, and communities. The Internet provides access to guidelines for screening and managing many health concerns.

STUDENT REFLECTION

At first, when I began assisting a faith community nurse, I was uncomfortable talking with patients about faith issues because I did not feel prepared by my college courses in how to do this. Once I realized that I did not have to have all the answers about religious issues, I relaxed about listening to how people's faith gave their life meaning. I finally got up the courage to ask whether the patient wanted to share a prayer at the end of a visit, and I found she was praying for me, too. That was a beautiful moment, and it did not matter what denomination we belonged to, which was different. I now feel comfortable including spiritual care in my intervention with patients.

Community-Level Outcomes and Documentation of Practice

Nurses need to evaluate outcomes for individual people, families, and communities. Did individuals, families, and groups meet the outcomes that were set for them? Did they maximize their rehabilitation following surgery? Did families successfully bond with their new babies? Did the shut-ins in the congregation feel the warmth of the holiday season through visits, calls, or cards? Documentation systems which report health status of clients or communities before and after faith community nursing interventions are able to show the difference nursing makes in this setting.

Faith community nurses have begun to document the outcomes of their practice, including its effect on costs of care (Brown, 2006; Miller & Carson, 2010; Rydholm, 2006; Rydholm et al., 2008). Rydholm reports on the work of faith community nurses in supporting community resources, and as informal caregivers who provide many of the services needed by elders and those with chronic illnesses. By gathering the stories of parish nurses, this researcher has documented "an interruption of downward-spiraling illnesses through rapid access to care" (Rydholm, 2006, p. 10). Some of the issues addressed were unsteadiness in movement, syncope, medication confusion, hypertensive crises, and shortness of breath. By coordinating care at an early stage, faith community nurses reduced more expensive hospitalizations. Brown (2006) reviewed parish nurse documentation and showed that healthcare costs were reduced by parish nurses who reduced emergency department visits through advocacy and referral.

Rydhom et al. (2008) reported a study of 1,061 notes by 75 faith community nurses who worked in Minnesota which were made during the care of 713 older adults. Researchers uncovered the needs of elders which were met by the faith community nurses, including end-of-life care, access and referral, guidance, providing adaptive equipment, and offering calm and motivating support. These elements are consistent with the case study at the beginning of the chapter. Without access to a faith community nurse, elders and people with chronic illness may develop serious complications, lose their ability to live independently, or enter the healthcare system through the emergency department, which is unnecessarily expensive.

EVIDENCE FOR PRACTICE

In addition to health promotion, parish nurses provide for the sick and dying. O'Brien (2006) conducted a qualitative research study of parish nursing for elders near the end of life. Using a theory of spiritual well-being in illness that she had developed, she observed a parish nurse care for 15 elders at the end of life. The nurse used the Spiritual Well-being Interview Guide and continued to visit the elders, two to four times over 8 months. The elders exhibited five identifiable nursing diagnoses: spiritual alienation, spiritual anxiety, spiritual anger, spiritual loss, and spiritual peace. Interventions offered included sharing prayer and scripture, spiritual presence, and pastoral counseling. By dealing with the meaning of their health and illness, the parish nurse was able to assist some of the elders who were in distress to in achieving some peace in their lives.

It is important to document faith community nursing, which allows people to see how this new specialty is actually practiced. One study (Burkhart & Androwich, 2004) reported that an existing documentation system, the NIC, was used to code free-form charts from 170 health records from 13 parish nurses at 7 sites, including urban, suburban, and rural settings. The investigators conducted this research to determine whether the system could capture the actions of parish nurses in 1,607 separate interactions. Experts coded notes separately and checked their accuracy by comparing their coding choices. Overall, 93% of interactions fit existing categories, with 117 different interventions identified. The study made several recommendations for new or modified interventions to fit the community practice of parish nursing.

In the Burkhart and Androwich (2004) study, the most frequently used interventions were surveillance, spiritual support, admission care, medication management, emotional support, referral, and vital sign monitoring. The interventions in NIC are organized into domains. The most frequently used domains were safety, behavioral, and health system activities. The NIC labels describing spiritual care worked well in this setting. The new interventions that were proposed included scheduling appointments, communication with patient, case closure, community transport, supply management (community), and dying care (community). Faith community nursing extends such care to the community, so recommendations were made to adjust the interventions as published by the research group which developed the NIC classification. This research showed that one published and accessible system was able to capture most of the faith community nurse activities recorded in parish nurse notes.

In a state of the science paper, Dyess, Chase, and Newlin (2010) reported that four main areas of evidence exist related to faith community nursing (1) the development of new faith community nursing practices, (2) actions and roles that were reported by faith community nurses, (3) the evaluation and documentation of faith community nursing practices, and (4) perceptions of faith community nursing by congregation members. The authors point out that further research is needed in the area of demonstrating the outcomes of faith community practices.

ETHICAL CONSIDERATIONS

All the ethical principles that guide nursing practice in general apply to nursing in faith communities. On the surface, it might seem that ethics would not be a problem where practice is independent, and where the community might be expected to share common values because of a common faith. In most cases, this is true. The parish nurse works to empower members of the congregation to take charge of their health. This can enhance their autonomy. The faith community nurse is also guided by beneficence, the act of doing good. This is an even more stringent requirement than nonmaleficence: the need to do no harm.

However, ethics do play a role in faith community nursing. One area where parish nurses can commit an ethical breach comes up often in the family context of a congregation. This area is the need to protect confidentiality. One member of the congregation might ask how another member, who is in the hospital, is doing. Because of the professional code requiring confidentiality, the parish nurse has more restrictions that the average person might have on what can be shared in everyday conversations in the congregation. The parish nurse is bound by professional confidentiality not to reveal information about the health of patients, even if they are known to members of the congregation. Refusing to share information in a way that does not seem cold is a delicate art. One way to avoid this conflict is to explain to congregants early in the program, and often thereafter, that confidentiality for each member will be maintained. Often, the nurse can simply say, "I am sure that she would appreciate a call or a card"; this relieves pressure to share much information. In annual reviews, and in meetings with the advisory committee, issues of confidentiality or other general ethical issues can be discussed, and annual reports use group or aggregate data only, so they are unlikely to betray a confidence.

Whoever seeks to set one religion against another seeks to destroy all religion.

Franklin D. Roosevelt

EDUCATION FOR FAITH COMMUNITY NURSING

Continuing education programs are often used to educate faith community nurses for their role. The IPNRC has developed a curriculum which can be delivered in a continuing education format, or through a more formal academic program for college credit. The curriculum for all participants is developed at the baccalaureate nurse level, even though many faith community nurses have diploma or associate degree preparation. Others may have master's degrees in community health, theology, or in advanced practice roles, such as nurse practitioner or clinical nurse specialist. The second edition of *Faith Community Nursing: Scope and Standards of Practice* (ANA, 2012) includes guides for advanced practice nurses as well as registered nurses. The scope of practice and breadth of faith community programs is in part determined by the educational preparation of the parish nurse. A study designed to compare activities of parish nurses who had, and had not, completed the endorsed education program from the IPNRC (Mosack, Medvene, & Wescott, 2006) found that for 265 nurses in a statewide network, those who had completed a particular educational program (53%) worked more hours per month and were more likely to provide health screening, health education, and referrals, especially referrals to those services which were nonmedical sources, such as social services and mental health services. The IPNRC is now a part of the Church Health Center based in Memphis, TN (Church Health Center, retrieved from http://www.parishnurses.org/). Among the roles of the Church Health Center are developing the curriculum for the preparation of faith community nurses, and identifying the seven specific functions that parish nurses perform in faith community work. These functions are derived from activities that all nurses may engage in, but some of these activities differ in faith community nursing (Table 23.4). Additionally, the Health Ministries Association offers a membership organization for nurses and others in health ministry, as well as training programs for prospective faith community nurses (https://hmassoc.org/).

In response to the need for community health experiences and in conjunction with faith community and other community initiatives, student nurses in academic programs can have clinical practice experiences in faith community settings (Kotecki, 2002). Students are not actually asked to function fully as faith community nurses. The role of the parish nurse includes spiritual care consistent with the faith and values of the congregation, which may be beyond appropriate expectations for the student, but many of the health screening and promotion activities can be performed by students with supervision.

table 23.4 **Functions of the Faith Community Nurse**

Function	Examples
Integrator of faith and health	Spiritual care Spiritual assessment Sharing scripture Therapeutic listening
Personal health counselor	Therapeutic communication Assessing for emotional distress Assessing for suicide risk
Health educator	Individual health teaching Group health teaching Provider of health resources
Health advocate	Empowerment of members of the congregation Empowerment of the congregation to improve the health of the community
Referral agent	Maintaining lists of local providers/agencies Communicating with referrals
Coordinator of volunteers	Assessing for needs for volunteer services Recruiting and training volunteers Scheduling and supporting volunteers Commissioning and recognizing volunteers
Accessing and developing support groups	Referring congregation members to existing support groups Developing support groups for congregation members

key concepts

- Faith community nursing provides health promotion, health screening, and health teaching as well as care for individual people and groups associated with the congregation.
- A variety of faith community nursing models exist. In the congregation-based model, the nurse is hired by the faith community to provide faith community nursing services.
- The steps of the nursing process are applied to the faith community.
- Values, cultural practices, and faith are a part of health.
- The body, mind, and spirit of community members are the primary focus of nursing in faith communities.

critical thinking questions

1. The congregation is happy to hear that a nurse wishes to establish a faith community nursing ministry in their setting. They are concerned about liability and require that the nurse not "write anything down" because they believe that any written documentation would provide the basis for legal suits. How should the parish nurse respond?
2. What sources of information are best for planning educational programs for parishioners? How does the parish nurse select materials?
3. An 86-year-old male parishioner is on hospice care at home, and his daughter, a nurse, has been trying to meet all his physical needs around the clock. The pastor, who had made a home visit, calls the faith community nurse to express his concern that the daughter is becoming "burned out." How can the faith community nurse engage the faith community as a whole to provide volunteer support to this family?
4. The faith community nurse decides to increase health awareness by holding a health fair. What types of exhibitors would be good to include? Would the health fair be any different when held in the congregational setting than in another community setting? In what ways?

community resources

- Go to the Web resources on thePoint for directories of churches, faith community programs, and training resources.
- Start with the International Parish Nurse Resource Center or the Health Ministry Association; they have directories of active programs. In your area, you could contact church offices to determine whether the individual congregations have health-related programs.
- Explore resources available at the Health Ministry Association website.
- If your college has a chaplain or ministry center, ask the staff there whether they know of programs in your area.
- Hospitals, particularly those with religious affiliations, may have an active faith community link.

references

American Nurses Association. (2012). *Faith community nursing: Scope and standards of practice* (2nd ed.). Silver Spring, MD: Author.

Bigby, J. (Ed.). (2003). *Cross-cultural medicine*. Philadelphia, PA: American College of Physicians.

Brown, A. (2006). Documenting the value of faith community nursing: 2. Faith nursing online. *Creative Nursing*, *12*(2), 13.

Bulechek, G. A., Butcher, H., & Dochterman, J. M. (Eds). (2008). *Nursing interventions classification (NIC)* (5th ed.). St. Louis, MO: Elsevier.

Burkhart, L., & Androwich, I. (2004). Measuring the domain completeness of the nursing interventions classification in parish nurse documentation. *Computers, Informatics, Nursing*, *22*(2), 72–82.

Catanzaro, A. M., Meador, K. G., Koenig, H. G., Kurchibhatla, M., & Clipp, E. C. (2006). Congregational health ministries: A national study of pastors' views. *Public Health Nursing*, *24*(1), 6–17.

Chase-Ziolek, M., & Iris, M. (2002). Nurses' perspectives on the distinctive aspects of providing nursing care in a congregational setting. *Journal of Community Health Nursing*, *19*(3), 173–186.

Dyess, S. M., & Chase, S. K. (2010). Caring for adults living with a chronic illness through communities of faith. *International Journal for Human Caring*, *14*(4), 38–44.

Dyess, S. M., & Chase, S. K. (2012). Sustaining health in faith community nursing practice: Emerging processes that support the development of a middle-range theory. *Holistic Nursing Practice*, *26*(4), 221–227.

Dyess, S. M., Chase, S. K., & Newlin, K. (2010). State of research for faith community nursing 2009. *Journal of Religion and Health*, *49*(2), 188–199. doi:10.1007/s10943-009-9262-x

Garity, J., & Ryan, A. (2002). The impact of an advisory board on a parish nurse program. *Journal of Nursing Administration*, *32*, 616–619.

references (continued)

Harr, J. (1995). *A civil action.* New York, NY: Random House.

King, M. A., & Tessaro, I. (2009). Parish nursing: Promoting healthy lifestyles in the church. *Journal of Christian Nursing, 26*(1), 22–24.

Kotecki, C. N. (2002). Incorporating faith-based partnerships into the curriculum. *Nurse Educator, 27*(1), 13–15.

Martin, K. S. (2005). *The Omaha system: A key to practice, documentation, and information management* (2nd ed.). Omaha, NE: Health Connections Press.

McGinnis, S. L., & Zoske, F. M. (2008). The emerging role of faith community nurses in prevention and management of chronic disease. *Policy, Politics & Nursing, 9*(3), 173–180.

Mendelson, S. G., McNeese-Smith, D., Koniak-Griffin, D., Nyamathi, A., & Lu, M. C. (2008). A community-based parish nurse intervention program for Mexican American women with gestational diabetes. *Journal of Obstetric, Gynecologic and Neonatal Nursing, 37*, 415–425.

Miller, S., & Carson, S. (2010). A documentation approach for faith community nursing. *Creative Nursing, 16*(3), 122–131.

Moorhead, S., Johnson, M., Maas, M. L., & Swanson, E. (Eds.). (2008). *Nursing outcomes classification (NOC)* (4th ed.). St. Louis, MO: Elsevier.

Mosack, V., Medvene, L. J., & Wescott, J. (2006). Differences between parish nurses and parish nurse associates: Results of a statewide survey of an ecumenical network. *Public Health Nursing, 23*(4), 347–353.

North American Nursing Diagnosis Association-International. (2012). *Nursing diagnoses: Definitions and classification 2012–2014* (H. Herdman, ed.). Philadelphia, PA: Author.

Newlin, K., Dyess, S. M., Allard, E., Chase, S., & Melkus, G. (2011). A methodological review of faith-based health promotion literature: Advancing the science to expand delivery of diabetes education to Black Americans. *Journal of Religion and Health, 51*(4), 1075–1097. doi:10.1007/s10943-011-9481-9

O'Brien, M. E. (2006). Parish nursing: Meeting spiritual needs of elders near the end of life. *Journal of Christian Nursing, 23*(1), 28–33.

Patillo, M. M., Chesley, D., Castles, P., & Sutter, R. (2002). Faith community nursing: Parish nursing/health ministry collaboration model in central Texas. *Family & Community Health, 25*(3), 41–51.

Rydholm, L. (2006). Documenting the value of faith community nursing: 1. Saving hundreds, making cents: A study of current realities. *Creative Nursing, 12*(2), 10–12.

Rydholm, L., Moone, R., Thornquist, L., Alexander, W., Gustafson, V., & Speece B. (2008). Care of community-dwelling older adults by Faith Community Nurses. *Journal of Gerontological Nursing,* 34(4), 18 -29.

Solari-Twadell, P. A. (2002). *The differentiation of the ministry of parish nursing practice within congregations* (Unpublished dissertation). Loyola University of Chicago.

Solari-Twadell, P. A., & Hackbarth, D. P. (2010). Evidence for a new paradigm of the ministry of parish nursing practice using the nursing intervention classification system. *Nursing Outlook, 58*, 69–75.

Solari-Twadell, P. A., & McDermott, M. (Eds). (1999). *Parish nursing: Promoting whole person health within faith communities.* Thousand Oaks, CA: Sage Publishing.

Tuck, I., & Wallace, D. C. (2000). Exploring parish nursing from an ethnographic perspective. *Journal of Transcultural Nursing, 11*(4), 290–299.

U. S. Department of Health and Human Services. (n.d.). *Healthy People 2020.* Retrieved April 28, 2009, from http://www.healthypeople.gov/

Wallace, D. C., Tuck, I., Boland, C. S., & Witucki, J. M. (2002). Client perceptions of parish nursing. *Public Health Nursing, 19*(2), 128–135.

Weis, D. M., Schank, M. J., Coenen, A., & Matheus, R. (2002). Parish nurse practice with client aggregates. *Journal of Community Health Nursing, 19*(2), 105–113.

web resources

Please visit thePoint® for up-to-date Web resources on this topic.

CHAPTER 24

Palliative and End-of-Life Care

Patricia Tabloski

DYING

The sun kept setting, setting still;
No hue of afternoon
Upon the village I perceived,—
From house to house 't was noon.
The dusk kept dropping, dropping still;
No dew upon the grass,
But only on my forehead stopped,
And wandered in my face.
My feet kept drowsing, drowsing still
My fingers were awake;
Yet why so little sound myself
Unto my seeming make?
How well I knew the light before!
I could not see it now.
'T is dying, I am doing; but
I'm not afraid to know.

Emily Dickinson

chapter highlights

- Social trends in aging and dying
- Palliative and hospice care for persons across the lifespan
- Caring for a person at the end of life
- Strategies for managing pain and common symptoms

objectives

- Describe the role of the community health nurse in providing quality end-of-life care for seriously ill patients and their families.
- Recognize changes in demographics, economics, and service delivery that require improved nursing interventions at the end of life.
- Identify the diverse settings for end-of-life care and the role of the nurse in each setting.
- Describe how pain and presence of adverse symptoms affect the dying process.
- Explore pharmacological and alternative methods of treating pain.
- Identify the signs of approaching death.
- Describe appropriate nursing interventions when caring for the dying.
- Describe postmortem care.
- Discuss family support during the grief and bereavement period.

key terms

Adjuvant drugs: Medications used along with analgesics to increase the effectiveness of the drugs to treat pain and associated symptoms.

Advance directives: Documents signed by the patient indicating his or her choice or wishes for medical treatment or naming of another to make choices if the patient is unable to do so.

Bereavement: A period of time or state of mind where feelings of loss, grief, or mourning are experienced by the survivor after the death of a loved one.

Breakthrough pain: Pain that is experienced despite the fact that a patient is receiving scheduled pain relief medication.

Comfort measures only (CMO): A plan of care that specifies nursing interventions designed not to treat disease but to improve pain, function, or quality of life.

Grief: Feelings of despair, sadness, and remorse in response to the loss of a loved one.

Healthcare proxy: A person designated to make healthcare decisions for another in the event that he or she is unable to make such decisions because of illness or disability.

Hospice home care: Care of patients and families who have 6 months or less to live in what they consider their home.

Mourning: The outward social expressions of loss often dictated by cultural norms, customs, rituals, and tradition.

Palliative care: Interdisciplinary team-based care for persons and family members experiencing life-threatening illness or injury that addresses their physical, emotional, social, and spiritual needs.

Postmortem care: Care provided by nurses to the body after death of the patient.

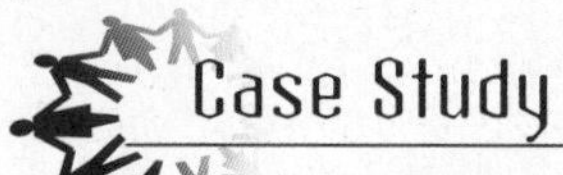

Case Study

References to the case study are found throughout this chapter (look for the case study icon). Readers should keep the case study in mind as they read the chapter.

Louise Clark is an 86-year-old woman who has just been discharged from a long-term care facility to her home. She spent 3 weeks at the facility after a 6-day acute care hospitalization for pneumonia and weight loss. Mrs. Clark, whose husband died 10 years ago, now lives alone with the help of her daughter, Mary, who lives nearby. Mary helps with cooking, shopping, and cleaning but is feeling overwhelmed; she is concerned that her mother may need more day-to-day assistance but does not want to consider permanent nursing home placement at this time.

Mrs. Clark has been diagnosed with several chronic conditions common to older persons, including macular degeneration, heart failure, and atrial fibrillation. The drugs and all the care related to these conditions were prescribed from primary care and emergency departments physicians from whom she has received care from over the last several years.

It is apparent to Mrs. Clark's family that she is failing and seems to be on a downhill trajectory, but her physician continues to state that "she is doing just fine for a woman her age." Mrs. Clark has named her daughter Mary as her healthcare proxy but has never given her specific information about the kind of care she would like as she gets older, other than to say she does not want to suffer needless pain and medical intervention near the end of her life as her husband did the year before he died.

Mrs. Clark received home care visits to assess and monitor her cardiovascular status. Her functional status has varied and at times she has been unable to leave her home without much effort. A home care nurse came to visit her for 2 months and then referred her to the local elder care services to acquire homemaker and home health aide assistance with bathing, meals, and light housekeeping. Mrs. Clark has had two emergency department visits and three admissions to the acute care hospital in the last year. These visits were related to falls, exacerbation of heart failure, and pneumonia. After each hospitalization, Mrs. Clark improved but never returned to her prehospitalization function.

Mary is concerned that it is less safe for her mom to live at home alone despite the help of her family and services; she needed to have more home health aide care for her safety. She was told that in order to qualify for more services she would need to become Medicaid eligible by "spending down" to $2,000 in order to receive the care she needed. Mrs. Clark is hesitant to spend down as she wanted to leave an inheritance to her daughter.

NURSING AND PATIENTS WITH CHRONIC DISEASE

Something began me
And it had no beginning
Something will end me
And it has no end.

Carl Sandburg

The number of adults of all ages in the United States with chronic progressive illness is growing dramatically. Greater numbers of vulnerable adults and children with multiple chronic conditions are residing in the community, resulting in such problems as strained caregiver systems, limited decision-making capacity, and dwindling financial resources (O'Mahony et al., 2008). Community- and home-based end-of-life palliative care and hospice services are necessary because of an increase in the aging population, an increase in the number of people who wish to receive care and die in their own homes, and a decrease in the number of available family caregivers (Aoun, Kristjanson, Oldham, & Currow, 2008).

In 2012, 83% of hospice patients were 65 years of age or older and more than 40% were 85 years of age or older. Pediatric patients (younger than 24 years of age) and younger adult population (25 to 64 years of age) accounted for less than 16% of hospice admissions (National Hospice & Palliative Care Organinization (NHPCO) (2013a). It is thought that younger adults and children with life-threatening or life-limiting conditions are often not referred for hospice care for a variety of reasons, including patient, family, and caregiver's fear of acknowledging the seriousness of the underlying condition, lack of knowledge regarding the services and benefits offered by a pediatric hospice, scarcity of hospices offering pediatric services, and lack of reimbursement by many insurance companies (Lindley, 2013). However, with the passage of the Patient Protection and Affordable Care Act of 2010, hospice care for children was expanded and children who are enrolled in the Mediciaid or Children's Health Insurance Program (CHIP) hospice benefit may continue to receive care for their terminal condition. This change in pediatric hospice eligibility signals a potential increase in demand for pediatric hospice services as currently only 28% of hospices provide services to children (Lindley, 2013).

Because of nursing's holistic focus, nurses in all settings, including community health nurses, are uniquely qualified to provide comprehensive, effective, compassionate, and cost-effective care to persons at the end of life. The Hospice and Palliative Nurses Association (HPNA, 2011c) has issued a position statement declaring that professional nursing care is critical to achieving goals of care at the end of life, and that support of hospice and palliative care research and education is necessary to ensure delivery of such care.

Among the members of the healthcare team, nurses spend the most time and have the most frequent and continuous contact with patients and families at the end of life (American Nurses Association [ANA], 2010; HPNA, 2011d). Patients of all ages and their families look to their nurse to educate, support, and guide them throughout serious illness and, if need be, the dying process. This intimate position allows the nurse to advocate for improved quality of life for the person with serious illness. According to HPNA (2011c), "when faced with serious illness, people turn to professional nurses for education, support, and guidance." Informed understanding of the patient's values, wishes, and goals allows the nurse to attend to the patient's physical, emotional, psychosocial, and spiritual needs.

EVIDENCE FOR PRACTICE

A systematic literature review surveying the unmet needs of palliative care patients and their caregivers who received home-based palliative care services was conducted to identify ways care can be improved. The most frequently reported unmet need was effective communication with and between healthcare professionals. The researchers found that lack of communication negatively impacted the psychosocial care received by patients and their caregivers. Physical care needs were met, indicating that the palliative home care services were delivering satisfactory care in this domain, but could improve communication to prevent or reduce suffering in areas such as psychosocial domains (Ventura, Burney, Brooker, Fletcher, & Ricciardelli, 2013). Quality of life issues that are crucial to address include self-esteem, adaptation to illness, social functioning, relationships, and spirituality.

Failure to acknowledge the presence and nature of distress experienced by seriously ill patients and their families may result in fragmentation of care, anxiety, and discomfort. Aggressive treatment of one condition may exacerbate the optimal functioning of other health problems. Through specialized end-of-life education with emphasis on therapeutic communication and pain and symptom management, the community health nurse can foster comfort and dignity for seriously ill patients, as well as for those with life-threatening illness; clarify goals of care; decrease unnecessary hospitalization; and prevent the administration of futile, aggressive end-of-life care.

Seriously ill patients and their families look to nurses to educate, support, and guide them throughout the illness trajectory. This intimate position allows nurses to advocate for improved quality of life for people with serious illness. According to HPNA (2011c), "achieving quality of life, especially at the end of life, is contingent upon competent, 'state of the art' professional nursing care." Informed understanding of patients' values, wishes, and goals allows nurses to attend to the physical, emotional, psychosocial, and spiritual needs of patients.

Let us live so that when we come to die even the undertaker will be sorry.

Mark Twain

STUDENT REFLECTION

I was assigned to visit Mrs. Clark during my community health rotation with my preceptor, Julie, an experienced home care nurse. At first I was frightened. I thought such a frail older person should be in the hospital, where she could be safe and nurses could look after her 24 hours a day. Julie explained to me that caring for patients at the end of their lives is complicated; nurses can provide physical care and manage pain and symptoms in the home while attending to the psychological, social, and spiritual needs of the patient and the family. Hospice and palliative care services can offer a number of benefits to frail patients living at home, including access to a multidisciplinary team skilled in the management of pain and symptoms that often accompany advanced disease. After Julie discussed the possibility of a hospice referral with Mrs. Clark and her daughter, everyone (including me) felt a lot better.

Nurses need to learn how to acknowledge and accept death as a natural process and realize that they can be instrumental in helping patients achieve the kind of death they desire. Obtaining the services needed to keep patients safe can help alleviate the fears of professional and lay caregivers, and home-residing patients in need of skilled nursing services will benefit from appropriate referrals and visiting nurse services. In addition, chronically ill persons may benefit from friendly visitor programs, home-delivered meals, community-based van or transportation services, and homemaker services. A hospice patient has access to additional services. Typically, hospice provides for home health aide five times a week for people with Medicare or who have private insurance with a hospice benefit in place. In 1982, the Medicare Hospice Benefit was enacted and authorized care in the patient's home, and in 2012 Medicare paid for 79% of all hospice care and Medicaid paid for slightly less than 4% (NHPCO, 2013a). The Centers for Medicare & Medicaid Services' definition of hospice is presented in Box 24.1. Patients can access Medicare hospice benefits if they meet *all* of the conditions listed in Box 24.2.

Generally, hospice care includes services that are reasonable and necessary for the comfort and management of a terminal illness. According to the National Hospice and

box 24.1 Definition of Hospice

- Hospice provides comfort and support services to people who are terminally ill. It helps them live out the time they have remaining to the fullest extent possible.
- Hospice care is provided by a specially trained team that cares for the "whole person," including his or her physical, emotional, social, and spiritual needs.
- Hospice provides support to family members caring for a terminally ill person.
- Hospice is generally given in the home.
- Hospice services may include drugs, physical care, counseling, equipment, and supplies for the terminal and related condition(s).
- Hospice is not only for people with cancer.
- Hospice does not shorten or prolong life.
- Hospice focuses on comfort, not on curing an illness.

Source: National Hospice & Palliative Care Organization. (2013a). *NHPCO facts and figures: Hospice care in America.* Alexandria, VA: NHCPO.

box 24.2 Conditions That Must Be Met to Obtain Medicare Hospice Benefits

- The patient is eligible for Medicare Part A (Hospital Insurance).
- A physician and the hospice medical director certify that the patient is terminally ill and has 6 months or less to live if the illness runs its normal course.
- The patient signs a statement choosing hospice care instead of other Medicare-covered benefits to treat the terminal illness. Medicare will still pay for covered benefits and treatment of any other health problems not related to the terminal illness.
- The patient receives care from a Medicare-approved hospice program.

Source: Medicare.gov. (2013). *Medicare hospice benefits.* Retrieved from http://www.medicare.gov/pubs/pdf/02154.pdf

Palliative Care Organization (NHPCO, 2013b), the following 10 components of quality in hospice care include:

- **Patient-and-Family-Centered Care**
  Providing care and services that are responsive to the needs and exceed the expectations of those served.
- **Ethical Behavior and Consumer Rights**
  Upholding high standards of ethical conduct and advocating for the rights of patients and their family caregivers.
- **Clinical Excellence and Safety**
  Ensuring clinical excellence and promoting safety through standards of practice.
- **Inclusion and Access**
  Promoting inclusiveness in the community by ensuring that all people—regardless of race, ethnicity, color, religion, gender, disability, sexual orientation, age, or other characteristics—have access to programs and services.
- **Organizational Excellence**
  Building a culture of quality and accountability within our organization that values collaboration and communication and ensures ethical business practices.
- **Workforce Excellence**
  Fostering a collaborative, interdisciplinary environment that promotes inclusion, individual accountability, and workforce excellence through professional development, training, and support to all staff and volunteers.
- **Standards**
  Adopting the NHPCO Standards of Practice for Hospice Programs and/or the National Consensus Project's Clinical Practice Guidelines for Quality Palliative Care as the foundation for an organization.
- **Compliance with Laws and Regulations**
  Ensuring compliance with all applicable laws, regulations, and professional standards of practice, and implementing systems and processes that prevent fraud and abuse.
- **Stewardship and Accountability**
  Developing a qualified and diverse governance structure and senior leadership who share the responsibilities of fiscal and managerial oversight.
- **Performance Measurement**
  Collecting, analyzing, and actively using performance measurement data to foster quality assessment and performance improvement in all areas of care and services (NHPCO, 2013b).

Hospice does not speed up or slow down the dying process. It does not prolong life and it does not hasten death.

National Hospice Foundation

Healthcare reform and benefits covered by Medicare are currently under debate in the U.S. Congress; therefore, it is wise to visit the Medicare website (http://www.medicare.gov) and/or consult with a knowledgeable social worker to obtain the most current and accurate information regarding services covered. The healthcare reform act has expanded services covered under the hospice benefit in an effort to improve care of the patient nearing the end of life. At present, a patient can get Medicare hospice benefits when they meet **all** of the following conditions:

- They are eligible for Medicare Part A (Hospital Insurance).
- The physician and the hospice medical director certify that the patient is terminally ill and has 6 months or less to live if the illness runs its normal course.
- The patient signs a statement choosing hospice care instead of other Medicare-covered benefits to treat the terminal illness. (Medicare will still pay for covered benefits for any health problems that are not related to the terminal illness.)
- The patient will receive care from a Medicare-approved hospice program (Medicare.gov, 2013).

Medicare covers the following hospice services when they are needed to care for the patient with terminal illness and related condition(s):

- Doctor services
- Nursing care
- Medical equipment (such as wheelchairs or walkers)
- Medical supplies (such as bandages and catheters)
- Drugs for symptom control or pain relief (may require a small co-payment)
- Hospice aide and homemaker services
- Physical and occupational therapy
- Speech-language pathology services
- Social worker services
- Dietary counseling
- Grief and loss counseling for the patient and family
- Short-term in-patient care (for pain and symptom management)
- Short-term respite care (may require a small co-payment)
- Any other Medicare-covered services needed to manage pain and other symptoms related to the terminal illness, as recommended by the hospice team (Medicare.gov, 2013)

Palliative care for children can reduce a child's pain, help manage other distressing symptoms, and provide important emotional support to the child and family throughout the course of an illness. Research has shown that pediatric palliative care services may also increase overall satisfaction with care for patients and their families. Yet, many healthcare providers continue to hesitate to recommend palliative care for their youngest patients, and parents and caregivers are often unaware of its benefits (National Institutes of Health, 2014). See Box 24.3 for Pediatric Palliative Care Referral Criteria.

Viewing death as a natural process, not a medical failure, is of utmost importance. Some caregivers consider that death is not normal and when it occurs, someone is at fault. Of course, nurses know that this is not true; in many serious progressive illnesses, death is an expected outcome. Nurses who help patients die comfortably and with dignity provide the following principles of quality patient-centered care (National Consensus Project [NCP] for Quality Palliative Care, 2013b):

- Providing care and services that are responsive to the needs and exceed the expectations of those we serve.
- The patient and family is the unit of care.
- The hospice interdisciplinary team, in collaboration with the patient, family, and caregiver, develops and maintains a patient-, family-, and caregiver-directed, individualized, safe and coordinated plan of palliative care.
- Addressing loss, grief, and bereavement needs begins with the initial assessment at the time of admission to the hospice and continues throughout the course of care.
- Anticipatory mourning services are provided to help patients, families, and caregivers cope with the multitude of losses that occur during the illness and eventual death of the patient. Bereavement services are provided after death and are based on a number of factors, including a bereavement risk assessment which assesses intensity of grief, coping and adapting abilities of the survivors and their individual needs, and the benefits and burdens of treatment.

To supply this care, nurses must be well educated, have appropriate supports in the clinical setting, and develop a close collaborative partnership with palliative care service providers and hospice programs.

box 24.3 Pediatric Palliative Care Referral Criteria

- Perinatal/neonatal: Life-threatening diagnoses made months to hours before birth of the neonate in the few days, weeks, or months of life
- Neurological conditions: Hypoxic injury, birth trauma, structural malformation of the CNS, metabolic diseases, genetic or congenital syndromes
- Congenital heart defects: Ventricle malformation, pulmonary vein stenosis, cardiomyopathy, pulmonary hypertension, coarctation of the aorta, posttransplant care
- Other diagnoses: Cystic fibrosis, solid organ transplant, oncology, primary immunodeficiency disorders, acquired immunodeficiency disorder, acute leukemia

Source: Adapted from Stroupe, L. M. (2013). Process improvement for pediatric supportive care. *Journal of Hospice & Palliative Nursing*, *15*(8), 479–484.

STUDENT REFLECTION

I was amazed at how quickly my home health nurse preceptor mobilized community-based resources. After making several phone calls to her professional colleagues (all of whom she knew by their first names!), she was quickly able to get the needed services in place. It really illustrated the importance of communication and teamwork.

Nurses must be confident in their clinical skills when caring for the dying—awareness of the ethical, spiritual, and legal issues they may confront while providing end-of-life care is essential. Many nurses believe that the first step in the process is confronting their own personal fears about death and dying. By addressing their own fears, nurses are better able to help patients and families when they are confronted with impending death. The nurse may then more objectively recognize and respect the patient and family's values and choices which guide their decisions at the end of life. Table 24.1 identifies common problems that interfere with quality end-of-life nursing care.

DEATH IN THE UNITED STATES

Stages in the Dying Process

Elisabeth Kübler-Ross, a psychiatrist at the University of Chicago, was also a pioneer for end-of-life care; the early hospice movement was supported by her research. Kübler-

table 24.1 **Problems That Interfere with Quality End-of-Life Community-Based Nursing Care**

Problem	Potential Outcomes
The community health nurse may hesitate to discuss a hospice referral.	Hospice services are not initiated in a timely manner may come too late to initiate advanced care planning and to support end-of-life choices.
The patient has not discussed his or her end-of-life preferences for care.	Professional caregivers and families may not have the appropriate information to institute a plan of care that meets the patient's expectations, including provision of appropriate interventions.
Financial matters and insurance approvals have not been obtained.	Needed services may be denied or delayed by a lengthy appeal process.
Funeral wishes, organ donation, and establishment of a will have not been specified.	Same-sex partners may be excluded from involvement, valuable organs are not available to others in need, and families may argue over inheritance and disposition of property.

Ross (1969) interviewed hundreds of dying patients and published her findings in *On Death and Dying: What the Dying Have to Teach Doctors, Nurses, Clergy and Their Own Families*. It was through her efforts that healthcare providers began to understand the needs of dying patients. Her work also emphasized the need for pain relief in terminally ill patients. The outcome of this research was the development of the "stages of dying." These stages include denial, anger, bargaining, and acceptance. It must be remembered that a dying person may not exhibit all of these stages, or may move quickly through a stage, only to return to it at a later time.

EVIDENCE FOR PRACTICE

Although Kübler-Ross' framework stimulated research and changed practice in the field of end-of-life care, the concept may not be as simple as described. Today, not all researchers agree with Kübler-Ross, and some claim that her research cannot be replicated (Konigsberg, 2011). Today, there are over 25 instruments widely used to measure grief, and each one differs from the other. It is difficult to categorize and synthesize all of the current research, most of which tends to describe complex and unique emotional responses to grief. Nurses will often find they need to think beyond the basic five stages.

Specialized Care at the End of Life

During the mid-1900s, technological advances dictated that sick people should go to hospitals where they could safely receive "high-tech" care. Surgery, antibiotics, and advanced testing techniques became the focus of healthcare, shifting away from the provision of care to the pursuit of cure. Table 24.2 illustrates the changing demographic and social trends surrounding the cause of death in the years 1900 and 2010. In 2010, the 10 leading causes of death, accounting for 80% of all death in the United States, include, in descending order, heart disease, malignant neoplasms, cerebrovascular disease, chronic lower respiratory disease, accidents, diabetes mellitus, influenza and pneumonia, Alzheimer disease, renal disease, and septicemia (Centers for Disease Control and Prevention, 2011). Often, the exact cause of death is difficult to determine in seriously ill adults. The patient with Alzheimer disease may fall, fracture a hip, and die shortly after the injury. However, the actual cause of the fall may have been a myocardial infarction that was not detected. The death certificate may indicate a fall or Alzheimer disease as the cause of death, whereas the true cause was the myocardial infarction. Some people think that these difficult-to-categorize deaths may be deemed "natural deaths" or deaths that occur because of numerous unspecified causes, including advanced age, organ failure, and impact of comorbidities.

table 24.2 **Cause of Death and Demographic/Social Trends**

	1900	2010
Focus of care	Comfort	Cure
Primary cause of death	Infectious diseases—e.g., pneumonia, influenza	Chronic illnesses—e.g., heart disease, cancer
Average life expectancy	50 years	78.3 years
Number of older persons (>65)	3.1 million	38.8 million
Place of death	Home	Institutions
Caregivers	Family	Professional healthcare providers
Disease trajectory	Short, downward trend	Prolonged, variable, peaks and valleys
Functional decline at the end of life	Short-term—expected and surprise	Lingering expected—frailty

Source: Centers for Disease Control and Prevention. (2009). *FastStats: Death and mortality*. Retrieved from http://www.cdc.gov/nchs/faststats.death.htm

In children, from 2000 to 2009, the overall annual unintentional injury death rate decreased 29%, from 15.5 to 11.0 per 100,000 population, accounting for 9,143 deaths in 2009. The rate decreased among all age groups except newborns and infants younger than 1 year; in this age group, rates increased from 23.1 to 27.7 per 100,000 primarily as a result of an increase in reported suffocations. The poisoning death rate among teens aged 15 to 19 years nearly doubled, from 1.7 to 3.3 per 100,000, in part because of an increase in prescription drug overdoses (e.g., opioid pain relievers). Childhood motor vehicle traffic-related death rates declined 41%; however, these deaths remain the leading cause of death by unintentional injury. Among states, unintentional injury death rates varied widely, from 4.0 to 25.1 per 100,000 in 2009. Malignant neoplasms, heart disease, congenital anomalies, sudden infant death syndrome, homicide, and suicide remain significant threats to the health of children and adolescents.

In the past century, social changes and technological advancements have shifted the goals of modern healthcare from care to cure. Over the decades, the experience of serious illness, death, and dying in the United States has evolved. What was once a short, rapid decline, which often occurred in the relative comfort of one's own home, now encompasses a trajectory of chronic illness with steady decline, periodic crises, the need for ongoing aggressive treatment, and finally death. Adults with chronic and progressive illnesses often lack coordinated care, with multiple episodic and unplanned emergency department visits which focus on single systems, quick diagnosis, and cure. As a result, seriously ill adults are at risk for polypharmacy, falls, functional decline, and institutionalization (O'Mahony et al., 2008).

NURSING CARE WHEN DEATH IS IMMINENT

Mrs. Clark has stated that she feels as if she is on a merry-go-round because she is in and out of the hospital so often. She says "I never want to go back to the cold, noisy hospital again. Please help me stay here in my home with my TV, my cats, and my memories."

Hospice care can be provided in many settings, including the patient's home, hospital, nursing home, assisted-living facilitiy, and in-patient hospice facility. When surveyed, most Americans express a preference to die in their own homes; however, most die in the institutional settings (Grunier et al., 2007). However, the past 20 years have seen a shift in the trends in place of death, with increasing numbers of people dying in their homes and long-term care settings, and decreasing numbers of people dying in the hospital. In 2007, 36% of Americans died in hospitals (down from 49% in 1989), 25% died in long-term care facilities, and 25% died at home (up from 17% in 1989) (CDC), 2011). Among the older adult population, race and ethnicity influence decisions about end-of-life care and place of death. Non-Hispanic White older adults are more likely to die in the nursing home, while older adults in other racial and ethnic groups are more likely to die in the hospital (Grunier et al., 2007; CDC, 2011).

Not only are fewer people dying in the hospital, older adults are spending less time in the hospital at the end of life. A recent report of the Dartmouth Atlas Project revealed that the average number of days older adults spend in the hospital before death, as well as the percentage of deaths associated with an intensive care stay, has declined in recent years (Dartmouth Atlas for Health Care & Clinical Practice, 2013). The report also demonstrated that increasing numbers of older adults are choosing hospice care at the end of life.

Data from numerous studies demonstrate high degrees of symptom distress in patients in hospitals and nursing homes; high use of burdensome technologies in seriously ill patients; caregiver burden on families; and communication problems among patients, families, and caregivers about the goals of care and medical decisions that should follow (Last Acts, 2002; NCP, 2013; Quill, 2000; SUPPORT Principal Investigators, 1995). Seriously ill patients who die at home avoid some of these problems. However, the reality of dying at home is often more complicated. Family caregivers are often stressed or may not be ever present; the home environment may be small, chaotic, or even unsafe, symptom control may be more difficulty; and the provision of basic nursing care such as bathing and grooming may be difficult for patients and caregivers. Additionally, some caregivers and patients may prefer more supportive in-patient care at the end of life (Lysaght & Ersek, 2013).

It requires more courage to suffer than to die.

Napoleon Bonaparte

EVIDENCE FOR PRACTICE

Research at the Dartmouth Atlas for Healthcare has provided evidence that populations living in regions with lower intensity of care in the last 6 months of life did not have higher mortality rates than those living in regions with higher care intensity. More than 80% of patients say that they wish to avoid hospitalization and intensive care during the terminal phase of illness, but those wishes are often overridden by other factors. If more intense intervention does not improve life expectancy, and if most patients prefer less care when more intensive care is likely to be futile, the fundamental question is whether the quality of care in regions with fewer resources and more conservative practice styles is more appropriate than in regions where more aggressive treatment is the norm (The Dartmouth Atlas for Health Care & Clinical Practice, 2013). All healthcare providers, including nurses, must work together and advocate for improvement in the quality of care provided at the end of life.

Decisions about Level of Care

Wherever patients spend their last days, these patients and their families face difficult decisions about end-of-life care. Uncertain prognoses may affect decision-making on the part of these patients, their families, and their healthcare providers, which perhaps leads to unnecessary interventions and treatments. Older people, especially, are at risk for overly aggressive care because they have high comorbidity rates and an increased likelihood of dementia (Derby & O'Mahony, 2006). For some patients, medical treatments offer little or no benefit, and at the same time may be painful or increase the burden of living; such care may be futile. Nurses, physicians, social workers, clergy, and others are responsible for counseling patients and families about making decisions regarding the type and level of care the patients wish to receive for the remainder of their lives. After the decision has been reached, it is usually noted in the patient's chart by the nurse or any other member of the healthcare team, so that the entire healthcare team is aware of the patient's wishes. Of course, the patient is always able to reverse these decisions.

Comfort Measures Only

A dying patient may decide to receive **comfort measures only (CMO)**—that is, allow death to occur naturally while maximizing comfort. CMO is the preferred choice when the patient confronts his or her mortality and considers less aggressive treatment. A nurse should review the use of life-sustaining technologies with the seriously ill patient. Those patients who wish to have CMO may receive traditional hospice care, with healthcare professionals focused on quality of life rather than on the length of life.

The physician or advanced practice nurse usually orders CMO when the patient, family, and staff are in agreement that the best care for the patient is not to prolong the dying process, but to keep the dying patient comfortable. Comfort becomes the focus of care when cure is no longer an attainable goal, expected quality of life is unacceptable, and comfort is a priority for the patient and family (Moneymaker, 2005). This does not mean that nursing care or treatments stop. Assessment and management of any physical conditions, activities of daily living, and behaviors, as well as pain, continue on a daily basis. Provision of excellent nursing care at the end of life can be a challenge, especially when the family has been told by the physician that "nothing more can be done." The designation of a patient as CMO does not signal the end of care, but rather shifts the focus of care from aggressive treatment of the disease to active nursing interventions to improve function, comfort, and quality of life.

Advance Directives

Many Americans are fearful of death and hesitate to discuss end-of-life preferences with their families and significant others. This can be problematic when the patient becomes very ill or incapacitated, and the healthcare professionals consult for assistance in medical decision-making. People of all ages should begin to discuss these issues with others who may be called on to make decisions in the case of serious illness or injury. This should occur in a noncrisis situation when the person has time to discuss the issue in depth, ask questions, and think about the risks and benefits of various interventions. Personal values, past experiences, cultural beliefs, religious preferences, medical knowledge, family orientation, and life experiences all help determine the end-of-life preferences. Each patient and his or her family should provide input into treatment decisions which are then based on goals of care, assessment of risk and benefit, best evidence, and personal preferences.

Advance directives are legal documents that allow people to convey their wishes for end-of-life care and include living wills, durable powers of attorney for healthcare, and healthcare proxies. Legal requirements for advance directives vary from state to state; some state laws mandate the use of living wills, and others require designation of a healthcare proxy or durable power of attorney for healthcare. All of these documents go into effect when the patient is no longer able to communicate his or her wishes. Living wills are documents in which patients describe their wishes regarding treatment intended to sustain life. This may include acceptance or limitation of life-sustaining treatment in the face of a life-threatening illness. It is necessary to copy a living will and share it with others; the physician, nurse, family members, and significant others should have copies and should indicate their willingness to comply with the terms stated therein. Many people place the living will in a safety deposit box so that others, who may not wish to honor it, cannot gain access to it. A **healthcare proxy** or durable power of attorney for healthcare is a person (and an alternate if the primary proxy is not available) designated to make decisions for the patient if he or she is unable to do so. The patient should then discuss his or her wishes with the proxy to ensure appropriate end-of-life care. The healthcare proxy is responsible for medical decisions only if the patient is unable to do this, and does not have legitimate input into any other areas of the patient's affairs (e.g., financial). It is necessary to make multiple copies of the proxy form, and healthcare providers and family members (including proxies) should keep them readily accessible.

Decision-making around the time of death raises many legal and ethical questions. Public debate and scrutiny help shape the ethical outcome of medical dilemmas. Healthcare professionals must work within the limits of the law and their professional standards of practice. Established ethical principles and moral norms play a vital role in determining healthcare issues.

In 1976, the Karen Ann Quinlan case brought life-sustaining medical treatment to the forefront of the U.S. legal system. A medical intervention, procedure, or administration of medicine to prevent the moment of death is seen as life-sustaining. This includes cardiopulmonary resuscitation (CPR), renal dialysis, use of ventilators, insertion of feeding tubes, total parenteral nutrition, chemotherapies, and other life-prolonging interventions. When questions regarding the initiation, ongoing use, and removal of life-sustaining technologies arise, and there are no advance directives in place, ethical and emotional issues arise. Many healthcare institutions have formed ethics committees to address these issues and to provide guidance and advice to the clinician, patient, and family. If the patient lacks a responsible family member, the courts may appoint a legal guardian. This is a cumbersome and difficult process, and naming a healthcare proxy or completing a living will prevent this process.

In 1990, the U.S. Supreme Court declared that all Americans have a right to make healthcare decisions. Even if a patient is deemed currently incompetent or unable to make his or her own decisions, the patient's previous wishes become the determining factor concerning care. The Patient Self-Determination Act became a federal law in 1991. This act states that the patient must understand that he or she may refuse medical treatment, care, procedures, medicines, and other similar procedures. It also states that patients must receive information about their right to prepare advance directives.

Most healthcare institutions have developed policies concerning self-determination which comply with specific state laws. In order to provide proper care as determined by the state statutes, it is necessary for the interdisciplinary team to form a collaborative relationship with the patient and family. When the patient is unable to make decisions, the healthcare team must consider the patient's diagnosis, the benefit or burden of treatment, the effect on the prognosis, and expressed verbal patient preference. Family members, other concerned people, or surrogates may take part in the decision-making process. Reevaluation must be ongoing because the patient's situation changes throughout the course of illness and treatment. Although a patient's decision-making capacity may be fluctuating or limited, the patient may sometimes be able to understand some aspects of the medical situation, and even express preferences through nonverbal communication.

ARTIFICIAL NUTRITION AND HYDRATION

The decision to institute artificial nutrition and hydration should take into account possible benefits and risks. It has traditionally been assumed that artificial nutrition and hydration meet several therapeutic goals: prolonging life, preventing aspiration pneumonia and "starvation," maintaining independence and physical function, improving nutritional status, assisting in healing of pressure ulcers, and decreasing suffering and discomfort at the end of life (HPNA, 2011d, ANA, 2003a; Lacey, 2005). However, the literature does not support this. Studies have shown that nursing home residents living with feeding tubes have similar survival rates to those living without these tubes, and that aspiration rates are higher in patients with feeding tubes (Lacey, 2005). Furthermore, artificial nutrition and nutritional supplements do not enhance the strength and physical function of frail elderly people (End-of-Life Nursing Education Consortium [ELNEC], 2006; Hallenbeck, 2005; HPNA, 2011a). Also contrary to expectations, most actively-dying patients do not experience hunger, even if they have inadequate caloric intake. In fact, risks such as increased infection, sensory deprivation, and restraint use have led researchers and palliative care experts to discourage the use of feeding tubes in dying patients and those with advanced dementia. To explore alternatives to artificial nutrition techniques, collaboration with other healthcare professionals (nutritionists and speech therapists) is indicated.

Dying patients, who feel strongly that they do not want feeding tubes inserted, should inform their healthcare proxies, and specify this in their living wills. Administration of artificial nutrition and hydration is a medical treatment, and thus a patient can accept or reject it. This right reflects respect for patient autonomy.

CARDIOPULMONARY RESUSCITATION

Cardiopulmonary resuscitation is the process of restarting the heart and/or lungs after one or both have stopped working. Traditionally, CPR is for people who are experiencing cardiac or respiratory arrest; simply put, CPR is most successful when it occurs in the hospital, specifically in the intensive care unit. However, when the seriously ill adult is frail, has multiple chronic conditions, and is nearing the end of life, CPR is significantly less effective. Current federal law mandates that long-term care facilities must ask residents (or their surrogates) whether they wish to receive CPR in the event of a cardiac or respiratory arrest. Research on CPR performed on elderly nursing home residents consistently shows very poor outcomes. Survival following CPR is less than 5% in this population, with most studies showing 0% survival. In such patients, the poor outcome of CPR in nursing home residents and those nearing the end of life is more likely a result of the irreversibility of the underlying diseases that end in cardiopulmonary arrest (American Medical Directors Association, 2013). Deciding to put a do-not-resuscitate (DNR) order in place usually involves the patient, his or her family, the nurse, physician, and others on the healthcare team. In most healthcare facilities, the physician or primary healthcare provider must write the DNR order in the chart for it to be legal; if no order is written, CPR is administered by default if the need arises. It can be very upsetting for the nurse to provide CPR to a dying patient, and the patient may suffer injury from anoxia, broken ribs, and aspiration.

When the nurse approaches the seriously ill patient and the family for clarification of the patient's "code" status, it is best to discuss the issue as fully and objectively as possible. It is necessary to present the facts with empathy, and express the idea that clinicians will support whatever reasonable decision is made. This conversation should be part of an ongoing discussion of the patient's wishes and goals for end-of-life care. According to the ANA, "the efficacy and desirability of CPR attempts, a balancing of benefits and burdens to the patient, and therapeutic goals should be considered" (ANA, 2003a, p. 1). The nurse should emphasize that the decision not to resuscitate is *not* condemning that person to death. Rather, the nurse is helping the person decide whether medical intervention *might* reverse the death process and even prohibit a peaceful death. The process of letting go may be painful for both the patient and the family.

Euthanasia and Physician-Assisted Suicide

Death is not the greatest of evils; it is worse to want to die, and not be able to.

Sophocles

Active euthanasia, or mercy killing, is the practice of ending the life of a terminally ill patient, at the request of the patient, for the purpose of limiting suffering. Active euthanasia is illegal throughout most of the United States, but legislators continue to sponsor bills in support of this action, and much public debate is ongoing concerning this issue. Rarely, a medication given for pain relief may have the unintended consequence of shortening the patient's life; however, because the intent of the medication is relief of pain and not the hastening of death, this is not considered euthanasia.

In 1994, Oregon voters approved physician-assisted suicide, which refers to a physician acting to aid a person in ending his or her life. Terminally ill residents of Oregon may receive prescriptions for lethal medications from their physician for self-administration. Currently (2013), it is legal in the states of Washington, Vermont, Oregon, and Montana, and to a limited extent, in Texas (Findlaw.com, 2013). The ANA (1994) does not endorse the concept of or participation of nurses in the process of euthanasia, mercy killing, or assisted suicide.

Cultural and Religious Issues

People of many cultural backgrounds reside in the United States. Culture encompasses dimensions such as race, ethnicity, gender, age, abilities/disabilities, sexual orientation, religion and spirituality, and socioeconomic status (Mazanec & Panke, 2006). An ever-changing system, culture is shaped over time as beliefs, values, and lifestyle patterns are passed from generation to generation. Sensitivity and empathy are essential when caring for a dying person from a different culture. Each person is a unique individual with cultural preferences which influence the specialized needs of the patient, the family, and their caregivers.

EVIDENCE FOR PRACTICE

Despite efforts to improve access to palliative care to all seriously ill patients, improvements are not reaching minority populations (Spruill, Mayer, & Hamilton, 2013). In a classic study, the SUPPORT Principal Investigators (1995) reported that the healthcare system expended fewer resources on African-American patients than on others with similar disease processes. Despite a higher incidence rate of cancer, shorter survival time after diagnosis, and higher cancer death rates, African-Americans made up only 8.7% of the population who used hospice in 2009, and they were less likely to use hospice services compared with other racial groups (Spruill, Mayer, & Hamilton, 2013). In general, minority patients often have an underlying mistrust of the healthcare system (Mazanec & Panke, 2006), and the literature has frequently described cases in which African-American patients desire aggressive life-sustaining interventions in the face of terminal disease. These patients may choose feeding tubes and CPR because of fears of being denied healthcare similar in scope to that of Caucasians.

Religion and spirituality play an important role in the forming of beliefs and practices which are paramount when death is imminent. Feelings of guilt, remorse, comfort, or peacefulness may all relate to religious beliefs. Religious customs are extremely important to many dying patients, and as death nears, concerns or fears may intensify. It is helpful to know a patient's religious preference; the nurse should remember that each patient's spiritual reactions are highly individualized. Requests by family or patients to seek spiritual counseling should be met with respect. Many healthcare facilities have chaplains, clergy, social workers, and others to assist staff. The nurse should ensure that spiritual care is made available to a patient at the end of life.

At times, a religious belief may help the patient determine the type of end-of-life care to request. The nurse must be aware of concerns the patient may have, and respond therapeutically. The age-old question of why this is happening may take on religious tones or thoughts. The patient may discuss or allude to punishment, atonement, God's will, or hope for a miracle. The nurse should follow the patient's lead in determining spiritual needs and beliefs. Serious illnesses frequently initiate a search for life's meaning, and questions may arise regarding the person's purpose in life. Religious or spiritual beliefs may even influence the emotional response to pain.

When discussing religion or spirituality with the patient, it is important to assist the patient in seeking meaning. Nurses who believe they are unable to assist patients in discussions of spirituality should make referrals to others on the team who have skills and knowledge in this area.

Specific rituals and practices are found in different faiths and religions. It is common for a patient of the Roman Catholic faith to wish to receive the Sacrament of the anointing of the sick to give spiritual strength and prepare for death. A religious item such as a rosary or medal may bring comfort. A patient who is Jewish may want to see a rabbi and participate in prayers. Burial takes place as soon as possible after death and before the Sabbath. A patient who is Muslim prefers that a family member be notified as soon as death occurs. It is best to wait for this person, since special washing and shrouding procedures should take place after death. According to Islam, the family should wash the body. Placement in a position that faces Mecca is necessary. If there is no family member to prepare the body, the staff may do so provided that they wear gloves. The burial of the body should occur as soon as possible, and cremation is not acceptable. Table 24.3 summarizes some religious beliefs and rituals practiced at the end of life.

table 24.3 **Religion and End-of-Life Care**

Religion	Belief	Ritual
Christian	Christians believe in an afterlife and the resurrection of Jesus Christ.	Catholic • Anointing the sick by a priest • Reconciliation and communion • Funeral held 2–3 days after death Protestant • No last rites • Anointing of the sick by some Others • Mormons will administer a Sacrament. • Jehovah's Witnesses will not receive blood transfusions. • Some sects have hands-on healing techniques.
Judaism	Death confers meaning to life.	Euthanasia is prohibited. Burial usually takes place within 24 hours. The funeral or shivah is held after the burial. Autopsy, organ donation, and cremation are not allowed. A rabbi is usually called when death is near.
Muslim	Muslims believe in an afterlife. The purpose of worldly life is to prepare for eternal life.	As death approaches, the patient is positioned supine facing Mecca. The room is perfumed, and anyone who is unclean leaves the room. Prayer occurs five times a day. Discussion of death and grief counseling are discouraged. Euthanasia is not allowed by law. Organ donation is allowed. Autopsy is discouraged.
Buddhist	Belief in the afterlife through the pursuit of perfection in worldly life.	End-of-life decisions are made with much family consultation. Families often do not want the patient to know the diagnosis to hide bad news. The elderly do not talk about funeral arrangements and often defer to physicians to make treatment decisions for them.

Source: Data from Cheng, B. (1997). Cultural clash between providers of majority culture and patients of Chinese culture. *Journal of Long-Term Health Care*, 16, 39–43; Kirkwood, N. (1993). *A hospital handbook on multiculturalism and religion*. Sydney, Australia: Millennium Books; Ross, H. (2000). Islamic tradition at the end of life. Unpublished manuscript.

PALLIATIVE CARE

Palliative care is interdisciplinary team-based care that is focused on the relief of suffering for patients with serious illness. It attempts to achieve the best possible quality of life, not only for patients but also for their families (Goldstein & Morrison, 2005). Nursing interventions which help enhance the quality of patients' lives, reduce pain and suffering, optimize functionality, and promote appropriate goal-setting and decision-making are integral to the provision of excellent palliative care (HPNA, 2008).

Regardless of the stage of the disease or the need for curative therapies, palliative care is appropriate for patients with life-limiting, serious illness. It may be concurrent with life-prolonging care, or may be the main focus of care (NCP, 2013). Although patients may be of any age, even children, palliative care is especially appropriate when provided to older people who have the following:

- Acute, serious, life-threatening illness (e.g., stroke, trauma, major myocardial infarction, and cancer, where cure or reversibility may or may not be a realistic goal, but the burden of treatment is high)
- Progressive chronic illness (e.g., end-stage dementia, congestive heart failure, renal or liver failure, and frailty)

Palliative care may occur in all settings, including hospitals, outpatient clinics, long-term care facilities, or the home. The patient and family are supported during the dying and **bereavement**, when they may experience feelings of loss after the death of a loved one. The care provided emphasizes quality of life and living as full a life as possible up until the moment of death.

The future and growth of palliative care will be largely determined by its acceptance within the medical model, and by reimbursement for palliative care services. The focus of palliative care includes the following:

- Controlling symptoms
- Coordinating care
- Reducing unnecessary tests and futile interventions
- Ongoing conversations with the patient and family (Kuebler, Heidrich, & Esper, 2007)

I am not afraid of death, I just don't want to be there when it happens.

Woody Allen

HOSPICE CARE

Through expert medical care, pain and symptom management, and emotional and spiritual support, **hospice care** provides support for people in the last phase of life-limiting illness, so that they may live as fully and comfortably as possible (NHPCO, 2013b). In 2011, an estimated 1.651 million patients received services from hospice. This estimate includes the following:

- 10,590,001 patients who died under hospice care in 2011
- 3,130,001 who remained on the hospice census at the end of 2011 (known as "carryovers")
- 2,780,001 patients who were discharged alive in 2011 for reasons including extended prognosis, desire for curative treatment, and other reasons (known as "live discharges") (NHPCO, 2013a)

The work of nurse leaders such as Florence Wald, Dame Cicely Saunders (also a physician), and Jeanne Quint Benoliel highlighted the need for "competent, expert, evidence-based care provided in a way that embodies compassion, respect for dignity, and an appreciation for the whole person and the family" (HPNA, 2011c). Another nurse leader, Harriet Goetz, published an approach to care for the dying in 1962, emphasizing therapeutic communication and symptom management techniques to provide comfort. Current standards of comprehensive and compassionate hospice and palliative nursing care are built upon the foundation of the work of these nurse leaders.

In 2008 in the United States, approximately 38.5% of the people who were dying received hospice services (Fig. 24.1). In the early 1980s, Congress added a hospice benefit to the Medicare program that was designed to support dying patients with an expected prognosis of less than 6 months to live if the disease ran its usual course. However, it is often difficult to predict with accuracy how long a patient will live, especially when the diagnosed disease is chronic (renal failure, congestive heart failure, cancer, or progressive dementia) (Centers for Medicare & Medicaid Services, 2008).

When two physicians determine that a seriously ill patient has 6 months or less to live, and the dying person and family agree to provide care and comfort as opposed to aggressive medical intervention, loved ones often seek hospice. Hospice care focuses on the whole person by caring for the body, mind, and spirit. The goal is for the patient to live his or her last days as fully and comfortably as possible. To achieve this goal, a multidisciplinary team of physicians, nurses, therapists, home health aides, pharmacists, pastoral counselors, social workers, and trained lay volunteers assist the family and caregivers in providing care (Fig. 24.2). The hospice nurse assumes the role of specialist in the management of pain and control of symptoms, and assesses the patient and family's coping mechanisms, available resources to care for the patient, the patient's wishes, and the support systems in place.

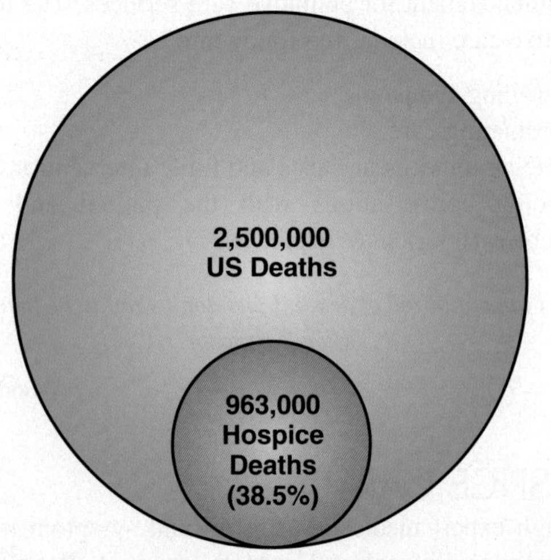

figure 24.1 Estimate of U.S. hospice use, 2008. (Adapted from National Hospice and Palliative Care Organization. [2013]. *NHPCO facts and figures: Hospice care in America*. Alexandria, VA: NHCPO.)

Hospice personnel may work with caregivers and patients in the home, nursing homes, other long-term care settings, and hospitals. Hospitals may have affiliated hospices, and some home health agencies promote their own home care hospices. Freestanding hospices that provide a homelike atmosphere in which care is provided by trained staff at the facility are also available, and these hospices may be a good option for patients who prefer a home death but do not have the necessary resources and support to safely remain in their homes. All hospices encourage family involvement and promote death with dignity. Because the experience of the dying and death of a loved one deeply affects the family, supportive care is provided to family and caregivers throughout the illness trajectory and for a period after the death has occurred.

CARING FOR PATIENTS AT THE END OF LIFE

The nurse providing quality end-of-life care to a seriously ill person and his or her family assumes the role of expert clinician. As an expert clinician, the community health nurse acts autonomously and completes physical, psychological, social, and spiritual assessments, and this nurse designs and implements plans of care (in collaboration with the patient, family, and interdisciplinary team) to meet the needs of the patient. Many validated instruments are available for use by healthcare professionals, including instruments for the assessment of pain and symptoms, mental health and mood, meaning in life and spirituality, functional assessment, quality of life, and caregiver strain. See the Toolkit of Instruments to Measure End-of-Life Care website for online copies and instructions for use of these various instruments.

Nurses who regularly assist patients and families to understand changes in their health status and the implications of these changes can alleviate many commonly held patient fears. Common fears and concerns of the dying include the following:

- Death itself
- Thoughts of a long or painful death
- Facing death alone
- Dying in a nursing home, hospital, or rest home

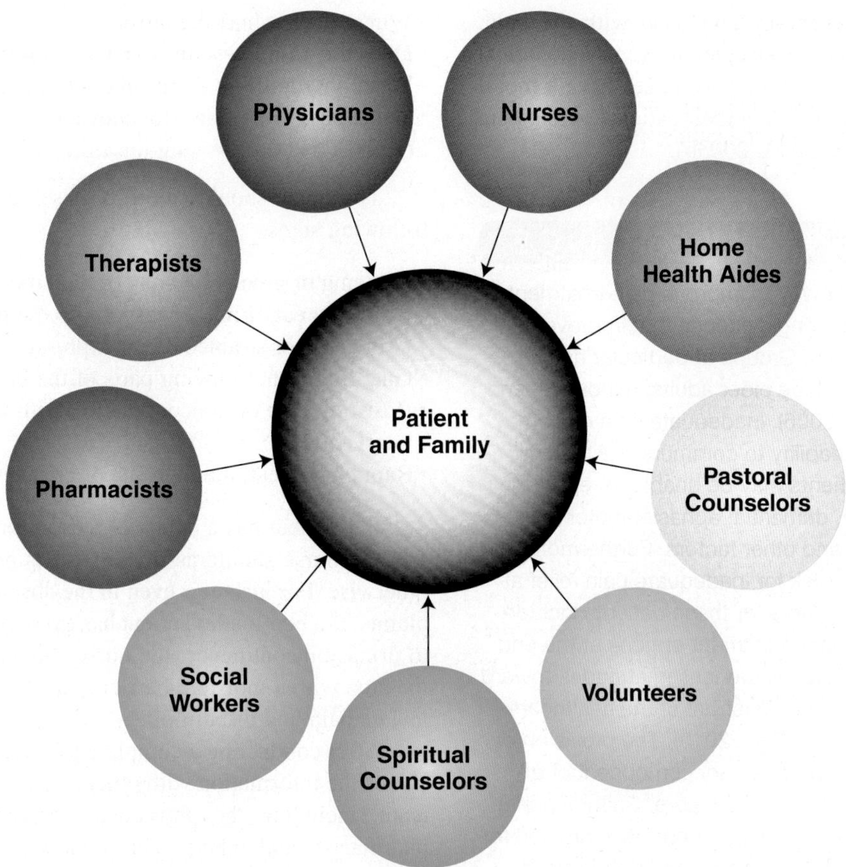

figure 24.2 Interdisciplinary hospice team.

- Loss of body control, such as bowel or bladder incontinence
- Not being able to make decisions concerning care
- Loss of consciousness
- Financial costs and becoming a burden on others
- Dying before having a chance to put personal affairs in order

The community health nurse can assist the patient to address some of these fears by ensuring patient comfort and support. Often, the nurse is present for the patient and family and can communicate compassion through caring acts. For instance, the small act of adjusting the patient's position so he or she can see the television a little better can be greatly appreciated by the patient and family. When a patient is diagnosed with a serious illness, life continues for an indefinite period; many patients live much longer than their prognosis predicts. The timing of a natural death is unpredictable, and it is difficult to predict exactly when death will occur. It is essential that each person have the opportunity to live life fully each day until the moment of death rather than engaging in a long, tedious dying trajectory. Therefore, accurate and timely deliverance of nursing care and addressing potential problem areas is of prime importance. The nurse's assessment guides the interdisciplinary team in providing individualized care with respect for the patient's wishes. The goal of the nurse is to help the seriously ill patient achieve the best possible quality of life through relief of suffering, control of symptoms, and restoration of functional capacity while remaining sensitive to personal values, cultural practices, and religious beliefs (NHPCO, 2013b).

Pain Management

Merciful relief of pain is essential for quality end-of-life care in dying patients, and nurses, including community health nurses, have a primary role in the assessment and management of pain at the end of life (ANA, 2003b). According to the ANA, "when the restoration of health is no longer possible, the focus of nursing care is assuring a comfortable, dignified death and the highest possible quality of remaining life" (p. 1). Patients and families fear pain during the dying process. However, through ongoing assessment of levels of pain, administration of pain medication, and evaluation of the effectiveness of the pain management plan, nurses may help alleviate the distress associated with untreated pain in dying patients.

Pain is associated with many negative outcomes in dying patients. It has the potential to hasten death and is associated with needless suffering at the end of life. People in pain do not eat or drink well, do not move around, cannot engage in meaningful conversations with others, and often become isolated to save energy and cope with the pain. Untreated pain is related to sleeplessness, psychological distress, fatigue, and restlessness, and nurses have a moral obligation to advocate on behalf of their patients so that pain is appropriately managed (ANA, 2003b).

EVIDENCE FOR PRACTICE

Although efforts are under way to improve pain treatment at the end of life, there is growing evidence that improvements are not reaching all patients. Groups at particular risk for undertreatment of pain include older adults, minorities, and women (Fine & MacLow, 2006). Inadequate pain relief may stem from the patient's inability to communicate pain; for example, some older patients may be unable to report their pain because of delirium, dementia, aphasia, motor weakness, language barriers, and other factors. Furthermore, minority patients are at high risk for inadequate pain relief at the end of life. Possible barriers for these patients include disparities in access to many treatment options at the end of life, insensitivity to cultural differences in attitudes toward death and end-of-life care, and mistrust of the healthcare system (Spruill, Mayer, & Hamilton, 2013). The provision of culturally-sensitive care is a necessary component of effective and comprehensive end-of-life care. Cultural preferences dictate how nurses assess and treat pain, provide for patient privacy, interact with the family, and deliver postmortem care after death.

PRACTICE POINT

At the end of life, assessing and managing pain, as well as relieving symptoms, is a primary responsibility of the hospice nurse. Untreated pain near the end of life is a nursing emergency and requires aggressive nursing intervention to ensure a comfortable and dignified death.

Pain Assessment

Pain assessment, including a thorough history, guides the development of a comprehensive pain management plan. Pain is a subjective experience, with self-report being the gold standard by which pain is measured. Accurate pain assessment is the basis of pain treatment, and physicians or nurses should perform it in a systematic and ongoing manner. Helpful questions may include the following:

- How bad is the pain? (It may help to use the facility pain indicator such as smiley face or rate the pain on a scale of 1 to 10.)
- How would you describe the pain (e.g., sharp, shooting, or dull)?
- Is the pain accompanied by other troublesome symptoms such as nausea or diarrhea?
- What makes the pain go away?
- Where does it hurt the most?
- Does the pain interfere with your ability to eat and sleep?
- What do you think is causing your pain?
- What have you done to alleviate the pain in the past? (ELNEC, 2006)

The nurse should carefully observe the patient for the following signs:

- Moaning or groaning at rest or with movement
- Failure to eat, drink, or respond to the presence of others
- Grimacing or strained facial expression
- Guarding or not moving parts of the body
- Resisting care or noncooperation with therapeutic interventions
- Rapid heartbeat, diaphoresis, or change in vital signs

If a patient has a potential reason for pain at the end of life, the nurse should assume that it is present until proven otherwise. For instance, even in the absence of patient complaints, if a bed-bound patient has excoriated skin secondary to urinary incontinence, the nurse should aggressively treat the area with a moisture barrier and a soothing cream to alleviate pain and discomfort.

After conducting a complete pain assessment, the nurse shares the information with other members of the healthcare team, including the physician, advanced practice nurse, pharmacist, and others. This collaboration is essential to achieve adequate pain control.

Types of Pain in Dying Patients

Pain at the end of life is complex and multifactorial, and prevalence varies according to diagnosis and other factors. Pain in the terminally ill may be both nociceptive and neuropathic (Fine & MacLow, 2006). It is important to differentiate between these types of pain for the pain to be appropriately managed. Nociceptive pain is the signal the brain imparts when there is tissue inflammation or damage. Cardiac ischemia and arthritis are examples of nociceptive pain. Nociceptive pain can be divided into two categories: somatic pain, which is characterized by aching, throbbing, or stabbing due to skin, muscle, or bone injury, and visceral pain, which is characterized by gnawing, cramping, or aching due to injury of the internal organs. Nociceptive pain usually resolves when the injury heals, and initial treatment involves nonopioid pain relievers. Acetaminophen is usually the first choice, followed by nonsteroidal anti-inflammatory drugs (NSAIDs); if no relief, then physicians and advanced practice nurses may choose opioids. Neuropathic pain, which occurs when nerves have been damaged, commonly affects older adults and takes the form of diabetic neuropathy, postherpetic neuralgia, or poststroke syndrome. The pain associated with these conditions is often described as burning, electrical, or tingling. Difficult to relieve with routine pain medications, neuropathic pain may be deep and severe. At times, anticonvulsants, antidepressants, and opioids are used for pain relief.

Mrs. Clark continues to become weaker and frailer at home, and she has developed severe pain in her left hip. You consult with the hospice physician, who recommends morphine. Mary fears that giving her mother morphine will hasten her death. What is your response?

Many healthcare providers, patients, and families believe that pain management with opioids shortens life; conversely, significant evidence exists to the contrary (Paice & Fine, 2006). Inadequate pain relief hastens death by increasing physiologic stress, potentially diminishing immunocompetency, decreasing mobility, worsening risk of pneumonia and thromboembolism, and increasing the work of breathing and myocardial oxygen requirements (Fine & MacLow, 2006). Unrelieved pain at the end of life can cause psychological distress and spiritual death and is often associated with negative outcomes, such as decreased quality of life (Paice & Fine, 2006). Nurses can play a key role by teaching patients and families that aggressive pain control and relief of pain is an indicator of quality nursing care.

Pain Relief During the Dying Process

Various nonpharmacologic and pharmacological methods of pain control may be implemented to control pain in the dying patient. Some nonpharmacologic approaches to reducing pain may include providing a glass of warm milk to promote sleep, a back rub, a change of position, a favorite peaceful musical selection, spending time listening to the patient, and/or visits from a priest, minister, or rabbi to meet spiritual needs. Nonpharmacologic methods can be used with pharmacologic therapy, and often augment the therapeutic effects of the drugs, resulting in the use of smaller doses.

Pharmacologic methods require close collaboration between the nurse, the physician, and the pharmacist to ensure the use of the correct medication, dosing regimen, and route of administration. These experts still use the model of pain relief developed by the World Health Organization (WHO) (1990) as the basis for the pharmacologic approach to pain management. It advocates a stepwise approach for pain treatment on the basis of the presence of mild, moderate, and severe or unrelenting pain. If the patient has neuropathic pain, mild pain (1–3 on the 0–10 scale) requires the use of **adjuvant drugs** (nonopioid medications such as antidepressants and muscle relaxants). Moderate pain (4–6 on the pain scale) necessitates the use of low doses of opioids; the use of nonopioids and adjuvants may continue. Severe pain (7–10 on the pain scale) requires the use of higher opioid doses. Patients presenting with severe pain should receive higher doses initially, rather than risking prolonged periods of uncontrolled pain while medications are titrated up from lower doses. It is necessary to titrate medications on the basis of patient goals, requirements for supplemental analgesics, pain intensity, severity of undesirable or adverse drug effects, measures of functionality, sleep, emotional state, and patient's or caregiver's report of the impact of pain on quality of life (ELNEC, 2006).

Whatever drugs are chosen, it is important to administer them routinely, and not on an as-needed (prn) basis, to prevent the unpleasant experience of the patient perceiving pain and then waiting for pain relief. Long-acting drugs (sustained-release formulations) are ideal because they provide consistent pain relief. Short-acting or immediate-release agents are excellent prn medications, and their only use should be for control of **breakthrough pain**. Breakthrough pain is defined as "intermittent episodes of moderate to severe pain that occur in spite of control of baseline continuous pain" (Paice & Fine, 2006, p. 144). Common in patients with advanced disease, breakthrough pain may occur with specific activities (physical therapy, activities of daily living) and end-of-dose failure (pain that occurs near the end of the usual dosing interval of regularly scheduled medications), and it may also be spontaneous. Breakthrough pain requires prompt treatment to avoid the fear or memory of pain and to prevent decreased functional ability. Dying patients who consistently experience breakthrough pain should have their physician increase the dosage of their regularly scheduled, long-acting pain medications.

Types of Drugs Used to Control Pain

NONOPIOID ANALGESICS

Common types of drugs in this category include acetaminophen and NSAIDs, which may be used alone or in combination with adjuvant drugs to enhance their effect. These drugs are very effective for the treatment of mild-to-moderate pain. Patients with normal liver function should take less than 4 g or less daily to avoid liver damage. It is essential to use these with caution in those with liver disease or have a history of significant alcohol use. NSAIDs can cause gastric irritation by inhibiting prostaglandin formation. Decreased prostaglandin synthesis results in thinning of the mucous lining that protects the stomach; this may result in gastrointestinal bleeding, especially in older adults. Other common side effects of NSAIDS are renal dysfunction and impaired platelet aggregation.

A newer class of NSAIDs selectively blocks the cyclooxygenase-2 (COX-2) enzyme, and there appears to be less risk of gastrointestinal bleeding with these drugs. However, studies have suggested that this benefit may not extend beyond 6 to 12 months (Paice & Fine, 2006). Furthermore, these drugs have been linked to increased risk of heart attack and stroke when used for prolonged periods. The U.S. Food and Drug Administration (FDA) has withdrawn several of these drugs, but others continue to be used cautiously.

OPIOIDS

Many experts consider opioids to be the most useful agents for pain management in patients with advanced illness (Paice & Fine, 2006). These medications block receptors in the central nervous system and prevent the release of chemicals involved in pain transmission. Examples are codeine, morphine, hydromorphone, fentanyl, methadone, and oxycodone. The WHO considers morphine to be the gold standard for the relief of cancer pain. Adverse effects are rare, and the only absolute contraindication for use is a history of a hypersensitivity reaction (rash, wheeze, or edema). Respiratory depression may occur with titration of opioid analgesics; however, this rarely occurs at the end of life (Paice & Fine, 2006). Most often, the respiratory rate becomes slower as the result of the dying process, not opioids. Constipation and sedation are two troublesome symptoms that are often associated with opioid use. Meperidine and propoxyphene are not recommended for use in older people because of their ineffectiveness in treating pain and their association with serious side effects. As disease progresses and organ function deteriorates, the potential for accumulation of the toxic metabolites of these drugs can lead to seizures, delirium, and tremors.

Some people with pain need higher levels of opioids than others and may fear reporting their pain is a sign of weakness. Others may fear addiction to opioid medications and refuse medication, resulting in needless suffering. When used as prescribed in seriously ill or dying patients, opioid medications improve activity levels and quality of life and ease suffering. Patients should be urged to use these medications without fear of addiction or feelings of guilt by interpreting their use as a sign of weakness.

Opioids often involve side effects such as nausea and feeling of lethargy that usually gradually resolve within 1 to 3 days. Other side effects, such as constipation, do not resolve without treatment. Over time, patients will become opioid-tolerant, meaning their bodies have adjusted to the medication and higher doses will be needed to relieve their pain. This is to be anticipated by the nurse, and the patient should be reassured that this does not mean they are addicted but rather their body has become adjusted to the medication and the same dose does not work as well as it once did.

ADJUVANT ANALGESICS

A wide array of nonopioid medications from several pharmacologic classes has been shown to improve pain relief when used concomitantly with pain medications. Such adjuvant medications include muscle relaxants, corticosteroids, anticonvulsants, antidepressants, and topical medications. Their use may enhance the effectiveness of other types of drugs, allowing improved treatment of pain at lower doses with decreased risk of side effects. Clinicians may prescribe them at any step of the "analgesic ladder" developed by the WHO (1990).

Routes of Administration

Usually, physicians prefer the oral route of administration because it is the easiest and most comfortable for the patient. However, many routes of administration are available at the end of life when the patient can no longer swallow. Pain medication may be administered by the following routes.

ORAL

Tablets, liquids, and capsules are administered orally to control pain. Long-acting or sustained-release tablets can control pain for up to 24 hours. Patients who are able to swallow can use this method until very close to the time of death. It is possible to mix liquid medications in juice and to open capsules and mix the contents in applesauce. For an oral medication, a higher dose of medication is usually necessary because of the first-pass effect (deactivation that occurs when medication passes through the liver).

ORAL MUCOSA

Even when the patient can no longer swallow, it is possible to deliver medication to the oral or buccal mucosa, from which it is absorbed. Placement of highly concentrated liquids such as morphine onto the mucosa involves using a dropper. Liquid morphine has a short half-life and duration of action; thus, more frequent administration may be necessary.

RECTAL

Some medications are available in suppository form, and the rectal route may be useful when the patient can no longer swallow or has problems with nausea and vomiting. The rectal route is invasive, and it may be difficult for family members to deliver medication using this route. In addition, if the patient cannot move easily, the positioning required for suppository insertion may be problematic.

TRANSDERMAL

Medications such as the fentanyl patch require placement on the skin of the upper body every 72 hours for relief of pain. However, because of changes in blood flow, metabolism, and fat distribution, some patients do not achieve or maintain stable drug levels and adequate pain relief. Peak onset may be delayed up to 24 hours, necessitating coverage with short-acting agents during the initial day of treatment.

TOPICAL

Topical capsaicin and local anesthetics (EMLA) can be useful for pain associated with postherpitic neuralgia and arthritis, and prior to invasive procedures such as insertion of IV lines or injections. When applied in small amounts to confined areas, as is recommended, topical medications usually result in little systemic absorption.

PARENTERAL

The IV and subcutaneous routes are useful when the patient is unable to swallow (intramuscular administration is inappropriate in the palliative care setting) (Paice & Fine, 2006). Pain may be associated with these methods of delivery. The IV route provides rapid drug delivery and pain relief, although risks of infection increase because of the need for vascular access. If the IV route is used, it is important to use the appropriate fluid delivery system and the smallest amount of fluid possible. This minimizes the risk of volume overload, which may lead to excess secretions and difficulty breathing. Subcutaneous administration is slower to take effect, with infusion of 2 to 3 mL/hour the easiest to absorb.

INTRASPINAL

The administration of drugs into or around the spinal cord via the epidural or intrathecal route is reserved for those patients who cannot achieve pain control in any other manner. The complexity of equipment used to deliver medications in this way leads to increased costs, and caregiver burden is a potential risk. Furthermore, risk of infection is a significant concern.

Tolerance

Patients who are managed with opioid analgesics over a period of time invariably develop tolerance or a "state of adaptation in which exposure to a drug induces changes that result in a diminution of one or more of the drug's effects over time" (Paice & Fine, 2006, p. 135). Medication dosages that were once therapeutic are no longer effective, especially as disease worsens. According to the ANA (2003b), "When pain and other distressing symptoms are present, the patient should have appropriate and sufficient medication by appropriate routes to control symptoms, in whatever dosage, and by whatever route is needed to control symptoms as perceived by the patient." It is imperative not to undertreat pain. As pain increases, it is essential to explore underlying causes, medicate the patient promptly, monitor the response to medication, and inform other team members about the effectiveness of the pain relief plan. The goal is to eliminate pain and help dying patients to improve the quality of their life through relief of suffering. Dying patients may need more pain medication than the normal range for the prescribed drug. Organic changes are occurring rapidly and systems are closing down; thus, absorption levels of drugs are also diminishing.

Preventing and Managing Adverse Effects

CONSTIPATION

Most opioid analgesics slow the movement of material in the intestinal tract and result in poor bowel elimination. Constipation may contribute to increased pain in dying patients, and it is extremely important that the nurse monitor the bowels carefully. It is necessary to initiate a prophylactic bowel regimen when using opioid analgesics. This includes the use of stool softeners (e.g., docusate sodium) and bowel stimulants (e.g., senna). Senna tea and fruits may also be helpful, and nurses should encourage patients to increase their fluid intake, if possible. Patients should avoid using bulking agents (e.g., psyllium) to prevent fecal impaction.

SEDATION

Many patients experience sedation when opioid analgesics are initiated; however, this effect should subside within 24 to 48 hours. If this condition continues after 24 to 48 hours, and clinicians have checked and managed other correctable causes, the patient may require a psychostimulant (Paice & Fine, 2006). Although sedation is commonly cited as a reason for avoiding opioids in older adults, evidence to support this claim is lacking (Bishop & Morrison, 2007).

RESPIRATORY DEPRESSION

As previously discussed, respiratory depression is often a concern for healthcare providers when using opioids for pain management; however, it is rarely a clinically significant problem for opioid-tolerant patients (Paice & Fine, 2006). Most patients develop a tolerance to respiratory depression within 5 to 7 days. If respiratory depression (respiratory rate <8 breaths/minute or O_2 saturation <90%) occurs, it usually has a multifactorial etiology.

NAUSEA AND VOMITING

Nausea and vomiting are common with the use of opioids in opioid-naive patients (those who have never used an opioid drug before) due to the activation of the chemoreceptor trigger zone in the medulla, vestibular sensitivity, and delayed gastric emptying (Paice & Fine, 2006; McPherson & Uritsky, 2011). Antiemetics that the patient has used successfully in the past may be scheduled for 2 to 3 days with a gradual tapering of the dose. Symptoms should subside within a few days if the underlying cause is the opioid analgesic (McPherson & Uritsky, 2011).

MYOCLONUS

Myoclonic jerking movements may be associated with high-dose opioid therapy (especially morphine). If this occurs, an alternate opioid should be used.

PRURITUS

Pruritus is most commonly associated with the use of morphine and is related in part to a release of histamine caused by the drug. Treatment with antihistamines (e.g., diphenhydramine) is effective but is very likely to cause sedation in older adults.

PRACTICE POINT

Control of pain and any related adverse effects of the pain medication is crucial to the delivery of quality end-of-life care.

Management of Distressing Symptoms at the End of Life

Secretions

At the end of life, it may not be easy to manage secretions. Painful xerostomia (dry mouth) can contribute to difficulty swallowing and impede clear speech; this is often exacerbated by the use of supplemental oxygen and reliance on open-mouthed breathing. Frequent mouth care at this time is crucial to making the patient comfortable. It is necessary to provide oral care using soft swabs several times a day, and whenever the mouth has a foul odor or appears to be causing problems for the patient. The nurse may instruct family members about the use of oral swabs or moistened cloths, allowing them to participate actively in their loved one's care. Alcohol-based products or those that contain perfume, lemon, or glycerin can be irritating and drying, and their use is discouraged. A salt-soda solution (1 teaspoon salt, 1 teaspoon baking soda, 1 quart tepid water) or artificial saliva used every 30 minutes may minimize dry mouth and the associated sensation of thirst (Emanuel, Ferris, von Gunten, & Von Roenn, 2006). It is acceptable to offer ice chips to relieve the feeling of dryness as long as the swallowing reflex is present. To prevent aspiration, the nurse should remind caregivers not to give oral fluids when the patient can no longer swallow. Soothing ointments or petroleum jelly may be applied to the lips to prevent painful cracking or drying. With increasing debility, oral thrush may appear, and clinicians should prescribe oral antifungal medications (e.g., nystatin swish and swallow).

As death approaches and the patient becomes increasingly sedated, the blink reflex decreases, resulting in dry eyes. Opened or half-opened eyelids become dry and irritated. When this occurs, the nurse or other caregiver provides frequent eye care to promote comfort. Artificial tears or ophthalmic saline solutions may be used to prevent drying of the eyes. The appearance of a loved one with half-open eyes, redness, or puffiness may be disturbing to family members and should be avoided if possible.

Anorexia and Dehydration

Most dying patients stop eating and drinking, and anorexia and dehydration are common and normal at the end of life. If the patient chooses to refuse food and drink, the nurse should consider this a rational decision and offer emotional and psychological support. Most experts believe that dehydration at the end of life does not cause distress and may actually initiate release of endorphins, resulting in a sense of well-being (Emanuel et al., 2006). Another benefit of dehydration is the decreased risk of lung congestion due to pulmonary edema, which leads to noisy, labored respirations, a sensation of breathlessness, and cough. By eliminating noisy respirations, the patient seems more comfortable, and quiet breath sounds decrease anxiety for family members. Oliguria (production of less than 15 cc of urine per hour) is another favorable outcome because the patient does not need to be positioned to use the bedpan or urinal frequently. When the patient stops eating, the nurse can reassure the family that anorexia may result in ketosis, leading to a peaceful state of mind and decreased pain. Furthermore, research has shown that initiation of parenteral or enteral nutrition at this time neither improves symptom control nor lengthens life (Emanuel et al., 2006).

Mrs. Clark has stopped eating, and her daughter is concerned that she is hungry. Mary asks you if a feeding tube would help her mother get stronger and live longer. How would you answer her?

Skin Integrity

It is necessary to monitor skin integrity carefully at the end of life because increased fatigue may result in decreased movement, resulting in pressure over bony prominences. Edema, bruising, dryness, and venous pooling may occur. Repositioning of the patient is essential, using lift or draw sheets, being careful to avoid shearing forces. Pressure-reducing surfaces, such as air mattresses or air beds, may help in alleviating pressure without needing to reposition the patient frequently. To promote comfort and reduce the risk of skin breakdown, the nurse or caregivers may provide gentle massage. Family members may feel comfortable applying lotion to the back or hands of the patient, again allowing participation in the care of their loved one. The nurse should tell them not to massage areas of nonblanching erythema and actual breakdown; this exacerbates ongoing tissue damage.

Incontinence

Bowel and bladder incontinence are frequent occurrences at the end of life. Seepage from body orifices may become uncontrolled, and it becomes necessary to have protective pads or briefs. It is extremely important to prevent decubitus ulcers from forming at this time because further breakdown is common due to contact with urine and feces. Barrier creams and change of position may also help maintain skin integrity. The nurse should discourage the use of in-dwelling urinary catheters if at all possible because they are often associated with distressing and painful urinary tract infections.

PRACTICE POINT

Confusion, restlessness, and agitation are common but distressing symptoms of terminal delirium.

Terminal Delirium

Terminal delirium can be a distressing phenomenon for families and caregivers. Typically, terminal delirium presents as "confusion, restlessness, and/or agitation, with or without day-night reversal" (Fine & MacLow, 2006, p. 8). Visual, auditory, and olfactory hallucinations may occur. It is important for the nurse to understand that this condition is often irreversible and that the patient's experience of the delirium may be very different from what is witnessed by caregivers (Fine & MacLow, 2006). In older adults, delirium is often a presenting aspect of acute illness or exacerbation of chronic illness. Further complicating the issue, delirium may exist concomitantly with dementia in older adults (Derby & O'Mahony, 2006).

Management of delirium includes identification and treatment of underlying causes (infection, electrolyte imbalances), reduction of environmental stimuli, provision of a safe environment, and reduction of anxiety. It is necessary to discontinue all nonessential medications (those not needed for comfort) when goals of care so dictate, and to continue pain medications and other agents used for comfort, such as benzodiazepines (lorazepam) and neuroleptics (haloperidol).

Eventually, neurologic changes occur in dying patients, and they slip from a lethargic state into an unconscious state (which may include periods of lucidness), then coma, and finally death. Family members frequently ask how much longer their loved one will live. The anxiety and distress of family and friends at this time may be great. Waiting for death is not an easy task, and time may pass slowly. This may be frustrating to those who are at the bedside. Extra support and encouragement at the crucial hours before death occurs is often necessary.

It is impossible to know exactly what unconscious patients at the end of life can hear; however, data from operating rooms and "near death" experiences suggest that persons near the end of life may be more aware of their environment than they are able to show (Emanuel et al., 2006). Although obtunded and comatose patients may not be able to communicate, it is believed that their sense of hearing is intact. People present at the bedside must not say or discuss anything they would not want the patient to hear. Nursing interventions at this time include encouraging family members to "let go" and give the terminal patient permission to die. Family members can assure their loved one that he or she will be "okay" and thank the person for loving them. The nurse should allow display of appropriate gestures of affection and provide privacy. Table 24.4 outlines suggested strategies for the management of common symptoms in dying patients.

PRACTICE POINT

Pleasant conversation or music at the bedside of the comatose patient may be therapeutic and reassuring to the dying patient.

table 24.4 **Suggested Strategies for the Management of Common Symptoms in Dying Patients**

Problem	Suggested Nursing Intervention
Constipation	Stimulants such as prune juice, senna, or lactulose. Avoid bulking agents (psyllium) in patients with inadequate fluid intake to avoid impaction. Monitor bowel function. Do not allow the patient to go longer than 3 days without a bowel movement. A mineral oil enema may be necessary to prevent impaction.
Delirium	Treat underlying cause if possible (fever, urinary tract infection, pain). Avoid use of physical restraints, sleep disruption, excessive medications. Urge family to remain with the patient, and have staff frequently visit and speak to and touch the patient. Use alternative interventions such as massage and music.
Dyspnea	Treat underlying cause if known (bronchospasm, hypoxia). Administer opioids to slow respiratory rate. Maintain the patient in a sitting position if possible. Minimize exertion by spreading out interventions and treatments. Provide humidified oxygen for comfort. Use alternative interventions such as massage and music.
Decubitus ulcers	Use appropriate positioning techniques, changing position every 2 hours. Keep the patient's skin clean and dry. Use special mattress pads to relieve pressure.
Cough	Assess and treat underlying cause such as postnasal drip or obstruction. Use chest physical therapy, cool humidified air, elevate head of the bed, and suction secretions as necessary. Cough suppressants may be used for comfort.
Anorexia and cachexia	The etiology of cachexia is rarely reversible in advanced disease, and aggressive nutritional treatment does not improve survival or quality of life and may create discomfort for the dying patient whose body is shutting down. Provide excellent mouth care. Treat oral problems such as candidiasis (thrush). Treat constipation, nausea, and vomiting, if present, as underlying causes. Assess the room for problem odors and try to minimize as much as possible. Generally, parenteral or enteral nutrition is useful only for patients with an appetite who cannot swallow. Offer the patient's favorite food and fluids as tolerated.
Nausea and vomiting	This occurs in up to 70% of patients at the end of life. Causes include metabolic disturbances, visceral disturbances, vestibular problems, medication side effects, emotional upset, and radiation. Assess cause and treat if possible (i.e., remove offending medication). Treatment medications include anticholinergics, steroids, benzodiazepines, and antiemetics (ondansetron and granisetron). Anticipate this and administer medications, if needed, before symptoms occur. Position the patient to prevent aspiration. Use complementary therapies such as music, relaxation, hypnosis, and acupuncture.
Fatigue	Fatigue is a subjective sense of tiredness or lack of energy that interferes with usual functioning. It may be disease-related, treatment-related, or psychological. If tolerated, exercise can improve function and sleep. Frequent rest periods and transfusions for very anemic patients may improve quality of life.
Anxiety	Anxiety may be a side effect of many medications such as stimulants and corticosteroids, or a paradoxical reaction to analgesics. Antidepressants and benzodiazepines may be beneficial.

Source: Data from Emanuel, L., Ferris, F. D., von Gunten, C. F., & Von Roenn, J. H. (2006). *The last hours of living: Practical advice for clinicians.* Retrieved July 31, 2007, from www.medscape.com; End-of-Life Nursing Education Consortium. (2006). *Promoting advanced practice nursing in palliative care.* Duarte, CA: City of Hope National Medical Center and Washington, DC: American Association of Colleges of Nursing.

NURSING CARE OF PATIENTS WHO ARE CLOSE TO DEATH

Preparing for Death

The knowledge or presumption that death is imminent may cause anxiety for the staff, family, and patient. Watching the body shut down life processes can bring feelings of helplessness and anxiety. Questions of an afterlife, unresolved emotional or social issues, concerns centered around family members and their acceptance of death, and financial matters are common issues generated at the end of life. It is part of the nursing role to attempt to allay the fears of patients and families at this time. Nurses must also remember to support themselves through this difficult period, recognizing and accepting an array of personal feelings. They may need individual support, as well as team support from outside the healthcare facility, to express and accept their true feelings. By doing this, it may be possible to prevent burnout.

In the context of terminal illness, hope is an ever-changing phenomenon. Healthcare professionals should never deny hope for the dying patient and family. Hope for a cure is not unusual for both the patient and family throughout the illness trajectory. As the disease progresses, the seriously ill patient may hope for small things to make the present situation more tolerable, such as a favorite meal or a visit from a family member. Hope for a dying patient may focus on living to see a grandchild graduate from college or the birth of a great-grandchild. Near the end of life, hopes may include such things as a comfortable death or death in the home. It is not unusual for patients to hope to speak with loved ones before they die.

Nurses should realize that the will to live is extremely strong in many persons confronting death, especially when there is a sense of unfinished business. Dying patients sometimes need reassurance from their families and caregivers that all is well and it is "OK" to let go.

Mary is able to obtain Visiting Nurse Association (VNA) care and grant her mother's wish to remain in her own home until the end of her life. As Mrs. Clark approaches the final moments of her life, Mary sits quietly at her mother's bedside. Mary notices that her mother is becoming dusky in color and that she seems to be having trouble breathing. Mary turns to you for advice and reassurance that her mother is not suffering. How would you respond?

The Dying Process

Under the wide and starry sky,
Dig the grave and let me lie. (from Requiem)

Robert Louis Stevenson, while dying from tuberculosis

Before death, the nurse must explain many physiologic processes to patients (if possible) and their families and caregivers. An expected set of physiologic changes typically occurs when death is imminent and is related to gradual hypoxia, respiratory acidosis, and renal failure. The nurse plays an integral role in assisting the family members who witness these changes to plan for the actual death. Expected changes include the following:

- Buildup of saliva and oropharyngeal secretions due to loss of the ability to swallow may lead to gurgling, crackling, or rattling sounds with breathing. This is sometimes referred to as the "death rattle," although this terminology should be avoided because it is often distressing to family members.
- Changes in respiratory patterns (shallow breaths with periods of apnea) may indicate significant neurologic declines, with Cheyne–Stokes respirations often heralding the impending death.
- Skin may appear dusky or gray and feel cold or clammy. Mottling of the lower extremities may take place days or hours before the actual death.
- Eyes may appear discolored, deeper set, or bruised.

Observing these body changes can be disturbing to family members. Although it is extremely difficult to assure the patient or family that death will happen within a certain time frame, the nurse's approach and explanations of the death process are reassuring to those present. Some family members may want to be present when death occurs, and others may want to be nearby but not physically present; it is important that the nurse support whatever decision is comfortable for the family and patient. Furthermore, patients may wish to be alone and die quietly with no one present because it may be difficult for the dying person to have loved ones near. Others find comfort in having family or professional caregivers in attendance. The dying process is as individual as living.

When respirations cease and a stethoscope does not detect breath sounds or heart sounds, the nurse should check the patient's carotid pulses with the stethoscope or fingers. Next, the nurse should check the eyes for pupillary light reflex. If the pupils are fixed and dilated and the heart has stopped beating, the clinician can pronounce that the patient is dead. Other signs of death include pale and waxen skin; lower body temperature; and relaxed muscles and sphincters, with released urine and stool (Emanuel et al., 2006). The nurse should note the time death occurred and put it on the patient's chart, notify the attending physician of the death, and make careful notes in the patient's chart to document the time the physician has been notified, and any directions received regarding postmortem care. There are certain settings where a nurse may make the death pronouncement, including long-term care. It is necessary to notify members of the interdisciplinary healthcare team of the death and express your condolences to the family. Even if the family is expecting the death, the actual occurrence of death comes as a shock and requires gentleness and empathy. If family members are present, the nurse should give them sufficient time to spend with the deceased before the body is removed.

STUDENT REFLECTION

Today, Mrs. Clark died quietly in her home. Even though her daughter, Mary, was there with her through every step of the process, she seemed shocked and sad when her mother took her last breath. She cried for a few minutes and then took my hand and smiled saying, "Thank you for helping me through this. I never could have done this for Mom without you." I cried a little bit also—tears of sadness, because I would miss Mrs. Clark, as well as tears of joy, because I knew I had helped her achieve the kind of death she wanted. I felt I had been a "good nurse."

Nursing Care after Death

One of the most difficult but essential parts of nursing is providing **postmortem care**. It is essential that the nurse does this promptly, quietly, efficiently, and with dignity, thereby communicating to the family that the deceased person was valued and respected. To promote comfort and ease anxiety at a time of stress, the nurse should honor the family's wishes about performing any religious or cultural rituals and practices. The nurse may also invite the family members to talk about their loved one and encourage the family members to touch and hold the person's body as they feel comfortable. If possible, before death occurs, the nurse should straighten the limbs and place the head on a pillow. If the death is suspicious or occurs outside of a healthcare facility, the coroner may request that the body be left undisturbed until an autopsy can be performed. However, the coroner does not investigate most deaths of seriously ill patients who die in their own homes.

After the pronouncement, the nurse should glove, remove all tubes, replace soiled dressings, pad the anal area in case of drainage, and gently wash the body to remove any discharges. The body should lie on its back, with head and shoulders elevated on a pillow. The nurse should grasp the eyelashes and gently pull the lids down. Insertion of dentures is necessary. It is important not to tie or secure any body parts because this may cause skin indentations. The nurse should place a clean gown on the body and pull a clean sheet up to the shoulders. When the body is moved or the extremities repositioned, the body may produce respiratory-type sounds or the chest may appear to rise and fall. Although this can be alarming, it is only the sound of air leaving the lungs. The nurse may want to check for respiration sounds again to be certain that the patient is dead. The nurse should prepare necessary paperwork for the removal of the body from the facility; call the funeral home, morgue, or other personnel for the removal of the body; and note the time in the chart, as well as who was called, and again chart when the body was released and to whom. It is advisable to also note whether eyeglasses, dentures, or any personal artifacts were released with the body and to whom they were given. If the facility requires that the body be identified with a tag, it is necessary to secure it properly.

Grief

The bitterest tears shed over graves are for words left unsaid and deeds left undone.

Harriet Beecher Stowe

Although the death may be expected, it may be met with shock by people who are left behind. Rationalizations (e.g., he lived a long life) may help ease the initial numbness of the actual death. Statements of relief, such as "he or she is no longer in pain," may help the bereaved cope with the immediate loss. The grieving process is considered difficult work that may last for years, and it is hard to endure at times. Past death experiences, emotional health, religious beliefs, and support of friends and family all are factors which may help ease the grief process. Bereavement is the process one undergoes after a loss. **Grief** is the emotion felt after the loss. The period of **mourning** is the recovery from the loss.

Several studies have shown that the accumulation of losses compounds the effects of grief and bereavement associated with death in older adults (Konigsberg, 2011). The widow or widower may experience grief for many years. Phases of grief may include some of the following:

Numb shock: The widow or widower cannot believe the spouse's death occurred. This phase is marked by shock, emotional dullness, and restless behavior that may include stupor and withdrawal. It may include physical characteristics such as nausea or insomnia. One wants to protect oneself from the feeling of loss.

Emotional turmoil or depression: Alarm or panic-type reactions occur. Emotional expression may include crying, low mood, sleep disturbance, and anorexia. Anger, guilt, or longing for the deceased may take place. The widow or widower may also become preoccupied with the meaning of the loss.

Reorganization or resolution: Reorganization eventually takes place, and coping strategies and positive outlooks emerge. A final resolution phase leads to acceptance of the loss. The widow or widower may return to prior levels of functioning.

When the full effects of death and its associated consequences set in, so do regret, self-doubt, and at times, despair. Life's purpose becomes confusing, and mood swings are prevalent. Being alone in the house may be a major problem. Research has shown that an active listener for reminiscence is helpful to the older adult during grief work. The nurse may also encourage the surviving spouse to focus on activities such as volunteer work. While actively participating in such activities, older adults often find the affection and companionship they need at this time.

Caring for the Caregiver

Most community health nurses not only care for the patient but also support and guide family caregivers. To prevent feelings of stress and burnout, those people who care for the dying need support and an opportunity to express emotional responses and grief. A periodic assessment might be beneficial for the caregivers who provide end-of-life care. Some questions may include the following:

- What have you done to meet your own needs today?
- Have you laughed today?
- Did you eat properly, rest enough, exercise, and play today?
- What have you felt today?
- Do you have something to look forward to?

Caregivers need to care for themselves to prevent anger, frustration, and anxiety. This makes it possible for the caregivers to continue to be sensitive to the needs of the dying patient.

I didn't attend the funeral, but I sent a nice letter saying I approved of it.

Mark Twain

COMPLEMENTARY AND ALTERNATIVE THERAPIES

Patients and families may request complementary and alternative medicine (CAM) concomitantly with hospice and palliative care. Use of CAM has great potential when integrated with traditional medical practices in end-of-life care. Traditional medicine may share the spotlight with such therapies as acupuncture, massage therapy, Reiki therapy, chiropractic care, and herbal medicine. In 1998, the National Institutes of Health initiated the National Center for Complementary and Alternative Medicine (NCCAM). NCCAM is dedicated to exploring complementary and alternative healing practices in the context of rigorous science, training CAM researchers, and disseminating authoritative information to the public and professionals. Patients who have used CAM at the end of life have reported that these therapies have physical, psychosocial, and spiritual benefits.

The Centers for Disease Control and Prevention reports that in 2007, 41.8% of hospice care providers offered CAM services, had a CAM provider on staff or under contract, or both. Among hospice care providers offering CAM, over one-half offered massage (71.7%), supportive group therapy (69.0%), music therapy (62.2%), pet therapy (58.6%), or guided imagery or relaxation (52.7%) (Berkovitz, Sengupta, Jones, Harris-Kojetin, 2011). Massage and mind-body interventions are cited as successful strategies for easing anxiety, emotional distress, nausea, and pain while improving overall comfort levels (Lafferty, Downey, McCarty, Standish, & Patrick, 2006).

Within the context of quality end-of-life care, the nurse must respect the unique needs of each seriously ill patient and his or her family. Several factors may cause patients with serious illness to seek complementary therapies: they may hope that these alternative methods will succeed where traditional medicine has failed, they may be attempting to regain control over life-threatening disease, or they may hope to achieve relief of suffering and improved quality of life (Lafferty et al., 2006). The HPNA (2011b) has developed a position statement regarding the use of complementary therapies in end-of-life care. According to this position statement, nurses working in end-of-life care need to learn about the many types of complementary therapies "because [they] may be particularly effective in managing symptoms and promoting wellness at the end of life" (p. 2). Nurses should also be aware of the increasing use of complementary therapies, recognize the role of CAM in symptom relief, and support the appropriate practice of complementary therapies to promote holistic end-of-life care (HPNA, 2011b).

key concepts

- Studies have documented that the American healthcare system has substantial shortcomings in the care of seriously ill patients and their families.
- Many patients die in pain or suffering from adverse symptoms.
- Aggressive care that carries a high burden of treatment is often delivered inappropriately to seriously ill patients because of communication barriers and lack of planning.
- The community health nurse can play a key role on the interdisciplinary team and serve as patient advocate, educator, care provider, and planner of quality end-of-life care.
- Pain and symptom control are crucial to the delivery of quality end-of-life care.
- Cultural and ethnic variations are key factors to be considered when providing end-of-life care.
- Palliative care and hospice programs can assist the nurse in the delivery of quality end-of-life care to seriously ill patients and their families.
- Families often rely on the nurse for support and assistance during the dying process and afterward in the mourning and grieving period.

critical thinking questions

1. Speak to nurses and nursing assistants who work in one of your clinical rotations about the assessment of pain in the dying patient. What factors do they identify as important?
2. Explain possible reasons caring for dying patients at the end of life may be difficult. Tell a story in a small group of fellow students and observe their reactions.
3. Keep a clinical journal of your feelings and experiences as you begin to become proficient in providing end-of-life care to seriously ill patients and their families.
4. Identify a few key people in your life who can help you as you struggle to become proficient in the provision of end-of-life care.
5. Identify key people in your life who helped you to come to terms with and understand death.

community resources

- Local hospitals that have hospital-based generic or hospice home care programs
- Local palliative care specialists
- Visiting nurse associations
- Volunteer church groups and friendly visitors
- Elder affairs
- Local and state health departments
- State offices of Medicare and Medicaid

references

American Medical Directors Association. (2013). *White paper on surrogate decision making and advance care planning in long term care*. Retrieved from http://www.amda.com/governance/whitepapers/surrogate/clinical.cfm?printPage=1&

American Nurses Association. (1994). *Position statement: Assisted suicide*. Washington, DC: American Nurses Association.

American Nurses Association. (2003a). *Position statement on nursing care and Do-Not-Resuscitate (DNR) decisions*. Washington, DC: American Nurses Association.

American Nurses Association. (2003b). *Position statement on pain management and control of distressing symptoms in dying patients*. Washington, DC: American Nurses Association.

American Nurses Association. (2010). *ANA position statement: Registered nurses' roles and responsibilities in providing expert care and counseling at the end of life*. Washington, DC: Author.

Aoun, S., Kristjanson, L., Oldham, L., & Currow, D. (2008). A qualitative investigation of the palliative care needs of terminally ill people who live alone. *Collegian, 15*, 3–9.

Berkovitz, A., Sengupta, M., Jones, A., & Harris-Kojetin, L. (2011). *Complementary and alternative therapies in hospice: The national home and hospice care survey–United States, 2007*. National Health Statistics Reports. Centers for Disease Control and Prevention. Retrieved from http://www.cdc.gov/nchs/data/nhsr/nhsr033.pdf

Bishop, T. F., & Morrison, R. S. (2007). Geriatric palliative care—part I: Pain and symptom management. *Clinical Geriatrics, 15*(1), 25–32.

Centers for Disease Control and Prevention. (2011). *FastStats: Death and mortality*. Retrieved from http://www. cdc.gov/nchs/faststats .death.htm

Centers of Medicare & Medicaid Services, U.S. Department of Health and Human Services. (2008). *Medicare hospice benefits*. Retrieved January 4, 2010, from http://medicare.gov/publications/Pubs/pdf/02154.pdf

Dartmouth Institute for Health Policy and Clinical Practice. (2013). *End of life care*. Retrieved from http://www.dartmouthatlas.org/data/topic/topic.aspx?cat=18

Derby, S., & O'Mahony, S. (2006). Elderly patients. In B. R. Ferrell & N. Coyle (Eds.), *Textbook of palliative nursing*, (pp. 635–659). Oxford: Oxford University Press.

Emanuel, L., Ferris, F. D., von Gunten, C. F., & Von Roenn, J. H. (2006). *The last hours of living: Practical advice for clinicians*. Retrieved July 31, 2007, from www.medscape.com

End-of-Life Nursing Education Consortium. (2006). *Promoting advanced practice nursing in palliative care*. Duarte, CA: City of Hope National Medical Center and Washington, DC: American Association of Colleges of Nursing.

Findlaw.com. (2013). *State euthanasia laws*. Retrieved from http://statelaws.findlaw.com/

Fine, P. G., & MacLow, C. (2006). *Principles of effective pain management at the end of life*. Retrieved July 31, 2007, from www.medscape.com

Goldstein, N. E., & Morrison, R. S. (2005). The intersection between geriatrics and palliative care: A call for a new research agenda. *Journal of the American Geriatrics Society, 53*, 1593–1598.

Gruneir, A., Miller, S. C., Intrator, O., & Mor, V. (2007). Hospitalization of nursing home residents with cognitive impairments: The influence of organizational features and state policies. *Gerontologist, 47*(4), 447–456.

Hallenbeck, J. (2005). *Fast facts and concepts #11: Tube feed or not tube feed?* End-of-Life Physician Education Resource Center. Retrieved October 30, 2007, from http://www.aahpm.org

Hospice and Palliative Nurses Association. (2008). *HPNA position statement: Pain management*. Retrieved from http://www .hpna.org

Hospice and Palliative Nurses Association. (2011a). *HPNA position statement: Artificial nutrition and hydration in advanced illness*. Retrieved from http://www.hpna.org

references (continued)

Hospice and Palliative Nurses Association. (2011b). *HPNA position statement: Complementary therapies in palliative care nursing practice.* Retrieved from http://www.hpna.org

Hospice and Palliative Nurses Association. (2011c). *HPNA position statement: Role of the nurse when hastened death is requested.* Retrieved from http://www.hpna.org

Hospice and Palliative Nurses Association. (2011d). *HPNA position statement: Value of the professional nurse in palliative care.* Retrieved from http://www.hpna.org

Konigsberg, R. D. (2011). *The truth about grief.* New York, NY: Simon and Schuster.

Kübler-Ross, E. (1969). *On death and dying: What the dying have to teach doctors, nurses, clergy, and their own families*. New York, NY: MacMillan.

Kuebler, K., Heidrich, D., & Esper, P. (2007). *Palliative and end-of-life care*. St. Louis, MO: Saunders Elsevier.

Lacey, D. (2005). Tube feeding, antibiotics, and hospitalization of nursing home residents with end-stage dementia: Perceptions of key medical decision-makers. *American Journal of Alzheimer's Disease and Other Dementias, 20*(4), 211–219.

Lafferty, W. E., Downey, L., McCarty, R. L., Standish, L. J., & Patrick, D. L. (2006). Evaluating CAM treatment at the end of life: A review of clinical trials for massage and meditation. *Complementary Therapies in Medicine, 14*(2), 100–112.

Last Acts. (2002). *Means to a better end: A report on dying in America*. Retrieved August 27, 2007, from www.lastacts.org

Lindley, L. (2013). Pediatric hospice care knowledge: A transaction cost perspective. *Journal of Hospice & Palliative Nursing, 13*(8), 485–490.

Lysaght, S. & Ersek, M. (2013). Settings of care within hospice: New options and questions about dying "At Home". *Journal of Hospice & Palliative Nursing, 15*(3), 171–176.

Mazanec, P., & Panke, J. T. (2006). Cultural considerations in palliative care. In B. R. Ferrell & N. Coyle (Eds.), *Textbook of palliative nursing* (pp. 623–633). Oxford: Oxford University Press.

McPherson, M. L., & Uritsky, T. J. (2011). Pharmacotherapy of pain in older adults: Opioid and adjuvant. In F. M. Gloth, III (Ed.), *Handbook of pain relief in older adults: An evidence-based approach* (pp. 83–95). New York, NY: Springer.

Medicaid.gov. (2013). *Seniors and medicare & medicaid enrollees.* Retrieved from http://www.medicaid.gov/Medicaid-CHIP-Program-Information/By-Population/Medicare-Medicaid-Enrollees-Dual-Eligibles/Seniors-and-Medicare-and-Medicaid-Enrollees.html

Moneymaker, K. (2005). Comfort measures only. *Journal of Palliative Medicine, 8*(3), 688.

National Consensus Project (NCP) for Quality Palliative Care. (2013). *Clinical practice guidelines for quality palliative care.* Retrieved from www.nationalconsensusproject.org

National Hospice and Palliative Care Organization. (2013a). *NHPCO facts and figures: Hospice care in America.* Alexandria, VA: NHCPO.

National Hospice and Palliative Care Organization. (2013b). *Ten components of quality care*. Alexandria, VA: NHPCO. Retrieved from http://www.nhpco.org/quality/10-components-quality-care

National Institutes of Health. (2014). NIH makes pediatric palliative care more attainable for children and their families. Retrieved from http://www.nih.gov/news/health/jan2014/ninr-08.htm

O'Mahony, S., Blank, A., Simpson, J., Persaud, J., Huvane, B., McAllen, S., … Selwyn, P. (2008). Preliminary report of a palliative care and case management project in an emergency department for chronically ill elderly patients. *Journal of Urban Health, 85*(3), 443–451.

Paice, J. A., & Fine, P. G. (2006). Pain at the end of life. In B. R. Ferrell & N. Coyle (Eds.), *Textbook of palliative nursing* (pp. 131–153). Oxford: Oxford University Press.

Quill, T. (2000). Perspectives on care at the close of life. Initiating end-of-life discussions with seriously ill patients: Addressing the "elephant in the room." *Journal of the American Medical Association, 284*(19), 2501–2507.

Spruill, A., Mayer, D., & Hamilton, J. (2013). Barriers in hospice use among African Americans with cancer. *Journal of Hospice & Palliative Nursing, 15*(3), 136–146.

SUPPORT Principal Investigators. (1995). A controlled trial to improve care for seriously ill hospitalized patients. The study to understand prognoses and preferences for outcomes and risks of treatment. *Journal of the American Medical Association, 274*(20), 1591–1598.

Ventura, A., Burney, S., Brooker, J., Fletcher, J., & Ricciardelli, L. (2013). Home-based palliative care: A systematic literature review of the self-reported unmet needs of patients and carers. *Palliative Medicine*. Retrieved from http://www.ncbi.nlm.nih.gov/pubmedhealth/PMH0062329/

World Health Organization. (1990). *Cancer pain relief and palliative care* (Technical Report Series, 804). Geneva, Switzerland: WHO.

web resources

Please visit thePoint® for up-to-date Web resources on this topic.

CHAPTER 25

Occupational Health Nursing

Christine Pontus and Gail A. Harkness

Everything that is really great and inspiring is created by the individual who can labor in freedom.

Albert Einstein

If you cannot work with love but only with distaste, it is better that you should leave your work.

Khalil Gibran

Oh, you hate your job? Why didn't you say so? There's a support group for that.
It's called everybody, and they meet at the bar.

Drew Carey

chapter highlights

- Characteristics of the worker and workplace
- Roles and responsibilities of occupational health nurses
- Models for occupational health practice
- Worker and workplace assessment
- Health promotion in workplace settings
- Use of epidemiologic techniques in occupational health
- Emergency preparedness and disaster management

objectives

- Explain the role of nursing in occupational health.
- State current trends in the U.S. workforce.
- Describe the four types of exposures and hazards in the workplace.
- Provide examples of common work-related injuries and illnesses.
- Explain the interaction of agent, host, and environment as applied to the workplace.
- Outline the steps involved in both worker and workplace assessment.
- Describe potential benefits to both workers and business in offering health promotion programs.
- Explain how principles of epidemiology are applied to occupational health.
- Assess specific components within an emergency preparedness plan that will vary from industry to industry based on risk.

key terms

American Association of Occupational Health Nurses (AAOHN): Professional association for nurses working in a business setting, dedicated to the health and safety of workers, worker populations, and community groups.

Biologic hazards: Hazards resulting from living organisms that cause adverse effects on people.

Chemical hazards: Generated from liquids, solids, dusts, fumes, vapors, and gases.

Ergonomics: Study of the relationship between people and their working environment.

National Institute of Occupational Safety and Health (NIOSH): The federal agency established to help ensure safe and healthy working conditions by conducting scientific research, gathering information, and providing education and training in occupational safety and health.

Occupational health history: An assessment of the characteristics of the workers' present jobs, a chronologic record of all past work and potential exposures, an occupational exposure inventory, and a list of other exposures in the home or community.

Occupational Safety and Health Administration (OSHA): The federal agency that sets exposure standards and is responsible for enforcement of safety and health legislation.

Physical hazards: Hazards that result from the transfer of physical energy to workers.

Psychosocial hazards: All organizational factors and interpersonal relationships in the workplace that may affect the health of the workers.

Root cause analysis: A process for understanding and solving a problem, with the goal of determining what happened, why it happened, and what can be done to prevent its reoccurrence.

Workplace walk-through: A complete survey of the workplace, inside and outside, compiling information as to the presence of hazards, the location of entries and exits, the availability of emergency equipment, and potential trouble spots.

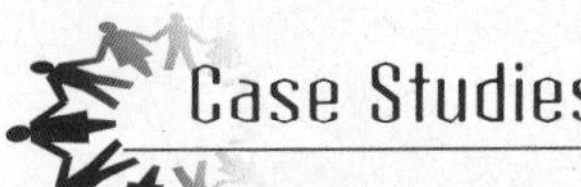

Case Studies

References to the case studies are found throughout this chapter (look for the case study icon). Readers should keep the case studies in mind as they read the chapter.

CASE 1

A 32-year-old female bank employee suddenly stops breathing while at work. A coworker calls rescue (911), and emergency medical technicians rush her to the hospital. Later, physicians determine that she suffered respiratory arrest related to an anaphylactic reaction. An occupational health nurse (OHN) investigates both the hospitalization and the workers' compensation claim because the incident occurred at the place of employment. This investigation clarifies the incident and identifies its underlying cause, so that measures can be taken to prevent it from happening to other workers.

On receiving the case briefing from both the loss prevention and the claims management departments, the OHN reviews the file and speaks to the worker and her supervisor. The worker said that she had an anaphylactic reaction and that her supervisor told her not to return to work until physicians discovered and medically confirmed the cause of her reaction. She has an appointment with an allergist about a possible allergy.

CASE 2

At the opening of business on a Friday morning, four people enter the occupational health clinic at a factory. The employees complain of nausea, vomiting, diarrhea, fatigue, and headache. The OHN, concerned that a common exposure caused these workers to become ill, discovers that all four attended the company picnic the day before. A phone call to human resources reveals that more employees who attended the picnic have called in sick with complaints of nausea, vomiting, and diarrhea. At the picnic, the food included hamburgers; sausage and pepper sandwiches; potato, chicken, and tossed salad; and beverages such as chocolate milk, soda, and water. The OHN talks to the kitchen manager. Apparently, there have been recent problems with heat regulators, a refrigeration unit, newly-hired help, and the training of cafeteria workers. The nurse immediately calls the Department of Public Health.

Occupational health nurses (OHNs) can be found in as many diverse settings as there are types of employment for workers. They observe and care for the community, group, business, or organization as a whole. This chapter presents an overview of the discipline, work, regulations, and conditions associated with the healthcare of the workforce, both nationally and internationally. It is hoped that this information will heighten an awareness of the kinds of care provided in the community workplace environment.

THE WORKER AND THE WORKPLACE

Work is an integral part of life for most people, providing challenging and worthwhile experiences that evolve and change over time. On average, employed adults spend about one-third of their time at work. Health risks are inherent in every industry, and as the workplace changes, the risk that workers will experience adverse health effects related to employment also changes. Although the potential for serious adverse health effects from exposure to dangerous substances or less-than-optimal conditions is associated with every occupation, the majority of workers do not experience hazards in the workplace. The common workplace exposures and hazards listed in Table 25.1 indicate that there are a wide variety of potential threats to health. The specialty of occupational health focuses on the identification and control of risks to health which occur as a result of physical, chemical, and other workplace hazards. The goal is to establish and maintain a safe and healthy environment for workers.

Occupational health is closely allied to the specialty of environmental health, a field of public health science that focuses on how the environment influences human health (see Chapter 19). **Ergonomics**, the study of the relationship between people and their working environment, emerged during the 20th century. Also called biotechnology and human engineering, ergonomics is the applied science of equipment design, intended to maximize productivity by reducing operator fatigue and discomfort.

Designing your product for monetization first and people second will probably leave you with neither.

Tara Hunt, marketing consultant

In 2010, there were approximately 125 million people in the workforce in the United States. In the civilian labor force, nearly 83% of people found employment in the service industries and another 11% found employment in manufacturing (U.S Department of Labor, Bureau of Labor Statistics [BLS], 2011). The U.S. Bureau of Labor Statistics also indicates that 3.8 of 100 workers in all industries, including state and local governments, have a reportable injury or illness. In contrast, in 2010, when state and local governments, which are responsible for protection of the public, were removed from the calculations, there were 3.5 cases per 100 workers in private industry. The trends illustrated in Figure 25.1 show that small companies have a lower rate of injury and illness over time, and companies with between 50 and 249 employees have consistently had the highest rates.

table 25.1 **Common Workplace Hazards and Exposures**

Biologic Hazards	Chemical Exposures	Physical Hazards	Psychosocial Factors
Infectious agents	Hazardous drug and toxin exposures	Electric and magnetic fields	Sexual harassment
Contaminated body fluids	Diesel exhaust	Ultraviolet radiation	Psychological stress
Poisonous plants	Aerosols	Cold stress	Interpersonal problems
Insects, scorpions, spiders	Respirable particulate matter and fumes	Heat stress	Assaults and violent acts
Venomous snakes	Take-home toxins (reached workers' home and families)	Noise	Bodily reaction and exertion
		Vibration	
		Lighting	
	Substances in cleaning solutions, for example, floor strippers, disinfection, and sterilization products	Falls	
		Fires and vibration	
		Particulate inhalation	
		Unsafe machinery and equipment	
		Abrasive blasting	
		Inadequate workstations	
		Transportation accidents	

The trends shown in Figure 25.2 indicate the private industries that had at least 50,000 nonfatal occupational injuries and illnesses in 2011, and showed that general medical and surgical hospitals were at the top of the list.

Table 25.2 shows the incidence rates of occupational injuries and illnesses by industry and case types in 2010. The case rate reflects the total number of reportable events that occurred, the majority of which are mild, such as strains and sprains. The case rate for days away from work indicates that a more serious injury or illness occurred that required time away from work. The resulting costs amount to billions of dollars each year. The injuries and illnesses occur at places of business; therefore, this spreads the costs to consumers in the form of higher prices, to workers in the form of lower wages, and to taxpayers.

Injuries were the most common result of workplace hazards. The majority of the 3 million nonfatal occupational injuries and illnesses recorded in 2011 were injuries. Seventy-five percent of these injuries occurred in service-providing industries such as healthcare and professional and

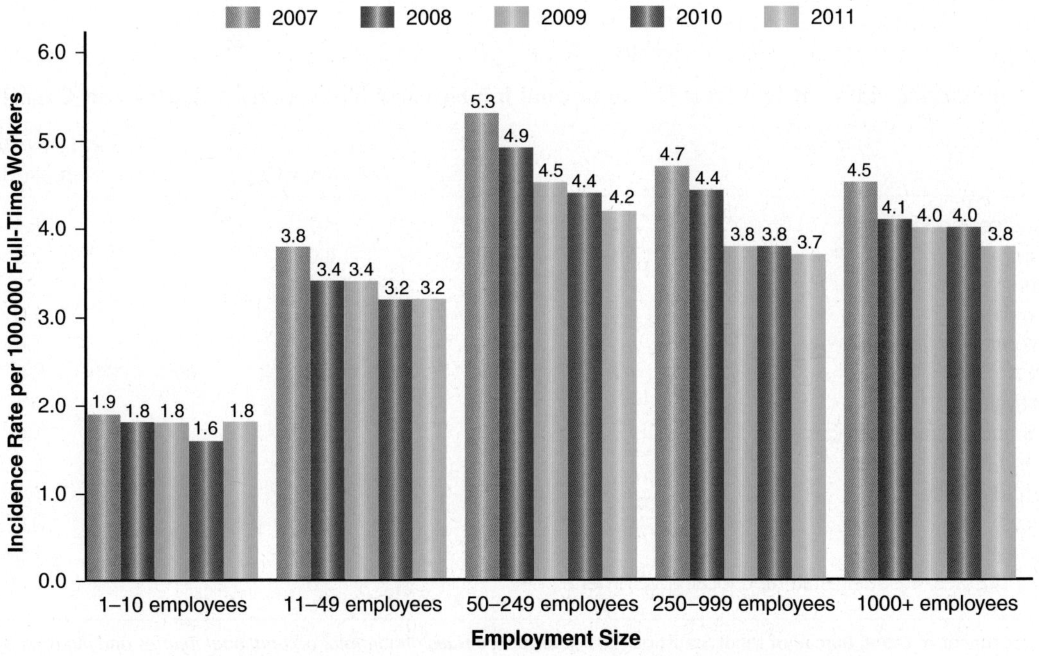

figure 25.1 Total recordable nonfatal occupational injury and illness incidence rates by employment size class, private industry, 2007–2011. (From Bureau of Labor Statistics, U.S. Department of Labor. [2012, October]. *Workplace Injuries and Illnesses—2011*. Retrieved from http://www.bls.gov/news.release/pdf/osh.pdf)

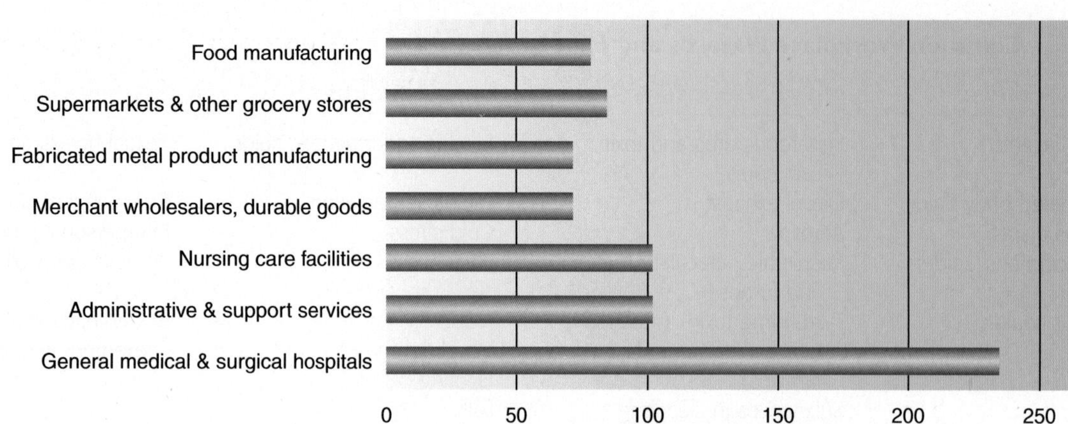

figure 25.2 Industries with at least 50,000 nonfatal occupational injuries and illnesses, private industry, 2011. (From U.S. Bureau of Labor Statistics, U.S. Department of Labor. [2012]. *Number of nonfatal occupational injuries and illnesses by industry and case type 2011*. Retrieved from http://www.bls.gov/iif/oshwc/osh/os/ostb3193.pdf)

technical businesses (U.S Department of Labor, BLS, 2012). Table 25.3 indicates that the highest incidence rate of injuries resulting in days away from work occurred from sprains, strains, and tears, followed by cuts and bruises. Workplace illnesses, most of which are associated with repetitive strain (i.e., carpal tunnel), accounted for only 1% of the total injury and illness cases in 2011 contributing to the most days away from work (BLS, 2012).

Unfortunately, deaths do occur in the workplace. In 2010, a total of 4,690 workers in the United States died as a result of injuries sustained at work. Figure 25.3 shows the number and rate of fatal occupational injuries, by industry sector, in 2010. Note that Figure 25.3 depicts that the number of fatal injuries related to transportation is the highest. Figure 25.4 shows the manner in which these occupational fatalities occurred. More work-related fatalities resulted from transportation incidents than from any other event. Although 3.5% of all workers in 2011 had an injury or illness related to the workplace, these statistics were consistent, reflecting no change for the first time in a decade (BLS, 2012).

Occupational health is a responsibility assumed by nurses worldwide. The World Health Organization (WHO) (2001) published a document describing the role of the OHN in workplace health management. This document reflects

table 25.2 **Incidence Rates of Nonfatal Occupational Injuries and Illnesses by Industry and Case Types, 2010**

Industry	Case Rate (%)	Case Rate for Days away from Work (%)
Natural resources and mining	3.7	1.4
Construction	4.0	1.5
Manufacturing	4.4	1.1
Service providing	3.4	1.0
Trade, transportation, and utilities	4.1	1.4
Information	1.8	0.8
Financial activities	1.3	0.4
Professional and business services	1.7	1.6
Education and health services	4.8	1.3
Leisure and hospitality	3.9	1.1
Other services	2.7	0.9
Public administration	4.2	1.8
Total for all industries, including state and local government	3.8	1.2

Source: U.S. Department of Labor, Bureau of Labor Statistics. (2011). *Incidence rates of non-fatal occupational injuries and illnesses by industry and case types, 2010*. Retrieved from http://www.bls.gov/iif/oshwc/osh/os/ostb2813.pdf

table 25.3 **Statistics on Occupational Injuries and Illnesses, Involving Days away from Work in Private Industry, State Government, and Local Government, 2011**

Characteristics	Incidence Rate per 10,000 Full-Time Workers	Median Days away from Work
Sprains, strains, tears	44.4	10
Cuts, lacerations, punctures	9.6	4
Bruises, contusions	10.2	5
Fractures	9.1	27
Multiple traumatic injuries	4.3	10
Heat (thermal) burns	1.5	5
Carpal tunnel syndrome	1.0	28
Amputations	0.5	25
Chemical burns	0.4	3
Tendonitis	1.0	28

Source: U.S. Department of Labor, Bureau of Labor Statistics. (2012). *Economic news release: Number, incidence rate, and median days away from work for non-fatal occupational injuries and illnesses involving days away from work by selected injury or illness characteristics and private industry, state government, and local government, 2011.* Retrieved from http://www.bls.gov/news.release/osh2.t05.htm

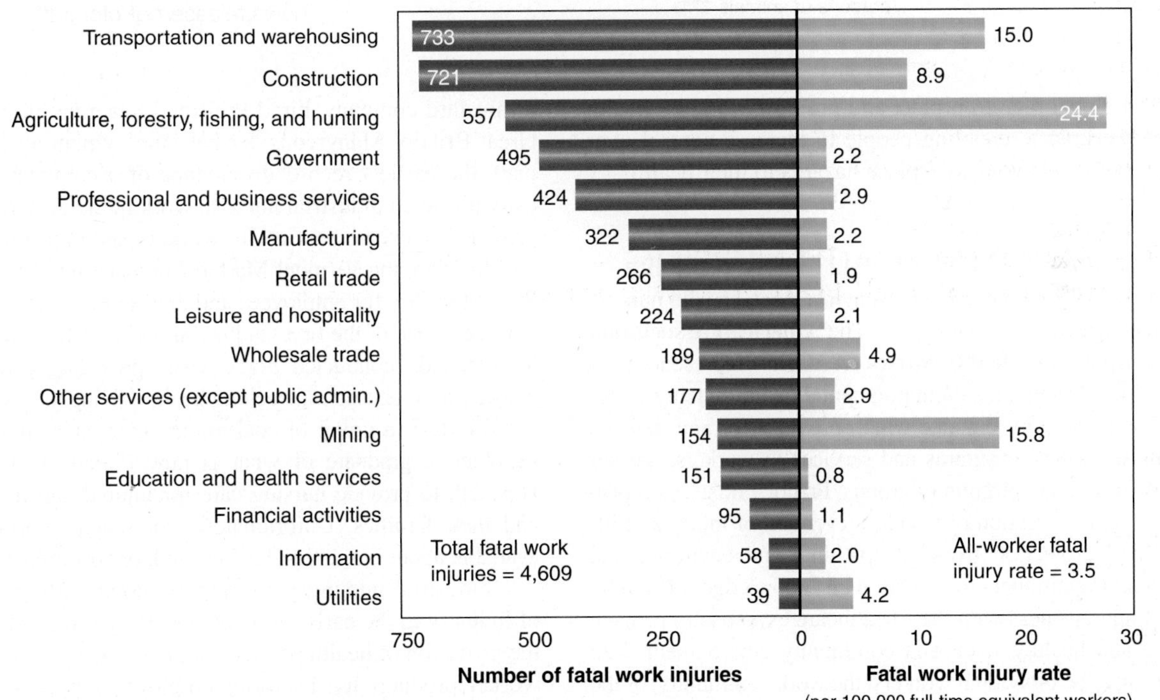

figure 25.3 Number and rate of fatal occupational injuries, by industry sector, 2011*
*Data for 2011 are preliminary. NOTE: All industries shown are private with the exception of government, which includes fatalities to workers employed by governmental organizations regardless of industry. Fatal injury rates exclude workers under the age of 16 years, volunteers, and resident military. The number of fatal work injuries represents total published fatal injuries before the exclusions. For additional information on the fatal work injury rate methodology changes please see http://www.bls.gov/iif/oshnotice10.htm.
SOURCE: U.S. Bureau of Labor Statistics, U.S. Department of Labor, 2012.

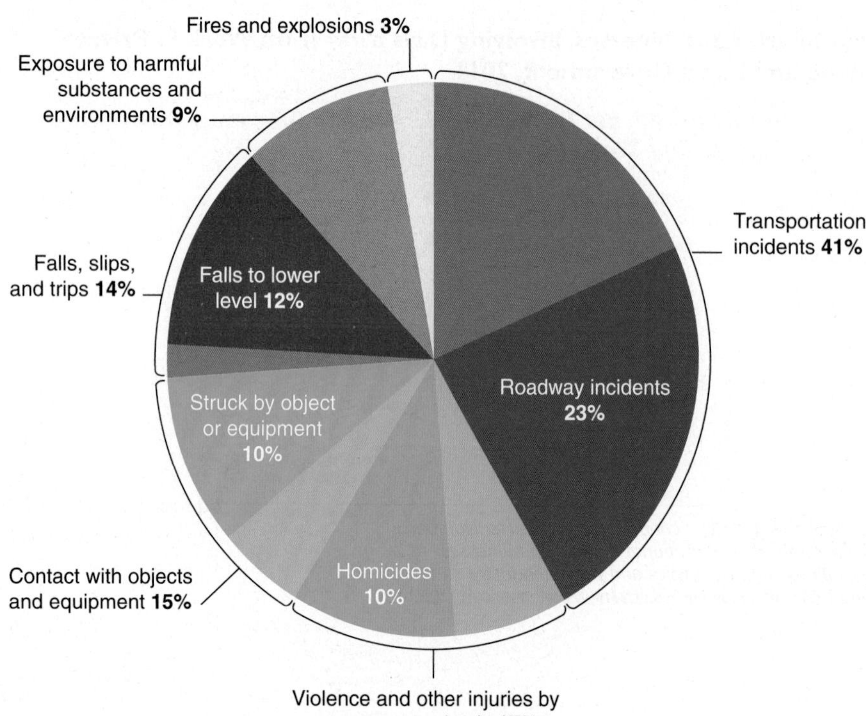

figure 25.4 Fatal Occupational Injuries in 2011 (National Census Preliminary Report) (Bureau of Labor Statistics, U.S. Department of Labor. [2012, September 20]. *National census of fatal occupational injuries in 2011* (preliminary report) [chart 1]. Retrieved from http://www.bls.gov/news.release/pdf/cfoi.pdf)

WHO's global plan to protect and promote workers' health in the workplace, enabling people to increase control over their health and avoid workplace hazards to their health.

OCCUPATIONAL HEALTH NURSING

Occupational health nursing and environmental health nursing are intertwined (see Chapter 19). The **American Association of Occupational Health Nurses** (AAOHN) represents both specialties. Occupational/environmental health nursing is defined as a specialty practice which provides for and delivers health and safety programs and services to workers, worker populations, and community groups. Practice focuses on promotion and restoration of health, prevention of injury and illness, and protection from occupational and environmental hazards. Practitioners combine their knowledge of public health and business with their healthcare expertise to provide a safe and healthy work and community environment. The clients may be individual workers, the work community, or the organization as a whole. This nursing specialty is multidisciplinary, practiced through the integration of knowledge from a variety of disciplines, including nursing, medicine, social and behavioral sciences, management, public health, and occupational health specialties such as toxicology, industrial hygiene, and ergonomics.

History

The earliest record of occupational health nursing, originally called industrial nursing, began a few years after Florence Nightingale opened the "Nightingale Training School for Nurses" in 1860. In 1867, J. & J. Colman, a mustard company, hired Phillipa Flowerday in Norwich, Great Britain. Many consider her employment at this company the earliest recorded evidence of a company specifically hiring an industrial nurse to work in the dispensary and provide home care services to workers and their families.

In 1885, the Vermont Marble Company hired Ada Mayo Stewart to care for employees and their families, and she may have been one of the first "industrial nurse." Often arriving by bicycle, Ada conducted home visits providing care for ill workers and focused on teaching healthy living habits to families. In 1888, a group of coal mining companies hired Betty Moulder, a graduate of what is now Philadelphia General Hospital, to provide nursing care for injured and ill workers and their families. Unfortunately, not much information is available about her duties, background, or accomplishments.

Industrial nursing grew rapidly along with the growth of industry in the early 20th century. People recognized that the provision of health services in the workplace led to more worker productivity. Factories employed nurses to combat the spread of infectious diseases such as tuberculosis, and to address health-related problems resulting from labor shortages during World War I. There were several thousand industrial nurses by World War II, and the establishment of educational programs along with professional organizations followed. The AAOHN formed in 1942, with 16 states represented by 300 nurses, and some member nurses created the American Association of Industrial Nurses (AAIN). The intent of AAOHN was to improve occupational health program services while enhancing career opportunities for occupational and environmental health nurses (Association of Occupational Health Nurses [AAOHN], n.d.a).

In the United States, Congress passed several laws in the 1960s and 1970s to protect the safety and health of workers, leading to an increased need for OHNs. The 1968 Mine Safety and Health Act required the first prevention programs for workers. In 1970 came the Occupational Safety and Health Act, which established two government agencies, the **Occupational Safety and Health Administration** (OSHA), and the **National Institute of Occupational Safety and Health** (NIOSH). The mission of OSHA is to prevent work-related injuries, illnesses, and fatalities by setting federal standards regulating workers' exposures to potentially toxic substances. Regulations, data, and information regarding compliance assistance, training programs, and consultation are available at the OSHA website. The purposes of NIOSH is to help ensure safe and healthy working conditions by conducting scientific research, gathering information, and providing education and training in occupational safety and health. The organization provides leadership worldwide by fostering the translation of new knowledge into products and services. The NIOSH website contains more information about its activities.

Standards of Practice

OHNs can be found in almost every industry, from manufacturing and construction to public administration and leisure and hospitality businesses. They collaborate with employees, employers, members of the occupational health and safety team, and other professionals to (1) identify health and safety needs, (2) prioritize interventions, (3) develop and implement interventions and programs, and (4) evaluate care and service delivery (AAOHN, 2012a). Their scope of practice encompasses a broad range of activities that are discussed later in this chapter.

As the professional association for occupational and environmental health nurses, the AAOHN establishes and promulgates standards to define and advance the practice within a framework for evaluation. These statements describe the accountability of the practitioner and reflect the values and priorities of the profession. AAOHN has identified 11 professional practice standards that describe a competent level of performance with regard to the nursing process and professional roles of the occupational and environmental health nurse. Criteria developed for each standard are key indicators of competent practice and permit occupational and environmental health nurses to evaluate their practice relative to the standards (AAOHN, 2012b). These standards can be accessed online.

The AAOHN identifies nine categories of competency in occupational and environmental health nursing. OHN competencies are associated with specific guidelines as they relate to all OHNs who function in various workplace settings. Different settings require different levels of competency and specific skill sets. Benner (1984) identified five stages of competency in clinical nursing practice: novice, advanced beginner, competent, proficient, and expert. Within each stage are levels of achievement that are expressed in measurable behavioral objectives. AAOHN has cross-referenced and stated behavioral objectives for the OHN in three of these stages: competent, proficient, and expert. This establishes criteria for individual nurses and those in management positions to use in their own professional development. AAOHN (2007) competency levels in occupational and environmental health nursing are listed in Box 25.1.

The nicest thing about standards is that there are so many of them to choose from.

Ken Olsen, founder, Digital Equipment Corporation

Environmental issues, conditions, and activities unique to OHN practice are addressed in the AAOHN Delivery of Occupational and Environmental Health Services position statement (AAOHN, 2012a). AAOHN makes the assertion that based on training, education, and experience, the licensed OHNs are in the best position to deliver comprehensive occupational and environmental health services and workplace programs. Today, the scope of practice is broad,

box 25.1 AAOHN Competency Levels in Occupational and Environmental Health Nursing

Competent—A nurse who is confident and a master with an ability to cope with specific situations. There is less of a need to rely on the judgment of peers and other professionals (Benner, 1984). Example: A competent occupational and environmental health nurse recognizes a range of practice issues and functions comfortably in roles as clinician, coordinator, and case manager following company procedures, utilizing assessment checklists and clinical protocols to provide treatment.

Proficient—A nurse with the ability to perceive client situations based on past experiences, with focus on relevant aspects of the situation. The nurse is able to predict expected events in certain situations and recognize that protocols must be altered at times to meet the needs of the client (Benner, 1984). Example: A proficient occupational and environmental health nurse quickly obtains the information needed for accurate assessment and moves quickly to the critical aspects of a problem, within priority setting and structural goals, in response to a client's situation. The nurse usually possesses sophisticated clinical or managerial skills in the work and/or community environment.

Expert—A nurse having extensive experience with a broad knowledge base that enables one to grasp a situation quickly and initiate action. The nurse has a sense of salience grounded in practice guiding actions and priorities (Benner, 1984). Example: An expert occupational and environmental health nurse provides leadership in developing occupational safety and health policy within the organization, functions in upper executive or management roles, serves as a consultant to business and government, and designs and conducts significant research.

Source: Used with permission. American Association of Occupational Health Nurses. (2007). Competencies in occupational and environmental health nursing. *American Association of Occupational Health Nurses, 55*(11), 442–447.

including disease management, environmental health, emergency preparedness, and disaster planning in response to natural, technologic, and human hazards in the work and community environment (AAOHN, n.d.a).

The OHN must also adhere to a code of ethics that is based on the belief that the goal of occupational and environmental health nurses is to promote workers' health and safety. The purpose of the AAOHN Code of Ethics is to serve as a guide for registered professional nurses to maintain and pursue professionally-recognized ethical behavior when providing occupational health services (AAOHN, 2012a).

Founded in 1972, the American Board of Occupational Health Nurses (ABOHN) is an independent nursing specialty certification board. ABOHN is the sole certifying body for OHNs in the United States. Standards of nursing practice are used to validate an individual registered nurse's qualifications, knowledge, and practice in specific areas of occupational health nursing. ABOHN awards four credentials: Certified Occupational Health Nurse (COHN), Certified Occupational Health Nurse–Specialist (COHN–S), and Case Management (CM), and Safety Management (SM). More information can be obtained from the ABOHN website (2012b).

CONCEPTUAL FRAMEWORKS

PRACTICE POINT

Applying the epidemiologic triad model to the specific workplace helps OHNs understand the interaction between hazards, workers, and the environment.

The Epidemiologic Triad

The epidemiologic triad, discussed in detail in Chapter 6, is very helpful in occupational health nursing practice as a means to understand the complex relationships among the workers, hazards in the workplace, and hazards in the environment (Fig. 25.5).

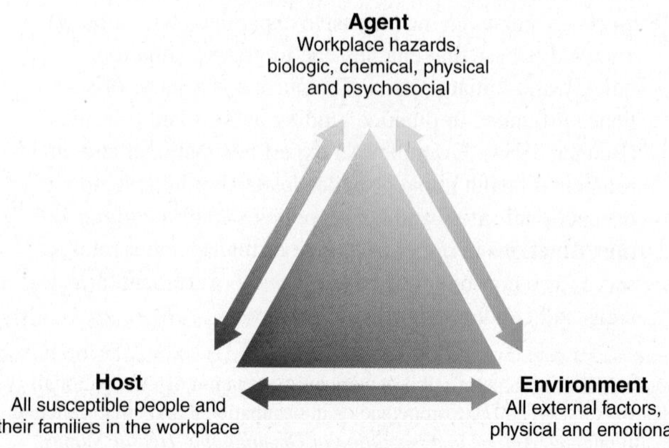

figure 25.5 The epidemiologic triad for the workplace.

Host

In the epidemiologic triad, each worker is a host within the work population. Each person (host) has his or her own innate, nonmodifiable characteristics, some of which put him or her at risk for workplace injury or illness. For example, age, gender, and ethnicity are nonmodifiable characteristics, whereas lifestyle, work practice, and to some degree, health status are modifiable characteristics. New workers with less than 1 year of experience are the most susceptible to injury. In contrast, older workers, who may have chronic illness, hearing loss, vision difficulties, or delayed reaction times, may adversely react to workplace hazards more frequently. Some workers are hypersusceptible, developing reactions, even though their exposure levels are below those determined to be safe.

Agent

The agents in the epidemiologic triad are workplace hazards classified as **biologic, chemical, physical,** or **psychosocial** agents (see Table 25.1).

BIOLOGIC AGENTS

Biologic agents include hazards from living organisms that have adverse effects. Although human illness often occurs from exposure to microorganisms, toxins released from microorganisms, insects, or animals are also biologic agents. Healthcare settings are particularly vulnerable to biologic hazards, and transmission of resistant infectious organisms is a major concern (see Chapter 14). Healthcare personnel are cognizant of potential exposures, but many workers such as maintenance workers, security personnel, and cleaners may be inadvertently exposed by trash, soiled linens, and contaminated equipment, which may result in illness.

CHEMICAL AGENTS

As industry grows, there is increasing general chemical contamination at work, at home, and in the community. Less than 1% of the 2 million chemicals used in industry have been studied for their effects on humans. Through ingestion, respiration, and injury, these environmental chemicals enter the body, and although exposure may be less than the maximal exposure standards (if they exist), the chemicals often accumulate, leading to a potentially chronic or life-threatening condition. There are many examples of illnesses resulting from chemical exposures. It has been known for decades that miners exposed to coal dust can suffer from pneumoconiosis, or black lung disease. Inhalation of asbestos may cause mesothelioma, a rare form of cancer found in the lining of the heart, lungs, abdomen, or the internal reproductive organs. Radiation exposure during pregnancy can result in congenital malformations, as can exposure to heavy metals and antineoplastic drugs. Interaction between the various chemicals entering the body also occurs, making it very difficult to predict the effects on health.

PHYSICAL AGENTS

Physical agents are sources of energy that may lead to injury or illness. Vibration produced through use of power tools may contribute to Raynaud phenomenon, which is vasoconstriction of the small arteries in fingers or toes, and which is triggered by cold or emotional upset. Vibrations associated with some power tools and trucks may adversely affect internal organs. Other common physical agents are radiation, temperature extremes, noise, lighting, falls, and unsafe equipment. Monitoring exposure to such agents and use of personal protective equipment such as preventive clothes, eye guards, and hearing protection are common practice in industry.

EVIDENCE FOR PRACTICE

Initial recognition of latex allergy occurred in the late 1970s. Healthcare workers are at risk through exposure to latex gloves or medical products containing latex. It is estimated that 8% to 12% of healthcare workers are latex-sensitive (Occupational Safety and Health Administration [OSHA], n.d.g). Hundreds of everyday products contain latex. Repeated exposure to the protein in natural latex can make a person more likely to develop a latex allergy. When the immune system detects the protein, a reaction can start in minutes, manifesting in a rash, asthma, and in rare cases shock from latex exposure (Mayo Foundation for Education and Research, 2011). Healthcare workers with suspected latex allergy may use nonlatex nitrile, synthetic rubber, or vinyl gloves.

PSYCHOSOCIAL AGENTS

Psychosocial agents include all organizational factors and interpersonal relationships in the workplace that may affect the health of the workers. Psychosocial hazards are as real as physical hazards, and if not recognized and controlled, they potentially can have a very negative impact. Studies have found that workers who have a high expectation for productivity, yet little or no control over their workplace and little reward for their efforts, are at risk for psychosocial distress. Stress, anger, and frustration can result in aggressive behavior, harassment, sabotage of the work or the work of others, poor physical and mental health, and disregard of safety measures. These feelings are enhanced if there is a perception of employer unfairness. Multiple studies have indicated that nurses have a wide range of occupational factors linked to stress (Box 25.2). Employers have increasingly developed strategies to manage the risks associated with psychosocial hazards. Examples include identifying the psychosocial hazards at the workplace, assessing ways to decentralize control, addressing workers' concerns about the workplace, and implementing systems to enable workers to report unacceptable behavior.

Of all man's miseries the bitterest is this, to know so much and to have control over nothing.

Herodotus

box 25.2 Occupational Factors Linked to Stress for Nurses

- Work overload
- Time pressure
- Lack of social support at work (especially from supervisors, head nurses, and higher management)
- Exposure to infectious diseases
- Needlestick injuries
- Exposure to work-related violence or threats
- Sleep deprivation
- Role ambiguity and conflict
- Understaffing
- Career development issues
- Dealing with difficult or seriously ill patients

Source: National Institute for Occupational Safety and Health. (2008). *NIOSH publication and products: Publication exposure to stress: Occupational hazards in hospitals.* (NIOSH Publication Number 2008-136). Retrieved from http://www.cdc.gov/niosh/docs/2008-136

EVIDENCE FOR PRACTICE

National Institute of Occupational Safety and Health (2008) defines occupational stress as "the harmful physical and emotional responses that occur when the requirements of the job do not match the capabilities, resources, or needs of the worker." Strategies recommended by NIOSH to reduce worker stress include distribution of workloads that are matched with workers capabilities and resources, clearly defined workers' roles and responsibilities, as well as methods to improve communication within the organization. NIOSH also suggests that workers be offered opportunities to participate in decisions and actions affecting their jobs. This process reduces uncertainty about career development and future employment prospects. OHNs should be cognizant of stress in the workplace and incorporate the strategies recommended by NIOSH in planning interventions.

Environment

The workplace exists within an external environment with specific geologic and atmospheric characteristics, air and water quality, and presence or absence of environmental pollution. Sometimes unanticipated results come from a difficult mix of agent, host, and environment characteristics. For example, patients in the intensive care unit of a major Chicago hospital were negatively affected by automobile exhaust from a highway a few hundred feet away. Replacing the air conditioning system solved the problem. Economic and political decisions can affect the public health infrastructure and, therefore, the health of a society. Factors such as adequate housing, literacy, crowding, culture, customs, and availability and accessibility of healthcare services are issues to be addressed. Social problems occurring from alcohol and substance abuse, infectious diseases, and poverty can have an impact on workforce productivity.

● PRACTICE POINT

There is a level of acceptable risk in any work setting. The primary goal is to lower the accepted level of risk of injury and illness associated with employment.

Practice Models

Figure 25.6 illustrates the Hanasaari model. This framework takes into account all the factors affecting people at work, a total environment concept. A group of OHNs developed this model at a workshop in Hanasaari, Finland, in 1989. Endorsed by the Federation of Occupational Health Nurses within the European Union (FOHNEU), it is now the basis for practice, education, and research throughout the European Union. The model presents an outer circle that represents the total global concept, covering all aspects of health and safety affecting the worker population in the general environment. Extending out from the center (occupational health nursing) are the social, political, ecologic, organizational, and economic factors that influence the global environment. The man-work-health triangle indicates that the total environment can have a significant effect on workplace health. Political and social policies, for example, either expand or contract the development of occupational health.

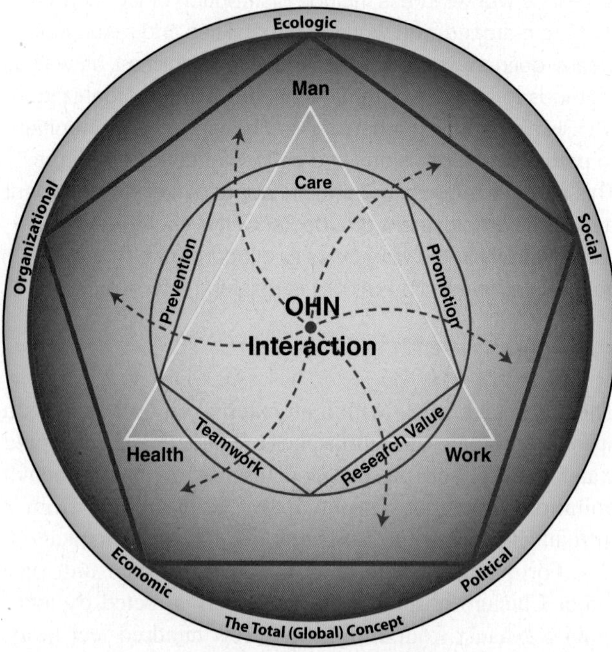

figure 25.6 The Hanasaari conceptual model for occupational health nursing (OHN). OHN is presented in the center of the model. The curving circle of arrows represents flexibility, influence, and eventual improvement in the health of people at work and in the total community environment. (From: Alston, R. M., et al. [1989]. *Workshop for Occupational Health Nurses, Hanasaari, Finland* [Unpublished manuscript]. Retrieved May 8, 2010, from http://www.fohneu.org/hanasaari_conceptual_model_for_o.htm)

A more recent model proposed by Thomason and Lagowski (2008) is one of collaboration and reciprocation while using the nursing process. Earlier models have not focused on the key concept of engaging clients in reciprocal relationships. This approach suggests that the OHN should use leadership and interpersonal relationship skills which foster communication and respect through continuous feedback from workers and community. The model provides a means of engaging and collaborating with clients in restoring and maintaining health, well-being, and workplace safety. Figure 25.7 illustrates the five steps of collaboration between the nurse and the client.

> *One of the tests of leadership is the ability to recognize a problem before it becomes an emergency.*
>
> **Arnold Glasgow, psychologist**

The OHN must deal with individual, family, and community issues that often involve medical, legal, and regulatory factors. Forces may contradict and hinder health and safety priorities unless the OHN can communicate and act to resolve the issues. For example, a system's approach can be very effective within a single department or division. However, the same system may fail when interfacing with other activities of the workplace within a community. It is often the workers who take the responsibility to correct an unplanned problem, and they may choose to put themselves at risk. Without recognition, support, and ongoing communication with workers, the risk may not be apparent. It is through reciprocation during these crucial moments of a worker's life that an OHN can help sustain and maintain worker and community health.

A large number of OHNs find employment in the field as individual, privately contracted professionals. It is common for many occupational and environmental health nurses to work in more than one designated role concurrently while employed by the same company (Zichello & Sheridan, 2008). One particular practice model includes corporate OHNs who often have a master's degree. They can be responsible for managing the implementation of occupational health goals and objectives for other nurses in various facilities

The ABOHN (2012b) conducted a 2011 Occupational Health Nursing Practice Analysis. Respondents revealed the majority of nurses are female (95.1%; male, 4.9%), and most do not have global responsibility. Nurses spend the greatest amount of time in two practice areas: health and wellness activities, and case management (ABOHN, 2012b). Midsize to larger companies may have more than one occupational and/or environmental health nurse on site. In large companies, there can be nurses and physicians, including advanced practice nurses, in nurse practitioner roles.

There are various ways nurses enter and function in OHN positions. Most employers conduct a job search for an

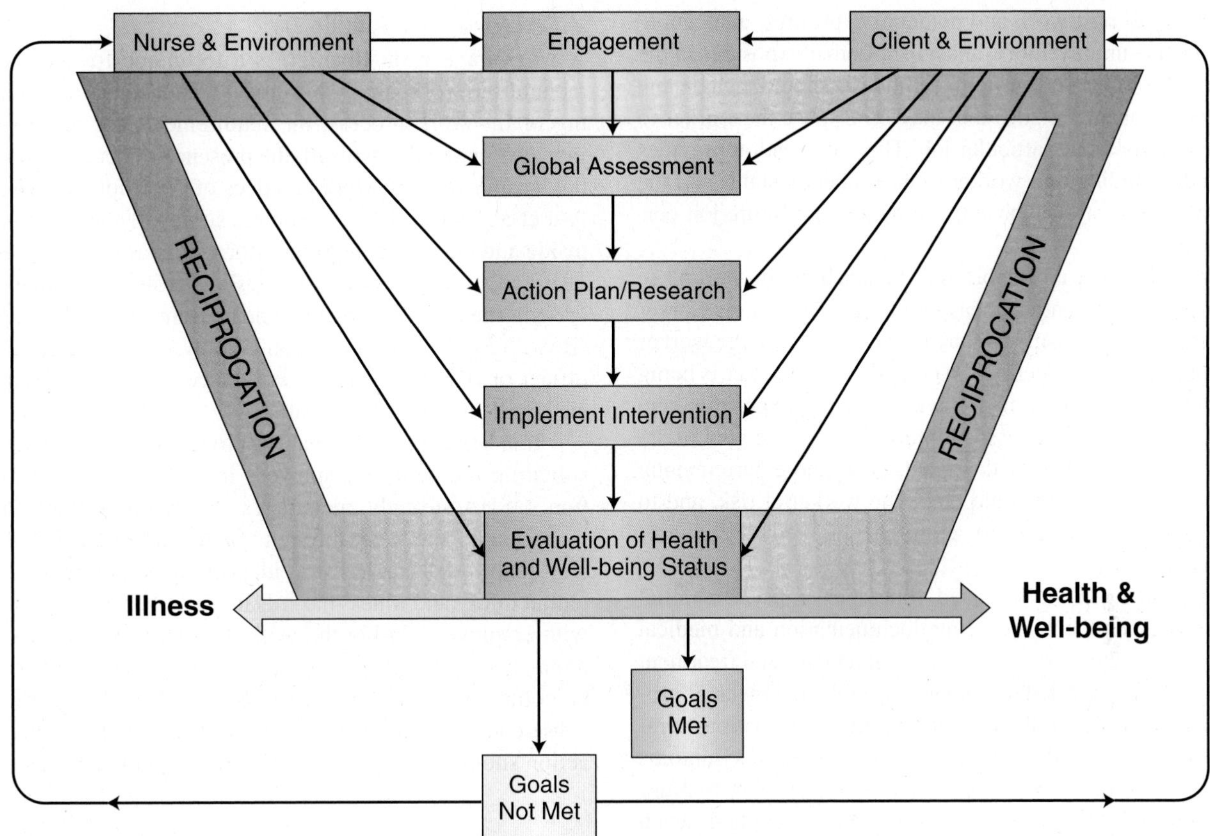

figure 25.7 Reciprocation model. (From Thomason, D. A., & Lagowski, L. R. [2008]. Sustaining a healthy work force in the 21st century—A model for collaborating through reciprocation. *Journal of American Association of Occupational Health Nursing*, *56*[12], 503–513.)

OHN, OHN manager, or a nurse practitioner and are specific about the education and experience required. Many employers look for a board-certified (ABOHN) nurse who has at least a bachelor of science in nursing, with 3 to 5 years' nursing experience. Some employers search for an advanced practice nurse or nurse practitioner who is prepared at the master's level. In recent years, licensed practical nurses (LPN) and licensed vocational nurses (LVN) are found to work in specific roles and function as a team member with other OHNs who may delegate and manage activity as necessary (AAOHN, 2012a).

OCCUPATIONAL HEALTH NURSING: PRACTICE

Following their job analysis study, the ABOHN determined and designated functional roles and responsibilities for the occupational and environmental health nurse. Occupational health nursing practice requires a wide variety of roles and functions, and specific responsibilities vary. Roles include clinician, case manager, counselor, health promotion specialist, manager/administrator, educator, and researcher (ABOHN, 2012a).

Clinician

The OHN acts as a clinician whose primary responsibilities are to prevent work and non-work-related health problems, and to restore as well as maintain the health of workers. Assessments of hazards, surveillance of the workers and workplace, investigation of illness, and monitoring events that lead to an injury are fundamental to achieving this goal.

As in the case of an outbreak of illness following the company picnic, frequent communication from employees brings a problem to a nurse's attention. What assessments should be performed as soon as the workers arrive at the clinic?

Worker Assessment

Along with the traditional history and physical assessment, an **occupational health history** of every worker is an essential component of OHN practice. Components include characteristics of the worker's present jobs, a chronologic record of all past work and potential exposures, an occupational exposure inventory, and a list of other exposures in the home or community. Particular emphasis should include any individual characteristics that may predispose the worker to increased risk in a particular job. This information provides an understanding of a worker's current health status and the potential impact of exposures on health and future job performance.

Nurses have an opportunity to teach about workplace hazards and prevention measures when performing worker assessments. Assessments may take place before the worker begins the job, on a periodic basis, when the worker is being transferred to a different job with different exposures, and when an exposure, illness, or injury occurs. The goal of assessments is to identify the agent, host, and environmental characteristics which could place the worker at risk, and to take preventive steps to eliminate or reduce adverse exposures.

Following a work-related illness or injury, an initial physical assessment, including documentation and medical case record initiation, is required. Direct care and treatment of injuries is provided, often using established medical protocols. Referrals are then made for further evaluation as required. However, illnesses and injuries are often symptoms of problems in the workplace. The concept of root cause analysis (RCA), discussed below, can be applied when performing an accident investigation after an injury.

In **Case 2**, the OHN conducts a telephone interview with the employee who had an anaphylactic reaction. What type of information should the OHN obtain?

The OHN discovers that the employee had been a nurse who left hospital employment 4 years earlier and began working in the bank. At the hospital, she had a good attendance record. She left the hospital because she was having difficulty doing her work; she had a rash on her hands and a general low energy level. Her hands would begin to heal and she felt better on long weekends and vacations. She was not asthmatic, had never experienced any respiratory problems, and had never received a diagnosis of an allergy. However, on further questioning and investigation, the OHN learns that the woman's mother was a nurse who could not work in a hospital setting because of a latex allergy. (She was also allergic to bananas and avocados.) This information confirms the possibility of an inherited type of sensitivity that a physician would need to further explore.

PRACTICE POINT

OHNs are more likely to notice the influence of work-health interactions if the worker assessment data are complete. The assessment involves continuous monitoring and surveillance of workers and their environment.

Workplace Assessment

A **workplace walk-through** is a technique for an assessment of the workplace. This process leads to an understanding of the work process, the requirements for the various jobs, the materials involved, the presence of actual or potential hazards, and the work practices of the employees (Peek-Asa et al., 2009). It is a complete survey of the workplace, inside and outside, compiling information as to the presence of hazards, the location of entries and exits, the availability of emergency equipment, and potential trouble spots (Box 25.3). If the organization employs a health and safety officer or risk manager, the workplace walk-through analysis will be a shared responsibility.

It is helpful to use a team approach during this process, soliciting the help of employees in gathering the information. OSHA strongly encourages maximum employee participation in the walk-through. Better-informed and more alert employees can assist in identifying and correcting potential injury and illness hazards in one's workplace. Talking with employees during the walk-through helps identify the nature and extent of specific hazards. The assessment should be comprehensive, thorough, and take place frequently because conditions may change daily. A system for corrective action should be in place when improvement is needed.

In **Case 1**, the OHN also finds that renovation and construction was occurring on the floors above the employee's office and in adjacent offices when the worker became ill. Fellow employees state that they noticed an odor on the day their coworker was rushed to the hospital. Five employees detected the odor, and two of them experienced a headache, with symptoms such as light-headedness and itchy, watering eyes. They became alarmed when their coworker started to have serious difficulty breathing.

The construction supervisor states that walls in the adjacent office space were being painted, carpets installed, seams glued, and general cleaning done in nearby areas the day of the incident. Immediately, the nurse asks the supervisor what type of paint was used the day of the incident. The OHN also wants to know what material the carpet was made of, and the type of glue, and what cleaning products were used. A combination of environmental factors such as chemicals, fumes, vapor, dust, heat, or moisture may create an adverse condition for some people.

Case Manager

Case manager responsibilities include coordination and management of services for ill or injured workers, including various aspects related to group health, workers' compensation, and regulations pertaining to the Family Medical Leave Act (FMLA) (AAOHN, n.d.a). Case managers are as concerned with prevention as they are with healthcare after an

box 25.3 Workplace Walk-Through—Evaluation of Workplace Hazards

Alarms and detection devices
Occupancy, building diagrams
Exits
Fire prevention plans
Procedures for processing, receiving, shipping, and storage
Condition of buildings and grounds
Housekeeping program for fall prevention
Heating, ventilation, air conditioning systems
Electricity
Lighting
Presence of guards for machine use
Worker training procedures
Hand and power tools
Hazardous materials
Maintenance and servicing of machines and equipment (control of hazardous energy)
Personal protective equipment use
Emergency action plans

accident. The overall goal is to do everything that can be done to prevent accidents and minimize illness.

The case manager tracks each incident that relates to employees' health and safety, beginning immediately after the onset of an illness or injury, and continuing through rehabilitation and return to work. Following the initial event, case managers gather case characteristics that provide detailed information about the circumstances of workplace injuries and illness that required one or more days away from work. There are four basic case characteristics: nature of the workplace incident, the part of the body involved, the source of the illness or injury, and the circumstances that resulted in the exposure or event. After case managers record this information for ongoing monitoring of the workplace, they perform an RCA.

Root Cause Analysis

Root cause analysis is a process for understanding and solving a problem, with the goal of determining what happened, why it happened, and what can be done to prevent its recurrence. Sometimes, determination of the problem is easy; however, the process can be more complicated.

There are usually three basic types of causes: (1) tangible physical causes where materials or machines have failed; (2) human causes where people did something wrong, either by commission or omission; or (3) organizational causes where the policies or procedures that are used to make decisions are faulty. RCA incorporates all three types of causes, and it is possible to apply this method in almost any situation. It involves investigating the patterns of negative effects, finding hidden flaws in the system, and discovering specific actions that contributed to the problem. This often means that RCA reveals more than one root cause. By tracing actions back to their origin, the person

box 25.4 Root Cause Analysis Process in Occupational Health

Define the problem
- Define the characteristics of the case.
- Determine the circumstances under which it occurred.

Collect data
- Determine whether similar illnesses or injuries occurred in the past.
- Compare similarities and differences.
- Create a time line related to the problem.
- Determine the impact of the problem.

Identify possible causal factors
- Convene people involved in the situation to discuss cause.
- Determine the sequence of events that led to the illness or injury.
- Identify the conditions that allowed the problem to occur.
- Identify other problems that could be related to the problem.
- Create a chart of possible causal factors.
- Identify causal factors and possible interrelationships.

Identify the root cause(s)
- Identify the true causes of the illness or injury.
- Determine why the causal factor(s) exist.
- Determine the real reason the problem occurred.

Recommend and implement solutions
- Identify ways to prevent the problem from happening again.
- Plan for implementation of solutions.
- Identify who will be responsible.
- Determine the risks of implementing the solution.

Evaluate the outcome
- Develop and implement an evaluation plan.

using RCA can determine where the problem started and how it contributed to the illness or injury that occurred. RCA is the application of the scientific method to a specific workplace problem when applied to occupational health settings. The steps of RCA are outlined in Box 25.4.

In Case 2, explain the steps that the OHN would take in initiating an RCA of the outbreak of illness following the company picnic. (Refer to Chapter 14 to review the steps in investigating an outbreak.)

Counselor/Consultant

The OHN acts as an advisor in selecting, developing, implementing, and evaluating occupational health and safety services, within both organizations and communities. As a clinician and nurse consultant, it is the role of the OHN to investigate all possible material and chemical exposures that could lead to an adverse reaction in workers. By law, workers and their advocates have a right to know the substances to which they may be exposed, and therefore, they may request the requisite information. A material safety data sheet (MSDS) provides information to employers from the manufacturer or producer of substances.

In addition to counseling people about work-related illnesses and injuries, OHNs also counsel groups regarding issues such as substance abuse, psychosocial needs, wellness/health promotion concerns, and work-related issues. The OHN may also assume primary responsibility for managing a variety of employee assistance programs. Often, an off-site provider or group is contracted to offer workers and their families counseling and other crisis intervention services. The nurse may also handle referrals to community resources while coordinating follow-up care for workers (AAOHN, n.d.a).

When we turn to one another for counsel we reduce the number of our enemies.

Khalil Gibran

In Case 1, after learning about the renovation, the OHN asks for a list of materials and the MSDSs for the substances used that day. The construction supervisor supplies names of the materials, a phone number to obtain a list of materials, as well as the MSDSs that addressed all the elements of the substances used during the renovation project.

Review of the MSDSs reveals that latex paint was used the day of the episode, along with cleaners and glues containing volatile organic compounds (VOCs). VOCs consist of a variety of chemicals that may have short- and long-term adverse health effects. Thousands of products emit VOCs, including paints, lacquers, paint strippers, adhesives, glues, cleaning supplies, pesticides, building materials, and furnishings. Concentrations of VOCs are consistently greater indoors than outdoors (U.S. Environmental Protection Agency [EPA], 2012a).

box 25.5 *Healthy People 2020* Occupational Health and Safety Objectives

OSH-1 Reduce deaths from work-related injuries.
OSH-2 Reduce nonfatal work-related injuries.
OSH-3 Reduce the rate of injury and illness cases involving days away from work due to overexertion or repetitive motion.
OSH-4 Reduce pneumoconiosis deaths.
OSH-5 Reduce deaths from work-related homicides.
OSH-6 Reduce deaths from work-related assaults.
OSH-7 Reduce the proportion of persons who have elevated blood lead concentrations from work exposures.
OSH-8 Reduce occupational skin diseases or disorders among full-time workers.
OSH-9 (Developmental) increase the proportion of employees who have access to programs that prevent or reduce employee stress.
OSH-10 Reduce new cases of work-related, noise-induced hearing loss.

Source: From Healthypeople.gov. (2013). *Healthy People 2020: Occupational safety and health.* Retrieved from http://www.healthypeople.gov/2020/topicsobjectives2020/objectiveslist.aspx?topicId=30

Health Promotion Specialist

As a health promotion specialist, the OHN participates in the development and management of a multidimensional, broad-range health promotion program that supports the business objectives of the organization. Health promotion and illness and injury prevention is a function that the OHN performs along a continuum for the worker population. The objective is to create an environment for the worker that provides a sense of balance among work, family, personal, health, and psychosocial concerns (AAOHN, n.d.a). *Healthy People 2020* Occupational Health and Safety Objectives for the United States are presented in Box 25.5.

Educating all employees and administrative staff regarding the exposures and hazards associated with the workplace is the foundation of health promotion efforts. Corporate nurse educators often design programs that are used to educate workers in multiple settings, with state, regional, national, or international audiences (Dirksen, 2006). Programs are conducted through a Webcast, satellite broadcast, Webinar, or the online use of Internet to an established website.

The health promotion frameworks discussed in Chapter 5 have a particular application in occupational health and safety. For example, the OHN has a unique opportunity to contribute toward the current *Healthy People* prevention agenda. He or she can use leading health indicators and national occupational health and safety objectives to assess the status of the workplace. This information is useful for identifying prevention objectives for the workplace, and implementation of specific interventions and action plans. The actual prevention activities performed at any given time are a result of many changing variables in the organization, and a balance among primary, secondary, and tertiary prevention efforts is essential. For example, the nurse who is concentrating on developing strategies to prevent work site injuries and disease (primary prevention) may have little time or resources for testing individual employees for risk factors that increase the potential for illness or injury (secondary prevention).

Historically, the OHN has been involved with workers in a supportive role to maintain health at the work site. In the 1989 work by Michael O'Donnell, the seminal definition of health promotion gave OHNs interested in the pursuit of wellness a relevant rationale to pursue this approach. According to O'Donnell (Fig. 25.8), optimal health includes a balance of physical, emotional, social, spiritual, and intellectual health. The nurse can contribute toward this end by creating an environment that develops awareness and encourages behavior change (O'Donnell, 2009).

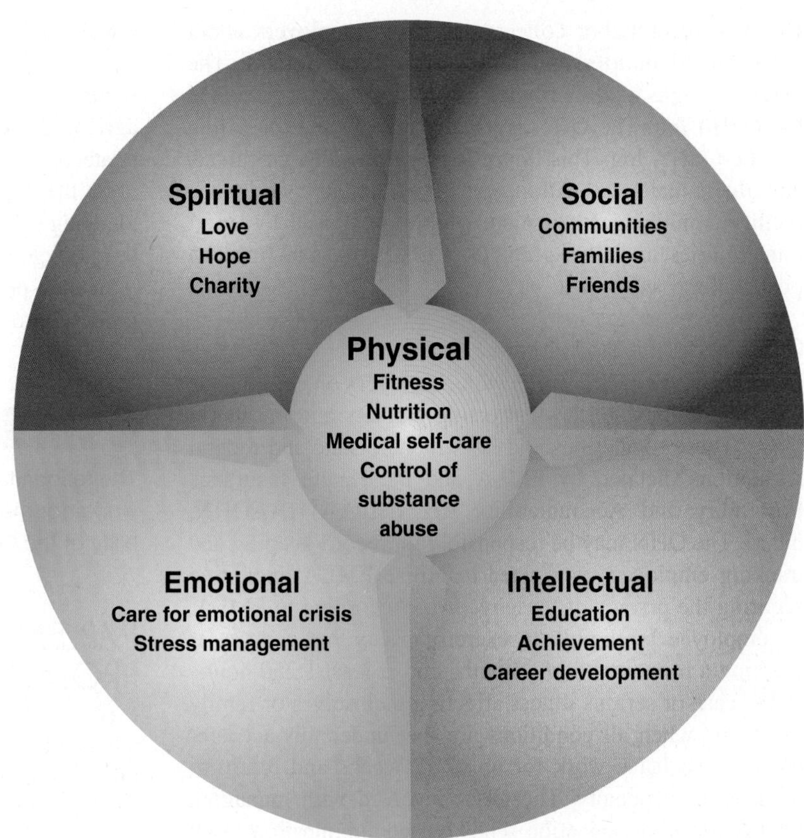

figure 25.8 O'Donnell health promotion model. (O'Donnell, M. P. [2009] Definition of health promotion 2.0: Embracing passion, enhancing motivation, recognizing dynamic balance, and creating opportunities. *American Journal of Health Promotion*, *24*[1], iv–iv.)

A common health and safety promotion program in occupational settings involves preservation of sight and hearing. Within a company eye protection program, the OHN often works collaboratively with the safety director and/or human resources personnel in the oversight of these programs. The OHN has a role in coordinating administration of eye examinations for those employees who need prescription safety eyeglasses. There are several approaches that a company can take when establishing and maintaining a hearing protection program. The OHN may become a certified hearing conservationist and carry out the required monitoring of noise levels within specific facilities, work areas, and departments. He or she may oversee or manage the distribution of hearing protection to workers, conduct education as needed, administer audiometric testing at the work site and manage the feedback of hearing tests results to employees, and ensure follow-up with a physician when needed.

Manager/Administrator

The responsibilities of the OHN frequently include participation in the development, management, and evaluation of the entire health and safety program of the organization, in conjunction with both the medical and safety directors. Written policies and procedures consistent with organizational goals and objectives are required to ensure compliance with legal, regulatory, and ethical standards. Often, a company may ask the OHN to prepare a business plan that justifies the cost for establishing health promotion programs. This plan, by necessity, justifies how the program will be implemented within the organizational culture by using key approaches such as working with teams and choosing relevant and sensitive interventions.

Constant surveillance, monitoring, and auditing of the safety conditions of the workplace is essential. This includes monitoring individual employees in their immediate work environment. A health record can be kept on the employees as part of their other employment records. This process often starts with an initial physical examination appropriate to the type of work that is going to be done. The physical examination helps ensure fitness for the job and provides a baseline for future comparison. Often, an employee's health and safety orientation and training follows, with issuance of proper personal safety protection. The OHN schedules routine safety meetings stressing health-related issues, such as safety gear and proper lifting techniques, on a proactive basis and conducts them thereafter on a need-to-know basis. An example of this is the introduction of a hazardous substance into the work area requiring more detailed information to ensure job safety. When injured employees do not return to work, the OHN may initiate or oversee a workers' compensation claim on behalf of the employee to ensure that the worker receives workers' compensation benefits.

OSHA Compliance

The need to comply with OSHA standards is often the starting point for initiation of safety measures. The U.S.

Department of Labor collects data from employers about occupational injuries and illness across the country. The OSHA designs and distributes record-keeping forms called the *OSHA log*. The OHN is usually responsible for filling out the OSHA log. This injury log is a record of accidents and illness that occur within a given year at every workplace facility employing 10 or more people. It is used to report total injuries and illness annually to OSHA and must be posted at the work site.

Other Legal Responsibilities

In addition, the OHN works with employers on compliance with regulations and laws affecting workers and the workplace. These regulations and laws include state and federal regulations dictated by FMLA and the Health Insurance Portability and Accountability Act (HIPAA) (AAOHN, n.d.a). The OHN may be responsible for record-keeping and tracking employees who need to utilize FMLA, including securing the privacy of these records. According to FMLA, an employee is eligible to exercise his or her right after working a minimum of 12 months and at least 1,250 hours. In the case of serious illness affecting themselves or family members, when all conditions are met under this act, employees can leave work for up to 12 weeks and return to work without penalty. The OHN involved with managing FMLA for an organization sends out communication to all employees who apply. The nurse helps ensure that the worker(s) or physician(s) is in compliance with the regulation by submitting the proper paperwork to the employer.

The OHN is also responsible for the privacy and record-keeping of occupational health and safety information as it relates to individuals at the workplace. The HIPAA mandates that all medical information be held in confidence. One way to ensure privacy is to keep all health-related information in a separate, secured file and storage area other than the business or human resource files.

Researcher

As researchers, OHNs contribute toward the future of the profession by identifying, analyzing, monitoring, measuring, and evaluating the effects of workplace exposures and hazards for workers and members of the community. They gather and use health and hazard data to select and implement preventive and control measures in a continual process. Examples include analysis of the effects of toxic chemical exposure, development of plans to prevent work-related accidents, and an analysis of groups, not just individual people, to detect patterns, trends, changes, and commonalities, as in pandemic situations (AAOHN, n.d.a; Dirksen, 2006).

The National Occupational Research Agenda (NORA) is a partnership program to stimulate innovative research and improved practices for safer, healthier workplaces. The program is directed toward the study of disease and injury, the work environment and the workforce, and the various research methods which are used to study occupational health. Released in 1996, NORA has become a research framework for NIOSH and the nation. Diverse parties collaborate to identify the most critical issues in workplace safety and health. NORA is composed of councils which focus on specific sectors of industry, such as construction, agriculture, or healthcare. The councils develop goals and strategies for the nation, and encourage partnerships to address the goals and promote improved workplace practices, all using open processes. The partners then work together to develop goals and objectives addressing these needs. All interested people have an opportunity to participate in this process through the CDC website.

PRACTICE POINT

The recognition of conditions that may harm the individual worker or members of the community is a crucial responsibility of the OHN.

IMPLEMENTING HEALTH PROMOTION IN THE WORKPLACE

It is imperative that management be involved in all stages of the health promotion effort. The company may give the OHN complete responsibility to create the initial vision and implement the plan, but constant communication with management is necessary to ensure that the plan is meeting the organization's expectations.

Balance theory is a systems approach that can be used by OHNs to help them organize a prevention model. The balance theory states that one element in the system influences other elements, having the potential to be positive or negative depending on the effect one part plays on another (Brunette, 2006). When using the balance theory, each workplace system is examined and categorized into five areas:

1. Organization
2. Tasks
3. Tools and technologies
4. Physical environment
5. People

The scenario in Case 2 illustrates the dynamic of the balance theory. The systems breakdown in this case involves operational and SM policy and procedure, machinery, and training of personnel. Identify several check-and-balance procedures that need to be in place to ensure a decreased health and safety risk for worker populations.

Developing a Team Approach

In creating a wellness team, it is essential to include key people, such as health professionals and interested parties in the workplace, who can help to identify company or organizational needs. Team members can contribute to the development of a plan of action based on national and local trends. They can also help with the distribution of surveys and answer questions.

Collecting data for presentation to management, such as projected healthcare costs based on current utilization trends, is one way to initiate a program. Insurance companies can provide reports of medical usage (utilization reviews) on the basis of diagnosis and/or categories of visits made to providers. The OHN may have the team review health insurance data; research national leading health indicators; or conduct interviews, workplace assessments, or on-site surveys to help determine the findings and outcome of the data.

Choosing Interventions

Interventions that are appropriate for a company or work site(s) through assessment of health promotion programs depend on the findings of an employee-needs assessment which is conducted by and for the organization. It is important that the team members who are involved know the purpose of the needs assessment prior to the actual method chosen, and the need for follow-up and future planning.

A good start for a small-to midsize company is to conduct a needs assessment with a general health promotion questionnaire. The questionnaire or survey can ask employees basic lifestyle questions, such as number of hours worked each week. Consumption of alcohol, diet, and smoking, exercise activity level, hours of sleep, and existing medical coverage is an excellent place to begin collecting data. The OHN should also watch for workers who take a second job to earn extra money, which may lead to fatigue and injury on and off the job.

It is important for a team to know what percentage of the working population has access to medical care because health promotion efforts depend on available resources. Some employees have medical coverage provided by a spouse or significant other working at another company. Others simply cannot afford medical insurance, and they are often referred to as the working poor (Shipler, 2004; Luhby, 2012).

The passing of the Massachusetts Health Care Reform Act made the Commonwealth the first state in the United States to address the problem of inadequate health insurance for all citizens. It is mandated by law that healthcare coverage be offered by all employers to workers. The state requires submission of proof of purchase or coverage for health insurance for both employer and employees to avoid a fine. Employers need to show they offered healthcare insurance, and if an employee declines, the employer must have the worker submit proof of healthcare insurance to be ready to present to the state if necessary. Workers must be ready to pay a fine on their state income tax return if they do not show proof of healthcare insurance (MassResources, 2013).

PRACTICE POINT

A proactive prevention approach in occupational health incorporates the belief that there are no accidents but only events that were not noticed or managed correctly with proper intervention.

IMPLEMENTING A PROGRAM: EXAMPLE, SMOKING CESSATION

Step I

The OHN makes a presentation to management to support offering a smoking cessation program. It is important to state the method that will be used to obtain the data (e.g., using a survey, questionnaire, or by direct interview). The OHN and/or the team could present the number of employees (by percentage) who smoke and the number of employees who say they would participate in a smoking cessation program if offered.

Step II

To initiate the program, the OHN sends out a memo calling appointed team members to attend a meeting. The team conducts an information-gathering meeting to point out why a smoking cessation program is needed, based on current smoking behaviors in the company. This includes statistics shared about smoking behaviors and risk at the local, state, and national level. It is best if the OHN is prepared with a meeting agenda and educational information to hand out to attendees for review.

Step III

The OHN and/or the team presents the following information to justify the cost involved with conducting a smoking cessation program. Statement of fact: It is documented that workplace smoking, and especially the secondhand smoke associated with it, causes death and long-term illness. Direct medical costs for employers and schools include the following:

- Increased absenteeism
- Higher cleaning costs
- Decreased productivity
- Higher insurance premiums (health, fire)
- Increased property damage resulting from tobacco use by smokers

Step IV

The OHN and/or the team should provide take-home information, such as a copy of U.S. Morbidity and Mortality Figures Related to Tobacco Use from the CDC Fact Sheet. It is also necessary to review handout material with the group for discussion.

Step V

The OHN and/or the team should review the economics of smoking. For example, each smoker in the United States costs $1,700 a year in extra medical bills, according to the CDC. Together with absenteeism and regular smoke breaks, the annual cost is estimated to be $3,400 per worker. The OHN can present the number of smokers currently working in the company and multiply that number by the projected cost of $3,400 per worker a year. An estimated dollar figure would show that the cost to initiate a smoking cessation program justifies the investment.

The following is an example of the initiation of a smoking cessation program and how it might progress once it is approved by management. A realistic goal would be to reach and help 4% of the smoking population become nonsmokers by the end of year one of the program. With more education and incentives for employees, the program could similarly affect an additional 1% after two more years.

Items such as cost of a program and incentives may be part of the program for those who need more support to quit smoking. The program is best offered when most workers are interested and can attend it. Time of day is important. Ideally, program times are set up during lunch time or directly after work, with experts who know how to work with people who may wish to discontinue smoking.

The OHN and/or team may send follow-up letters to participants periodically to offer continued support and information, and to provide tips about diet and activities that support the employee's new nonsmoking behavior. Invitations to join activities, such as baseball, rowing, or bowling leagues, to help people replace old behaviors, may help. Finally, program planners should anticipate that there will be those who relapse, and they should provide reassurance for continuing with the program. It is necessary to establish a plan of action to support these workers who want to begin the process again.

Much of what the OHN does in health promotion is to support employees in their choice of behaviors that are more life-enhancing. C-Change is a group of individuals and member organizations that are the key cancer leaders from government, business, and nonprofit sectors in the United States. This group of the nation's cancer experts has made health promotion the focus of their efforts. It has concluded that only 5% of cancers are caused by genetics, one-third are caused by tobacco, and one-third by nutrition (C-Change, 2010). Creating an opportunity to affect people and the quality of their lives at the work site is a logical place to begin.

STUDENT REFLECTION

After working several years in the hospital, I realized that many patients were there because of needless accidents and diseases that could be prevented. Knowing how devastating the consequences of acute and chronic diseases can be, I decided to focus on health promotion and prevention of disabilities in the community when I returned to the university. I really enjoyed my experience in a health promotion program in the workplace. It allowed me to apply both my nursing and previously-acquired knowledge while learning something new.

The project required tracking, quantifying, and systematically measuring the outcome of a simple nursing intervention, monitoring the employees' blood pressure (BP). The key to the success of this program had to do with consistent follow-up, continued monitoring, and referral for medical treatment as needed.

The first step was to conduct a facility-wide volunteer BP screening. All employees who were being screened received a questionnaire that contained general history questions such as the following:

Have you had high BP in the past?
Are you currently under a doctor's care?
Are you being treated for high BP?
Are you taking medication?
Are you overweight?
Do you exercise?

Advertisements for the program appeared in the company newsletter. Employees who participated for five consecutive weeks of BP monitoring received stipends for use in the company cafeteria. Individuals who were interested signed up and had their BP taken systematically, department by department, in the building where they worked. Workers with extremely elevated BP received an immediate referral to a healthcare provider for follow-up care. Nurses asked workers with no known history of elevated BP, but who showed two out of three moderately elevated readings at week three, to return periodically to continue their screenings. With the workers' consent, nurses also gathered weight information and further investigated diet and medical history. At this point, the nurses recommended that workers who continued to show consistent moderate elevations see their physician.

The process continued with workers who showed slight elevations while working on goals involving exercise and diet. This experience showed me that most workers respond well when given the education and the support associated with the BP screening and monitoring program. Throughout this project, I was able to track progress and demonstrate the potential to increase quality of life, reduce medical costs, and prevent further disease such as stroke, heart attack, and kidney disease. The workplace does indeed have a captive audience; when approached in the right manner, these workers are very interested in maintaining and pursuing their health.

EPIDEMIOLOGY AND OCCUPATIONAL HEALTH

The use of epidemiology as a tool for assessing the hazards of workers has a long and productive history. Ancient Egyptian documents told about the difficult life of workers, and other early historical publications addressed the hazards of working with heavy metals and mining. In the 17th century, the Italian physician Ramazzini outlined the health hazards of chemicals, dust, metals, repetitive or violent motions, odd postures, and other disease-causative agents encountered by workers in 52 occupations. The first physician to clearly recognize the relationship between healthy workers and economic productivity, he is now considered the father of occupational medicine.

Occupational epidemiology today deals specifically with the study of distribution and determinants of states of health related to hazardous exposures and conditions found in the workplace. In other words, epidemiologic methods are applied to populations of workers. The nurse needs to explain trends and potential or real hazards, based on epidemiologic reports, to workers, managers, and community representatives (Lukes, 2007). The epidemiologic data, plus the documented need in the workplace, are the rationale for recommending health promotion programs.

Epidemiologic Surveillance

Health surveillance is an essential concept in occupational health. The need to carefully monitor both the employee and the work environment to detect any health risk and thereby be able to initiate health protective behaviors is critical. Workplace health surveillance includes physical examinations and the tracking of injuries, illness, hazards, and exposures both in individual people and for groups of workers. Every industry should have monitoring procedures in place that are specific to the setting. For example, biomonitoring assesses the total body burden of a hazardous chemical in a worker through laboratory tests of body fluid specimens. The best practice is to use noninvasive procedures as much as possible.

EVIDENCE FOR PRACTICE

In 1991, the CDC developed procedures that require state and local health departments to investigate healthcare personnel with HIV/AIDS who had no known risk of HIV infection. More recently in 2011, the CDC released surveillance data reflecting documented and possible cases of occupationally acquired HIV/AIDS in healthcare personnel. Information from 1981 to 2010 showed a total of 57 actual reported and documented cases among healthcare workers, with a possible actual number recorded as 143. As shown in Table 25.4, nurses constituted 24 of the actual documented cases, with a possible number of 34 cases (Centers for Disease Control and Prevention [CDC], 2010). Nurses and other healthcare personnel should report any possible occupational exposure to HIV.

Incidence

Workers often come to an OHN with symptoms. If there happens to be more than one worker from the same department with consistent symptoms and objective findings, the OHN may immediately begin to suspect that a cluster or cohort is forming. Clusters are aggregations of disease diagnoses collected from a specific population within a distinct period of time or space. Documenting the number of cases of an injury or disease is an important responsibility of the OHN (Eisen, Wegman, & O'Neill, 2006).

The calculation of incidence rates is a helpful tool in understanding the severity of a workplace problem. For example, the nurse can tally the number of workers whose

table 25.4 Healthcare Personnel with Documented and Possible Occupationally Acquired HIV Infection, by Occupation, 1981–2010

Occupation	Documented	Possible
Nurse	24	36
Laboratory worker, clinical	16	17
Physician, nonsurgical	6	13
Laboratory technician, nonclinical	3	-
Housekeeper/maintenance worker	2	14
Technician, surgical	2	2
Embalmer/morgue technician	1	2
Health aide/attendant	1	15
Respiratory therapist	1	2
Technician, dialysis	1	3
Dental worker, including dentist	-	6
Emergency medical technician/ paramedic	-	12
Physician, surgical	-	6
Other technician/therapist	-	9
Other healthcare occupation	-	6
Total	57	143

Source: Centers for Disease Control and Prevention. (2010). *Surveillance of occupationally acquired HIV/AIDS in healthcare personnel, as of December 2010*. Retrieved from http://www.cdc.gov/HAI/organisms/hiv/Surveillance-Occupationally-Acquired-HIV-AIDS.html#table

scores on a hearing test change when compared with the previous year's results. The yearly occurrence rate of hearing loss among workers is determined by dividing the number of workers who have changes in their recorded hearing test(s) by the number of workers at risk during that year. If 56 of 1,000 employees have more difficulty hearing at certain frequencies this year than last, then the yearly incidence rate for hearing loss is 56 divided by 1,000, or 0.056%. It is 5.6% for the current year (see Chapter 7).

The OHN should calculate specific rates for population subgroups, often by age, sex, or exposure. For example, it may be beneficial to calculate an injury rate during several different activities. The OHN might find it helpful to calculate a rate for hearing loss among workers who perform a work-related activity such as operating loud machines in a specific department at the workplace (Lukes, 2007).

Prevalence

Prevalence reflects the total burden of the injury or illness that exists in the population—in this case, the workplace. It includes both new cases and existing cases. Using the example of hearing loss, the prevalence rate indicates the extent of hearing loss in the workplace. When hearing loss has occurred, it is imperative that people be protected through a hearing conservation program. In most cases, once the damage begins, the person without protective equipment or a transfer to a quieter environment is at greater risk for more hearing loss at an increasing rate. Prevalence rises over time if working conditions are not corrected (Lukes, 2007).

Ratios

Ratios can compare and involve groups of workers in settings. Hearing tests may be given to workers from different departments within the same facility, or to workers who do the same type of work in another facility or building in another state or country. This approach adds clarity when comparing the number of affected workers in an organization that employs workers located in various geographic locations. The ratio of workers who incurred the greatest hearing loss from the previous year may be compared by facility, department, or task. This can provide information about different groups and how noise, injury, or disease affects them over a specific period of time (Lukes, 2007).

Epidemiologic Studies

Two types of epidemiologic studies are common in investigating occupational health issues in the workplace: cohort and case-control studies. First, prospective, cohort epidemiologic studies investigate workers who have been exposed to a variety of chemical, biologic, or physical agents (see Table 25.1). The purpose of these follow-up studies is to determine whether the risk of adverse health outcomes is increased after the event. Second, epidemiologic studies may involve the evaluation of workers who have already experienced a common adverse health outcome. In this case, the outcome has already occurred, so the purpose of these case-control studies is to investigate, retrospectively, what agent or set of agents may explain their condition. Chapter 8 discusses these methods in more detail.

Ecologic studies are types of epidemiologic studies that compare the rates of exposures and diseases in different populations. Aggregate data on exposure and disease are gathered, rather than data pertaining to individuals. This could be data from a group of workers within an organization, facility, community, state, or nation. Average exposures and disease rates are compared between two groups in different locations during the same time (Eisen et al., 2006). Ecologic studies are the fastest and easiest of epidemiologic studies related to the OHN practice. These approaches study the relationships between variables when research or funds are limited.

Case 2 demonstrates that actions lead to an outcome and that actions further unfold in a sequence of related events. The OHN learns that at the time of the outbreak, one of the refrigerator units was about to be replaced because of higher-than-normal holding temperatures. Also, there had been a turnover of kitchen staff in the last few weeks. Apparently, the department was short on kitchen help on the day of the picnic, and there was no record of the daily temperatures required that morning.

Holding food at correct temperatures is essential to avoid food-borne illness. For hot food, this temperature must be 140° F (60°C). For cold food, this temperature must be 40° F (4°C) or colder. Keeping food within the recommended temperatures is necessary to prevent microbial growth (U.S. Department of Agriculture, 2013).

By calculating attack (incidence) rates associated with the various foods, the OHN determines that the sausage was contaminated. Most of the people who ate the sausage manifested symptoms of food poisoning, establishing the relationship between ingestion and sickness (Aschengrau & Seage, 2003; Lukes, 2007).

EMERGENCY PREPAREDNESS PLANNING AND DISASTER MANAGEMENT

As a member of the emergency planning committee in the workplace, the OHN contributes to the design and implementation of the emergency preparedness plan. The plan ensures a line of communication with emergency management teams. Having an emergency planning committee composed of representatives from all departments is the best way to establish emergency planning in business environments. Committee members meet on a regular basis and have access to all relevant health and safety information, so that they can make responsible, informed decisions. The committees annually review documentation and update the existing emergency plans. This includes all state and federal laws that apply to the facility and type of business operation (OSHA, 2010).

Components of an Emergency Preparedness Plan

The goals of an emergency plan are to anticipate emergencies and to establish clear reporting instructions for employees. The plan names key personnel who will assume necessary tasks. It establishes emergency escape routes, and procedures to identify workers and visitors with and without disabilities. The plan ensures that predesignated areas have been arranged and employees have participated in actual drills (OSHA, n.d.b).

The committee is responsible for conducting a vulnerability analysis best utilizing an all-hazards approach. Committee members review the types of emergencies that are likely to occur at the facility and what resources will be needed to respond. Major natural emergencies are fires, floods, hurricanes, tornadoes, earthquakes, and winter storms. Human-made or technologic events include fires, violence, bomb threats, transportation accidents, industrial accidents, civil disturbance, radiation, and unintentional or intentional release of chemicals or infectious organisms (bioterrorism) (Federal Emergency Management Agency [FEMA], 2013b).

Next, the committee reviews existing internal resources such as personnel, security systems, sprinkler and alarm systems, transportation and heavy equipment, shelters (for providing shelter in place), and firefighting apparatus (OSHA, n.d.d; n.d.e). If a facility is located near a river or body of water, it is necessary to have a plan to deal with flooding, one of the most common hazards in the United States (FEMA 2013a).

Key components of the emergency plan involve alarms, reporting, communication, evacuation, a system for counting the occupants, procedures for staff who do not immediately evacuate, and rescue and medical services. (A list of key personnel, training for all staff, drills, with an approach to conduct an assessment following an emergency evacuation plan, must identify escape routes that are clearly marked and meet the criteria within the key components.) It is essential that the plan discuss how workers and visitors with and without disabilities will be assisted through the evacuation routes and where they will reassemble for verification of safe evacuation (OSHA, n.d.c, n.d.d).

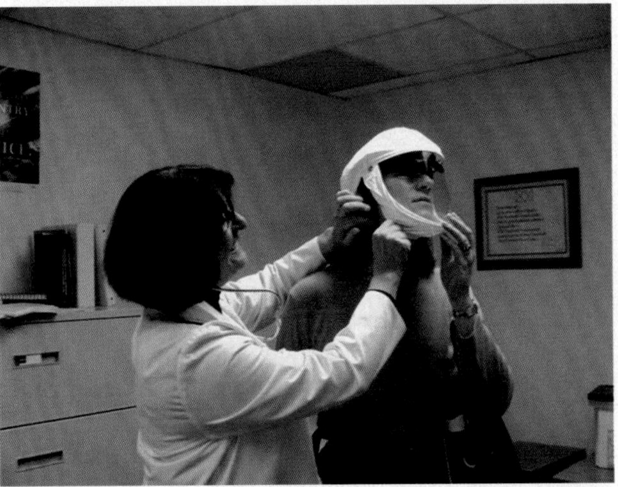

figure 25.9 **Personal protective equipment: Personal fit testing for emergency preparedness.**

Critical Functions of the Plan

The OHN helps ensure that procedures are established for people who attend to critical functions in the facility and who do not leave the building immediately. Floor captains are responsible for making sure everyone gets out of the building. This includes people who administer first aid and those trained to use fire extinguishers (OSHA, n.d.c).

Internal rescue and medical services depend highly on the location of the facility and its proximity to police, fire, and external rescue services. According to the hazard communication standard (OSHA, n.d.a), employers must have personal protective equipment available for those who work with and around hazardous material and chemicals (Fig. 25.9). They also must have procedures to decontaminate workers who work with and around hazardous material and chemicals. Another important aspect of every plan is *shelter in place*. A shelter-in-place policy and procedure must be established for emergencies such as hurricanes, tornadoes, high winds, or chemical releases in buildings such as healthcare and correctional facilities. Having drills on a regular basis helps ensure that workers know what they are to do in an emergency. When alarms go off, evacuation needs to occur quickly and in an orderly manner. The intent of the drill is to reduce confusion and panic (OSHA, n.d.b, n.d.c). Chapter 20 discusses emergency preparedness in further detail.

A plan for resuming operations following an emergency is necessary. The OHN may conduct a needs assessment that identifies the immediate and ongoing needs of the staff and the organization following an emergency. It is essential that counseling services are available for employees who may suffer from symptoms of post-traumatic stress. The committee periodically evaluates and modifies the plan to update key personnel lists, emergency contacts, and telephone numbers. Floor plans, changes of department location, and ongoing work in the building should be kept current (OSHA, 2010, n.d.b).

key concepts

- The primary responsibility of the OHN is that of injury prevention and health promotion, including recognition of conditions that may harm the individual worker or the community.
- The occupational health nursing process begins with assessment of both the worker and the workplace.
- Disciplines that guide the occupational nurse in understanding the agent, host, and environment relationship are epidemiology, toxicology, industrial hygiene, and safety principles.
- Advocating for patients, clients, or groups is a continual process in occupational health nursing.
- The knowledge base generated through epidemiologic studies is used to identify and prevent injury and disease.
- The recognition of adverse conditions, and the initiation of proven practice interventions, supports individuals and groups in both their work and community environments.
- With good occupational health surveillance programs in place, it is possible to proactively identify employees at risk by tracking incidence and prevalence of injuries and illness and their causes.
- The nurse must have the autonomy and skills to take action and reduce possible exposure or harm to workers.
- An understanding of regulatory, legal, and economic functions and their relationship to business production, workers, and the community environment is an essential component of occupational health nursing practice.

critical thinking questions

1. When the population's rate is unknown, the OHN may want to use a national or state rate to compare information that is being obtained at the work site. For example, if 10% of those who participate in a company's health screening indicate they are smokers, what generalizations, if any, can be made by the OHN about the smoking rate of the company's population if a smoking assessment has not been done? Does 10% represent the true percentage of smokers? Does the company have the same or higher smoking rate as the rest of the state (e.g., approximately 25%). What percentages of workers who smoke avoid health screening?
2. Choose an occupational setting and describe the process of risk assessment you would initiate in that setting.
3. Review Figures 25.1, 25.2, and 25.3 and Table 25.3. What are some of the factors that contributed to the decline in rates of injury and illness at the workplace? What confounding factors might be present?
4. In Case 1, the OHN deduced possible substances (agents) to which workers could be exposed. The next steps are to determine how the substances are delivered to the workers (host) and to investigate the characteristics of the workplace which lead to transmission of the substances (environment). The OHN inquires about the heating, ventilation, and air conditioning (HVAC) system at the bank. One of the questions asked concerned the position of the air vents which deliver air into the office space, and its relationship with the renovation work. The OHN learns that neither an extra exhaust system was provided for the project nor was any provision made to deal with particulates of construction materials which may have been in the air. Use this information to develop an epidemiologic triangle that identifies the interactions between the harmful substances (agent), the workers (host), and the workplace (environment).

references

American Association of Occupational Health Nurses. (2007). Competencies in occupational and environmental health nursing. *American Association of Occupational Health Nurses*, *55*(11), 442–447.

American Association of Occupational Health Nurses. (2012a). *Code of ethics*. Retrieved from http://www.aaohn.org/component/content/article/12-practice/10-code-of-ethics.html

American Association of Occupational Health Nurses. (2012b). *Delivery of occupational and environmental health services*. Retrieved from http://www.aaohn.org/practice/position-statements.html

American Association of Occupational Health Nurses. (n.d.a). *Careers: Profession of occupational and environmental health nursing*. Retrieved from http://www.aaohn.org/careers/profession-of-occupation-environmental-health-nursing.html

American Board of Occupational Health Nurses, Inc. (2012a). *Eligibility*. Retrieved from http://www.abohn.org/eligibility.cfm

American Board of Occupational Health Nurses, Inc. (2012b). *Occupational health nursing 2011 practice analysis*. Retrieved from http://www.abohn.org/documents/ABOHN2011PracticeAnalysisReport.pdf

Aschengrau, A., & Seage, G. R., III. (2003). *Essentials of epidemiology in public health*. Sudbury, MA: Jones and Bartlett.

Benner, P. (1984). *From novice to expert: Excellence and power in clinical nursing practice*. Menlo Park, CA: Addison-Wesley.

Brunette, M. J. (2006). Safety. In B. S. Levy, D. H. Wegman, S. L. Baron, & R. K. Sokas (Eds.), *Occupational and environmental health: Recognizing and preventing disease and injury* (pp. 218–237). Philadelphia, PA: Lippincott Williams & Wilkins.

C-Change. (2010). *Publications & reports*. Retrieved from http://c-changetogether.org/publications-reports

Centers for Disease Control and Prevention. (2010). *Surveillance of occupationally acquired HIV/AIDS in healthcare personnel, as of December 2010*. Retrieved from http://www.cdc.gov/HAI/organisms/hiv/Surveillance-Occupationally-Acquired-HIV-AIDS.html

Dirksen, M. E. (2006). Occupational and environmental health nursing: An overview. In M. K. Salazar (3rd ed.), *Core curriculum for occupational & environmental health nursing* (pp. 3–34). St. Louis, MO: Saunders.

Eisen, E. A., Wegman, D. H., & O'Neill, M. S. (2006). Epidemiology. In B. S. Levy, D. H. Wegman, S. L. Baron, & R. K. Sokas (Eds.), *Occupational and environmental health: Recognizing and preventing disease and injury* (pp. 172–179). Philadelphia, PA: Lippincott Williams & Wilkins.

Federal Emergency Management Agency. (2013a). *National flood insurance plan*. Retrieved from http://www.fema.gov/hazard/flood/index.shtm

Federal Emergency Management Agency. (2013b). *Incident command system*. Retrieved from http://www.fema.gov/incident-command-system

Luhby, T. (2012, October 24). America's near poor: 30 million and struggling. *CNN Money*. Retrieved from http://money.cnn.com/2012/10/24/news/economy/americans-poverty/index.html

Lukes, E. (2007). Epidemiology basics for occupational health nurses. *American Association of Occupational Health Nurses*, *55*(1), 26–31.

MassResources. (2013). *Massachusetts health insurance requirements—Health Care Reform Act*. Retrieved from http://www.massresources.org/health-reform.html

Mayo Foundation for Education and Research. (2011). *Latex allergy symptoms*. Retrieved from http://www.mayoclinic.com/health/latex-allergy/DS00621/DSECTION=symptoms

National Institute for Occupational Safety and Health. (2008). *NIOSH publication and products: Publication exposure to stress: Occupational hazards in hospitals*. (NIOSH Publication Number 2008-136). Retrieved from http://www.cdc.gov/niosh/docs/2008-136

O'Donnell, M. (2009). *Definition of health promotion* 2.0: Embracing passion, enhancing motivation, recognizing dynamic balance, and creating opportunities. *American Journal of Health Promotion*, *24*(1), iv–iv. doi: http://dx.doi.org/10.4278/ajhp.24.1.iv

Occupational Safety and Health Administration. (2010). *Getting started–General preparedness and response*. Retrieved from http://www.osha.gov/SLTC/emergencypreparedness/gettingstarted.html

Occupational Safety and Health Administration. (n.d.a). *Evacuation plans and procedures: Employee alarm systems*. Retrieved from http://www.osha.gov/SLTC/etools/evacuation/alarms.html

Occupational Safety and Health Administration. (n.d.b). *Hazard communication standard final rule*. Retrieved from http://www.osha.gov/dsg/hazcom/HCSFactsheet.html

Occupational Safety and Health Administration. (n.d.c). *Evacuation plans and procedures: Develop and implement an emergency action plan*. Retrieved from http://www.osha.gov/SLTC/etools/evacuation/implementation.html

Occupational Safety and Health Administration. (n.d.d). *Evacuation plans and procedures: Fire, rescue and medical services*. Retrieved from http://www.osha.gov/SLTC/etools/evacuation/fire_med_service.html

Occupational Safety and Health Administration. (n.d.e). *Evacuation plans and procedures: Maintenance, safeguards, and operational features for exit routes*. Retrieved from http://www.osha.gov/SLTC/etools/evacuation/egress.html

Occupational Safety and Health Administration. (n.d.g). *Guidance on preparing workplaces for an influenza pandemic*. Retrieved from http://www.osha.gov/Publications/OSHA3327pandemic.pdf

Peek-Asa, C., Casteel, C., Allareddy, V., Nocera, M., Goldmacher, S., OHagan, E., ... Harrison, R. (2009). Workplace violence prevention programs in psychiatric units and facilities. *Archives of Psychiatric Nursing, 23*(2), 166–176.

Shipler, D. (2004). *The working poor: Invisible in America*. New York, NY: Alfred A. Knopf.

Thomason, D. A., & Lagowski, L. R. (2008). Sustaining a healthy work force in the 21st century; a model for collaborating through reciprocation. *Journal of American Association of Occupational Health Nursing, 56*(12), 503–513.

U.S. Department of Agriculture. (2013). *Food safety and inspection services: Regulations and policies*. Retrieved from http://www.fsis.usda.gov/Regulations_&_Policies/index.asp

U.S. Department of Labor, Bureau of Labor Statistics. (2011). *Incidence rates of non-fatal occupational injuries and illnesses by industry and case types, 2010*. Retrieved from http://www.bls.gov/iif/oshwc/osh/os/ostb2813.pdf

U.S. Department of Labor, Bureau of Labor Statistics. (2012). *Economic news release: Occupational injuries and illnesses news release*. Retrieved from http://www.bls.gov/news.release/osh.htm

U.S. Environmental Protection Agency. (2012a). *An introduction to indoor air quality*. Retrieved from http://www.epa.gov/iaq/voc.html

U.S. Environmental Protection Agency. (2012b). *National pollutant discharge elimination system compliance monitoring*. Retrieved from http://www.epa.gov/compliance/monitoring/programs/cwa/npdes.html

U.S. Environmental Protection Agency. (2012c). *Pollutants and sources*. Retrieved from http://www.epa.gov/ttn/atw/pollsour.html

U.S. Environmental Protection Agency. (2013a). *The origins of EPA*. Retrieved from http://www.epa.gov/history/origins.html

World Health Organization. (2001). *The role of the occupational health nurse in workplace health management*. Retrieved from http://www.who.int/occupational_health/regions/en/oeheurnursing.pdf

Zichello, C., & Sheridan, J. (2008). Occupational health nurses and workers' compensation insurance programs. *Journal of the American Association of Occupational Health Nurses, 56*(11), 455–458.

web resources

Please visit thePoint® for up-to-date Web resources on this topic.

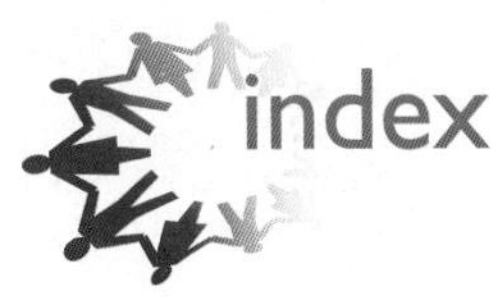

index

Page numbers followed by italicized *b*, *f*, and *t* refer to boxes, figures and tables

A

abandoned buildings, 393*t*
abstinence, 325, 326
abuse, 317–319. *See also* violence
  assessing for, 218–219
  child maltreatment, 317–318
  of disabled people, 318–319
  elder, 317
  mandatory reporting of, 317–319
  model of care for victims, 320
acamprosate, 348
accidental disasters, 408
accountability, 168, 504
Accountable Care Organization (ACO) model, 221
acetaminophen, 514
acids, 426*t*
acquired immunodeficiency syndrome. *See* HIV/AIDS
Act for the Relief of Sick and Disabled Seamen, 14
Action for Healthy Kids Program, 58
active euthanasia, 510
active immunity, 89–90
adaptive model, 64
Adderall, 346*t*
addiction, 68, 325, 326
adjusted rate, 121, 124–125
adjuvant analgesics, 516
adjuvant drugs, 501, 515
Adolescent Family Life (AFL) program, 477
adolescents
  alcohol abuse in, 329, 338–340, 475
  cannabis use in, 330
  illicit drug use in, 330–331, 475
  motivational interviewing with, 337, 351*b*
  nutrition, 478–479
  obesity in, 478
  school violence, 310, 479–482
  sexual behavior, 476–478
  smoking in, 475–476
  substance abuse in, 329–331, 334–338
  teenage pregnancy, 476–478
adult respiratory distress syndrome, 254
advance directives, 501, 508–510
advocacy, 11*t*, 57–58
Affordable Care Act (ACA), 221, 315, 460
after-action report, 405, 433
age-adjusted death rates, 125*f*, 132*f*
age-specific mortality rate, 126*t*
agencies, 208–209
  hospital-based, 208
  official, 209
  private, 208
  proprietary, 209
  voluntary, 208
Agency for Healthcare Research and Quality (AHRQ), 5, 57–58
agents, 532–533
  biologic, 532
  chemical, 532
  of infectious diseases, 256
  physical, 532–533
  psychosocial, 533
aggregate, 3
AIDS. *See* HIV/AIDS
air quality, 402
airborne transmission, 258
alcohol abuse, 338–340. *See also* substance abuse
  in adolescents, 329–330, 475
  AUDIT-C and CAGE screening instruments for, 344*b*
  nursing assessments and implications, 346–347*t*
  in older adults, 340–342
  pharmacologic treatments, 348
    acamprosate, 348
    disulfiram, 348
    naltrexone, 348
  self-help programs, 341–342
Alcoholics Anonymous (AA), 341–342
Alma Alta Declaration for Primary Healthcare, 71
alprazolam, 346*t*
alternative medicine, 522
ambient air, 393*t*
American Association of Occupational Health Nurses (AAOHN), 525, 531
American Board of Occupational Health Nurses (ABOHN), 431*b*
American College of Medical Toxicologists, 392*b*
American Public Health Association (APHA), 9
American Recovery and Reinvestment Act (ARRA), 55
Americans with Disabilities Act (ADA), 469, 482
amphetamines, 346*t*
analgesics, 516
analytical studies, 139, 142–145
  case-control studies, 143–144
  cohort studies, 142–143
  definition of, 137
ANA's Principles of Environmental Health for Nursing Practice with Implementation Strategies, 382
animals, 394*t*
anorexia, 518, 519*t*
anthrax, 421–424, 422*t*
  spores, 386*t*
anti-psychotics, 447
  first-generation, 440, 447
  metabolic syndrome and, 447
  second-generation, 440, 447
antigenic drift, 281, 283
antigenic shift, 281, 283
anxiety, 519*t*
Army Nurse Corps, 17, 18
arranged marriage, 236
arsenic, 389*t*
artemisinin-based combination therapies (ACTs), 449
artemisinin-based combination therapies (ACTs), 68
artificial nutrition, 509
asbestos, 387*t*
ASSERT project screening, 350*b*
assessment, 114–116
  asset-based, 187, 200–201
  community, 117–118
  family, 225–245
  health, 472–473
  health impact, 160
  individual, 114–117
  interventions and, 116
  population-based, 472–473
asset-based assessment, 187, 200–201
assimilation, 235
assisted living, 204, 214–215
association, 137, 142
Association of Community Health Nurse Educators (ACHNE), 9
Association of Occupational and Environmental Clinics (AOEC), 392*b*
Association of State and Territorial Directors of Nursing (ASTDN), 9
attack rate, 121, 125–126
attention deficit/hyperactivity disorders (ADHDs), 455–456
attributable risk, 121, 133
Australia, health care measures in, 31*t*
autism, 456–458
  public health initiatives in, 457–458
autism spectrum disorders (ASDs), 439, 457
avian influenza A virus H5N1, 254, 289–291. *See also* infectious diseases
  fatality rate, 290
  infection control for prevention of avian A (H5N1) influenza transmission, 290–291
  outbreaks, 290
  reassortment of, 290, 290*f*
  transmission, 258
azithromycin, 268, 269

B

"baby boomers," 340
Bacillus anthracis, 386*t*, 421
Balanced Budget Act, 204, 208
Barton, Clara, 16
behavior models, 92–98
  definition of, 83, 93
  ecological model, 97–98
  health belief model, 94–95
  learning model, 93–94
  relapse prevention model, 96–97
  social learning theory, 83, 96
  social support, 96
  theory of reasoned action, 95–96
  transtheoretical model, 95
Behavioral Risk Factor Surveillance System (BRFSS), 116–117, 140, 153
benzene, 387*t*
benzodiazepines, 341, 455
bereavement, 501, 511
bilateral agencies, 26, 41–42
Bill and Melissa Gates Foundation, 42
Bills of Mortality, 108
binge drinking, 330, 338–340, 475
bioavailability, 378, 390
biologic hazards, 525, 527*t*, 532
biomedicine, 180
biomonitoring, 378, 390–391
bioterrorism, 419–425. *See also* disaster management
  advantages of biological weapons, 420*b*
  agents, 422–423*t*
    anthrax, 421–424, 422*t*
    biosafety levels for, 425*b*
    botulism, 422*t*, 424
    categories of, 420, 421*b*
    plague, 422*t*, 424
    smallpox, 423*t*, 424
    tularemia, 423*t*, 424
    viral hemorrhagic fevers, 423*t*, 425
  attacks, 420*b*
    clues of, 421*b*
  detection of event, 420
  history of, 420
biotoxins, 426*t*
bird flu, 254, 292
birth rate, 126*t*
bisexuals, 371–373, 373*b*
"Black Box" warnings, 439, 456
blast injuries, 430
blister agents, 426*t*
blood agents, 426*t*, 427*t*

botulism, 422*t*, 424
bovine spongiform encephalopathy (BSE), 254
breakthrough pain, 501, 515
Breckinridge, Mary, 17
Buddhism, 511*t*
built environment, 159
bullying prevention, 480*b*
buprenorphine, 342, 349
Bush, George W., 19

C

cachexia, 519*t*
Cadet Nurse Corps, 18
Campbell, Jacquelyn, 312
Campylobacter enteritis, 263
Canada
  health care measures in, 31*t*
  health care system in, 34–36
cannabis, 330
  effects of, 347*t*
  schizophrenia and, 446
capsaicin, 516
cardiopulmonary resuscitation (CPR), 509–510
cardiovascular disease, 196
care
  access to, 58
  and health insurance, access to, 51–52
  quality of, 54–55
care delivery value chains (CDVCs), 75
care management, 204, 205
caregivers
  burden, 225
  caring for, 521–522
  family, 204
  nurses as, 11*t*
Carlson, Rachel, 380
carriers, 251, 257
case-control studies, 137, 143–144, 544
case-fatality rate, 121, 126*t*, 133
case-finding, 11*t*
case management, 11*t*, 204, 206–207, 221–222
case manager, 536–537
case studies, 137, 139–140
Catholic Relief Services, 42
causality, 137, 143*b*
cause-specific mortality rate, 121, 126*t*, 133
caustics, 426*t*
ceftriaxone, 269
Centers for Disease Control and Prevention (CDC), 4–5, 152, 254, 310, 522
Centers for Medicare and Medicaid Services (CMS), 54, 153
cephalosporin, 269
certification, 12
Cervarix, 271
change
  community readiness for, 162–164
  levers of, 162
change theory, 161–164
changing, 162
chemical disasters, 425–430. *See also* disaster management
  evacuation, 428–429
  hazardous chemicals, 426*t*
  roles of nurses in, 427–428
  shelter in place, 428
  stay or go decision, 428–429
  treatment guidelines, 427*t*
chemical exposure, 405
chemical hazards, 525, 527*t*, 532
Chemical Weapons Convention, 426
child abuse, 317–318
Child Abuse Prevention and Treatment Act (CAPTA), 317
Child Protection Team, 320
childbearing, 243
children
  attention deficit/hyperactivity disorders, 455–456
  emotional disorders in, 455–456
  health schools and, 400–401
  homicide, 309
  maltreatment, 317–318
  nutrition, 478–479
  obesity in, 478
  undernutrition, 68
  vulnerability to environment, 399–400
Children at Risk Team, 320
Children's Defense Fund (CDF), 368, 368–369*b*
Children's Health Insurance Program (CHIP), 57, 502
Chinese-American children, 235
chlamydia, 268
Chlamydia trachomatis, 268
chloral hydrate, 346*t*
choking agents, 426*t*
cholesterol, 196, 196*t*
Christianity, 511*t*
Church Health Center, 498
Clean Air Act (CAA), 380*b*
clean water, 402
Clean Water Act, 380*b*
client-centered health care, 5–6
client outcomes, 204, 210
climate, 394*t*
climate change, 402–403
clinical excellence, 504
Clinical Institute Withdrawal Assessment-Alcohol (CIWA-A), 345*f*
clinical model, 63
clinical trials, 137, 145
clinicians, 184, 535–536
clonazepam (Klonopin), 346t, 457
Clostridium botulinum, 424
Clostridium perfringens, 262
clozapine, 447
coalition, 156
coalition builder, 11*t*, 151
cocaine, 346*t*
Code of Ethics for Nurses, 56
codeine, 346*t*
cohabiting couples and families, 228
cohort studies, 137, 142–143, 544
collaboration, 11*t*, 166–167
collaborative models, 187, 201
Collaborative Oncological Gene-Environment Study (COGS), 360
Collaborative Studies on Genetics of Alcoholism (COGA), 334
colonization, 251, 257
comfort measures only (CMO), 501, 508
Coming Plague, The (Garrett), 282
Commission on Social Determinants of Health (CSDH), 152
common source outbreak, 251, 259
Commonwealth Fund Commission on a High Performance Health System, 54
communicable diseases, 262–276. *See also* infectious diseases
  food-borne, 262–264
  sexually transmitted diseases, 266–276
  waterborne diseases, 264–266
communication, 181–182
  nonverbal, 181
  styles, 181–182
  verbal, 181
communities, 187, 189
  -acquired MRSA, 257
  faith communities as, 490–492
  geopolitical, 187, 189
  international, 191–192
  national, 191–192
  as partner, 187, 197
  phenomenological, 189–190
  societal, 191–192
  stakeholders, 156–157
  working with, 155–157
community assessment, 154–155, 187–202
  assets-based approach, 200–201
  collaborative model, 201
  defining communities and boundaries in, 189–192
  epidemiologic approach to, 117–118, 193–197
  frameworks for, 192–201
  resources for, 195*t*
  steps in, 189*b*
community benefit programs, 169–170
community concerns, 395*t*
Community Connections for Families program, 460
community environment, 380–381
Community Health Assessment and Group Evaluation (CHANGE), 154
community health improvement planning, guideline and template for, 154*b*
community health interventions, 164*b*
community health nursing
  challenges, 19–24
    community change planning, 21
    cultural competence, 20–21
    disaster preparedness, 22
    eliminating health disparities, 20
    evidence-based practices, 19–20
  family assessment in, 230, 233
  responsibility to families, 244–245
community health planning, models and tools for, 154*b*
community health workers (CHWs), 167
community mental health, 439–465
  centers, 439, 458–459
  evolution of, 458–459
  insurance benefits, 459–460
  levels of prevention in, 460*b*
  mental illness, 440–458
  practitioners, 460–461
community organizing, 11*t*
community readiness model (CRM), 162–164
community report card indicators, 194*t*
community school health, 469
community school model, 469, 483
community toolbox, 154*b*
Community Transformation Grant (CTG) program, 56, 169
complementary and alternative medicine (CAM), 522
compliance with laws and regulations, 504
Comprehensive Environmental Response, Compensation and Liability Act, 380*b*
Concerta, 346*t*
congregation, 486, 488
congregation-based model, 486
Congress on Nursing Practice and Economics (CNPE), 9
constipation, 517, 519*t*
consultants, 537–538
consultation, 11*t*
consumer rights, 504
contagious diseases, 251, 256
contaminant exposure, 405
contaminants, 382–395
  environmental media, 383
  exposure pathways, 384–389*t*
  point of exposure, 383
  receptor population, 383, 390
  route of exposure, 383
  source of contamination, 383
  transport mechanisms, 383
controls, 137
convergence model, 281, 282, 284*f*
Cooperative State Research, Education and Extension Service (CSREES), 366
Core Competencies for Public Health Nurses (CCPHN), 10
correctional health, 367–371
cost–benefit analysis, 46, 51
  healthcare finances and, 50–51
costs of health care, 31*t*
cough, 519*t*
council on school health, 469
counseling, 11*t*
  and psychology services, 472*t*
counselor, 537–538
"crack babies," 333
CRAFFT drug screening, 335, 335*b*
craving, 325, 348
Crime Victims with Disabilities Awareness Act, 318
cross-cultural nursing, 174, 176
cross-sectional studies, 137, 140–142
crude birth rate, 126*t*
crude mortality rate, 126*t*
crude rate, 121, 124
Cryptosporidium, 262

cultural brokerage, 181
cultural competence, 20–21, 174, 176–179
  institutional, 177
  principles of, 177–178
cultural competency, 46, 52
cultural health assessment, 184
cultural humility, 178
cultural practices and traditions, 394*t*
cultural safety, 174, 178–179
culturally competent mental health services, 439, 460
culture, 175–179, 409
  communication, 181–182
  definition of, 174, 175
  diversity and, 234
  dynamic, 175–176
  ethnocentrism, 178–179
  health, 180–184
  healthcare and, 180–184
  learning, 176
  and nursing, 175–179
  properties of, 175–176
  race, 179
  religion, 182–184
  roles, 182
  sharing of, 176
  subculture, 179
  time orientation, 182
cyberbullying, 469, 480
  for educators, 480–481*b*
  suggestions for parents and caregivers, 481*b*
Cyclospora, 262

D
Daughters of Charity, 12, 14
death, 505–507
  causes of, 506*t*
  demographic/social trends, 506*t*
  nursing care after, 521
  nursing care of patients who are close to, 520–522
  preparing for, 520
  stages of dying, 505–506
  in workplace, 528
death houses, 12
death of family member, 241–242
Declaration for Human Rights, 71
decontamination, 405, 426
decontamination tent, 428*f*
decubitus ulcers, 519*t*
deer tick, 296
dehydration, 518
deinstitutionalization, 439, 448
delegation, 11*t*
delirium, 518–519, 519*t*
demographic data, 121, 127
demographic transition, 62, 64–65
Department of Health and Human Services, 26, 28, 29, 33, 54, 57–58
Department of Homeland Security (DHS), 19
depression, 521
descriptive studies, 139–142
  case studies, 139–140
  cross-sectional studies, 140–142
  definition of, 137
developmental models, 187, 198
diabetes, type 2, 447–448
Diagnostic and Statistical Manual, 5th edition (DSM-5), 439, 441
diazepam, 346*t*
diet, 180
direct contact, 258
directly observed therapy (DOT), 281, 299
"dirty bombs," 429–430
disability, 242–243
  describing, 193–195
disability-adjusted life year (DALY), 68
disabled people, abuse of, 318–319
disaster management, 410–419
  competencies, 415*b*
  continuum, 411*f*
  evaluation, 414
  mitigation, 412
  occupation health and, 544
  preparedness, 22, 409–412
    in culturally diverse society, 409–410
    hazard identification, 410
    national response framework, 411–412
    risk assessment, 411
    vulnerability analysis, 411
  public health, 431–433
    after-action evaluation, 433
    communication, 432
    recovery, 433
    scope and magnitude, 431–432
  recovery, 413–414
  response, 412–414
  roles of nurses in, 414–419, 414*t*
    documentation, 418–419
    field triage, 416–417
    just-in-time training, 415–416
    personal protective equipment, 418
    point of distribution plans, 417–418
    public health nurses as first responders, 415
    skill building, 419
  vs. public health practices, 414*t*
disasters, 407–409
  accidental, 408
  bioterrorism, 419–425
  chemical, 425–430
  natural, 408
  populations traumatized by, 461
  public health response, 431–433
    after-action evaluation, 433
    communication, 432
    recovery, 433
    scope and magnitude, 431–432
  radiological, 429–430
  relief assistance, 41
diseases
  attribution of, 180
  communicable, 262–276
  contagious, 251, 256
  describing, 193–195
  endemic, 251, 258
  epidemic, 105, 107, 258
  infectious, 251–277
  vaccine-preventable, 89*b*
disparities, 359
displaced families, 244
district nursing, 12
  definition of, 3
  duties, 14*b*
disulfiram, 348
diverse families, 234–235
diverse society, disaster preparedness in, 409–410
diverse workforce, 52
diversity, 234–235
  arranged marriage, 236
  culture and, 234
  diverse families, 234–235
  intergenerational, 236–237
  interracial marriage, 235–236
divorce, 242
Dix, Dorothea, 15–16
documentation, 418–419
domestic violence. *See* intimate partner violence (IPV)
Domestic Violence Enhanced Home Visitation (DOVE) Program, 319
doxycycline, 270–271
drinking water, 264–266
droplet transmission, 258
Durkheim, Emile, 450
dyspnea, 519*t*

E
early intervention programs, 440
Early Periodic Screening, Diagnosis, and Treatment (EPSDT), 469, 470
Ebola hemorrhagic fever, 254, 302
Ebola virus disease (EVD), 302–303
  infection prevention and control of, 303
  signs, symptoms, and diagnosis of, 303
ecological model, 83, 97–98
  disease prevention and, 100
  exosystem, 99
  health promotion and, 100
  macroculture, 99–100
  microsystem, 99
  ontogenic system, 98
ecomap, 225, 228, 230
Economic Resource Service (ERS), 361*b*
economics, 194*t*
  defined, 46, 50
ecosystem, 281, 285
ecstasy, 330
education, 58, 194*t*
Education for All Handicapped Children Act of 1975, 471
effectiveness, 54
elder mistreatment, 317
elderly, 365–366
  abuse of, 317
  substance abuse in, 340–342
electroconvulsive therapy (ECT), 454
electronic health records (EHRs), 55
emergencies, 22
emergency operations plan (EOP), 411
Emergency Planning and Community Right-To-Know (EPCRA), 425
emergency preparedness, 475, 544–545
  plan, 544–545
    critical functions of, 545
emerging infectious diseases, 281–304
  convergence model, 282, 284*f*
  definition of, 281
  factors, 282–287, 283*b*
    breakdown of public health infrastructures, 286–287
    changing ecosystem, 285
    climate, 285
    human behavior, 285
    human susceptibility to infection, 284
    industry, 285–286
    lack of political will, 286–287
    microbial adaptation and change, 283–284
    technology, 285–286
    travel, 285–286
  geographic distribution of, 286*f*
  recent emerging and reemerging infectious diseases, 287–303
    avian influenza A virus H5N1, 289–291
    Ebola virus disease, 302
    Escherichia O157:H7, 296
    H1N1 influenza, 291–292
    H7N9 influenza, 292
    Lyme disease, 293–296
    middle east respiratory syndrome coronavirus, 288–289
    novel avian influenza A virus (H7N9), 292
    severe acute respiratory syndrome, 287–288
    tuberculosis, 297–302
    West Nile virus, 292–293
emotional turmoil, 521
end-of-life care, 501–522
  artificial nutrition and hydration, 509
  cardiopulmonary resuscitation, 509–510
  caring for clients, 512–519
  cultural issues, 510
  distressing symptom management, 517–519, 519*t*
    anorexia, 518
    dehydration, 518
    incontinence, 518
    secretions, 517–518
    skin integrity, 518
    terminal delirium, 518–519
  dying process, 520–521
  hospice care, 511–512
  imminent death and, 507–510
  level of care decisions, 508–510
    advance directives, 508–510
    comfort measures only, 508
    healthcare proxy, 508
  pain management in, 513–517
    drugs, 515–516
    pain assessment, 514
    types of pain, 514
  palliative care, 511
  patients with chronic disease, 502–505
  postmortem care, 521
  preparing for death, 520

end-of-life care (*continued*)
problems in, 506*t*
religious issues, 510, 511*t*
specialized care, 506–507
endemic disease, 251, 258
English Poor Law of 1601, 12
environmental epidemiology, 378, 397–398
environmental health, 378–403
air quality, 402
assessment of contaminants, 382–395
environmental media, 383
exposure pathways, 384–389*t*
point of exposure, 383
receptor population, 383, 390
route of exposure, 383
source of contamination, 383
transport mechanisms, 383
assessment of individuals, 395
behavioral factors, 381
chemical and contaminant exposure, 405
children's health and, 399–401
clean water and sanitation, 402
climate change, 402–403
community environment, 380–381, 392, 393–395*t*
completed exposure pathway, 390–392
definition of, 378, 379
evaluation, 397
exposure history, 395, 396*t*
genetic factors, 381
global challenges, 401–403
healthy communities, 399
healthy homes, 399
healthy schools, 400–401
history of, 379–380
human health and, 379–382
interventions, 395–397
nursing practice and, 381–382, 382*b*
public health nursing and, 366–367
environmental health nursing
challenges in, 22
competency in, 531*b*
environmental justice, 378, 401
Environmental Protection Agency (EPA), 265, 380
epidemic, 105, 107, 258
epidemic curve, 121, 129, 251–252
epidemiologic descriptive studies, 121, 135
epidemiologic models, 110–113
definition of, 187
epidemiologic triad, 110–111, 111*f*
natural history of disease, 112–113
prevention and, 87–88
web of causation, 111–112
wheel of causation, 111
epidemiologic research, 137
epidemiologic studies, 544
epidemiologic transition, 62, 64–65
epidemiologic triad, 105, 110–111, 111*f*, 532–533
epidemiology, 105
community assessment, 117–118
definition of, 3, 19, 105, 107–108
development of, 108–110
epidemiologic models, 110–113
individual assessment, 114–117
milestones in, 109–110*t*
occupational health and, 542–544
epidemiologic studies, 544
incidence, 543
prevalence, 543–544
ratios, 544
surveillance, 543–544
scope of, 107
equality, 54
equity, 46
defined, 55
in healthcare access and quality, 55–56
ergonomics, 525, 526
erythema migrans, 295
Escherichia, 254
Escherichia O157:H7, 264, 296
ethambutol, 299
ethical behavior, 504
ethnocentrism, 174, 178–179
eudaimonistic model, 64
euthanasia, 510
evacuation, 405, 428–429
evaluation, 414
evidence-based approach, 141–142
evidence-based nursing, 3, 19
evidence-based nursing practice, 137
evidence-based psychological interventions, 464*t*
evidence-based public health, 3, 19
exosystem, 99
expenditures, 33
experimental studies, 145
experimenter effect, 145*b*
exposure, 379
definition of, 378
estimate, 378, 390
history, 378, 395, 396*t*
pathway, 378, 382
external validity, 145*b*
eye contact, 181

F

faith communities, 489–492
as community, 490–492
relationship with clergy, 490
faith community nursing, 486–499
definition of, 486, 487–488
education for, 498
ethical principles, 497–498
history, 488
home visits in, 216
institution-based model, 489
models, 488–489, 489*b*
nursing process in, 494–497
assessment and diagnosis, 494–495
community-level interventions, 496
community-level outcomes, 496–497
documentation of practice, 496–497
interventions and outcomes, 495–497
roles of nurses in, 492
scope of, 493–494
standards of practice in, 493–494, 493*t*
Faith Community Nursing: Scope and Standards of Practice, 498
falls, risk of, 217–218
families, 225
cohabiting couples and families, 228
definition of, 227
disharmony within, 235
diversity and, 234–235
gay and lesbian, 228
members, 236
health risks, 237–244
nontraditional, 227–228
nurses working with, 226–227
stressful life events, 240–244
childbearing, 243
death of a family member, 241–242
disability, 242–243
divorce, 242
illness, 242–243
intrafamily strain, 242–243
legal issues, 242
marital/partner strain, 242
pregnancy, 243
work–family interface, 243–244
family assessment, 225–245, 227
conceptual models, 232
definition of, 225
family interview, 230–232
key points, 230*b*
nontraditional families, 227–228
nursing models, 232*t*
nursing perspectives on, 228–234
questions and considerations, 233*b*
tools, 228
ecomap, 228
genogram, 228, 229*f*
family caregiver, 204
Family Educational Rights and Privacy Act of 1974 (FERPA), 482
family health, routines and rituals, 232–233
family interview, 230–232
family risk reduction, 225, 237–238
family spirit, 335*b*
family systems, 232*t*
Family Violence Prevention Fund, 307
family/community involvement, 472*t*
Farr, William, 108
fatigue, 519*t*
Federal Emergency Management Agency (FEMA), 19, 412
federal government, 27–28
femicide, 307, 311
fentanyl, 346*t*, 516
fertility rate, 126*t*
fetal alcohol syndrome (FAS), 243, 331, 333*b*
fetal mortality rate, 126*t*
field triage, 416–417
flesh-eating bacteria, 254
Fliedner, Theodore, 12
fluoxetine (Prozac), 450
folk medicine, 184
follow-up, 11*t*
Food Allergy and Anaphylaxis Management Act (FAAMA), 469
food-borne diseases, 262–264. *See also* waterborne diseases
Campylobacter enteritis, 263
Escherichia O157:H7, 264
incidence of, 262
Listeria monocytogenes, 263
nontyphoid *Salmonella*, 263–264
noroviruses, 263
prevention and control of, 276
Food-Safe Schools Action Guide (FSSAG), 474
force field analysis, 162, 163*f*
forensic nursing, 320–321
frameworks, 187, 192–201, 225
France
health care measures in, 31*t*
health care system in, 36–37
functional health patterns, 187, 198, 199–200*t*, 232*t*, 233

G

Gardasil, 271
Garrett, Laurie, 282
gastroenteritis, 263
gateway effect theory, 336
gay families, 228
gender-based violence, 307, 311
genogram, 225, 228, 229*f*, 230
genomics, 357, 359
underserved populations, 359–360
geographic information systems (GIS), 196
geopolitical communities, 187, 189
geriatric scholar program (GSP), 364
Germany
health care measures in, 31*t*
health care system in, 37–38
Global Autism Public Health Initiative, 457
global burden of disease (GBD), 65–68
by age and income, 67*f*
definition of, 62, 65
noncommunicable diseases, 65–67
risk factors, 70–71
Global Code of Practice of the Recruitment of Health Personnel, 76
global health, 62–77
definition of, 62, 64
demographic transition, 64–65
determinants of health, 64
economic and political factors, 74
epidemiological transition, 64–65
health care systems and, 74–77
leading causes of death, 66*f*
role of nurses in, 77
Global Initiative on Primary Prevention of Substance Abuse, 327
Global Outbreak Alert and Response Network, 262
Gonococcal Isolate Surveillance Project (GISP), 269
gonorrhea, 268–270
government
agencies, 27–29, 169
healthcare spending, 31*t*
role in healthcare, 4–5
grand nursing theory, 225, 230, 231*t*
Graunt, John, 108

green spaces, access to, 393*t*
Grey Sisters, 12
grief, 501, 521
gross domestic product (GDP), 46, 50
Guide to Community Preventive Services, 164
guns, 309–310, 309*t*

H
H1N1 influenza, 254, 291–292
H5N1 influenza. *See* avian influenza A virus H5N1
H7N9 influenza, 292
hallucinogens, 347*t*
Hanasaari conceptual model, 534, 534*f*
hantavirus pulmonary syndrome, 254, 257
Hawthorne effect, 145*b*
hazard identification, 410
hazardous chemicals, 426*t*
HAZMAT experts, 427, 428, 430
health, 62, 194*t*
  advocacy, and healthcare reform, 57–58
  advocate, 498*t*
  appraisal, 225, 238
  assessment, 472–473
  and culture, 180–184
  definitions of, 63–64, 83, 85
  determinants of, 62, 64
  as expanding consciousness theory, 231*t*
  models of, 64
  occupational, 366–367
  personal responsibility for, 8–9
  right to, 71
  risks, 358–360
  social determinants of, 4, 159–161, 359
  status, 32, 195–196
health-adjusted life expectancy (HALE), 69*b*
Health Alert Network, 431
Health and Human Services (HHS), 152
health belief model, 83, 94–95
health disparities, 160–161. *See also underserved populations*
  definition of, 3, 26, 33, 225, 238
  eliminating, 20
  social determinants of, 359
Health Education Curriculum Analysis Tool (HECAT), 474
health educator, 498*t*
health equity, 160–161
Healthy Homes Initiative, 399
health impact assessment (HIA), 160
health impact pyramid, 157–158, 158*f*
health indicators, 62, 68–70, 69*b*, 193*t*
health information network, 7*f*
health information technology, 3, 7–8
health insurance, 459–460
Health Insurance Portability and Accountability Act (HIPAA), 540
health maintenance organizations (HMOs), 169
health planning, 152–154
  at global level, 152
  at national and state levels, 152–153
health policy, 46, 47–48
health professional shortage area (HPSA), 357, 362, 363*b*
Health Promoting Lifestyle Profile (HPLP-II), 496
health promotion, 85–86
  ecological model, 98–100
    exosystem, 99
    macroculture, 99–100
    microsystem, 99
    ontogenic system, 98
  epidemiologic model, 87–88
  interventions, 541
  levels of prevention, 88–92
  smoking cessation program, 541–542
  specialist, 538–539
  team approach, 540–541
  for women living with HIV/AIDS, 100
  in workplace, 540–541
health services research, 58
healthcare
  access to, 394*t*
  per capita spending, 31*t*
  community change and, 21
  and culture, 180–184
  in developed countries, 31*t*
  evaluation of, 118
  government role in, 4–5
  home. *See* home healthcare
  patient/client-centered, 5–6
  reform, 221–222
    health advocacy and, 57–58
  shortcomings in delivery of, 70*b*
  social determinants of, 4
  technology and, 6–8
  utilization of resources, 32–33
  vulnerable populations and, 33
healthcare access and quality, equity in, 55–56
healthcare-associated infections (HAIs), 252, 260–261. *See also* infectious diseases
healthcare finances, and cost–benefit, 50–51
healthcare organizations, 184
healthcare policy
  nursing's role in, 53–54
  and political process, 47–50
healthcare proxy, 501, 508
healthcare reform act, 504
healthcare systems
  Canada, 34–36
  factors, 74–77
  France, 36–37
  Germany, 37–38
  global health and, 74–77
  information management of, 55
  Netherlands, 38–39
  steps to improve, 58
  United Kingdom, 39–40
  workforce migration, 76, 76*t*
  workforce shortages, 76
healthcare workers, 56, 76
healthcare workforce diversity, 52–53
healthy and safe school environment, 472*t*
healthy communities, 379, 399
  design, 159
healthy foods, access to, 394*t*
healthy homes, 399
Healthy People 2000, 86–87
Healthy People 2010, 86–87, 141, 294, 442*f*, 474
  description of, 8–9
  goals of, 351–352
  ranking of rural health priorities, 365*b*
Healthy People 2020, 26, 31, 86–87, 86*b*, 116, 141, 152, 153, 154, 160, 164*b*, 205, 238, 244, 273, 359, 406, 457
  assessment of, 141*t*
  food safety objectives, 262*b*
  HIV objectives, 273, 274*b*
  immunization and infectious disease objectives, 253*b*
  injury and violence prevention, 308, 314
  occupational health nursing and, 538*b*
  overarching goals, 9*b*
  priorities, 492–493
  ranking of rural health priorities, 365*b*
  sexually transmitted disease objectives, 267*b*
  studies that relate to, 239*t*
  suicide and, 451*f*, 452*f*
  water quality objectives, 265*b*
Hemenway, David, 309
hemolytic-uremic syndrome (HUS), 296
Henry Street Settlement, 16
hepatitis B, 257
hepatitis viruses, 275–276
herd immunity, 281, 284
herpes simplex virus (HSV), 275
highly active antiretroviral therapy (HAART), 99
Hippocrates, 106
history, 143*b*
HITECH, 55
HIV/AIDS, 254, 272–275. *See also* sexually transmitted diseases (STDs)
  in African-American women, 98
  AZT therapeutic trials, 146
  families of infected women, 243
  health promotion and, 100
  heterosexual transmission, 273
  infection with, 257
  mortality/morbidity rate, 32
  new infections, 272–273
  number of infected people, 272, 272*t*
  prevention of, 100, 273–274
  substance abuse and, 328
  syphilis and, 271
  testing for infection, 91, 274
  transmission, 273
  tuberculosis and, 297–298
holistic care model, 488
home healthcare, 207–222
  agencies, 209
  chronic conditions in, 220–221
  definition of, 204
  financing of, 209–210
  history of, 207–208, 207*b*
  interdisciplinary collaboration, 213–214
  models, 214–216
    assisted living, 214–215
    home visits to homeless, 215–216
    parish nursing, 216
  nurse–family interactions in, 219–220
    confidentiality, 220
    contracting, 219–220
    culture, 219
    privacy, 220
    security, 220
  quality improvement in, 220–221
  regulation of, 209–210
  role and scope of, 212–213
home monitoring devices, 8
home visits, 216–219. *See also* home healthcare
  assessing for, 217–219
    risk of abuse and neglect, 218–219
    risk of falls, 217–218
    risk of medication errors, 217
  directions, 216
  equipment, 216
  in-home, 217–219
  initiating, 216
  personal safety, 216–217
  postvisit planning, 219
  preparation, 216–217
  termination of, 219
  to the homeless, 215–216
homebound, 204, 209
homeless
  children, 244
  families, 244
  home visits to, 215–216
  mothers, 244
  populations, 373–374
homicide, 309
hospice care, 503–504, 511–512. *See also* end-of-life care
hospice home care, 501, 512
hospital-based agencies, 204, 208
host, 532. *See also* infectious diseases
housing, access to, 393*t*
human immunodeficiency virus. *See* HIV/AIDS
human-made hazards, 395*t*
human papillomavirus (HPV), 271–272
human rights, 307, 311
Hurricane Katrina, 401
hypothesis, 138, 139

I
illicit drugs, 330–331, 331*f*
  nursing assessments and implications, 346–347*t*
  in schools, 475
illness, 242–243
  attribution of, 180
  mental, 440–458
imiquimod, 271
immigrants, 235
immunity, 90
immunization, 90
immunogenicity, 256*b*
Improving the Health of Adolescents and Young Adults: A Guide for States and Communities, 474
in-home visits, 217–219
incapacitating agents, 426*t*, 427*t*
incidence, 307, 315
incidence density, 121, 133

incidence rate, 121, 126*t*, 133–134
attributable risk, 133
definition of, 125–126
in exposed group, 134
incidence density and, 133
mortality rate, 133
in nonexposed group, 134
relative risk ratio, 134
incident command system (ICS), 405, 412–413
incontinence, 518
incubation period, 252, 256–257
indirect contact, 258
individual assessment, 114–115
Individual Education Plan (IEP), 469
Individuals with Disabilities Education Act (IDEA), 469, 471
indoor air, 393*t*
Industrial Revolution, 14–15
industry, 285–286
infant mortality, 31*t*
rate, 126*t*
infectious agents, 256, 256*b*
infectious diseases, 251–277. *See also* communicable diseases
agent, 256
definition of, 252
emerging, 281–304
convergence model, 282, 284*f*
factors, 282–287
geographic distribution of, 286*f*
recent emerging and reemerging infectious diseases, 287–303
environment, 257
epidemiology, 255–258
food-borne, 262–264
health care-associated infections, 260–261
host, 256–257
incubation period, 256–257
portals of entry and exit, 256
human susceptibility to, 284
outbreak investigation, 258–260
prevention and control of, 276–277
public health surveillance, 261–262
sexually transmitted disease, 266–276
transmission, 257–258
airborne, 258
direct contact, 258
droplet, 258
indirect contact, 258
waterborne, 264–266
infectivity, 256*b*
influenza, incubation period for, 256
informant, 225, 230, 233*b*
information management, of healthcare system, 55
inhalants, 336, 347*t*
injection drug users, 342
inmates, 357, 367–371
insecticide-treated bed nets (ITNs), 68
Institute of Medicine (IOM), 19
institution-based model, 486, 489
instrumentation, 143*b*
integrator, of faith and health, 498*t*
Interagency Autism Coordinating Committee (IACC), 457
interdisciplinary collaboration, 204, 213–214
interferon gamma (IFN-g), 301
intergenerational diversity, 225, 236–237
intermittent care, 204, 210
internal validity, 143*b*
international communities, 191–192
International Council of Nurses (ICN), 26, 42
international health organizations, 41–42
International Health Regulations (IHR), 40
international public health, 22–23, 40–42. *See also* public health
refugee and disaster relief assistance, 41
interracial marriage, 235–236
intervention studies, 138, 146. *See also* observational studies
preventive trials, 145
therapeutic trials, 146
interventions, 319–320, 541
community-level, 164–166
evaluation of, 167–168
developing and testing, 196
funding, 168–170
history and, 145*b*
multilevel, 158–159
selection and, 145*b*
setting and, 145*b*
intimate partner violence (IPV), 311–317
consequences in children exposed to, 315
definition of, 307
extent of, 311–315
inquiry and assessment for, 316
lethality risks, 312*b*
prevalence of, 311
risk factors, 312*t*, 312*b*
safety assessment and planning, 316–317
screening for, 315–316
women's health problem, 311
intoxication, 325, 336
intrafamily strain, 225, 242–243
invacuation, 405, 428
invasiveness, 256*b*
Ixodes pacificus, 293
Ixodes scapularis, 294

J
jails, 367–371
Japan, health care measures in, 31*t*
Judaism, 511*t*
just-in-time training, 415–416
juvenile-onset recurrent respiratory papillomatosis, 271

K
K-12 health education, 472*t*
K-12 physical education, 472*t*
key informant, 151

L
Ladies' Benevolent Society, 14
lead, 384*t*
learning model, 83, 93–94
legal issues, 242
Legionella pneumophila, 266
Legionnaires' disease, 266
lesbian families, 228
lesbian, gay, bisexual and transgender people (LGBT), 371–373, 373*b*
lethality assessment, 307, 312
levo-a-acetylmethadol (LAAM), 349
Lewin, Karl, 161–162
life events, 240–244
childbearing, 243
death of a family member, 241–242
disability, 242–243
divorce, 242
illness, 242–243
intrafamily strain, 242–243
legal issues, 242
marital/partner strain, 242
pregnancy, 243
work–family interface, 243–244
life expectancy, 31*t*, 32, 69*b*
life span development, 232*t*
LifeSkills Training (LST), 337*b*
lifestyle, 116–119
management, to lower blood pressure, 142*t*
liquid morphine, 516
Listeria, 262
Listeria monocytogenes, 263
Living Proof Project, 42
local health department, 29–30
local resources, 169
logic model, 151, 164–166
long-acting coagulants, 426*t*
long-term change, 131
low-term change, 121
lung agents, 426*t*
lyme borreliosis, 254
Lyme disease, 293–296. *See also* infectious diseases
emergence of, 257
epidemiology, 293–294
incidence rate, 294, 295*t*
prevention of, 296, 296*t*
signs and symptoms, 295
surveillance, 295
lysergic acid diethylamide (LSD), 347*t*

M
macroculture, 99–100
Making it Happen!, 474
managed care, 204, 208
managed care organizations (MCOs), 367
manager/administrator, 539–540
manners, 230
MAP-IT, 154*b*
marijuana, 330, 475
Marine Hospital Service, 14
marital strain, 225, 242
marriage, 235
arranged, 236
interracial, 235–236
Massachusetts Health Care Reform Act, 541
Maternal and Infancy Act, 18
maternal and infant rates, 126*t*
maternal mortality rate, 126*t*
maternal undernutrition, 68
maturation, 143*b*
means restriction, 453
Medicaid, 18, 57, 58, 210, 502
hospice benefits, 503
services reimbursable by, 471*b*
medical devices, 6–7
medically underserved area (MUA), 357, 362, 363*b*
medically underserved population (MUP), 357, 362, 363*b*
Medicare, 18, 57, 210
Medicare Hospice Benefit, 503
Medicare Payment Advisory Committee (MedPAC), 221–222
medication errors, 217
Mental Health Parity Act (MHPA), 459
Mental Health Parity and Addiction Equity Act of 2008, 350, 459
mental illness, 440–458. *See also* community mental health
attention deficit/hyperactivity disorders, 455–456
autism, 456–458
cultural context, 440
definitions of, 441
mood and anxiety disorders, 450–458
prevalence of, 443*t*
schizophrenia, 443–449
scope of, 441
meperidine, 516
meprobamate, 346*t*
mercury, 384*t*, 400
mercy killing, 510
mescaline, 347*t*
metabolic syndrome, 447
metals, 426*t*
methadone, 342, 349
methamphetamine, 342–343
Methamphetamine Anti-Proliferation Act, 343
methicillin-resistant *Staphylococcus aureus* (MRSA) infection, 257
3,4-methylenedioxy-N-methylamphetamine (MDMA), 347*t*
microbial adaptation, 281, 283–284
microsystem, 99
middle east respiratory syndrome coronavirus (MERS-CoV), 288–289
infection control for prevention of transmission, 288–289
migrant workers, 244
Millennium Declaration, 152, 160
Millennium Development Goals (MDGs), 26, 40–41
achievements and challenges, 72*t*
goals and targets, 70*b*
impact of, 71–73
right to health, 71
mitigation, 412
Mobilizing for Action through Planning and Partnership (MAPP), 154*b*
modifiable risk, 83
mold, 386*t*

mood and anxiety disorders, 450–458. *See also* community mental health; mental illness
biological theories, 450
epidemiology, 450
nursing interventions, 454–455
social factors, 450
suicide, 450–454, 451*f*, 452*f*
morbidity, 121
rates, 32, 121, 126
Morbidity and Mortality Weekly Report, 32
morphine, 346*t*, 516
mortality, 143*b*
rate, 32, 126*t*, 133
motivational interviewing, 83, 93
with adolescents, 337, 351*b*
mourning, 501, 521
multidrug-resistant TB (MDR-TB), 301
multilateral agencies, 26, 41
multilevel interventions, 158–159
Muslims, 182, 511*t*
Mycobacterium tuberculosis, 297
myoclonus, 517

N

naloxone, 349
naltrexone, 348
Narcotics Anonymous (NA), 341–342
National Association of County and City Health Officials (NACCHO), 154*b*
National Center for Complementary and Alternative Medicine (NCCAM), 522
National Center on Health Statistics (NCHS), 152–153
national communities, 191–192
National Comorbidity Survey, 441
National Consensus Project's Clinical Practice Guidelines for Quality Palliative Care, 504
National Health and Nutrition Examination Survey (NHANES), 154
national health expenditure, 46, 50
National Health Expenditure Accounts (NHEA), 26, 33
National Health Interview Survey (NHIS), 153
National Health Service (NHS), 39
National Healthcare Disparities Report (NHDR), 5
National Healthcare Quality Report (NHQR), 5
National Healthcare Safety Network (NHSN), 261
National High Blood Pressure Education Program, 141
national incident management system (NIMS), 405, 412
National Institute of Occupational Safety and Health (NIOSH), 525, 531
National Institute on Alcohol Abuse and Alcoholism (NIAAA), 330
National Occupational Research Agenda (NORA), 540
National Organization for Public Health Nursing, 16
National Prevention Council, 153
National Prevention Strategy (NPS), 152, 153
National Registry of Evidence Based Programs and Practices (NREPP), 475
national response framework (NRF), 405, 411–412
National Select Agent Registry Program, 287
National Strategy for Suicide Prevention (NSSP), 453
Nationwide Health Information Network (NwHIN), 7–8
natural disasters, 408
natural hazards, 395*t*
natural history, 105
of disease, 112–113
naturally occurring retirement communities (NORCs), 215
nausea, 517, 519*t*
Navy Nurse Corps, 17, 18
necessity (home care criterion), 204, 210
necrotizing fasciitis, 254
neglect, assessing for, 218–219
Neisseria gonorrhoeae, 268–269
neonatal mortality rate (NMR), 69*b*, 126*t*
nerve agents, 426*t*, 427*t*
Netherlands, health care system in, 38–39
neuropathic pain, 514
NHPCO Standards of Practice for Hospice Programs, 504
Nightingale, Florence, 12, 14, 110, 406, 530
No Child Left Behind Act of 2003, 58, 471, 483
nociceptive pain, 514
noise, 394*t*
non-steroidal anti-inflammatory drugs (NSAIDs), 515
nonadherence, 440, 446
noncommunicable diseases, 62
factors in rise of, 67*t*
global burden of disease and, 65–67
nongovernmental organizations (NGOs), 26, 42
nonskilled care, 212*t*
nonsteroidal anti-inflammatory drugs (NSAIDs), 514
nontyphoid *Salmonella*, 263–264
nonverbal communication, 181
noroviruses, 263
North American Nursing Diagnosis Association-International (NANDA-I), 494
novel avian influenza A virus (H7N9), 292
novelty, 145*b*
nucleic acid amplification tests (NAATs), 268
null hypothesis, 138, 146
numb shock, 521
Nurse Family Partnership program, 319
nurse-managed health centers (NMHCs), 170–171
Nurse–Family Partnership (NFP), 334, 334*b*
nurses
as change agent, 161
ethical consideration for, 56–57
nursing
cross-cultural, 174, 176
culture and, 175–179
district, 3, 12
evidence-based, 19
forensic, 320–321
occupational health, 525–545
policy-making and, 54
role in healthcare policy, 53–54
Nursing Emergency Preparedness Education Coalition (NEPEC), 414
nutrition, 58, 478–479
services, 472*t*

O

O'Donnell health promotion model, 539*f*
Obama, Barack, 5, 56, 57
Obamacare, 5
obesity, 116, 118*f*, 478
obesogenic environment, 159–160
observational studies, 138, 139–144. *See also* intervention studies
analytical studies, 142–145
case-control studies, 143–144
case studies, 139–140
cohort studies, 142–143
cross-sectional studies, 140–142
descriptive studies, 139–142
occupational hazards, 532–533
biologic, 532
chemical, 532
environment, 533
physical, 532–533
psychosocial, 533
occupational health, 366–367
disaster management, 544
emergency preparedness, 544–545
epidemiologic studies, 544
epidemiologic surveillance, 543–544
prevalence, 543–544
ratios, 544
occupational health nursing, 525–545
competency in, 531, 531*b*
conceptual frameworks, 532–535
epidemiologic triad, 532–533
practice models, 534–535
epidemiology and, 542–544
epidemiologic studies, 544
incidence, 543
prevalence, 543–544
ratios, 544
surveillance, 543–544
health promotion, 540–541
history, 530–531
overview, 530
practice, 535–540
case manager, 536–537
clinician, 535–536
counselor/consultant, 537–538
health promotion specialist, 538–539
manager/administrator, 539–540
researcher, 540
root cause analysis, 537
standards of practice, 531–532
workplace walk-through, 536, 537*b*
occupational injuries, 527, 528*f*
fatal, 529–530*f*
incidence rate, 528*t*
nonfatal, 527, 527–528*f*, 528*t*
statistics on, 529*t*
Occupational Safety and Health Administration (OSHA), 531, 539–540
occurrence rate, 125–126
odds ratio, 138, 225, 237
Office of Autism Research Coordination (OARC), 457
Office of Management and Budget (OMB), 361*b*
Office of the National Coordinator for Health Information Technology (ONC), 7
official agencies, 204, 209
Omaha System, 210, 211*b*
opinion leaders, 156–157
opioid substitution treatment, 341, 348–349
buprenorphine, 349
methadone, 349
naloxone, 349
opioids, 515–516
oral mucosa, 516
organic solvents, 426*t*
Organization for Economic Cooperation and Development (OECD), 26, 27
organizational ethics, 56
organizational excellence, 504
oseltamivir, 292
outbreaks, 258–260. *See also* infectious diseases
common source, 259
definition of, 105
investigation of, 258–260
establishing existence of, 258–259
steps in, 259*b*
preventing and controlling, 118
propagated, 259, 260*f*
Outcome and Assessment Information Set (OASIS), 209, 233
overweight children, 235
Oxfam International, 42
oxycodone, 346*t*

P

P value, 138, 146
pain, 513–514
adjuvant drugs, 515
assessment, 514
breakthrough, 515
in dying clients, 514–515
neuropathic, 514
nociceptive, 514
somatic, 514
visceral, 514
pain drugs, 515–516
adjuvant analgesics, 516
nonopioid analgesics, 515
opioids, 515–516
routes of administration, 516–517
intraspinal, 517
oral, 516
oral mucosa, 516
parenteral, 516–517
rectal, 516
topical, 516
transdermal, 516
side effects of, 517
constipation, 517
myoclonus, 517

pain drugs (*continued*)
nausea, 517
pruritus, 517
respiratory depression, 517
sedation, 517
vomiting, 517
tolerance, 517
palliative care, 501, 511. *See also* end-of-life care
pandemic, 281, 290, 291–292
parish nursing, 204, 216, 486, 488
paroxetine (Paxil), 450
participant effect, 145*b*
passive immunity, 90
pathogenicity, 252, 256*b*
patient-and-family-centered care, 504
patient-centered medical home (PCMH), 215
patient-centeredness, 54
Patient Protection and Affordable Care Act (PPACA), 5, 74, 153, 406, 477, 502
Patient Self-Determination Act, 509
patient/client-centered health care, 5–6
pauper nurses, 12
Pediatric Environmental Health Specialty Units (PEHSU), 392*b*
pediatric palliative care referral criteria, 505
penicillin G, 270
perchloroethylene, 385*t*
performance measurement, 504
perinatal mortality rate, 126*t*
period prevalence, 121, 126
periodic change, 121, 131
perpetrate, 311
personal health counselor, 498*t*
personal protective equipment (PPE), 405, 418, 427, 431
personal responsibility, 8–9
personal space, 181
pesticides, 388*t*, 401
pests, 394*t*
peyote, 347*t*
phencyclidine (PCP), 347*t*
phenomenological communities, 189–190
philanthropic organizations, 26, 27, 42
physical activity, access to, 394*t*
Physical Education Curriculum Analysis Tool (PECAT), 474
physical hazards, 525, 527*t*, 532–533
picaridin, 293
plague, 422*t*, 424
plan of care, 204, 209
Planet Health, 85
podofilox, 271
point of distribution (POD), 405, 417–418
point prevalence, 121, 126
policy, 46, 47, 49*f*
policy adoption, 49
policy assessment, 49
policy development, 11*t*
policy enforcement, 11*t*
policy formulation, 49
policy implementation, 49
policy-making process, 54
events in, 49, 49*f*
nurses and, 54
policy modification, 49
political process, health care policy and, 47–50
politics, 46, 48
polychlorinated biphenyls (PCBs), 385*t*, 391–392
population aggregate, 151, 153
population at risk, 121, 122. *See also* vulnerable populations
population-based assessment, 472–473
population of interest, defining, 155–156
post-traumatic stress disorder (PTSD), 450
postmortem care, 501, 521
potable water, 264–266
access to, 393*t*
precautionary principle, 378, 381
precede–proceed model, 154*b*
pregnancy, 243
cocaine use and, 333
fetal alcohol syndrome, 331
prevention, 477–478
substance abuse and, 331–334
with syphilis, 270
T-ACE alcohol screening questionnaire for use in, 332*b*
teenage, 476–478
President's New Freedom Commission on Mental Health, 440, 459, 460
prevalence, 308, 311
rate, 121, 126
prevention
epidemiologic model and, 87–88
levels of, 88–92
natural history of disease and, 88*f*, 93*f*
primary, 83, 88–90
in public health, 85–86
role of nurses in, 100
secondary, 83, 90–92
tertiary, 85, 92
Prevention and Public Health Fund, 169
Prevention Research Centers, 84
preventive trials, 138, 145
primary healthcare, 62, 63
primary prevention, 88–90
definition of, 83
examples of, 89*b*
prisons, 367–371
private agencies, 208
private foundations, 169
Private Guns, Public Health, 309
prodromal stage, 440, 444
program replication, 168
Program to Encourage Active Rewarding Lives for Seniors (PEARLS), 84
project ASSERT screening, 350*b*
project funding, 169
propagated outbreak, 252, 259, 260*f*
proportion, 122, 123, 124
proportional mortality ratio (PMR), 122, 126*t*, 133
propoxyphene, 516
proprietary agencies, 204, 209
prospective studies, 138, 142–143
pruritus, 517
psychological first aid, 461–463
defined, 461
in different cultures, 463*b*
populations at risk for psychological trauma, 461–463
populations traumatized by disasters, 461
SAMSHA, 462*f*
psychological trauma, populations at risk for, 461–463
psychosocial hazards, 525, 533
psychosocial treatments, 349–351
public facilities, location of, 394*t*
public health, 27–42
in 20th century, 16–19
achievements in 1900-1999, 5*b*
definition of, 3, 62, 63
in developed countries, 34–42
Canada, 34–36
France, 36–37
Germany, 37–38
Netherlands, 38–39
United Kingdom, 39–40
disaster response, 431–433
after-action evaluation, 433
communication, 432
recovery, 433
scope and magnitude, 431–432
in early America, 14–16
evidence-based, 3, 19
expenditures, 33
federal agencies, 30*f*
federal government and, 27–28
functions of, 30–32
government agencies and, 27–29
international, 40–42
milestones in, 13*t*
models for populations at risk, 343–348
principles of, 9*b*
problem solving, 20*f*
state departments of, 154
state government and, 28
surveillance, 89*b*, 261–262
trends, 32–33
public health nursing, 9, 10–11, 11*t*
certification for specialty practice, 12
challenges, 19–24
community change planning, 21
cultural competence, 20–21
disaster preparedness, 22
eliminating health disparities, 20
evidence-based practices, 19–20
competencies, 9–10
daily practice vs. disaster response, 414*t*
definition of, 3–4
in disaster management, 414–419
documentation, 418–419
field triage, 416–417
just-in-time training, 415–416
personal protective equipment, 418
point of distribution plans, 417–418
public health nurses as first responders, 415
education, 11–12
history, 12–19
interventions, 10*f*, 11*t*
milestones in, 13*t*
principles of, 9*b*
Public Health Nursing: Scope and Standards of Practic', 9
public health policy, 46, 47
components of, 48
public transportation, location of, 394*t*
pulmonary agents, 426*t*, 427*t*
pyrazinamide, 299

Q
Quad Council of Public Health Nursing Organizations, 9
quality of care, 46, 48, 54–55
QuantiFERON-TB Gold In-Tube test (QFT-GIT), 301
Quinlan, Karen Ann, 508

R
race, 179
radiological disasters, 429–430. *See also* disaster management
"dirty bombs," 429–430
role of nurses in, 430
radon, 385*t*
rates, 123–127
adjusted, 124–125
attributable risk, 133
calculation of, 124*b*, 125*t*
crude, 124
definition of, 105, 122, 124
incidence, 125–126, 126*t*, 133–134
mortality, 133
prevalence, 126
relative risk ratio, 134
specific, 127–133
Rathbone, William, 12, 14
ratios, 122, 123, 126*t*, 544
RE-AIM framework, 168
reactivity, 145*b*
real-time, 405
reasoned action, theory of, 85, 95–96
reciprocation model, 535*f*
recovery, 413–414, 433
recreational water, 265, 395*t*
Red Cross, 42
referral, 11*t*
referral agent, 498*t*
reform, 57–58
defined, 46
healthcare, 221–222
refreezing, 162
refugees, 26, 41
registered nurses, employment statistics, 9
reimbursement, 204, 208
relapse prevention model, 83, 96–97
relationship, 138, 140
relative risk (RR), 138
relative risk ratio, 122, 134
religion, 182–184
remission, 325

reorganization (grief phase), 521
researcher, 540
reservoir, 252, 257
resolution (grief phase), 521
respiratory depression, 517
retrospective studies, 138, 143–144
rifampin, 299
right to health, 62, 71
riot control agents, 426*t*
risk, 105, 114
risk assessment, 379, 382, 411
risk factors, 62, 68, 105, 114, 116
risk reduction, 83, 84, 85–86
rituals and routines, 232–233, 232*t*
role-performance model, 64
roles, 182
Roll Back Malaria, 68
root cause analysis (RCA), 525, 537, 537*b*
Roy adaptation model, 231*t*
rural areas, 361*b*, 361*t*
rural geopolitical areas, 364*b*
rural populations, 360–367

S

Safe Motherhood Initiative, 71
safety, 54, 194*t*, 504
Salmonella, 262, 263–264, 264*f*
Salmonella typhimurium, 130*f*
salutogenic environment, 159–160
same-sex parents, 228
samples, 138, 140
sanitation, 393*t*, 402
scenario, 406
schizophrenia, 443–449. *See also* community mental health; mental illness
  cannabis use and, 446
  community mental health teams, 449–450
  early intervention programs, 444–446, 445*t*
  epidemiology, 443–444
  first-episode psychosis, 444–446
  high-risk populations, 448–449
  primary prevention programs, 446
  prodromal stage, 444
  screening tools, 446
  treatment adherence in, 446–448
school-based health centers (SBHCs), 474
school health council, 474
School Health Index, 469, 473
school health nursing, 469–484
  child advocacy and, 482–483
  common health concerns, 475–482
    alcohol use, 475
    illicit drugs, 475
    nutrition, 478–479
    sexual behavior, 476–478
    sexually transmitted infections, 478
    smoking, 475–476
    teenage pregnancy, 476–478
    violence, 479–482
  community school model, 483
  definition of, 469
  history of, 470–471
  roles of school nurse, 471–475
    assessment of school health needs, 473–475
    emergency preparedness, 475
    health education, 474
    health promotion, 473–475
    individual health assessment, 472
    population-based assessment, 472–473
  screening program, 473*b*
school health programs, 472*t*
school violence, 310, 479–482
schools, 400
  location of, 394*t*
science of unitary beings, 231*t*
screening, 11*t*, 90–91
secondary
  immunity, 90–92
  infections, 252, 259
  prevention, 83, 90–92
sedation, 517
selection, 143*b*
selective serotonin reuptake inhibitors (SSRIs), 450, 455
self-care agency, 231*t*
sensitivity, 91*b*, 122, 134–135
sertraline (Zoloft), 450
Seton, Elizabeth Ann, 14
severe acute respiratory syndrome (SARS), 287–288. *See also* infectious diseases
  outbreaks, 288–289
  superspreading event, 287
  transmission, 254
sexual and reproductive health, 68
Sexual Assault Nurse Examiner (SANE), 320
sexual behavior, 476–478
sexually transmitted diseases (STDs), 266–276. *See also* HIV/AIDS; infectious diseases
  in adolescents, 478
    epidemiology, 478
    school relevance, 478
  chlamydia, 268
  gonorrhea, 268–270
  hepatitis B infection and, 275–276
  herpes simplex virus, 275
  HIV/AIDS, 272–275
  human papillomavirus, 271–272
  prevention and control of, 276–277
  syphilis, 270–271
  transmission, 257–258
  urinary tract infections and, 261
Shattuck, Lemuel, 15
shelter in place, 406, 428
Sheppard-Towner Act, 18
Shiga toxin–producing *Escherichia coli* (STEC), 262
Shigella, 262
shock, 521
short-term change, 122, 129
silencing the self, 100
"silent" infection, 268
Silent Spring (Carson), 380
simple triage and rapid treatment (START), 417
simulation, 406
sinecatechins, 271
Sisters of Charity, 12, 14
skilled care, 204, 210, 212*t*
skilled needs, 204, 210
skin integrity, 518
smallpox, 423*t*, 424
SMART objectives, 166, 166*b*
smoking, 475–476
  in adolescents, 475–476
  cessation program, 541–542
  epidemiology, 475–476
  prevention, 476, 476*b*
Snow, John, 108–109, 259
social cognitive theory, 96
social ecological model, 157
social justice, 160–161
social learning, 83
  theory, 96
social marketing, 11*t*, 170
Social Security Act of 1935, 18
social support, 83
  theory, 96
societal communities, 191–192
somatic pain, 514
Spanish flu, 289
Spanish–American War of 1898, 17
Special Supplemental Nutrition Program for Women, Infants, and Children (WIC and SNAP), 58
specialty practice, 12
specific rates, 122, 127–133
specificity, 91*b*, 122, 134–135
spillover, 226, 244
spiritual care, 486, 488
stakeholders, 151, 156–157
Staphylococcus aureus, 262
state government, 28
state health department, 29–30
Steere, Alan, 293
stewardship, 504
Stewart, Ada Mayo, 530
stray animals, 394*t*
Streptococcus pyogenes, 254
subculture, 174, 179
subsistence food, 394*t*
substance abuse
  in adolescents, 329–331, 334–338, 475–476
  alcohol, 329–330, 475
  at an early age, 334–338
  binge drinking, 338–340
  cannabis, 330
  evidence-based psychosocial treatments, 349–351
  gateway effect theory, 336
  illicit drugs, 330–331, 475
  impact on the community, 343
  injection drugs, 342
  international aspects of, 326–331
  methamphetamine, 342–343
  nursing assessments and implications, 346–347*t*
  in older adults, 340–342
  pharmacologic treatments, 348–349
  in pregnant women, 331–334
  prize incentives contingency management for, 350*b*
  psychosocial treatments, 349–351
  public health models for populations at risk, 343–348
  smoking, 475–476
  tobacco, 330
Substance Abuse and Mental Health Services Administration (SAMHSA), 328, 460
substance use, 325–353, 326, 328*f*
  definition of, 325
  national scope of, 328–331
  public health policies to minimize harms from, 326–328
  scope of, 326
substance use disorders, 325, 328
suicide, 450–454
superfund, 380
superspreading event, 287
supplemental food, 394*t*
support groups, 498*t*
suppositories, 516
surveillance, 11*t*, 252, 262, 406
survey research, 138, 140
sustainability, 151, 162, 168
Sweden, health care measures in, 31*t*
swine flu, 254, 291–292
syphilis, 270–271
syringe-exchange programs, 342
system, 226, 227
  theory, 155

T

T-ACE screening, 331, 332*b*
Tai Chi, 182
Tamiflu, 292
tardive dyskinesia, 440, 447
Task Force on Community Preventive Services (TFCPS), 164
teaching, 11*t*
teamwork, 166–167
tear gas, 426*t*
technology, 285–286
  health care and, 6–8
teenage pregnancy, 476–478
  prevention, 477–478
telehealth, 8, 204, 214
terminal delirium, 518–519
terrorism, 22, 406, 409
tertiary prevention, 85, 92
testing, 143*b*
tetrachloroethylene, 385*t*
tetracycline, 270
Theodore Roosevelt, 57
theory (definition), 226, 230
theory of reasoned action, 85, 95–96
therapeutic conversation, 230
therapeutic questions, 230
therapeutic trials, 138, 146
time orientation, 182
timeliness, 54
tobacco, 330
tobacco companies, 476
tolerance, 326, 341
toxic alcohols, 426*t*
toxic shock syndrome, 254

toxicity, 256*b*
toxicology, 379, 390
transcultural nursing, 174, 176
transdermal drugs, 516
transgender people, 371–373, 373*b*
transmission, 257–258. *See also* infectious diseases
  airborne, 258
  definition of, 252
  direct contact, 258
  droplet, 258
  indirect contact, 258
transtheoretical model, 85, 95
trauma, 98
travel, 285–286
Treponema pallidum, 270
TRICARE, 209
tricyclic antidepressants, 454
trimorbidity, 357, 374
tuberculosis, 297–302. *See also* infectious diseases
  contact investigation, 299–300
  diagnostic tests, 300–302
  directly observed therapy, 299
  epidemiology, 297
  geographic distribution of, 297
  HIV infection and, 297–298
  infection control guidelines for healthcare settings, 301–302
  latent vs. active, 298*t*
  multidrug-resistant, 301
  prevention and control of, 298–302
  QuantiFERON-TB Gold In-Tube test, 301
  signs and symptoms, 297–298
  targeted tuberculin testing, 298–299
  treatment of active infection, 299
  treatment of latent infection, 298–299
tularemia, 423*t*, 424
type I error, 138, 146
type II error, 138, 146

U

ultraviolet radiation, 394*t*
undernutrition, 68
underserved populations, 357–375, 359
  definition of, 357
  elderly people, 365–366
  environmental health problems, 366–367
  genomics and, 359–360
  health professional shortage areas, 362, 363*b*
  health risks, 358–360
  homeless populations, 373–374
  inmates, 367–371
  lesbian, gay, bisexual and transgender people, 371–373
  morbidity issues, 363
  mortality issues, 363
  occupational health problems, 366–367
  rural populations, 360–367, 364*b*
unfreezing, 161–162
United Kingdom
  health care measures in, 31*t*
  health care system in, 39–40
United Nations High Commissioner for Refugees (UNHCR), 41
United Nations Millennium Declaration, 41
United Nations Office on Drugs and Crime (UNODC), 327
United States
  health care measures in, 31*t*
  public health in, 30–32
United States Committee on the Prevention of Weapons of Mass Destruction Proliferation and Terrorism, 419
urban areas, 361*b*, 361*t*
urinary tract infections, 261
U.S. Agency for International Development (USAID), 42
U.S. Census Bureau, 361*b*
U.S. Department of Health and Human Services (USDHHS), 261
U.S. President's Emergency Plan for AIDS Relief (PEPFAR), 254
U.S. Preventive Service Task Force (USPSTF), 314, 343–348
U.S. Public Health Service (USPHS), 17–18
U.S. Safe Drinking Water Act, 265
Utilization Review Accreditation Commission (URAC), 205

V

vacant lots, 393*t*
vaccination, 90
variables, 138, 139
vectors, 394*t*
verbal communication, 181
vesicants, 426*t*, 427*t*
Veterans Administration, 209
Vibrio cholerae, 287
violence, 308–311. *See also* abuse
  definition of, 308
  guns, 309–310, 309*t*
  homicide, 309
  intimate partner, 311–317
  model of care for victims, 320
  school violence, 310, 482
viral hemorrhagic fevers (VHFs), 423*t*, 425
virulence, 256*b*
visceral pain, 514
Visiting Nurse Association of New York City, 16
voluntary agencies, 204, 208
volunteers, coordinator of, 498*t*
vomiting, 517, 519*t*
  agents, 426*t*
vulnerability, 358–359
  analysis, 411
vulnerable populations, 33. *See also* population at risk

W

Wald, Lillian, 16
ward maids, 12
waste removal, 393*t*
waterborne diseases, 264–266. *See also* food-borne diseases
  from drinking/potable water, 276–277
  prevention and control of, 276–277
  from recreational water, 265
web of causation, 105, 111–112
Weight Watchers, 94
well-being, 85
West Nile virus (WNV), 292–293. *See also* infectious diseases
  incidence of, 292
  outbreaks, 292–293
  prevention of infection, 293
  symptoms, 293
  transmission of, 292–293
Western biomedicine, 180
wheel of causation, 105, 111
white blood cells, 448
WHO World Health Statistics Report, 69*b*
windshield survey, 187
withdrawal symptoms, 326, 341
women's health problem, 311
worker assessment, 535–536
work–family interface, 243–244
workforce, 526
  employment size class, 527*f*
  migration, 76, 76*t*
workforce diversity, 46
workforce excellence, 504
workplace, 526–530
  assessment, 536
  hazards, 527*t*, 532–533
    biologic, 532
    chemical, 532
    environment, 533
    physical, 532–533
    psychosocial, 533
  health promotion in, 540–541
  injuries, 527, 528*f*
    fatal, 529–530*f*
    incidence rate, 528*t*
    nonfatal, 527, 527–528*f*, 528*t*
  walk-through, 525, 536, 537*b*
workplace assessment, 536
World Bank, 26, 27, 41
World Health Assembly, 40
World Health Organization, 26, 27, 40–41, 152
World Summit for Children, 71
World War I, 18

X

xerostomia, 517–518

Y

Yersinia, 262
Yersinia pestis, 424
yoga, 182
Youth Risk Behavior Surveillance Survey (YRBSS), 469, 473, 473*b*, 478
Youth Risk Behavior Survey (YRBS), 141, 154

Z

zidovudine, 146
zoonoses, 257